Diagnostic Medical Sonography

OBSTETRICS AND GYNECOLOGY

Diagnostic Medical Sonography

OBSTETRICS AND GYNECOLOGY

Third Edition

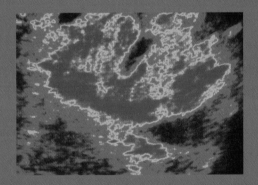

Susan Raatz Stephenson, MAEd,
RDMS (OB)(AB)(BR), RVT, RT(R)(C), CIIP
Sonographer
Sandy, Utah

Wolters Kluwer | Lippincott Williams & Wilkins

Philadelphia • Baltimore • New York • London
Buenos Aires • Hong Kong • Sydney • Tokyo

Publisher: Julie K. Stegman
Senior Product Manager: Heather Rybacki
Product Manager: Kristin Royer
Marketing Manager: Shauna Kelley
Design Coordinator: Joan Wendt
Art Director: Jennifer Clements
Manufacturing Coordinator: Margie Orzech
Production Services: Absolute Service, Inc.

351 West Camden Street
Baltimore, MD 21201

Two Commerce Square
2001 Market Street
Philadelphia, PA 19103

Third Edition

Printed in China.

Library of Congress Cataloging-in-Publication Data
  Diagnostic medical sonography. Obstetrics and gynecology. — 3rd ed. / edited by Susan Raatz Stephenson.
    p. ; cm.
  Obstetrics and gynecology
  Rev. ed. of: Obstetrics and gynecology / edited by Mimi C. Berman, Harris L. Cohen. 2nd ed. c1997.
  Includes bibliographical references and index.
  ISBN 978-1-60831-117-0 (alk. paper)
  I. Stephenson, Susan Raatz. II. Obstetrics and gynecology. III. Title: Obstetrics and gynecology.
  [DNLM: 1. Genital Diseases, Female–ultrasonography. 2. Fetal Diseases–ultrasonography. 3. Pregnancy Complications–ultrasonography. 4. Ultrasonography, Prenatal. WP 141]
  618.1'07543–dc23
                                    2011043624

To purchase additional copies of this book, call our customer service department at (800) 638-3030 or fax orders to (301) 223-2320. International customers should call (301) 223-2300.
Visit Lippincott Williams & Wilkins on the Internet **at LWW.com** Lippincott Williams & Wilkins customer service representatives are available from 8:30 AM to 6:00 PM, EST.

10 9 8 7 6 5 4 3 2 1

To the men in my life, none of whom wanted this dedication. Beginning with my father who nurtured the personality, to my brother with whom I compete, the son who has become a great person, the man I chose to spend my life with and has to put up with me, and finally, to my nephew who I look forward to getting to know better.

Susan Raatz Stephenson

And to students and professionals who will use this book: In my own journey to this point, there were many times when I wished the technology changes would slow down. Through the years, it became evident that the development and use of modes, such as Doppler and now Volume Imaging, require lifelong learning. My advice to you is to endeavor to understand the why and when we use the facets of sonography. Remember, "Curiosity is the very basis of education and if you tell me that curiosity killed the cat, I say only the cat died nobly."

—Arnold Edinborough

A final note from B.B. King, "The beautiful thing about learning is nobody can take it away from you."

Contents

Acknowledgments

Three years ago when Diane Kawamura contacted me about this project, I had no idea how much I would learn in the process. Contributing authors provided an amazing amount of information, some formatted content in a manner adopted for subsequent chapters. All provided some aspect of women's health imaging that was new to this editor. The support of fellow editors, Anne Marie Kupinski (vascular) and Diane M. Kawamura (abdomen), in creating the three volumes of *Diagnostic Medical Sonography* were invaluable. Their input and ideas were a significant contribution to the project.

The image contributions became just as valuable. We thank the many sonographers and physicians for their assistance. A special thank you and recognition for ongoing support in image acquisition includes Philips Medical Systems, Bothell, WA; GE Healthcare, Wauwatosa, WI; Joe Antony, MD, Cochin, India; Robin Davies, Ann Smith, and Denise Raney, Derry Imaging Center, Derry, NH; Barbara Hall-Terracciano; the sonographers at the Intermountain Medical Center, Murray, UT; Darla Matthew, Doña Ana Community College; and Pamela M. Foy at The Ohio State University Medical Center.

Many thanks to the production team at Lippincott Williams & Wilkins who helped edit, produce, promote, and deliver this textbook. We especially thank in the development of this edition Peter Sabatini, acquisitions editor, and Kristin Royer, associate product manager, for their patience, follow-through, support, and encouragement.

To our colleagues, students, friends, and family, who provide continued sources of encouragement, enthusiasm, and inspiration, thank you.

**Susan Raatz Stephenson MAEd,
RDMS (OB)(AB)(BR), RVT, RT(R)(C), CIIP**

Preface

The third edition of *Diagnostic Medical Sonography: Obstetrics and Gynecology* is a major revision. Educators and colleagues encouraged us to produce a third edition to incorporate the new advances used to image, to refresh the foundational content, and to continue to provide information that recognizes readers have diverse backgrounds and experiences. The result is a textbook that can be used as either an introduction to the profession or as a reference for the profession. The content lays the foundation for a better understanding of anatomy, physiology, pathophysiology, and complementary imaging expanding the sonographer practitioner, sonographer, sonologist, or student when caring for the patient.

The first chapter "Principles of Scanning Technique in Obstetric and Gynecologic Ultrasound" contains information on patient care and the process of beginning the imaging exam. Technology in the form of the picture archiving and communication systems (PACS) and interconnected computer systems within a clinic or hospital have revolutionized our profession.

The remainder of the textbook arrangement groups the gynecologic and obstetric chapters together. Throughout the chapters, we have tried to incorporate instrumentation and complementary imaging modalities when appropriate. This allows for integration of sonographic physics as well as other imaging modality findings that sonographers often follow.

We made every attempt to produce an up-to-date and factual textbook, at the same time presenting the material in an interesting and enjoyable format to capture the reader's attention. To do this, we provided detailed descriptions of anatomy, physiology, pathology, and the normal and abnormal sonographic representation of these anatomical and pathologic entities with illustrations, summary tables, and images, many of which include valuable case study information.

Our goal is to present as complete a text as possible, and recognizing that by tomorrow, the textbook must be supplemented by current journal readings. With every technological advance made in equipment, the sonographer's imagination must stretch to create new applications. With the comprehensive foundation available in this text, the sonographer can meet that challenge.

**Susan Raatz Stephenson MAEd,
RDMS (OB)(AB)(BR), RVT, RT(R)(C), CIIP**

Contributors

Lisa M. Allen, BS, RDMS (AB)(NE)(OB), RDCS (FE), RVT, FAIUM
Department of Obstetrics and Gynecology
Division of Maternal-Fetal Medicine
The Regional Perinatal Center
State University of New York
Upstate Medical University
Syracuse, NY

Amanda Auckland, RDMS (AB)(NE)(OB), RDCS (FE), RVT
Department of Ultrasound
University of Colorado Hospital
Aurora, CO

Sue Benzonelli-Blanchard, BS, RDMS (AB)(OB), RDCS (AE)
Issaquah, WA

Danielle M. Bolger, RT(R), RDMS (AB)(OB), RVT, RDCS
Department of Ultrasound
University of Colorado Hospital
Aurora, CO

Tonya N. Brathwaite, MBA, BS, RDMS
Supervisor, The Perinatal Diagnostic
  Testing Center
Department of Obstetrics and Gynecology
Jamaica Hospital Medical Center
Jamaica, NY
Adjunct Instructor
Diagnostic Medical Ultrasound Program
Sanford-Brown Institute
Garden City, NY

Allison A. Cowett, MD, MPH
Assistant Professor of Clinical Obstetrics
  and Gynecology and Associate Director,
  Fellowship in Family Planning
University of Illinois at Chicago College of
  Medicine
Director, Center for Reproductive Health
  and Director, Gynecologic Ultrasound
University of Illinois Medical Center at
  Chicago, IL

Meredith O. Cruz, MD
Division of Maternal Fetal Medicine
Department of Obstetrics and Gynecology
University of Illinois at Chicago
Chicago, IL

Molina Dayal, MD
Associate Professor
Department of Obstetrics and Gynecology
Fertility and IVF Center
George Washington Medical Facility
  Associates
Washington, DC

Julia A. Drose, BA, RDMS, RDMS (AB) (OB), RDCS (AE)(FE), RVT
Department of Ultrasound
University of Colorado Hospital
Aurora, CO

Marium Holland, MD, MPH
Department of Obstetrics, Gynecology, &
  Reproductive Sciences
Division of Maternal-Fetal Medicine
University of Texas Medical School
  at Houston
Houston, TX

Faith Hutson, BS, RT(R), RDMS (AB) (OB), RVT
Doña Ana Community College
Las Cruces, NM

Catheeja Ismail, Ed.D. RDMS (AB)(OB)
Director, Sonography Program
The George Washington University
Washington, DC

Susan Johnston, RDMS (AB)(FE)(OB)
GE Healthcare - Ultrasound
Lebanon, TN

Michelle Kominiarek, MD
Assistant Professor of Obstetrics and
  Gynecology
Department of Obstetrics and Gynecology
University of Illinois at Chicago
Chicago, IL

Sanja Plavsic Kupesic, MD, PhD
Clinical Professor of Obstetrics and
    Gynecology and Radiology
Department of Medical Education
Paul L. Foster School of Medicine
El Paso, TX

**Gertrude Alfonsin Layton, RDMS (AB)
(BR)(OB), RVT**
Woodland Park, CO

**Bridgette M. Lunsford, MAEd, RDMS
(AB)(OB), RVT**
Clinical Applications Specialist
GE Healthcare - Ultrasound
Arlington, VA

**Robert G. Magner, Jr., RDMS (AB)(BR)
(NE)(OB), RDCS (FE), RVT**
Penrose-St. Francis Health Services
Colorado Springs, CO

Jennifer Martin, RDMS (AB)(OB)
North Prairie, WI

Joan M. Mastrobattista, MD
Department of Obstetrics, Gynecology, &
    Reproductive Sciences
Division of Maternal-Fetal Medicine
    Baylor College of Medicine
University of Texas Medical School
    at Houston
Houston, TX

Roa M. Qato, MD
Administrative Chief Resident,
    Department of Ob/Gyn
University of Illinois at Chicago
Chicago, IL

**Dea Shatterly, BS, RDMS (OB)(AB),
RT(R)**
Ultrasound Department
Scott & White Healthcare
Temple, TX

**Molly Siemens, BS, RT (R), RDMS (AB)
(OB), RVT**
Hutch Clinic
McPherson, KS

**Tammy Stearns, MSAS, BSRT (R),
RDMS (AB)(NE)(OB), RVT**
CoxHealth School of Diagnostic Medical
    Sonography
Springfield, MO

**Susan Raatz Stephenson, MAEd,
RDMS (OB)(AB)(BR), RVT, RT(R)(C), CIIP**
University of Utah, George Washington
    University
Sandy, UT

**Malka Stromer, MAEd, BS,
RDMS (AB)(OB)**
Professor
Diagnostic Medical Sonography
GateWay Community College
Phoenix, AZ

John F. Trombly, BS, RT
Red Rocks Community College
Arvada, CO

Tricia Turner, BS, RDMS (AB)(OB), RVT
Assistant Program Coordinator
Diagnostic Medical Sonography
South Hills School of Business and
    Technology
State College, PA

**Cheryl A. Vance, MA, RDMS (AB)(BR)
(OB), RVT, RT(R)(M)**
Women's Health & Specialty Education
    Program Manager
GE Healthcare - Ultrasound
San Antonio, TX

Isabelle Wilkins, MD
Professor of Obstetrics and Gynecology
Interim Head, Department of Obstetrics
    and Gynecology
Department of Obstetrics and Gynecology
University of Illinois at Chicago
Chicago, IL

Michelle Wilson, MS, RDMS
Kaiser Permanente Medical Center at
    Vallejo
Sonography Session LLC
University of Southern Indiana
Napa, CA

**Paula Woletz MPH, RDMS (AB)(OB),
RDCS (AE)(FE)**
Director of Accreditation and Clinical Affairs
American Institute of Ultrasound in Medicine
Laurel, MD

Linda Woolpert, RDMS
Jenison, MI

Using This Series

The books in the *Diagnostic Medical Sonography* Series will help you develop an understanding of specialty sonography topics. Key learning resources and tools throughout the textbook aim to increase your understanding of the topics provided and better prepare you for your professional career. This User's Guide will help you familiarize yourself with these exciting features designed to enhance your learning experience.

18 Abnormalities of the Placenta and Umbilical Cord

Lisa M. Allen

OBJECTIVES

Recognize the sonographic appearance of placental and umbilical cord anomalies

Discuss developmental variations in placental size, shape, and configuration

Identify placenta previa classifications

Explain placental abruption and the associated risk factors

List placenta accreta classifications and known risk factors

Name the various abnormalities of umbilical cord insertion into the placenta

Describe cystic and solid masses of the umbilical cord

KEY TERMS

succenturiate lobe | circummarginate placenta | circumvallate placenta | placenta previa | placental abruption | placenta accreta spectrum | chorioangioma | amniotic band syndrome | uterine synechiae | marginal insertion | battledore placenta | velamentous insertion | true knot | false knot | nuchal cord | cord prolapse | vasa previa | single umbilical artery | cord entanglement | umbilical cord hemangioma | umbilical cord coiling | umbilical coiling index

GLOSSARY

Aneurysm Focal dilatation of an artery

Bilobed placenta Placenta where the lobes are nearly equal in size and the cord inserts into the chorionic bridge of tissue that connects the two lobes

Body stalk anomaly Fatal condition associated with multiple congenital anomalies and absence of the umbilical cord

Breus' mole Very rare condition where there is massive subchorionic thrombosis of the placenta secondary to extreme venous obstruction

Extrachorial placenta Attachment of the placental membranes to the fetal surface of the placenta rather than to the underlying villous placental margin

False knot Bending, twisting, and bulging of the umbilical cord vessels mimicking a knot in the umbilical cord

Gastroschisis Periumbilical abdominal wall defect, typically to the right of normal cord insertion, that allows for free-floating bowel in the amniotic fluid

Limb–body wall complex Condition characterized by multiple complex fetal anomalies and a short umbilical cord

Marginal insertion (a.k.a. battledore placenta) Occurs when the umbilical cord inserts at the placental margin instead of centrally

Mickey Mouse sign Term used to describe the cross-section of the three-vessel umbilical cord or the portal triad (portal vein, hepatic artery, common bile duct)

Omphalocele Central anterior abdominal wall defect of the umbilicus where abdominal organs are contained by a covering membrane consisting of peritoneum, Wharton's jelly, and amnion

Placentomegaly Term that refers to a thickened placenta

Synechia (Asherman's syndrome) Linear, extra amniotic tissue that projects into the amniotic cavity with no restriction of fetal movement

Thrombosis Intraplacental area of hemorrhage and clot

True knot Result of the fetus actually passing through a loop or loops of umbilical cord creating one or more knots in the cord

425

CHAPTER OBJECTIVES

Measurable objectives listed at the beginning of each chapter help you understand the intended outcomes for the chapter, as well as recognize and study important concept within each chapter.

GLOSSARY

Key terms are listed at the beginning of each chapter and clearly defined, then highlighted in bold type throughout the chapter to help you to learn and recall important terminology.

PATHOLOGY BOXES

Each chapter includes tables of relevant pathologies, which you can use as a quick reference for reviewing the material.

CRITICAL THINKING QUESTIONS

Throughout the chapter are critical thinking questions to test your knowledge and help you develop analytical skills that you will need in your profession.

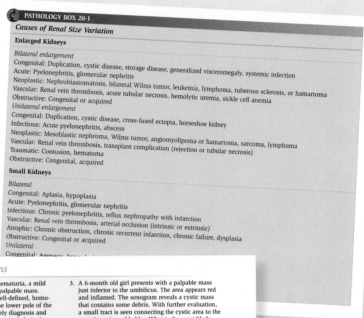

PATHOLOGY BOX 20-1

Causes of Renal Size Variation

Enlarged Kidneys

Bilateral enlargement
Congenital: Duplication, cystic disease, storage disease, generalized visceromegaly, systemic infection
Acute: Pyelonephritis, glomerular nephritis
Neoplastic: Nephroblastomatosis, bilateral Wilms tumor, leukemia, lymphoma, tuberous sclerosis, or hamartoma
Vascular: Renal vein thrombosis, acute tubular necrosis, hemolytic uremia, sickle cell anemia
Obstructive: Congenital or acquired

Unilateral enlargement
Congenital: Duplication, cystic disease, cross-fused ectopia, horseshoe kidney
Infectious: Acute pyelonephritis, abscess
Neoplastic: Mesoblastic nephroma, Wilms tumor, angiomyolipoma or hamartoma, sarcoma, lymphoma
Vascular: Renal vein thrombosis, transplant complication (rejection or tubular necrosis)
Traumatic: Contusion, hematoma
Obstructive: Congenital, acquired

Small Kidneys

Bilateral
Congenital: Aplasia, hypoplasia
Acute: Pyelonephritis, glomerular nephritis
Infectious: Chronic pyelonephritis, reflux nephropathy with infarction
Vascular: Renal vein thrombosis, arterial occlusion (intrinsic or extrinsic)
Atrophic: Chronic obstruction, chronic recurrent infarction, chronic failure, dysplasia
Obstructive: Congenital or acquired

Unilateral
Congenital: Agenesis, hypoplasia

Critical Thinking Questions

1. A 3-year-old boy presents with hematuria, a mild fever, and a left upper quadrant palpable mass. The sonogram demonstrates a well-defined, homogeneously solid, 3-cm mass in the lower pole of the left kidney. What is the most likely diagnosis and where else should the sonographer include in the examination?

2. The sonographer receives a requisition to perform an abdominal sonogram on a 2-day-old infant with a right upper quadrant abdominal mass following a difficult delivery. The examination reveals a large echogenic mass superior to the right kidney and appears separate from the right kidney. What is the most likely diagnosis and what would help to confirm the diagnosis?

3. A 6-month old girl presents with a palpable mass just inferior to the umbilicus. The area appears red and inflamed. The sonogram reveals a cystic mass that contains some debris. With further evaluation, a small tract is seen connecting the cystic area to the superior urinary bladder. What is the most likely diagnosis?

4. What is the most common cause of hydronephrosis in infants?

5. While scanning a newborn patient for a renal examination, the sonographer notices both kidneys are enlarged and echogenic with hyperechoic foci scattered throughout both kidneys. What is the most likely diagnosis?

RESOURCES

You will also find additional resources and exercises online, including a glossary with pronunciations, quiz bank, sonographic video clips, and weblinks. Use these interactive resources to test your knowledge, assess your progress, and review for quizzes and tests.

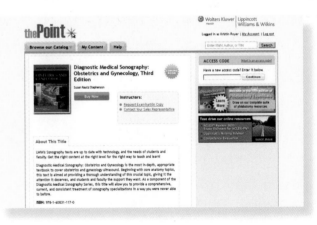

1 Principles of Scanning Technique in Obstetric and Gynecologic Ultrasound

Susan Raatz Stephenson

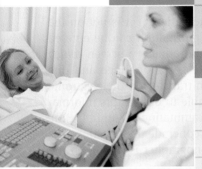

OBJECTIVES

Describe preparation of the patient for an obstetric or gynecologic sonogram

Identify the appropriate transducer for an examination

Explain ultrasound safety and the basic premise of as low as reasonably possible (ALARA)

Discuss the safety of 2D, 3D, and Doppler imaging

List the certification options available to a practicing sonographer

Explain the need for laboratory accreditation

KEY TERMS

patient preparation | transabdominal | endovaginal | exam protocol | ALARA | certification | registry

GLOSSARY

Adnexa Area around an organ

Aortocaval compression syndrome (supine hypotensive syndrome) Compression of the aorta and inferior vena cava (IVC) by the gravid uterus resulting in symptoms of nausea, hypotension, lightheadedness, and syncope

Ascites Fluid within the abdominal or pelvic cavity

Bioeffects Biophysical results of the interaction of sound waves and tissue

Ectopic pregnancy Pregnancy outside of the uterus

Electronic medical record (EMR) Electronic database containing all the patient information

Endocavity Inside a cavity such as the abdomen or pelvis

Fundus Top portion of the uterus

Hospital information system (HIS) Paper-based or computerized system designed to manage hospital data, such as billing and patient records

Lithotomy position Position of the patient with the feet in stirrups often used during delivery

Modality worklist (MWL) Electronic list of patients entered into a modality, such as ultrasound, which helps reduce data entry errors

Nongravid Nonpregnant

Perivascular Around the vessels

Picture archiving and communication system (PACS) Database that stores radiologic images

Placenta previa Condition where the placenta implantation is low in the uterus and will deliver before the fetus

Radiology information system (RIS) Physical or electronic system designed to manage radiology data, such as billing, reports, and images

Scanning protocol List of images required for a complete examination

Transabdominal Imaging through the abdomen

Transducer footprint Area of the transducer that comes in contact with the patient and emits ultrasound

Transvaginal/endovaginal Within the vagina

Vasa previa Condition where the umbilical cord becomes trapped between the presenting fetal part and the cervix

The goal of any sonographic examination is to produce a diagnostic study through the use of proper technique and patient preparation. Optimization of the examination reduces costs, adheres to the ALARA[1] principle of reducing exposure to ultrasound energy, and decreases patient discomfort. A protocol-driven approach help ensure complete imaging of the pelvic organs or fetus. This systematic imaging includes two-dimensional (2D) real-time, spectral, color or power Doppler, and increasingly, three-dimensional (3D) and four-dimensional (4D) imaging.

Manipulation of the technical factors such as overall gain, persistence, and output power has increasingly become linked to automated image adjustment. Obtaining the required images for a study requires knowledge of not only the physics of ultrasound but also a thorough knowledge of normal and abnormal anatomy, and the disease processes being imaged.

In this chapter, you will find descriptions of basic techniques and protocols of scanning in obstetrics and gynecology along with emerging imaging technologies. Routines specific to the topics discussed are explained in greater detail in subsequent chapters.

PATIENT PREPARATION

GETTING SET UP

When the patient arrives for her sonographic examination, she first must be entered into the hospital information system (HIS). A patient number assignment identifies the patient's electronic medical record (EMR), to which all laboratory, pathology, and imaging studies are attached. Each visit generates a separate number to help identify procedures. Upon entry into the radiology information system (RIS), the sonographer is able to search the modality worklist (MWL), and the patient study information automatically populates on the ultrasound machine. Although this sounds quite complicated, the connected hospital makes our lives much easier through the elimination of errors and the use of film.[2]

The sonographer should introduce himself or herself when meeting the patient. To confirm the patient's identification, use two identifiers such as the name and the date of birth. Some facilities attach an arm band to the patient that can be used for identification purposes. At this time, ask the patient what she is scheduled for to confirm the correct order and her perception of the upcoming examination (Table 1-1). Upon completion of patient identity and exam confirmation, explain the procedure, the length of the examination, what she may expect to feel, and where and how the transducer will be moved.

All pertinent clinical information should be included on the ultrasound report. This includes patient age, date of the last menstrual period (LMP; also whether it is normal), gravidity, parity, symptoms such as pain or bleeding, history of pelvic procedures, and any other pertinent medical or surgical history. This information

TABLE	1-1
Patient Identifiers[a]	

- Ask patient his or her name
- Have the patient state his or her date of birth (DOB)
- Exam type
- Ordering clinician
- Armband

[a]To ensure the proper patient, use two different identifiers.[40]

should be obtained from the patient if it is not on the examination request. This information can be entered into the equipment in an introductory screen *which in many cases can* calculate gestational age and due dates. This information then transfers to the electronic report (Fig. 1-1). It is desirable to obtain this information before beginning the examination to minimize the chance that the patient will conclude the questions are related to something the sonographer is seeing on the screen.

Knowing the patient's reproductive history gives the sonographer information with which to design and interpret the sonographic examination. For example, if the patient is small for gestational age (SGA), the exam might reveal growth problems or low fluid levels. Although variations of the obstetric coding system may be used, the following is the most common: *Gravidity* (G) refers to the number of previous pregnancies and includes the current gestation. A pregnant woman who had a nonviable ectopic pregnancy and later gave birth to twins would be G3. If the patient is currently nongravid but has had four previous pregnancies, she is said to be G4. *Parity* (P) refers to the number of pregnancies the patient has carried to term; thus, an ectopic pregnancy would be recorded as P0 and a twin gestation would be P1. The numbers used after P refer, in order, to the number of term pregnancies, abortions (spontaneous or induced), and living children. Thus, the currently pregnant patient would be classified as a G3P1A1T2, which would mean the woman has had three pregnancies, one full-term pregnancy, one abortion (the ectopic pregnancy in this case), and two full-term births, (in this case, a set of twins).[3] If the patient is not currently pregnant, she would be a G2P1A1T2 (Table 1-2).

It is generally accepted that the first day of the LMP is used to date pregnancies. The LMP usually occurs about 2 weeks before conception. The LMP is chosen because women can document this date. Still, 20% to 40% of pregnant women are uncertain of their LMP, making dating of a pregnancy unreliable. Ultrasound can narrow the estimated date of delivery (EDD), also referred to as estimated date of confinement (EDC), to as little as ±2.7 days by using the average of at least three first-trimester crown-rump length (CRL) measurements.[4]

Figure 1-1 The patient data entry (PDE) screen allows entry of the accession number or the patient visit number, LMP, and patient pregnancy information. If you work in a facility that does not have a connected workflow, the patient information may be manually entered on this screen.

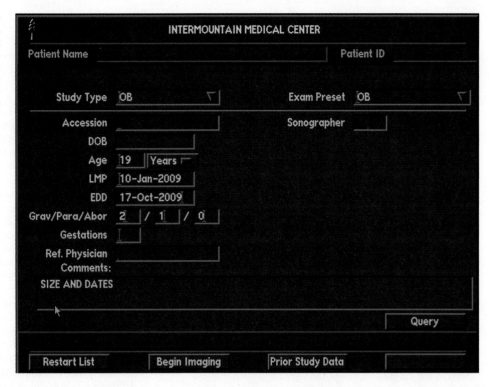

After obtaining all pertinent clinical information, assist the patient onto the examination table, making her as comfortable as possible. A pillow or two under the patient's knees relieves back strain. For a transabdominal examination, apply gel liberally to the lower abdomen to provide an effective medium for sound transmission. To minimize patient discomfort, warm the gel to body temperature. If a laboratory is not equipped with a gel warmer, the gel may be warmed in a sink of warm water. Do not use a microwave, as the gel heats unevenly and may explode. If an endovaginal examination is to be performed, give the patient privacy while she undresses from the waist down and drapes herself with a sheet.

Every laboratory should develop scanning protocols for each type of examination and include these in a printed reference manual. Suggested protocols have been developed for obstetric and gynecologic scanning by the American Institute of Ultrasound in Medicine (AIUM; Displays 1-1 and 1-2).[5,6] The Society of

TABLE	1-2	
Gravida/Parity Definitions		
Term/Abbreviation	**Definition**	
Gravida (G)	Number of pregnancies	
Para (P)	Number of pregnancies over 36 weeks (term)	
Abortion (A)	Number of failed pregnancies	
Term (T)	Number of live births	

DISPLAY 1-1

Guidelines for the Performance of the Antepartum Obstetrical Ultrasound Examination

Guidelines for First-Trimester Sonography

Indications: Confirm intrauterine pregnancy; evaluate for suspected ectopic pregnancy; determine the cause of vaginal bleeding or pelvic pain; estimate gestational age; diagnose or evaluate multiple pregnancies; confirm viability, adjunct to chorionic villus sampling (CVS), embryo transfer, and localization and removal of an intrauterine device (IUD); assess for fetal anomalies such as anencephaly; evaluate maternal uterine anomalies and/or pelvic masses; measure the nuchal translucency (NT); and evaluate for suspected hydatidiform mole.

Overall Comment. Scanning in the first trimester may be performed abdominally, vaginally, or using both methods. If an abdominal examination fails to provide diagnostic information, perform a vaginal or transperioneal examination. Similarly, if a vaginal scan fails to image all areas needed for diagnosis, an abdominal scan should be performed.

1. Evaluate the uterus and adnexa for the presence of a gestational sac. Document any visualized gestational sac and determine the location. Note the presence or absence of an embryo and record the CRL.

   Comment. (1) CRL is a more accurate indicator of gestational age than gestational sac diameter. If the embryo is not identified, evaluate the gestational sac for the presence of a yolk sac. The estimate of gestational age would be based on either the mean diameter of the gestational sac or on the morphology and contents of the gestational sac. (2) Identification of a yolk sac or an embryo is definitive evidence of a gestational sac. Use caution in making a definitive diagnosis of a gestational sac prior to the development of these structures. The lack of a yolk sac and embryo raises suspicion of an intrauterine fluid collection, which often coexists with the pseudogestational sac associated with an ectopic pregnancy. (3) During the late first trimester, biparietal diameter (BPD) and other fetal measurements also may be used to establish fetal age.

2. Record the presence or absence of cardiac activity with M-Mode or Cineloop.

Comment. (1) Real-time observation is critical for this diagnosis. (2) With vaginal scans, an embryo with a CRL of 5 mm or greater should demonstrate cardiac motion. If an embryo less than 5 mm in length is seen with no cardiac activity, a follow-up scan may be needed to evaluate for fetal life.

3. Document fetal number.

Comment. Report multiple pregnancies only when imaging multiple embryos. Incomplete amnion and chorion fusion, or elevation of the chorionic membrane by intrauterine hemorrhage, often mimic a second sac in the first trimester, leading to an incorrect diagnosis of a multiple pregnancy.

4. Evaluate the uterus, adnexal structures, and cul-de-sac.

Comment. (1) This allows recognition of incidental findings of potential clinical significance. Record the presence, location, and size of myomas and adnexal masses. Scan the cul-de-sac for presence or absence of fluid. If there is fluid in the cul-de-sac, image the flanks and subhepatic space for intra-abdominal fluid. (2) Correlate serum hormonal levels with ultrasound findings to help in differentiation of a normal, abnormal, or ectopic pregnancy.

5. Evaluate the nuchal region in the presence of a live fetus.

Comment. (1) The NT measurement is a very specific measurement obtained at laboratory-determined intervals. (2) Use the NT measurement in conjunction with serum biochemistry to determine the patient risk for trisomy 13 or 18, or other defects such as heart or spine malformations. (3) NT certification ensures consistent quality and examination performance between sonographers.

Guidelines for Second- and Third-Trimester Sonography

Indications: Evaluation of gestational age and fetal growth; determination of the cause of vaginal bleeding, pelvic pain, or cervical insufficiency; determination of fetal presentation; diagnosis or evaluation of multiple pregnancies; confirmation of viability, adjunct to amniocentesis; determination of cause of uterine size and clinical date discrepancies; assessment for fetal anomalies; evaluation of maternal uterine anomalies, pelvic masses, or suspected ectopic pregnancy; evaluation of fetal well-being; determination of amniotic fluid levels, suspected placental abruption, placement of cervical cerclage, adjunct to external cephalic version, premature rupture of membranes (PROM), abnormal biochemical markers; follow up to a fetal anomaly and placental location, history of a congenital anomaly; evaluation of fetal condition in patients with late prenatal care; assessment of findings that increase the risk of aneuploidy; and evaluation for suspected hydatidiform mole.

1. Document fetal life, number, presentation, and activity.

Comment. (1) Report an abnormal heart rate and/or rhythm. (2) Multiple pregnancies require the documentation of additional information: number of gestational sacs, number of placentas, presence or absence of a dividing membrane, fetal genitalia (if visible), comparison of fetal sizes, and comparison of amniotic fluid volume (AFV) on each side of the membrane.

2. Report an estimate of AFV (increased, decreased, normal).

Comment. When determining the appropriateness of AFV, consider the physiologic variation that occurs with each stage of pregnancy.

3. Record the placental location and appearance, as well as its relationship to the internal cervical os. Document the umbilical cord insertion sites into both the placenta and fetus. Include a cross-section of the free floating cord for three vessel confirmation as well as color Doppler images of the umbilical vessels coursing lateral to the fetal bladder.

Comment. (1) It is recognized that apparent placental position early in pregnancy may not correlate well with its location at the time of delivery. (2) An overdistended maternal urinary bladder or a lower uterine contraction can give the examiner a false impression of placenta previa. (3) Abdominal, transperineal, or vaginal views may be helpful in visualizing the internal cervical os and its relationship to the placenta.

4. Obtain fetal measurements to assess gestational age using a combination of cranial measurement such as the BPD or head circumference (HC), and limb measurement such as the femur length (FL).

Comment. (1) Third-trimester measurements may not accurately reflect gestational age due to morphologic differences in individuals (i.e., short, tall). Base the current exam dates on the earliest examination as the CRL, BPD, HC, and FL have a greater accuracy earlier in the pregnancy. To determine the current fetal age, use an OB wheel, enter data into the equipment or use the following calculation: CRL, BPD, HC, and/or the FL by the equation: current fetal age = estimated age at time of initial study + number of weeks elapsed since first study.

4A. The standard reference level for measurement of the BPD is an axial image that includes the thalamus.

Comment. If the fetal head is dolichocephalic or brachycephalic, the BPD measurement may be misleading. Occasionally, computation of the cephalic index (CI), a ratio of the BPD to the fronto-occipital diameter, is needed to make this determination. In such situations, other measurements of head size, such as the HC, may be necessary.

4B. Measure the HC at the same level as the PBD, around the outer perimeter of the calvarium at the level of the thalamus.

4C. Routinely measure and record the FL after the 14th week of gestation.

Comment. As with head measurements, there is considerable biologic variation in normal FLs late in pregnancy.

5. Obtain a fetal weight estimate in the late second and in the third trimesters. This measurement requires an abdominal diameter or circumference.

Comment. (1) Check appropriateness of growth from previous studies at least 2 to 4 weeks previous. (2) Fetal weight estimations may be as much as ±15% from actual delivery weights. This may be due to the patient population, sonographer measuring techniques, and technical factors.

5A. Measure the abdominal circumference (AC) on a true transverse view, preferably at the level of the junction of the left and right portal veins and fetal stomach.

Comment. An AC measurement helps estimate fetal weight and may allow detection of growth retardation and macrosomia.

5B. Estimate interval growth from previous fetal biometric studies.

6. Evaluate the uterus (including the cervix) and adnexal structures.

   Comment. This allows recognition of incidental findings of potential clinical significance. Record the presence, location, and size of myomas and adnexal masses. It is frequently not possible to image the maternal ovaries during the second and third trimesters. Vaginal or transperineal scanning may be helpful in evaluating the cervix when the fetal head prevents visualization of the cervix from transabdominal scanning.

7. The study should include, but not necessarily be limited to, assessment of the following fetal anatomy: cerebral ventricles, posterior fossa (including cerebellar hemispheres and cisterna magna), choroid plexus, lateral cerebral ventricles, midline falx, cavum septi pellucid, upper lip, views of the heart to include the four-chambers (including its position within the thorax), left ventricular outflow, and right ventricular outflow along with aortic arch and ductal arch images, spine, stomach, kidneys, urinary bladder, color Doppler or Color Power Angio images of the umbilical vessels lateral to the bladder, fetal umbilical cord insertion site, and intactness of the anterior abdominal wall and placenta. Also include images of the limbs, along with the presence or absence of the long bone and the fetal sex determination. Although not considered part of the minimum required examination, when fetal position permits, it is desirable to examine all areas of the anatomy.

   Comment. (1) It is recognized that not all malformations of the previously mentioned organ systems can be detected using ultrasonography. (2) Consider these recommendations as a minimum guideline for the fetal anatomic survey. Occasionally, some of these structures may not be well visualized, as occurs when fetal position, low amniotic volume, or maternal body habitus limit the sonographic examination. When this occurs, the report of the ultrasound examination should include a notation delineating structures that were not well seen. (3) Suspected abnormalities may require a targeted evaluation of the area(s) of concern. (4) In the patient with an increased risk of aneuploidy, perform a nuchal fold measurement.

(American Institute of Ultrasound in Medicine. *Guidelines for Performance of the Antepartum Obstetrical Ultrasound Examination.* Laurel, MD: AIUM; 2007.)

DISPLAY 1-2

Guidelines for Performance of the Ultrasound Examination of the Female Pelvis

Indications: Pain; painful menses (dysmenorrhea); lack of menses (amenorrhea); excessive menstrual bleeding (menorrhagia); irregular uterine bleeding (metrorrhagia); excessive irregular bleeding (menometrorrhagia); follow-up of previous detected abnormality; evaluation, monitoring, and/or treatment of infertility patients; delayed menses, precocious puberty, or vaginal bleeding in a prepubertal child; postmenopausal bleeding; abnormal or technically limited manual examination; signs and symptoms of a pelvic infection; further imaging of an anomaly found during another imaging study; congenital anomaly evaluation; excessive bleeding; pain or signs of infection after pelvis

surgery; delivery or abortion; localization of an intrauterine device (IUD), malignancy screening for high-risk patients; urinary incontinence or pelvic organ prolapse; and guidance for interventional or surgical procedures.

The following guidelines describe the examination to be performed for each organ and anatomic region in the female pelvis. All relevant structures should be identified by the abdominal and/or vaginal approach. If an abdominal examination is performed and fails to provide the necessary diagnostic information, a vaginal scan should be done when possible. Similarly, if a vaginal scan is performed and fails to image all areas needed for diagnosis, an abdominal scan should be performed. In some cases, both an abdominal and a vaginal scan may be needed.

GENERAL PELVIC PREPARATION

For a pelvic sonogram performed through the abdominal wall, the patient's urinary bladder should, in general, be distended adequately to displace the small bowel and its contained gas from the field of view. Occasionally, overdistention of the bladder may compromise evaluation. When this occurs, imaging should be repeated after the patient partially empties the bladder.

For a vaginal sonogram, the urinary bladder is preferably empty. The vaginal transducer may be introduced by the patient, the sonographer, or the physician. A female member of the physician's or hospital's staff should be present, when possible, as a chaperone in the examining room during vaginal sonography.

UTERUS

The vagina and uterus provide anatomic landmarks that can be used as reference points when evaluating the pelvic structures. In evaluating the uterus, document the following: (1) uterine size, shape, and orientation; (2) the endometrium; (3) the myometrium; and (4) the cervix.

Evaluate the uterine length on a long-axis view as the distance from the fundus to the cervix. The depth of the uterus (anteroposterior dimension) is measured on the same long-axis view from its anterior to posterior walls, perpendicular to its long axis. Measure the width on the axial or coronal view. Exclude the cervix when performing volume measurements of the uterus.

Document abnormalities of the uterus to include of contour changes, echogenicity, masses, and cysts. Measure findings on at least two dimensions, acknowledging that it is not necessary to measure all fibroids.

Analyze the endometrium for thickness, focal abnormality, and the presence of any fluid or masses in the endometrial cavity. Measure the endometrium on a midline sagittal image, including anterior and posterior portions of the basal endometrium and excluding the adjacent hypoechoic myometrium and any endometrial fluid. Assessment of the endometrium should allow for normal variations in the appearance of the endometrium expected with phases of the menstrual cycle and with hormonal supplementation. Sonohysterography helps evaluate the patient with abnormal dysfunctional uterine bleeding or with an abnormally thickened endometerium. Document an IUD and the location within the uterus. When available, obtain a 3D volume for coronal reconstruction of the uterus.

ADNEXA (OVARIES AND FALLOPIAN TUBES)

When evaluating the adnexa, an attempt should be made to identify the ovaries first since they can serve as a major point of reference for assessing the presence of adnexal pathology. Although their location is variable, the ovaries are most often situated anterior to the internal iliac (hypogastric) vessels, lateral to the uterus, and superficial to the obturator internus muscle. Measure the ovaries and document any ovarian abnormalities. Determine the ovarian size by measuring the ovary in three dimensions (width, length, and depth) on views obtained in two orthogonal planes. To ensure measurement of three orthogonal planes, utilize the dual-imaging format. It is recognized that the ovaries may not be identifiable in some women. This occurs most frequently after menopause or in patients with a large leiomyomatous uterus.

The normal fallopian tubes are not visualized in most patients. Survey the para-adnexal regions for abnormalities, particularly fluid-filled or distended tubular structures that may represent dilated fallopian tubes.

Reference any adnexal masses to its relationship to the uterus. Document the ipsilateral ovary. Determine the ovary size and echo pattern (cystic, solid, or mixed; presence of septations). Doppler ultrasound may be useful in select cases to identify the vascular nature of pelvic structures.

CUL-DE-SAC

The cul-de-sac and bowel posterior to the uterus may not be clearly visualized. This area should be evaluated for the presence of free fluid or mass. When free fluid is detected, its echogenicity should be assessed. If a mass is detected, its size, position, shape, echo pattern (cystic, solid, or complex), and its relationship to the ovaries and uterus should be documented. Peristalsis is held to differentiate bowel from a pelvic mass. In the absence of peristalsis, differentiation of normal or abnormal loops of bowel from a mass may, at times, be difficult. An endovaginal examination may be helpful in distinguishing a suspected mass from fluid and feces within the normal rectosigmoid. An ultrasound water enema study or a repeat examination after a cleansing enema may also help distinguish a suspected mass from bowel.

(American Institute of Ultrasound in Medicine. *Guidelines for Performing of the Ultrasound Examination of the Female Pelvis.* Laurel, MD: AIUM; 2009.)

Diagnostic Medical Sonography (SDMS) Guidelines for Obstetrics and Gynecology Review includes a section on scanning techniques[7] as do the American College of Radiology (ACR) guidelines. A sonographer developing his or her own protocols should keep in mind that the sonographic examination must clearly demonstrate the normality or abnormality of each anatomic structure through a series of representative images.

Developing an examination protocol ensures performance of all studies in a consistent and complete manner, thereby reducing the likelihood of missing pathology. Many articles have discussed the weaknesses of the Routine Antenatal Diagnostic Imaging with Ultrasound Study (RADIUS),[8] which concluded that routine obstetric ultrasound was not cost-effective. Of interest to sonographers is that the study illustrated the difference in the rate of fetal anomaly detection between tertiary care centers and nontertiary care centers.[6,7] The rate of detection was 60% lower in nontertiary care centers than in tertiary care centers, which presumably

had more experienced sonographers and physicians. This study illustrated the importance of being thorough and optimizing image quality when performing a sonographic study.

GYNECOLOGIC EXAMINATIONS

A full urinary bladder is the hallmark of obstetric and gynecologic scanning (Fig. 1-2). Instructions on how to prepare for an examination should be tailored to the patient, the examination objectives, and the transducer type. A premenopausal woman who is to be examined for a possible ovarian cyst can be instructed to eat normally, void, and then finish drinking four 8-oz glasses of water 1 hour *before* the examination and not void until after the examination. These directions should ensure that she will be properly prepared for the transabdominal pelvic sonogram. A postmenopausal woman in her 60s or 70s who is scheduled because of uterine bleeding may have decreased bladder capacity or may suffer from incontinence. The directions for this patient could be modified by asking her to drink only three 8-oz glasses of water. If a patient is scheduled for an endovaginal examination, the bladder must be empty unless the abdominal scan occurs during the same examination.

An adequately filled bladder usually extends slightly beyond the fundus of a nongravid uterus. If the uterus and adnexa are clearly delineated, the bladder is full enough; if not, the patient should be instructed to drink more water or wait for her bladder to fill more. Patient positioning techniques may be particularly helpful with a less than optimally filled bladder. Ask the patient to lie in a left or right posterior oblique position so that the bladder drapes over the structure of interest, such as the lateral section of the uterus, the adnexa, or a mass.

If the patient's bladder is so distended that it compresses and displaces the pelvic viscera, or the patient cannot tolerate the examination, have her partially empty by giving her a cup and telling her how many cups she may void. Many patients are skeptical of their ability to stop the flow of urine, but most are successful.

In many cases, it is possible to evaluate most of the low-lying pelvic structures with an empty urinary bladder by using a endovaginal transducer. The transabdominal approach is used primarily to rule out pelvic masses that are beyond the imaging range of the endovaginal transducer.

Performing the Gynecologic Examination

Regardless of clinical indication, a gynecologic examination should include the following images: sagittal midline of the uterus, including the cervix and vagina; right and left parasagittal views of the uterus and both adnexa; and transverse views of the uterine fundus with cornua, the uterine corpus, cervix, vagina, and each ovary. Demonstrate and record characteristics of

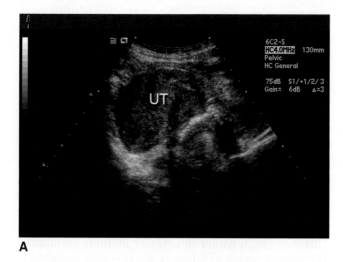

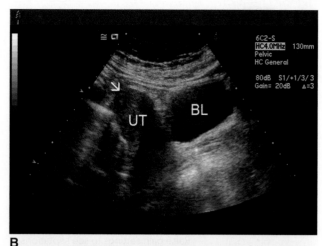

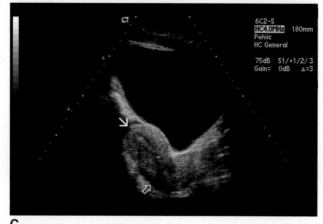

Figure 1-2 A: This sagittal transabdominal scan through an empty bladder presents a suboptimal image of the uterus *(UT)*. The adnexa does not visualize. **B:** This image demonstrates a partially filled bladder (BL). Although the UT visualizes better, the BL is not filled enough to allow complete evaluation of the fundal region *(arrow)*. **C:** With the BL adequately filled, the fundus *(arrow)* can be evaluated, as can the echogenicity of the myometrium and endometrium. A small amount of free fluid images in the posterior cul-de-sac *(open arrow)*.

any suspected pathology in addition to the standard views. Include several sagittal and transverse views of any suspected abnormality in the sonographic record. Documentation should include images with and without measurements and a demonstration of the echogenicity of the abnormal structure. Every attempt should be made to delineate clearly the mass and its relationship to surrounding organs and structures. If results of the sonographic examination are negative, the area of interest should be imaged to prove that no pathology was seen.

The sonographer must also be aware of associated findings of a particular disease. For instance, when imaging a solid ovarian mass, the sonographer also will carefully examine the cul-de-sac, Morison's pouch, the liver edge, and the flanks for ascites. Also examine the liver, kidneys, and perivascular areas for evidence of metastases. Every examination must be performed thoroughly; the additional time required is minimal when using real-time scanners and the findings may be critical to the patient's well-being. Although sonographic images of gynecologic masses often are frustratingly nonspecific, with optimal technique, characteristics related to particular masses can be visualized (Table 1-3).

It is also important to understand when Doppler and color Doppler may enhance diagnosis. Several chapters in this textbook describe specific techniques for imaging pelvic masses.

A good understanding of the physical principles of ultrasound enables the sonographer to solve imaging problems. Many excellent textbooks explain these principles.[9,10]

Every sonographer should make efforts to minimize sonographic artifacts produced during imaging. The following basic scanning principles help achieve diagnostic images:

1. To optimize the superior axial resolution of the transducer, keep the sonographic beam as close to perpendicular as possible to the area of interest
2. The best resolution occurs within the focal zone of the transducer
3. Higher-frequency transducers provide better resolution
4. Lower-frequency transducers provide greater depth of penetration
5. Fluid-filled structures enhance the transmission of sound
6. Solid structures attenuate sound to varying degrees

TABLE 1-3	
General Principles of Gynecologic Scanning Techniques	
Characteristics of Mass	**Scanning Technique**
Size	Measure three longest dimensions: length, height, width
Mobility	Turn patient, empty bladder, apply transducer pressure
Tissue composition	Change transducer: high to low frequency
	Compare to urine, which is fluid and anechoic
	Raise gain settings to see septations, lower gain to see shadows from calcifications
	Look for edge shadowing and anterior reverberation artifacts in fluid-filled structures
	Check for peristalsis in mass to determine whether it is bowel
Extension	Examine bladder wall, which should appear as clean, echogenic line measuring 3 to 6 mm
	Examine cul-de-sac, flanks, Morison's pouch for ascites
	Examine liver for metastases
	Examine kidneys for hydronephrosis and metastases
	Examine perivascular area for enlarged nodes

OBSTETRIC EXAMINATIONS

The degree of bladder filling required depends on the stage of gestation. In the first trimester, a full bladder is needed for transabdominal scanning to push the air-filled intestines out of the false pelvis and allow for an unobstructed view of the uterus (Fig. 1-3). Once the second trimester begins, it is usually not necessary for the patient to have as full of a bladder because the uterus fills the pelvic cavity and displaces the intestines.

A moderately filled bladder enhances visualization of the internal os by providing an unobstructed view of that area. This is useful when assessing competency of the internal os, in determining placental position relative to the os when there is a low-lying placenta, and in displacing a low fetal head upward into a position where the BPD can be measured. Endovaginal or perineal studies enable the sonographer to evaluate the cervix or presenting fetal part in more detail than may be possible by the transabdominal approach.

Performing the Obstetric Examination

Imaging a pregnant patient before the 15th week of gestation requires basically the same technique as a gynecologic ultrasound examination. The protocol detailing the number of examinations and measurements that need to be taken is summarized in Display 1-1 and is described more fully in subsequent chapters.

If the patient had a previous examination and you are using the same piece of equipment, the exam may still be on the hard drive. In this case, the previous examination may be accessed along with the measurements. This becomes important when performing serial exams for fetal growth problems. If the data is not on the equipment, you are able to manually enter the information.

After about 20 weeks' gestation, some women suffer from aortocaval compression syndrome, the cause of supine hypotensive syndrome, which results in the inability of mothers to lie on their back for long periods. This may begin earlier in cases of multiple gestations. The patient begins to fidget as she becomes uncomfortable and may complain that she is hot, nauseous, or feels like she is going to faint. At the first sign of these symptoms, the patient should be turned to a side or have her back elevated. A drink of cold water or a cold, wet washcloth to the forehead will enable her to recover more quickly. Once she has recovered, the examination may resume after putting a pillow under one side of the patient so that her body is tilted. This provides the patient with relief from her symptoms while providing the sonographer with access to her pelvis. Scanning in the most efficient manner possible minimizes the time the patient lies on the table.

The sonographer should establish an organized routine for scanning; for example, begin the scan with the fetal environment, fluid, placenta cord, and cervix. Do not forget to search for any ovarian masses. When imaging the fetus, begin at the fetal head and neural tube structures. Then image the internal organs and limbs. Record representative images as they are obtained through this survey. Consistency in performing or adhering to a protocol saves the sonographer from having to design a new approach for each patient, makes doing complete examinations habitual, and alerts the sonographer very quickly when something is unusual or abnormal. Having a checklist of fetal anatomy and measurements is also helpful in ensuring that each study is complete.

TRANSDUCER SELECTION

The choice of transducer should be based on patient habitus, stage of pregnancy, and examination objectives. Each laboratory should have a selection of transducers of varying frequencies with M-mode, Doppler, and color Doppler capabilities. Many transducers are now duplex: a 2D image is seen on the screen with a simultaneous M-mode or Doppler spectral display. Imaging with 2D, color, and spectral Doppler is called triplex imaging. Most transducers are electronically focused, enabling the sonographer to optimally image the structure of interest by changing the depth of the

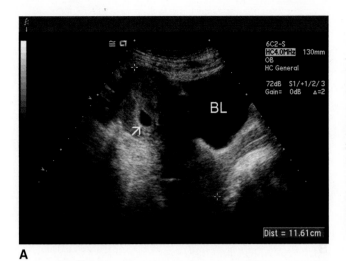
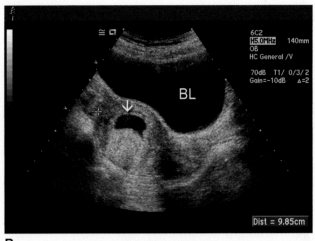

A   **B**

Figure 1-3 A: The urinary bladder *(BL)* is partially full, but not enough to determine whether the gestational sac *(arrow)* contains a viable embryo. **B:** The uterus with the fundal gestational sac *(arrow)* can now be clearly delineated because the bladder is full.

focal point, and the number of focal points. Broadband transducers enable the operator to change imaging frequencies to optimize resolution at different depths.[9,10]

The small scanning surface or footprint of sector transducers make them easily maneuverable and, therefore, effective in most gynecologic and early gestation applications. Linear transducers in a variety of sizes and shapes provide various fields of view related to their length and produce more accurate measurements of linear structures (e.g., femur), making them particularly useful in late pregnancy. Curved linear array transducers combine the wider field of view of sector transducers with greater near-field visualization and increased linear measurement accuracy.

Patient body habitus affects the choice of transducer frequency. Large patients may require the use of a 2.5-MHz transducer, whereas 5.0 MHz provides excellent resolution on slender women and on children. Infants are often best imaged with 7.5-MHz transducers. In pregnant women, the stage of gestation also influences the choice of frequencies. A 5-MHz transducer may provide optimal images well into the third trimester on a slender patient. In later pregnancy and in heavier women, a 3.5-MHz transducer usually provides better depth penetration. Improvement in image processing has enhanced resolution, thereby allowing patients to be studied with higher-frequency transducers than was previously feasible. To optimize image quality, the sonographer should change transducers depending on the depth of the structure being imaged. For example, if the fetal spine is up, and the kidneys appear suspect, change to a higher-frequency transducer to improve resolution. If a patient is obese, and therefore the fetus is far from the transducer face, change to a lower-frequency transducer.

The utility of the endovaginal transducer and the superior imaging it provides in most gynecologic and some obstetric applications make it an essential addition to the transducer arsenal of any laboratory doing gynecologic and obstetric ultrasound. Endovaginal transducers range from 3.0 to more typically 6.0 to 7.5 MHz. Selection of frequency is determined by the distance from the cervix of the structure to be evaluated. Endovaginal transducers produced by different manufacturers vary in size, shape, orientation of the imaging plane in relation to the shaft of the transducer, whether the shaft has an angle to it, and the addition of duplexed M-mode (simultaneous display of M-mode with 2D images), Doppler, color Doppler, and color Power Angio capabilities. Some machines and transducers also have the capability of beam steering.[9,10]

Endovaginal transducers are used primarily for evaluating the nongravid female pelvis and the first trimester fetus. Later in pregnancy, the endovaginal transducer may be useful in the evaluation of presenting fetal parts and the cervix, and to rule out a placenta previa or vasa previa. Endovaginal transducers have also been found to be useful in delineating fetal anatomy in obese pregnant patients when imaging through the maternal umbilicus, where the subcutaneous fat thickness is significantly reduced. When selecting equipment, the laboratory should consider the applications for which various transducers may be used.

ENDOVAGINAL SCANNING

Endovaginal scans are often performed in conjunction with transabdominal scans. The endovaginal transducer images anatomy within a focal range of 2 to 7 cm and cannot be inserted past the area of the vaginal fornices, limiting visualization to the uterus and adnexa in the nongravid patient without an enlarged leiomyomatous uterus, and the lower uterine segment in a gravid patient. Most clinical situations require an extensive view of the pelvis and abdomen, which cannot be provided

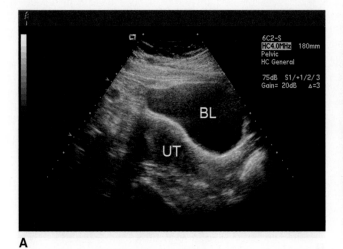

A

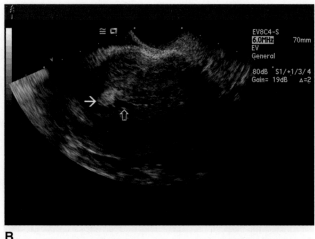

B

Figure 1-4 A: An abdominal scan demonstrates a relatively normal appearing uterus *(UT)* posterior to a relatively full bladder *(BL)*. The reverberation artifact is due to patient obesity; however, a decrease of dynamic range or overall gain helps remove some of the scattering artifact. **B:** The endovaginal scan allows better imaging of the endometrium revealing an echogenic *(arrow)* polyp and fluid *(open arrow)*.

by the endovaginal transducer alone (Fig. 1-4). A few applications for endovaginal sonography include ectopic pregnancy evaluation; uterine, ovarian, and pelvic inflammatory disease; placenta previa or accrete; fetal anatomy and cardiovascular systems; and monitoring ovulation. It may also be used to guide procedures such as ova aspiration, embryo transfer, drainage or aspiration of pelvic fluid, and treatment of ectopic pregnancies. The SDMS publication *Sonography Examination Guidelines*[11] provides a good overview of the technique, and the AIUM's Ultrasound Practice Committee has issued recommendations[12] for cleaning endocavitary transducers.

TECHNIQUE

Carefully explain the procedure to the patient before beginning the examination procedure. In some institutions, the patient is asked to sign an informed consent form before the examination.

1. Scan the patient with an empty bladder, as a distended bladder may distort pelvic anatomy and push organs of interest out of the transducer range. Patients being examined for low-lying placenta should have a half-full bladder to help outline the internal os and anterior portion of the cervix.
2. The lithotomy position is used or a pillow may be placed under the supine patient's buttocks. The patient's upper body should be positioned higher than the pelvis to permit pooling of any fluid in the cul-de-sac.
3. Cover the transducer with a cover designed for this purpose. The cover reduces the patient's risk of infection. If a transducer cover is not available, substitute a condom or a digit of a surgical glove. Place a small amount of gel on the face of the transducer before covering to provide a fluid contact between

the scanning face and the cover. Take care to remove all air bubbles between the transducer face and the cover to optimize image quality.
4. Lubricate the transducer cover with K-Y jelly to minimize patient discomfort. If the patient is being treated for infertility, no coupling gel should be used because of its spermicidal effect; instead, lubricate the transducer with saline.
5. Depending on institutional policy, the patient, physician, or sonographer inserts the transducer into the vagina. It is advisable for a female chaperone to be present during the performance of the examination.
6. The sonographer manipulates the transducer to image sagittal, coronal, and transverse sections of the uterus and adnexa. This is done by pushing or pulling the transducer and by tilting or rotating the handle. Advance the transducer while imaging to avoid advancing the transducer too far. As with standard scanning, enlarging the image enhances visualization.
7. Because the orientation of the images differs from transabdominal scans, it is important to indicate the location and directions on each scan. Orientation and labeling have not been standardized; therefore, referencing images by using anatomic landmarks is recommended (e.g., demonstrating the ovaries in relationship to the iliac vessels).
8. At the completion of the examination, remove the condom carefully and disinfect the transducer as recommended by the manufacturer of the transducer.[12]

TRANSPERINEAL SCANNING

In some cases, endovaginal scanning may be contraindicated. If there is a concern about introducing infection, for example, in the case of ruptured membranes, or if the patient refuses an endovaginal scan, the transperineal approach may enable the sonographer to obtain images of the cervix and the lower uterine segment. The patient is positioned as for an endovaginal scan. The study is done by using a conventional ultrasound transducer that has been covered with a transducer cover (as described in the section on endovaginal technique) and scanning between the labia on the perineum. Occasionally, the view may be obstructed by bowel gas. To improve visualization, the patient's buttocks may be elevated onto a pillow or towels, shifting the bowel and changing the angle of the ultrasound beam relative to the cervix.[13,14] (Fig. 1-5).

COMPLETION OF THE EXAMINATION

Obtaining the needed images for the examination is only a portion of the required steps for the examination. The measurements obtained during the exam display on an electronic report contained within the equipment (Fig. 1-6). These, along with the patient information screens, are often included as images in the patient record. The report pages may be printed on a paper printer or a standalone printer.

If your equipment is set up to batch send, this is the time to review your images, deleting any that you repeated or felt were technically inadequate. If the images are sent as acquired, the only method to delete images is from the picture archiving and communication system (PACS).

Although it sounds complicated, when you end the examination, the images are sent to the PACS, stored, and then attached to the patient's EMR. This allows the electronic report to appear with both the main record and the one contained within the radiology department. This allows access to the approved people, including the clinician, to the images and reports contained within the patient chart. Often, the dictated report is sent electronically within a day or two, reducing the time a patient must wait for results.

SAFETY OF ULTRASOUND

The patient will undoubtedly ask questions about the findings of the examination and the safety to the fetus and herself of exposure to diagnostic ultrasound. The sonographer must answer these questions accurately and clearly. Extensive research has been done

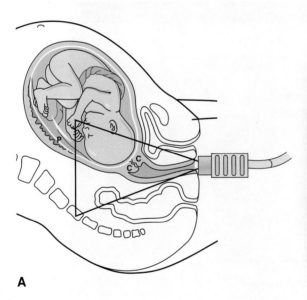

A

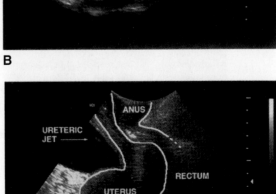

B

C

Figure 1-5 A: Schematic diagram of transperineal scanning plane. (Hertzberg BS, Bowie JD, Carroll BA, et al. Diagnosis of placenta previa during the third trimester: role of transperineal sonography. *Am J Roentgenol.* 1992;159:83–87). **B:** Transperineal sonogram of normal uterus, **(C)** with machine-generated outline of structures. (Sonograms courtesy of Susan Schultz, RDMS, Technical Coordinator of Education, The Jefferson Ultrasound Institute, Philadelphia, PA.)

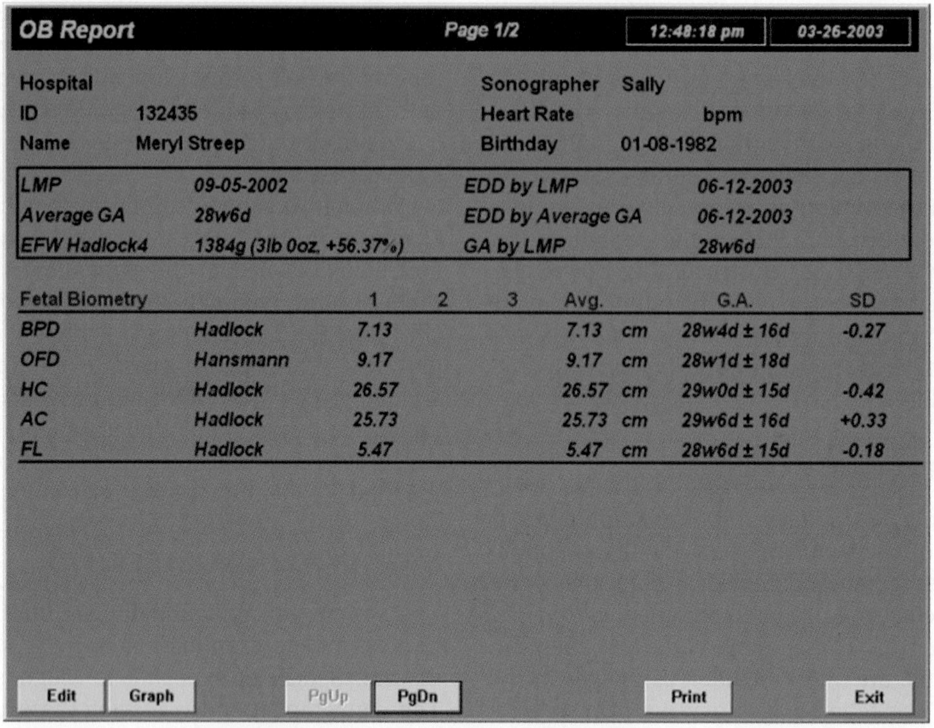

OB Report   Page 1/2   12:48:18 pm   03-26-2003

Hospital		Sonographer	Sally
ID	132435	Heart Rate	bpm
Name	Meryl Streep	Birthday	01-08-1982

LMP	09-05-2002	EDD by LMP	06-12-2003
Average GA	28w6d	EDD by Average GA	06-12-2003
EFW Hadlock4	1384g (3lb 0oz. +56.37%)	GA by LMP	28w6d

Fetal Biometry		1	2	3	Avg.		G.A.	SD
BPD	Hadlock	7.13			7.13	cm	28w4d ± 16d	-0.27
OFD	Hansmann	9.17			9.17	cm	28w1d ± 18d	
HC	Hadlock	26.57			26.57	cm	29w0d ± 15d	-0.42
AC	Hadlock	25.73			25.73	cm	29w6d ± 16d	+0.33
FL	Hadlock	5.47			5.47	cm	28w6d ± 15d	-0.18

Edit   Graph   PgUp   PgDn   Print   Exit

A

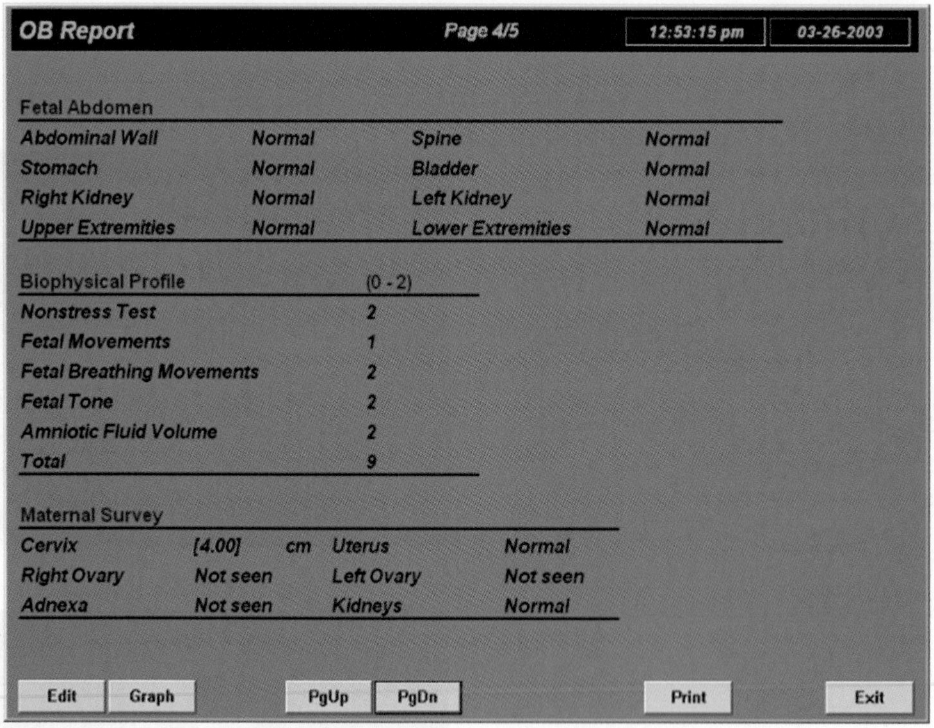

OB Report   Page 4/5   12:53:15 pm   03-26-2003

Fetal Abdomen			
Abdominal Wall	Normal	Spine	Normal
Stomach	Normal	Bladder	Normal
Right Kidney	Normal	Left Kidney	Normal
Upper Extremities	Normal	Lower Extremities	Normal

Biophysical Profile	(0 - 2)
Nonstress Test	2
Fetal Movements	1
Fetal Breathing Movements	2
Fetal Tone	2
Amniotic Fluid Volume	2
Total	9

Maternal Survey			
Cervix	[4.00] cm	Uterus	Normal
Right Ovary	Not seen	Left Ovary	Not seen
Adnexa	Not seen	Kidneys	Normal

Edit   Graph   PgUp   PgDn   Print   Exit

B

Figure 1-6 A,B: These two report pages for an OB examination demonstrate the fetal measurements, anatomy, biophysical profile, and the maternal survey. *(continued)*

on the potential deleterious effects of diagnostic ultrasound. The AIUM, the SDMS, the National Institutes of Health (NIH), and the U.S. Food and Drug Administration (FDA) carefully monitor results of epidemiologic and biologic studies. In 1984, the NIH and the FDA convened a Consensus Development Conference on Diagnostic Ultrasound Imaging in Pregnancy. It is the consensus of the panel that ultrasound examination in pregnancy should be performed for a specific medical indication. The data on clinical efficacy and safety do not allow a recommendation for routine screening at this time.

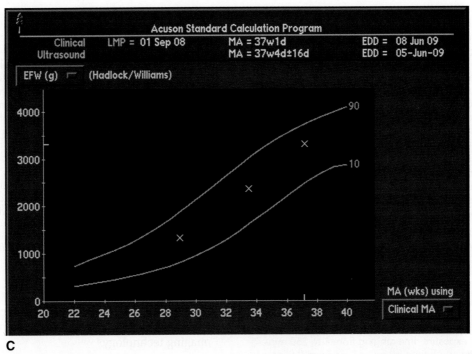

C

Figure 1-6 *(continued)* **C:** This graph displays the estimated fetal weight (EFW) of multiple examinations performed on this fetus. The *yellow* X indicated the weight at different stages of the pregnancy. Their position between the graph lines indicates a normal growth pattern.

Although the ultrasound community continues to uphold the rationale for this guideline, nearly every pregnant woman now receives at least one sonogram. The AIUM regularly publishes statements and reports informing the ultrasound community of the most recent information regarding safety issues and epidemiologic information.[15–22] The statements presented in Displays 1-3, 1-4, 1-5, and 1-6 continue to reinforce the NIH's conclusion that no deleterious effects have been demonstrated as resulting from the use of diagnostic ultrasound, either 2D or 3D, but that it should continue to be used prudently.

These conclusions and statements apply equally to the use of Doppler ultrasound, although output from Doppler instruments tends to be higher than for gray-scale imaging.[18] The FDA has established guidelines that restrict the power levels used in Doppler fetal scanning to those used before 1976. Recently, the FDA approved some devices that use higher-output data if power output information is displayed in real time on the equipment's monitor. The AIUM, FDA, the National Electrical Manufacturers Association, and 38 other professional organizations have developed an output display standard for all ultrasound equipment that requires mechanical and thermal indices (the mechanisms relating to bioeffects) be visible on the monitor.[23] By knowing the mechanical and thermal indices values, the sonographer can adjust power levels to minimize the patient's exposure to diagnostic ultrasound. It is incumbent on the sonographer to always minimize the patient's exposure to ultrasound energy by efficient scanning and by using the lowest exposure levels possible (ALARA).[1]

DISPLAY 1-3

American Institute of Ultrasound in Medicine Official Statement on Clinical Safety

Diagnostic ultrasound has been in use since the late 1950s. Given its known benefits and recognized efficacy for medical diagnosis, including its use during human pregnancy, the American Institute of Ultrasound in Medicine herein addresses the clinical safety of such use:

No independently confirmed adverse effects caused by exposure from present diagnostic ultrasound instruments have been reported in human patients in the absence of contrast agents. Biological effects (such as localized pulmonary bleeding) have been reported in mammalian systems at diagnostically relevant exposures but the clinical significance of such effects is not yet known. Ultrasound should be used by qualified health professionals to provide medical benefit to the patient.

(American Institute of Ultrasound in Medicine. *Bioeffects and Safety of Diagnostic Ultrasound.* Laurel, MD: AIUM; 2007.)

DISPLAY 1-4

Conclusions Regarding Epidemiology

Based on epidemiologic evidence to date and on current knowledge of interactive mechanisms, there is insufficient justification to warrant a conclusion that there is a causal relationship between diagnostic ultrasound and adverse effects.

(American Institute of Ultrasound in Medicine. *Conclusions Regarding Epidemiology.* Laurel, MD: AIUM; 2005.)

DISPLAY 1-5

AIUM Statement on Mammalian In Vivo Ultrasonic Biologic Effects

Information from experiments using laboratory mammals has contributed significantly to our understanding of ultrasonically induced biologic effects and the mechanisms that are most likely responsible. The following statement summarizes observations relative to specific diagnostic ultrasound parameters and indices.

In the low-megahertz frequency range, there have been no independently confirmed adverse biologic effects in mammalian tissues exposed in vivo under experimental ultrasound conditions, as follows:

1. Thermal Mechanisms
   a. No effects have been observed for an unfocused beam having free-field spatial-peak temporal-average (SPTA) intensities[a] below 100 mW/cm², or a focused[b] beam having intensities below 1 W/cm², or thermal index values of less than 2.
   b. For fetal exposures, no effects have been reported for a temperature increase above the normal physiologic temperature, ΔT, when $\Delta T < 4.5 - (\log 10t/0.6)$, where t is exposure time ranging from 1 to 250 minutes, including off time for pulsed exposure (Miller et al. 2002).
      For postnatal exposures producing temperature increases of 6° C or less, no effects have been reported when $\Delta T < 6 - (\log 10t/0.6)$, including off time for pulsed exposure. For example, for temperature increases of 6° C and 2° C, the corresponding limits for the exposure durations t are 1 and 250 minutes (O'Brien et al. 2008).
   c. For postnatal exposures producing temperature increases of 6° C or more, no effects have been reported when $\Delta T < 6 - (\log 10t/0.3)$, including off time for pulsed exposure. For example, for a temperature increase of 9.6° C, the corresponding limit for the exposure duration is 5 seconds (=0.083 minutes) (O'Brien et al. 2008).
2. Nonthermal Mechanisms
   a. In tissues that contain well-defined gas bodies (e.g., lung), no effects have been observed for in situ peak rarefactional pressures below approximately 0.4 MPa or mechanical index values less than approximately 0.4.
   b. In tissues that do not contain well-defined gas bodies, no effects have been reported for peak rarefactional pressures below approximately 4.0 MPa or mechanical index values less than approximately 4.0 (Church et al. 2008).

[a]Free-field SPTA intensity for continuous wave and pulsed exposures.
[b]Quarter-power (−6-dB) beam width smaller than 4 wavelengths or 4 mm, whichever is less at the exposure frequency.
(American Institute of Ultrasound in Medicine. *Statement on Mammalian In Vivo Ultrasonic Biological Effects.* Laurel, MD: AIUM; 2008.)

DISPLAY 1-6

3D Technology

Currently, 2D gray-scale real-time sonography is the primary method of medically indicated anatomic imaging with ultrasound. The term 3D ultrasound refers to the acquisition of imaging data from a volume of tissue. This volumetric data can be displayed as slabs of varying thickness, multiplanar reconstruction or as a rendered image. The 2D display remains the primary method of image presentation regardless of the method of acquisition. While 3D ultrasound may be helpful in diagnosis, it is currently an adjunct to, but not a replacement for 2D ultrasound. As with any developing technology, its clinical value may improve and its diagnostic role will be periodically re-evaluated.

(American Institute of Ultrasound in Medicine. *Official Statement 3D Technology.* Laurel, MD: AIUM; 2005.)

---

fetal vessels, the fetal cardiovascular system and to image flow in these structures using color flow imaging technology.[1]

If the patient asks, the sonographer should convey the gist of these statements to allay any immediate fears but should also indicate that examinations should not be performed indiscriminately.

Sharing the results of the examination with the patient depends on many factors, most of them involving common sense. The physician who ordered the sonographic examination is the best person to explain and discuss the findings with the patient. Whether patients are given immediate reassurance and are allowed to view the images, especially in a normal pregnancy, depends on the philosophy of the ultrasound laboratory. The impact on the patient of seeing the images should be the primary consideration.

NEW DEVELOPMENTS IN DIAGNOSTIC MEDICAL ULTRASOUND

Sonohysterography is a technique in which 25 to 30 mL of sterile saline is infused into the endometrial cavity to enhance visualization by either the transabdominal or endovaginal approach. The saline is infused through a fine, flexible catheter that is placed through the cervix. Patient preparation may include testing for *Chlamydia, Ureaplasma,* and gonorrhea and the use of prophylactic antibiotics. As in endovaginal examinations, the patient is in the dorsal lithotomy position. A speculum is inserted into the vagina to expose the cervix, the external os is cleaned with Betadine, and then the catheter is inserted.[24] Patients tolerate the procedure well, reporting little or no pain. The endometrial cavity is delineated by the anechoic saline that often initially appears echogenic because of contained microbubbles of air. Passage of the saline through the fallopian tubes can be demonstrated by imaging fluid in the cul-de-sac. The

---

The AIUM's position statement on the use of Doppler ultrasound is as follows:

AIUM feels that there is currently sufficient information to justify clinical use of continuous wave, pulsed and color flow Doppler ultrasound to evaluate blood flow in uterine, umbilical and

technique has proven superior to endovaginal sonography alone in characterizing the thickened endometrium for contained polyps, submucous myomas, synechiae, endometrial hyperplasia, and signs of cancerous masses, and in investigating tubal patency.[24]

Contrast agents such as saline have been used in gynecologic scanning to enhance visualization of the endometrial cavity and fallopian tubes. Coupled with the acquisition of a 3D data set, saline injected through an inserted catheter through the vagina and cervical os has successfully demonstrated patent and blocked tubes.[25,26] The use of saline in the hysterosalpingogram (HSG) has proven diagnostic validity. What role the sonographer has depends on the setting in which he or she practices. Usually, the sonographer acts as an assistant to the physician instilling the saline. However, as sonographers begin developing the role of the advanced practitioner, that person might be considered qualified to perform the entire examination.

3D ultrasound, an outgrowth of computer technology, is one of the most dynamic new developments in sonographic imaging. Several types of 3D ultrasound are being investigated, such as 2D serial scanning,[10] volume imaging,[27,28] and the use of a defocusing lens.[9] Studies of the efficacy of 2D serial scanning (commonly referred to as 3D imaging) in obstetric scanning, particularly in the evaluation of the first-trimester embryo,[29] fetal face, limbs, and digits, have shown it to add important detail to the study. Spatio-temoporal image correlation (STIC) is a 3D imaging method to image the fetal heart that results in the display of three orthogonal planes of the heart in a multiplanar reconstruction (MPR) format.[30]

Scanning technique for 3D or 4D imaging does not change appreciably. The volume transducer mechanically obtains sequential images, which are stored as volume data. At some time after the scan, the data may be recalled and volumetric reconstructions produced that may be rotated approximately 360 degrees. The clinician is able to evaluate entire organs in a dynamic manner, rather than in static sections. The technique enables the user to study an infinite variety of orthogonal views through an area of interest at any time after storage of the volume data.

3D data is said to have three dimensions, the X, Y, and Z plane, whereas 4D or real-time imaging has the fourth dimension of time. This allows for viewing of fetal movements even though the slower frame rates make the image appear less smooth than conventional 2D imaging. This technique enables the user to view the surface or internal structure of an object in three dimensions. To image the surface of a structure, a fetal face, for example, fluid must surround the area of interest. Some of the anomalies that are being detected more easily with this type of evaluation include facial features (Fig. 1-7), ear anomalies, finger and toe numbers and positions, neural tube defects, and limb malformations.

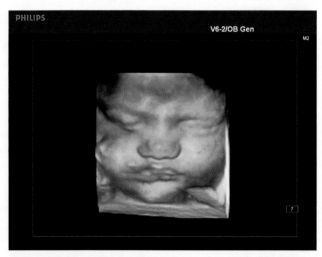

Figure 1-7 3D surface rendered image of a 20-week fetal face. (Image complements of Philips Medical Systems, Bothell, WA.)

Internal anomalies identified with the skeletal processing method include hemivertebrae, boney limb malformations, and myelomeningoceles (Fig. 1-8).

PROFESSIONAL RESPONSIBILITIES OF THE SONOGRAPHER

In March of 2002, sonography became a unique professional classification by the Bureau of Labor Statistics[31] and became listed in the Occupational Outlook Handbook.[32] It is essential that sonographers be familiar with the Sonographer's Code of Professional Conduct[33] (Table 1-4), Code of Ethics,[34] The Scope of Practice,[7] that they abide by the Patients' Bill of Rights, and that they practice infection control techniques to protect their patients and themselves.

Individuals choosing diagnostic ultrasound as a profession should take certifying examinations. There are currently several testing bodies, such as the American

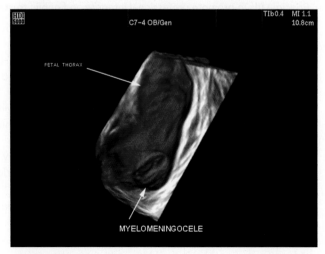

Figure 1-8 A 3D surface rendering of a sacral myelomeningocele. (Image complements of Philips Medical Systems, Bothell, WA.)

TABLE 1-4

Code of Professional Conduct for Diagnostic Medical Sonographers

The goal of this code of ethics is to promote excellence in patient care by fostering responsibility and accountability among diagnostic medical sonographers. In so doing, the integrity of the profession of diagnostic medical sonography will be maintained.

Objectives

To create and encourage an environment where professional and ethical issues are discussed and addressed.

To help the individual diagnostic medical sonographer identify ethical issues.

To provide guidelines for individual diagnostic medical sonographers regarding ethical behavior.

Principles

Principle I: In order to promote patient well-being, the diagnostic medical sonographer shall:

   A. Provide information to the patient about the purpose of the sonography procedure and respond to the patient's questions and concerns

   B. Respect the patient's autonomy and the right to refuse the procedure

   C. Recognize the patient's individuality and provide care in a nonjudgmental and nondiscriminatory manner

   D. Promote the privacy, dignity, and comfort of the patient by thoroughly explaining the examination and patient positioning and implementing proper draping techniques

   E. Maintain confidentiality of acquired patient information and follow national patient privacy regulations as required by the Health Insurance Portability and Accountability Act of 1996 (HIPAA)

   F. Promote patient safety during the provision of sonography procedures and while the patient is in the care of the diagnostic medical sonographer

Principle II: To promote the highest level of competent practice, diagnostic medical sonographers shall:

   A. Obtain appropriate diagnostic medical sonography education and clinical skills to ensure competence

   B. Achieve and maintain specialty specific sonography credentials. Sonography credentials must be awarded by a national sonography credentialing body that is accredited by a national organization that accredits credentialing bodies, that is the National Commission for Certifying Agencies (NCCA), http://www.noca.org/ncca/ncca.htm; or the International Organization for Standardization (ISO), http://www.iso.org/iso/en/ISOOnline.frontpage.

   C. Uphold professional standards by adhering to defined technical protocols and diagnostic criteria established by peer review

   D. Acknowledge personal and legal limits, practice within the defined scope of practice, and assume responsibility for his or her actions

   E. Maintain continued competence through lifelong learning, which includes continuing education, acquisition of specialty specific credentials, and recredentialing

   F. Perform medically indicated ultrasound studies, ordered by a licensed physician or a designated health care provider

   G. Protect patients and/or study subjects by adhering to oversight and approval of investigational procedures, including documented informed consent

   H. Refrain from the use of any substances that may alter judgment or skill and thereby compromise patient care

   I. Be accountable and participate in regular assessment and review of equipment, procedures, protocols, and results. This can be accomplished through facility accreditation.

Principle III: To promote professional integrity and public trust, the diagnostic medical sonographer shall:

   A. Be truthful and promote appropriate communications with patients and colleagues

   B. Respect the rights of patients, colleagues, and yourself

   C. Avoid conflicts of interest and situations that exploit others or misrepresent information

   D. Accurately represent his or her experience, education, and credentialing

   E. Promote equitable access to care

   F. Collaborate with professional colleagues to create an environment that promotes communication and respect

   G. Communicate and collaborate with others to promote ethical practice

   H. Engage in ethical billing practices

   I. Engage only in legal arrangements in the medical industry

   J. Report deviations from the Code of Ethics to institutional leadership for internal sanctions, local intervention, and/or criminal prosecution. The Code of Ethics can serve as a valuable tool to develop local policies and procedures.

(The Society of Diagnostic Medical Sonographers. *Code of Professional Conduct for Diagnostic Medical Sonographers.* Dallas, TX: SDMS; 2006.)

Registry of Radiologic Technologists (ARRT); however, the gold standard is still the test given by the American Registry of Diagnostic Medical Sonographers (ARDMS). The ARRT test contains general topics, whereas the ARDMS specifies specialty areas such as Obstetrics/Gynecology. A newer certification for first-trimester imaging is the Nuchal Translucency Quality Review (NTQR), which provides testing to ensure quality and consistency in measuring the nuchal translucency and the nasal bone.[35] When deciding which test to take, be sure they are accepted by your facility's accrediting body.

Passing a credentialing examination attests that the sonographer has a practicing level of knowledge in the specialties in which he or she is registered. The sonographer registered through the ARDMS can use the designation RDMS (registered diagnostic medical sonographer), whereas the ARRT allows the use of RT(S) (Sonography) for the general imaging test and the designation of RT(BS) for Breast Sonography[36] after his or her name. Several states require regional licensure to practice, which requires presentation of ARDMS or ARRT credentialing. To maintain this status, the sonographer must compile 30 to 36 hours of continuing medical education (CME) credits every 3 years depending on the credential held. In a field as dynamic as diagnostic ultrasound, keeping informed of innovations is imperative. Without CME maintenance, none of the testing bodies list the registrant on the web page directory search as an active member.

The AIUM accredits practices that image obstetric, gynecologic, abdominal, and breast ultrasound areas.[37] Another governing body, the ACR, also accredits imaging laboratories. The AIUM requires the ARDMS registry in the accrediting specialty areas; however, they do accept the ARRT Breast certification.[38] The ACR accepts either the ARDMS or the ARRT credential.[39] Each requires the proper education and credentialing of sonographers in the practice. Add to this the increasing requirements by third-party payers, such as Medicare—which will only reimburse for examinations performed in accredited labs with certified sonographers—and it becomes clear that anyone performing the sonographic examination has to have credentialing.

The sonographer should become a member of a professional society in his or her area of practice, in this case, General and Women's Health Imaging. Examples of societies include the SDMS, the AIUM, or even the International Society of Ultrasound in Obstetrics and Gynecology (ISUOG). Membership in a society brings with it the benefits of being part of a professional organization whose mission is to keep its members informed and competent. Among the resources the SDMS and AIUM provides are educational guidelines, profiles of sonographer characteristics (including salary levels), peer-reviewed journals (*The Journal of Diagnostic Medical Sonography, Journal of Ultrasound Medicine, Ultrasound in Obstetrics and Gynecology*), and annual national and regional scientific meetings. It also keeps its membership informed of legislation and current societal trends that can affect the practice of ultrasound at the local, national, and international level.

SUMMARY

- The sonographic examination begins with entry of patient data into the EMR, RIS, and, if available, the MWL on the equipment.

Critical Thinking Questions

1. You have been asked to be part of a hiring committee for the sonography department. After reviewing the applicants' application material, you want to verify CME, ARDMS, and ASRT registry status. What resources would you use to perform this task?

   ANSWER: A visit to the ARDMS Directory of Registrants lists most sonographers, whereas the ARRT Directory Search lists applicants with radiology and a sonography registry. Current CME status results in a current status for sonographers registered with the ARDMS or ARRT. It is unadvisable to use copies of certificates or cards for verification as these can easily be altered.

2. As a newly appointed CME coordinator, it is your responsibility to find and provide educational opportunities for your fellow sonographers. What resources would you use to set up your own program? How would you locate independent study activities at little or no cost?

   ANSWER: A visit to the SDMS and ASRT website to locate the procedure for departmental CME award would be the first step. These websites also provide links to other CME providers. Equipment manufacturers offer complementary or low-cost credits. If your department has purchased new equipment, the vendor may provide CME credit as part of a package.

3. An obstetrician's office would like to become accredited to ensure quality sonographic examinations. This office images from the first trimester to term, performing early pregnancy screening for aneuploidy. What is the first step in becoming accredited?

   ANSWER: Check with the ACR and AIUM for the accreditation requirements and choose one that best matches the clinic's needs. Since the clinicians perform early screening for aneuploidy, sonographers will need to pass the NTQR certification.

- The performing sonographer introduces himself or herself, confirms patient identity through multiple methods (name, date of birth, exam, armband), and takes a history.

- Each imaging laboratory must develop an imaging protocol to ensure completeness of the exam and consistency between examinations.

- A transabdominal examination of the female reproductive organs, either in a gravid or nongravid state, begins with an adequately full bladder.

- Transducer selection depends on the transducer footprint, body habitus, examination, and stage of pregnancy.

- Endovaginal and transperoneal examinations require covering of the transducer.

- There is general consensus of multiple entities, such as the FDA and NIH, that ultrasound examination should only be performed for a specific medical condition.

- Sonographers will always minimize the patient's exposure to ultrasound energy by efficient scanning and by using the lowest exposure levels possible (ALARA).

- Professionalism is partially determined through obtaining certification and maintaining registries through CME completion.

REFERENCES

1. American Institute of Ultrasound in Medicine. *Official Statement As Low As Reasonably Achievable (ALARA) Principle*. Laurel, MD: AIUM; 2008.
2. Shortliff EH, Cimino JJ. *Biomedical Informatics: Computer applications in health care and biomedicine*. 3rd ed. New York, NY: Springer; 2006.
3. Hacker NF, Moore JG. *Essentials of Obstetrics and Gynecology*. Philadelphia, PA: WB Saunders; 1986.
4. Hansman M, Hackeloer BJ, Staudach A. *Ultrasound Diagnosis in Obstetrics and Gynecology*. Berlin, Germany: Springer-Verlag; 1985.
5. American Institute of Ultrasound in Medicine. *Guidelines for Performance of the Antepartum Obstetrical Ultrasound Examination*. Laurel, MD: AIUM; 2007.
6. American Institute of Ultrasound in Medicine. *Guidelines for Performance of the Ultrasound Examination of the Female Pelvis*. Laurel, MD: AIUM; 2009.
7. Society of Diagnostic Medical Sonographers. *The Scope of Practice for the Diagnostic Medical Sonographer*. Dallas: SDMS; 2009.
8. American Institute of Ultrasound in Medicine. Bioeffects committee reviews RADIUS study. *AIUM Reporter*. 1994;10:2–4.
9. Kremkau F. *Diagnostic Ultrasound: Principles and Instruments*. 7th ed. Philadelphia, PA: Saunders Elsevier; 2006.
10. Hedrick WR, Hykes DL, Starchman DE. *Ultrasound Physics and Instrumentation*. 4th ed. St. Louis, MO: Mosby; 2004.
11. Society of Diagnostic Medical Sonographers. *Sonography Examination Guidelines*. 2nd ed. Plano: SDMS; 2006.
12. American Institute of Ultrasound in Medicine. Guidelines for cleaning and preparing endocavitary ultrasound transducers between patients. AIUM Official statement. 2003.
13. Jhobta A, Kaur R, Jhobta R, et al. Fistula in Ano: role of transperineal and transvaginal sonography. *J Diagn Med Sonogr*. 2006;22:375–381.
14. Meijer-Hoogeveen M, Stoutenbeek P, Visser GH. Transperineal versus transvaginal sonographic cervical length measurement in second- and third-trimester pregnancies. *Ultrasound Obstet Gynecol*. 2008;32(5):657–662.
15. American Institute of Ultrasound in Medicine. *Bioeffects and Safety of Diagnostic Ultrasound*. Laurel, MD: AIUM; 2008.
16. Kremkau FW. Bioeffects and safety: III. Output indices and bioeffects statement. *J Diagn Med Sonogr*. 1993;9:336–338.
17. American Institute of Ultrasound in Medicine. *Position statement on 3D Technology*. Laurel, MD: AIUM; 2005.
18. American Institute of Ultrasound in Medicine. Position statement on fetal Doppler. AIUM Newsletter. October 1993:3.
19. American Institute of Ultrasound in Medicine. *Performance Criteria and Measurements for Doppler Ultrasound Devices: Technical Discussion*. Laurel, MD: AIUM; 2007.
20. American Institute of Ultrasound in Medicine. *Statement on Mammalian In Vivo Ultrasonic Biological Effects*. Laurel, MD: AIUM; 2008.
21. American Institute of Ultrasound in Medicine. *Medical Ultrasound Safety*. Laurel, MD: AIUM; 1994.
22. American Institute of Ultrasound in Medicine. *Conclusions Regarding Epidemiology*. Laurel, MD: AIUM; 2005.
23. Kremkau FW. Bioeffects and safety: III. Output indices and bioeffects statement. *J Diagn Med Sonogr*. 1993; 9:336–338.
24. Elsayes KM, Pandya A, Platt JF, et al. Technique and diagnostic utility of saline infusion sonohysterography. *Int J Gynaecol Obstet*. 2009;105(1):5–9.
25. Chan CC, Ng EH, Tang OS, et al. Comparison of three-dimensional hysterosalpingo-contrast-sonography and diagnostic laparoscopy with chromopertubation in the assessment of tubal patency for the investigation of subfertility. *Acta Obstet Gynecol Scand*. 2005;84(9):909–913.
26. De Felice C, Porfiri LM, Savelli S, et al. Infertility in women combined sonohysterography and hysterosalpingography in the evaluation of the uterine cavity. *Ultraschall Med*. 2009;30(1):52–57. *Erratum in: Ultraschall Med*. 2009;30(2):195.
27. Andrist L, Katz V, Elijah R, et al. Developing a plan for routine 3-dimensional surface rendering in obstetrics. *J Diagn Med Sonogr*. 2001;17:16–21.
28. Ballard-Taraschi K, Roberts D, Thompson S. Utilizing 3D ultrasound to visualize trisomy 18 abnormalities in the first trimester. *J Diagn Med Sonogr*. 2003;19:110–113.
29. Fauchon DE, Benzie RJ, Wye DA, et al. What information on fetal anatomy can be provided by a single first-trimester transabdominal three-dimensional sweep? *Ultrasound Obstet Gynecol*. 2008;31(3):266–274.
30. Hata T, Dai SY, Inubashiri E, et al. Real-time three-dimensional color Doppler fetal echocardiographic features of congenital heart disease. *J Obstet Gynaecol Res*. 2008;34(4 pt 2):670–673.
31. Government Recognizes Diagnostic Medical Sonography as Independent Profession [press release]. Society of Diagnostic Medical Sonography; March 18, 2002. http://www.sdms.org/news/release03182002.asp. Accessed August 2009.
32. The U.S. Department of Labor. Occupational Outlook Handbook, 2008–2009 Edition. http://www.bls.gov/oco/ocos273.htm. Accessed August 2009.

33. The Society of Diagnostic Medical Sonographers. *Code of Professional Conduct for Diagnostic Medical Sonographers.* Plano: SDMS; 2006.

34. The Society of Diagnostic Medical Sonographers. *Code of Ethics for the Profession of Diagnostic Medical Sonography.* Plano: SDMS; 2006.

35. Nuchal Translucency Quality Review. www.ntqr.org. Accessed August 2009.

36. American Registry of Radiologic Technologists. *Sonography Primary Pathway: Certification and Application Materials.* St. Paul, MN: ARRT; 2008.

37. American Institute of Ultrasound in Medicine. *Standards and Guidelines for the Accreditation of Ultrasound Practices.* Laurel, MD: AIUM; 2005.

38. American Institute of Ultrasound in Medicine. *Ultrasound Practice Accreditation: The Measure of Excellence.* Laurel: AIUM; 2009.

39. American College of Radiology. Ultrasound Accreditation Program Requirements. Reston, VA: ACR; 2009.

40. National Patient Safety Goals. The Joint Commission. http://www.jointcommission.org/PatientSafety/National-PatientSafetyGoals/. Accessed December 2009.

2 Embryonic Development of the Female Genital System

Susan Raatz Stephenson

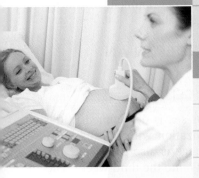

OBJECTIVES

Order the appearance of embryonic structures

Describe the first-trimester Carnegie staging

Relate embryonic structures to the resultant adult organs

List the development stages of the female reproductive system

Explain the interconnectivity of the urinary and reproductive systems

KEY TERMS

embryogenesis | urogenital | primordial germ cells | mesonephros | pronephros | inducer germ cells | mesonephric ducts | paramesonephric ducts | müllerian ducts | external genitalia | wolffian ducts

GLOSSARY

Allantois Saclike vascular structure that lies below the chorion and develops from the hindgut

Atretic Blockage or absence of a structure

Broad ligament Fold of peritoneum that connects the uterus to the pelvis

Embryogenesis Formation of an embryo

Cloaca Cavity that is part of the development of the digestive and reproductive organs

Diploid Normal number of paired chromosomes

Gonadal ridges Structure that appears at approximately 5 weeks' gestation and becomes either ovaries or testes

Hydrometrocolpos Accumulation of secreted fluid resulting in distention of the uterus and vagina due to obstruction

Hydronephrosis Urine collection in the kidneys due to distal obstruction

Hydroureter Large, sometimes tortuous, ureter due to distal blockage

Mesonephric ducts Connection between the mesonephros and the cloaca

Mesonephros Second stage of kidney development (aka wolffian body)

Mesovarium Section of the uterine broad ligament that covers the ovary

Müllerian ducts (paramesonephric ducts) Paired ducts that become the oviducts, uterus, cervix, and upper vagina

Oocytes Female germ cells

Oogonia Immature oocytes

Paramesonephric ducts see müllerian ducts

Primordial germ cells Precursor of germ cells, become oocytes or spermatozoa in the adult

Pronephros Primary or first kidney, which develops in the embryo

Wolffian ducts see Mesonephros

Urogenital Pertaining to the urinary and genital system

Understanding female reproductive anatomy begins with a thorough knowledge of pelvis structure embryogenisis. Imaging of the uterus and ovaries becomes complicated in the presence of developmental anomalies due to changes in the normal sonographic anatomy. Understanding the developmental relationship between the urinary and reproductive systems requires a normal and abnormal development of both organ systems.

Commonly, anomalies in either system result in coexisting malformations in the other. The urogenital system easily images in utero and throughout a woman's life. This allows for diagnosis of morphologic anomalies in all stages of life from fetal, neonatal, pediatric, reproductive, and postmenopausal.

Carnegie staging, a method used to classify the embryo, places the embryo into categories depending on the age, size, and morphologic characteristics. The embryo develops structures in a specific order that remains constant. Since, as with any organism, each develops at a different rate, the segmentation of development allows for consideration of morphologic development, regardless of dates.[1]

Carnegie staging applies to the first 8 weeks of the gestation and pertains to the organogenesis of the embryo. The resulting 23 stages end after the 8th week when the fetal period begins. Carnegie stages will be included with each organ development chapter. This chapter covers the normal development of the female urogenital structures, including the correlating Carnegie stages. Abnormalities of development are further discussed in the next chapter.

FETAL PERIOD

The genitourinary system encompasses two systems: reproductive (genito-) and urinary. These systems develop in tandem in the embryo and retain the close association in the adult.

Most congenital anomalies discovered in fetuses in utero occur in the genitourinary system, with urinary tract abnormalities accounting for about 50% of the total.[2] These anomalies represent a wide range, from complete agenesis of the kidney and ureters to partial malformations, duplications, and obstructions with concomitant cyst formation. Prenatal ultrasound may also detect congenital anomalies in the ovaries, uterus, and vagina, especially when they enlarge and produce a pelvic mass. Cloacal anomalies, which can result in hydrometrocolpos, are the result of obstruction of vaginal outflow in the female fetus.[3] This hypoechoic mass posterior to the bladder compresses the urinary tract, causing obstructive uropathy demonstrated by hydronephrosis or hydroureter.[3]

NEONATAL PERIOD

As in the fetal period, the most common mass lesions in neonates are of renal origin[4]; however, ovarian cysts are known to be the most common intra-abdominal lesion in the neonate.[5] Identify the normal urinary bladder, uterus, vagina, and (whenever possible) ovaries when imaging the pelvis in a newborn girl to rule out masses and obstructions.

PREMENARCHE THROUGH ADULTHOOD

The onset of puberty results in menstrual irregularities and, thus, a visit to the sonography lab. This often is the first time any developmental abnormalities become apparent. For example, in the patient with a duplicated uterus with one septate vagina, obstruction to menstrual flow from one side can present as unilateral hematocolpos.[6] In these patients, imaging of the kidneys becomes important as there are often associated anomalies.[6] Asymptomatic patients may not be aware

of the congenital anomalies unless other conditions require sonographic imaging.

These anomalies occur early in embryonic life. The following sections review the development of the female internal and external genitalia.

EXPRESSION OF GENDER IN AN EMBRYO

THE PRIMORDIAL GERM CELLS

The chromosomal gender or sex is determined in the first Carnegie stage at fertilization with the fusion of the sperm and egg.[1] This stage is also called the *pre-embryonic phase*, which lasts into the third week.[1] The female gamete (the ovum) always contains the X sex chromosome. The male gamete (the spermatozoon) contributes either an X (female) or Y (male). If the sperm contributes an X to the ovum's X, the result is a female zygote (XX). If the male contributes a Y chromosome, the result is a male zygote (XY).[6] Fertilization results in a diploid chromosome count of 46 with two sex chromosomes (XX or XY).

The primordial germ cells that express or produce femaleness or maleness are first discernible in the embryo late in the third week to early in the fourth week (approximately the 17th day[1]) after conception. This stage, the embryonic phase, begins in the fourth week and extends into the eighth.[1] The appearance of the primordial germ cells along with the primitive groove, streak, and node indicate Carnegie stage 6.[1] These germ cells differentiate from cells in the caudal part of the yolk sac, close to the allantois (a small diverticulum of the yolk sac that extends into the connecting stalk) (Fig. 2-1A). In the sixth week during Carnegie stage 17,[2] the primordial germ cells migrate from the yolk sac along the allantois and into the gonadal cords.[6,7] The genital or gonadal ridges form simultaneously and are the precursors to the female ovaries and to the male testes. These ridges are located on the anteromedial sides of the mesonephros, the embryonic regions where the kidneys develop (Fig. 2-1B).[7] The urinary system and the reproductive system are intimately associated in origin, development, and certain final relations. Both arise from mesoderm that initially takes the form of a common ridge (mesonephros) located on both sides of the median plane. This tissue appears during the sixth Carnegie stage at about 13 days postovulation.[2] Both systems continue to develop in close proximity; they drain into a common cloaca and slightly later into a urogenital sinus, which is a subdivision of the cloaca. Some parts of the urogenital system disappear after a transitory existence.[8] For example, by the fifth developmental week, the first-stage kidney (pronephros) has differentiated and has already disappeared.[9] The final set of kidneys forms at about days 31–38, during the 14th and 15th Carnegie stage.[3] Certain common primordia transform differently in males and females.

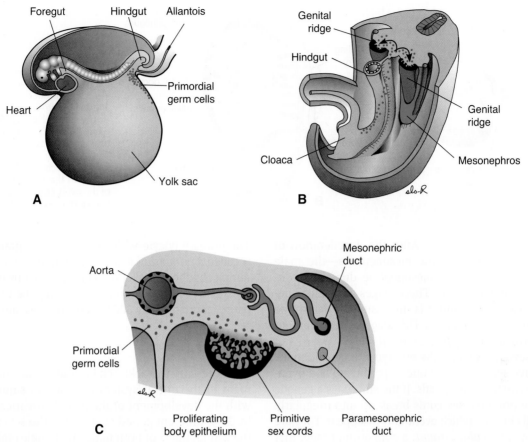

Figure 2-1 Future sperm and egg cells gather in the genital ridge. Gametes arise in the gut tube endoderm **(A)** and migrate through the dorsal mesentery **(B)** to receptive primitive sex cords that are proliferating in the genital ridge **(C)**. (From Sadler TW. Langman's Medical Embryology. 10th ed. Baltimore, MD: Lippincott Williams & Wilkins, 2006. Figure 15.18a,b, p. 240; Figure 15.19, p. 249.)

INDUCER GERM CELLS

During the fifth week of development, the primordial germ cells migrate by ameboid movement from their origin in the yolk sac along the dorsal mesentery. In the sixth week, they invade the gonadal ridges (Fig. 2-1B). If by chance they do not reach the ridges, the gonads cease to develop. Thus, these primordial germ cells act as inducers of the gonads. Note that at this time in development (the sixth week), the mesonephros (previously named wolffian bodies) or second-stage kidney and its mesonephric duct (previously named wolffian ducts) have developed lateral to the gonadal ridges.[7,10]

As the primordial cells are invading the ridges, an outer layer of fetal tissue called *coelomic epithelium* grows into the underlying mesenchymal tissue, or embryonic connective tissue. Active tissue growth here forms a network, or rete, called the *primitive sex cords* (Fig. 2-2). This rete forms anastomoses with a portion of the mesonephric duct, thus establishing the first urogenital

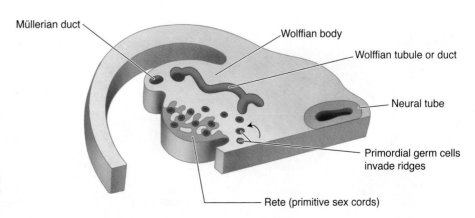

Figure 2-2 Development of embryo on one side. Indifferent gonad stage; formation of primitive sex cords.

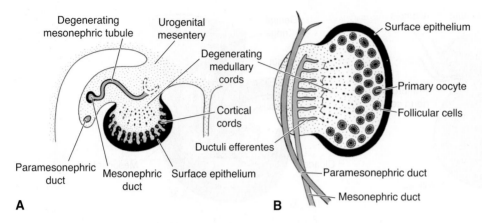

Figure 2-3 **A:** Transverse section of the ovary at the seventh week, showing degeneration of the primitive (medullary) sex cords and formation of the cortical cords. **B:** Ovary and genital ducts in the fifth month. Note degeneration of the medullary cords. The excretory mesonephric tubules (efferent ductules) do not communicate with the rete. The cortical zone of the ovary contains groups of oogonia surrounded by follicular cells.

connections in the embryo. After the degeneration of the second-stage kidney, the mesonephros—the male embryo—appropriates its mesonephric duct and converts it into genital canals. These stages are similar between the two sexes, and it is impossible to determine gender through morphology. This stage of development is often termed the *indifferent gonad stage*.[6,7,10]

In the seventh week, if the embryo is a genetic male, the primitive sex cords continue to proliferate and eventually give rise to the rete testis. If the embryo is a genetic female, the primitive sex cords break up into irregularly shaped cell clusters, which eventually disappear. They are replaced by a *vascular stroma*, a supporting tissue, that later forms the ovarian medulla (Fig. 2-3).[6,7] In a female gonad (the ovary), the outer layer of epithelium continues to proliferate, giving rise to a second group of cords, which eventually occupy the cortex of the ovary. These are the cortical cords, or Pluger's tubules (Fig. 2-4).[10]

In the fourth month, the cortical cords split into isolated cell clusters, each surrounding one or more primitive germ cells. Now, the primitive germ cells differentiate into oogonia, which divide repeatedly by mitosis to reach a maximum number of 7 million by the fifth month of prenatal life. Many oogonia subsequently degenerate, so at birth, their number is approximately 1 million (Fig. 2-5).[7]

The surviving oogonia differentiate into primary oocytes during prenatal life and are surrounded by a single layer of granulosa cells derived from the cortical cords.

The primary oocyte with its surrounding granulosa cells is called a *primordial follicle*. Many undergo degeneration during childhood and adolescence, so that by puberty, approximately 500,000 remain. Between puberty and menopause, approximately 300 to 400 fertile ova are produced.[7]

GENITAL DUCTS

It is necessary to backtrack in time to trace the development of the ductal system that occurs simultaneously with the development of the gonads (ovaries or testes). In the indifferent gonad stage (until the seventh week), the genital tracts of both male and female embryos have the same appearance and comprise two pairs of ducts. The mesonephric ducts arise from the second-stage kidney, the mesonephros. The müllerian ducts (or paramesonephric ducts) arise from an invagination or pocket of coelomic epithelium lateral to the cranial end of each mesonephric duct. Growth progresses caudad, eventually hollowing out to form an open duct.[10] Development of the embryonic ductal system and external genitalia occurs under the influence of circulating hormones in the fetus. In males, fetal testes produce an inducer substance that causes differentiation and growth of the mesonephric ducts and inhibition of the müllerian ducts. In females, because the male inducer substance is absent, the mesonephric ducts regress while the müllerian ductal system, influenced by maternal and placental estrogens, develops into the fallopian tubes and uterus.[10,11]

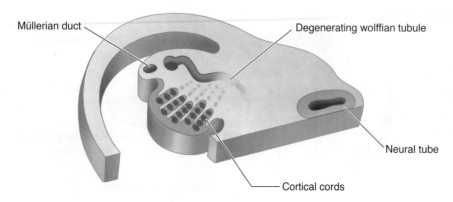

Figure 2-4 Formation of the cortical cords.

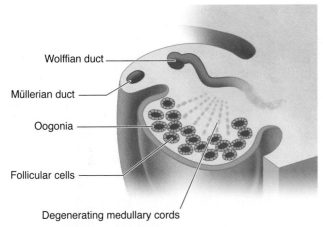

Figure 2-5 Differentiation of primitive germ cells into oogonia in the fourth month.

- Wolffian duct
- Müllerian duct
- Oogonia
- Follicular cells
- Degenerating medullary cords

The müllerian ducts first extend downward parallel to the mesonephric ducts, then turn medial in the lower abdomen, crossing anterior to the mesonephric ducts and fusing together in the midline to form a single duct, the uterovaginal canal (Fig. 2-6). This fusion begins caudally and progresses up to the site of the future fallopian tubes. In normal development, the midline septum disappears by the end of the third month and the uterine corpus and cervix are formed. They are surrounded by a layer of mesenchyme, which eventually forms the muscular coat of the uterus (the myometrium) and its peritoneal covering (the perimetrium).[7,10]

FORMATION OF THE FALLOPIAN TUBES

After the formation of the uterovaginal canal, the segment of each müllerian duct positioned above the junction of the inguinal ligament becomes a fallopian tube. The cranial orifice of the müllerian duct, which stays open to the peritoneal cavity, becomes the fimbriae of the

fallopian tube. Initially, the fallopian tube lies in a vertical position. As development proceeds, it moves to the interior of the abdominal cavity to lie horizontally. This causes the ovary, which is attached to the fallopian tube by the mesovarium, to descend and finally to assume a position dorsal to the fallopian tube (Table 2-1, Fig. 2-7).[7]

FORMATION OF THE BROAD LIGAMENT

As the müllerian duct fuses medially and the ovary is successfully located cranial and finally dorsal to the fallopian tubes, the mesenteries follow these positional changes.[10] This movement causes the folds of the peritoneum to be elevated from the posterolateral wall, thus creating a large transverse pelvic fold called the *broad ligament*, which extends from the lateral sides of the fused müllerian ducts toward the wall of the pelvis. The fallopian tube will be located on its superior surface and on its posterior surface, the ovary (Fig. 2-7). The ovary is suspended by several structures: (1) the *mesovarium* is a double-layered fold of peritoneum that is continuous with the posterosuperior layer of the broad ligament. (2) The *proper ligament of the ovary* is a band of connective tissue that lies between the two layers of the broad ligament and connects the lower pole of the ovary with the lateral uterine wall. (3) The *suspensory ligament* is a triangular fold of peritoneum that actually forms the upper lateral corner of the broad ligament. This ligament suspends both the ovary and the fallopian tube by its confluence with the parietal peritoneum at the pelvic brim.[11]

FORMATION OF THE VAGINA

The vagina has a dual origin: its upper region is derived from the mesodermal tissue of the müllerian ducts and its lower region is derived from the urogenital sinus. The urogenital sinus is the ventral half of the primitive cloaca (hindgut) after it has been divided by the

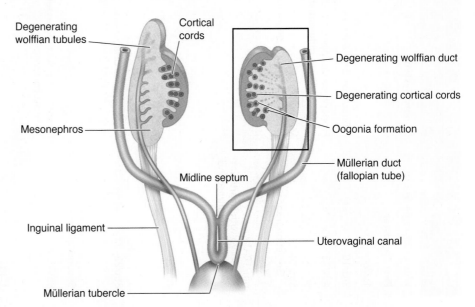

- Degenerating wolffian tubules
- Cortical cords
- Mesonephros
- Midline septum
- Inguinal ligament
- Müllerian tubercle
- Degenerating wolffian duct
- Degenerating cortical cords
- Oogonia formation
- Müllerian duct (fallopian tube)
- Uterovaginal canal

Figure 2-6 Formation of uterovaginal canal, eighth week. *Inset:* ovary at fourth month, forming the oogonia.

TABLE 2-1

Embryonic Development Chart for Female Urogenital System[1,2,7]

Week/Carnegie Stage	Urinary System	Gonads	Ducts	Mesenteries	Embryo Size
First Trimester					
1st/6		Primordial germ cells appear			NA
3rd/10	Pronephros differentiates	Primordial cells seen in allantois			0.2–3.5 cm
4th/13	Pronephros disappears and mesonephros differentiates	Formation of genital ridges			0.4–0.6 mm
5th/14–16 Gestational sac seen with ultrasound	Metanephros (permanent kidney) starts to differentiate	Migration of primordial germ cells			0.5–0.11 cm
6th/18–19 Embryo with heartbeat images with ultrasound		Primitive germ cells invade gonadal ridges Genital tubercle appears Formation of primitive sex cords: "indifferent stage"	Two sets of ducts exist: mesonephric (kidney) and müllerian (genital ridge)		0.16–0.18 cm
7th/20		Primitive sex cords disappear Testes or ovaries form Cortical cords arise			0.18–0.22 cm
8th/22–23	Mesonephros disappears, only its duct (mesonephric) remains	External genitalia form but difficult to differentiate			0.27–0.31 cm
Second trimester					
8th–12th	Mesonephric duct regresses almost completely		Müllerian ducts fuse to form uterovaginal canal and fallopian tubes		
12th		Male/female genitalia characteristics become evident Ovary descends	Median septum disappears		
12th–5th month	Metanephros—third-stage kidney	Cortical cords split up and surround primitive germ cells to produce 7,000,000 oogonia		Formation of mesosalpinx, mesovarium, broad ligament, proper ovarian ligament, and suspensory ligament	

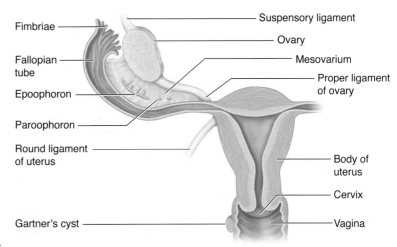

Figure 2-7 Fully developed female reproductive organs.

urorectal septum. The upper portion of the urogenital sinus becomes the urinary bladder, and the lower portion is divided into two portions: the pars pelvina, which is involved in the formation of the vagina, and the pars phallica, which is related to the primordia (developing organs) of the external genitalia. This can best be understood by following the development of the vagina step by step. First, the distal end of the uterovaginal canal makes contact with the posterior wall of the urogenital sinus (Fig. 2-8A). As these structures fuse, a solid group of cells called the *vaginal plate* is formed (Fig. 2-8B). From the vaginal plate, two outgrowths (sinovaginal bulbs) surround the uterovaginal canal and fuse on opposite sides (Fig. 2-8C). If the sinovaginal bulbs do not fuse normally, a vagina with two outlets, or a vagina with one normal outlet and one atretic one, may result.[7,10]

After normal development, the center core of cells hollows out to form a lumen in the vagina. The vagina is now separated from the urogenital sinus only by a thin tissue plate, the *hymen* (Fig. 2-8D). The vaginal fornices, which surround the ends of the uterus (cervix), are thought to be of müllerian duct origin.

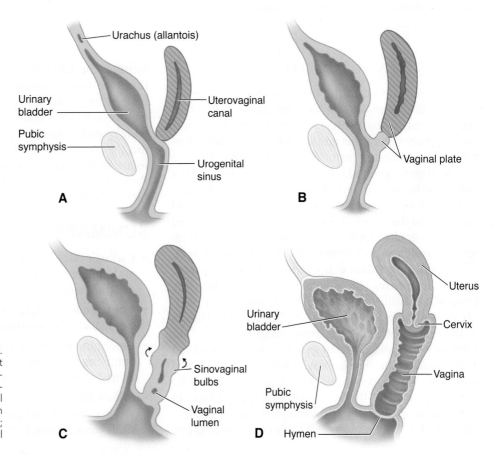

Figure 2-8 Formation of the vagina. **A:** Uterovaginal canal makes contact with wall of urogenital sinus. **B:** Formation of vaginal plate. **C:** Sinovaginal bulbs encircle the vaginal plate and elongate. **D:** Canalization of vaginal plate to form the vagina; separation of vagina and urogenital sinus by the hymen.

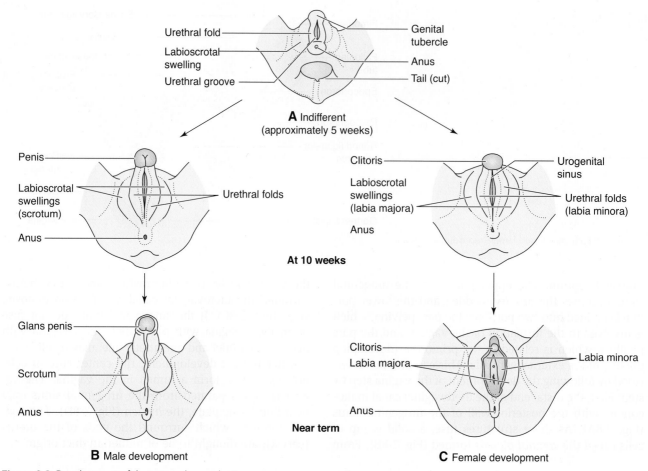

Figure 2-9 Development of the external reproductive organs.

EXTERNAL GENITALIA DEVELOPMENT

As discussed earlier, in the first few months of development, the genitalia are undifferentiated. External development of the genitalia is similar in both sexes until approximately the ninth week.[12] Maternal estrogen is the promoting factor in the development of the female external genitalia. External genitalia include the lower portion (vestibule) of the vagina, vestibule, Bartholin and Skene glans, the clitoris, labia minora and majora, and the mons pubis.[10,11] In the undifferentiated stage, the genital tubercle elongates while the labioscrotal swellings and urogenital folds develop lateral to the cloacal membrane at 44 to 48 days during stage 18.[2] In both sexes, the genital tubercle becomes the primordial phallus. At this point, the primordial phallus discontinues development to become the clitoris in the female, which is relatively large until the 18th week of gestation.[7] Gonadal gender can be determined in the male embryo at approximately the 44th day of gestation, which correlates with Carnegie stage 18.[1] Gonadal gender for the female embryo appears later in Carnegie stage 20, which correlates to approximately the 49th day.[1] The labioscrotal folds continue to grow,

forming the labia minora through fusion of the posterior portion resulting in the frenulum. These folds fuse in the posterior area to form the posterior labial commissure with anterior fusion forming the anterior labial commissure and mons pubis. The labia majora are the result of nonfused labioscrotal folds and correlate to the male scrotum (Table 2-2, Fig. 2-9).[7,10,12,13] By stage 23 (56 days), the external genitalia are completely formed.[1]

SUMMARY

- Carnegie stages classify the embryo by age, size, and appearance of structures in the first 8 weeks of development.
- The reproductive (genital) and urinary systems develop simultaneously, resulting in coexisting malformations.
- Determination of chromosomal gender or sex occurs at the time of fertilization and is either female (46XX) or male (46XY) in the normal configuration.
- Primordial germ cells appear in the third to fourth week during Carnegie stage 6 and migrate in the sixth week during Carnegie stage 17.

TABLE	2-2	
Embryonic Origin of Adult Structures[7,8,10,11]		
Embryonic Structure	**Intermediate Structure**	**Adult Structure**
Indifferent gonad/ primitive sex cords	Genital/ gonadal ridges	Ovary/testies
Cortical cords/ Pluger's tubules		Cortex of the ovary/ primary oocytes
Mesonephros	Wolffian ducts	Genital canals
Coelomic epithelium	Müllerian ducts	Fallopian tubes, uterus, myometrium, perimetrium
Upper urogenital sinus		Urinary bladder
Müllerian ducts/ lower urogenital sinus		Vagina
Primordial phallus		Glans of clitoris
Urogenital membrane	Urogenital groove/ folds	Labia minora
Labioscrotal swellings		Labia majora

- Gonadal ridges (mesoderm), located on the anteromedial sides of the mesonephros, are precursors to the female ovaries and male testes, developing during Carnegie stage 6 approximately 2 weeks postovulation.

- The first-stage kidney (pronephros) forms during the fifth week, and second-stage kidneys (mesonephros) form in the sixth week; the final set of kidneys develops during Carnegie stages 14 and 15.

- Migration of the primordial germ cells into the gonadal ridge results in development of the gonads.

- Rete form the primitive sex cords and the first anastomoses with the mesonephric duct (second-stage kidneys), establishing urogenital connections in the embryo.

- In the seventh week, the primitive sex cords change and either proliferate (male) or degenerate (female).

- Müllerian ducts fuse to develop the normal uterus, also giving rise to the fallopian tubes; the broad ligament is a fold of the peritoneum.

- The vaginal formation occurs through development of the urogenital sinus and the primitive cloaca.

- Genitalia are undifferentiated until Carnegie stage 18 at approximately 44–48 days.

- During Carnegie stage 23, the external genitalia form.

Critical Thinking Question

A 25-year-old patient presents to her clinician with the inability to become pregnant after a year of trying. The initial sonogram revealed what appears to be a bicornuate uterus. Explain the development of this malformation and how this discovery would change your imaging procedure. ANSWER: Uterine malformations are due to improper fusion of the müllerian ducts. The reproductive (genital) and urinary systems develop simultaneously, resulting in coexisting malformations. If there is a uterine fusion malformation, it is quite probable that the kidneys also have some type of congenital anomaly.

REFERENCES

1. Swiss Virtual Campus. Module 8 Embryonic phase. University of Fribourg, Lausanne, and Bern (Swizerland). http://www.embryology.ch/anglais/iperiodembry/carnegie01.html. Accessed 2009.
2. Ahmadzadeh A, Tahmasebi M, Gharibvand MM. Causes and outcome of prenatally diagnosed hydronephrosis. *Saudi J Kidney Dis Transpl.* 2009;20(2):246–250.
3. Hung YH, Tsai CC, Ou CY, et al. Late prenatal diagnosis of hydrometrocolpos secondary to a cloacal anomaly by abdominal ultrasonography with complementary magnetic resonance imaging. *Taiwan J Obstet Gynecol.* 2008;47(1):79–83.
4. The Visible Embryo. http://www.visembryo.com/. Accessed 2009.
5. Papaioannou G, McHugh K . Investigation of an abdominal mass in childhood. *Imaging.* 2004;16:114–123.
6. Wilhelm D, Palmer S, Koopman P. Sex determination and gonadal development in mammals. *Physiol Rev.* 2007;87:1–28.
7. Moore KL, Persaud TVN. *The Developing Human; Clinically Oriented Embryology.* 8th ed. Philadelphia, PA: Saunders; 2007.
8. Tsai CH, Chen CP, Chang MD, et al. Hematometrocolpos secondary to didelphic uterus and unilateral imperforated double vagina as an unusual case of acute abdomen. *Taiwan J Obstet Gynecol.* 2007;46(4):448–452.
9. Khong PL, Cheung SCW, Ooi CGC. Ultrasonography of intra-abdominal cystic lesions in the newborn. *Clin Radiol.* 2004;58(6):449–454.
10. Sadler T. Langman's medical embryology: North American edition. 11th ed. Philadelphia, PA: Lippincott Williams & Wilkins; 2009.
11. Rey R. Anti-Müllerian hormone in disorders of sex determination and differentiation. *Arg Bras Endocrinol Metabol.* 2005;49(1):26–36.
12. Tanagho EA, Smith DR, McAninch JW. Smith's General Urology. 17th ed. New York, NY: McGraw Hill Medical; 2007.
13. Moore KL, Dalley AF, Agur AM. Clinically oriented anatomy. 6th ed. Philadelphia, PA: Lippincott Williams & Wilkins; 2009.

3 Congenital Anomalies of the Female Genital System

Faith Hutson

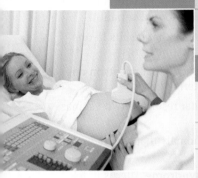

OBJECTIVES

Discuss normal and abnormal paramesonephric (müllerian) and mesonephric (wolffian) duct development

Identify criteria to differentiate a bicornuate from a septate uterus

Compare different uterine fusion anomalies on sonographic, radiographic, and magnetic resonance imaging (MRI) studies

Explain treatment options for uterine anomalies

Relate uterine anomalies to possible renal positional and structural changes

Recognize the characteristic uterine appearance of a patient exposed to diethylstilbestrol (DES)

Summarize fertility and pregnancy outcomes for the patient with congenital anomalies of the uterus

KEY TERMS

arcuate uterus | bicornuate bicollis uterus | bicornuate unicollis uterus | diethylstilbestrol-related anomalies | hysterosalpingography | Mayer-Rokitansky-Küster-Hauser syndrome | mesonephric ducts | müllerian duct anomalies | paramesonephric ducts | septate uterus | subseptate uterus | T-shaped uterus | unicornuate uterus | uterine agenesis | uterus didelphys | vaginal agenesis | wolffian duct | Wunderlich-Herlyn-Werner syndrome

GLOSSARY

Apoptosis Mechanism by which the uterine septum regresses

Cervical incompetence Medical condition in which a pregnant woman's cervix begins to dilate and efface before her pregnancy has reached term. Cervical incompetence may cause miscarriage or preterm birth during the second and third trimesters.

Congenital Mental or physical traits, anomalies, malformations, or diseases present at birth

Diethylstilbestrol (DES) Nonsteroidal drug administered between the late 1940s and the early 1970s to pregnant women. This drug was the first demonstrated transplacental carcinogen responsible for clear-cell vaginal carcinoma in girls born to mothers who took the drug during pregnancy to prevent miscarriage. Uterine malformations associated with DES exposure include uterine hypoplasia and T-shaped endometrium.

Hematocolpos Accumulation of menstrual blood in the vagina resulting from a lower vaginal obstruction or imperforate hymen

Hematometra Retention of blood in the uterine cavity

Hematometrocolpos Accumulation of menstrual blood in the uterus and vagina caused by either an imperforate hymen or other obstruction

Hydrometra Accumulation of watery fluid in the uterine cavity

Hymen Ringlike area of tissue that represents the opening to the vagina

Hysterosalpingography Radiographic imaging of the uterus and fallopian after injection of radiopaque material

Imperforate hymen Usually congenital due to the failure of degeneration of central epithelial cells of the hymenal membrane. An imperforate hymen is visible upon examination as a translucent thin membrane just inferior to the urethral meatus that bulges with the Valsalva maneuver and completely covers the vagina; it must be surgically corrected.

Klippel-Feil syndrome Characterized by congenital fusion of the cervical spine, a short neck, a low posterior hairline, and a limited range of cervical spine motion; associated with Mayer-Rokitansky-Küster-Hauser syndrome

Metroplasty Reconstructive surgery on the uterus used primarily to correct a septate uterus

Ostium (pl. ostia) A small opening, especially one of entrance into a hollow organ or canal

Paramesonephric (müllerian) ducts Paired embryonic tubes roughly parallel to the mesonephric ducts that empty into the urogenital sinus; in the female, the upper part of these ducts form the fallopian tubes and the lower parts fuse to form the uterus

Renal agenesis Absence of one or both kidneys

Septate uterus Complete failure of the median septum to be reabsorbed

Sinovaginal bulb Part of the vaginal plate of the urogenital sinus, which forms the lower 20% of the vagina

Subseptate uterus Partial failure of the median septum to be reabsorbed

Uterine aplasia Complete absence of the uterus

Uterus arcuatus Mildest fusion anomaly, resulting in a partial indentation of the uterine fundus with a normal endometrial cavity; considered a normal variant

Uterus bicornis bicollis Anomaly that results in one vagina, two cervices, and two uterine horns

Uterus bicornis unicollis Anomaly that results in one vagina, one cervix, and two uterine horns

Uterus didelphys Anomaly that results in two vaginas, two cervices, and two uteri

Uterus unicornis unicollis Anomaly that results in one cervix and one uterine horn

Wunderlich-Herlyn-Werner syndrome Uterus didelphys with obstructed unilateral vagina and associated ipsilateral renal and ureter agenesis

Congenital anomalies of the female reproductive organs are rare, accounting for less than 5% of all women.[1] Because uterine abnormalities are usually not recognized at birth, the actual incidence and prevalence of müllerian duct anomalies in the general population are not known. Most cases are diagnosed in the infertility or recurrent pregnancy loss populations. Other factors contributing to the unknown incidence include non-standardization of classification systems, differences in diagnostic criteria of study populations, and nonuniformity in diagnostic procedures.[2]

Uterine and vaginal malformations occur from any of the following complications:

1. Arrested development of the paramesonephric (müllerian) ducts
2. Failure of fusion of the müllerian ducts
3. Failure of resorption of the median septum[3]

In 1979, Buttram and Gibbons proposed a classification system based on the configuration of the anomaly, its clinical symptoms, the treatment options, and prognosis. This classification system, which has been adapted by the American Fertility Society, provides a useful reference system when discussing congenital anomalies (Table 3-1).

EMBRYOLOGY

In the fetus, the undifferentiated gonads are induced to develop by germ cells that migrate from the yolk sac to the gonadal region at about 5 weeks' gestation. These germ cells form the genital ridges, which become the sex cords. If the germ cells do not migrate to the gonadal region of the pelvis, the gonads and ovaries will not form.[4]

At 6 weeks, gestational age, both male and female embryos have two sets of paired genital ducts: the paramesonephric (müllerian) and the mesonephric

(wolffian) ducts. At this phase in embryo development, the genital systems are identical, although there are cellular differences. Wolffian duct development precedes müllerian duct development and, for a brief period, the wolffian ducts drain the primitive mesonephric kidney into the cloaca. In the absence of testosterone in the female fetus, the wolffian ducts degenerate, while the müllerian ducts develop bidirectionally along the lateral aspects of the gonads.[2] The remaining vestiges of the wolffian ducts provide a template for the developing müllerian ducts. Renal anomalies are associated with abnormal differentiation of the wolffian and developing müllerian ducts. Renal agenesis is the most commonly associated anomaly, but duplicated collecting systems, cystic renal dysplasia, and crossed renal ectopia have all been described.[4] The proximal segments of the müllerian ducts remain unfused and open into the peritoneal cavity to form the fallopian tubes. The distal ductal segments join together to create the uterovaginal canal that forms the uterus, cervix, and upper four-fifths of the vagina.

Although initially separated by a septum, by 10 weeks, the müllerian ducts fuse at the inferior margin and the septum regresses to form the unified body of the uterus and cervix (Fig. 2-3; Fig. 3-1). Regression of the septum occurs because of apoptosis, which is mediated by the Bc12 gene. In the absence of this gene, the septum persists.[5] Recently reported cases range from a partial uterine septum limited to the uterine fundus to a complete septum extending from the fundus into the cervical canal. Occasionally, a longitudinal vaginal septum is also present. Even rarer are the cases of cervical duplication in conjunction with complete uterine and vaginal septa.[5] All these various case presentations confound attempts at clinical diagnosis, make classification difficult, and change pregnancy outcome predictions.

TABLE	3-1
Classification System of Müllerian Duct Anomalies	

Class I

Hypoplasia or agenesis of:

- A. Vagina
- B. Cervix
- C. Fundus
- D. Tubal
- E. Combined

Class II

Unicornuate:

- A1a. Communicating
- A1b. Noncommunicating
- A2. No cavity
- B. No horn

Class III

Uterus didelphys

Class IV

Bicornuate:

- A. Complete
- B. Partial
- C. Arcuate

Class V

Septate uterus:

- A. Complete
- B. Partial

Class VI

DES- and drug-related anomalies or Arcuate

(From Buttram VC, Gibbons WE. Müllerian anomalies: a proposed classification [an analysis of 144 cases]. *Fertil Steril.* 1979;32:40–46.)

Because of newly reported cases, the classic theory of unidirectional (caudal to cranial) müllerian duct development was challenged and the alternative theory of bidirectional development was proposed. According to this theory, fusion and resorption begin at the isthmus and proceed simultaneously in both the cranial and caudal directions.[5] This theory could explain anomalies such as a complete uterine septum with a duplicated cervix or an isolated vertical upper vaginal septum with a normal uterus.[4]

While the uterovaginal canal develops, the sinusal tubercle begins to thicken, forming the sinovaginal bulbs of the urogenital sinus; this in turn forms the lower one-fifth of the vagina. The uterovaginal canal is separated from the sinovaginal bulb by a horizontal vaginal membrane or plate; this plate elongates during the third to fifth months, and its interface with the urogenital sinus produces the hymen. The hymen typically ruptures during the perinatal period[4]; if it does not, an imperforate hymen results. The diagnosis of an imperforate hymen is usually made at menarche, when a tense, bulging membrane is palpated. Sonography is very useful in imaging hematometrocolpos, a combination of menstrual blood, fluid, and secretions in the distended vagina and uterus (Fig. 3-2).

The ovaries are not associated with müllerian duct anomalies because they are formed from the mesenchyme and the epithelium of the gonadal ridge and therefore are not affected by formation errors of the mesonephric and paramesonephric ducts.

ARRESTED DEVELOPMENT

Arrested development of the müllerian ducts can be either bilateral or unilateral. Arrested bilateral development is quite rare and produces agenesis or hypoplasia of the vagina and/or uterus. If the arrested development is unilateral, then there is development of a uterus unicornis unicollis (one uterine horn and one cervix).[6]

AGENESIS/HYPOPLASIA OF THE UTERUS AND VAGINA

Approximately 5% to 10% of müllerian duct anomalies are attributed to arrested development of the paramesonephric ducts; this produces either hypoplasia (partial arrestment) or agenesis of the vagina and uterus (complete arrestment).[4]

The most common manifestation of complete agenesis of the vagina and uterus is Mayer-Rokitansky-Küster-Hauser (MRKH) syndrome, with a related 15% to 40% incidence of urologic abnormalities in diagnosed cases. Skeletal anomalies such as an absence of or fusion of the vertebra occur in 12% to 50% of cases, resulting in an association between MRKH and Klippel-Feil syndrome.[2,7] Hypoplasia (partial arrestment) is more rarely encountered and is characterized by a normal uterus and small vaginal pouch (Fig. 3-3).

Clinical signs present at puberty include primary amenorrhea with severe cyclic pelvic pain. Physical examination will probably reveal an obstructed uterus, resulting in hematometra (Fig. 3-4). Secondary sexual characteristic are present, indicating normal ovarian function.

Treatment

Both surgical and nonsurgical methods of treatment have been used. The nonsurgical techniques involve graduated dilators to progressively widen an opening, creating a neovagina; this process can take months or years before a functional vagina is formed. In the case of vaginal agenesis, vaginoplasty is used to create a vagina. Various surgical methods can be used depending on the surgeon's preference and level of experience as well as the patient's preference. One successful method involves using the distal sigmoid colon to create a vagina.[2]

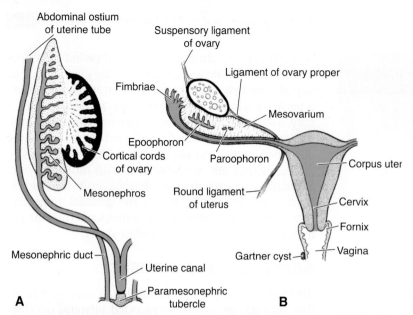

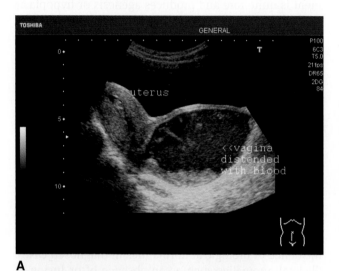

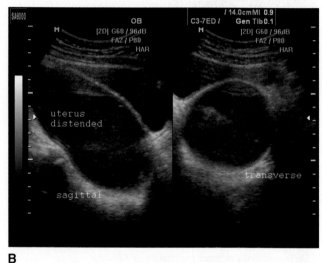

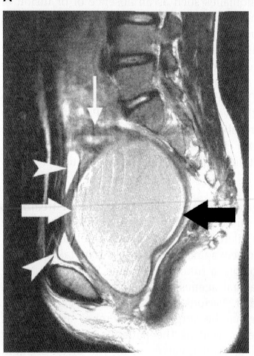

Figure 3-1 A: Genital ducts in the female at the end of the second month. Note the paramesonephric (müllerian) tubercle and formation of the uterine canal. **B:** Genital ducts after descent of the ovary. The only parts remaining from the mesonephric system are the epoophoron, paroophoron, and Gartner cyst. Note the suspensory ligament of the ovary, ligament of the ovary proper, and round ligament of the uterus.

Figure 3-2 A: This image demonstrates hematocolpos with the vagina distended with hemorrhagic material. The uterus is not involved. **B:** This young patient presented with primary amenorrhea and an abdominal mass. Ultrasound images reveal hypoechoic fluid distending the uterus and vagina. Fine particulate debris is seen within the fluid (blood). These findings suggest vaginal outflow obstruction due to imperforate hymen. Nearly 800 mL of blood was drained during surgery on this patient. (Images courtesy of Joe Antony, MD, Cochin, India. From the website at: http://www.ultrasound-images.com/fetus-general.htm.) **C:** Hematocolpos in a patient with uterus didelphys. Sagittal T2-weighted image of pelvis demonstrates large fluid-filled vagina *(arrows)* compressing bladder *(arrowheads)*. Note continuity of fluid with superiorly displaced uterine horn *(thin arrow)*.

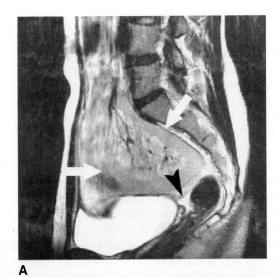

A

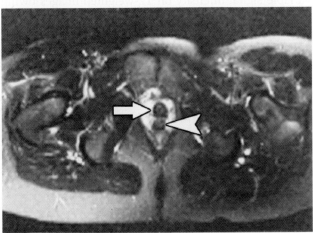

B

Figure 3-3 Mayer-Rokitansky-Küster-Hauser syndrome. **A:** Sagittal T2-weighted image through the pelvis of a female patient with amenorrhea reveals absence of uterus with only small amount of fluid occupying space between bladder and rectum *(arrowhead)*. Solitary pelvic kidney *(arrows)* is noted. **B:** Axial fat-suppressed T2-weighted image through lower pelvis in same patient as **(A)** shows normal urethra *(arrow)* surrounded by high-signal-intensity periurethral veins. Vagina *(arrowhead)* lacks normal "H" shape.

Pregnancy Outcomes

Pregnancy is incompatible with uterine agenesis. There is little possibility of reproduction for patients with uterine hypoplasia; this, however, depends on the degree of hypoplasia and amount of functional endometrial tissue present. Since the ovaries are normal, oocyte harvesting can be done in women who want to have children with a surrogate.

Imaging Techniques

Hysterosalpingography (HSG) is not useful in the evaluation of vaginal agenesis and hypoplasia.

With müllerian agenesis, there is no uterus or vagina identified with transabdominal sonography, although the ovaries can typically be seen. Evaluation of a hypoplastic uterus or uterine remnant may be difficult due to peristalsing bowel loops.

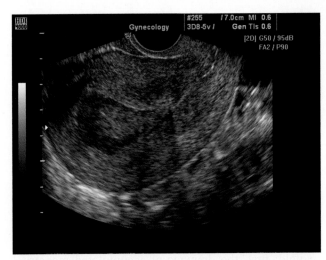

Figure 3-4 A sagittal endovaginal image of a uterus with hematometra. (Image courtesy of Philips Medical Systems, Bothell, WA.)

MRI is often a compliment to sonography. Uterine agenesis and hypoplasia are best imaged in a sagittal plane, whereas vaginal agenesis is more easily demonstrated in a transverse plane (Fig. 3-5). With müllerian agenesis, no identifiable uterus is seen on MRI; uterine hypoplasia demonstrates abnormal low-signal-intensity myometrium on T2-weighted images, with poorly delineated zonal anatomy. Both the endometrial cavity and the myometrium are small.[4]

VAGINAL SEPTUM

In addition to obstruction from vaginal agenesis, defects of vertical vagina fusion can result in the formation of a transverse vaginal septum, which can also cause obstruction and produce hematocolpos in patients having a uterus with functional endometrial tissue.[4] The most frequent location for this transverse septum is at the

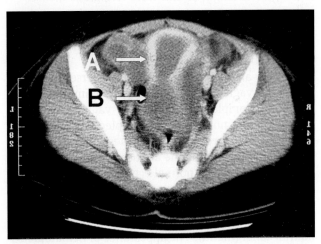

Figure 3-5 Congenital absence of the lower one-third of the vagina. MRI demonstrates that a uterus is present **(A)** as well as an upper vaginal pouch **(B)**. The upper vagina has formed a hematocolpos, which began soon after menarche and presented as a pelvic mass.

junction of the upper and middle third of the vaginal canal. An imperforate hymen can mimic a low transverse septum with resultant hematocolpos; however, imperforate hymen is not a müllerian duct anomaly, resulting in necessitating different treatment upon diagnosis. A transverse septum can occur with any type of müllerian duct anomaly, although it is most often associated with uterus didelphys.

Defects of lateral fusion produce longitudinal septa that are most often associated with septate and duplication anomalies; if there is obstruction, it is usually unilateral.[4]

Treatment

With the presence of a uterus, surgical therapy is twofold: first, the drainage of accumulated menstrual blood; and second, the preservation of a perineal space of adequate size to function as a normal vagina.[8] Most often, the septum can be excised through the vagina. In cases of high transverse septum, the septum is much thicker, making the surgical procedure more difficult.[9]

Pregnancy Outcomes

Pregnancy outcomes for complete transverse vaginal septum are hard to ascertain because there has been little follow-up of the reproductive capacity of many of these patients.[9] Successful pregnancy outcomes on whether the anomaly is just in the vagina or if there is also uterine involvement, and also on the location of the transverse septum. Patients with a transverse septum in the middle or upper vagina are less likely to conceive than are those with a lower vaginal transverse septum.[9] One theory is that retrograde menstrual flow through the uterus and fallopian tubes would occur earlier in patients with a middle or upper transverse septum, making them more asymptomatic and predisposing them to endometriosis, whereas patients with a lower vaginal septum would have more vaginal distention and therefore a greater length of time from retrograde menses.[9]

Imaging Techniques

HSG has no role in evaluating a transverse septum, given the inability to catheterize the cervix.

Vaginal anomalies, including transverse septa and duplicated vagina, can be challenging to image with sonography. Complete absence of the vagina is apparent by the missing normal central coapted vaginal echoes. When there is partial vaginal agenesis, ultrasound can be useful in identifying the atretic area by mapping out the section where no normal echoes are visualized.

Visualization of a discrete attenuated transverse septum is not always possible but can be inferred by the accumulations of blood in the vagina (colpos) or endometrial canal (metra). The appearance of hematometrocolpos is variable; most often, it is seen as a cystic mass with low-level echoes distending the endometrium and the vagina.

With transabdominal scanning, the vaginal canal and the surrounding vaginal muscles should appear continuous with the cervix in a longitudinal plane. Absence of this continuity could indicate atresia, which can be further documented in the transverse plane.

The endovaginal approach should be performed with caution if there is suspicion of an atretic or absent vagina. The transperineal approach is also helpful in determining vaginal absence or obstruction.

Because of the complexity of these anomalies, MRI is an important diagnostic imaging tool, especially since ultrasound can be limited by field of view and distortion of anatomy due to hematometrocolpos. MRI can visualize the vaginal septum and resultant hematometra or hematometrocolpos. The trapped blood demonstrates increased signal intensity on T1-weighted images and variable signal intensity on T2-weighted images owing to the variable age of the retained blood.[4] MRI multiplanar capability is very effective at delineating complex anomalies, any resultant distortion of the uterovaginal anatomy, and any secondary processes that can involve the ovaries and adnexa, such as endometriosis.[4]

UTERUS UNICORNIS

This anomaly occurs when there is complete or incomplete failure of one müllerian duct to elongate while the other duct develops normally; this accounts for

---

PATHOLOGY BOX 3-1

Sonographic Appearance of Congenital Vaginal Anomalies

Anomaly	Sonographic Appearance
Hydrocolpos or hematocolpos	Anechoic to hypoechoic pear-shaped mass with no normal vaginal echoes located adjacent and posterior to the bladder
Vaginal septa	Normal vaginal echoes
Double vagina	Either no significant change in appearance of normal vagina or enlarged vagina; endovaginal scanning may demonstrate second vagina
Absent vagina	Absence of normal vaginal echoes
Duplicated uterus with unilateral imperforate vagina	Vagina appears normal; lateral to normal uterus, ananechoic or echo-filled mass might be seen. Kidney ipsilateral to mass is usually absent
Intact hymen	In postmenarchal symptomatic patient, possible finding of hematocolpos or hematometrocolpos
Gartner duct cyst	Anechoic small mass in anterolateral vagina

between 2.4% and 13% of all müllerian duct defects. In three unrelated studies, researchers have reported a unicornuate uterus and ipsilateral ovarian agenesis leading to speculation that in some situations the uterus unicornis may be the result of agenesis involving all structures derived from the urogenital ridge rather than just the müllerian duct[2] (Fig. 3-6).

Although this defect may occur alone, it is frequently associated with a rudimentary horn on the opposite side. The rudimentary horn can have a uterine cavity with functional endometrium, and in some cases, there may be communication between the endometrium of the main horn and the rudimentary horn. If the noncommunicating rudimentary horn has functional endometrial tissue, there will be either retrograde menses (often increasing the likelihood of endometriosis[3]) or retention of menstrual blood (leading to hematometra[6]), depending on whether an opening into the pelvic cavity is present or not. Unexplained is the predominance of the unicornuate uterus to be on the right side.[4] Associated urologic anomalies are common (44%), especially with an obstructed horn. Urological anomalies include ipsilateral renal agenesis (67%), horseshoe kidneys, and ipsilateral pelvic kidney (15%)[2,10] (Fig. 3-7).

Treatment

With noncommunicating horns, resection is advisable for both symptomatic relief and because of the possibility of ectopic pregnancies through transperitoneal sperm migration.[4] Additionally, there is an increased incidence of endometriosis with the noncommunication subgroup. Consideration should be given to the resection of a communicating rudimentary horn as well because

pregnancies that develop in there rarely produce viable offspring. Rudimentary horns without endometrial tissue typically do not require surgical intervention.[4]

Pregnancy Outcomes

Numerous studies have all concluded that the unicornuate uterus has the poorest overall productive outcomes of all the uterine anomalies. Reported spontaneous abortion rates range from 41% to 62%, whereas premature birth rates range from 10% to 20%. Reproductive problems are attributed to abnormal uterine vasculature and diminished myometrial mass. Other common obstetric complications include ectopic pregnancy (4.3%), missed abortion, uterine rupture, intrauterine growth restriction, and abnormal fetal lie or maternal death (0.5%).[4]

Imaging Techniques

Upon instillation of contrast medium with HSG, the endometrium appears fusiform, draining into a solitary fallopian tube. The uterus typically is shifted away from midline. HSG is unable to delineate noncavitary and noncommunication rudimentary horns[8] (Fig. 3-8).

Two-dimensional (2D) vaginal sonography without HSG is less sensitive in identifying the unicornuate uterus, probably because the single cavity of the unicornuate uterus can be confused with a normal uterine cavity.[8] Recent studies have found that three-dimensional (3D) sonography with multiplanar imaging is very effective in the diagnosis and classification of müllerian duct defects.[11] With major müllerian duct defects, various authors reported the sensitivity and specificity of endovaginal 3D ultrasound were both 100%, compared with 100% sensitivity and 95% specificity for endovaginal

---

PATHOLOGY BOX 3-2

Sonographic Appearance of Uterine Anomalies

	Sonographic Appearance	
Anomaly	**Nonpregnant Uterus**	**Pregnant Uterus**[a]
Cervical atresia	No cervical echoes but corpus of uterus appears as echogenic mass	
Uterine agenesis	Absence of echoes in area of uterus or small remnant of apparently fibrous tissue	
Unicornuate uterus	Normal to slightly asymmetric uterus, loss of pear shape, lateral displacement	In advanced pregnancy, no abnormalities
Didelphic uterus	Double cervix, uterine corpora, enlarged uterus, two endometrial canal echoes visualized	Pregnancy in one uterus; decidual reaction and enlarged other
Bicornuate uterus	Dependent on degree of cleft between horns; broad uterine fundus, two distinct cornua, with a cleft between them of over 1 cm and angle between horns of over 75 degrees, two endometrial cavity echoes or normal-looking uterus	Eccentric implantation of gestational sac
Subseptate uterus	Depends on extent of septum (partial or complete). Undivided and widened fundus, convex or flat in contour. Two endometrial echoes might be seen until fusion of endometrium	Thick septum might be seen in early pregnancy. Sac might extend across septum. Differentials include large ovarian cyst, degenerated cystic fibroid, ectopic gestation

[a]After 22 weeks' gestation, most anomalies cannot be visualized.

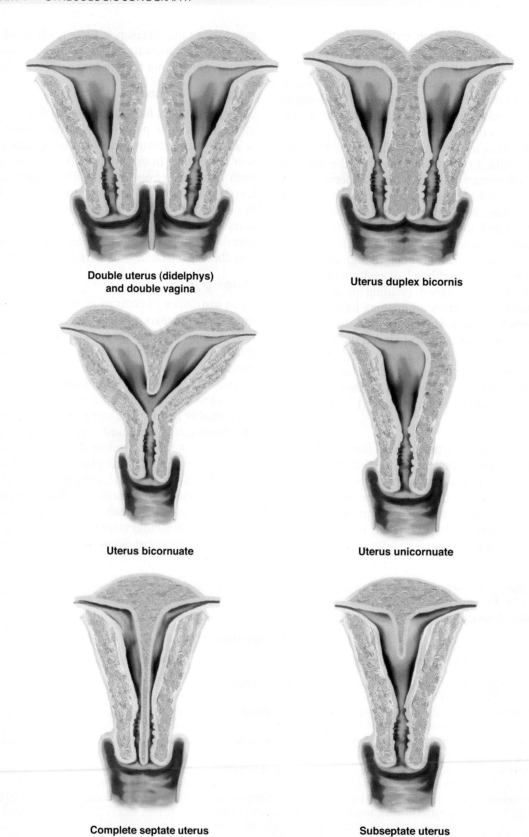

Double uterus (didelphys) and double vagina

Uterus duplex bicornis

Uterus bicornuate

Uterus unicornuate

Complete septate uterus

Subseptate uterus

Figure 3-6 Uterine anomalies. Uterine fusion abnormalities include double uterus, double cervix, double vagina, uterine duplex bicornis, bicornuate uterus single cervix, unicornuate uterus, septated uterus, and subseptate uterus.

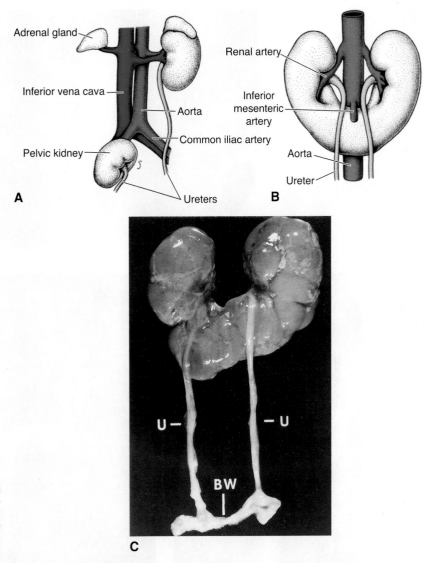

Figure 3-7 A: Unilateral pelvic kidney showing the position of the adrenal gland on the affected side. **B,C:** Illustration and photomicrograph, respectively, of horseshoe kidneys showing the position of the inferior mesenteric artery. *BW,* bladder wall; *U,* ureters.

2D ultrasound. However, the largest difference was the positive predictive value, with 100% for 3D compared with 50% for 2D sonography.[6] 3D sonography can image in the coronal plane, which 2D sonography cannot since there is limited mobility of transducer without the confines of the vagina. This coronal plane can show the relationship of the myometrium and the endometrium at the uterine fundus, delineate the entire endometrial and cervical canals, and visualize the cornual angles and external uterine contours.[4] Since all potential imaging planes are captured within the volume data set on 3D sonography, there is no loss of information, which is a possibility with selected static 2D images (Fig. 3-9).

Sonohysterography, also called *saline-infused sonography* (SIS), uses a saline injection to distend the uterine cavity, separating the walls of the uterus and highlighting any defects. Using 3D coronal imaging while the uterine cavity is distended with saline reduces the time the uterus is distended, thereby reducing pain for the patient. It also facilitates visualization of endometrial irregularities and provides immediate acquisition

and storage of volume data, which can be reviewed retrospectively. Coronal views record the relationship of the myometrium and the endometrium.

On MRI, the unicornuate uterus is curved and elongated, with the external uterine contour having a banana-shaped appearance. Uterine volume is reduced, although there is normal zonal anatomy of the myometrium. The endometrium may be uniformly narrow or it may taper at the apex, giving a bullet shape. If present, the appearance of the rudimentary horn is variable. When the endometrium is absent, the horn has low signal intensity, with a loss of normal zonal anatomy. If the rudimentary horn has endometrial tissue, normal zonal anatomy may be preserved.[4]

FAILURE OF FUSION

Partial fusion failure results in either a uterus bicornis bicollis (one vagina, two cervices, and two uterine horns) or a uterus bicornis unicollis (one vagina, one cervix, and two uterine horns). A uterus arcuatus is

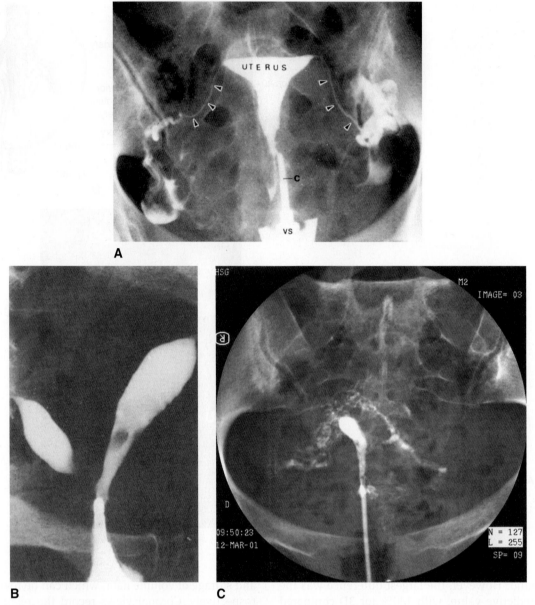

Figure 3-8 A: Radiograph of the normal uterus and uterine tubes (hysterosalpingogram). Radiopaque material was injected into the uterus through the external os of the uterus. The contrast medium has traveled through the triangular uterine cavity and uterine tubes *(arrowheads)* and passed into the pararectal fossae of the peritoneal cavity (lateral to the arrowheads). *(C)* Catheter in the cervical canal. **B:** The hysterogram is suggestive of a unicornuate malformation. The exam reveals nonsymmetrical horns with the left horn developed more than the right horn. **C:** Hysterogram suggestive of a unicornuate uterus.

considered either a very mild form of the bicornuate uterus or a normal variant. It results in a partial indentation of the uterine fundus with a normal endometrial cavity. Complete fusion failure produces a uterus didelphys (two vaginas, two cervices, and two uterine horns).

BICORNUATE UTERUS

The bicornuate uterus accounts for approximately 10% of all the müllerian duct anomalies. Troiano et al. lists at least six variations of the bicornuate uterus with longitudinal upper vaginal septa coexisting in 25% of bicornuate uteri.[4] The two cornua are fused caudad,

usually at the isthmus with communication of the endometrial cavities. In the bicornuate unicollis, the intervening muscular septum extends to the internal cervical os, while the cleft of the bicornuate bicollis can be of variable length.[4]

It is extremely important to distinguish between a bicornuate and a septate uterus because the pregnancy outcomes and treatment techniques differ considerably.

Treatment

Generally, surgical intervention is not indicated; however, Strassmann metroplasty has been advocated for women with a history of recurrent miscarriage (RM)

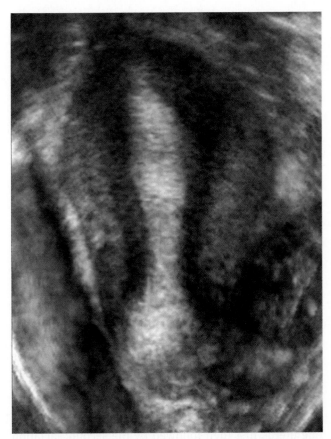

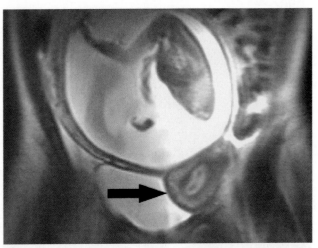

Figure 3-10 Gravid bicornuate uterus. Coronal Half-Fourier Acquired Single-shot Turbo spin Echo (HASTE) image demonstrates second uterine horn (arrow) in pregnant patient with bicornuate uterus.

Figure 3-9 Failure of one of the müllerian ducts to form properly results in the development of a unicornuate uterus. A rudimentary horn may accompany this malformation. The small horn may have a cavity containing endometrial tissue. Usually the rudimentary horn remains separate but may have access to the main body of the uterus. (Image courtesy of GE Healthcare, Wauwatosa, WI.)

who have no other infertility issues. The Strassmann procedure removes the muscular septum by wedge resection to unify the two cavities. Few studies have demonstrated the benefits of metroplasty with this type of anomaly. Cervical incompetence has been reported in about 38% of bicornuate uterus anomalies, and the placement of a cervical cerclage has been reported to increase fetal survival rates.[4]

Pregnancy Outcomes

Women with bicornuate uterus but no other extrauterine infertility issues usually have no difficulty conceiving; however, maintaining a healthy pregnancy is another issue. The reported spontaneous abortion rates for bicornis bicollis uteri range from 28% to 35%. Premature birth rates range from 14% to 23%, and fetal survival rates range from 57% to 63%. In women with bicornis unicollis uteri, the rates of spontaneous abortion and premature delivery are even higher[4,12](Fig. 3-10).

Imaging Techniques

HSG cannot reliably distinguish bicornuate from septate uteri because the radiographic appearance has a great degree of overlap and because the external uterine contour cannot be evaluated (Fig. 3-11).

Sonographic imaging should be performed during the secretory phase of the endometrial cycle, when the endometrial echo pattern is more easily identified. Correct classification depends on identification of a large fundal cleft with divergence of the uterine horns. 3D endovaginal sonography is very useful for all the müllerian duct anomalies but especially in making the distinction between bicornuate and septate anomalies (Fig. 3-12).

MRI can definitively make the distinction when bicornuate uterus is suspected. There is increased intercornual distance, usually greater than 4 cm, and a concave cleft in the external fundal uterine contour measuring deeper than 1 cm (Fig. 3-13). The fundal contour is best visualized in an oblique coronal plane, along the long axis of the uterus. Typically, the septum exhibits signal characteristics identical to the myometrium.[3]

UTERUS DIDELPHYS

Uterus didelphys is defined as the complete midline failure of müllerian duct fusion. The result of failure of fusion is the production of two hemiuteri each with their own endometrium and vagina. Each hemiuteri is associated with one fallopian tube and there is no communication between the duplicated endometrial cavities. Ovarian malposition may also be present.[2] Uterus didelphys comprises approximately 5% of uterine anomalies.

Women with nonobstructive uterus didelphys are typically asymptomatic, although it may be diagnosed at menarche with tampon use if these fail to obstruct menstrual flow. With obstructive uterus didelphys, the most common presenting symptoms are onset of dysmenorrhea after the onset of menses and progressive pelvic pain. Physical examination may detect a unilateral pelvic mass seen twice as often on the right side.[2]

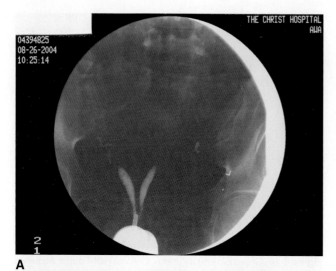

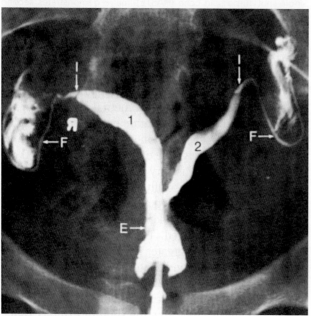

B

Figure 3-11 **A:** Hysterosalpingogram demonstrating a large uterine septum. This cannot be distinguished from a bicornuate uterus in the absence of careful evaluation of the external contour of the uterus. (Courtesy of Sherif G. Awadalla, MD.) **B:** Hysterosalpingogram showing a bicornate uterus. *1 and 2,* uterine cavity; *I,* isthmus of tube; *E,* cervical canal; *F,* uterine tube. (Courtesy of C.E. Stuart and David F. Reid. In Copeland LJ. *Textbook of Gynecology.* Philadelphia, PA: WB Saunders; 1993.)

Endometriosis and pelvic adhesions are secondary to vaginal obstruction and retrograde menstrual flow.

Uterus didelphys, more than any other müllerian anomaly, is associated with renal agenesis. The reported incidence of renal anomalies is 20%. Uterus didelphys with obstructed unilateral vagina is more frequently associated with ipsilateral renal and ureter agenesis; this condition is called Wunderlich-Herlyn-Werner syndrome. Numerous case reports of this syndrome have been published between 2000 and 2004 due to the increased use of MRI.[2]

Treatment

Resection of the vaginal septum is indicated for an obstructed unilateral vagina. Unless removed after diagnosis, hematometra is present and possibly retrograde menses leading to hematosalpinx, endometriosis, and possibly pelvic adhesions. Without obstruction, there is little indication for surgical unification of the uteri; cervical unification is difficult and can result in cervical incompetence or stenosis.

Pregnancy Outcomes

Given the low incidence of uterine didelphys, less data are available about the reproductive outcomes; however, they are reported to be better than for women with unicornis uterus. Compiled data from two studies revealed the following information from 86 pregnancies: 21 (24.4%) preterm deliveries, 59 (68.6%) live births, 2 (2.3%) ectopics, and 18 (20.9%) spontaneous abortions.[2,4]

An unusual finding of uterus didelphys is the ability to have intercourse in both vaginas. Simultaneous pregnancies can occur in each uterus and, although it is rare, it is well documented. The twins are always dizygotic, and each pregnancy should be regarded as a separate entity since the delivery of twins can be widely spaced apart, ranging from 3 hours to 8 weeks between the deliveries.[1] It is speculated that labor is complete in one uterus first then followed by the second; lactation is reported to occur after the birth of the second twin. Delivery management also varies with some authorities believing that vaginal delivery is safe, whereas others advocate cesarean delivery. Some reported complications include unilateral premature labor and unilateral placental abruption.[2]

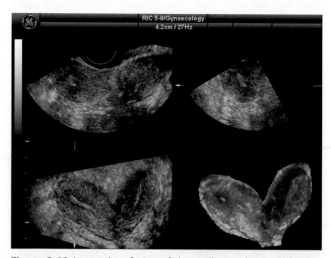

Figure 3-12 Incomplete fusion of the müllerian ducts results in a bicornuate uterus. This anomaly has communication of the two uterine cavities with fusion of the lower uterine segment and cervix. Note the characteristic midsaggital indentation of the fundus on the Z plane and 3D reconstruction on this multiplanar image. This image represents a bicornuate bicollis uterus. (Image courtesy of GE Healthcare, Wauwatosa, WI.)

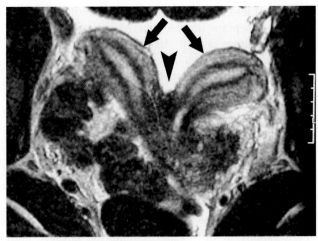

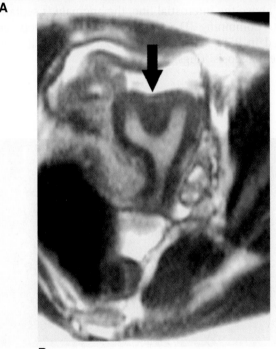

B

Figure 3-13 Uterine variants. **A:** Bicornuate uterus. Note large separation between uterine horns *(arrows)* and deep fundal cleft *(arrowhead)*. **B:** Subseptate uterus. Note lack of fundal cleft *(arrow)* at site of thick septum.

Imaging Techniques

With uterus didelphys, HSG demonstrates two separate endocervical canals, each opening into separate endometrial cavities. There is no communication between the uterine horns. Each endometrial cavity ends in a single fallopian tube. If there is unilateral obstruction, only one cervical os may be visualized.

With sonography, especially 3D endovaginal imaging, separate diverging horns are visualized with a large fundal cleft. The endometrial cavities are separate with no communication; two separate cervices should be documented. Transverse images best visualize duplications of the cervix and uterus. Optimal visualization of the endometrial and cervical echoes is best during the

late secretory phase when the endometrium is at its thickest and most echogenic. Hematometrocolpos will be visualized if there is unilateral obstruction.

MRI also demonstrates two separate uteri, two separate endometria, two separate cervices, and many times, an upper vaginal septum. Each uterus has normal zonal anatomy, and the endometrial-to-myometrial ratio is intact. An obstructed unilateral vaginal septum shows variance of deformity depending on the degree of hematometrocolpos.[4]

FAILURE OF RESORPTION

The resultant failure of median septum resorption is a septate uterus (complete failure) or subseptate uterus (partial failure). This leads to complete or partial duplication of the uterine cavities without duplication of the uterine horns, since complete fusion of the müllerian ducts has already taken place. Failure of resorption is the most common, occurring in approximately 55% of all müllerian anomalies.[4]

The septum is composed of poorly vascularized fibromuscular tissue. Numerous variations of septum formation exist. There is the complete septum, which extends from the fundus to the internal os, dividing the endometrium into two halves; this is associated with a longitudinal vaginal septum. There is the partial septum, which typically does not extend down to the internal os. Another variant consists of the triad of complete septum, duplicated cervix, and vaginal septum and may be more common than previously reported. Additionally, some septa have segments and may permit partial communication between the endometrial cavities.

The most common presenting symptoms are dyspareunia, dysmenorrhea, and infertility—either primary or secondary.[2] A very rare variant is the Robert uterus, which is characterized by a complete septum and noncommunicating hemiuteri with a blind horn. This anomaly presents with hematometra and dysmenorrhea.[2]

Treatment

The septate uterus is typically treated by hysteroscopic resection of the septum. The decision for surgical correction should be based on poor reproductive outcome rather than just on the presence of a septum.[2] Candidates for septal resection are women having recurrent spontaneous abortions, second-trimester loss, or history of preterm delivery. Controversy surrounds surgical management for women with complete septate uterus, duplicate cervix, and septal defects of the vagina. Some specialists advocate the removal of the vaginal septum, whereas others argue that this will increase the risk of cervical incompetence and likelihood of surgical complications.[2]

Pregnancy Outcomes

Although fertility with the septate uterus is not typically compromised, this anomaly is associated with the poorest reproductive outcomes of all the mülleri-an duct anomalies. Compilation of data from several sources indicates that the spontaneous abortion rate is between 26% and 94%,[2,4] premature birth rates range from 9% to 33%, and fetal survival rate ranges from 10% to 75%.[4] Numerous septal biopsies demonstrate large amounts of muscular tissue rather than the previously thought connective tissue. Troiano et al. and Dabirashrafi et al. theorize that the decreased connective tissue may result in poor decidualization and implantation, while the increased muscular tissue could result in increased contractibility and thus the propensity for spontaneous abortions.[4,8] Narrowing of the uterine cavity by the septum is also an implication in poor pregnancy outcomes.

Imaging Techniques

The accuracy of differentiating septate uterus from bi-cornuate uteri with HSG alone is only 55%. In general,

an angle of less than 75 degrees between uterine horns suggests a septate uterus, whereas an angle of more than 105 degrees is more definitive of bicornuate uteri. Unfortunately, there is considerable overlap between these two anomalies, and the presence of myomas or adenomyosis within the septum can widen the angles of divergence, making the correct diagnosis more difficult.[11] Tubal patency and the length and thickness of the septum can, however, be assessed with HSG.[2]

With the sonographic orthogonal view, a line can be drawn between the apices of the endometrium at the level of the ostia. If the fundal indentation of the external uterine contour is below the interostial line or less than 5 mm above the line, the uterus is either didelphic or bicornuate. If the fundal indentation is more than 5 mm above the interostial line, the anomaly is septate uterus.[4] Combining 3D sonography with color Doppler resulted in 95% sensitivity and 99.3% specificity for septate diagnosis[2] (Figs. 3-14 and 3-15).

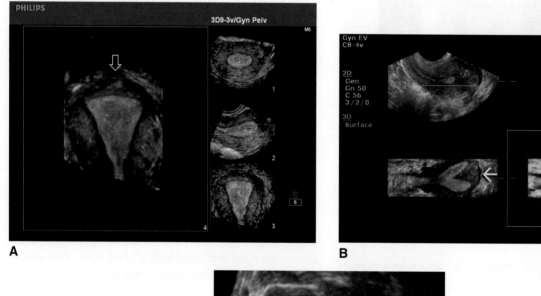

A

B

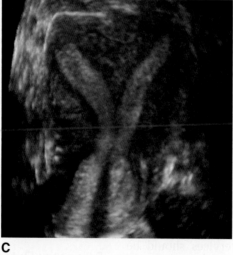

C

Figure 3-14 A: A multiplanar reconstruction of a normal uterus. Notice the triangular endometrial shape and the smooth outer contour *(open arrow)*. **B:** The triangular septation extending into the endometrium *(arrow)* and the maintenance of the rounded outer contour of the uterus would result in a diagnosis of a partial septation or subseptate uterus. (Images courtesy of Philips Medical Systems, Bothell, WA.) **C:** A septation extending from the fundus to the cervix is considered a complete septate uterus. (Image courtesy of GE Healthcare, Wauwatosa, WI.)

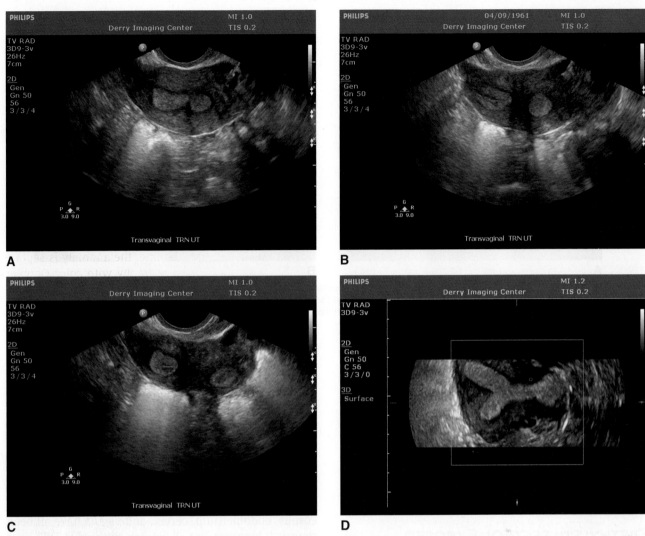

Figure 3-15 A–C: Serial transverse images from the lower uterine segment to the fundus demonstrate the characteristic appearance of the two endometria seen with the septate or didelphic uterus. **D:** If the coronal reconstruction of the uterus has less than a 1 cm indentation, then the malformation is considered septate rather than bicornuate. (Images courtesy of Derry Imaging Center, Derry NH Robin Davies, Ann Smith, and Denise Raney.)

On MRI, the septate uterus has a normal fundal contour with outward fundal convexity, but each endometrial cavity appears smaller than a normal cavity. There is low signal intensity for the septum[2] (Fig. 3-16).

ARCUATE UTERUS

With this anomaly, there is only a mild indentation of the endometrium at the fundus because of near complete resorption of the uterovaginal septum. Buttram and Gibbons originally classified the arcuate uterus as a subclassification of the bicornuate; the American Fertility Society reclassified the arcuate under a separate classification because of its complete fundal unification; however, classification remains problematic, since it is unclear whether this is a true anomaly or an anatomic variant of normal[4](Fig. 3-17).

Treatment

As with the bicornuate, no surgical treatment is indicated.

Pregnancy Outcomes

There is a great amount of conflicting data concerning the reproductive outcomes of the arcuate uterus. Both negative and positive obstetric outcomes have been reported. In the RM population, the arcuate uterus is approximately 12%, more than threefold the prevalence of the general fertile population.[8] According to a study by Woelfer et al., women with arcuate uteri tend to miscarry more often during the second trimester, whereas women with septate uteri more often miscarry during the first trimester.[8]

According to Troiano et al., when there is a ratio of less than 10% between the height of the fundal indentation and the distance between the lateral apical horns, a good pregnancy outcome is expected.[4]

Imaging Techniques

HSG demonstrates a single uterine cavity with a broad saddle-shaped indentation of the uterine fundus.

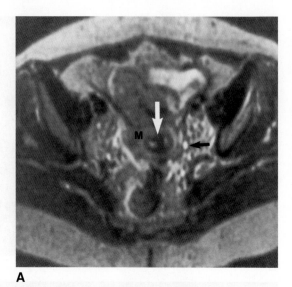

A

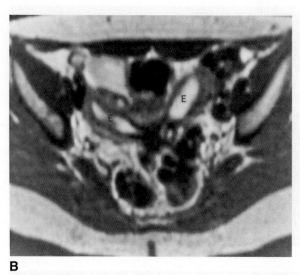

B

Figure 3-16 A: This axial MRI T2-weighted image demonstrates a septate uterus. Taken at the mid uterine *(small arrow)* level, the image shows a single uterine horn with two endometrial canals divided by a septum *(large arrow) M,* myometrium. **B:** Compare to the bicornuate uterus axial T2-weighted image showing two uterine horns of similar size with functioning endometrium *(E)*.

A broad smooth indentation on the fundal portion of the endometrium can be discerned with sonography. The fundal indentation is best demonstrated in the transverse view (Figs. 3-18 and 3-19).

A normal external uterine contour is appreciated with MRI. The fundal indentation is smooth and broad, and the signal is isointense to the normal myometrium. MRIs can sometimes show a subtle indentation of the peripheral subserosal arcuate vessels at the level of the fundus.[4]

DIETHYLSTILBESTROL-EXPOSED UTERUS

DES is an estrogen that was first introduced in 1948 and prescribed to women experiencing pregnancy complications, including premature deliveries and repeat spontaneous abortions. The drug was discontinued in 1971 after it was proven that in utero exposure caused clear cell carcinoma of the vagina. The incidence of clear cell carcinoma development is 0.14 to 1.4 per 1,000 women exposed.[4] DES daughters over age 40 are nearly twice as likely as unexposed women to get breast cancer,

and for DES daughters older than 50 the relative risk is estimated to be even higher.[13] A common structural malformation associated with this drug exposure is the T-shaped endometrium. It is estimated that 2 to 3 million women received DES, exposing 1.0 to 1.5 million offspring in utero; the negative repercussions on reproductive potential will probably continue for the next 10 to 15 years.[4]

DES interferes with embryonic development of the mesenchyme of the genital tract. Anomalies of the uterine corpus, endometrium, cervix, and vagina have all been reported; however, not all women exposed to DES have reproductive problems. Reproductive complications depend on the amount of DES ingested and the gestational age of the fetus at exposure. If the drug was

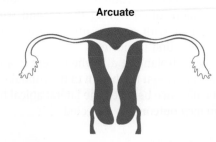

Arcuate

Figure 3-17 Müllerian duct anomaly, arcuate—Schematic representation of developmental anomaly of the müllerian duct involving an arcuate uterus.

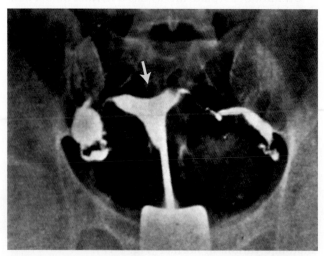

Figure 3-18 This image demonstrates bilateral hydrosalpinx obstructing the fallopian tubes at the fimbriated ends. The characteristic saddle-shaped indentation *(arrow)* indicates an arcuate uterus.

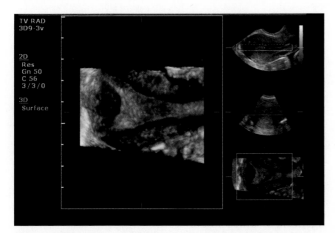

Figure 3-19 A 3D multiplanar reconstruction of a uterus demonstrating an arcuate uterus. (Image courtesy of Philips Medical Systems, Bothell, WA.)

administered very early in the first trimester or after 22 weeks' gestation, structural anomalies are not likely to occur[4] (Fig. 3-20).

TREATMENT

The author found no sources recommending surgical repair of a small, T-shaped, DES-exposed uterus since the benefits have not been established and the risks are high. The risk factors include severing of a major uterine artery branch, resulting in hemorrhage putting the woman at a high risk for hysterectomy and significant morbidity or even mortality.

PREGNANCY OUTCOMES

There is little evidence that women exposed to DES in utero have decreased conception rates; rather, they have a twofold increased risk of spontaneous abortions and a ninefold increased risk of ectopic pregnancy. Numerous studies also show increased risk of premature labor and perinatal mortality.[4] There are reports of cervical incompetence from both structural

changes and histologic changes such as abnormal smooth muscle-to-collagen ratio and decreased cervical elastin.[4]

IMAGING TECHNIQUES

Approximately 69% of DES-exposed women have uterine anomalies visualized with HSG; perhaps the most commonly associated anomaly is a T-shaped endometrial cavity, which is seen in 31% of exposed women. Other uterine abnormalities include constriction bands, small hypoplastic uterus, widened lower uterine segment, irregular endometrial margins (including a narrowed fundal segment of the endometrial canal), and intraluminal filling defects. Cervical anomalies occur in 44% of patients and include hypoplasia, anterior cervical ridge, cervical collar, and pseudopolyps. Cervical hypoplasia and cervical stenosis can make cannula insertion for HSG difficult. Fallopian tube anomalies are also visualized with HSG, including foreshortening of the tube, sacculations and fimbrial stenosis, and deformities[4] (Fig. 3-21).

3D multiplanar endovaginal sonography is valuable in imaging the hypoplastic uterus and T-shaped uterine cavity. 3D ultrasound can also evaluate the internal and external uterine contours, which HSG cannot.[3,6] Doppler ultrasound studies have shown an increased uterine artery pulsatility index (PI), which indicates decreased uterine perfusion[4] (Fig. 3-22).

MRI is extremely good at visualization of uterine hypoplasia, T-shaped uterine canal, and constriction bands. Imaging parallel to the long axis of the uterus gives the best views of the T-shaped configuration. Constriction bands are seen as focal thickening of the junctional zone.[4]

POTENTIAL PITFALLS

Normal sonographic findings of pregnancy can mimic many of the uterine anomalies: an ectopic gestational sac in a fallopian tube may look like a pregnancy in a

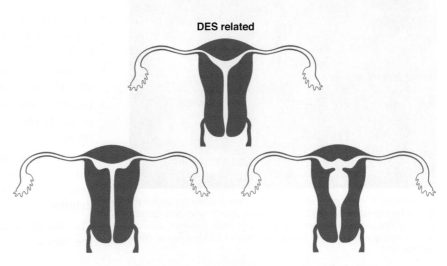

Figure 3-20 Schematic representation of müllerian duct developmental anomalies related to DES.

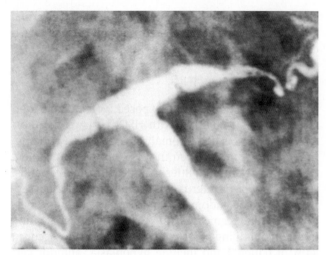

Figure 3-21 Hysterosalpingogram demonstrating T-shaped uterus in patient exposed to DES in utero.

uterine horn; a cornual uterine fibroid may look like a nonpregnant horn; the decidual reaction in the nonpregnant bicornuate uterus may suggest a twin gestation. Knowledge of the patient's clinical symptoms and the sonographic characteristics of each müllerian duct anomaly helps avoid any pitfalls.

FALLOPIAN TUBES

In extreme rare cases, both fallopian tubes are absent in müllerian duct anomalies. More typical is unilateral absence in association with uterus unicornis. Isolated anomalies of the fallopian tubes are quite rare and include accessory ostia, duplication of the tubes, an absent muscular layer, luminal atresia, absent ampulla with blind fimbria, or ectopic location. Rare doubling of the tube can also occur on one side.[2] Atresia of a portion of

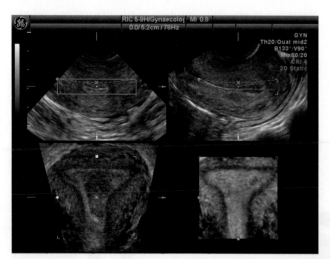

Figure 3-22 A multiplanar reconstruction demonstrating the characteristic hypoplastic T-shaped uterine cavity seen in women exposed to DES. The external uterine contour is normal; however, cervical defects may also be present. (Image courtesy of GE Healthcare, Wauwatosa, WI.)

a tube can cause infertility or tubal pregnancy. Fallopian tube patency can be established with HSG or sonohysterography using a contrast agent or saline, respectively.

OVARIES

Congenital agenesis of the ovaries is very rare since they arise from the epithelium and mesenchyme of the gonadal ridge, which is not associated with the formation of the mesonephric and paramesonephric ducts[4]; however, it has been reported that ovaries are frequently malpositioned above the iliac vessels in patients with congenital uterine anomalies, particularly in uterine agenesis or unicornuate uteri.[14]

Supernumerary ovaries are occasionally found remotely located in the omentum and retroperitoneum. This condition probably results from development of separate primordia in an ectopic portion of the gonadal ridge. Benign teratomas and dermoid cysts can occasionally be found in supernumerary ovaries.[15]

Occasionally, an ovary may be split into separate portions. This accessory ovarian tissue can be found in the broad ligament near the normal ovary or near the cornua of the uterus.[15] Ectopic ovarian tissue may also be found near the kidney or elsewhere in the retroperitoneum.

SUMMARY

- Malformations of the female genital tract are due to lack of müllerian duct development, fusion, or reabsorbtion.
- Germ cell migration from the yolk sac into the gonadal region results in formation of the gonads and ovaries.
- Abnormal differentiation of the embryonic wolffian and müllerian ducts results in renal, uterine, cervix, and vaginal malformations.
- Arrested development of the paramesonephric ducts results in hypoplasia or agenesis of the vagina and uterus.
- HSG, MRI, CT, and sonography help diagnose and monitor patients with congenital anomalies of the genital tract.
- A transverse vaginal septum is not the same as the imperforate hymen.
- Uterus unicornis is the result of normal development of half of the uterus with no or rudimentary development of the rest.
- Partial fusion failure of the müllerian duct results in either a uterus bicornis bicollis or a uterus bicornis unicollis. Complete fusion failure results in uterus didelphys.
- The septate and subseptate uterus is due to lack of the median septum reabsorbtion.

Critical Thinking Questions

1. During the sonographic examination of a 15-year-old patient, the sonographer finds a large uterus filled with complex-appearing material. Since the patient is currently virginal, an endovaginal examination cannot be performed. The patient denies the start of her menses and complains of lower abdominal pain and pressure. What is a possible differential diagnosis for these findings?

   ANSWER: Hematocolpos due to an intact hymen

2. A primiparous patient presents to your department for a routine first trimester size and dates. The sonographic examination reveals a uterus with a lobular appearance on the transverse plane with an eccentric implantation of a 6-week viable embryo. The sagittal images reveal an echogenic thick endometrium. The cervix appears normal. List the differentials for these findings. How can the sonographer help in differentiating between your differential diagnoses?

   ANSWER: Bicornuate uterus or a sebseptate uterus. To differentiate between the bicornuate and subseptate uterus, obtain a coronal image of the uterine fundus. If there is a 1 cm or greater cleft between the horns, this is a bicornuate uterus.

- A mild indentation of the superior portion of the endometrium is called an *arcuate uterus*.
- Women exposed to DES in utero before 22 weeks often develop a T-shaped uterus.

REFERENCES

1. Allegrezza RT, Danielle M. Uterus didelphys and dicavitary twin pregnancy. *J Diagn Med Sonogr.* 2007;23:286–289.
2. Amesse L, Pfaff-Amesse T. "Müllerian Duct Anomalies." *emedicine* http://emedicine.medscape.com. Updated February 16, 2009.
3. Callen P. *Ultrasonography in Obstetrics and Gynecology.* 5th ed. Philadelphia, PA: Saunders Elsevier; 2008.
4. Trojano RN, McCarthy SM. Müllerian duct anomalies: imaging and clinical issues. *Radiology.* 2004; 233:19–34.
5. Ribeiro SC, Tormena RA, Peterson TV, et al. Müllerian duct anomalies: review of current management. *Sao Paulo Med J.* 2009;127(2):92–96.
6. Rumack C, Wilson S, Charboneau JW. *Diagnostic Ultrasound.* Vol 1. 3rd ed. St. Louis, MO: Mosby; 2005.
7. Morcel K, Camborieux L, Guerrier D. *Mayer-Rokitansky-Küster-Hauser (MRKH) syndrome. Orphanet J Rare Dis.* 2007;14;2:13.
8. Saravelos SH, Cocksedge KA, Li TC, et al. Prevalence and diagnosis of congenital uterine anomalies in women with reproductive failure: a critical appraisal. *Hum Reprod Update.* 2008;14(5):415–429.
9. Rock JA, Zacur HA, Dlugi MD, et al. Pregnancy success following surgical correction of imperforate hymen and complete transverse vaginal septum. *Obstet Gynecol.* 1982;59(4):448–451.
10. Yen TH, Lai PC, Huang CC, et al. Single kidney eliciting a search for associated genital tract anomaly. *Nephrol Dial Transplant.* 2004;19(3):731–732.
11. Kupesic S. Clinical implications of sonographic detection of uterine anomalies for reproductive outcome. *Ultrasound Obstet & Gynecol.* 2001;18:387–400.
12. Chaudhry S. AJR teaching file: infertility in a young woman. *AJR Am J Roentgenol.* 2007;189(3 suppl):S11–S12.
13. Palmer JR. Prenatal diethylstilbesterol exposure and risk of breast cancer. *Cancer Epidemiol Biomarkers Prev.* 2006;15:1509.
14. Dabirashrafi H, Mohammad K, Moghadami-Tabrizi N. Ovarian malposition in women with uterine anomalies. *Obstet Gynecol.* 1994;83:293–294.
15. Durfee RB. Congenital anomalies in female genital tract. In: Benson R, ed. *Current Obstetrics and Gynecology: Diagnosis and Treatment.* 2nd ed. Los Altos, CA: Lange; 1978:147–156.

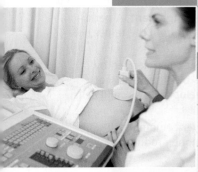

4 The Female Cycle

Sue Benzonelli-Blanchard

OBJECTIVES

Describe the physiology of the menstrual cycle

Identify the hormonal changes that occur during the various ovulatory and endometrial phases

Explain ovum development and its passage from the ovary to the uterus

Discuss the function of the female cycle

KEY TERMS

corpus luteum | estrogen | follicle-stimulating hormone (FSH) | gonadotropin-releasing hormone (GnRH) | luteinizing hormone (LH) | oocyte | ovum | progesterone

GLOSSARY

Amenorrhea Absence of menstruation

Androgens Male hormones produced in small quantities by the female ovaries and adrenal glands, with the greatest quantities occurring at the midpoint of a woman's menstrual cycle

Anteflexed Uterus angled forward toward the cervix

Anteverted Forward-tipped uterus with the cervix and vaginal canal forming a 90-degree angle or less

Antrum (follicular) The portion of an ovarian follicle filled with liquor folliculi. Spaces formed by the confluence of small lakes of follicular liquid in the ovary

Broad ligament The broad ligament is a peritoneal fold that also supports the fallopian tubes, uterus, and vagina. It connects the sides of the uterus to the walls and floor of the pelvis[1]

Cardinal ligament The cardinal ligament attaches to the uterus at the level of the cervix and from the superior part of the vagina to the lateral walls of the pelvis.[1] The cardinal ligament provides support to the uterus.

Corpus luteum (Latin for "yellow body") Formed in the ovary when a follicle has matured and released its egg (ovum) after ovulation. The follicle becomes the corpus luteum that produces progesterone. Progesterone causes the lining of the uterus to thicken for egg implantation[2]

Dysmenorrhea Painful menstruation

Endocrine system A system of glands and cells that produce hormones released directly into the circulatory system

Estrogen General term for female steroid sex hormones secreted by the ovary and responsible for female sexual characteristics

Follicle-stimulating hormone (FSH) Hormone produced by the anterior pituitary, which stimulates ovarian follicle production in females and sperm production in males[1]

Gonadotropins Hormones produced by the anterior pituitary that affects the female and male gonads[1]

Gonadotropic Protein hormones secreted by gonadotrope cells of the pituitary gland

Graafian follicle A mature, fully developed ovarian cyst containing the ripe ovum

Luteinization The transformation of the mature ovarian follicle into a corpus luteum

Negative feedback When concentration of a hormone rises above a certain level, a series of actions take place within a system to cause the concentration to fall. Conversely, steps are taken to increase concentration when the level is too low

Menorrhagia Abnormally heavy or prolonged menstruation

Mesometrium The mesentery of the uterus. It constitutes the majority of the broad ligament of the uterus, excluding only the portions adjacent to the uterine tube and ovary

Oligomenorrhea Abnormally light or infrequent menstruation. Opposite of menorrhagia

Perimetrium The outer serosa layer of the uterus, equivalent to the peritoneum

Positive feedback loop Steps taken to increase concentration when the level is too low

Polymenorrhea (poly = many, menorrhea = bleeding) Frequent irregular periods

Progesterone A steroid hormone produced by the corpus luteum, whose function is to prepare and maintain the endometrium for the reception and development of the fertilized ovum

Rectouterine recess (pouch) An area in the pelvic cavity between the rectum and the uterus that is likely to accumulate free fluid; also known as the posterior cul-de-sac and the pouch of Douglas

Retroflexed A backward angle of the uterine fundus in relation to the cervix

Retroverted A uterus tilted posterior toward the rectum

Suspensory (infundibulopelvic) ligament A peritoneum ligament extending upward from the upper pole of the ovary

Theca interna An ovarian layer characterized by polyhedral cells and numerous blood vessels that secrete estrogen. The cells develop from stromal cells, which produce steroid hormones.

Theca externa An ovarian layer containing spindle-shaped cells incapable of hormone production

A female baby is born with approximately one million immature eggs or **oocytes** in each one of her ovaries. At birth, the female baby's oocytes stop development and will not restart until puberty. At this time, the ovaries contain approximately 300,000 oocytes. When the first menses begins, several oocytes restart their development each month but usually only one matures. About 400 oocytes actually ovulate during a woman's lifetime with immature oocytes degenerating.[5-7]

The menstrual cycle is a series of changes in the endometrium of the uterus in preparation for the arrival of a fertilized **ovum** that will develop in the uterus until birth. If fertilization does not occur, the lining of the endometrium sheds during menstruation. In general, the term "female reproductive cycle" includes the ovarian and uterine cycles, the hormonal changes that regulate them, and related cyclical changes in the breasts and cervix.

The female reproductive cycle is an intricate series of chemical secretions, reactions, and changes in physical anatomy. Understanding the physiology of the female cycle is important for understanding the pathophysiology of the female pelvis. This chapter describes the different parts of the female reproductive system: the hormones that regulate a woman's body, the menstrual cycle, ovulation, and postmenopause.

ANATOMY

The female reproductive internal organs include the uterus, fallopian tubes, two ovaries, cervix, vagina, and the mammary glands. The uterus is shaped like an upside-down or inverted pear, with a thick lining and muscular walls lying between the urinary bladder and rectum. The anatomic sections of the uterus are the fundus (dome-shaped portion above the uterine tubes), the central portion called the body, and the inferior narrow portion opening into the vagina called the cervix.[8]

The uterus contains three layers:
- Perimetrium: The serous outer layer of the uterus
- Myometrium: The muscular middle layer. Smooth muscle that forms the walls of the uterus
- Endometrium: Mucous membrane that lines the uterus. See Figure 5-37 for endometrial layers.

The uterus is hollow to allow a blastocyte, or fertilized egg, to implant and grow. It also allows for the inner lining of the uterus to build up until a fertilized egg implants, or it is sloughed off during menses.

At the upper corners of the uterus are the fallopian tubes. There are two fallopian tubes, called the "uterine tubes" or the "oviducts." The fallopian tubes have different segments. These segments are:
- Isthmus: The narrow portion of the tube that connects the fallopian tube to the uterus
- Ampulla: The wide portion of the fallopian tube that curves around the ovary. Fertilization usually occurs in the ampulla, which ends at the infundibulum
- Infundibulum: The distal funnel-shaped portion of the fallopian tube. It contains ciliated, finger-like projections called fimbriae, which catch the released egg from the ovary

Each fallopian tube attaches to one side of the uterus and connects to an ovary positioned between the ligaments that support the uterus. When an ovary releases an egg, it is swept into the lumen of the fallopian tube by fimbriae. Once the egg is in the fallopian tube, tiny hairs in the fallopian tube's lining help push the egg down the narrow passageway toward the uterus.

The ovaries are oval or almond-sized organs located on each side of the uterus in relation to the lateral wall of the pelvis. Normal ovaries (after menarche) are approximately 3 to 5 centimeters in length, 1.5 to 3 centimeters in width, and about 0.5 to 1.5 centimeters thick. They attach to the posterior border of the uterine broad ligament, behind and below the uterine tubes. The ovaries attach to the uterus by the ovarian ligament and to the pelvic wall by the suspensory ligament.[8,9] The first pregnancy displaces the ovaries, which do not often return to the original location after the pregnancy.

The lower portion of the uterus is the cervix. The cervix (from Latin "neck") is the portion of the uterus that joins with the top end of the vagina; where they join together forms an almost 90-degree curve. The vagina is the canal that leads from the uterus to the outside (Fig. 4-1). Mammary glands are the organs that produce milk for the nourishment of the baby.

PHYSIOLOGY

The endocrine system controls the ovarian and uterine cycles by chemical messengers or "hormones." These hormones are secreted by the hypothalamus (**gonadotropin**

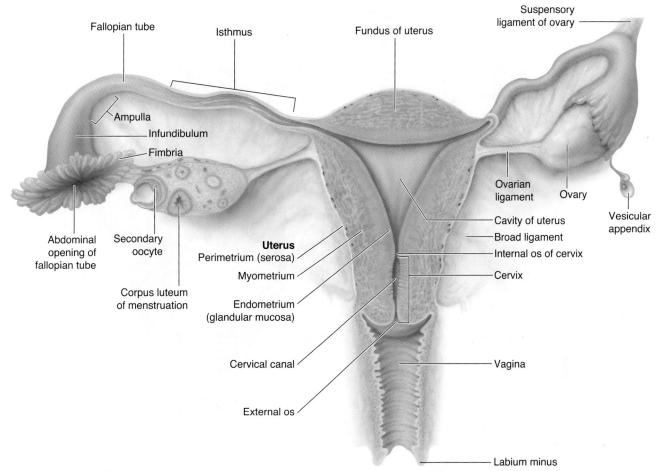

Figure 4-1 Anatomy of the female reproductive system.

releasing hormone [**GnRH**]), anterior pituitary gland (**follicle-stimulating hormone [FSH]** and **luteinizing hormone [LH]**), and ovaries (**estrogen, progesterone,** and inhibin) and control the female reproductive events.

FEMALE REPRODUCTIVE ENDOCRINE GLANDS

This section describes the endocrine glands necessary for the control of the female reproductive system.

Hypothalamus

The hypothalamus is sometimes called the control center of the endocrine system. This is because the hypothalamus collects and integrates a variety of information from the body and organizes neural and endocrine responses in order to maintain a stable internal environment (homeostasis).[10]

The hypothalamus is part of the diencephalon located at the center of the base of the brain, below the thalamus and directly above the pituitary gland. It makes up the floor of the third cerebral ventricle. This small cone-shaped structure projects downward from the brain, ending in the pituitary (infundibulum) stalk.[11]

About ten or eleven small nerve cell groups are located in the hypothalamus. Cells located in the anterior and posterior areas of the hypothalamus monitor blood temperature and adjust abnormal body temperature.

Neural activity in the anterior area controls heat loss by dilating blood vessels and inducing sweating. In the posterior hypothalamus, neurons help to preserve heat by constricting blood vessels, activating shivering, and slowing breathing. In addition, other hypothalamic nuclei work together to balance food intake. Activity in the lateral hypothalamic area stimulates the appetite, while the ventromedial nucleus (VMN) suppresses appetite. In the preoptic area are cells that use several hormonal mechanisms to stimulate and regulate the menstrual cycle and other reproductive functions.[12]

The hypothalamus secretes hormones that stimulate or suppress the release of hormones in the pituitary gland. Many of these hormones are "releasing hormones," which are secreted into an artery (the hypophyseal portal system) that carries the hormones directly to the anterior pituitary gland. The anterior pituitary gland receives releasing and inhibitory hormones in the blood via the hypophyseal portal system (Fig. 4-2).

The Hypophyseal Portal System

The hypophyseal portal system facilitates endocrine communication between the two structures. The hypophyseal portal system, also known as the hypothalamo-hypophyseal portal system, is a group of blood vessels that link the hypothalamus to the anterior

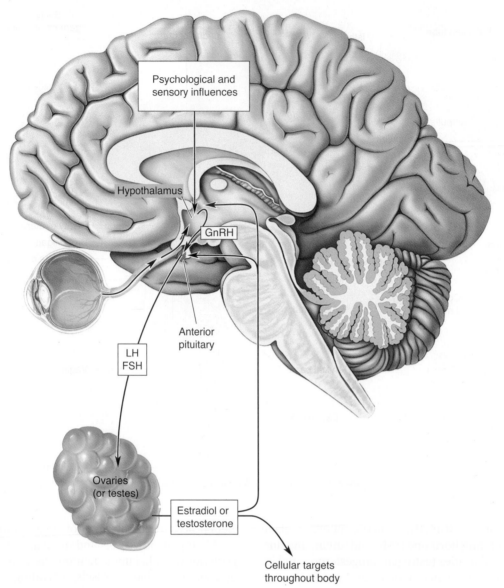

Figure 4-2 Bidirectional interactions between the brain and the gonads. The hypothalamus is influenced by both psychological factors and sensory information, such as light responses from the retina. GnRH from the hypothalmus regulates gonadotropin (LH and FSH) release from the anterior pituitary. The testes secrete testosterone and the ovaries secrete estradiol, as directed by the gonadotropins. The sex hormones have diverse effects on the body and also send feedback to the pituitary and hypothalamus.

pituitary gland. This unique group of blood vessels passes from the hypothalamus through the pituitary stalk to the anterior pituitary gland. Instead of a direct neural link to the anterior pituitary gland, the hypothalamus uses the hypophyseal portal system, which is a "capillary to capillary" connection. The hypophyseal portal system is one of the few portal systems in the body that involves two capillary beds connected by a series of venules.[13,14]

The hypothalamic hormones reach the anterior pituitary by the following path:

1. A branch of the hypophyseal artery diverges into a capillary bed in the lower hypothalamus, and the hypothalamic hormones secrete into that capillary blood
2. Blood from those capillaries drains into the hypothalamic-hypophyseal portal veins, which branch again into another series of anterior pituitary capillaries

3. The anterior pituitary capillaries, which carry anterior pituitary hormones, turn into veins that drain into the systemic venous blood (Fig. 4-3)

The utility of this unconventional vascular system is that minute quantities of hypothalamic hormones are carried in a concentrated form directly to their target cells in the anterior pituitary and are not diluted out in the systemic circulation (Fig. 4-4).[13]

Pituitary Gland

The pituitary gland, also known as the "hypophysis," lies immediately beneath the hypothalamus, resting in a pocket of bone called the sella turcica ("Turkish saddle") at the base of the brain. It is about the size of a pea and it connects to the hypothalamus by the pituitary stalk, which contains nerve fibers and blood vessels.[10]

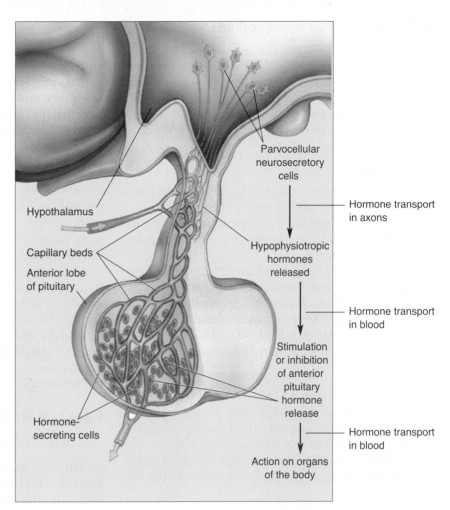

Parvocellular
neurosecretory
cells

Hormone transport
in axons

Hypophysiotropic
hormones
released

Hormone transport
in blood

Hypothalamus

Capillary beds

Anterior lobe
of pituitary

Stimulation
or inhibition
of anterior
pituitary
hormone
release

Hormone transport
in blood

Hormone-
secreting cells

Action on organs
of the body

Figure 4-3 Parvocellular neurosecretory cells of the hypothalamus. Parvocellular neurosecretory cells secrete hypophysiotropic hormones into specialized capillary beds of the hypothalamo-pituitary portal circulation. These hormones travel to the anterior lobe of the pituitary, where they trigger or inhibit the release of pituitary hormones from secretory cells.

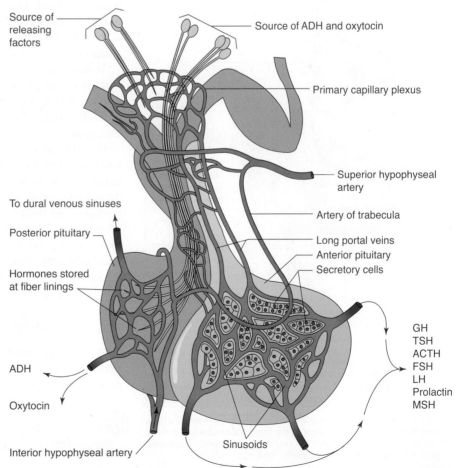

Source of
releasing
factors

Source of ADH and oxytocin

Primary capillary plexus

Superior hypophyseal
artery

To dural venous sinuses

Artery of trabecula

Posterior pituitary

Long portal veins
Anterior pituitary
Secretory cells

Hormones stored
at fiber linings

ADH

GH
TSH
ACTH
FSH
LH
Prolactin
MSH

Oxytocin

Interior hypophyseal artery

Sinusoids

Figure 4-4 The hypothalamus and the anterior and posterior pituitary. The hypothalamic-releasing or -inhibiting hormones are transported to the anterior pituitary by way of the portal vessels. ADH and oxytocin are produced by nerve cells in the supraoptic and paraventricular nuclei of the hypothalamus and then transported through the nerve axon to the posterior pituitary, where they are released into the circulation.

The pituitary gland actually functions as two separate but distinctive tissues, an anterior portion (adenohypohysis-hormone producing) and the posterior gland (neurohypophysis).

Each lobe of the pituitary gland produces distinctive hormones.

Anterior Lobe

- Growth hormone—Controls growth and development; promotes protein production
- Prolactin—Stimulates milk production after birth
- Adrenocorticotropic hormone (ACTH)—Stimulates the adrenal glands
- Thyroid-stimulating hormone (TSH)—Stimulates the production and secretion of thyroid hormones
- FSH—Stimulates ovarian follicle growth and maturation, estrogen secretion, and endometrial changes
- LH—Main function is to cause ovulation as well as the secretion of androgens and progesterone.

Posterior Lobe

- Antidiuretic hormone (ADH)—helps the body to retain water by decreasing urine production
- Oxytocin—contracts the uterus during childbirth and stimulates milk production (Fig. 4-5)[15]

The anterior pituitary gland secretes important endocrine hormones. These hormones are released from the anterior pituitary under the direct influence of the hypothalamus. Hypothalamic hormones secrete to the anterior lobe through a special capillary system called the hypothalamic-hypophyseal portal system (discussed above). The anterior pituitary hormones that are most important to the female reproductive system are FSH and LH.

Ovaries

Ovaries are both gonads and endocrine glands, which produce eggs (ova) and are the main source of female hormones, such as estrogen and progesterone. The ovaries perform dual and interrelated functions of oogenesis (producing ova) and the endocrine function of producing hormones. The ovaries produce small quantities of testosterone, releasing the hormone into the bloodstream via the ovaries and adrenal glands.

Ovarian endocrine functions control the development of female body characteristics, for example, the breasts, body shape, and body hair. They also regulate the menstrual cycle and pregnancy (Table 4-1).[16]

FEMALE REPRODUCTIVE HORMONES

GONADOTROPIN-RELEASING HORMONE

GnRH, also known as luteinizing-hormone-releasing hormone (LHRH), is secreted by the hypothalamus and stimulates the release of FSH and LH from the anterior pituitary gland. GnRH is a neurohormone, which is a hormone produced in a specific neural cell and released at its neural terminal. The preoptic area of the hypothalamus contains most of the GnRH-secreting neurons.[18,19]

When GnRH reaches the anterior pituitary gland, it stimulates the formation and secretion of the gonadotropins, which are controlled by the size and frequency of GnRH "pulses" and by feedback from androgens and estrogens.

GnRH is secreted into the hypophyseal portal system and transported to the anterior pituitary in a "pulsatile" manner. The pulses vary in frequency and amplitude depending upon different physiologic conditions. On average, the frequency of GnRH secretion is once per 90 minutes during the early follicular phase, increases to once per 60 to 70 minutes, and decreases with increased amplitude during the luteal phase. GnRH induces the release of both FSH and LH; however, LH is much more sensitive to changes in GnRH levels.[20,21]

FOLLICLE-STIMULATING HORMONE

FSH is a glycoprotein (molecule that contains a carbohydrate and a protein) gonadotropin secreted by the anterior pituitary gland in response to GnRH. FSH is

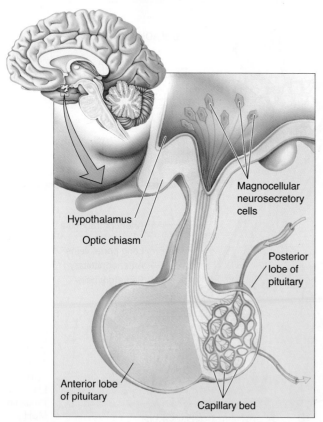

Figure 4-5 Magnocellular neurosecretory cells of the hypothalamus. Shown here is a midsagittal view of the hypothalamus and pituitary. Magnocellular neurosecretory cells secrete oxytocin and vasopressin directly into capillaries in the posterior lobe of the pituitary.

Magnocellular neurosecretory cells

Hypothalamus

Optic chiasm

Posterior lobe of pituitary

Anterior lobe of pituitary

Capillary bed

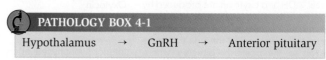

PATHOLOGY BOX 4-1

| Hypothalamus | → | GnRH | → | Anterior pituitary |

TABLE 4-1

Female Reproductive Endocrine Glands

Endocrine Glands Affecting Female Reproductive System	Hormone	Target Cells	Major Function (Is in Control of:)
Hypothalamus	GnRH	Anterior pituitary	Secretes hormones that control the secretion of anterior pituitary hormones
Anterior pituitary	Gonadotropic hormones (FSH and LH)		Stimulate gonads (gamete production and sex hormone secretion)
	FSH	Ovarian follicles	• Promotes follicular growth and development • Stimulates estrogen production
	LH	Ovarian follicles and corpus luteum	Stimulates: • Ovulation • Corpus luteum development • Estrogen production • Progesterone production
Ovaries	Estrogen Progesterone	• Breast, vagina, uterus, bone, fallopian tubes, placenta • LH and FSH • Endometrium • LH • Myometrium • Vaginal epithelium and cervical mucus	• Reproductive system, growth and development • Negative feedback reducing the production of GnRH, LH, FSH • Prepares the endometrium for implantation • Inhibits the secretion of LH, thus inhibiting ovulation • Desensitizes the myometrium to oxytocic activity • Modifies the secretory activity

primarily responsible for promoting follicle development within the ovary and spermatogenesis in men. FSH is responsible for the maturation of the egg, the cells surrounding the egg that produce the hormones (estrogen) needed to support a pregnancy, and the fluid around the egg.[20,22]

As the follicle grows, cells in the follicle produce an increasing amount of estrogen that is released into the bloodstream. Estrogen stimulates the endometrium to thicken before ovulation occurs. The higher estrogen blood levels signal the hypothalamus and pituitary gland to slow the production and release of FSH.[22]

LUTEINIZING HORMONE

LH is a gonadotropic hormone secreted by the anterior pituitary. LH is required for both the growth of preovulatory follicles and the luteinization and ovulation of the dominant follicle. LH controls the duration and progression of the female menstrual cycle, including ovulation, preparation of the uterus for implantation of a fertilized egg, and the ovarian production of both estrogen and progesterone. Theca cells (connective tissue surrounding the follicle) in the ovary respond to LH stimulation by secretion of testosterone, which is converted into estrogen by adjacent granulosa cells.[23]

The "LH surge" or "preovulary LH surge" is a sharp rise in LH that triggers ovulation. LH is responsible for the maturing or ripening of the Graafian follicle, which contains the matured ovum. After ovulation, the group of hormone-producing follicle cells becomes the corpus luteum. The **corpus luteum** produces estrogen and large amounts of progesterone. Progesterone causes the endometrium to mature so that it can support implantation of the fertilized egg or embryo. If implantation of a fertilized egg does not occur, the levels of estrogen and progesterone decrease, the endometrium sloughs off, and menstruation occurs.[24]

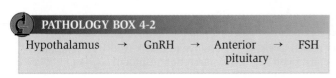

PATHOLOGY BOX 4-2

Hypothalamus → GnRH → Anterior pituitary → FSH

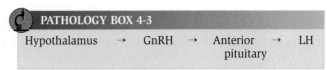

PATHOLOGY BOX 4-3

Hypothalamus → GnRH → Anterior pituitary → LH

PATHOLOGY BOX 4-4

| Hypothalamus | → | GnRH | → | Pituitary | → | LH | → | Theca interna | → | Androgens | → | Estrogen |

THECA INTERNA

The theca folliculi is a cover of condensed connective tissue surrounding a developing follicle within the ovary. The theca folliculi are divided into two layers, the theca interna and the theca externa. The theca interna responds to LH by synthesizing and secreting androgens, which are processed into estrogen. Theca cells do not begin secreting estrogen until puberty.[25]

ESTROGEN

Estrogen (or oestrogen) is the name for a class of naturally occurring steroid hormones that primarily regulate the growth, development, and function of the female reproductive system. The main sources of estrogen in the body are the ovaries, but the corpus luteum and the placenta also produce small amounts of estrogen. The three major naturally occurring estrogens are estradiol, estriol, and estrone, all of which promote the development of female body characteristics. Some of the female body characteristics are:

- development of breasts
- uterus and vagina
- pubic and axillary hair growth
- the distribution of adipose tissue
- broadening of the pelvis
- voice pitch

Estradiol is the principal estrogen formed from developing ovarian follicles, the adrenal cortex, and placenta. Estradiol is responsible for female characteristics, sexual functioning, and the growth of the uterus, fallopian tubes, and vagina. It promotes breast development and the growth of the outer genitals. In addition, estradiol is important to women's bone health. However, estradiol contributes to most gynecologic problems such as endometriosis and fibroids and even female cancers.[26,27] Estriol is made from the placenta and is only produced during pregnancy.[26] Estrone is widespread throughout the body. It is the only estrogen present in any amount in women after menopause.[26]

During the menstrual cycle, estrogen stimulates the endometrium to thicken before ovulation. This produces an environment acceptable for fertilization, implantation, and nutrition of the early embryo. In addition to regulating the menstrual cycle, estrogens also help promote blood clotting and help minimize the loss of calcium from the bones. Estrogen affects many organ systems, including the musculoskeletal and cardiovascular systems and the brain.[28]

Estrogen is the principal modulator of the "hypothalamus-pituitary axis." This involves complex interactions between pituitary and ovarian hormones that are involved with forward control, positive feedback, and negative feedback mechanisms. The higher blood levels of estrogen also tell the hypothalamus and pituitary gland to slow the production and release of FSH. The ability of estrogens to suppress secretion of FSH and thereby inhibit ovulation makes estrogen and estrogenlike compounds major components in oral contraceptives.

CONTROL OF GNRH (POSITIVE AND NEGATIVE FEEDBACK)

High levels of estrogen in the bloodstream result in the placement of negative feedback on LH and FSH secretion, resulting in inhibition of the secretion of these hormones. The opposite, low estrogen levels, results in a positive feedback on LH and FSH secretion, resuming production.[29,30]

PROGESTERONE

Progesterone is a steroid that belongs to a group of hormones called "progestogens" and is the major naturally occurring human progestogen. Its production is stimulated by the corpus luteum, which is stimulated by LH, which in turn is stimulated by GnRH.

When a LH surge occurs (remember that a LH surge is a sharp increase in LH in the blood that triggers ovulation), it causes the follicle to rupture. The residual cells within ovulated follicles develop to form the corpus luteum, which then starts to secrete the hormones progesterone and estradiol.[31] Small amounts of progesterone are also produced in the adrenal glands.

Progesterone prepares the body for pregnancy and maintains it until birth. Progesterone is a hard-working hormone, as it:

- Prepares the endometrium for implantation
- Desensitizes the myometrium to oxytocic activity (oxytocin is produced in the posterior pituitary gland and stimulates rhythmic contractions of the uterus); in other words, it decreases the contractility of the uterine smooth muscle

PATHOLOGY BOX 4-5

| Increased levels of estrogen | → | Negative feedback (GnRH, LH, and FSH secretion stopped) | → | Decreased levels of estrogen | → | Positive feedback (GnRH, LH, and FSH secretion resumed) |

- Blocks the development of new follicles (inhibits the secretion of LH, thus inhibiting ovulation)
- Modifies the secretory activity of the vaginal epithelium and cervical mucus (makes it thick and impenetrable to sperm)
- Increases the basal body temperature
- Stimulates the development of the alveolar system
- Inhibits lactation during pregnancy. The decrease in progesterone levels following delivery is one of the triggers of the mammary glands for milk production.
- Decreases the maternal immune response and prepares the lining of the uterus for the fertilized ovum implantation.[32,33]
- Stimulates the growth of the uterine wall and the uterine blood vessels.[33]

If implantation occurs, the placenta will begin to secrete progesterone near the end of the first trimester and will continue until the end of the pregnancy. One of progesterone's most important functions is to stimulate the endometrium to secrete special proteins during the second half of the menstrual cycle, preparing it to implant and nourish the fertilized egg. If there is no implantation, estrogen and progesterone levels drop, the corpus luteum begins to break down, the endometrium breaks down, and menstruation occurs.[29,33]

Progesterone Feedback

Elevated levels of progesterone are controlled by the same positive and negative feedback loop used by estrogen. High levels of progesterone also inhibit the secretion of GnRH and LH, just like high estrogen levels.[29]

OVARIAN CYCLE

The ovarian cycle is a series of ovarian physiologic events involved in ovulation. This cycle covers oocyte maturation, ovulation, and the release of the mature ovum into the fallopian tube. The ovarian cycle contains three phases, the follicular phase, ovulatory phase, and the luteal phase.

OOGENESIS

During fetal development, the primitive germ cells or oogonia (singular is oogonium) go through numerous mitotic divisions during the first 7 months. After the seventh month, the oogonia stop dividing, with most oogonia dying during this period. The remaining oogonia (called primary oocytes) begin the first meiotic division until they reach the diplotene stage (completion of DNA replication). At this stage the primary oocytes enter into meiotic arrest until puberty.[35,36]

The first part of meiosis begins in the fetus and does not resume until roughly 12 years later, when puberty begins. With the onset of puberty, there is renewed activity in the ovary. The first meiotic division is completed just before the oocyte is about to be released from the ovary.[16,36]

After the maturing primary oocyte completes meiosis I, it divides into two haploid cells. Each of the haploid cells receives half the chromosomes (23) and two chromatids. One cell is called the "polar body." It is the smaller of the two cells and receives very little cytoplasm. The other cell is now a secondary oocyte and enters meiosis II. This larger cell (dominant follicle) is in meiotic arrest until fertilization.[16]

At around day 14, the secondary oocyte bursts from the ovary. The fallopian tube contains microscopic cilia that beat and draw the released oocyte. Thus, the secondary oocyte enters the fallopian tube where it waits for fertilization and completion of the meiosis process.[16]

Upon fertilization, the second meiotic division occurs in the fallopian tube right after ovulation. The oocyte divides into two daughter cells with each cell receiving 23 chromosomes with a single chromatid. One daughter cell is the mature ovum (or fertilized ovum) and it retains almost all the cytoplasm. The second small nonfunctional daughter cell is called a "second polar body"[16] (Fig. 4-6).

FOLLICLE STAGES

Oocytes exist in follicles. The ovary contains either primordial follicles or primary (more developed follicle) follicles. Both follicle types consist of a primary oocyte with a single layer of surrounding cells (called granulosa cells). As the primary follicle develops, the oocyte siza and granulosa cells increase. As the granulosa cells increase, they secrete a thick layer of material called the zona pellucida, which forms a layer around the granulosa cells and oocyte. As the follicle continues to grow, new layers form such as the outer layer, which

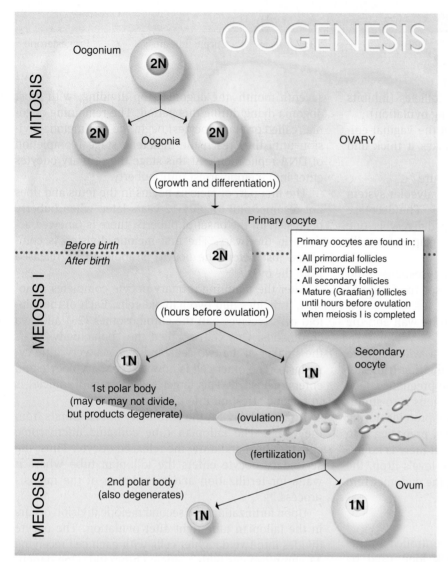

OOGENESIS

MITOSIS

Oogonium 2N

Oogonia 2N 2N

OVARY

(growth and differentiation)

Primary oocyte

MEIOSIS I

Before birth
After birth

2N

Primary oocytes are found in:
• All primordial follicles
• All primary follicles
• All secondary follicles
• Mature (Graafian) follicles until hours before ovulation when meiosis I is completed

(hours before ovulation)

1N

1st polar body (may or may not divide, but products degenerate)

(ovulation)

Secondary oocyte 1N

(fertilization)

MEIOSIS II

2nd polar body (also degenerates)

1N

Ovum 1N

Figure 4-6 The female embryo ovaries contain primordial germ cells which undergo mitosis to form oogonia (singular is oogonium). By the 7th month of fetal development, the primary oocytes become surrounded by a layer of flattened cells and become known as primordial follicles. At this point the oogonia stop dividing, with most oogonia dying during this period. The remaining oogonia (called primary oocytes) begin the first meiotic division until they reach the diplotene stage (completion of DNA replication). At this stage the primary oocytes enter into meiotic arrest until puberty. With the onset of puberty, the first meiotic division is completed just before the oocyte is about to be released from the ovary.

After the maturing primary oocyte completes meiosis I, it divides into two haploid cells. One cell is called the "polar body." The other cell is now a secondary oocyte and enters meiosis II. This larger cell (dominant follicle) is in meiotic arrest until fertilization. Upon fertilization, the second meiotic division occurs in the fallopian tube right after ovulation. Theoocyte divides into two daughter cells with each cell receiving 23 chromosomes with a single chromatid.

is called the "theca." When the theca layer forms, the follicle is at the "preantral" stage. When the follicle has almost reached its full size, a fluid-filled space called the antrum starts to form in the granulosa cells. The granulosa cells secrete a fluid into this space and at this point going forward, the growth of the follicle will be due to the expanding antral space. The follicle is now in the antral stage.[16]

Approximately 1 week in the menstrual cycle, a selection process begins. The largest, most mature follicle continues to develop and other follicles go through a degeneration process called "atresia." The mature follicle or Graafian follicle bulges out of the surface of the ovary. Ovulation occurs when the Graafian follicle and ovarian wall rupture to release the oocyte (Fig. 4-7).[16] *Note: In 1% to 2% of all menstrual cycles, two or more*

follicles may reach maturity and more than one oocyte will be released from the ovary.

Follicular Phase

The follicular phase (or preovulatory phase) starts when the menstrual cycle begins with the first day of menstrual bleeding (day 1). Menstrual bleeding occurs with the fall of estrogen and progesterone levels. The decrease in these two hormones causes the thickened endometrial lining to break down and slough off, as it is no longer needed to sustain a possible pregnancy. The follicular phase lasts from day 1 of the menstrual cycle and ends when the LH surge occurs and ovulation begins (typically on day 14).[37] The main purpose of the follicular phase is to develop a viable follicle capable of surviving ovulation.

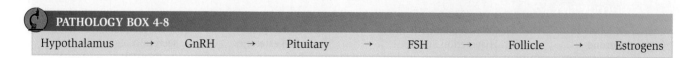

PATHOLOGY BOX 4-8

| Hypothalamus | → | GnRH | → | Pituitary | → | FSH | → | Follicle | → | Estrogens |

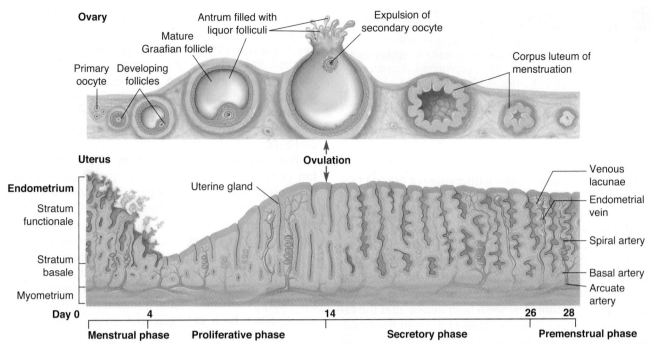

Figure 4-7 This diagram demonstrates the interconnectivity between the ovarian and endometrial cycle throughout the menstrual cycle.

Remember what happens when the estrogen levels in the blood decrease? The positive feedback mechanism triggers the secretion of GnRH, FSH, and LH. When the FSH levels start to rise, FSH then stimulates the development of several ovarian follicles, each containing an egg. Every month, FSH initiates and promotes the growth of a group of follicles. Soon, one or two follicles assume dominance, continuing to grow, mature, and produce estrogen. The follicle will start to secrete estrogen (estradiol) by increasing the secretion of androgens by the theca externa. Estrogen will then stimulate the cervix to produce mucus, allowing sperm to pass through the cervix and reach the ovum. In addition, as estrogen levels rise, menses begins to slow and stop, with the endometrial lining of the uterus beginning to thicken and develop progesterone receptors.[34]

Estrogen levels peak toward the end of the follicular phase of the menstrual cycle. This rise in estrogen is a signal that a mature follicle (Graafian follicle) is ready to ovulate. At this critical moment, estrogen exerts positive feedback on LH, generating a dramatic preovulatory LH surge.[38,39] The LH level will start to rise rapidly 24 to 36 hours before ovulation.[40] Under the influence of LH, the primary oocyte enters the final stage of the first meiotic division and divides into a secondary oocyte (Fig. 4-8).

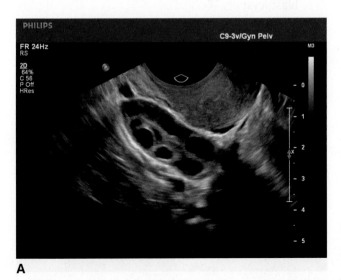

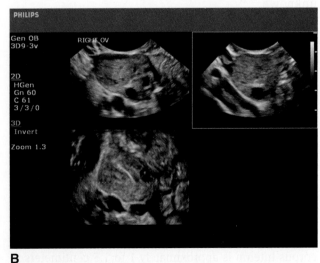

A   B

Figure 4-8 A: Early follicular phase ovary in an endovaginal exam. **B:** 3D multiplanar reconstruction (MPR) of a follicular phase ovary.

PATHOLOGY BOX 4-9

Rising levels → Estrogen	• Cervical mucus is produced • Endometrium starts to thicken and develops progesterone receptors • Triggers LH surge • Negative feedback (GnRH, FSH secretion stopped)

Ovulatory Phase

The ovulatory phase begins with a surge of LH and FSH levels, usually occurring on day 14 of the menstrual cycle (it may differ among some women). The release of the mature ovum ends this phase. The LH surge induces release of enzymes that degrade the cells on the surface of the Graafian follicle. It stimulates angiogenesis (development of new blood vessels) in the follicular wall. The LH effects on the follicle cause it to swell and rupture. Within a 24- to 36-hour period after the LH surge, the mature ovum is expelled through the Graafian follicle and ovarian wall and a small amount of fluid collects in the posterior cul-de-sac.[41] At this time, a urine test can detect the amount of LH in a woman's urine (about 12 to 24 hours after release of the ovum). The amount of LH in the urine helps determine when a woman is fertile, as the egg will need to be fertilized within a 12-hour period after its release.[37] After the egg has been expelled from the ovary, contractions of the fallopian tube bring the oocyte into contact with the epithelium of the fallopian tube to initiate migration through the oviduct.

At ovulation, some women experience a dull pain/ache or a sudden sharp pain on one side of the lower abdomen. Occurring on the same side as ovulation, this dull pain is called mittelschmerz. The word "mittelschmerz" actually means "middle pain," because of mid-cycle pain occurring in conjunction with ovulation. It can last anywhere from a few hours up to days. The cause of mittelschmerz is unknown.[38,41]

Luteal Phase

The luteal phase begins after ovulation, lasting on average approximately 14 days (unless fertilization occurs), and ends just before a menstrual period. The luteal phase needs to be at least 10 days in order to have a successful implantation. The main hormone associated with this phase is progesterone.

In the luteal phase, the ruptured Graafian follicle closes after releasing the egg, and FSH and LH stimulate the remaining parts of the Graafian follicle to form a structure called a corpus luteum (Latin for "yellow body"). The corpus luteum forms from the zona granulosa and theca cells left after ovulation and some of the surrounding capillaries and connective tissue.[38] The corpus luteum is approximately 1 to 1.5 centimeters in diameter.[42]

One important effect of the LH surge is the conversion of the granulosa cells from predominantly androgen-converting cells to mostly progesterone-synthesizing cells. The corpus luteum secretes mostly progesterone and some estrogen. Following ovulation, the corpus luteum responds to continued elevated LH levels by synthesizing high concentrations of progesterone and estrogen (Figs. 4-9, 5-48, and 5-70).

The progesterone secreted by the corpus luteum peaks at around 5 to 7 days postovulation. The high progesterone levels trigger a negative feedback on GnRH and as a result the GnRH pulse frequency stops. After ovulation, the corpus luteum only lasts for about 12 to 14 days unless it begins receiving human chorionic gonadotropin (hCG) from a developing embryo. If the egg is not fertilized, the corpus luteum starts to degenerate and begins to evolve into the "corpus albicans," and progesterone production stops. Since both estrogen and progesterone levels decrease, the negative feedback control on the GnRH pulse frequency is removed. Positive feedback initiates and FSH and LH start to rise to begin the next menstrual cycle.[34,38] See Figure 4-10.

Progesterone

- Causes the mucus in the cervix to thicken so that sperm or bacteria are less likely to enter the uterus
- Causes body temperature to increase slightly during the luteal phase and remain elevated until a menstrual period begins (this increase in temperature can be used to estimate whether ovulation has occurred)
- With estrogen, causes milk ducts in the breasts to widen (dilate). As a result, the breasts may swell and become tender
- With estrogen, causes the endometrium to thicken and develop additional blood vessels to accept the blastocyst

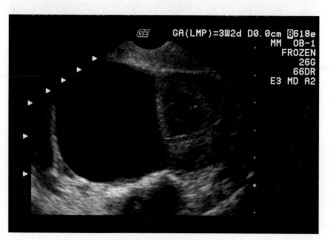

Figure 4-9 Anechoic corpus luteal cyst.

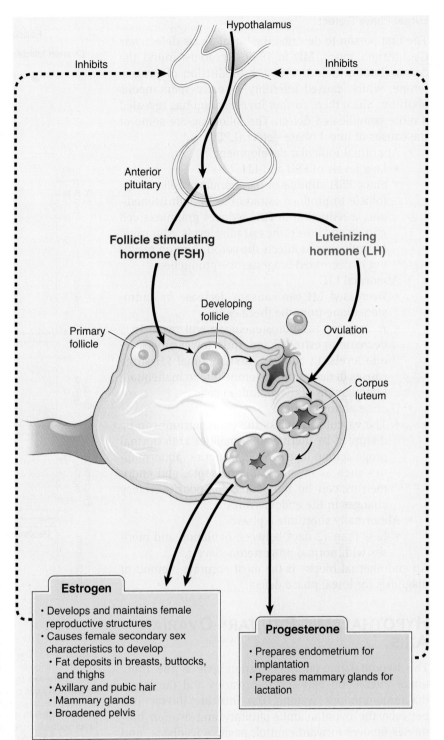

Figure 4-10 Effects of pituitary FSH and LH in ovulation. The hypothalamus stimulates the pituitary gland first to release FSH, then LH. FSH stimulates ovarian follicle development, ovulation, and follicular estrogen secretion, which in turn stimulates the endometrium to grow (the proliferative phase). Next, LH stimulates formation of the corpus luteum from the ruptured follicle after ovulation. The corpus luteum secretes progesterone, stimulating endometrial glandular development and glycogen accumulation and readying the endometrium for implantation. If pregnancy does not occur, the corpus luteum atrophies to become a corpus albicans, and menstruation occurs.

The corpus luteum produces progesterone until the placenta begins to take over production at around the tenth week of gestation. When a pregnancy occurs and the developing blastocyst burrows into the endometrium, the cells around the developing zygote produce a hormone called human chorionic gonadotropin (hCG). This hormone maintains the corpus luteum, which continues to produce progesterone and estrogen until the placenta takes over, after approximately 3 months. Pregnancy tests are based on detecting an increase in hCG level (Fig. 4-7).[38]

PATHOLOGY BOX 4-10

| Hypothalamus | → | GnRH | → | Pituitary | → | LH | → | Corpus luteum | → | Progesterone |

Luteal Phase Defect

The first person to describe the luteal phase defect was Georgeanna Jones, MD in 1949. Dr. Jones found the corpus luteum defective in the production of progesterone, which caused infertility or early spontaneous abortion. Since then, further investigation has revealed a more complicated defect. The following are some of the causes of luteal phase defect (LPD):

- Abnormal follicular development
  - Low levels of FSH and LH
  - Since FSH stimulates the granulosa cells in the follicle to produce estradiol from androstenedione, a reduction in FSH reduces granulosa cell growth and lowers the estradiol levels. Abnormal folliculogenesis affects the corpus luteum resulting in decreased progesterone production
- Abnormal LH
  - Decreased LH can cause a decrease in androstenedione from the theca cells
  - A decrease in androstenedione will result in a decrease in estradiol and, thus, lower progesterone levels. In addition, a suboptimal LH surge causes deficient progesterone due to inadequate luteinization of the granulosa cells
- Uterine abnormalities
  - The vascularization of the endometrium can be disrupted by uterine abnormalities with normal progesterone levels. Several uterine abnormalities such as myomas, uterine septa, and endometritis can be the source for poor secretory changes in the endometrium
- Abnormally short luteal phase
  - Less than 12 days between ovulation and menses with normal progesterone levels.[43]

An endometrial biopsy is the most accurate method of diagnosis for luteal phase defect.

HYPOTHALAMIC-PITUITARY-OVARIAN AXIS

The hypothalamic-pituitary-ovarian axis is the functional interaction between the ovaries and the hypothalamus-pituitary system. The intricate interactions between the hypothalamus-pituitary and ovarian hormones involve forward control, positive feedback, and negative feedback mechanisms.

One of the most important functions of the hypothalamic-pituitary-ovarian axis is to regulate reproduction and sustain a self-perpetuating, monthly endocrine cycle. By controlling the uterine and ovarian cycles, the brain and ovaries are able to regulate reproduction.[44]

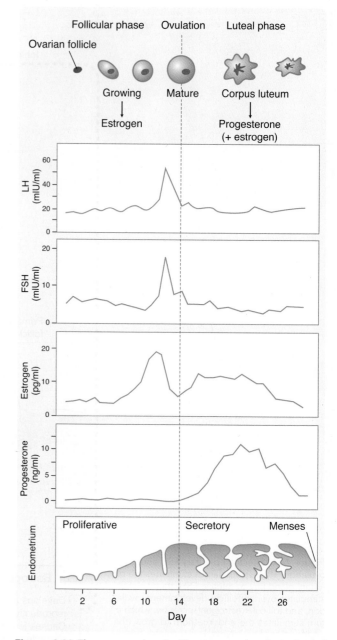

Figure 4-11 The menstrual cycle. The menstrual cycle is divided into the follicular and the luteal phase. Ovulation defines the transition between these two phases. During the follicular phase, gonadotroph cells of the anterior pituitary gland secrete LH and FSH in response to pulsatile GnRH stimulation. Circulating LH and FSH promote growth and maturation of ovarian follicles. Developing follicles secrete increasing amounts of estrogen. At first, the estrogen has an inhibitory effect on gonadotropin release. Just before the midpoint in the menstrual cycle, however, estrogen exerts a brief positive feedback effect on LH and FSH release. This is followed by follicular rupture and release of an egg into the fallopian tube. During the second half of the cycle, the corpus luteum secretes both estrogen and progesterone. Progesterone induces a change in the endometrium from a proliferative to a secretory type. If fertilization and implantation of a blastocyst does not occur within 14 days after ovulation, the corpus luteum involutes, secretion of estrogen and progesterone declines, menses occurs, and a new cycle begins.

PATHOLOGY BOX 4-11					
Hypothalamus	→ GnRH	→ Anterior pituitary	→ FSH	→ Follicles activate the theca externa into androgen synthesis	→ Secretion of estrogen

| Increased levels of estrogen | → | Negative feedback mechanism is activated | → | Hypothalamus is inhibited from producing GnRH secretion | → | Decreased FSH and LH secretion |

The glands and hormones involved in the hypothalamic-pituitary-ovarian axis are:

- The hypothalamus, which produces GnRH
- The anterior pituitary gland, which produces LH and FSH
- The ovaries (gonads), which produce estrogen and testosterone (Fig. 4-11)[44]

INCREASED FOLLICLE STIMULATING HORMONE

The anterior pituitary gland is stimulated by GnRH to secrete FSH. FSH stimulates the follicles to activate androgen synthesis by the theca externa, which in turn produces estrogen. Estrogen secretion peaks during days 10 to 13 in the menstrual cycle.

INCREASED ESTROGEN SECRETION

A negative feedback will be placed on the hypothalamus when circulating estrogen reaches a high level. The hypothalamus will inhibit GnRH secretion; if GnRH secretion stops, the anterior pituitary will not be stimulated to produce FSH and LH.

THE LH SURGE

The LH surge occurs when estrogen reaches a peak level. How can this be? We just discussed how an increase in estrogen levels activates the negative feedback mechanism, which in turn decreases LH and FSH production. How do peak estrogen levels exert a positive feedback? When a follicle reaches its mature stage and begins to produce a higher level of estrogen within a specific "critical" threshold and duration, the opposite effect takes place. A positive feedback mechanism then activates and the pituitary releases a preovulatory surge of LH and, to a lesser extent, FSH.

The LH surge stimulates the Graafian follicle and ovarian wall to rupture and release the mature ovum.[16] The remaining granulosa cells, theca cells, and surrounding connective tissue of the Graafian follicle form into the corpus luteum. The corpus luteum begins to produce progesterone while LH and FSH levels decrease.

PROGESTERONE AND ESTROGEN

The corpus luteum secretes progesterone and estrogen until it starts to degenerate during the luteal phase. When the corpus luteum undergoes atresia to become the corpus albicans, progesterone and estrogen production stops and their levels decrease.

DECREASED PROGESTERONE AND ESTROGEN

Diminished estrogen and progesterone levels initiate, removing the negative feedback control on the GnRH pulse frequency. FSH and LH start to rise upon initiation of the positive feedback beginning the next menstrual cycle.

MENSTRUAL AND/OR ENDOMETRIAL CYCLE

The female reproductive years begin around 11 to 13 years of age with the start of menstruation and end around the age of 50 with the end of menstruation. Menstruation is the periodic discharge of blood, mucus, tissue, fluid, and epithelial cells. It is a rhythmic approximately 28-day cycle and is tightly coordinated with the ovarian cycle. Cycles can range anywhere from 21 to 35 days in adults and from 21 to 45 days in young teens. When a menstrual cycle length is less than 21 days, it is called "polymenorrheic" (poly = many, menorrhea = bleeding). When a menstrual cycle is longer than 35 days it is called "oligomenorrheic" (oligo = having little, menorrhea = bleeding).

ULTRASOUND EVALUATION OF THE ENDOMETRIUM IN PREMENOPAUSAL WOMEN

Ultrasound evaluation and measurements of the endometrium vary with phases of the menstrual cycle. Measurements also vary depending upon menopausal status, age, parity, and gravidity. The endometrial thickness measurement is important, as it can help detect a number of benign and malignant abnormalities. Changes in endometrial thickness can be associated

| Hypothalamus | → | GnRH | → | Pituitary | → | LH | → | Corpus luteum | → | Progesterone and estrogen are secreted |

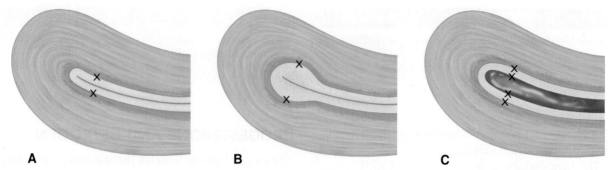

Figure 4-12 A: Measurement of the thin uniform endometrium from a sagittal approach. **B:** Caliper placement for a focally thickened endometrium on a sagittal view. **C:** In the presence of intrauterine fluid, measure each endometrial layer on a sagittal plane.

with endometrial polyps, hyperplasia, or carcinoma. In general, the normal endometrium should be uniform in thickness, homogeneous in echotexture, and not displaced by any submucosal, myometrial abnormality.

The American Institute of Ultrasound in Medicine (AIUM) in its practice guidelines for the performance of pelvic ultrasound examinations states that the endometrium is to be measured as follows:

> "The endometrium should be measured on a midline sagittal image, including anterior and posterior portions of the basal endometrium and excluding the adjacent hypoechoic myometrium and any endometrial fluid"[68] (Fig. 4-12).

ULTRASOUND EVALUATION OF THE OVARIES

According to the AIUM practice guidelines for the performance of pelvic ultrasound examinations, "ovarian size may be determined by measuring the ovary in three dimensions (width, length, and depth), on views obtained in two orthogonal planes."[68]

MENSTRUAL CYCLE

The menstrual cycle is regulated by the complex interaction of hormones: LH, FSH, estrogen, and progesterone. The menstrual cycle has three phases: menses phase, proliferative phase, and the secretory phase.

Menses or Menstruation Phase

Days One to Five (Early Follicular Phase)

The menstrual cycle begins with menstrual bleeding and lasts, on average, five days. Some women may have a shorter menses phase and some may have a longer phase. Menses coincides with day 1 of the ovarian follicular phase. At this time, estrogen and progesterone are at their lowest levels. The low levels of estrogen and progesterone initiate menstrual bleeding and stimulate positive feedback. The low levels of estrogen and progesterone stimulate the hypothalamus to secrete GnRH, which in turn simulates the pituitary to secrete FSH and LH. As the secretions of FSH and LH reach the ovary via the bloodstream, the follicles in the ovaries are stimulated to start developing, and the primary follicles begin to grow. Each follicle consists of an oocyte surrounded by cells that produce estrogen.

Endometrium During Days One to Five

During menstruation, two layers of the endometrium are shed, the stratum compactum and the spongiosum. The stratum basal layer is not shed during menstruation and is responsible for the regeneration of the endometrium. The decrease in estrogen and progesterone levels triggers a constriction of the spiral arteries, which leads to tissue necrosis in the stratum compactum and spongiosum. It must be noted that the network of blood vessels in the endometrium has a selective process with hormonal changes. The radial and basal arterioles do not react to hormonal changes, but the spiral arteries do. They are very sensitive to hormone changes and will constrict when progesterone diminishes (Figs. 4-13 and 4-14).[45]

ULTRASOUND EVALUATION:

Sonographic Appearance

Uterus

During late menstruation, the endometrium images as a thin hypoechoic to echogenic line measuring less than 1 millimeter in thickness.[48] Intraluminal blood or sheets of sloughed endometria may be identified. In the postmenstruation time, the endometrium consists of a superficial functional layer and a deep basal layer. As a result, the superficial functional layer appears as the thin echogenic line (Table 4-2).

PATHOLOGY BOX 4-14

| Hypothalamus | → | GnRH | → | Anterior pituitary | → | FSH and LH secreted into the bloodstream to stimulate follicle growth |

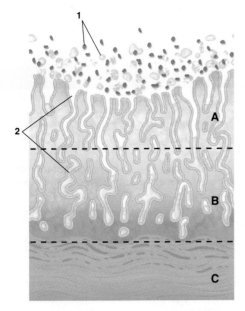

0.5 mm

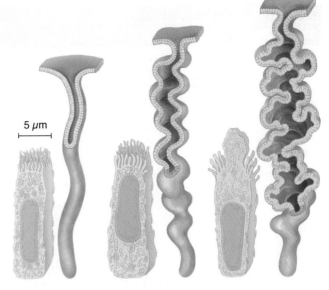

A   Functional layer

B   Basal layer

C   Myometrium

1   Uterine cavity with epithelial cells, blood corpuscles, and remainders of the expulsed mucosa

2   Intact and partially expulsed uterine glands

Figure 4-13 Endometrium during the menstruation phase.

| End of proliferative phase 14 days | Initial secretory phase 15-21 days | Late secretory phase 22-28 days |

Figure 4-14 Changes in the uterine glands and gland cells during the menstrual cycle.

5 μm

TABLE 4-2

Menstruation Phase: Days 1–5[46,48]

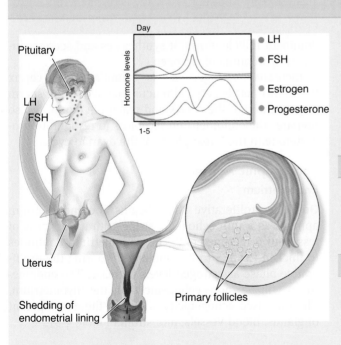

Endocrinology

- Estrogen and progesterone levels are low (see hormone graph)
- Low levels of estrogen and progesterone trigger the hypothalamus to secrete GnRH. GnRH signals the pituitary to secrete FSH and LH
- FSH and LH start to travel in the bloodstream from the pituitary to the ovaries
- FSH begins to stimulate the maturation of several follicles
- FSH and LH stimulate the development of estrogen

Uterine Cycle

- Decrease of estrogen and progesterone trigger the uterine endometrium to break down and shed the endometrial lining. Menstrual bleeding starts on day 1
- The thin endometrium measures <4 millimeters thick at the end of the menstrual phase

- Coincides with early ovarian follicular phase
- Primary follicles begin development
- Each follicle contains an oocyte surrounded by granulosa cells
- FSH initiates and promotes the growth of a group of follicles
- As the follicles begin to mature, the theca starts to produce low levels of estrogen
- The theca interna responds to LH by synthesizing and secreting androgens that process into estrogen

TABLE 4-3

Proliferative Phase: Days 6–10[47,48]

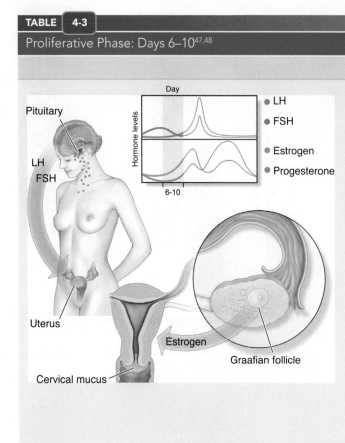

Endocrinology

- Estrogen levels continue to rise as follicles develop
- FSH continues to stimulate maturation of several ovarian follicles
- Synthesis and release of estrogen occurs predominantly from a single dominant follicle (Graafian follicle) around the mid-to-late proliferative phase
- Estrogen starts to prepare the endometrium receptors to respond to progesterone in the luteal phase

Ovarian Cycle

- Coincides with the late ovarian follicular phase
- The selection process begins and one becomes dominant and continues to grow and mature. The rest of the follicles undergo atresia
- Usually one mature follicle grows to the antral state (two if there are twins). As the dominant follicle matures, it will secrete increasing amounts of estrogen (see the hormone chart)

Uterine Cycle

- The estrogens that follicles secrete stimulate the formation of a new layer of endometrium lining in the uterus (proliferative endometrium). Blood vessels and glands supply the thickening endometrium
- Maximum thickness is 11 millimeters late in the follicular phase/proliferative phase
- Increased estrogen levels stimulate the cervix to produce fertile cervical mucus, allowing the sperm to pass through the cervix and reach the ovum

Proliferative Phase/Postmenstrual Phase (Late Follicular Phase): Days Six to Thirteen

The proliferative phase begins when menstrual bleeding stops. At this point, the endometrium appears as a thin central stripe. The positive feedback mechanism stimulates the secretion of FSH and LH. FSH stimulates the maturation of several ovarian follicles. As they increase in size, they produce more estrogen. As the estrogen levels increase, the endometrium starts to thicken and form a new endometrium layer in the uterus (proliferative endometrium). As the endometrium becomes thicker, it becomes supplied with more blood vessels and glands.

During the mid to late proliferative phase, one (sometimes two) follicle(s) become(s) dominant. The rest of the follicles start to die off (atresia). The dominant follicle continues to grow to maturation from a preantral to antral follicle or Graafian follicle. As the dominant follicle grows, it synthesizes and secretes increasing amounts of estrogen.

Increased estrogen levels stimulate the cervix to produce fertile cervical mucus that allows the sperm to pass through the cervix and reach the ovum. It also prepares the endometrium receptors to respond to progesterone in the luteal phase of the ovarian cycle.

Sonographic Appearance

Endometrium

Once the proliferative phase begins, the endometrium appears as a thin echogenic stripe with a thickness of less than 6 millimeters.[39] The endometrium continues to thicken (from 5 to 7 millimeters)[48] during the proliferative phase as estrogen levels increase. The endometrium will be more echogenic than the myometrium. The increased echogenicity is due to the development of glands, blood vessels, and stroma (Table 4-3).

PATHOLOGY BOX 4-15

Increased levels of estrogen	→	Negative feedback mechanism is activated	→	Hypothalamus is inhibited from producing GnRH	→	Decreased FSH and LH secretion

TABLE	4-4

Proliferative Phase: Days 11–12

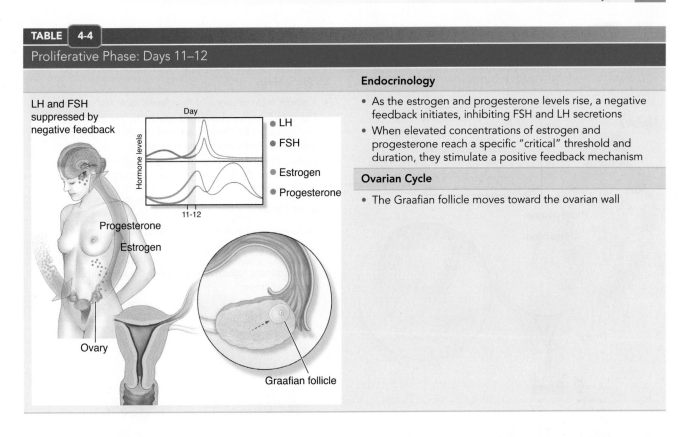

LH and FSH suppressed by negative feedback

- LH
- FSH
- Estrogen
- Progesterone

Progesterone

Estrogen

Ovary

Graafian follicle

Endocrinology

- As the estrogen and progesterone levels rise, a negative feedback initiates, inhibiting FSH and LH secretions
- When elevated concentrations of estrogen and progesterone reach a specific "critical" threshold and duration, they stimulate a positive feedback mechanism

Ovarian Cycle

- The Graafian follicle moves toward the ovarian wall

Days 11–12 of the Proliferative Phase

Starting at around days 11 to 13, the prolonged duration of elevated estrogen levels triggers the negative feedback mechanism. The hypothalamus is stimulated to inhibit GnRH production, which in turn inhibits FSH and LH secretions (Table 4-4).

Day 13 of the Proliferative Phase (Preovulation or Periovulatory Phase): Sonographic Appearance

Endometrium

In the late proliferative (preovulatory) phase, the endometrium develops the "three line sign" or becomes multilayered. A thin echogenic layer separates the echogenic basal layer and hyperechoic inner functional layer. At this stage, the endometrium may measure as much as 5 to 11 millimeters in thickness. The three line sign usually disappears 48 hours after ovulation (Table 4-5).[48]

Secretory Phase (Premenstrual) Day 14 (Ovulation)

When the Graafian follicle matures, it secretes enough estrogen to trigger a positive feedback. The pituitary gland releases a surge of LH. The rise in LH stimulates the developing ovum within the follicle to complete the first meiotic division (meiosis I). The mature ovum now forms into a secondary oocyte and meiosis II division occurs. LH weakens the wall of the Graafian follicle, which leads to the release of the mature ovum. Which of the two ovaries (right or left) ovulates is entirely random. The mature ovum is then swept up into the fallopian tube by the fimbria.[46,49] With ovulation, the external os opens slightly and fills with mucus; in the cervix, the mucus thins to become more permeable to sperm.[46,49]

Sonographic Appearance

Endometrium

The endometrium becomes its thickest during the secretory phase (9 to 14 millimeters).[47] It also becomes more echogenic in appearance with posterior enhancement. The increase in endometrial echogenicity is believed to be caused by stromal edema and glands distended with mucus and glycogen. The posterior acoustical enhancement is considered to be caused by stromal edema.[48]

During the secretory phase, the endometrium will
- Appear uniformly hyperechoic
- Lose its three layer structure and hypoechoic border
- Appear increasingly hyperechoic to the myometrium[51] (Table 4-6)

Secretory Phase: Days 15 to 22

The Graafian cavity collapses with the release of the follicular fluid, and the corpus luteum phase of development begins. The corpus luteum becomes a site of concentrated angiogenesis, resulting in the formation of

TABLE	4-5

Proliferative Phase: Day 13[40]

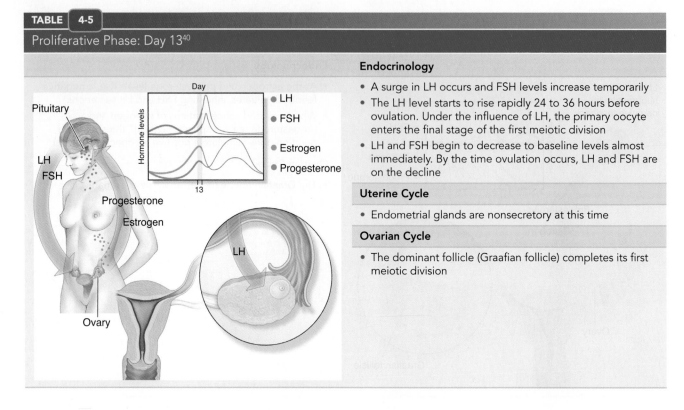

Endocrinology

- A surge in LH occurs and FSH levels increase temporarily
- The LH level starts to rise rapidly 24 to 36 hours before ovulation. Under the influence of LH, the primary oocyte enters the final stage of the first meiotic division
- LH and FSH begin to decrease to baseline levels almost immediately. By the time ovulation occurs, LH and FSH are on the decline

Uterine Cycle

- Endometrial glands are nonsecretory at this time

Ovarian Cycle

- The dominant follicle (Graafian follicle) completes its first meiotic division

a dense capillary network. This enables the hormone-producing cells to obtain the oxygen, nutrients, and hormone precursors necessary to synthesize and release large amounts of progesterone and, to a lesser extent, estrogen. Progesterone has an important role in converting the proliferative endometrium into a secretory lining receptive to implantation and supportive of the blastocyst.[45,46]

The rising levels of estrogen and progesterone in the blood trigger the negative feedback control and inhibit the production of FSH and LH from the pituitary. The levels of FSH and LH begin to fall.

TABLE	4-6

Secretory Phase (Premenstrual) Day 14 (Ovulation)[47]

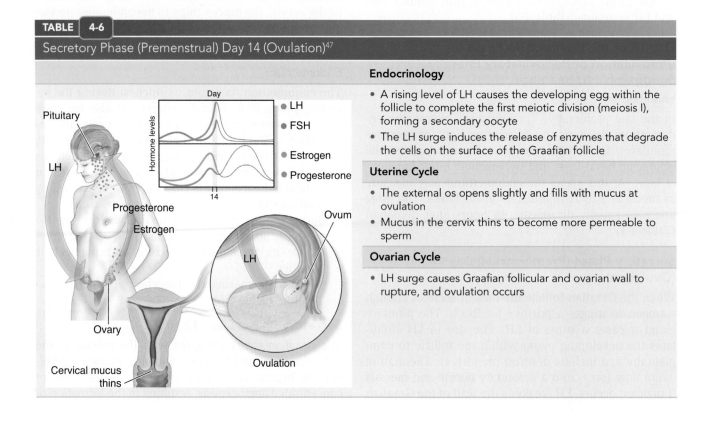

Endocrinology

- A rising level of LH causes the developing egg within the follicle to complete the first meiotic division (meiosis I), forming a secondary oocyte
- The LH surge induces the release of enzymes that degrade the cells on the surface of the Graafian follicle

Uterine Cycle

- The external os opens slightly and fills with mucus at ovulation
- Mucus in the cervix thins to become more permeable to sperm

Ovarian Cycle

- LH surge causes Graafian follicular and ovarian wall to rupture, and ovulation occurs

If the released mature ovum is fertilized by sperm in the fallopian tube, the developing blastocyst implants into the endometrium approximately 7 days after ovulation. The implantation of the blastocyst stimulates the endometrium to produce hCG, which supports the corpus luteum so that it will continue to secrete progesterone and estrogen.[50] Progesterone thickens the endometrium during the pregnancy until it forms the placenta. It also triggers the mucus in the cervix to thicken so that sperm or bacteria are less likely to enter the uterus (Table 4-7).

If the released mature ovum is not fertilized the corpus luteum starts to degenerate and begins to evolve into the corpus albicans, which is a mass of fibrous scar tissue. Progesterone and estrogen production stops. When estrogen and progesterone levels drop to a certain level, it initiates a positive feedback control and FSH and LH will start to rise to begin the next menstrual cycle.[38] Without a high level of progesterone, the endometrium starts to degenerate, which will lead to menses. Decreasing levels of progesterone initiate menstrual shedding.

Secretory Phase: Days 23 to 28

If the released mature ovum is not fertilized the corpus luteum starts to degenerate and begins to evolve into the "corpus albicans" (which is a mass of fibrous scar tissue). Progesterone and estrogen production stops. When estrogen and progesterone levels drop to a certain level it will initiate a positive feedback control and

FSH and LH will start to rise to begin the next menstrual cycle.[38] (Tables 4-8, 4-9, and 4-10).

Abnormal Menstrual Cycle

Amenorrhea

Amenorrhea is an absence or cessation of menstruation. It is a condition that can be transient, intermittent, or permanent. It can be the result of a dysfunction of the hypothalamus, pituitary, ovaries, uterus, or vagina. It is divided into two categories: primary and secondary amenorrhea.

Primary Amenorrhea

Primary amenorrhea is when menstruation fails to take place. Menarche does not occur in a young girl age 16.[52]

Secondary Amenorrhea

Secondary amenorrhea occurs in women who have started menstruation, but have had the absence of menses for the equivalent of three menstrual cycles or 6 months.[52]

Oligomenorrhea

Oligomenorrhea is infrequent or very light menstruation. When a woman has menstrual periods that occur at intervals of greater than 35 days, with only four to nine periods in a year, she is considered to have oligomenorrhea.

TABLE	4-7

Secretory Phase: Days 15–22

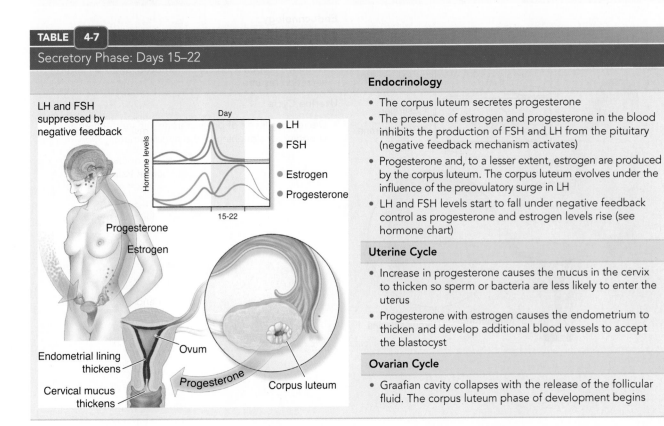

Endocrinology

- The corpus luteum secretes progesterone
- The presence of estrogen and progesterone in the blood inhibits the production of FSH and LH from the pituitary (negative feedback mechanism activates)
- Progesterone and, to a lesser extent, estrogen are produced by the corpus luteum. The corpus luteum evolves under the influence of the preovulatory surge in LH
- LH and FSH levels start to fall under negative feedback control as progesterone and estrogen levels rise (see hormone chart)

Uterine Cycle

- Increase in progesterone causes the mucus in the cervix to thicken so sperm or bacteria are less likely to enter the uterus
- Progesterone with estrogen causes the endometrium to thicken and develop additional blood vessels to accept the blastocyst

Ovarian Cycle

- Graafian cavity collapses with the release of the follicular fluid. The corpus luteum phase of development begins

TABLE 4-8

Secretory Phase—Days 23–25

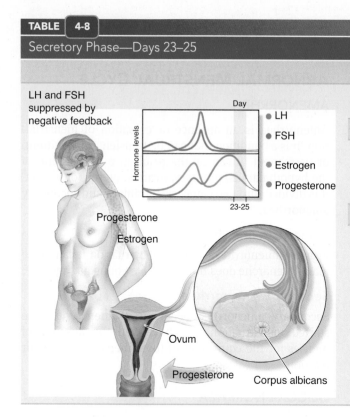

LH and FSH suppressed by negative feedback

Progesterone
Estrogen
Ovum
Progesterone
Corpus albicans

Day
● LH
● FSH
● Estrogen
● Progesterone
23-25

Endocrinology

- If fertilization does not occur, the corpus luteum degenerates and progesterone and estrogen levels fall

Uterine Cycle

- As progesterone and estrogen levels decrease with the degeneration of the corpus luteum, the endometrium starts to break down
- Endometrial blood vessels start to necrose

Ovarian Cycle

- If fertilization does not occur, the corpus luteum undergoes atresia, evolving into the corpus albicans

TABLE 4-9

Secretory phase—Days 26–28

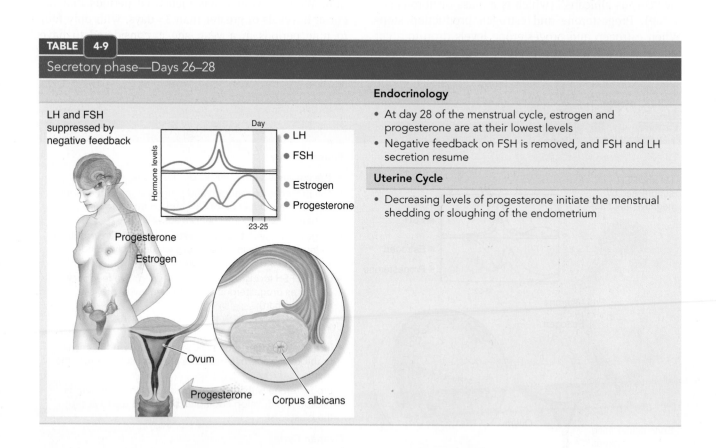

LH and FSH suppressed by negative feedback

Progesterone
Estrogen
Ovum
Progesterone
Corpus albicans

Day
● LH
● FSH
● Estrogen
● Progesterone
23-25

Endocrinology

- At day 28 of the menstrual cycle, estrogen and progesterone are at their lowest levels
- Negative feedback on FSH is removed, and FSH and LH secretion resume

Uterine Cycle

- Decreasing levels of progesterone initiate the menstrual shedding or sloughing of the endometrium

TABLE 4-10

Cyclic Endometrial and Ovarian Changes

Uterine Phase	Ovarian Phase	Day	Endometrial Thickness (mm)	Endometrial Appearance	Uterine Images	Ovarian Images
Late Menstrual	Follicular	1–5	1–4			
Proliferative	Follicular	6–13	5–8			
Late Proliferative	Follicular		11			
Secretory	Ovulatory	~ 14				
Luteal	Luteal	14–25	9–16			

The late menstrual endometrium images as a thin echogenic line on both the transabdominal and endovaginal images. In the early proliferative phase, the endometrium begins to demonstrate the characteristic three-layer appearance. These layers become more distinct in the late proliferative phase. A dominant follicle develops, which demonstrates peripheral hyperemic flow. The secretory phase of the menstrual cycle shows a thickened, echogenic endometrium with posterior enhancement (arrows). Ovulation occurs at approximately day 14, evident by the collapsed follicle (arrow); afterward the corpus luteum forms.

POLYCYSTIC OVARIAN SYNDROME/OVARIAN FAILURE (DYSFUNCTION) OR PREMATURE OVARIAN FAILURE

Premature ovarian failure (POF) is a primary ovarian defect characterized by a lack of menarche (primary amenorrhea) or premature depletion of ovarian follicles before the age of 40 years (secondary amenorrhea). This heterogeneous disorder affects approximately 1% of women under 40, 1:10,000 women by age 20, and 1:1,000 women by age 30.[53] POF puts women at risk for some other health conditions, such as

- Osteoporosis
- Low thyroid function
- Addison's disease
- Heart disease risk[54]

According to the Mayo Clinic, polycystic ovarian syndrome (PCOS) is the most common hormonal disorder among women of reproductive age. Women who have PCOS do not ovulate. They have infrequent menstrual periods, excess hair growth, acne, obesity, and a much higher risk of high blood pressure and stroke. In some cases, women with the disorder have enlarged ovaries containing multiple small cysts. These cysts are usually located on the outer edge of the ovary.[55] See Chapter 8 for a detailed discussion of PCOS.

MENOPAUSE

Menopause is the transition period in a woman's life usually (but not always) occurring during her late 40s or early 50s. The ovaries slowly cease to produce ova, and less estrogen and progesterone are produced. During the menopausal stage, the hormone levels are unstable. Estrogen and progesterone keep surging and then reach a low point, until finally estrogen and progesterone levels become permanently low. The constant fluctuation in hormone levels is the cause of the many symptoms of menopause. The ovaries slowly stop responding to FSH and LH. Menstruation becomes less frequent and eventually stops altogether. With the cessation of ovarian function, no ovum is released, there is no growth of the endometrium, and no menses occurs.[56] The transition from reproductive to nonreproductive is normally not sudden or abrupt, tends to occur over a period of years, and is a natural consequence of aging. Once the menopausal stage is over, the woman enters the postmenopausal stage where estrogen and progesterone levels are constantly low.

TABLE	4-11				

Uterine Size[64–67]

	Length (cm)	Width (cm)	AP (cm)	Cervix/Corpus Ratio
Infantile	2–3	0.5–1	0.5–1	1:2
Neonate	2–5	0.8–2	0.8–2	1:1
Pediatric	5–7	2–3	2–3	1:1
Nulliparous adult	6–8	3–5	3–5	2:1
Parous adult	8–10	5–6	5–6	3:1
Postmenopausal	3–5	2–3	2–3	1:1

POSTMENOPAUSE

Postmenopause is the stage that the body enters after menopause.

Postmenopausal Uterus

The uterus becomes small and fibrotic because of atrophy of the muscles after menopause. Since the ovaries fail to produce any follicles after menopause, the estrogen level in the blood is reduced and the endometrial lining becomes thin and atrophic. The normal uterus size in an ovulating adult is approximately 6 to 8 centimeters in length, 3 to 5 centimeters wide, and 3 to 5 centimeters deep (anteroposterior dimension). During the postmenopausal years, the uterus decreases in size and the endometrium atrophies. The postmenopausal uterus measures approximately 3 to 5 centimeters in length, 2 to 3 centimeters wide, and 2 to 3 centimeters deep (anteroposterior dimension).[39] The decrease in uterine size is based on how many years a woman has been postmenopausal (Table 4-11).[48]

Postmenopausal Ovaries

The postmenopausal ovary is a hypoechoic, well-defined ovoid echo complex and may be difficult to identify because of the absence of follicles. Postmenopausal ovaries undergo changes such as a decrease in size and decreased to absent folliculogenesis. There is an inverse relationship between ovarian size and the time since menopause. As the length of the postmenopausal period increases, the ovarian size decreases. The exception to this inverse relationship is when a patient is receiving hormone replacement therapy (HRT). The ovary may demonstrate no changes in ovarian volume at all.[57] The volume size of a postmenopausal ovary depends upon the investigator (Table 4-12).

PATHOLOGY BOX 4-16

Ovaries cease to produce ova	→	No ova is released	→	Estrogen production is decreased	→	Endometrium is not stimulated to proliferate or grow	→	No menses occurs

TABLE 4-12				
Postmenopausal Ovarian Volumes[58,59]				
	Schoenfeld et al.	**Fleischer et al.**	**Aboulghar et al.**	**Goswamy et al.**
Normal average Postmenopausal ovary volume	1.3 ± 0.7 cm³	2.6 ± 2.0 cm³	3.4 ± 1.7 cm³	Calculated right ovarian volume at 3.58 ± 1.40 cm³ (range 1.00–14.01) and left ovarian volume at 3.57 ± 1.37 cm³ (range 0.88–10.90)

According to Fleischer et al., the size of the normal, sonographically visualized postmenopausal ovary is 2.2 ± 0.7 centimeters in transverse, 1.2 ± 0.3 centimeters in anteroposterior, and 1.1 ± 0.6 centimeters in longitudinal axis.

Postmenopausal Endometrium

The normal postmenopausal atrophic endometrium (without HRT) appears as a thin, homogeneous, and echogenic linear echo within the uterus. It should measure less than 4 millimeters in double-layer thickness and less than 2.5 millimeters in single-layer thickness in a sonohysterography. It should also appear smooth and uniform in echotexture and not be displaced by any submucosal, myometrial abnormalities.[60] The exception is in women on estrogen therapy. The endometrium in an HRT patient may vary up to 3 millimeters when using cyclic estrogen and progestin therapy. The normal postmenopausal endometrium measures 7 millimeters or less (Fig. 4-15).[48]

Postmenopausal Bleeding

Postmenopausal bleeding can occur when a patient experiences endometrial atrophy, endometrial polyps, submucosal fibroids, endometrial hyperplasia, endometrial carcinoma, or estrogen withdrawal. The best time to image a postmenopausal patient that is bleeding is directly after the bleeding has stopped. Presumably, the endometrium is at its thinnest, and it will be easier to spot irregularities. Generally, if the endometrial thickness is less than 4 to 5 millimeters, cancer can be excluded. If the endometrial thickness is greater than 5 millimeters, or if the endometrium appears irregular and inhomogeneous, further investigation may be needed either by a sonohysterography, biopsy, or hysteroscopy.[49]

Postmenopausal Hormonal Changes Due to Estrogen Deficiency

Estrogen deficiency produces changes in the female reproductive system. The vaginal mucous membrane becomes thin and loses its rugosity (typical wrinkles in the mucosa). The depth of the vaginal vault disappears while decreased secretions make the vagina dry. Sexual intercourse becomes painful and difficult because of a "dry vagina." The fat in the labia majora and the mons pubis decreases and pubic hair becomes sparse. The vaginal opening becomes narrower. Endocervical cells produce less cervical mucus and the cervix becomes smaller and appears to flush with the vagina. The breast also changes with a decrease in estrogen. The glandular structure of the breasts will start to atrophy, but not the breast fat.[61]

Postmenopausal Hormone Replacement Therapy

HRT was thought to be able to ward off heart disease, osteoporosis, and cancer while improving a woman's quality of life. Doctors prescribed HRT to relieve the symptoms resulting from low levels of female hormones. But beginning in July 2002, findings emerged from clinical studies that showed long-term use of HRT posed serious risks and may increase the risk of heart attack and stroke. HRT can involve the use of either estrogen alone, or it can be combined with progesterone or progestin in its synthetic form. Estrogen plus progestin actually increases the chance of a first heart attack, as well as breast cancer, and it increases the risk for blood clots.[62]

HRT Is Beneficial for

1. Reducing "hot flashes"
2. Helping to keep bones strong; it can help prevent osteoporosis
3. Decreasing pain and irritation caused by vaginal dryness
4. Raising high-density lipoprotein ("good cholesterol") and lowering low-density lipoprotein ("bad cholesterol")

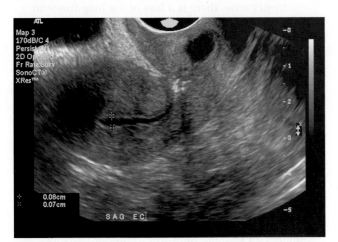

Figure 4-15 This figure demonstrates a typical postmenopausal fluid collection. The one-sided measurements of the endometrium measure 0.8 millimeters anteriorly and 0.7 millimeters posteriorly (1.5 millimeters in aggregate).

HRT Risks

1. Increased chance of uterine cancer. When estrogen therapy is used, it stimulates the endometrium to grow and increases the risk of endometrial cancer
2. Both estrogen and progestin increase the risk of breast cancer
3. Increased risk of blood clots
4. Both estrogen and progestin increase the risk of a heart attack[62,63]

Postmenopausal Endometrial Lining in HRT Patients

In HRT patients, both uterine size and cyclical endometrial changes may stay the same as those seen in a premenopausal patient. In general, estrogen therapy in the postmenopausal endometrium creates the same effect as natural estrogens in the normal cycle.[56]

Postmenopausal Ultrasound

Ultrasound is important in the management of the postmenopausal patient. One of its most important uses is in diagnosing and managing endometrial cancer. About 90% of patients diagnosed with endometrial cancer have abnormal vaginal bleeding, such as bleeding between periods or after menopause, so obtaining a patient history is important.[64]

To determine how far an endometrial carcinoma has advanced, the ratio of the anteroposterior (AP) diameter of the total measured endometrial thickness to the AP diameter of the uterine corpus is calculated. If it is less than 50% the tumor has invaded less than half of the myometrium. If the ratio is greater than 50%, the tumor has invaded all the way to the outer half of the myometrium.[65] For more information on endometrial carcinoma, see Chapter 9.

SUMMARY

- A complex interaction of hormones regulates the menstrual cycle.
  - GnRH
  - LH
  - FSH
  - estrogen
  - progesterone
- GnRH stimulates the pituitary to synthesize and secrete FSH and LH.

Critical Thinking Questions

1. Explain the difference between a positive and negative feedback loop. What is the importance of these processes? Give examples of these systems from the chapter and other obstetric physiologic processes.

   ANSWER: Feedback loops are the interaction between opposing physiologic functions where the amount of one hormone influences changes in another hormone. When the system responds to changes in the same direction, this is called positive feedback. In this chapter this occurs when hormone concentrations are low, resulting in an increase in hormone production. Changes in the opposite direction are called negative feedback and result in a decrease in hormone production. Positive feedback results in an increase in hormone production while negative feedback results in a decrease in hormone production. If there is no counteraction (negative feedback), systemic hormone levels become abnormal.

   The following are a few of the many examples of physiologic feedback loops:

   a. During parturition, oxytocin levels increase, resulting in uterine contractions. As labor continues, oxytocin levels increase, also increasing the strength and duration of the contractions. This positive feedback loop continues the process of childbirth.

   b. As estrogen blood levels increase, the release of LH and FSH inhibits secretion (negative feedback). In the case of low estrogen levels, LH and FSH levels decrease, resulting in an increase of estrogen production (positive feedback).

   c. During menopause, estrogen and progesterone levels decrease because of low production by the ovaries, resulting in constant FSH and LH production. This is a positive feedback system due to the lack of estrogen production to counteract LH/FSH production. Remember, a positive feedback system goes in one direction and the negative feedback counteracts that direction. In the case of menopause, there is a loss of the loop function.

2. Describe the appearance of the endometrium in the late proliferative phase. Discuss the importance of this finding in patients tracking ovulation. How does the endometrium change upon ovulation?

   ANSWER: The late proliferative or preovulatory phase endometrium images with three layers representing the echogenic basal, hyperechoic inner functional layer, and the echogenic separating layer. At this phase, the double-layer endometrium measures as much as 11 millimeters. The three line sign disappears within 48 hours after ovulation. In the postovulatory period, the secretory endometrium thickens up to 14 millimeters and begins to lose the characteristic three layer appearance. Sonography images an endometrium with posterior enhancement uniformly hyperechoic, and the myometrium increases in echogenicity.

- FSH stimulates follicle growth.
- Growing follicles produce estrogen.
- Reversal of negative feedback occurs when estrogen rises to the threshold level and an LH surge occurs.
- The LH surge breaks down the Graafian follicle and ovarian walls and ovulation occurs, releasing the mature ovum.
- The corpus luteum forms after ovulation.
- The corpus luteum synthesizes and secretes estrogen and progesterone.
- Serum levels of estrogen and progesterone climb steadily, suppressing LH output.
- If the ovum is not fertilized, the corpus luteum starts to degenerate and begins to evolve into the corpus albicans.
- The atresia of the corpus luteum leads to a decline in estrogen and progesterone secretions.
- When estrogen and progesterone levels are low, the negative feedback control on the GnRH pulse frequency is removed.
- Positive feedback begins and FSH and LH rise to begin the next menstrual cycle.
- If a pregnancy does occur and the developing blastocyst burrows into the endometrium, the cells around the developing zygote will produce hCG, which maintains the corpus luteum, which in turn produces progesterone and estrogen until the placenta takes over (approximately 3 months).

REFERENCES

1. Marieb E. *Human Anatomy and Physiology*. Redwood City: The Benjamin/Cummings Publishing Company Inc.; 1989.
2. Encyclopedia Britannica eb.com. Corpus Luteum. Available at: http://www.britannica.com/EBchecked/topic/138543/corpus-luteum. Accessed Sept. 2010.
3. What is the corpus luteum? Available at: http://www.justmommies.com/articles/corpus-luteum.shtml. Accessed Sept. 2010.
4. Google's Definitions of estrogen on the Web. Available at: http://www.google.com/search?hl=en&rlz=1T4ADBF_enUS230US231&defl=en&q=define:estrogen&sa=X&ei=2eNFTOulBIu6sQOPmszZAg&ved=0CBEQkAE. Accessed Sept. 2010.
5. Berkeley University: The Reproductive System. Available at: http://mcb.berkeley.edu/courses/mcb32/Miller%20notes-Reproduction. Accessed Sept. 2010.
6. Kimball's Biology Pages. Sexual Reproduction in Humans by John W. Kimball. Available at: http://users.rcn.com/jkimball.ma.ultranet/BiologyPages/S/Sexual_Reproduction.html. Accessed Sept. 2010.
7. The Merck Manuals Online Medical Library. Internal Genital Organs by Peter L. Rosenblatt. MD. Last full review/revision July 2007. Available at: http://www.merck.com/mmhe/sec22/ch241/ch241c.html. Accessed Sept. 2010.
8. Tortora GJ. *Principles of Human Anatomy*. 5th ed. New York: Harper Collins Publishers Inc.; 1989.
9. Marrinan, Greg, MD, Stein, Marjorie, MD. Polycystic Ovarian Disease (Stein-Leventhal Syndrome). Updated: Aug 11, 2009. Available at e-medicine: http://emedicine.medscape.com/article/404754-overview. Accessed Sept. 2010.
10. Colorado State University: Bowen, RA. Functional Anatomy of the Hypothalamus and Pituitary Gland. Last updated on September 4, 2001. Available at: http://www.vivo.colostate.edu/hbooks/pathphys/endocrine/hypopit/anatomy.html. Accessed Sept. 2010.
11. Encyclopedia Britannica eb.com Science and Technology: Hypothalamus: Available at: http://www.britannica.com/EBchecked/topic/280044/hypothalamus. Accessed Sept. 2010
12. Biology Reference. Hypothalamus. Available at: http://www.biologyreference.com/Ho-La/Hypothalamus.html. Accessed Sept. 2010.
13. Science, Natural Phenomena and Medicine, Hypophyseal Portal System. (posted Wednesday, April 7, 2010). Posted by Homo Sapiens at 3:10 pm. Available at: http://sciencenaturalphenomena.blogspot.com/2010/04/hypophyseal-portal-system.html. Accessed Sept. 2010.
14. Sherwood L. Human Physiology: From Cells to Systems. 7th edition—2010 Brooks/Cole, Cengage Learning; Brooks/Cole 10 Davis Drive, Belmont, CA 94002 (on-line book). Available at: http://books.google.com/books?id=gOmpysGBC90C&printsec=frontcover&dq=inauthor:%22Lauralee+Sherwood%22&hl=en&ei=3iRsTIjKJITCsAPW99SMCA&sa=X&oi=book_result&ct=result&resnum=2&ved=0CDEQ6AEwAQ#v=onepage&q&f=false. Accessed Sept. 2010.
15. University of Maryland Medical Center. Endocrinology Health Guide: The Pituitary Gland. Available at: http://www.umm.edu/endocrin/pitgland.htm. Accessed Sept. 2010.
16. Vander AJ, Sherman JH, Luciano DS. *Human Physiology*. 5th ed. New York: McGraw-Hill Publishing Company; 1990.
17. The Merck Manuals Online Medical Library. Endocrine function. Last full review/revision May 2006 by John E. Morley, MB, BCh. Available at: http://www.merck.com/mmhe/sec13/ch161/ch161c.html. Accessed Sept. 2010.
18. Campbell RE, Gaidamaka G, Han S-K, et al. Dendro-dendritic bundling and shared synapses between gonadotropin-releasing hormone neurons. Proceedings of the National Academy of Sciences of the United States of America (PNAS). Neuroscience, published online 2009, June 17. Available at: http://www.ncbi.nlm.nih.gov/pmc/articles/PMC2705602/?tool=pmcentrez. Accessed Sept. 2010.
19. Wikipedia the free encyclopedia: Gonadotropin-releasing hormone. Available at: http://en.wikipedia.org/wiki/Gonadotropin-releasing_hormone#cite_note-pmid19541658-0. Accessed Sept. 2010.
20. MM Student Projects/McGill Medicine. Endocrinology of the Menstrual Cycle. Available at: http://sprojects.mmi.mcgill.ca/menstrualcycle/endocrinology.html. Accessed Sept. 2010.
21. Kaiser UB, Jakubowiak A, Steinberger A, et al. Differential effects of gonadotropin-releasing hormone (GnRH) pulse frequency on gonadotropin subunit and GnRH receptor messenger ribonucleic acid levels in vitro. *Endocrinology*. 1997;138(3):1224–1231.

22. Mayo Clinic.com. Follicle Stimulating Hormone and Luteinizing Hormone (Intramuscular Route, Subcutaneous Route). Portions of this document last updated: Nov. 1, 2009. Available at: http://www.mayoclinic.com/health/drug-information/DR600403. Accessed Sept. 2010.

23. Medical.WebEnds.com is a free online medical terminology dictionary. Theca Cells. Available at: http://medical.webends.com/kw/Theca%20Cells. Accessed Sept. 2010.

24. University of South Wales, Sidney, Australia (UNSW). Embryology: Corpus Luteum by Dr. Mark Hill 2010. Available at: http://embryology.med.unsw.edu.au/notes/week1_3d.htm. Accessed Sept. 2010.

25. Women's health (Web MD). Women's Health. Normal Testosterone and Estrogen Levels in Women. Reviewed by Mikio A. Nihira, MD on March 07, 2010. Accessed Sept. 2010. http://women.webmd.com/normal-testosterone-and-estrogen-levels-in-women?page=3. Accessed Sept. 2010.

26. Medline Plus, U.S. National Library of Medicine. Estradiol test. Available at: http://www.nlm.nih.gov/medlineplus/ency/article/003711.htm. Accessed Sept. 2010.

27. New York Presbyterian Hospital. Estrogen Effects on the Female Body. Available at: http://nyp.org/health/estrogen-effects.html. Accessed Sept. 2010.

28. Ovarian Cycle and Hormonal Regulation by Judyth Sassoon. Available at: http://science.jrank.org/pages/4950/Ovarian-Cycle-Hormonal-Regulation.html. Accessed Sept. 2010.

29. Gonadotropins: Luteinizing and Follicle Stimulating Hormones by Author: R. Bowen. Last updated on May 13, 2004. Available at: http://www.vivo.colostate.edu/hbooks/pathphys/endocrine/hypopit/lhfsh.html. Accessed Sept. 2010.

30. Progesterone by Kimball JW (2007-05-27). Kimball's Biology Pages. Available at: http://users.rcn.com/jkimball.ma.ultranet/BiologyPages/P/Progesterone.html. Accessed Sept. 2010.

31. Progesterone. Wikipedia. Available at: http://en.wikipedia.org/wiki/Progesterone. Accessed Sept. 2010.

32. MM Student Projects/ McGill Medicine. Menstrual Cycle Home Page. Available at: http://sprojects.mmi.mcgill.ca/menstrualcycle/home.html. Accessed Sept. 2010.

33. Gilbert SF. Oogenesis—Oogenic meiosis. Biology Development, 6th ed. Sinauer Associates, 2000. Available at: http://www.ncbi.nlm.nih.gov/bookshelf/br.fcgi?book=dbio. Accessed Sept. 2010.

34. About.com Women's health: Follicular Phase of the Menstrual Cycle By Tracee Cornforth. Updated November 22, 2006. Available at: http://womenshealth.about.com/od/womenshealthglossary/g/follicular_phas.htm. Accessed Sept. 2010.

35. The Merck Manuals Online Medical Library. Menstrual Cycle. Last full review/revision July 2007 by Peter L. Rosenblatt, MD. Available at: http://www.merck.com/mmhe/sec22/ch241/ch241e.html Accessed Sept. 2010.

36. Brown JB. Emeritus Professor. Pituitary and Ovarian Hormones of a Woman's Reproductive Cycle. Available at: http://www.billings-ovulation-method.org.au/act/physiolo.shtml. Accessed Sept. 2010.

37. Hangen-Ansert, SL. Textbook of Diagnostic Ultrasonography, 6th edition, volume 2. St. Louis: Mosby Elsevier; 2006.

38. American Pregnancy Association: Understanding Ovulation. Available at: http://www.americanpregnancy.org/gettingpregnant/understandingovulation.html. Accessed Sept. 2010.

39. eMedicine health. Mittelschmerz Author: Frederick B Gaupp, MD, et al. Last Editorial Review: 9/22/2005. Available at: http://www.emedicinehealth.com/mittelschmerz/article_em.htm Accessed Sept. 2010.

40. WebMD; Medical Dictionary: Corpus Luteum. WEB MD referenced: Stedman's Medical Dictionary 28th Edition, Copyright© 2006_Lippincott Williams & Wilkins. Available at: http://dictionary.webmd.com/terms/corpus-luteum. Accessed Sept. 2010.

41. Thomas L Alderson, DO. Luteal Phase Dysfunction. Medscape. Updated: Oct 8, 2008. Available at: http://emedicine.medscape.com/article/254934-overview Accessed Sept. 2010.

42. Alonso R., Marín F., González M., Guelmes P., et.al. The Hypothalamus-Pituitary-Ovarian Axis as a Model System for the Study of SERM Effects. An Overview of Experimental and Clinical Studies—2006 Springer Berlin Heidelberg. Available at: http://www.springerlink.com/content/978-3-540-24227-7/contents/. Accessed Sept. 2010.

43. Novak E. Gynecology and Female Endocrinology. Little, Brown, 1941.

44. The Merck Manuals Online Medical Library. Female Reproductive Endocrinology. by Robert G. Brzyski, MD, PhD and Jani R. Jensen, MD. Last full review/revision March 2007. Available at: http://www.merck.com/mmpe/sec18/ch243/ch243a.html. Accessed Sept. 2010.

45. Goldberg BB., McGahan JP. Atlas of ultrasound measurements. Elsevier Health Sciences, 2006.

46. Kenneth M. Nalaboff, MD, John S. Pellerito, MD, Eran Ben-Levi MD. Imaging the Endometrium: Disease and Normal Variants. Radio Graphics. Available at: http://radiographics.rsna.org/content/21/6/1409.full. Accessed Sept. 2010.

47. Science.jrank.org. Menstrual Cycle-Secretory Phase, page: 4233. Available at: http://science.jrank.org/pages/4233/Menstrual-Cycle-Secretory-phase.html#ixzz0zXqK9u4U. Accessed Sept. 2010.

48. Embryology.ch. Developed by the universities of Frebourg, Lausanne and Bern (Switzerland)Human Embryology; Module 6.1 Role and functional anatomy of the endometrium. Available at: http://www.embryology.ch/anglais/gnidation/role02.html. Accessed Sept. 2010.

49. Werner Schmidt, Asim Kurjak. Color Doppler Sonography in Gynecology and Obstetrics. 2005 Georg Thieme Verlag, Stuttgart, Germany.

50. Corrine K Welt, MD, Robert L Barbieri, MD. Etiology, diagnosis, and treatment of primary amenorrhea, Last literature review version 18.2: May 2010. This topic last updated: April 14, 2009. Available at: http://www.uptodate.com/patients/content/topic.do?topicKey=~7MdcWOax0pABxb7. Accessed Sept. 2010.

51. Paolo Beck-Peccoz and Luca Persani. Premature ovarian failure. Received March 2, 2006; Accepted April 6, 2006. *Orphanet Journal of Rare Diseases*. 2006,; 1: 9. Published online 2006 April 6. Available at: http://www.ojrd.com/content/1/1/9. Accessed Sept. 2010.

52. Eunice Kennedy Shriver National Institute of Child Health and Human Development. Premature Ovarian Failure. Last Update: 05/22/2007. Available at: http://www.nichd.nih.gov/health/topics/premature_ovarian_failure.cfm Accessed Sept. 2010.

53. Wikipedia. Menopause. Available at: http://en.wikipedia.org/wiki/Menopause. Accessed Sept. 2010.

54. Mayo Clinical Staff. Polycystic ovary syndrome. 1998–2010 Mayo Foundation for Medical Education and Research (MFMER) Available at: http://www.mayoclinic.com/health/polycystic-ovary-syndrome/DS00423. Accessed Sept. 2010.

55. Sit AS, Modugno F, Hill LM, et al. Transvaginal ultrasound measurement of endometrial thickness as a biomarker for estrogen exposure. *Cancer Epidemiol Biomarkers Prev.* 2004 Sep;13(9):1459–1465. Available at: http://cebp.aacrjournals.org/content/13/9/1459.full. Accessed Sept. 2010.

56. Michael Applebaum, MD, JD, FCLM. Ultrasound and the Menopause Web Booklet. Available at: http://www.drapplebaum.com/menopause.htm#THE%20OVARIES. Accessed Sept. 2010.

57. Fleischer AC, McKee MS, Gordon AN, et al. Transvaginal sonography of postmenopausal ovaries with pathologic correlation. *J Ultrasound Med.* 1990;9(11):637–644. Copyright © 1990 by American Institute of Ultrasound in Medicine. Available at: http://www.jultrasoundmed.org/cgi/content/abstract/9/11/637. Accessed Sept. 2010.

58. Davis PC, O'Neil MJ, Yoder IC, et al. Sonohysterographic findings of endometrial and subendometrial conditions. *RadioGraphics.* 2002 July;22(4):803–816. Available at: http://radiographics.rsna.org/content/22/4/803.abstract. Accessed Sept. 2010.

59. GynaeOnline. Symptoms of Menopause. Available at: http://www.gynaeonline.com/menopause.htm. Accessed Sept. 2010.

60. American College of Gastroenterology. Postmenopausal Hormone Therapy. Facts about menopausal hormone therapy. Available at: http://www.acg.gi.org/patients/women/menop.asp. Accessed Sept. 2010.

61. Dept. of Health and Human Services, National Institute of Health, National Heart, Lung and Blood Institute. Important Facts About Post Menopausal Hormone Replacement Therapy (HRT). Available at: http://www.nhlbi.nih.gov/health/women/pht_facts.htm. Accessed Sept. 2010.

62. American Cancer Society. How is endometrial cancer diagnosed? Last Medical Review: 10/22/2009. Last Revised: 08/18/2010. Available at: http://www.cancer.org/Cancer/EndometrialCancer/DetailedGuide/endometrial-uterine-cancer-diagnosis. Accessed Sept. 2010.

63. Merz E. Ultrasound in obstetrics and gynecology: Gynecology. Vol 2: Gynecology, 2nd ed. New York, NY: Thieme; 2007.

64. Salem S, Wilson S. Gynecologic ultrasound. In: Rumack CM, Wilson SR, Charboneau JW, Johnson JM, eds. *Diagnostic Ultrasound*, 3rd ed. St. Louis: Elsevier Mosby; 2005.

65. Baggish MS. Anatomy of the uterus. In: Baggish MS, Valle RF, Guedj H. Hysteroscopy: *Visual Perspective of Uterine Anatomy, Physiology and Pathology*. 3rd ed. Baltimore: Wolters Kluwer | Lippincott Williams & Wilkins; 2007.

66. Salsgiver TL, Hagen-Ansert SL. Normal Anatomy and Physiology of the Female Pelvis. In: Haga-Ansert S. *Textbook of Diagnostic Ultrasonography*. 6th ed. St. Louis: Mosby Elsevier; 2006.

67. Hagan-Ansert SL. Pediatric Congenital Anomalies of the Female Pelvis. In: Haga-Ansert S. *Textbook of Diagnostic Ultrasonography*. 6th ed. St. Louis: Mosby Elsevier; 2006.

68. AIUM Practice Guideline for the Performance of Pelvic Ultrasound Examinations; Original copyright 1995; revised 2009, 2006; http://www.aium.org/publications/guidelines/pelvis.pdf

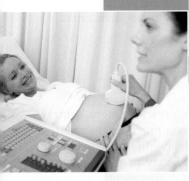

5 Normal Anatomy of the Female Pelvis

Sanja Plavsic Kupesic and Tricia Turner

OBJECTIVES

Identify the bony structures within the pelvic skeleton, pelvic muscles, and pelvic organs

Differentiate between the true and false pelvis

Discuss the sonographic techniques used for pelvic evaluation

List the segments, muscle layers, size and shape, and positional variants of the uterus

Explain the location of the fallopian tubes, ovaries, suspensory ligaments, ureters, and vasculature within the pelvis

Describe the normal sonographic appearance of the gynecologic, bowel, and vascular structures

Summarize transabdominal sonography (TAS) and endovaginal sonography (EVS) examination techniques for pelvic imaging

Explain the use of color, power and spectral Doppler, as well as 3D image data set acquisition of the pelvic organs.

KEY TERMS

false pelvis | true pelvis | sacrum | coccyx | innominate | rectus abdominis muscle | psoas major muscle | iliopsoas muscle | linea terminalis | obturator internus muscle | piriformis | puborectalis muscle | levator ani muscles | transperoneal | bladder trigone | posterior enhancement | myometrium | endometrium | retroflex | anteflex | anteversion | retroversion | cardinal ligaments | uterosacral ligaments | round ligaments | broad ligament | posterior cul-de-sac | pouch of Douglas | recto-uterine pouch | Graafian follicle | follicle-stimulating hormone (FSH) | internal iliac artery | uterine artery | ovarian arteries | bimanual maneuver

GLOSSARY

Anterior cul-de-sac aka vesicouterine recess. Potential space between the uterus and urinary bladder

Contralateral On the opposite side

Corpora albicantia Fibrous tissue that replaces the corpus luteum

False pelvis aka greater or major pelvis. Area superior to and anterior to the pelvic brim

Follicle-stimulating hormone (FSH) Hormone that stimulates growth and maturation of the ovarian Graafian follicle. The anterior pituitary gland secretes the hormone

Follicular atresia Degeneration and reabsorption of the follicle before maturity

Fundus Latin anatomic term referring to the portion of an organ opposite from its opening

Iliopectineal line aka pelvic brim or linea terminalis. The inner surface of the pubic and ilium bones contains a bony ridge, which serves as the line dividing the true and false pelvis

Iliopsoas muscle Combination of the psoas major, psoas minor, and iliacus muscles

Hypertrophy Increase in size

Ipsilateral On the same side

Linea terminalis aka innominate line. Line drawn from the pubic crest to the arcuate line dividing the true and false pelvis

Orthogonal At right angles (perpendicular)

Pouch of Douglas aka posterior cul-de-sac or rectouterine recess. Potential space between the rectum and uterus

Serosa Serous membrane enclosing an organ that often excretes lubricating serous fluid

Space of Retzius aka properitoneal space. Space between the pubic symphysis and urinary bladder

True pelvis aka lesser or minor pelvis. Portion of the pelvic cavity inferior and posterior to the pelvic brim

Ultrasound is one of the most popular imaging modalities used to evaluate the female pelvis. Modern ultrasound units provide high-resolution images of pelvic anatomy and pathology without the need for extensive prescan preparation or use of ionizing radiation.

The use of diagnostic ultrasound began in the mid-1970's. The two most common techniques are transabdominal sonography (TAS) and transvaginal sonography (TVS), also known as endovaginal sonography (EVS). These techniques are complementary, and ultrasound laboratories perform both examinations.

TAS provides a global view of the pelvic anatomy and enables the sonographer to visualize the true and false pelvis, allowing imaging of physiological and pathological changes. TAS also permits evaluation of anatomy and pathology related to the urinary bladder and abdominal wall muscles. TAS utilizes lower frequency settings, which results in a greater depth of anatomic coverage. The use of lower frequencies results in a trade-off in a decrease in anatomic resolution.

A filled urinary bladder and a curvilinear broadband transducer in the 3 to 5 MHz range provide optimal imaging for the transabdominal exam. The full bladder displaces the gassy bowel away from the field of view, providing an acoustic window to visualize pelvic structures. Drinking approximately 32 ounces of fluid prior to the exam hydrates the patient, with dehydrated patients requiring more fluids to adequately fill the bladder. An alternate filling method is via a pre-existing Foley catheter. The scanning technologist must be considerate of the pressure applied on the full bladder, as this may be uncomfortable. The presence of free fluid in the pelvis enhances visualization of the uterine borders and possibly reveals the broad ligament and fallopian tubes.

Limitations of TAS include a decrease in anatomic resolution due to use of lower ultrasound frequencies, patient discomfort from a full bladder, and possible time constraints due to bladder filling.

Endovaginal techniques allow a more direct assessment of the pelvic anatomy with shorter scanning distances and less interference from the bowel. The distance between the transducer and the ovary using EVS is half of that for TAS. Endovaginal imaging allows for the use of a higher frequency transducer, thus increasing detail due to the close proximity of the pelvic organs. Most endovaginal transducers supply a broadband frequency range between 5 and 9 MHz.

The routine EV exam requires an empty urinary bladder. In the case of placenta previa assessment, a slight residual of urine helps identify and image the internal os of the cervix. EVS may be used not only as a diagnostic, but also as a therapeutic modality to guide the invasive procedures. Tables 5-1 and 5-2 summarize various applications of EVS. Limitations of EVS include a smaller field of view and possible patient discomfort due to transducer manipulation. Contraindication of EVS includes premature rupture of membranes, as this may introduce an infection, and in prepubertal virgins. Table 5-3 provides a summary of the advantages and disadvantages of both transabdominal and endovaginal sonographic techniques.

A thorough knowledge of the gross and cross-sectional anatomy of the female pelvis is essential for the sonographer who is examining the pelvis. Understanding pelvic anatomy begins by building a mental picture of pelvic layers, beginning with the osseous structures.

TABLE 5-1
Diagnostic Applications of Transvaginal Ultrasound
Early detection of intrauterine pregnancy
Direct and indirect signs of ectopic pregnancy
Detection of early pregnancy failure and pathology
Detection of embryonal and early fetal anomalies
Location, numeration, and chorionicity in multiple gestations
Early dating by biometry
Diagnosis of placenta previa
Monitoring cervical dynamics to rule out cervical incompetence
Evaluation of the presenting fetal part in patients with oligohydramnios
Scanning of fetal head in cephalic presentations
Diagnosis of uterine disease
Detection of uterine malformations
Detection and scoring of ovarian lesions
Evaluation of posterior cul-de-sac
Monitoring follicular growth
Periovulatory monitoring of endometrial, cervical, and pelvic changes
Evaluation of nongynecologic lesions (i.e., urinary bladder and tract, and bowel)
Evaluation of urodynamics

TABLE	5-2			
Procedures Guided With Transvaginal Ultrasound (TVS)				
TVS-Guided Procedure	**Indication**	**Alternative Procedures**	**Observations**
Puncture of ovarian cyst	Ovum retrieval Histology	Laparoscopy Laparotomy	
Treatment of ectopic pregnancy	Tubal, cornual, ovarian, or cervical ectopic	Laparotomy Laparoscopy	
Reduction of multifetal pregnancy	Super-multifetal pregnancy Twin with major anomaly		Timely reduction compared to transabdominal sonography
Drainage of pelvic content	Pelvic abscess Peritoneal cysts Postoperative collection of blood or lymph	Laparotomy Laparoscopy	
Culdocentesis	Ectopic pregnancy Corpus luteum rupture	Blind culdocentesis	
Early amniocentesis			Rarely performed
Chorionic villus sampling (CVS)	Multiple anterior uterine fibroids	Abdominal CVS Cervical CVS	Rarely performed
Coelocentesis	Early extra amniotic cytogenetics		Rarely performed
Hysterosonography	Pathology of the endometrial cavity	Dilatation and curettage Hysteroscopy	

Salpingosonography
Saline
  Contrast medium
  Air
	Pathology of the fallopian tube	Laparoscopy
		Hysterosalpingography	

THE PELVIC SKELETON

In adults, the osseous pelvis is a ring composed of four bones: the sacrum, the coccyx, and the two large innominate bones, which result from fusion of the ilium, ischium, and pubic bones (Fig. 5-1).[1] The sacrum and coccyx form the posterior wall of the pelvis, and the innominate bones form the lateral and anterior walls (Fig. 5-2). The innominate bones join posteriorly at the sacrum and anteriorly in the midline at the symphysis pubis. The outer surface of each of the innominate bone forms the acetabulum, the socket for the femoral head.

The sacrum and coccyx are modified segments of the vertebral column. The sacrum consists of the five sacral vertebrae, and the coccyx (vestigial tail of the humans) consists of four fused coccygeal vertebrae (Fig. 5-3). Between the sacrum and coccyx is an articulation that permits antero-posterior (AP) minimal motion.

The female pelvis serves three principal functions. First, it provides a weight-bearing bridge between the spine and the bones of the lower limbs through the sacrum and the innominate bones. Second, it directs the pathway of the fetal head during childbirth (parturition). Third, it protects reproductive and other pelvic organs.

Pelvic bones define two distinct spaces, the true pelvis and the false pelvis, which are separated by an imaginary line (the linea terminalis) extending from the sacral prominence (promontory) along the inner surface of the innominate bone down to the symphysis

TABLE	5-3		
Advantages and Disadvantages of Transabdominal and Endovaginal Ultrasound			
Exam Type	**Advantages**	**Disadvantages**
Endovaginal	Use of higher frequency Better resolution Proximity to area of interest Empty bladder	Smaller field of view Discomfort for patient Limited patient population
Transabdominal	Global view Perform on everyone Applicable to all patient populations	Lower frequency requirement Anatomic resolution Discomfort due to bladder filling

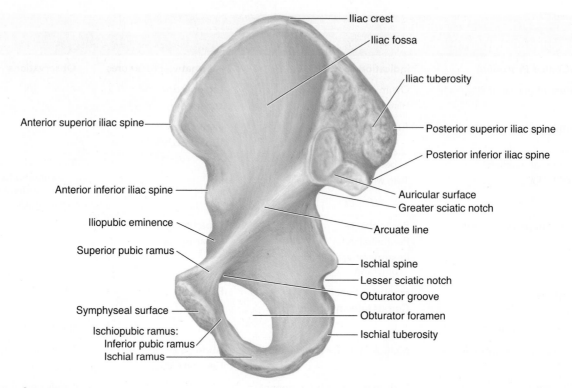

Iliac crest
Iliac fossa
Iliac tuberosity
Anterior superior iliac spine
Posterior superior iliac spine
Posterior inferior iliac spine
Anterior inferior iliac spine
Auricular surface
Greater sciatic notch
Iliopubic eminence
Arcuate line
Superior pubic ramus
Ischial spine
Lesser sciatic notch
Obturator groove
Symphyseal surface
Obturator foramen
Ischiopubic ramus:
Inferior pubic ramus
Ischial tuberosity
Ischial ramus

A Medial view

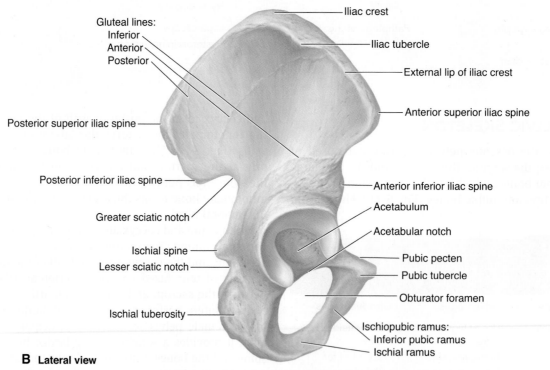

Gluteal lines:
Inferior
Anterior
Posterior
Iliac crest
Iliac tubercle
External lip of iliac crest
Posterior superior iliac spine
Anterior superior iliac spine
Posterior inferior iliac spine
Anterior inferior iliac spine
Greater sciatic notch
Acetabulum
Acetabular notch
Ischial spine
Pubic pecten
Lesser sciatic notch
Pubic tubercle
Obturator foramen
Ischial tuberosity
Ischiopubic ramus:
Inferior pubic ramus
Ischial ramus

B Lateral view

Figure 5-1 Medial and lateral view of the pelvis.

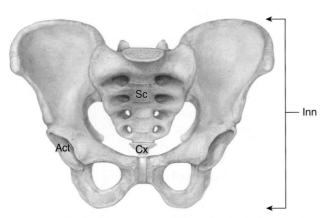

Figure 5-2 The female pelvis viewed from the front. *Act*, acetabulum; *Inn*, innominate bone; *Sc*, sacrum; *Cx*, coccyx.

pubis anteriorly (Figs. 5-4 to 5-6).[1] The true pelvis, situated below the linea terminalis, has a horizontally oriented inlet and a vertically oriented outlet (Fig. 5-7). The inlet of the true pelvis is entirely, and the outlet only partially, walled by bone (Figs. 5-2, 5-5, and 5-6). It is apparent that other structures fill in the gaps, and these include the membranes, ligaments, and muscles of the pelvic floor.

THE PELVIC MUSCLES

Muscles forming much of the abdominal body wall and lining the osseous framework of the pelvis easily image with ultrasound. Most are bilaterally symmetric paired structures. The pelvic skeletal muscles, along with the osseous pelvis, define the limits of the space examined with pelvic sonography. The sonographer should be able to recognize these pelvic muscles to avoid confusing them with masses. Skeletal muscles appear hypoechoic compared to fat or smooth muscle and exhibit linear internal echoes outlining the muscle bundles (Fig. 5-11). Echogenic fascia and retroperitoneal fat outline the muscle borders.

Two muscles commonly demonstrated on transverse pelvic scans, the rectus abdominis and psoas, also extend through the abdominal region. The rectus abdominis muscles form much of the anterior body wall. They extend from the costal cartilages of the fifth, sixth, and seventh ribs, and the xiphoid process to the symphysis pubis and the pubic crest (Fig. 5-8).[2] On cross-sectional imaging, the rectus muscle has an ovoid or lens shape, most pronounced in the lower abdomen.

The psoas major muscle originates from the lower thoracic and the lumbar vertebrae.[2] This cylindrical muscle then courses laterally and anteriorly as it descends through the lower abdomen (Fig. 5-9). Above the level of the fourth lumbar vertebra (L4), the psoas closely attaches to the lateral margins of the spine. At about L5, it separates from the spine and changes the course more laterally, creating a gutter or troughlike space with the spine. The common iliac vessels run through this space. Below the level of the iliac crest, fibers of the psoas major lie adjacent to or begin to interdigitate with the fibers from the medial aspect of the iliacus muscle, thus creating the iliopsoas. This composite muscle continues its lateral and anterior course through the false pelvis, passing over the pelvic brim to insert on the lesser trochanter of the femur.

Through most of the false pelvis, the cross-sectional shape of the iliopsoas is that of an oddly shaped hook with *(text continued on page 91)*

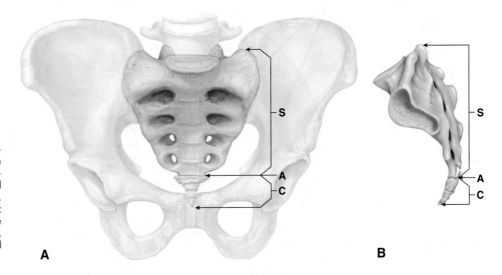

Figure 5-3 A: Ventral and **(B)** lateral surfaces of the adult sacrum *(S)* and coccyx *(C)*. Five fused vertebral bodies form the sacrum, and four fused bodies form the coccyx. The shallow S-shaped curve that these bones create establish the posterior wall of the pelvis. (*A*, articulation between sacrum and coccyx.)

A   B

PATHOLOGY BOX 5-2

The Pelvis Muscles

Region	Muscle	Location
Abdominopelvic	Rectus abdominis	Anterior wall
	Psoas major	Posterior wall
False pelvis	Iliacus	Iliac fossa
True pelvis	Obturator internus	Lateral wall
	Piriformis	Posterior wall
	Coccygeus	Posterior floor
	Levator ani	Middle and anterior floor

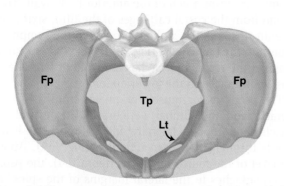

Figure 5-4 The true and false pelvic cavities. The wide but shallow false pelvis *(Fp)* surrounds the deep central true pelvis *(Tp)*. The dividing line between the two spaces is the linea terminalis *(Lt)*.

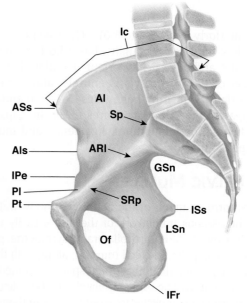

Figure 5-5 Pelvis viewed from the side with the left innominate bone removed. The linea terminalis (innominate line) is made up of the pectineal line and the arcuate line. *Sp*, sacral protuberance; *Al*, ala (wing) of the ilium bone forming iliac fossa; *Ic*, iliac crest; *ASs*, anterior superior iliac spine; *Als*, anterior inferior iliac spine; *Pt*, pubic tubercle; *ISt*, ischial tuberosity; *ISs*, ischial spine; *Gsn*, greater sciatic notch; *LSn*, lesser sciatic notch; *IFr*, inferior ramus of pubis; *Of*, obturator foramen; *SRp*, superior ramis of pubis; *IPe*, iliopubic eminence; *Pl*, pectineal line; *ARI*, arcuate line.

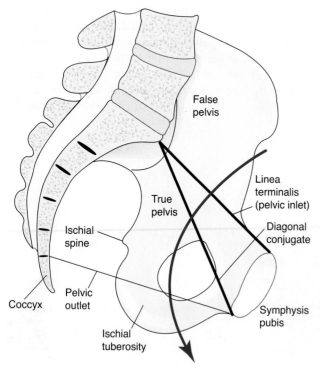

Figure 5-6 True and false pelvis. Portion above linea terminalis is false pelvis; portion below is true pelvis. Arrow shows "stovepipe" curve that the fetus must follow to be born.

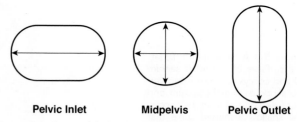

Figure 5-7 Shape of the true pelvis at its inlet, midpelvis, and outlet. Although the inlet and outlet are similar in shape, their axes differ by 90 degrees, which affects the orientation of the fetal head during parturition.

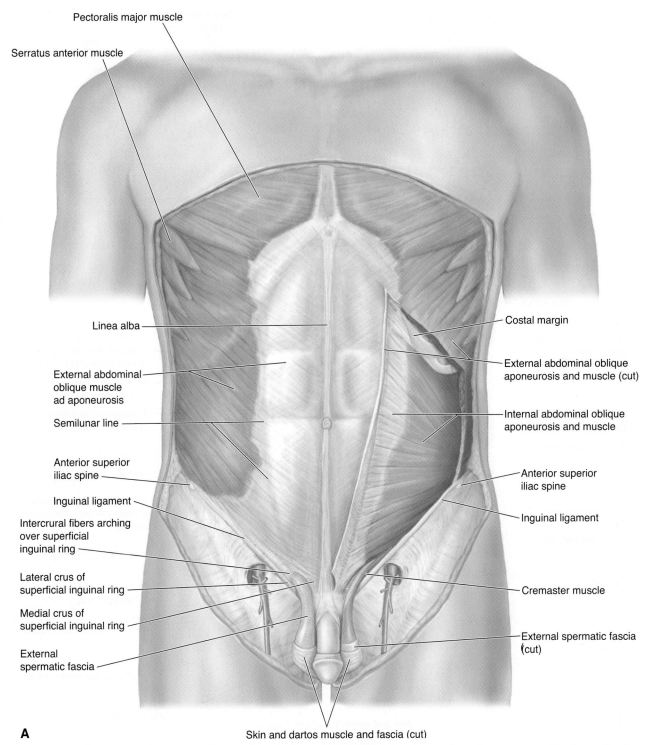

Pectoralis major muscle

Serratus anterior muscle

Linea alba

External abdominal
oblique muscle
ad aponeurosis

Semilunar line

Anterior superior
iliac spine

Inguinal ligament

Intercrural fibers arching
over superficial
inguinal ring

Lateral crus of
superficial inguinal ring

Medial crus of
superficial inguinal ring

External
spermatic fascia

Costal margin

External abdominal oblique
aponeurosis and muscle (cut)

Internal abdominal oblique
aponeurosis and muscle

Anterior superior
iliac spine

Inguinal ligament

Cremaster muscle

External spermatic fascia
(cut)

A

Skin and dartos muscle and fascia (cut)

Figure 5-8 A,B: The rectus abdominis muscles seen from the front. The left and right columns of muscle are separated by the midline linea alba and are interrupted by transverse tendinous intersections at the level of the umbilicus, between the umbilicus and the xiphoid, and at the xiphoid process. *(continued)*

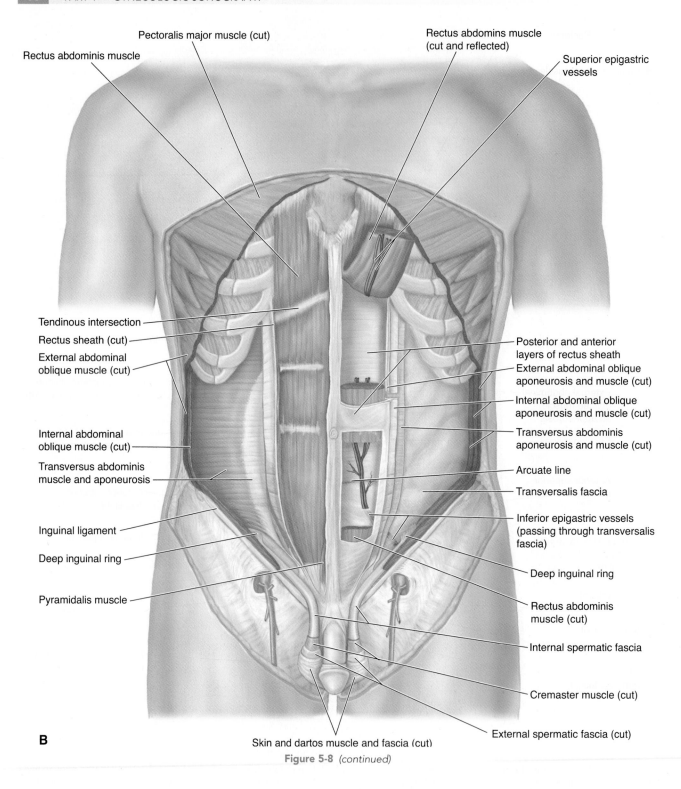

Pectoralis major muscle (cut)

Rectus abdominis muscle

Rectus abdomins muscle
(cut and reflected)

Superior epigastric
vessels

Tendinous intersection

Rectus sheath (cut)

External abdominal
oblique muscle (cut)

Internal abdominal
oblique muscle (cut)

Transversus abdominis
muscle and aponeurosis

Inguinal ligament

Deep inguinal ring

Pyramidalis muscle

Posterior and anterior
layers of rectus sheath

External abdominal oblique
aponeurosis and muscle (cut)

Internal abdominal oblique
aponeurosis and muscle (cut)

Transversus abdominis
aponeurosis and muscle (cut)

Arcuate line

Transversalis fascia

Inferior epigastric vessels
(passing through transversalis
fascia)

Deep inguinal ring

Rectus abdominis
muscle (cut)

Internal spermatic fascia

Cremaster muscle (cut)

External spermatic fascia (cut)

B

Skin and dartos muscle and fascia (cut)

Figure 5-8 (continued)

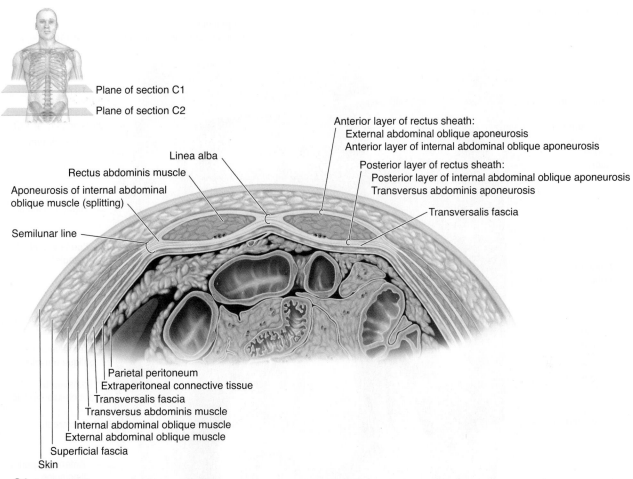

Plane of section C1

Plane of section C2

Linea alba

Rectus abdominis muscle

Aponeurosis of internal abdominal oblique muscle (splitting)

Semilunar line

Anterior layer of rectus sheath:
External abdominal oblique aponeurosis
Anterior layer of internal abdominal oblique aponeurosis

Posterior layer of rectus sheath:
Posterior layer of internal abdominal oblique aponeurosis
Transversus abdominis aponeurosis

Transversalis fascia

Parietal peritoneum
Extraperitoneal connective tissue
Transversalis fascia
Transversus abdominis muscle
Internal abdominal oblique muscle
External abdominal oblique muscle
Superficial fascia
Skin

C1 Cross-section superior to arcuate line

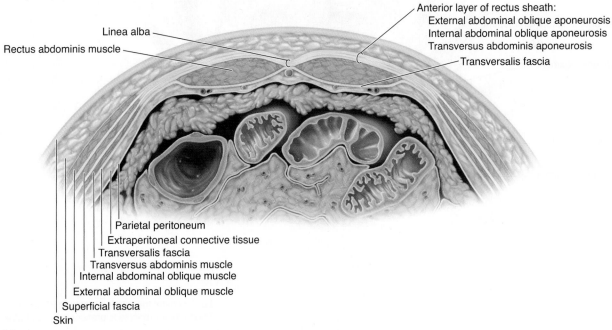

Linea alba

Rectus abdominis muscle

Anterior layer of rectus sheath:
External abdominal oblique aponeurosis
Internal abdominal oblique aponeurosis
Transversus abdominis aponeurosis

Transversalis fascia

Parietal peritoneum
Extraperitoneal connective tissue
Transversalis fascia
Transversus abdominis muscle
Internal abdominal oblique muscle
External abdominal oblique muscle
Superficial fascia
Skin

C2 Cross-section inferior to arcuate line

Figure 5-8 *(continued)* **C:** Cross-section views of the abdominal muscles at the upper and lower abdominal areas.

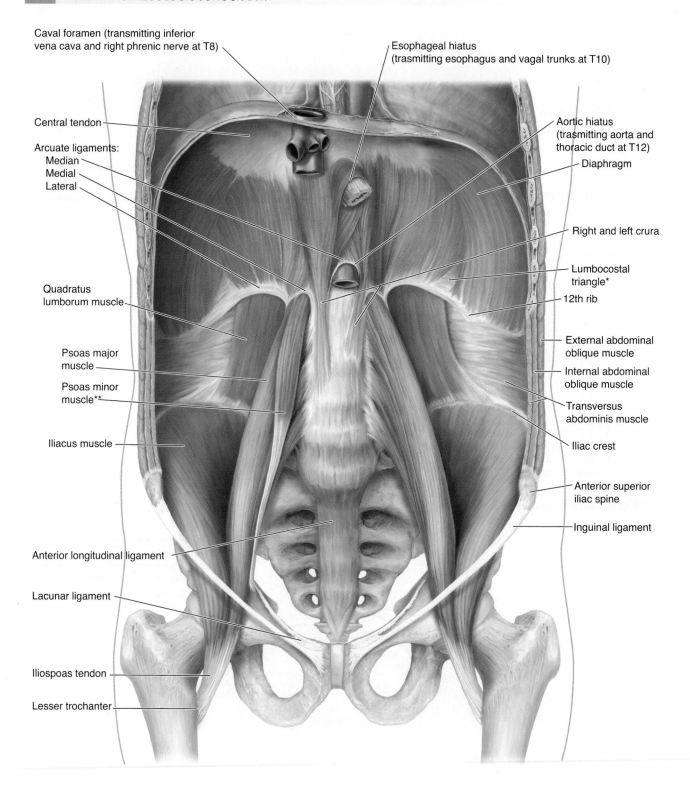

Caval foramen (transmitting inferior vena cava and right phrenic nerve at T8)

Esophageal hiatus (trasmitting esophagus and vagal trunks at T10)

Central tendon

Arcuate ligaments:
Median
Medial
Lateral

Aortic hiatus (trasmitting aorta and thoracic duct at T12)

Diaphragm

Right and left crura

Lumbocostal triangle*

12th rib

Quadratus lumborum muscle

External abdominal oblique muscle

Psoas major muscle

Internal abdominal oblique muscle

Psoas minor muscle**

Transversus abdominis muscle

Iliacus muscle

Iliac crest

Anterior superior iliac spine

Inguinal ligament

Anterior longitudinal ligament

Lacunar ligament

Iliospoas tendon

Lesser trochanter

* Lumbocostal triangle is present in 80% of cases
** Psoas minor muscle is present in 50% of cases

Figure 5-9 Muscles of the posterior body wall and the false pelvis, viewed from the front.

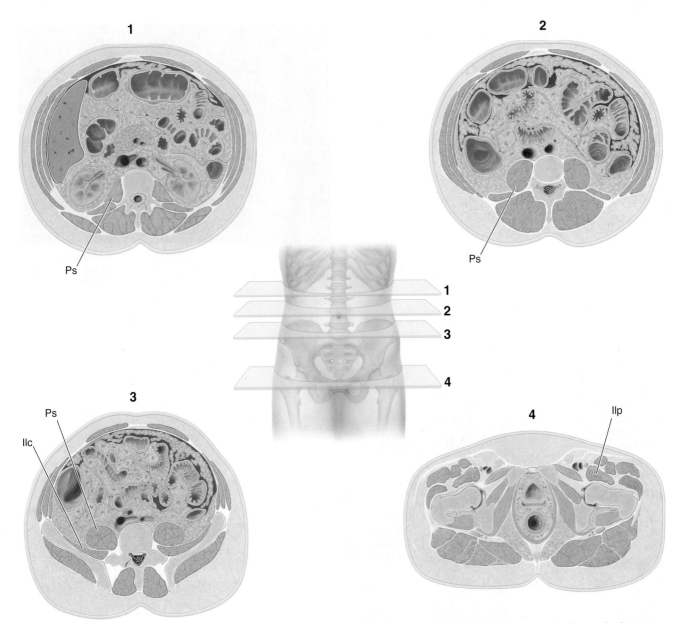

Figure 5-10 Shape of the iliopsoas muscles on cross-section at various levels in the abdomen and pelvis. *Ps*, psoas; *Ilc*, Iliacus; *Ilp*, iliopsoas.

a bulbous medial limb (Fig. 5-10, section 4). On sagittal ultrasound scans, these muscles appear as a long, dark strip with a posterior margin coursing upward toward the anterior wall as the body muscle complex descends through the pelvis (Fig. 5-11). The iliopsoas does not enter the true pelvis. In the false pelvis, its medial margin crosses the linea terminalis and thus marks the border between the true and false pelvis (Fig. 5-12).

Within the true pelvic space is the obturator internus muscle (Fig. 5-13). This triangular sheet of muscle originates as bands of fibers anchored along the brim of the true pelvis and from the inner surface of the obturator membrane, which closes the obturator foramen.[2] The muscle extends posteriorly and medially along the sidewall of the true pelvis, passing beneath the levator ani muscles to exit from the pelvic space through the lesser sciatic foramen. Because it lies parallel and adjacent to the lateral pelvic

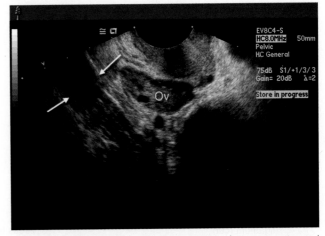

Figure 5-11 Endovaginal image demonstrating the psoas major and iliac muscles *(between arrows)* in the true pelvis adjacent to the ovary *(Ov)*. Faint lines within the muscle arise from the fiber bundles and fascial planes. Note the upward slant of the posterior wall of the muscle group.

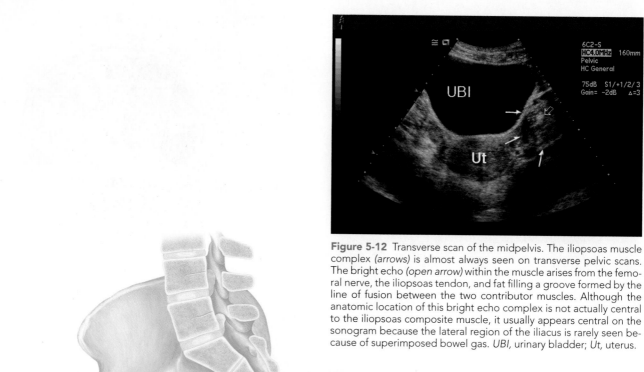

Figure 5-12 Transverse scan of the midpelvis. The iliopsoas muscle complex *(arrows)* is almost always seen on transverse pelvic scans. The bright echo *(open arrow)* within the muscle arises from the femoral nerve, the iliopsoas tendon, and fat filling a groove formed by the line of fusion between the two contributor muscles. Although the anatomic location of this bright echo complex is not actually central to the iliopsoas composite muscle, it usually appears central on the sonogram because the lateral region of the iliacus is rarely seen because of superimposed bowel gas. *UBI,* urinary bladder; *Ut,* uterus.

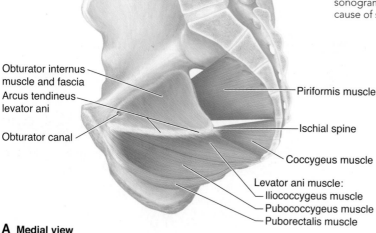

Obturator internus
muscle and fascia

Arcus tendineus
levator ani

Obturator canal

Piriformis muscle

Ischial spine

Coccygeus muscle

Levator ani muscle:
— Iliococcygeus muscle
— Pubococcygeus muscle
— Puborectalis muscle

A Medial view

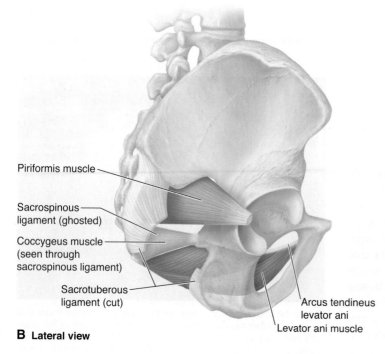

Piriformis muscle

Sacrospinous
ligament (ghosted)

Coccygeus muscle
(seen through
sacrospinous ligament)

Sacrotuberous
ligament (cut)

Arcus tendineus
levator ani

Levator ani muscle

B Lateral view

Figure 5-13 A: Lateral view of pelvis with the deep pelvic sidewall muscles. The piriformis muscle exits the true pelvis through the greater sciatic foramen; the obturator internus exits the true pelvis through the lesser sciatic foramen. These foramina are defined by the sacrospinous and the sacrotuberous ligaments. **B:** The obturator internus muscle exhibits a tendinous band that runs anterior to posterior across the muscle. This band is the point of attachment for the pelvic diaphragm, which is in part suspended from the surface of the obturator internus muscle.

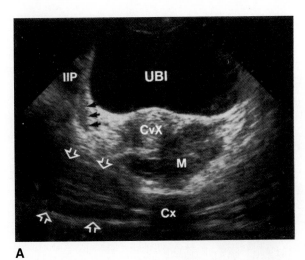
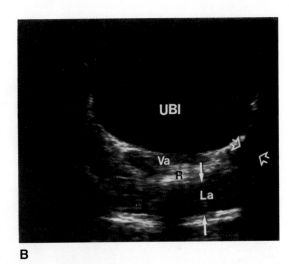

A   **B**

Figure 5-14 A: Transverse scan of the pelvis demonstrates the obturator internus muscle as a thin, hypoechoic strip *(black arrows)* adjacent to the lateral pelvic wall. The upper margin of the muscle is just below the brim of the pelvis. The levator ani muscle group is also well seen *(open arrows)*. *UBI,* urinary bladder; *CvX,* cervix; *Cx,* coccyx; *M,* mass adjacent to cervix; *Ilp,* iliopsoas muscle. **B:** Forming the floor of the true pelvic space is the levator ani muscle group *(arrows)*, which attaches to the medial surface of the obturator internus muscle *(open arrows)*. *UBI,* urinary bladder; *La,* levator ani muscle; *R,* rectum; *Va,* vagina.

wall, the obturator internus is difficult to identify on a sagittal ultrasound image. At normal gain levels it is often obscured on transverse scans as well; however, when it is visible, the obturator appears as a thin, hypoechoic, vertical strip lining the wall of the pelvis (Fig. 5-14).

Deeply posterior in the true pelvis is another roughly triangular muscle, the piriformis, which originates from the sacrum and then courses laterally through the greater sciatic foramen and inserts on the greater trochanter of the femur (Fig. 5-15).[2] Unless the urinary bladder is very full, the piriformis is usually obscured by overlying bowel gas in the sigmoid colon.

A complex group of mutually similar muscles collectively forms a two-layered pelvic diaphragm forming the floor of the true pelvis. The outermost layer is composed of the muscles of the perineum, which are rarely identifiable in transabdominal ultrasound images. In contrast, the innermost layer of the pelvic diaphragm commonly visualizes in transverse ultrasound images. The named muscles of the innermost group include, from posterior to anterior, the coccygeus, the iliococcygeus, and the pubococcygeus, a part of which is classified as the puborectalis muscle (Figs. 5-15 and 5-16).[2] The iliococcygeus, pubococcygeus, and puborectalis are more correctly described as the levator ani muscles. Most authors include the coccygeus as part of the levator ani, but some do not because it functions only to support the sacrum.

The levator ani is similar to a hammock stretched between the pubis and the coccyx. Its lateral margins attach to a thickened band of the fascia that covers the obturator internus muscle, thus anchoring the levator ani to the lateral pelvic walls.[2] In the midline, fibers from the levator ani insert on the walls of the rectum, vagina, and urethra as they pass through the pelvic diaphragm.

The levator ani and the gravity resist increased intraabdominal pressure, such as in coughing or straining,

holding the pelvic organs in place (Fig. 5-17).[2] If these muscles fail in their function, one of the results is prolapse of the pelvic organs through the pelvic floor.

THE PELVIC ORGANS

The pelvic organs are (1) the external genitalia, (2) the urinary bladder and urethra, (3) the uterus, fallopian tubes, and vagina, (4) the ovaries, and (5) the colon and rectum.

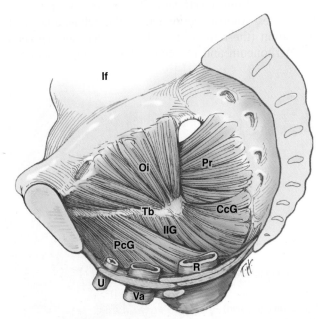

Figure 5-15 A more detailed view of the pelvic muscles with the pelvic diaphragm in place. The ragged edges along the tendinous band of the obturator internus are the cut edges of the fascial membrane that covers these muscles. The major orifices that pass through the pelvic diaphragm are also shown. *Oi,* obturator internus muscle; *Pr,* piriformis muscle; *Tb,* tendinous band; *CcG,* coccygeus muscle; *IlG,* iliococcygeus; *PcG,* pubococcygeus; *U,* urethra; *Va,* vagina; *R,* rectum; *If,* iliac fossa.

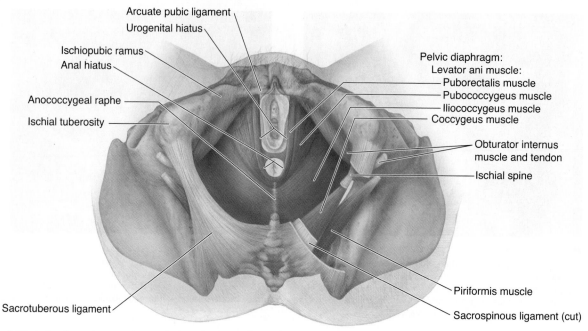

Arcuate pubic ligament
Urogenital hiatus
Ischiopubic ramus
Anal hiatus
Anococcygeal raphe
Ischial tuberosity

Pelvic diaphragm:
Levator ani muscle:
Puborectalis muscle
Pubococcygeus muscle
Iliococcygeus muscle
Coccygeus muscle
Obturator internus muscle and tendon
Ischial spine
Piriformis muscle
Sacrospinous ligament (cut)

Sacrotuberous ligament

Figure 5-16 A view from above and posterior into the true pelvis. Relate the position of the muscles in this view to the view shown in Figure 5-15.

Before beginning a detailed examination of the organs of the female pelvis, the reader should take a moment to conceptualize the various layers of the pelvic walls formed by the bones, muscles, aponeuroses, and tendons. Like the walls of a house, this wall provides a relatively rigid framework that supports a layer of fascia composed of loose connective tissue through which runs the "plumbing" (arteries, veins, and lymphatics) and the "electrical and communication lines," the nerves. Almost everywhere in the pelvis, a layer of insulation (the retroperitoneal fat, which lies between the peritoneum and the endopelvic fascia) covers the

membranous fascia. The peritoneum covers the surface and the organs reside within the pelvis. Most of the organs of the female pelvis—the urinary bladder, uterus, and rectum—are extraperitoneally located. From a practical standpoint, however, the pelvic organs should be conceptualized as being inside the area defined by the pelvic walls. These organs constantly change size as the urinary bladder and rectum expand and contract. The uterus also expands during pregnancy, contracting after the birth of the fetus.

The arrangement of the organs within the pelvic space (Fig. 5-18) facilitates dimensional changes, but it

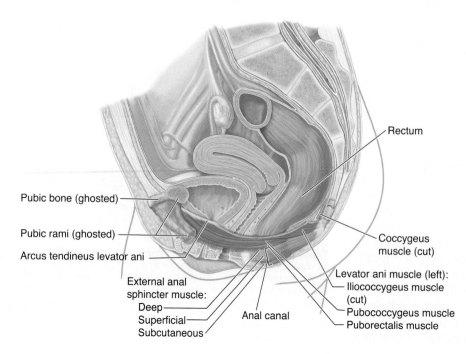

Pubic bone (ghosted)
Pubic rami (ghosted)
Arcus tendineus levator ani

External anal
sphincter muscle:
Deep
Superficial
Subcutaneous

Anal canal

Rectum

Coccygeus muscle (cut)

Levator ani muscle (left):
Iliococcygeus muscle (cut)
Pubococcygeus muscle
Puborectalis muscle

Figure 5-17 Relationship of the pubococcygeus muscle of the levator ani to the orifices that pass through the pelvic diaphragm.

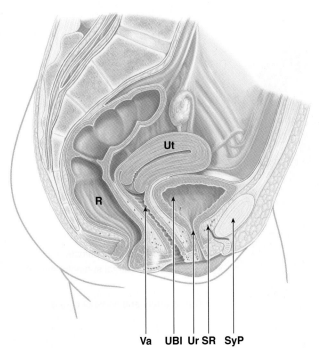

Figure 5-18 Midline view of the female pelvis. *Va,* vagina; *UBl,* urinary bladder; *Ur,* urethra; *SR,* space of Retzius; *SyP,* symphysis pubis; *Ut,* uterus; *R,* rectum.

also means that the position and contour of each organ varies in response to the degree of filling of the other organs that share the same space. These variations dramatically affect the ultrasound image, as is described later in this chapter.

THE EXTERNAL GENITALIA

Before insertion of the endovaginal transducer, the sonographer should carefully inspect the female perineum, the area located between the vulva and the anus. The female pubic hair forms a triangle with its base located on the superior surface of the mons pubis. The labia majora are easily visible. The clitoris and its hood are visible at the superior end of the labia majora. In young females, the labia minora may not be visible between the labia majora. The labia minora open to flank the vestibule of the vagina, which receives the urethral caruncle and ostium of the vagina. Sonography also allows imaging of the female labia, perineum, and urethra via transperitoneal ultrasound.

THE URINARY BLADDER AND URETHRA

The urinary bladder is a thick-walled, highly distensible muscular sac that lies between the symphysis pubis and the vagina. When empty, its shape on a sagittal section is an inverted triangle with the apex, which is posterior to the pubic bones, at the orifice of the urethra.

The anterior surface of the bladder is loosely anchored to the pubic arch by fibrous connective tissue (the pubovesical ligament) but is separated from the symphysis pubis by an interposed pad of extraperitoneal fat in the space of Retzius, or preperitoneal space.[3] The posterior wall is composed largely of the trigone region, which is defined by the orifices of the two ureters and the urethra (Fig. 5-19). A thin layer of fat and connective tissue separates the anterior vaginal wall from the bladder, with a thicker, rigid area indicating the trigone region. The superior wall, the dome of the bladder, is covered by the parietal peritoneum and usually is in contact with the anterior wall of the uterus, which folds forward to rest on the dome (Fig. 5-18).

The walls of the urinary bladder are composed of three layers, but only two are visible on sonography. The thick middle muscularis layer or detrusor muscle is composed predominantly of smooth muscle fibers, which give the bladder its contractility. The outer serosal layer is not visible in ultrasound scans because it is thin and in intimate contact with adjacent layers of fascia and fatty tissues that cover most of the anterior and posterior walls. The inner layer of the bladder is the mucosa, which is very echogenic. Sonographic demonstration of the muscularis and mucosa depends on the degree of bladder filling. When the urinary bladder is empty, the bladder mucosa is quite thick and easily demonstrated (Fig. 5-20A). The distended bladder stretches the mucosal lining, resulting in thinning and the inability to identify the mucosa as a discrete layer.

Extending from the kidneys are the two ureters, which carry urine from the kidneys into the bladder. The urethra conducts urine from the bladder, crossing into the pelvic inlet anterior to the common iliac artery bifurcation, coursing posterior to the ovary, and lateral to the vagina to terminate at the urethral orifice. The urethra lies between the labia minora of the external female genitalia. The thickened muscular internal sphincter surrounds the urethra marking the urethral exit. Sagittal sonographic images of this area often visualize this structure (Fig. 5-20B).

Peristaltic contraction of the ureter walls transports urine into the bladder. As the contraction reaches the bladder, back pressure from the bladder must be overcome; the ureteral valve pops open and a bolus of urine enters the bladder in a brief jet (Fig. 5-21). Urine jets routinely image on sonography with high gain in gray-scale imaging or with color Doppler, but the jet is transient and the echoes disappear quickly. The cause of these echoes is the subject of debate, but it is probable that the pressure differential between the jet and the surrounding urine is sufficient explanation. Urine in the renal calyces, pelvis, ureters, and urinary bladder is normally sterile and completely anechoic.

The contour of the urinary bladder does not change uniformly as it expands with filling. The dome is the most distensible region of the bladder, so it might be expected to expand uniformly in the cephalad direction, but two factors dictate nonuniform expansion of

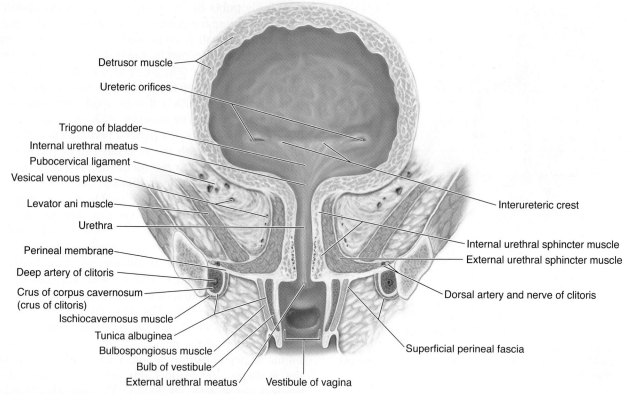

Detrusor muscle
Ureteric orifices
Trigone of bladder
Internal urethral meatus
Pubocervical ligament
Vesical venous plexus
Levator ani muscle
Urethra
Perineal membrane
Deep artery of clitoris
Crus of corpus cavernosum (crus of clitoris)
Ischiocavernosus muscle
Tunica albuginea
Bulbospongiosus muscle
Bulb of vestibule
External urethral meatus
Vestibule of vagina
Interureteric crest
Internal urethral sphincter muscle
External urethral sphincter muscle
Dorsal artery and nerve of clitoris
Superficial perineal fascia

Figure 5-19 Cutaway view of the posterior wall of the urinary bladder. The ureters enter the bladder at the level of the cervix and on the posterior and inferior wall of the bladder. Their passage through the bladder wall is oblique, forming a passive valve system that resists urine reflux. Orientation of the bladder has the base anterior to the vagina, neck resting on the urogenital diaphragm, and the apex posterior to the pubic bones.

the bladder walls. First, the trigone is thicker and more rigid; second, the bladder must accommodate the space requirements of the other organs in the pelvis, chiefly the uterus. Because the uterus is normally anteverted and rests on the posterior and midregions of the dome, the anterior bladder wall has the least resistance to expansion. This region needs to displace only highly mobile loops of small bowel, which normally fill any unoccupied space in the true pelvis. The anterior part of the urinary bladder expands upward, resulting in the typical asymmetric shape of the distended bladder on sagittal section (Fig. 5-22).

Because the bladder contour molds to or "reflects" structures with which it is in contact, the examiner

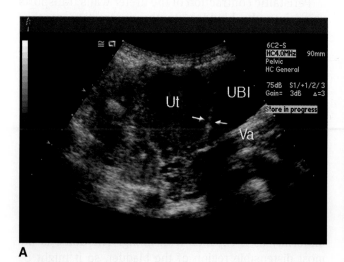

A

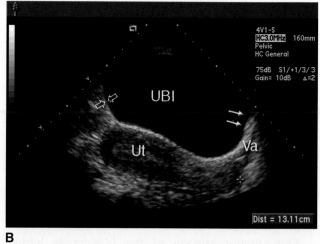

B

Figure 5-20 A: Sagittal scan in midline. When the urinary bladder contains only a small amount of urine, the bladder walls *(arrows)* are thick and easily demonstrated. **B:** Sagittal scan in midline. When fully distended, the bladder walls *(open arrows)* nearly disappear from the image. The "urethral hump" formed by the internal sphincter is clearly visible in this scan *(solid arrows)*. *UBl*, urinary bladder; *Ut*, uterus; *Va*, vagina.

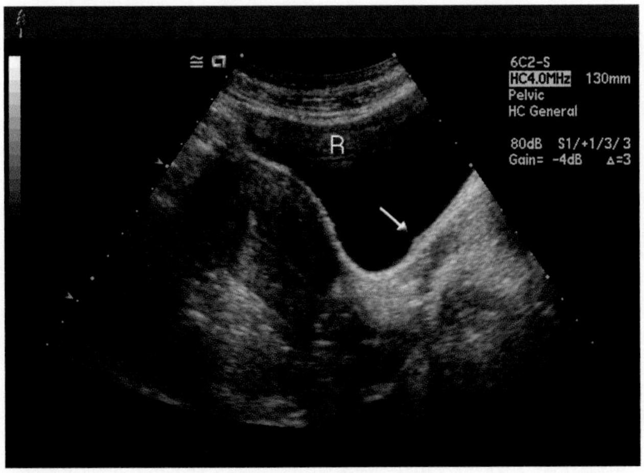

A

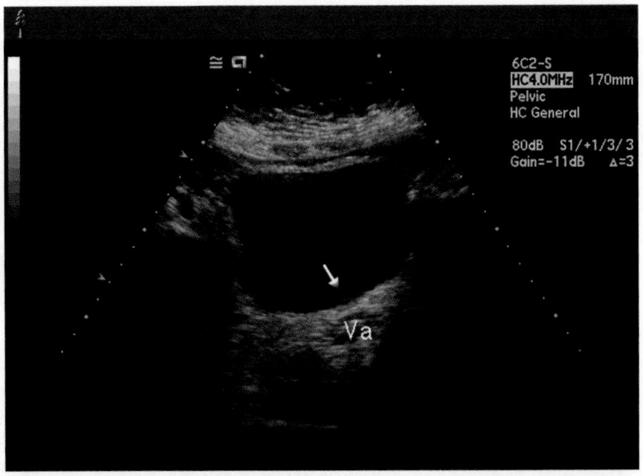

B

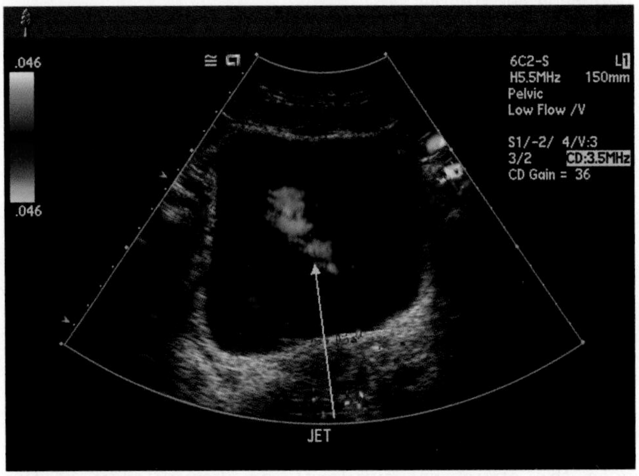

C

Figure 5-21 **A:** Sagittal scan slightly to the left of midline. The ureteric valve is visible occasionally as a small projection *(arrow)*. When the valve structure is normal, this projection appears only briefly as the valve pops open. If persistent, it may represent a ureterocele. This image is also a good example of the typical reverberation artifact *(R)*, which occurs as a result of the repeated reflection of the acoustic beam between the tissue layers. **B:** A slightly oblique transverse scan shows the left urtric valve *(arrow)* anterior to the vagina *(Va)*. **C:** Color Doppler of the region of the ureteric orifices often shows dramatic plumes of color when the jets enter the urinary bladder.

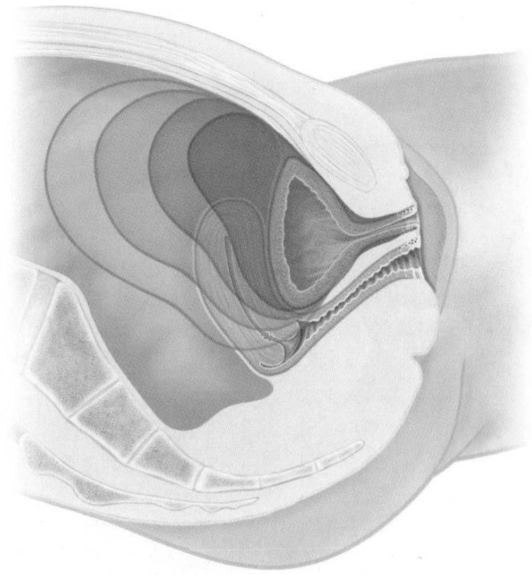

Figure 5-22 Contours of the urinary bladder with progressive filling. The uterus is shown in its initial position, folded forward over the dome of the empty urinary bladder. For clarity, the corresponding positions of the uterus are not shown, although the indentation of the posterior bladder wall by the uterus is indicated for each stage of filling.

should carefully examine the urinary bladder before trying to determine the identity and relationship of other structures in the pelvis. The urinary bladder contours provide a "reverse map" of the pelvis (Figs. 5-23 and 5-24). In addition, urine in the bladder provides both a window and a reference standard. Like water, urine attenuates ultrasound frequencies only slightly, permitting transmission deep into the pelvis with minimal attenuation. If there are echoes in the urine (with the exception of the normal anterior wall reverberation artifact seen on transabdominal sonography), then either the gain setting is too high or the urine is abnormal.

Cell casts from the renal tubules and uric acid crystals can cause punctate echoes in the urine, but sonographers encounter these only rarely. More often, echoes in the urine represent "noise" associated with a high gain or power output level. If such false echoes appear in the urine, they will also appear in soft tissues, making identification difficult. The most common technical error in gynecologic sonography is excessive gain obscuring subtle details within the soft

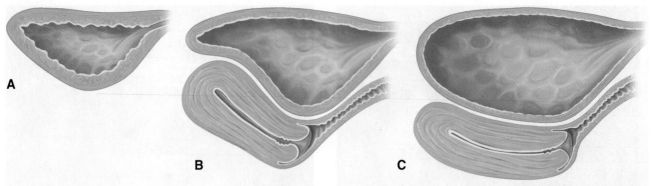

Figure 5-23 The urinary bladder contour is directly influenced by the presence of the uterus within the defined space of the pelvis. When the uterus has been surgically removed or is congenitally absent, the bladder contour is distinctly deltoid **(A)**. The normal anteflexed uterus creates a gentle indentation of the moderately distended bladder **(B)**. The degree of indentation is influenced by the size of the uterus and the degree of bladder filling. If overdistended, the bladder can compress the uterus excessively, altering the uterine shape and echo pattern **(C)**. The ideal degree of filling results in extension of the bladder one to two centimeters above the fundus of the uterus, while preserving the normal uterine contour.

tissues. A good rule of thumb is to use the minimum output and gain level consistent with adequate demonstration of tissue echo patterns. The second way in which urine serves as a reference standard is for comparison with other echo patterns in pelvic structures. The appropriate gain level results in the same anechoic appearance in cystic structures of the ovary (such as follicles) (Fig. 5-25).

By comparing the echogenicity of the urine with the echogenicity of the unknown structure at various gain levels, the sonographer can qualitatively assess the structural similarity or dissimilarity of the two. Echogenicity is not a definitive criterion for the presence of fluid. Homogeneous solid uterine fibroids can be anechoic at normal gain levels and fluids (e.g., blood, pus) can be echogenic. Distinguishing fluid from

solid tissue requires the use of both echogenicity and through-transmission characteristics.

THE VAGINA

The vagina is a relatively thin-walled, 7- to 10-centimeter-long muscular tube that extends from the cervix of the uterus to the vestibule of the external genitalia and lies between the urinary bladder and the rectum.[4] Half lies within the perineum, while the lower half lies above the pelvic floor. The walls contain smooth muscle and elastic connective tissue and are lined with stratified squamous epithelium, similar to skin, hence its name; the vagina is essentially an invagination of the skin. The outer surface of the vagina (the adventitial coat) is a thin, fibrous layer that is continuous with the

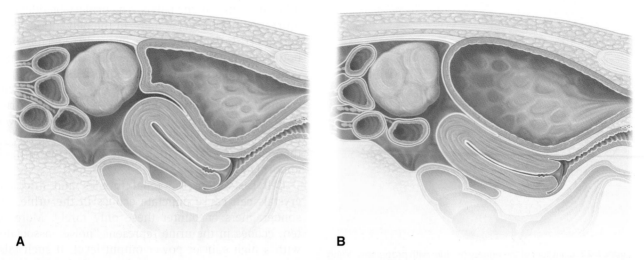

Figure 5-24 The cephalad margin of the urinary bladder can provide an important clue to the presence of a mass superior to the urinary bladder and uterine fundus **(A)**. If the bladder is only moderately distended, it can respond to the weight of a mass by forming a gentle curve around the mass **(B)**. As the bladder wall becomes tense with overdistention, the weight of a cephalad mass may be insufficient to alter the bladder contour. Because masses cephalad to the urinary bladder and uterine fundus may be surrounded by loops of small bowel, the bladder contour may be the only indication of the presence of the mass.

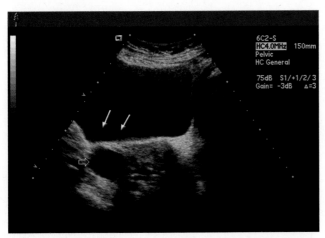

Figure 5-25 A side lobe artifact appears as false echoes *(straight arrows)* in the posterior area of the bladder while reverberation occurs in the anterior portion. These artifactual echoes also appear in the follicular cyst in the ovary *(open arrow)*.

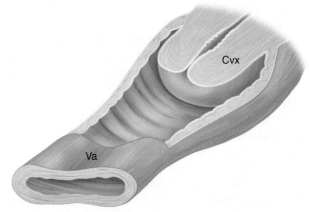

Figure 5-27 Cutaway view of vagina. Note cross-section when collapsed and relationship of uterine cervix *(Cvx)* to vaginal *(Va)* walls.

surrounding endopelvic fascia (Fig. 5-26). Normally, the vaginal canal is a potential space, because the anterior and posterior walls are in apposition. When collapsed, the vagina assumes a rounded "H" shape on cross-section, and the inner mucosal surface of the wall wrinkles up to form transverse ridges (rugae), which largely disappear when the vaginal wall is stretched (Fig. 5-27).

The posterior wall of the vagina is longer than the anterior wall. The upper end of the vagina attaches to the cervix of the uterus along an oblique line about halfway up the length of the cervix.[3] This form of attachment creates a ring-shaped, blind pocket (the fornix) between the outer wall of the cervix and the inner surface of the vaginal wall. By convention, this continuous ring-shaped space divides the anterior, lateral, and posterior fornices (Fig. 5-28). Because of the oblique attachment of the vagina to the cervix, the posterior fornix is deeper than the anterior, and its posterior location causes it to be the site of pooling of urine, pus, blood, or other fluid that originates in the vagina.

The length and wall thickness of the vagina vary in response to filling of the urinary bladder. The vagina attaches to the displaced uterus, thus stretching and reducing the thickness of the vaginal wall as the bladder expands. The combined thickness of the normal anterior and posterior vaginal walls should not exceed

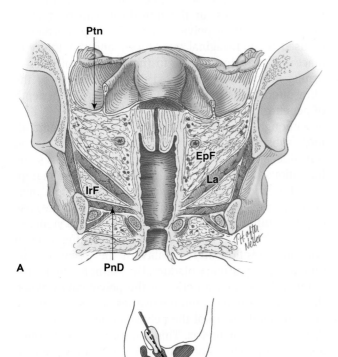

Figure 5-26 A: Oblique section through lower uterus and vagina. The plane of section is indicated in **(B)**. The uterus has been elevated to stretch the vagina and align it with the plane of section. Note the relationship between the perineal diaphragm and the levator ani muscle group. *PnD*, perineal diaphragm; *La*, levator ani; *EpF*, endopelvic fascia; *Ptn*, peritoneum; *IrF*, ischiorectal fossa.

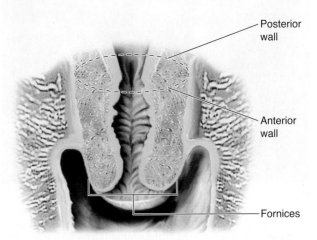

Figure 5-28 Relationship between uterus and vagina. The posterior vaginal wall attaches higher on the cervix than the anterior wall. The fornices are the blind pockets formed by the inner surface of the vaginal walls and the outer surface of the cervix. These spaces are normally collapsed or contain only a small amount of mucus.

one centimeter when measured from a transabdominal scan with the urinary bladder distended.[5]

On sonograms, the muscular walls of the vagina produce a moderately hypoechoic pattern typical of smooth muscle (Fig. 5-29). The mucosa of the vagina is highly echogenic, but it may be difficult to visualize when the walls of the vagina are stretched by a distended bladder (Fig. 5-30). Although the vagina can move laterally in response to pressure from a distended rectum, it is most commonly at or near the sagittal midline of the pelvis. Its anteroposterior position, however, varies substantially in response to the degree of filling of the urinary bladder and the rectum. In addition, the upper part of the vagina follows the cervix if the uterus displaces laterally by a pelvic mass or a distended rectum or sigmoid colon.

The introduction of endovaginal ultrasound imaging has placed new emphasis on the importance of a

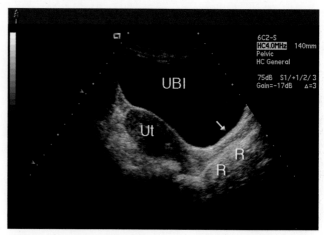

Figure 5-30 Echo pattern of the vagina when the bladder is fully distended. The vaginal walls can be identified readily (arrow). Ut, uterus; UBl, urinary bladder; R, rectum.

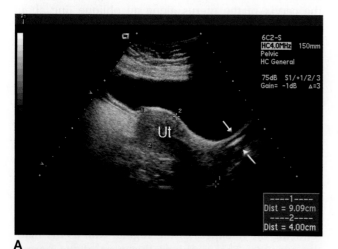

A

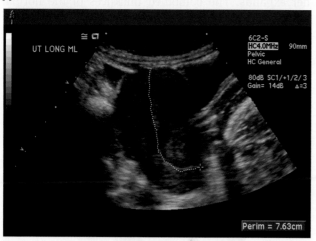

B

Figure 5-29 A: Median sagittal scan with the bladder filled. Note the thickness (arrows) and cephalocaudad length of the vaginal walls. The vaginal canal is indicated by the interrupted bright line separating the anterior and posterior walls. (Ut, uterus) Demonstrated is the usual method of measuring the uterus for length and AP dimension in a patient with a full bladder. **B:** If the patient presents with a partially full or empty bladder, the normal anteverted position of the uterus makes an accurate longitudinal measurement difficult. This image demonstrates an alternate method using the trace function.

complete understanding of the anatomy of the vagina and its relationship to the surrounding organs. The typical endovaginal exam requires an empty or nearly empty urinary bladder (Fig. 5-31). A specially designed transducer inserts into the vagina with the footprint of the transducer positioned at the tip of the cervix or in the fornix. The ultrasound beam may then be directed anteriorly and cephalad to image the uterus, fallopian tubes, and ovaries, or the transducer can be rotated to view the lateral pelvic walls.[6] The higher frequency used by endovaginal transducers and the ability to place the transducer close to the structure of interest results in markedly improved detail resolution of the ultrasound image (Fig. 5-31B,C) at the sacrifice of depth of penetration.

Although the remarkable flexibility of the vagina affords substantial latitude in positioning the ultrasound transducer, the shape of the pelvic cavity imposes some limitations. In addition, the transducer must be manipulated judiciously. The patient may have limited tolerance for transducer movement, particularly in the case of pelvic inflammation, adhesions, or vaginal stenosis. The examiner also must be aware of the differences in anatomic position and mobility of the pelvic organs with an empty urinary bladder. For example, the uterus is much lower and anterior in the pelvic cavity when the bladder is empty, and the ovaries are usually in the posterolateral region of the pelvis and may lie at some distance from the uterus. This is in contrast with transabdominal pelvic scans, on which the ovaries are usually deeper in the true pelvic space and press against the lateral or superior margins of the uterus.

THE UTERUS

In nulliparous women the uterus is a small, pear-shaped muscular organ suspended in the true pelvis. In one sense, the uterus is only a prominent bulge in

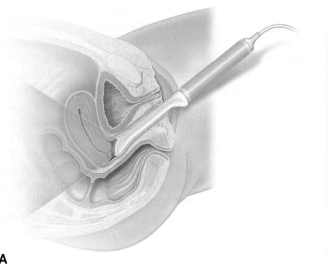

A

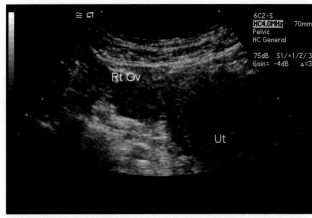

B

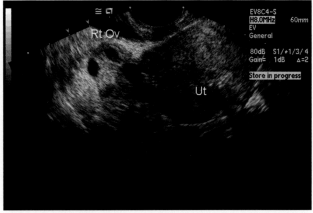

C

Figure 5-31 A: Endovaginal sonography permits the specially adapted transducer to be placed close to the organs of interest. These transducers generate higher acoustic frequencies, increasing the detail of imaged anatomy. **B:** A transverse transabdominal view of the right ovary. **C:** A endovaginal image of the same ovary. Note the improved visualization of the internal structure of the ovary. (*Rt Ov*, right ovary; *Ut*, uterus.)

the middle section of a continuous muscular canal that begins with the fallopian tubes and ends with the external orifice of the vagina (Fig. 5-32), but, because its structure and size are so different from the fallopian tubes and the vagina, the uterus is usually considered a separate organ. Its sole function is reproductive; it receives the fertilized egg and nourishes the developing conceptus, and ultimately expels the fetus.

Segments of the Uterus

The uterus has four segments: the fundus, corpus, isthmus, and cervix. The arbitrarily defined regions

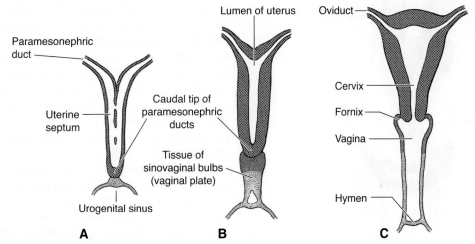

Figure 5-32 Paramesonephric ducts merge to form a uterus. The paramesonephric ducts from each side merge into themselves at their bottoms and erode their walls to form a single chamber, the future uterus, as seen in schematic frontal view **(A).** The merger still abuts the back wall of the bladder (shown here as the urogenital sinus), but eventually the duct draws up the back wall **(B)** and evacuates it to form a canal at the bottom end of the uterus **(C).** Importantly, as seen in the far right **(C),** this canal is still closed to the outside world because it never did break down the back wall of the bladder. (From Sadler TW. Langman's Medical Embryology, 9th Edition Image Bank. Baltimore: Lippincott Williams & Wilkins, 2004.)

use the uterine contour and structure as landmarks (Fig. 5-33).

Fundus

The most cephalad portion of the uterus is the fundus ("bottom"), which begins at the point where the fallopian tubes arise from the uterine walls. The fundus is a rounded or dome-shaped area above the level of the uterine cavity. It narrows at its outer and lateral margins to form the cornu, i.e., horn of the uterus,[7] through which passes the interstitial portion of the fallopian tube (Fig. 5-33).

Corpus and Isthmus

The corpus (body) is the largest portion of the uterus within which is the uterine cavity. On cross-section, the corpus appears rounded or ovoid (Fig. 5-34). In both sagittal and coronal sections, the corpus usually appears cylindrical or slightly tapered, narrowing as it approaches the isthmus, or the waist, of the uterus. The isthmus marks the transition from the corpus to the cervix, or neck. The isthmus is the most flexible portion.

Cervix

The cervix is the cylindrical neck of the uterus which projects into the vagina (Fig. 5-35). It contains more

fibrous and less muscular tissue and has a distinctive endothelium. This barrel-shaped cylinder is slightly wider in the middle and 2 to 3 centimeters long in nulliparous women.[7] The hyperechoic mucosa images as a spindle-shaped endocervical canal, sometimes referred to as the endocervix, and extends from the internal to the external os. Oblique ridges or palmate folds slant downward toward the external os.[7] The endocervical mucosa has a rich supply of mucous glands on the anterior and posterior surfaces (Fig. 5-36A,B). The mucus serves to impede upward migration of bacteria from the vagina into the uterus. In pregnancy, the mucosa of the endocervical canal undergoes hypertrophy and the glands produce a dense, sticky mucous plug (the mucous plug of pregnancy) which effectively seals the uterus.

The Uterine Cavity

The uterine cavity has an inverted triangle shape with the basal angles defined by the fallopian tube ostia and the cervical internal os defining the apex. The cavity is widest at the fundus and narrowest at the isthmus, and it narrows in AP direction, so that the anterior and posterior endometrial surfaces are normally separated only by a thin layer of mucus.

Layers of the Uterus

The walls of the uterus are composed of three tissue layers (Fig. 5-37). The outermost layer is the serosa or perimetrium, which is quite thin and not visible on sonography. The serosa is continuous with the pelvic fascia. The thick middle layer, the myometrium, is composed of smooth muscle cells and interspersed connective tissue fibers. Lining the inner surface of the uterus is a mucosa known as the endometrium, which forms the walls of the uterine cavity.

Myometrium

The muscular middle layer of the uterus forms most of the bulk of the uterine body. The myometrium may be subdivided into three rather indistinct layers: an outer layer characterized by longitudinal muscle fibers, a richly vascularized thick middle layer (Fig. 5-37B,C, Fig. 5-38), and a denser inner layer of which predominantly spiral muscle fibers are arranged both longitudinally and obliquely.[7] Throughout a woman's reproductive years, the muscles of the uterus demonstrate a low-amplitude contractile activity to maintain the muscle tone of the uterus. Just before and during the menstrual flow, contractile activity results in slow, ripplelike contractions originating in the fundus and sweeping in the caudal direction to the internal os. These contractions are of low amplitude and slow, requiring several seconds to progress from fundus to the isthmus. The progressive focal rippling distortion of the endometrial echo pattern images during endovaginal imaging. During ovulation, EVS images contractions sweeping in the opposite direction, cephalad from the internal os to the fundus. These contractions may assist the migration

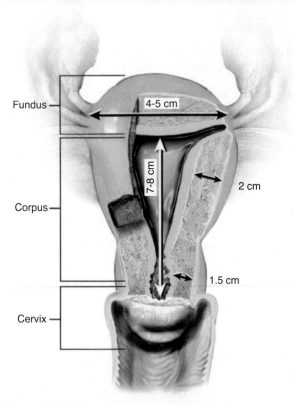

Figure 5-33 The anterior wall of the uterus has been cut out. The three major subdivisions of the uterus are clearly identified: cervix, corpus, and fundus. The thickest musculature is seen in the corpus and fundus. The narrowed area between the internal os of the cervix and the wider corpus is the isthmus.

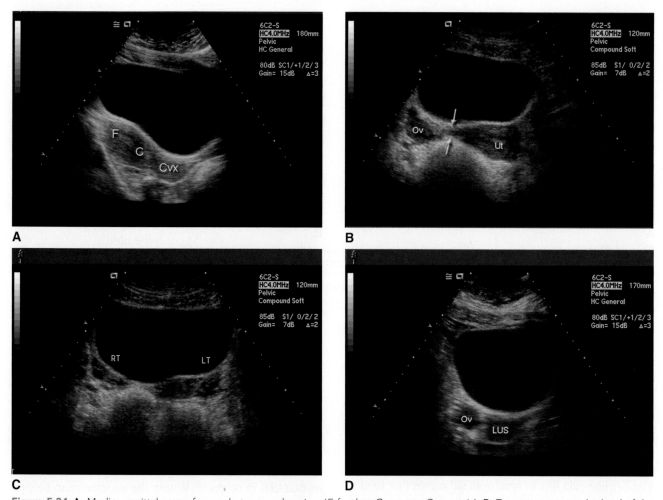

Figure 5-34 A: Median sagittal scan of normal uterus and vagina. (*F*, fundus; *C*, corpus; *Cvx*, cervix). **B:** Transverse scan at the level of the fundus. The right ovary *(OV)* is demonstrated. The broad ligament and/or fallopian tube *(arrows)* bridge the space between the uterine fundus *(Ut)* and the ovary. **C:** Transverse scan demonstrating both ovaries. **D:** Transverse scan at the level of the lower uterine segment *(LUS)*. The right ovary *(OV)* is adjacent to the uterus.

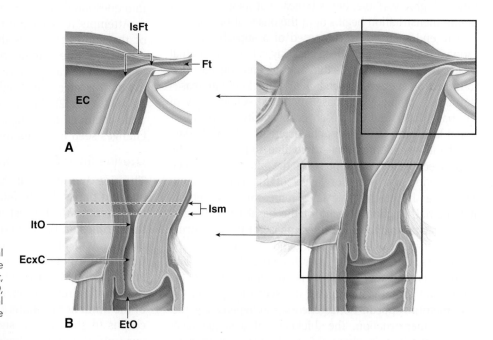

Figure 5-35 Structure of the cornual **(A)** and cervical **(B)** regions of the uterus. *EC,* endometrial cavity; *Ft,* fallopian tube; *ItO,* internal os; *EtO,* external os; *EcxC,* endocervical canal; *IsFt,* interstitial portion of the fallopian tube; *Ism,* isthmus.

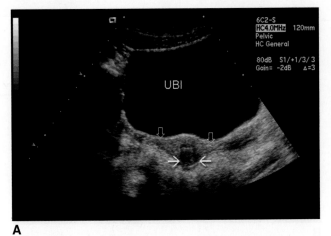

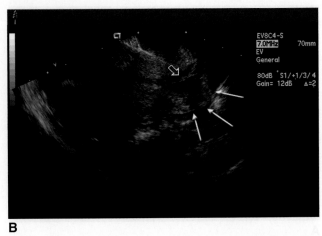

A   **B**

Figure 5-36 A: Transverse scan of a cervix that is shifted to the right side of the pelvic cavity. Note the lateral extensions of the cervical echo pattern *(open arrows)*. These ill-defined "wings" are the transverse cervical ligaments. Also note the shadows *(solid arrows)*, which bracket a central zone of decreased echoes. This pattern is characteristic of the cervix. *(UBI, urinary bladder)*. **B:** Endovaginal sagittal image of the cervix. Note the posterior vaginal wall *(long arrows)*, which extends around the cervical tip to insert on the posterior wall. The prominent endocervical canal *(open arrow)* visualizes throughout the length of the cervix.

of sperm upward through the uterus to the fallopian tubes, with uncoordinated, reverse contractions resulting in fertility problems.[8]

Endometrium

The endometrium is a specialized mucosa that varies in echogenicity, thickness, and composition through the menstrual cycle. Covering the surface are ciliated cells interrupted at intervals by the orifices of mucous glands.[4] The hairlike cilia flex in synchronized waves that tend to force surface mucus toward the cervix. This steady downward flow of a sticky tide of mucus impedes bacteria from migrating upward into the uterine cavity. Although bacteria richly colonize the vagina, the endometrium and the endocervical canal are normally free of foreign microorganisms. The amount of mucus present at any given time is highly variable, but is typically at its greatest just before menstruation begins or at the onset of pregnancy.

The endometrium is composed of a superficial layer (zona functionalis) and a deep basal layer. In the menstrual phase, the endometrium is thin and hyperechogenic. Due to the estrogen effect, the endometrial thickness increases during the proliferative phase. Increased echogenicity of the basal layer and decreased echogenicity of the functional layer lead to the most characteristic sign of the late proliferative endometrium—triple line appearance. The central echogenic line represents the interface between the anterior and posterior layers of the endometrium. The outer hyperechogenic lines represent endometrial–myometrial junction or echo of the basal layer. Progesterone secretion during the luteal phase of the menstrual cycle differentiates endometrial glands for secreting glycoproteins. The functional layer becomes thickened and edematous, and the spiral arteries become tortuous. On ultrasound examination during the secretory phase, the endometrium appears homogeneous and hyperechogenic.

After menstruation, the thickness of a single layer of endometrium is about 0.5 to 1 cubic millimeters,

increasing to a maximum of five to seven millimeters at the onset of the next menstrual flow. Sonographic measurements of the endometrium on the longitudinal axis of the uterus include the anterior and posterior endometrial layers. When measured this way, endometrial thickness ranges from approximately 1 millimeter immediately after menstruation to about 14 millimeters immediately before menstruation. When measuring the endometrium, exclude the outermost, hypoechoic layer, because it is myometrial in origin.[9,10] Within the endometrium proper, up to three layers image (Fig. 5-39A). Their exact clinical significance is a matter of debate; however, it was noted that a thin hypoechoic layer may sometimes be seen lining the innermost surface of the endometrial cavity at the time of ovulation or immediately afterward (Fig. 5-39).[9,10] Inconsistent identification of this "inner ring" sign brings into question this sign as a confirmation of ovulation.[10]

Attempts to correlate the echo pattern or thickness of the endometrium with the stage of the menstrual cycle failed due to menstrual cycle variations from cycle to cycle. The range of variation from individual to individual is great, and only generalizations may safely be made. The 28-day division of the average menstrual cycle includes four stages related to the morphologic changes seen in the endometrium.

Uterine Size, Shape, and Position

The size and shape of the uterus vary markedly with age and parity. In the fetus, the uterus grows at a rate consistent with the rest of the body until early in the third trimester. For the remainder of the gestational period, growth of the uterine corpus accelerates due to high levels of maternal estrogen. As a result, the uterus is larger and has a more "adult" contour in newborns than in children.[11] Immediately after birth, withdrawal of the influence of maternal estrogen causes the uterine corpus to shrink, and significant growth does not occur until the ovaries begin to produce hormones as a

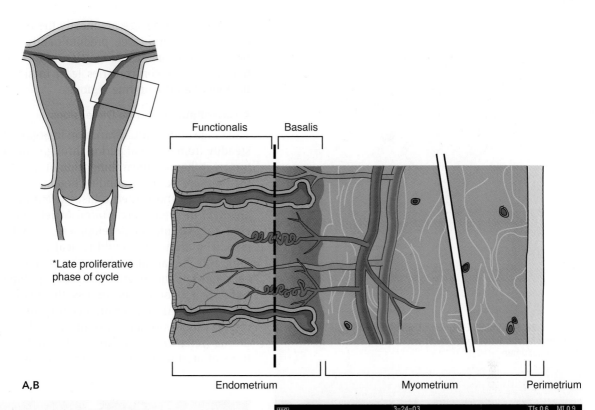

*Late proliferative phase of cycle

Functionalis | Basalis

A,B

Endometrium | Myometrium | Perimetrium

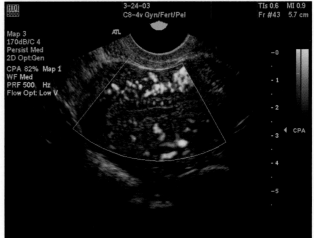

Figure 5-37 A: Frontal plane schematic of the uterus with an enlarged view of tissues that form the uterine wall. **B:** An endovaginal sagittal view of the uterus with a color Doppler sample box placed over the fundus and midcorpus region. Note the rich vascularization of the middle layer of the myometrium, indicated by the bright spots of color in areas of detected flow. **C:** A power Doppler image of the same uterus. Power Doppler has less dependency on flow direction and is more sensitive to the presence of flow. These vessels are normally not visible on gray scale imaging alone. (Images courtesy of Philips Medical Systems, Bothell, WA.)

C

prelude to puberty.[11] In infants, the uterus is cylindrical, high in the pelvis, and located along the same axis as the vagina. In young girls, the uterus remains nearly cylindrical (Fig. 5-40B), but the body (corpus and fundus) becomes more globular as it matures. By puberty, the uterus has assumed the characteristic inverted pear shape. With each pregnancy the corpus and fundus grow thicker, increasing the globularity of the multiparous uterus (Fig. 5-40E). After menopause the corpus and fundus shrink and regress to the prepubertal state (Fig. 5-40F), and in elderly women it may appear as little more than a cap above the cervix. Throughout life,

PATHOLOGY BOX 5-3

The Endometrium

Phase	Days of Cycle	Thickness (double layer/mm)	Endometrial Echo Pattern
Menstrual	1–5	<1	Thin echogenic line
Postmenstrual	6–9	2–4	Mostly anechoic
Proliferative	10–13	5–8	Slightly echogenic
Secretory	14–28	9–14	Highly echogenic

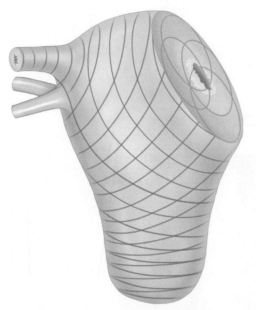

Figure 5-38 Schematic diagram of spiral smooth muscle fibers of the uterus. Contraction of these fibers tends to increase pressure in the uterine lumen.

changes in uterine size are mostly the result of changes in the muscularis layer, predominantly in the corpus. Because of its smaller proportion of muscle to connective tissue, the cervix varies least in size and is least flexible of all the uterine regions.

A Caveat about Uterine Dimensions

The range of individual variation in organ size increases steadily from the fetal period through adulthood. Many factors influence linear dimension of the uterus, including pressure from surrounding organs, stage of the menstrual cycle, and obstetric history. Normal dimensions given for the uterus are arbitrarily defined points on the continuum of uterine development, growth, and regression. The uterus of a child typically is 2.5 centimeters long and has an anteroposterior diameter of about 1 centimeter.[12] The length of the adult nulliparous uterus typically is 8 centimeters or less, the width 5.5 centimeters, and the AP dimension 3 centimeters.[11] The sonographer should use a consistent method to measure the uterus (refer to the example in Fig. 5-41). Small variations of uterine size are not clinically significant.

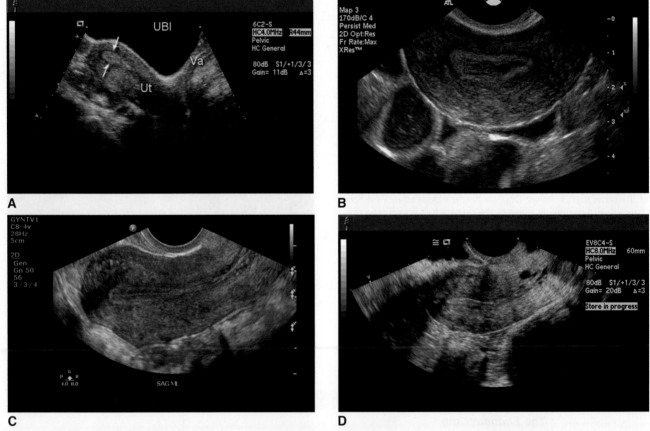

Figure 5-39 A: Sagittal transabdominal image of the uterus (*Ut*) and vagina (*Va*). This immediately premenstrual (day 27) endometrium (*arrows*) produces abundant mucus, which has outlined the uterine cavity. Four distinct echo layers can be identified. The outermost dark layer is myometrium and should not be included in measurement of the endometrium. This layer abuts on the thick, echogenic glandular layer that forms the bulk of the endometrium. A hypoechoic inner layer separates the echogenic glandular layer from a thin, highly echogenic line formed by mucus and the surfaces of the endometrium. (*UBI*, urinary bladder). **B:** In this transverse endovaginal scan of a midsecretory-phase endometrium, the layers are more difficult to identify, and the echo pattern in the glandular layer is patchy. **C:** The distinct layers are more easily appreciated in this endovaginal sagittal scan of the uterine corpus during the late proliferative stage. **D:** Endovaginal sagittal scan of the uterus immediately postmenstruation. The endometrium is not visible through most of the uterus.

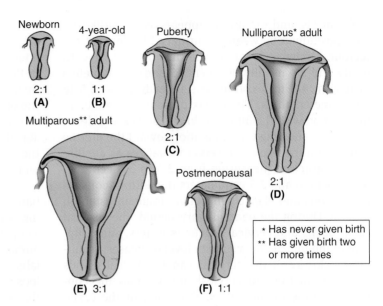

Figure 5-40 Anterior views of coronally sectional uteri.

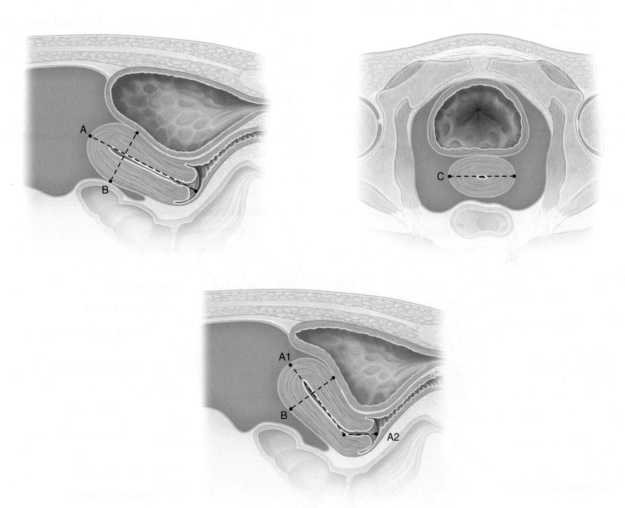

Figure 5-41 Measurement technique for the uterus. The long axis of the uterus should be measured from the fundus to the tip of the cervix (*line A*). When making this measurement, carefully identify the true long axis of the uterus, because it is seldom parallel to the pelvic midline. Gain and scan plane are then adjusted to optimally demonstrate the tip of the cervix. The posterior wall of the vagina serves as a guide; its curve can be followed around the posterior lip of the cervix to identify where the cervix ends and the vaginal wall begins. On the same image, the greatest anteroposterior diameter of the uterus should be measured along a line perpendicular to line A at a point where the uterus appears widest. Then the midpoint of the field of view is centered on the same line used to measure the anteroposterior diameter and the transducer is rotated 90 degrees, maintaining a constant tilt. This ensures that the transverse diameter (*line C*) is measured in the same plane as the anteroposterior diameter (*line B*), which increases accuracy and consistency of uterine measurements. If the uterus is strongly anteflexed, two measurements of the long axis (*lines A1 and A2*) should be made and added together to obtain the true length.

On ultrasound the uterus appears as a pearlike organ, positioned between the urinary bladder and the rectum. Dimensions of the uterine body vary with parity and are usually between 7.5 and 9 centimeters in length, 4.5 to 6 centimeters in width, and 2.5 to 4 centimeters thick. The cervix presents uterine communication with the outer world and serves as a depot for sperm, allowing their migration toward the uterine ostia. On ultrasound, the cervix visualizes as a cylinderlike structure measuring from 2.5 to 3.5 centimeters in length and 2.5 centimeters in width. It consists of a fibrous and elastic connective tissue and smooth muscle. During the periovulatory period, the cervical canal opens and cervical mucus is watery. After rupture of the follicle, the estrogen level decreases, resulting in closure of the cervical canal. Cervical glands extend from the endocervical mucosa into the connective tissue of the cervix. Occlusion of the cervical glands leads to formation of the cervical retention cysts, known as Nabothian cysts.

The Uterine Ligaments

The urinary bladder and rectum have close attachments to the pelvic walls. This contrasts to the loose uterine attachment within the pelvic cavity. The cardinal ligaments (also called transverse cervical ligaments) are ill-defined, wide bands of condensed fibromuscular tissue that originate from the lateral region of the cervix and along the lateral margin of the uterine corpus. These bands insert over a broad region of the lateral pelvic wall and extend posteriorly to the margins of the sacrum.[3] The posterior edge of the cardinal ligaments is denser than other regions and is identified as the uterosacral ligaments (Fig. 5-42). They extend from the posterior-lateral margin of the cervix to the sacrum. Together, the cardinal and uterosacral ligaments anchor the cervix and orient its axis so that it is roughly parallel to the central axis of the body.

The round ligaments (Fig. 5-42) are fibromuscular bands originating from the uterine cornua and extending across the pelvic space from posterior to anterior. They cross over the pelvic brim, pass through the inguinal ring, and then disperse as fibers anchored in the labia majora of the external genitalia.[3] These ligaments loosely tether the uterine fundus and tilt it forward in the pelvis, aiding in the normal anteflexion of the uterus at the isthmus.

Of all the ligaments of the pelvis, the broad ligament is the most difficult to define because it is not a true ligament but simply a double fold of peritoneum. The parietal peritoneum is a thin, glistening serous membrane that forms a sac that lines the abdominopelvic cavity. The visceral peritoneum is investing the organs within the peritoneal cavity. The peritoneum produces the layer of serous fluid, which decreases friction as organs move within the abdominal cavity.

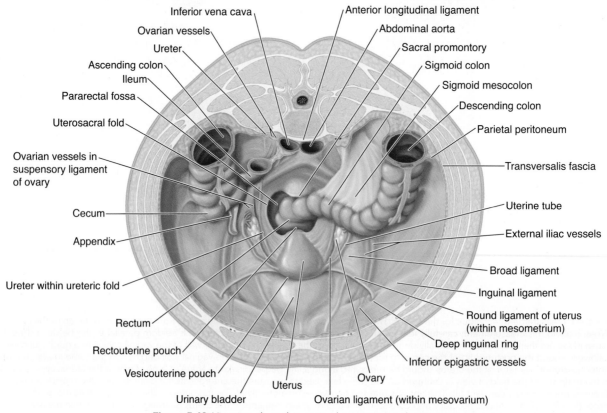

Figure 5-42 View into the pelvic cavity demonstrating the organs.

The broad ligament is simply the double layer of peritoneum, with fat, vessels, and nerves between the two layers. This arrangement probably has only minimal function in suspending the uterus; however, the broad ligament incompletely divides the true pelvis into anterior and posterior pelvic compartments. The ovaries attach to the posterior surface of the broad ligament, thus constraining their movements to the posterior pelvic compartment.

Spaces Adjacent to the Uterus

In addition to its anatomic function of coating, isolating, and lubricating the surfaces of organs, the peritoneum also forms particular spaces in the pelvis. The peritoneum reflects, or folds back, from the anterior wall of the pelvic cavity to cover the dome of the bladder, and then folds more sharply to cover the anterior surface of the uterus. This fold forms the relatively shallow anterior cul-de-sac (vesicouterine pouch), which lies between the anterior wall of the uterus and the urinary bladder.[3] This space virtually disappears as the urinary bladder fills; it is not of great significance to the sonographer. In contrast, the similar pocket formed by reflection of the peritoneum from the posterior wall of the pelvis, which covers the rectum, to the posterior wall of the uterus is very important. The posterior cul-de-sac (pouch of Douglas or rectouterine pouch) is the most posterior and dependent portion of the peritoneal sac lining the peritoneal cavity.[13] Fluid originating anywhere in the peritoneal sac tends to accumulate into the posterior cul-de-sac. This space is relatively complex in its configuration. The inferior portion consists of a deep, narrow pocket that extends inferiorly between the rectum and the cervix, with the upper margins defined by the uterosacral ligaments. Above these ligaments, the cul-de-sac widens out and is continuous with the broad, shallow spaces to the side of the uterus. The peritoneum lines these shallow adnexal spaces, forming the broad ligament.

Variants of Uterine Position

In some women, the uterus does not maintain the anteflexed position, instead bending backward with the fundus extending into the posterior cul-de-sac (Fig. 5-43).[4] This retroflexion of the uterus is relatively common, rarely has clinical significance, and may be transient or persistent in a particular individual.

Retroflexion of the uterus is responsible for significant alterations in the echo pattern of the uterus when demonstrated by transabdominal scanning. Normally, the uterus lies in a plane roughly perpendicular to an ultrasound beam entering through the full urinary bladder. Most of the uterus lies at a relatively constant depth from the transducer, so the echo pattern is uniform throughout the myometrium. In contrast, the corpus and fundus of a retroflexed uterus tilts back into the posterior pelvic cavity, and the acoustic beam must traverse the muscle tissue of the corpus to reach the fundus. As a result, the fundus of a retroflexed uterus often appears echo-poor compared with the corpus (Fig. 5-44).[11] This difference is due to absorption of the ultrasound beam by the muscle of the corpus. The resulting hypoechoic fundus increases the risk of misidentification of the uterus as a mass in the cul-de-sac.

THE FALLOPIAN TUBES

The fallopian tubes (oviducts or salpinges [singular: salpinx]) are paired musculomembranous tubes that extend from the fundus of the uterus to the ovary and lateral pelvic wall. Most of the length of the fallopian tube lies within the free edge of the fold of peritoneum that forms the broad ligament. Like the uterine wall, the wall of the fallopian tube consists of three layers: an

---

PATHOLOGY BOX 5-4

Variants in Uterine Position

Term	Definition
Anteflexion	Bending of the fundus toward the abdominal wall
Antevered	Tipping of the uterus toward the anterior abdominal wall. This is the usual position of the uterus with an empty bladder.
Dextroflexed	Flexed to the right
Dextroposition	Displacement to the right
Levoflexed	Flexed to the left
Levoposition	Displacement to the left
Prolape	Dropping of the uterus into the vaginal canal
Retroflexed	Bending of the fundus toward the rectum
Retrocession	Backward displacement of the entire uterus
Retroverted	Tipping of the entire uterus toward the sacrum
Retroversioflexion	Combination of retroversion and retroflexion

Note: All in relation to the pelvic axis

Anteflexed

Anteverted

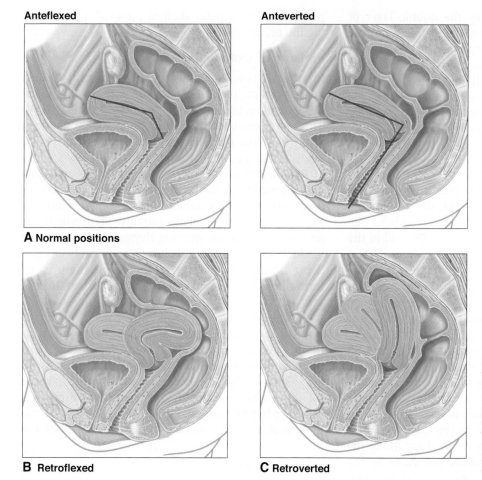

A Normal positions

B Retroflexed

C Retroverted

Figure 5-43 Variants of uterine position within the pelvis. **A:** Anteflex and anteverted positions of the uterus. **B:** Retroflexion of the uterus. The cervix maintains a normal position but the corpus and fundus flex backward into the posterior pelvic compartment. Note that the point of flexion is at the isthmus. **C:** Retroversion of the uterus occurs at the cervix.

outer serosal coat (which is continuous with the overlying peritoneum over the isthmic portion of the tube), a middle muscular layer, and an inner mucosa. The fallopian tube division includes intramural, isthmic, and ampullary portions (Fig. 5-45). The total tubal length in an adult, 7 to 14 cubic centimeters, is usually greater than the distance from the uterus to the lateral pelvic

wall, so in its normal state the tube is more tortuous than its wall structure alone would impose. The tubal lumen widens as it moves away from the uterus. The intramural portion is the narrowest (~1 millimeter), and the third portion or ampulla is the widest (~6 millimeters).[7] The ampullary portion terminates in the trumpet-shaped infundibulum, which is open toward

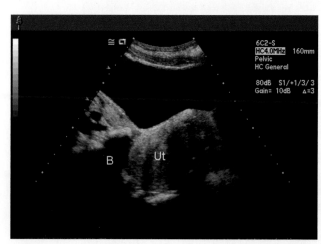

Figure 5-44 Sagittal scan of a retroflexed multiparous uterus. Note the bowel at the fundus of the uterus. *Ut,* uterus; *Bm,* bowel.

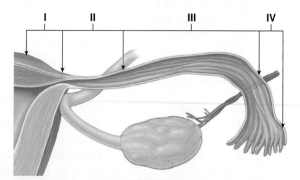

Figure 5-45 Regions of the fallopian tube. For this illustration, the tube has been stretched horizontally. The intramural (interstitial) portion *(I)* is relatively straight and is located within the uterine wall. The isthmic portion *(II)* is longer and slightly wavy in its course. The ampullary portion *(III)* is the longest section of the tube and is quite tortuous in vivo. It terminates in the trumpet-shaped infundibulum *(IV),* which is fringed with fingerlike projections, the fimbriae.

the peritoneal cavity. This trumpet-shaped opening is about 1 centimeter wide and ends in delicate, finger-like projections called fimbriae. Usually one of these, the fimbria ovarica, attaches to the ovary and serves to maintain a close relationship between the opening of the tube and the ovarian surface.[3] The vascular supply to the fallopian tube originates from the anastomoses of the uterine and ovarian arteries.

The similarity of the fallopian tube echo pattern makes it difficult to separate from surrounding abdominal structures. Although commonly demonstrated, recognition of the fallopian tube often only occurs when it is distended by fluid. A typical pattern images at the infundibulum at the lateral pole of the ovary (Fig. 5-46A). Because of the relative thinness of its wall, the characteristic echo pattern of the fallopian tube is that of a thin layer of hypoechoic muscle tissue lined by the hyperechoic mucosa surrounding a crescentic or cylindrical lumen. The fallopian tube easily images during endovaginal scanning, where it

appears as a tubular extension of the myometrium, often with high-amplitude echoes representing the tubal mucosa (Figs. 5-46 C, D). Color Doppler imaging helps locate the tube via the accompanying vessels (Fig. 5-46 B). The fallopian tube is the final element of a channel that connects the interior of the peritoneal cavity with the exterior of the female body. This channel is composed of the external genitalia, uterus, and the fallopian tubes.

THE OVARIES

In many respects the ovary is unlike any other organ of the female pelvis. It is a solid, parenchymatous structure, it secretes hormones, has no peritoneal covering, and is the only organ that is entirely inside the peritoneal sac..

In a term infant, the ovary is an elongated structure shaped like a round-edged prism and located in the posterior segment of the false pelvis, directly adjacent to the posterior uterine surface. This smooth surfaced

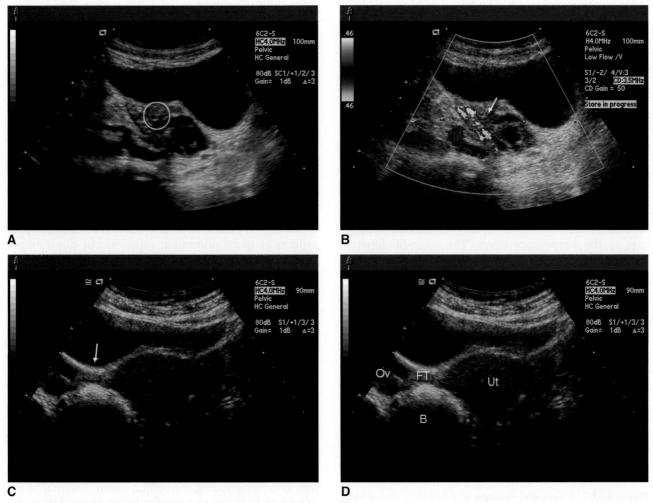

Figure 5-46 A: Sagittal scan of the left ovary with the fallopian tube (circle) seen over the upper pole. Without the small amount of fluid that defines the crescentic lumen, it would not be possible to positively identify these echoes as representing the tube. **B:** Color Doppler aids in locating the vessels surrounding the fallopian tube (arrow). **C,D:** An image of the uterus at the cornua shows the fallopian tube extending from the uterine body to the ovary. Beneath the tube is a loop of small bowel. Differentiation of these structures is more easily performed in real-time imaging because the small bowel is actively peristaltic. Note that a short section of tubal lumen is seen as a linear high-amplitude echo pattern *(arrow)* within the isthmic portion. *Ov,* ovary; *B,* bowel; *FT,* fallopian tube; *Ut,* uterus.

organ measures approximately 2.5 × 1.5 × 0.5 centimeters.[11] By menarche, the ovary moves into the true pelvic space and has assumed its almond-shaped adult contour and location.

The normal size of the oval or almond-shaped adult ovary is a length of 2.5 to 5 centimeters, a width of 1.5 to 3 centimeters, and an anteroposterior thickness of 0.6 to 2.2 centimeters.[14] Individual variation for a single linear dimension of the ovary is greater than either the average of the three linear dimensions or the volume. Short ovaries tend to be thicker, and thin ovaries tend to be longer. For this reason, a single linear dimension of the ovary cannot assess normality of size. Instead, a volume calculation should be used (length × width × height/2 = volume in cm³). With this approach, the upper normal value for the prepubertal ovary is 1 cubic centimeter. During the reproductive years, the ovarian volumes average 6 to 9 cubic centimeters.[15] For ovarian volumes by life stage, refer to Chapter 10.

The anterior margin of the ovary is relatively thin and attaches to the posterior surface of the broad ligament by the mesovarium. The posterior or free edge of the ovary is thicker and bows outward, giving the ovary its characteristic asymmetric almond shape.

Three anchoring structures suspend the ovary in the pelvic space (Fig. 5-47). The ovarian ligament, which is also known as the utero-ovarian ligament, is a flattened fibromuscular band, which extends from the uterine cornu, where the fallopian tube exits the uterine wall, to the inferior (medial or uterine) pole of the ovary. The infundibulopelvic ligament consists of fibromuscular strands intertwined with the ovarian vessels and lymphatics as they pass from the brim of the pelvis to the lateral pole of the ovary. These vessels and their supporting fibers form a ridge in the overlying peritoneum, which is thicker in this region and contributes to the suspensory effect. The infundibulopelvic

ligament suspends the superior (lateral or pelvic brim) pole of the ovary from the posteriolateral pelvic wall at the brim of the true pelvic space. The mesovarium is a short double layer of peritoneum extending from the posterior surface of the broad ligament. The mesovarium provides only a minimal suspensory effect in comparison with the fibromuscular ovarian ligament, but it does provide the primary route of access for vessels entering the ovarian hilum.

The outer layer of the ovary is composed of so-called germinal epithelium, which is neither germinal nor a true epithelium. The term originates from the early anatomists who have made some incorrect assumptions. It is actually a modified form of the peritoneum but sufficiently different to result in the ovary's being considered "nude," that is, not covered by the coelomic peritoneum.[3] Immediately beneath the germinal epithelium is a thin layer of fibrous tissue, which forms the tunica albuginea, meaning the white coat, or capsule of the ovary.

The bulk of the ovarian substance consists of a thick layer of ovarian parenchyma, the cortex, containing a large number of primordial follicles (Fig. 5-48A). This surface becomes markedly pitted or puckered after years of ovulation. In the center of the ovary is the medulla, which contains blood vessels (Fig. 5-48B,C) and connective tissue but no follicles.[3] Along the margins of the ovarian hilum, the ovarian germinal epithelium is continuous with the peritoneum that forms the broad ligament. Occasionally the hilum also contains vestigial remnants of the primitive mesonephros, which persist in the adult ovary as a cluster of tubules known as the epoöphoron.[3] These are of some interest to the sonographer because they occasionally give rise to simple cysts called parovarian cysts, which, when very large, can be mistaken for the urinary bladder.

Each ovary of a newborn infant contains about a million or more primordial follicles, but this number substantially reduces through spontaneous follicular regression as the infant matures. Only 300 to 400 of the many thousands of follicles that persist into adult life will actually progress through development and ovulation over the 30 or more reproductive years.[14]

Follicular Development

The stages of follicular development (Fig. 5-49) have been of particular interest to sonographers since the advent of fertility therapy using ultrasound monitoring of follicular growth. A complex cycle of chemical interchanges between the hypothalamus, the anterior pituitary gland, and the ovary control these stages. The early developing follicle is a solid mass consisting of granulosa cells surrounding the central ovum. External to the granulosa layer are two thinner layers of theca cells, the theca interna, which is richly vascularized, and the theca externa, which is composed mostly of connective tissue. With further development, a fluid-filled crescentic cavity forms eccentrically within the granulosa layer. As this

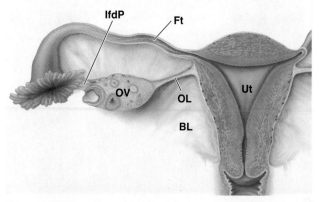

Figure 5-47 The ovary and its suspensory structures. This view of the posterior surface of the broad ligament shows the relationship of the ovary to the broad ligament, fallopian tube, infundibulopelvic ligament, and ovarian ligament. The fallopian tube has been lifted up to expose the ovary and its ligaments. *Ft*, fallopian tube; *OL*, ovarian ligament; *IfdP*, infundibulopelvic ligament; *OV*, ovary; *Ut*, uterus; *BL*, broad ligament.

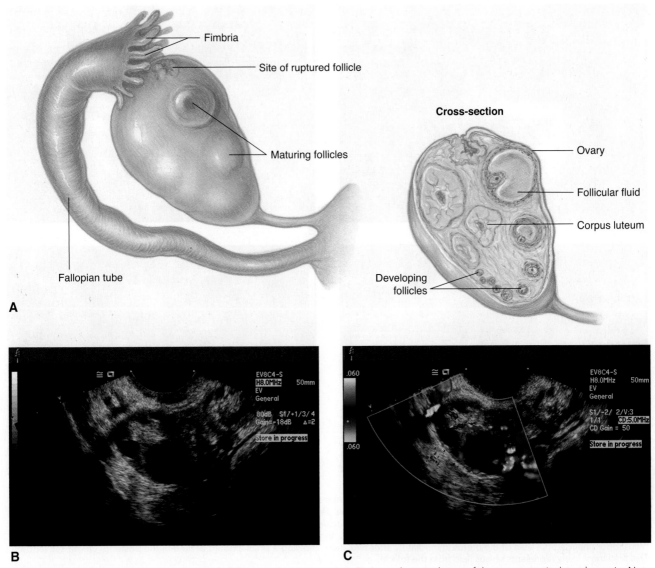

Figure 5-48 A: Diagrammatic representation of the ovary in cross-section. **B:** An endovaginal scan of the ovary near its lateral margin. Note the anechoic developing follicles. **C:** A color Doppler image of the same ovary, in a slightly more medial plane. The color highlights blood flow in the abundant vessels in the ovary.

cavity (known as the antrum) enlarges, the ovum contained within a surrounding mound of granulosa cells projects into the cavity, forming a structure known as the cumulus oöphorus (discus proligerus).[14] As the follicle continues to develop, it enlarges and becomes a mature follicle, eventually impinging on the tunica albuginea of the ovarian surface. Typically, a mature follicle reaches 20 millimeter in size before rupturing.

The ripening follicle is referred to as a Graafian follicle. Each month during the reproductive years, follicle-stimulating hormone (FSH) triggers rapid growth of multiple ovarian follicles. In a normal ovulatory cycle, only one of these follicles becomes dominant and ruptures through the tunica albuginea, releasing its contained egg, resulting in ovulation. The other follicles undergo atresia,[14] while the corpus luteum rapidly shrinks becoming an amorphous mass of hyaline scar

tissue known as the corpus albicans. Artificial stimulation of follicular development (i.e., fertility therapy) can result in simultaneous development of multiple follicles.

At ovulation, the combination of the discharged follicular fluid and hemorrhage associated with follicular rupture results in accumulation of 5 to 10 milliliters of fluid in the posterior cul-de-sac, where it can be observed as a crescentic anechoic collection behind the cervix.[16] The process of ovulation may be associated with midcycle pain (mittelschmerz). The stigma (the opening through which the egg was discharged) is sealed by a blood clot, thus reestablishing a closed cystic structure filled with clotted blood. The theca interna layer of the ruptured follicle undergoes rapid proliferation and luteinization through deposit within the cells of golden or reddish brown pigment and fat.[14] The follicle thus becomes the corpus luteum, which means yellow or golden body. In

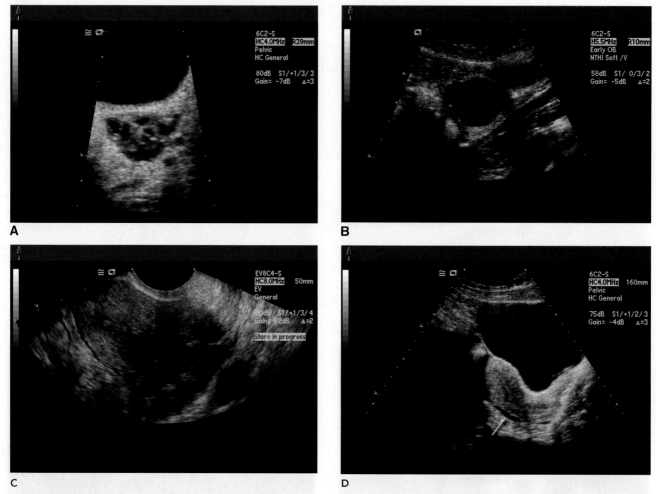

Figure 5-49 A: Transabdominal transverse scan of a normal adult ovary on day 7 of the menstrual cycle. Several small follicles are seen within the ovary. Note the decrease of the sector size, which increases line density and image resolution. **B:** Sagittal image of a dominant follicle immediately after its rupture at ovulation. Note the partially collapsed walls resulting from loss of most of the liquor folliculi. **C:** Endovaginal scan of an ovary that has been artificially stimulated during fertility therapy. Multiple follicles are seen in this scan plane. **(D)** Transvesical (transabdominal) sagittal scan of the uterus immediately after ovulation, showing a small amount of fluid in the posterior cul-de-sac *(arrows)*. This fluid most likely represents serous fluid from the follicle.

the normal development of the corpus luteum, the blood clot is gradually absorbed, sometimes forming strands of fibrin within the liquefied center of the corpus luteum.[6]

Fertilization of the discharged egg results in maintenance of the corpus luteum throughout the first trimester of pregnancy and sometimes forming the corpus luteum cyst of pregnancy. This cystic structure may grow up to the size of 5 to 6 centimeters and persists through the early stages of pregnancy. If fertilization does not occur, the corpus luteum undergoes regression, involuting to become the corpus albicans. The surface of the ovary where rupture of the follicle occurred puckers inward as the scar forms, giving the aging ovary a quilted or cobbled surface. At menopause, the remaining follicles undergo atresia over the subsequent 4 or 5 years, although occasionally a postmenopausal follicle may undergo development, ovulation, and corpus luteum formation.[14] This, however, is rare, and any persistent cyst in the postmenopausal ovary must be regarded with suspicion. After menopause the ovary shrinks steadily until it is less than one-third of its

mature size.[14] Occasionally, dilated veins can mimic follicles in postmenopausal women, and the sonographer may misinterpret the persistent fluid-filled structure as a persistent follicle. Doppler ultrasound helps differentiate a true cyst from a dilated vessel.

Ultrasound measurements of the follicle are most often performed using an average of the follicular diameter in three planes, but when precise measurements are required, the follicle measurement procedure is similar to the ovary. A volume can be calculated using (length × width × height)/2 = volume in cubic centimeters. If only two diameters are available, the formula is (diameter A × diameter B × diameter B)/2.

Location and Acoustic Patterns of the Ovary

When the urinary bladder is empty, the ovary rests in the ovarian fossa, a shallow depression on the posterior-lateral pelvic wall just beneath the brim of the pelvis and formed by the external iliac vessels and the ureter. With the uterine fundus in its normal position, resting on the dome of the urinary bladder, the ovary is substantially superior and posterior to the fundus of the uterus. As the bladder fills, the uterus is physiologically retroverted and pushed upward toward the sacral protuberance. As filling progresses, the uterus moves upward, while the ovaries tend to remain stationary in their fossae and lie at the sides of the uterine fundus (Fig. 5-50). With further filling of the bladder, the ovaries are subjected to increasing pressure from the bladder and are usually forced in the caudad direction. Frequently one may slip farther down into the posterior cul-de-sac. Excessive filling of the bladder often forces the ovaries out of the lower regions of the posterior pelvic compartment. The ovaries come to rest cephalad to the fundus of the uterus in the axial position.

The ovary may be found in any of three regions of the posterior pelvic compartment: the posterior cul-de-sac, the adnexal space to the side of the uterus, or above (cephalad to) or behind the fundus of the uterus. The attachment by the mesovarium to the posterior surface of the broad ligament prevents an ovary location anterior to the broad ligament (in front of the uterus, between the uterus and the urinary bladder, or in the anterior cul-de-sac).

The relationship of the true pelvic space, the degree of filling of the rectum and urinary bladder, and uterine size govern ovarian movement. When meticulous scanning with gain variations does not reveal the ovary, the sonographer should consider having the patient void partially, especially if the bladder is highly distended. This usually increases ovarian visibility due to a change in position, most commonly adjacent to the uterine fundus. Another method to move the ovary is to have the patient roll on her side. This may move the ovary out of loops of bowel, allowing visualization.

Endovaginal imaging is the method of choice when the primary interest is detailed visualization of the ovaries. The advantages of endovaginal imaging is a balance between depth and transducer position limitations. For the initial evaluation of the pelvic organs, especially with a suspected pelvic mass, transabdominal imaging is the method of choice. Endovaginal imaging supplements this examination through acquisition of detailed images of specific structures. Endovaginal

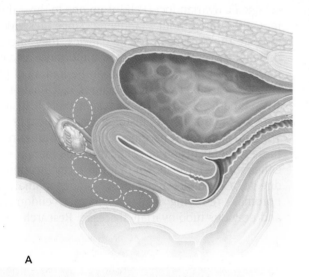

A

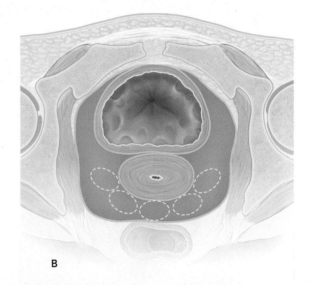

B

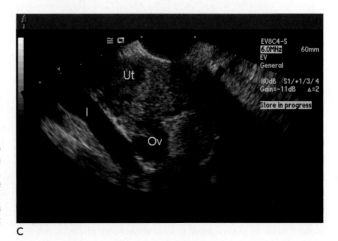

C

Figure 5-50 A: Positions of the ovary. Because of its attachment to the posterior surface of the broad ligament, the ovary may be found in the posterior pelvic compartment or above the fundus of the uterus, in the adnexal spaces or in the posterior cul-de-sac, but not in the anterior cul-de-sac or between the urinary bladder and the uterus. **B:** Endovaginal sagittal scan slightly to the right of midline shows a normal ovary located in the posterior cul-de-sac. *Ov,* ovary; *Ut,* uterus; *I,* iliac.

imaging alone can be used for follow-up examinations, in cases in which only the ovaries are to be evaluated (e.g., in fertility therapy or post hysterectomy), and for a few cases in which the patient is unable to maintain a distended urinary bladder.

The normal echo pattern of the adult ovary, compared with homogeneously echogenic myometrium, consists of low-amplitude echoes of the follicles. Corpora albicantia in the ovarian cortex and small vessels in the ovarian medulla most likely cause the bright reflections. On both transabdominal and endovaginal ultrasound, the ovary may be identified by its characteristic "Swiss cheese" pattern of anechoic follicles against the low-amplitude gray of the ovarian cortex.

Ovaries of infants and postmenopausal women become difficult to detect, as they are isoechoic with the surrounding parametrial tissues. During the reproductive age, the echo patterns of the uterus and the ovary are subtly different (Fig. 5-51). In difficult cases, an acoustic property of the ovary may provide the only clue to its location. To locate a "difficult" ovary, the examiner should reduce gain levels so that most of the echoes from the uterus and the parametrium disappear. The ovary will be revealed by the burst of acoustic enhancement (increased through-transmission) seen beneath it as a column of brighter echoes (Fig. 5-52).

The increased resolution of endovaginal imaging allows for imaging of previously discounted or nonimaged ovarian details. Commonly, sonographers find echogenic ovarian foci (EOF) from one to three millimeters with and without shadowing. Since these foci may indicate the presence of malignancies, they have come under close scrutiny due to their importance as a cancer marker. Early studies suggest that the finding of peripheral EOF is merely psammomatous calcifications seen with superficial epithelial inclusion cysts.[39] In a study done by Muradali et al., histologic assessment of ovaries with nonshadowing peripheral echogenic areas revealed these to be inclusion or solitary corpus luteum cysts. [40] Other studies have shown that these calcifications were due to a dermoid, mucinous cystadenenoma, adenofibromas, resolving hemorrhagic cyst, endometriosis, and previous tubo-ovarian abscess.[41] Research seems to

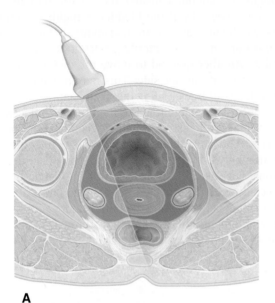

A

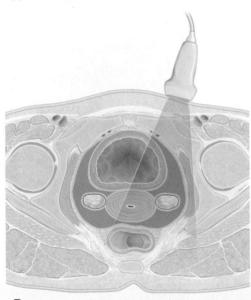

B

Figure 5-51 A: The ovary can be differentiated from the obturator internus muscle by scanning in a transverse plane and angling the beam in from the side of the pelvis opposite the ovary to be demonstrated. This steep angle brings the ultrasound beam more perpendicular to the surface of the obturator internus muscle and usually demonstrates the thin layer of fat overlying the muscle, thus separating the dark echo pattern of the ovary from the similar dark pattern of the muscle. **B:** A more difficult task is to separate the ovary from the myometrium when the two are in opposition. Scanning in a transverse plane with the transducer positioned on the same side of the pelvis as the ovary of interest and angled slightly back toward the midline often permits demonstration of a thin line between the ovary and the uterus, which confirms that the structure is an ovary and not a small subserosal fibroid. Careful attention to matching ovarian position with the focal zone of the ultrasound beam also helps. Placing the patient in a decubitus position may make it easier to obtain certain steeply angled scan planes.

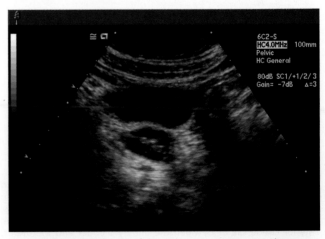

Figure 5-52 Sagittal scan of the right ovary at an optimal gain setting. Note posterior enhancement that "marks" the position of the overlying ovary.

confirm that with a normal ovary, peripherally located EOF are a benign process; however, there has been little study of EOF within the medulla of the ovary.[40,41]

THE BOWEL

The degree of filling of the rectum influences the uterine position. Bowel may be easily mistaken for a pelvic mass, particularly when peristalsis is not readily evident in the real-time image. The descending colon becomes the sigmoid colon and enters the pelvic space through the left iliac fossa. The sigmoid typically forms one or more S-curves, which loop back and forth through the pelvis (Fig. 5-53).

Peritoneum covers the sigmoid, which forms a short suspensory membrane known as the mesocolon, which contains vessels and nerves. The flexibility of the mesocolon permits the sigmoid colon to move over a relatively wide area of the posterior pelvic compartment. When the urinary bladder is full, the sigmoid and the loops of small bowel occupy the posterior cul-de-sac. This location of the sigmoid can create some difficulties during the endovaginal sonographic exam. Transducer placement in the posterior fornix results in imaging of sigmoid colon loops that may lie between the transducer and the ovaries. In such cases, transfer of the transducer to the lateral fornix may permit better visualization. This is not a problem in transabdominal scanning because the distended urinary bladder forces the sigmoid and loops of small bowel upward so that they move above and behind the fundus of the uterus.

The fecal-filled sigmoid colon runs from the left posterolateral brim of the pelvis down to the cul-de-sac. At about the midpoint of the sacral curve, the sigmoid moves posterior to the peritoneum and, like the descending colon, becomes partially buried, so that only its anterior surface and part of its lateral surfaces are covered by peritoneum. From this point to the anus, the large bowel

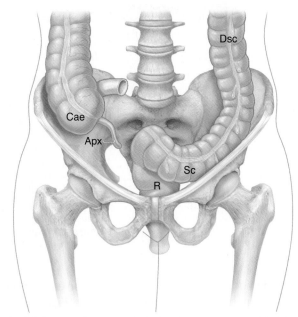

Figure 5-53 Schematic diagram of the large bowel and its relationship to the false pelvis. The false pelvis is usually filled with loops of small bowel. The cecum and appendix are found on the right side of the false pelvis, and the pelvic portion of the descending colon and the proximal (upper) part of the sigmoid colon are found on the left. The location of the appendix is highly variable, and it may be found virtually anywhere in the right false pelvis, or even in the true pelvis. *Cae,* cecum; *Apx,* appendix; *Dsc,* descending colon; *Sc,* sigmoid colon; *R,* rectum.

is the rectum. This portion demonstrates characteristic thick and muscular walls.

The rectum walls are usually not visible, but rectal contents image easily. Fecal material in the rectum causes irregular shadows and produces a pattern of very dense, bright echoes typical of material containing gassy areas. Fluid in the rectum or fecal material containing little gas permits visualization of the anterior surface of the sacrum lying deep to the rectum (Fig. 5-54A). On real-time observation, loops of small

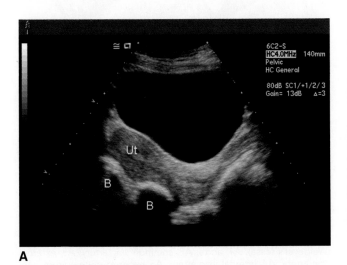

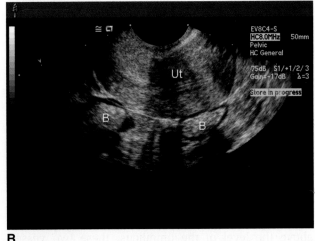

A   **B**

Figure 5-54 A: A sagittal transabdominal image of the uterus demonstrating bowel (*B*) with typical "dirty" shadows. **B:** Endovaginal scan of the uterus. Loops of bowel (**B**) are seen posterior to the uterus (*Ut*).

PATHOLOGY BOX 5-5

Echo Pattern of Bowel

	Echo Pattern	Shadows
Small bowel	Variably echogenic content with thin, anechoic ring representing the muscular wall	Shifts with movement of bowel and content
Cecum	Variably echogenic content with thin, anechoic ring representing the muscular wall	Constant except when peristalsis occurs
Sigmoid	Echogenic content with thin, anechoic ring representing the muscular wall	Constant except when peristalsis occurs
Rectum	Echogenic content with thin, anechoic ring representing the muscular wall	Constant and nearly complete: only top surface of fecal boluses can be seen

bowel demonstrate peristalsis allowing for easy differentiation, particularly if filled with fluid (Fig. 5-54B). In contrast, rectal peristalsis is infrequent and is identified by its location and echo pattern, rather than by its motion.

The cecum and appendix can usually be identified in the right iliac fossa. The appendix is one of the most variable structures in the human body, and although technically it is an abdominal structure, sonographers often locate it in the pelvis.[17]

In most cases the bowel is relatively easy to differentiate from other pelvic organs and from the muscle. If it is not clear whether the posterior cul-de-sac harbors a mass versus a bowel loop, a water enema administered with simultaneous real-time imaging helps establish a diagnosis. Movement of water through the rectum and sigmoid should permit positive identification of these structures.

THE PELVIC VASCULAR SYSTEM

Until the early 1990s, information about the pelvic vascular system had little direct value for sonographers. Occasionally, they encountered dilated pelvic veins mimicking a complex mass, but these were rare. Spectral, color, and power Doppler examinations of the pelvic vessels is becoming increasingly important in obstetric ultrasound and are promising to have applications in gynecologic sonography, as well.

The pelvic vascular system consists of three distinct components: the arteries, the veins, and the lymphatics. The lymphatic channels usually have no significance in pelvic sonography.

The spatial relationship of the great vessels (aorta and vena cava) changes as they descend through the abdomen. In the upper abdomen, the vena cava is located closer to the abdominal wall than the aorta. Just above the level of the umbilicus, these two vessels come to lie side by side, and then at their bifurcation the veins come to lie posterior to the arteries.[16]

ARTERIAL SYSTEM OF THE PELVIS

The aorta usually bifurcates at a point slightly higher than the inferior vena cava, giving rise to the common iliac arteries, which are quite short, extending only for a few centimeters. They bifurcate into the large external iliac artery and the smaller internal iliac artery (Fig. 5-55). The external iliac artery runs along the medial border of the iliopsoas muscle at the brim of the

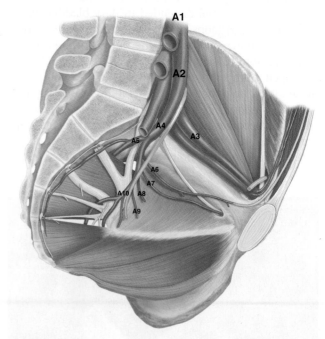

Figure 5-55 The pelvic vascular system. Although only the arteries are shown in detail, the veins follow the same pattern but lie posterior to the arteries. The one exception to the pattern of naming the vessels is the internal iliac artery, whose companion vein is named the internal iliac vein rather than the internal iliac artery. Note the triangular space defined by the vessels at the bifurcation of the common iliac vessels. This open-based triangle is the ovarian fossa (Waldeyer's fossa). *A1*, aorta; *A2*, common iliac artery; *A5*, external iliac artery; *A4*, internal iliac artery; *A5*, superior gluteal artery; *A6*, obturator artery; *A7*, umbilical artery; *A8*, uterine artery; *A9*, superior vesical artery; *A10*, internal pudendal and inferior gluteal arteries.

true pelvic space. When it reaches the lower margin of the pelvis, the external iliac artery passes beneath the inguinal ligament to enter the thigh, becoming the common femoral artery.

The internal iliac artery, also known as the hypogastric artery, courses from the bifurcation at the upper and posterior margin of the true pelvic space down into the pelvic cavity along the lateral wall for a distance of only one or two centimeters. It then gives rise to the relatively large and posteriorly directed superior gluteal artery. The internal iliac artery continues downward along the pelvic wall, giving rise to four small branches that course anteriorly along the pelvic wall: the obturator artery, the umbilical artery, the uterine-vaginal artery, and the superior vesical artery. Finally, the internal iliac terminates in two posteriorly directed branches: the internal pudendal and the inferior gluteal arteries. Except for these last two posteriorly directed branches, the branches of the internal iliac artery and their many subdivisions fan out along the lateral wall of the pelvis, descending to the pelvic floor to pass over the pelvic diaphragm to reach their target organs or muscles.[18] The internal iliac artery is the primary blood supply for the uterus, vagina, urinary bladder, and most of the muscles of the pelvic floor. Remember, branching patterns of blood vessels are highly variable.

Most of the smaller branches of the internal iliac artery are not individually identifiable in the ultrasound image, but one branch, the uterine artery, is important to sonographers. The uterine artery extends across the pelvic floor to reach the uterus at approximately the level of the tip of the cervix (Fig. 5-56A). At this point, it bifurcates into a uterine branch and a descending vaginal branch. Its uterine component turns upward to run along the lateral margin of the uterus (Fig. 5-56B) to the fallopian tube, where it again makes a sharp turn to run along the fallopian tube. Just past the cervical "right-angle" turn, the uterine artery is relatively straight as it ascends alongside the cervix. At this point the artery is most accessible for Doppler evaluation with an endovaginal transducer. As it courses upward along the lateral border of the uterus, the uterine artery becomes very tortuous.

The reproductive organs, like the brain, have an elaborate fail-safe blood supply. In addition to terminating in capillaries embedded in the target organ, the internal pudendal artery, vaginal artery, and uterine artery all have anastomotic branches that form a complex network of interconnected channels around the vagina and most of the uterus. This anastomotic network ensures that compromised flow through any one of these arteries does not result in tissue damage in the target organ. Other feeder vessels of the network provide an immediate compensatory flow, thus preserving tissue function. An even more elaborate system exists to supply the ovary.

The embryonic ovaries originate in the abdominal region from a common mesenchymal tissue, which also gives rise to the adrenal glands. This explains tumors with adrenal characteristics forming in the pelvis and adrenal gland tumor production of sex hormones. In the later stages of embryonic life, the ovaries descend into the pelvis, guided by a ligamentous band called the gubernaculum. As the embryonic ovaries descend, they bring along their original blood supply derived from the aorta and draining into the vena cava. These vessels persist in adult life as the ovarian artery and vein. The ovarian arteries, sometimes called the gonadal arteries, originate as lateral branches of the aorta at about the level of the lower margin of the renal pelvis (Fig. 5-57). These arteries course downward over the psoas muscles and along the same path followed by the ureters, crossing over the common iliac artery just superior to its bifurcation into the external and internal iliac arteries. The ovarian artery then bridges across from the upper margin of the pelvis to the ovary through the infundibulopelvic ligament. From the infundibulopelvic ligament it passes through the mesovarium to reach the ovarian hilum, where it supplies the ovarian parenchyma. In addition, the ovarian artery forms anastomoses with the ovarian branches of the uterine artery, thus providing a closed-loop or fail-safe blood supply originating from two widely divergent points in the arterial system.

VENOUS SYSTEM OF THE PELVIS

The venous system of the pelvis follows a pattern virtually identical to that of the arterial system. The inferior vena cava bifurcates slightly below the level of the aortic bifurcation, giving rise to the common iliac veins, which run beneath the common iliac arteries. These short vessels in turn give rise to the large external iliac veins, which drain the legs, and the internal iliac veins, which drain the pelvic organs and muscles. The ovarian veins follow the same course as the ovarian arteries until they reach the midabdomen, where the right ovarian vein drains directly into the vena cava and the left ovarian vein drains into the left renal vein.

Because the veins are thin walled, they are highly distensible and vary in size with certain conditions, most notably pregnancy. After parturition, the venous channels usually shrink, but they may remain prominent and easily visible. If venous congestion occurs, the veins may form pelvic varices, which are readily identifiable in the ultrasound image. In some women, particularly after parturition, the venous channels in the outer regions of the myometrium are clearly visible.

The Ureter

The ureters course along the lateral pelvic wall posterior to the ovary. These musculomembranous tubes move urine by peristalsis and enter the pelvis at a point just caudad to the bifurcation of the common iliac vessels. The ureter is posterior and lateral to the ovary with the most common position lateral to the uterus (Fig. 5-58).

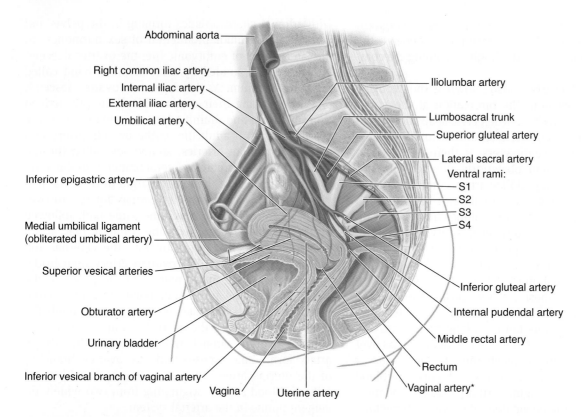

Abdominal aorta

Right common iliac artery

Internal iliac artery

External iliac artery

Umbilical artery

Inferior epigastric artery

Medial umbilical ligament
(obliterated umbilical artery)

Superior vesical arteries

Obturator artery

Urinary bladder

Inferior vesical branch of vaginal artery

Vagina   Uterine artery

Iliolumbar artery

Lumbosacral trunk

Superior gluteal artery

Lateral sacral artery
Ventral rami:
S1
S2
S3
S4

Inferior gluteal artery

Internal pudendal artery

Middle rectal artery

Rectum

Vaginal artery*

A   *Vaginal artery arises from uterine artery in 11% of cases

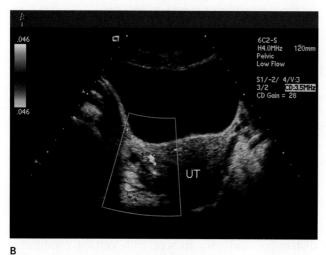

B

Figure 5-56 A: Arterial supply to the uterus. The broad ligament has been removed to expose the uterine artery as it courses upward from the level of the cervix to the cornu of the uterus, where it makes a sharp turn to run along the underside of the fallopian tube. The uterine artery forms an anastomosis with the ovarian artery beneath the fallopian tube. Thus, although the uterine artery is the principal supplier of blood to the uterus, it is not the sole supplier. Anastomotic connections are not limited to the uterine-ovarian arteries. They are found throughout the pelvis, providing an elaborate fail-safe network of alternate channels to each of the organs. **B:** This transverse endovaginal image of the region of the uterine isthmus (*Ut*) uses color Doppler to demonstrate the abundant vessels that lie along the lateral uterine margins. Blood flow is indicated by the presence of color.

PATHOLOGY BOX 5-6

Arterial Vasculature of the Pelvis

Vessel	Pelvic Organ Supplied	Branches Supplying Pelvic Organs
Aorta	All via branches	External and internal iliac
Internal iliac artery (aka hypogastric artery)	All via branches	Uterine, ovarian, bladder, rectum, umbilical artery in the fetus
Uterine Artery	Uterus, fallopian tube, ovary, vagina	Arcuate, vaginal
Ovarian (aka gonadal artery)	Ovary, ureters, fallopian tube	

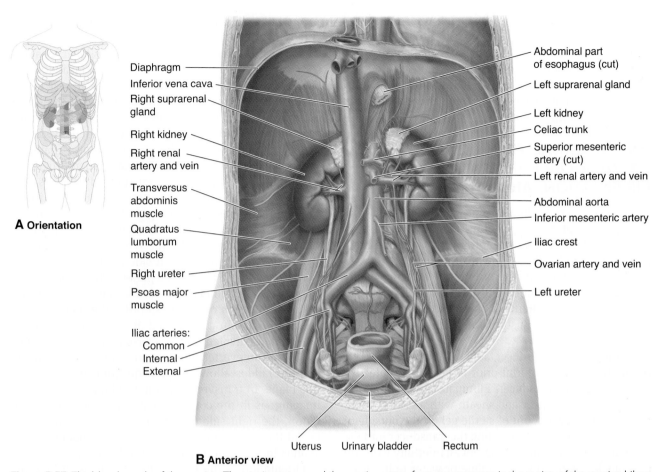

A Orientation

Diaphragm

Inferior vena cava

Right suprarenal gland

Right kidney

Right renal artery and vein

Transversus abdominis muscle

Quadratus lumborum muscle

Right ureter

Psoas major muscle

Iliac arteries:
Common
Internal
External

Abdominal part of esophagus (cut)

Left suprarenal gland

Left kidney

Celiac trunk

Superior mesenteric artery (cut)

Left renal artery and vein

Abdominal aorta

Inferior mesenteric artery

Iliac crest

Ovarian artery and vein

Left ureter

Uterus   Urinary bladder   Rectum

B Anterior view

Figure 5-57 The blood supply of the ovaries. The uterine artery and the ovarian artery form anastomoses in the region of the ovarian hilum. Note the difference in the pattern of ovarian artery origin versus ovarian vein termination. Because lymphatics follow the gonadal (ovarian) vessels, tumor spread from the pelvis to the para-aortic nodes at the level of the renal pelvis is common.

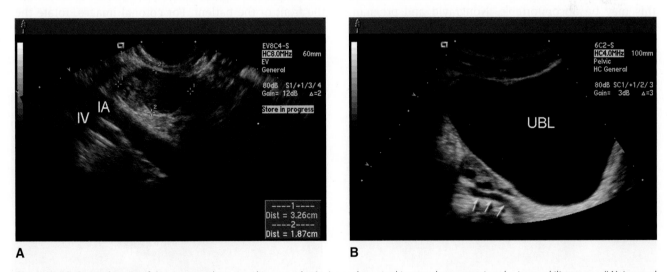

A

B

Figure 5-58 Sagittal scans of the ovary and surrounding vessels. **A:** An endovaginal image demonstrating the internal iliac artery (*IA*), internal iliac vein (*IV*), and a normal ovary. **B:** A transabdominal image on a more medial scan plane demonstrates mostly ovarian tissue, with the ureter (*arrows*) running posterior to the ovary. *UBL*, urinary bladder.

As the ureter descends into the pelvic space, it moves medially to reach the trigone of the urinary bladder, and therefore oblique scan planes are usually required to demonstrate long segments of the ureter in the pelvis. Real-time sonography images ureteral contractions, with endovaginal images identifying the ureter easier than transabdominal imaging.

ENDOVAGINAL TECHNIQUE, TRANSDUCER PREPARATION, ORIENTATION, AND MANIPULATION

A female chaperone should be present when a male sonographer or physician performs a endovaginal examination. Explain the examination to the patient before a procedure to help alleviate anxiety.

Place the patient in the lithotomy position, ideally on a gynecologic examination table. If such a table is not available, the patient's hips can be elevated with a foam pad or pillow. Ensure complete coverage of the pelvis and legs.

To prepare the transducer, apply scanning gel directly on the transducer footprint prior to placing a protective sheath over the transducer. Eliminate any air bubbles between the transducer and sheath with a gloved hand. Place a generous amount of sterile gel on the outside of the sheath before gently inserting the transducer into the vaginal canal. If the study is part of an infertility work-up or follicular monitoring, use saline or water to lubricate the sheath, as gel may inhibit sperm motility. If using commercial condoms, ensure they are free of spermicide. The sonographer, the physician, or the patient herself can then insert the transducer.

Avoid extreme angling of the transducer because this may be uncomfortable. Nongravid and pregnant patients easily tolerate a well-performed endovaginal examination. Endovaginal sonography images have a different orientation compared to conventional transabdominal images because of the transducer location. The typical orientation for a pelvic transabdominal image demonstrates that the structures closest to the footprint of the transducer are at the top of the image screen. Figure 5-59 illustrates a typical TAS sagittal view demonstrating the anterior aspect (patient's belly) at the top of the screen, the posterior aspect (patient's back) at the bottom, superior (toward patient's head) to the left of the image and inferior (toward patient's feet) at the right side of the image. As a result, when in the longitudinal plane performing a EVS examination, the bottom of the screen is oriented toward the patient's head (superior); the top of the screen is toward the patient's feet (inferior); the left side is the patient's belly (anterior) and the right is the patient's back (posterior), as demonstrated in Figure 5-60. The organ-to-image orientation depends on the position of the uterus within the pelvis. Obtain coronal and oblique coronal images, which are equivalent of transverse images produced by TAS. The anteverted uterine position occurs with an empty bladder allowing for acquisition of images on this plane. In transverse (coronal/oblique coronal) EVS imaging, as in the conventional transabdominal orientation, the right side of the patient corresponds to the left of the screen and the left side of the patient corresponds to the right of the screen (Fig. 5-61).

Orientation of the image often begins with how the sonographer holds the transducer. The EV transducer, like any other transducer, has a notch or raised portion to indicate the orientation. Most transducers orient this marker with the manufacturer logo next to the top of the image. For sagittal images, the marker is up toward the front of the patient. For coronal images, rotate the notch counterclockwise (toward the patient's right).

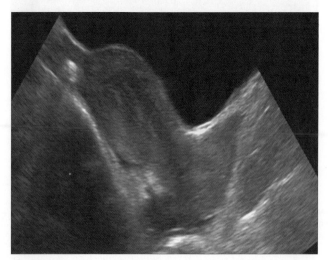

Figure 5-59 A TAS in sagittal view demonstrates the anterior aspect (patient's abdomen) at the top of the screen, the posterior aspect (patient's back) at the bottom, superior (toward patient's head) is to the left of the image and inferior (toward patient's feet) is at the right of the image.

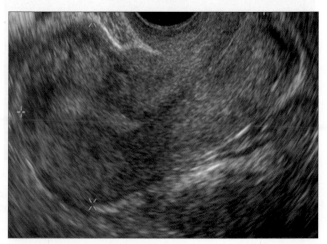

Figure 5-60 An EVS examination. The bottom of the screen is oriented toward the patient's head (superior); the top of the screen is toward the patient's feet (inferior); the left side is the patient's belly (anterior) and the right is the patient's back (posterior).

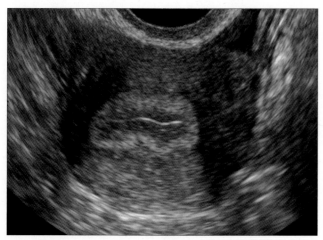

Figure 5-61 EVS image in oblique transverse view.

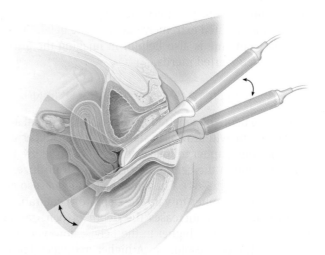

Figure 5-62 Schematic diagram demonstrating the movement of the transducer to produce sagittal views of the uterus in the same plane. The transducer handle is moved anterior and posterior to view all the sections of the uterus in the sagittal plane. (From DuBose TJ. Fetal Sonography. Philadelphia: WB Saunders; 1996:61–64; illustration by Victoria Vescovo Alderman, MA, RDMS.)

Some endovaginal transducers have a slanted face, requiring a little different technique for the coronal views. Rotation of the transducer in the above method works well for the right ovary; however, to image the left ovary, the marker must be rotated clockwise. This results in reversal of the image. To remedy this, locate the invert function to flip the image. Obtain the left ovary images and do not forget to orient the image to the original plane.

Many authors found it easier to use "organ-oriented" scanning rather than trying to locate traditional anatomic planes. This approach entails scanning the target organ from axial, longitudinal, as well as other planes.[19,20,21]

The technique of EVS examination and image interpretation becomes easier to discuss upon understanding the basic concept of image orientation. The most common transducer/patient manipulations are the following:

1. Anteroposterior angulation (belly-to-back)
2. Lateral (side-to-side) angulation
3. Depth of penetration (push-pull)
4. Rotation
5. Bimanual maneuvers

ANTEROPOSTERIOR ANGULATION

In the longitudinal plane, anteroposterior angulation allows the operator to optimize imaging of the uterus (Fig. 5-62). A slight and gradual downward movement of the transducer's handle angles the transducer upward, allowing better visualization of an anteverted uterus. Conversely, an upward motion of the handle angles the transducer toward the patient's back, allowing better visualization of a retroverted uterus.

LATERAL ANGULATION

Side-to-side manipulation of the transducer improves visualization of a uterus deviated to the right or left of midline, the cornua of the uterus, and the ipsilateral

ovary, fallopian tube, pelvic vasculature, ligaments, bowel, and other organs or structures (Fig. 5-63).

Many pieces of equipment allow for steering of the beam without the need for transducer manipulation. Upon decreasing the sector width, quite often the sonographer is able to steer the beam to the right or left

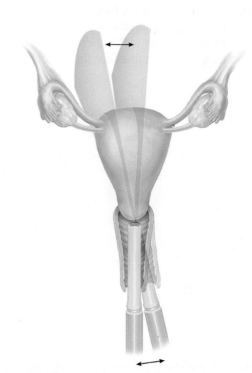

Figure 5-63 Schematic diagram demonstrating the movement of the transducer to view sagittal images in different planes. As the transducer is angled from one side to the other, parallel slices of the uterus are imaged. (From DuBose TJ. Fetal Sonography. Philadelphia: WB Saunders; 1996: 61–64; illustration by Victoria Vescovo Alderman, MA, RDMS.)

of the central beam. This becomes helpful in the patient with ovaries located extremely lateral in the pelvis. This steering technique is also helpful in imaging the anteverted or retroverted uterus.

DEPTH OF PENETRATION VS. RESOLUTION

Changes in depth of penetration created by a gradual advancement or withdrawal of the vaginal transducer allows the sonographer to image an organ or structure by placing it within the central portion of the transducer's field of view (Fig. 5-64). Changing the frequency also allows the sonographer to vary the depth of penetration. A lower frequency increases the depth of penetration to include structures higher in the pelvis; however, this comes with lower resolution. A higher frequency limits the depth to the structures in the true pelvis. The higher resolution increases the image resolution.

Decreasing the sector size also changes the resolution through changes in line density. The smaller sector size results in more lines within the sector, thus increasing the resolution. To obtain the optimal image resolution, use the highest frequency, shallowest depth, and the smallest sector size.

ROTATION

A 90-degree counterclockwise rotation of the transducer allows for imaging in the "semicoronal" or oblique transverse planes (Fig. 5-65). This rotation, coupled with slow maneuvering of the transducer handle up and down (anteroposterior angulation), produces a sweep of the pelvic anatomy from the superior to the inferior regions. Lateral angulation provides focus to either the left or right side

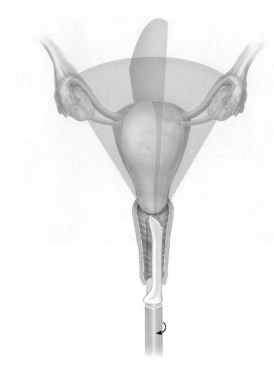

Figure 5-65 Schematic diagram demonstrating the movement of the transducer to view semicoronal/transverse images of the uterus. Beginning in a sagittal plane, the transducer is rotated 90 degrees counterclockwise to image the uterus in transverse, with the right adnexa appearing on the right side of the screen. (From DuBose TJ. Fetal Sonography. Philadelphia: WB Saunders; 1996:61–64; illustration by Victoria Vescovo Alderman, MA, RDMS.)

in the "semicoronal" transverse plane of the adnexa and its contents.

BIMANUAL MANEUVER

Another aid in optimizing endovaginal imaging is the bimanual maneuver. The sonographer places his or her free hand on the patient's pelvic area and gently applies pressure over the site of interest. This maneuver displaces bowel and moves organs or structures located higher in the pelvis into the EVS transducer's field of view. The bimanual maneuver can also help the examiner discriminate between a uterine and nonuterine mass. A uterine mass moves with the rest of the uterus, whereas a non-uterine mass slides past the uterine wall. This is also beneficial in ovarian masses.

The EVS examination of the female pelvis should begin by imaging the cervix, with the transducer incompletely inserted, increasing the distance between it and the cervix. Image the entire uterus sagitally by angling the transducer from one side to the other (lateral angulation). View the transverse planes by rotating the transducer 90 degrees counterclockwise and angle it anterior to posterior to visualize all sections of the uterus and the cul-de-sac. Image the ovaries in both planes, using the same landmarks as in TAS. In postmenopausal women the lack of follicles may make the ovaries more difficult to locate.

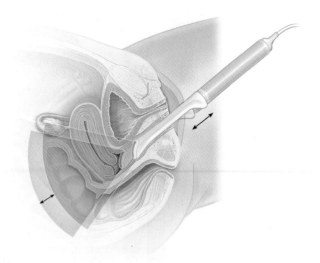

Figure 5-64 Schematic diagram demonstrating the movement of the transducer to view structures at various distances from the fornix. Pushing the transducer deeper into the fornix brings more distant structures into the field of view, whereas withdrawing the transducer permits visualization of the cervix. (From DuBose TJ. Fetal Sonography. Philadelphia: WB Saunders; 1996:61–64; illustration by Victoria Vescovo Alderman, MA, RDMS.)

The American College of Radiology (ACR) and the American Institute of Ultrasound in Medicine (AIUM) provides a pelvic sonogram guideline for sonographers.[22] The protocol may be adapted for specific needs of a department, doctor, and/or patient. The representative images obtained and required may vary between facilities. The following protocol contains the minimum views for a normal pelvic exam. Visit the ACR or AIUM web site for a detailed protocol.[22]

1) Image the cervix in the sagittal and coronal planes. Use the vaginal canal as a landmark for the cervix

2) Advance the transducer to the fornix of the vagina to examine the uterus in both the long and short axis planes. Be sure to evaluate and scan through the entire organ. Measure on three orthogonal planes

3) Image and measure the endometrium on the midline sagittal plane

4) Proceed to evaluate both adnexa by sweeping through each side in the longitudinal and transverse planes

5) Use spectral, color, and/or power Doppler to identify vascular structures within the pelvis

6) Capture images of the ovaries demonstrating both long and short axis of each organ, documenting any abnormalities detected in both planes as well. Measure each ovary on three planes

7) Finally, examine and image the pelvic cul-de-sac for the presence of fluid. Normal anatomic structures such as the ovaries and fallopian tubes, and/or pathology, may be present in this area as well

PRACTICAL TIPS: HOW TO IMPROVE ENDOVAGINAL SCANNING

Sometimes it is hard to obtain a clear image of the object remote from the transducer head because the endovaginal transducer uses high-frequency ultrasound with poor tissue penetration. The solution to this problem is to bring the transducer head as close as possible to the object. For example, if the ovary is in the cul-de-sac, the transducer should be positioned in the posterior vaginal fornix.

When using a frequency-selectable transducer, choose the frequency that allows for adequate penetration and the best detail. When the object is near the vaginal fornix, a high-frequency setting is used. To image a structure further from the transducer face, use a low-frequency setting. A closer structure requires less penetration, thus allowing for use of a higher-frequency setting.

Consider the pressure to the object by the transducer head. The pressure by the transducer head easily transmits to the object because there is no hard tissue like the abdominal wall in transabdominal sonography.

The pressure of endovaginal ultrasound transducers may temporarily deform soft objects such as an ovarian cyst. In patients complaining of lower abdominal and pelvic pain, palpate the uterus and adnexa with the transducer head. This is an efficient way to detect the cause and location of the pain. In patients presenting with abnormal uterine bleeding, for outlining the uterine cavity a negative contrast medium such as saline is used.

When the object is far from the vaginal fornix, use bimanual maneuver and push the object toward the vaginal fornix. If it does not work satisfactorily or the object is too big, use transabdominal sonography or other modalities such as CT or MRI. Endovaginal sonography is powerful in gynecologic examination but not universal.

COLOR AND SPECTRAL DOPPLER IMAGING

Doppler ultrasound can determine the presence or absence of flow, flow direction, and flow character.[23] One of the fundamental limitations of flow information provided by the Doppler effects is that it is angle dependent. Furthermore, artifacts in Doppler ultrasound can be confusing and lead to misinterpretation. The Doppler effect consists of a change in frequency of waves that reflect from moving reflectors. The amount of the change of frequency is called Doppler shift and is measured in Hz. Velocity can be calculated when the angle between ultrasound beam and flow direction is known. Apart from absolute velocity measurement, one can define relative indices, which are particularly useful for flow evaluation without known angle between the flow and ultrasound beam. Because of inherent difficulties in quantitatively evaluating blood flow, the blood flow velocity waveform has commonly been interpreted to distinguish patterns associated with high and low resistance in the distal vascular tree. Three indices are in common use, the systolic/diastolic ratio (S/D ratio), the pulsatility index (PI, also called the impedance index), and the resistance index (RI, also called the Pourcelot ratio). The S/D ratio is the simplest, but it is irrelevant when diastolic velocities are absent and the ratio becomes infinite. An "extremely high" value would be above 8.0.

Definitions of RI and PI are as follows:

Resistance index (RI) = S − D / S

Pulsatility index (PI) = S − D / mean

Spectral Doppler or pulsed Doppler display the peak velocity of flow in a vessel. Spectral Doppler presents as either a positive or a negative shift above or below the baseline, indicating the direction of flow within the evaluated vessel. Direction of flow is more important when evaluating larger blood vessels and can be quite challenging for smaller vessels. Each vessel in the body has a spectral waveform expected during the examination. Pulsed Doppler of the pelvic vasculature may and can vary depending on the menstrual phase of the patient, as will be discussed later in this chapter.

Color Doppler demonstrates the average flow frequencies, displayed as a velocity, over time within the specific area examined. Color Doppler also provides directional information, determining whether the flow is toward or away from the transducer.

Power Doppler is another option available if color Doppler is not producing the desired effects. Power Doppler is another mode which displays the Doppler shift as color. Unlike color Doppler, where a slow or low flow states result in a poor signal, power Doppler uses the strength or amplitude of the signal. This results in an increased sensitivity to low blood flow; thus vessels that produce lower Doppler shifts image with power Doppler. Newer equipment now has the ability to display what is called directional power Doppler; however, standard power Doppler does not represent direction. Power Doppler used as an adjunct to color supplies the sonographer with more valuable diagnostic information.

The preset for the pelvic exam is a good starting point for Doppler settings; however, the sonographer has the capability to adjust the pulse repetition frequency (PRF) or scale, color or pulsed Doppler gain, wall filter, and baseline.

Transabdominal and endovaginal imaging may both benefit from the implementation of spectral, color, and power Doppler. Apply these techniques to situations such as ovarian torsion evaluation, adnexal masses, retained products of conception (RPOC), and ectopic pregnancies. Use of the various Doppler modes have improved the diagnosis of many pelvic abnormalities and emergencies.

FOLLICULAR AND LUTEAL BLOOD FLOW

With endovaginal sonography and color flow imaging, it is possible to study subtle vascular changes during the ovarian cycle in physiological and

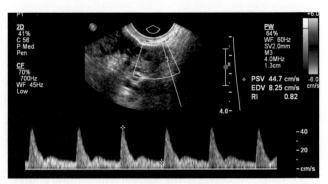

Figure 5-66 Blood flow velocity waveforms obtained from the ovarian artery during the luteal phase of the menstrual cycle. Note continuous diastolic flow and RI of 0.82, reflecting increased flow to the dominant ovary.

pathophysiological conditions.[24,25] The ovary receives arterial blood flow from two sources: the ovarian artery and the utero-ovarian branch of the uterine artery. These arteries anastomose and form an arch parallel to the ovarian hilum. Characteristic flow signals from the ovarian artery demonstrate low Doppler shifts and blood velocity (Fig. 5-66). The waveform varies with the state of activity of the ovary. Studies of the ovarian artery blood flow velocity waveforms demonstrated a difference in the vascular impedance between the two ovarian arteries, depending on the presence of the dominant follicle or corpus luteum.[24,25] Decreased pulsatility and resistance indices reflect decreased vascular impedance and increased flow to the ovary containing the dominant follicle or corpus luteum.[24] The ovarian artery of the inactive ovary shows low enddiastolic flow or absence of diastolic flow. A rise in end-diastolic flow velocity of the active ovary is most obvious during the midluteal phase.

From the ovarian hilum, arterial branches penetrate the stroma and acquire a tortuous and helicoid pathway. Spiral or helical artery naming is due to their characteristic shape. This type of vascularity demonstrates a high resistance to blood flow. Such vessel structure also facilitates accommodation to changes in ovarian size due to development of the follicle and the corpus luteum. As they grow, the arteries unwind

---

PATHOLOGY BOX 5-7

Tips for Endovaginal Sonography

- Ensure removal of all air between the sheath and transducer
- Use the highest frequency possible for the best detail
- Reduce the sector width to increase detail
- Image the organ of interest in the central beam
- Position the transducer footprint close to the area of interest
- Decrease the depth to fill the image with the target organ
- Use external maneuvers such as bimanual manipulation or rolling the patient to bring the area of interest into range
- Color or power Doppler helps identify surrounding vessels and thus the organ (i.e., ovary)
- Ask for help

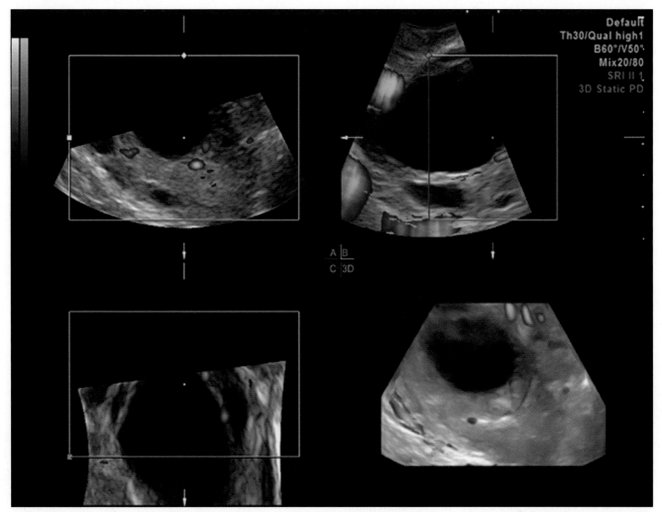

Figure 5-67 3D power Doppler image of a preovulatory follicle. Perifollicular flow is easily obtained by power Doppler imaging.

and become larger, returning to the basal state during follicular atresia or luteal regression. Routine clinical practice uses follicular growth assessment starting from the ninth or the tenth day of a regular 28-day menstrual cycle. The dominant follicle images as an anechoic cystic structure with sharp borders usually measuring 8 to 10 millimeter in diameter. As stated, it grows at a rate of 2 to 3 millimeters per day. Detection of follicular rim flow velocity patterns occur when a dominant follicle attains 10 millimeters in diameter (Fig. 5-67).[24,25] A few days preceding ovulation, the resistance index (RI) is about 0.54 (Fig. 5-68). A decline in resistance to flow usually starts 2 days prior to ovulation, resulting in an RI of approximately 0.44 ± 0.04 at ovulation. Blood flow velocity increases before ovulation probably because of both hormonal factors and angiogenesis. A significant increase in the peak systolic blood flow velocity also helps determine imminent ovulation even in the presence of a relatively constant RI. This may be due to angiogenesis and dilatation of these newly formed vessels between the vascular theca cell layer and the hypoxic granulosa cell layer of the follicle. Disruption of these vascular changes may have profound effects on oxygen concentration across the follicular epithelium. In luteinized unruptured follicles, there is a failure of blood velocity to peak during the preovulatory period.[25] These data support the hypothesis that changes in oxygen tension within the follicular wall may be necessary for follicular rupture.

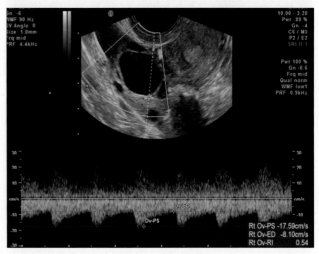

Figure 5-68 Pulsed Doppler waveform analysis of follicular flow shows RI of 0.54.

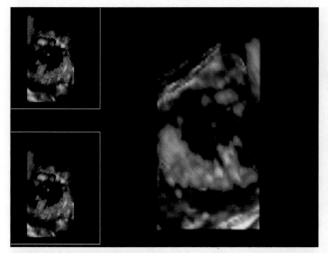

Figure 5-69 Demonstration of increased intraovarian vascularity during the luteal phase as demonstrated by 3D power Doppler ultrasound.

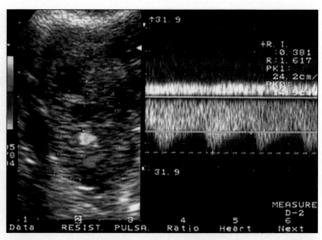

Figure 5-71 Pulsed Doppler waveform analysis shows high velocity (24.2 cm/s) and low impedance (RI = 0.38), both indicative of normal corpus luteum function.

In patients with polycystic ovarian syndrome, there are no changes in the ovarian arteries and intra-ovarian vascular resistance during the menstrual cycle.

Following ovulation, the corpus luteum forms as the result of many structural, functional, and vascular changes in the former follicular wall (Fig. 5-69). Endovaginal color Doppler may detect luteal flow early in the second half of the ovarian cycle and also during the first trimester of pregnancy.[26,27] The mature corpus luteum demonstrates increased blood flow velocity in relation to the preovulatory follicle, with a mean RI of 0.43 ± 0.04 (Figs. 5-70 and 5-71).[24] In the nonpregnant state the regression of the corpus luteum begins at about the 23rd day of the menstrual cycle and is recognized by an increased RI of 0.49 ± 0.02. In pregnancy, the corpus luteum is maintained by the secretion of human chorionic gonadotropin (hCG) produced by the trophoblast.

UTERINE BLOOD FLOW

The majority of the blood supply to the uterus is from the uterine arteries with minimal contribution from the ovarian arteries. The uterine arteries give rise to the arcuate arteries, which orient circumferentially in the outer third of the myometrium (Fig. 5-72). These vessels give rise to the radial arteries, which after crossing the myometrial-endometrial border further branch and give rise to the basal arteries and the spiral arteries. The basal arteries, which are relatively short, terminate in a capillary bed that serves the stratum basale of the endometrium. The spiral arteries, on the other hand, project further into the endometrium and terminate in a vast capillary network that serves the functional layer of the endometrium.

Only the spiral arteries undergo substantial anatomic changes during the menstrual cycle (Fig. 5-73).[24,25]

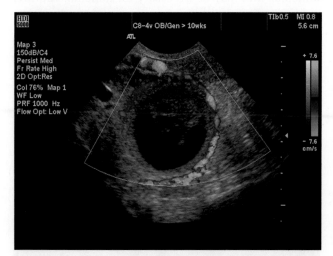

Figure 5-70 Endovaginal color Doppler scan of a hemorrhagic corpus luteum. Color coded area represents corpus luteum angiogenesis. (Image courtesy of Philips Medical Systems, Bothell, WA.)

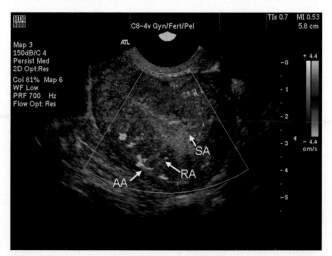

Figure 5-72 Endovaginal color Doppler scan of the uterus demonstrating arcuate (AA), radial (RA), and spiral arteries (SA). (Image courtesy of Philips Medical Systems, Bothell, WA.)

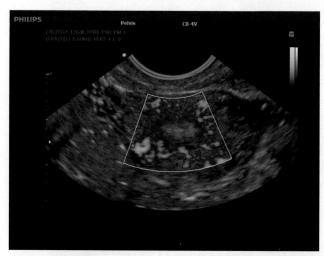

Figure 5-73 Endovaginal power Doppler scan demonstrating thickened, early secretory transformed endometrium. Spiral arteries are demonstrated at the periphery of the endometrium. (Image courtesy of Philips Medical Systems, Bothell, WA.)

Rhythmic changes in uterine blood flow during the estrous cycle in different species are associated with the daily ratio of estrogen to progesterone in systemic blood. The higher the estrogen-progesterone ratio, the greater the quantity of blood flow through the uterine vascular bed.[25] Progesterone antagonizes the uterine vasodilatory effect of estrogen and the magnitude of this inhibition relates to the ratio of the two steroids.

Color Doppler signals from the main uterine arteries image lateral to the cervix at the level of the cervicocorporal junction of the uterus (Fig. 5-74).[24] Waveform analysis demonstrates high to moderate velocity of the flow. The RI depends on age, phase of the menstrual cycle and special conditions (pregnancy, uterine fibroid etc.). During the proliferative phase of the menstrual cycle, there is a small amount of end-diastolic flow in the uterine arteries.[24,25] The RI is about 0.88 ± 0.04 until day 13 of the 28-day menstrual cycle. Reports reveal a further increase in uterine artery impedance 3 days after the luteinizing hormone (LH) peak. Increased uterine contractility and compression of the vessels traversing the uterine wall, which decrease their diameter and cause consequently higher resistance to blood flow, may explain these findings. During the normal menstrual cycle there is a sharp increase in end-diastolic velocities between the proliferative and secretory phases of the menstrual cycle. The lowest blood flow impedance occurs during the time of peak luteal function, during which implantation is most likely to occur.[24,25] In anovulatory cycles these changes are not present, and the RI shows a continuous increase. The persistently lower RI in the luteal phase suggests that the relaxation effects on the uterine arteries persist until the onset of menstruation. Sonographers should also be aware of the circadian rhythm in uterine artery blood flow during the periovulatory period, which appears to be independent from hormonal changes.[28]

The quality of endometrial perfusion is highly dependent upon the uterine, arcuate, and radial artery blood flow. The characteristic spiral artery flow has a lower velocity spectral tracing when compared to the uterine artery.[24,25] It is hypothesized that the features of endometrial blood flow might be used to predict the implantation success rate and reveal unexplained infertility problems.

THREE-DIMENSIONAL ULTRASOUND

The introduction of three-dimensional (3D) ultrasound into a routine practice has enabled storage of complete sets of volume data (Fig. 5-75). Once stored, these data sets allow access and image reconstruction at any time without deterioration in quality. Any desired image plane within the acquired volume can be restored, and the entire dataset manipulated to render the mulitplanar, surface, or transparent views. The 3D ultrasound examination has four main steps: data acquisition, 3D visualization, volume/image processing, and storage of the volume or image data.[29]

The acquisition of the gynecologic 3D data set deviates from the procedure for the routine two-dimensional (2D) examination. The transducers used for 2D image acquisition double as a 3D acquisition tool using a freehand method. Since this is nonquantitative, a mechanical transducer is often preferred. For a complete discussion of these methods of obtaining the 3D data set, refer to Chapter 32.

There are many advantages to using 3D ultrasound in evaluating female pelvic anatomy. The sonographer can navigate through the stored volume in all three planes with tomographic precision. Visualization

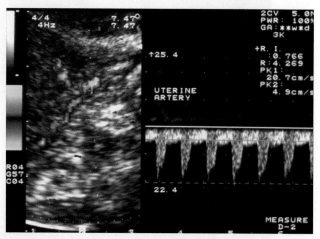

Figure 5-74 Blood flow velocity waveforms extracted from the uterine arteries during the secretory phase demonstrate increased end-diastolic velocity and RI of 0.77.

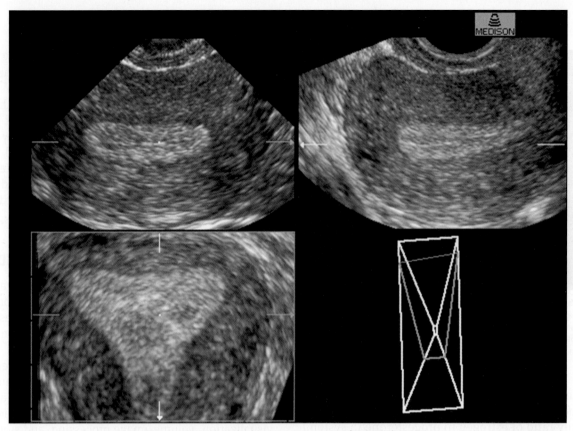

Figure 5-75 3D multiplanar reconstruction of a normal uterus.

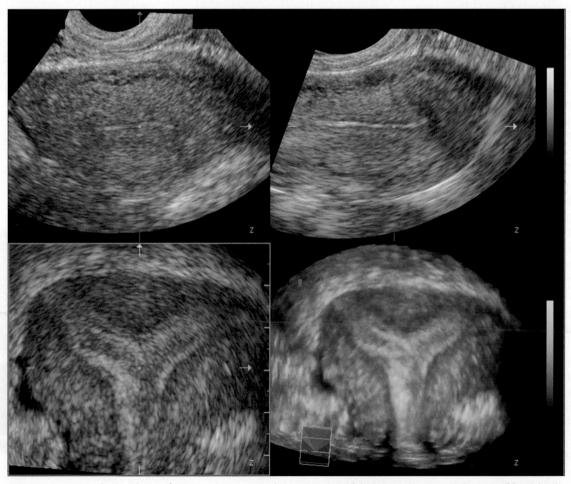

Figure 5-76 Three perpendicular planes of septate uterus. Note clear separation of the uterine cavity and absence of fundal indentation.

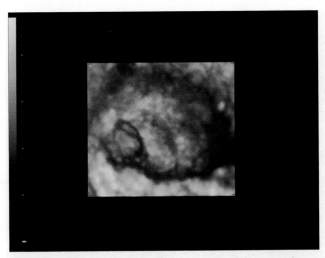

Figure 5-77 3D ultrasound (surface rendering) of the preovulatory follicle. Cumulus oophorus is suggestive of imminent ovulation.

of a coronal plane enables instantaneous visualization of the uterine cavity, myometrium, and fundus, which facilitates diagnosis of uterine anomalies (Fig. 5-76).[30,31,32] Accurate volumetry has made precise estimations of follicular, ovarian, and endometrial volumes feasible (Figs. 5-77 and 5-78).[33,34] Ovarian volume assessment contributes to accurate diagnosis of polycystic ovarian syndrome and prediction of the response to ovulation induction (Fig. 5-79). By providing multiple tomographic sections of the uterine cavity, uterine polyps, submucosal fibroids, and intrauterine synechiae become easily visible (Fig. 5-80).[35] Quantification of the endometrial volume in combination with blood flow studies contributes to the assessment of the endometrial receptivity and may have the potential to predict pregnancy rate in assisted reproductive techniques (Fig. 5-81).[36] Combined evaluations of

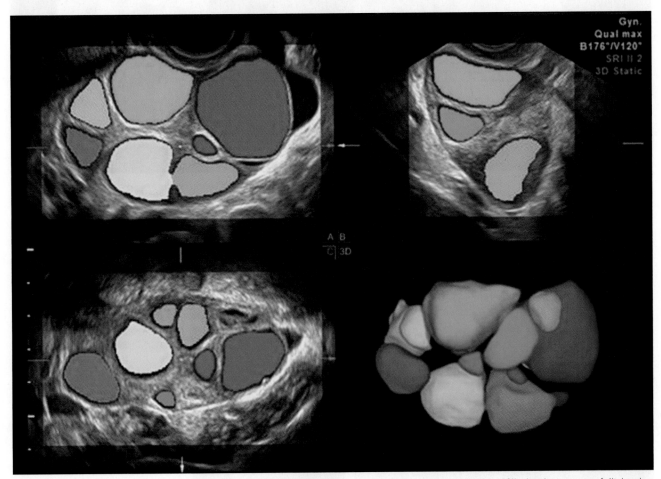

Figure 5-78 3D ultrasound of the hyperstimulated ovary after ovulation induction. The ovary is enlarged and filled with numerous follicles that are coded in different colors.

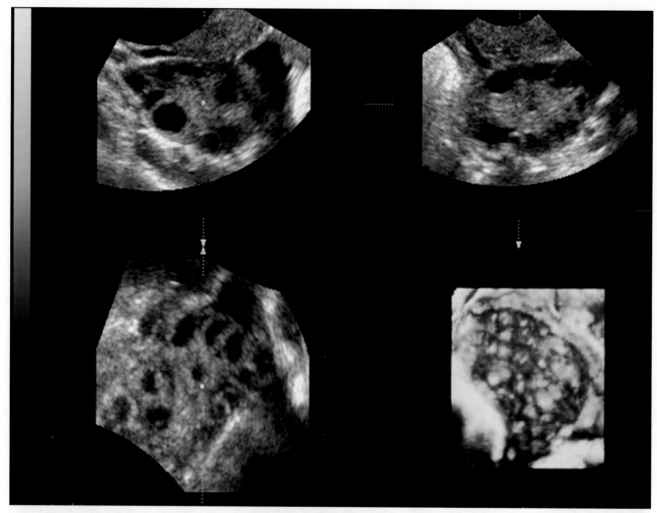

Figure 5-79 General pattern of polycystic ovary as seen by 3D ultrasound.

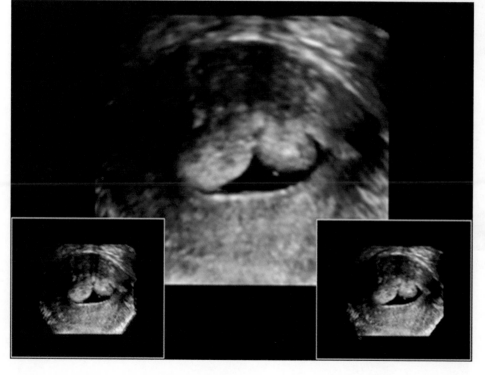

Figure 5-80 Frontal reformatted section of the uterus, demonstrating two focal areas of increased echogenicity. Histeroscopy confirmed two endometrial polyps.

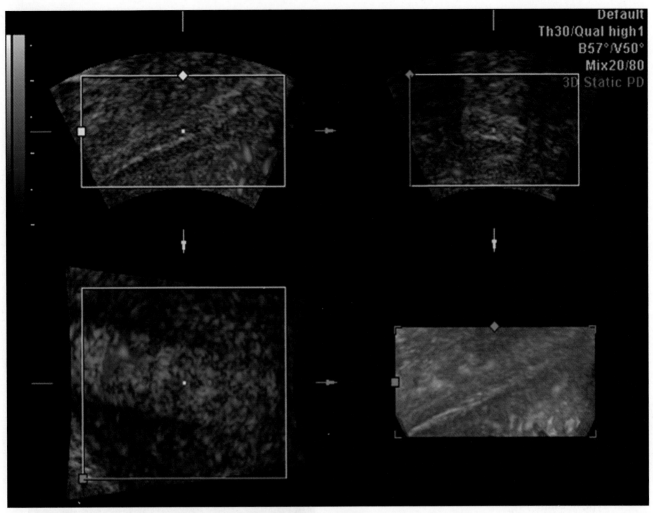

Figure 5-81 3D power Doppler scan of the periovulatory endometrium.

morphology and neovascularity by 3D power Doppler may improve detection of ovarian and uterine malignancy.[37,38]

Digital volume storage allows retrospective analysis of the volumes and independent review by a second examiner or expert. De-identified datasets allow efficient use of images and data for training purposes.

SUMMARY

- TAS imaging provides a global view of the pelvic structures
- EVS provides close-up detailed imaging of the pelvic organs
- The pelvic skeleton of the pelvis include the sacrum, coccyx, and two innominate bones
- The true pelvis contains the organs of reproduction
- Fat or smooth muscles are more echogenic than the skeletal muscles
- The bladder has three portions; the apex, base, and neck

- Ureters insert into the bladder at the trigone
- Segments of the uterus include the fundus, corpus, and cervix
- The three tissue layers of the uterus are the serosa, myometrium, and endometrium
- Uterine and ovary size vary with age, menstrual cycle, and hormone status
- Uterus location is posterior to the bladder and vesicouterine pouch and anterior to the pouch of Douglas and rectum
- Uterine vessels, broad ligaments, fallopian tubes, and ovaries are lateral to the uterus
- Bowel produces "dirty shadows" within the pelvis and may or may not demonstrate peristalsis
- Arterial supply for the pelvic organs originate from the aorta
- Venous supply of the pelvis mimics the arterial except for the ovarian/gonadal veins, with the right terminating into the inferior vena cava and the left into the left renal vein

Critical Thinking Questions

1. This image is from a normal pelvic exam. Critique the image for improvements.

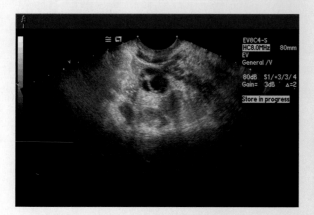

ANSWER:
- Time gain compensation (TGC) high in near field and low in the far field
- Overall gain to high
- Depth to shallow for imaging the ovary
- Decrease the sector width to increase the line density and thus the detail

2. A 43-year-old patient presents to your department with a history of ovarian cysts seen on a CT scan done last month. Her clinician ordered the exam for pelvic pain, which has since resolved. Identify the following:
   a. Type of exam
   b. Endometrial phase
   c. Structures indicated by the arrows and how to confirm your identification

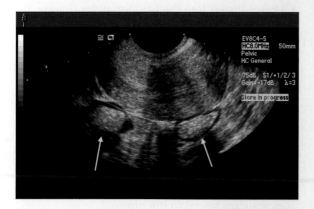

ANSWER: This is a midline, sagittal, endovaginal image of the uterus in the proliferative phase. The structures indicated by the yellow arrows are loops of bowel. They can be identified by the characteristic shadowing and peristalsis.

3. A 23-year-old patient presents to the department with complaints of menstrual irregularity. Unfortunately, she voided before her exam. After viewing the images:
   a. Describe the position of the uterus using both images.
   b. Identify the structures indicated by the star on the transverse image of the uterus.

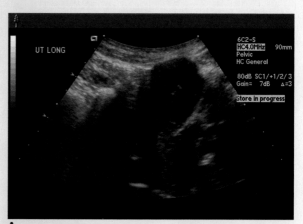

A

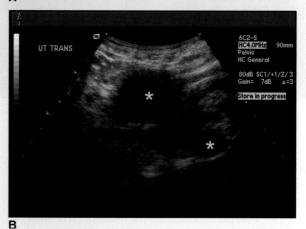

B

ANSWER: The anteflexed uterus has a dextroflexed deviation from midline. Since the bladder is empty and the uterus is in the anteflexed postion, a transverse image results in an image slice through both the fundus and lower uterine segment.

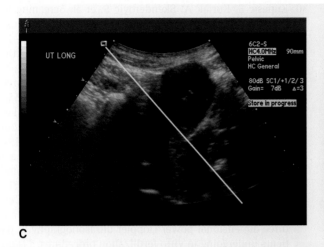

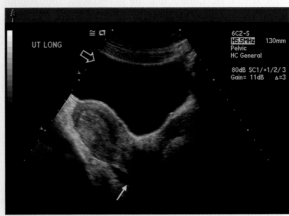

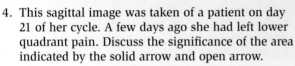

C

4. This sagittal image was taken of a patient on day 21 of her cycle. A few days ago she had left lower quadrant pain. Discuss the significance of the area indicated by the solid arrow and open arrow.

ANSWER: The solid arrow indicates free fluid. The day of her cycle and the pain in the left lower quadrant indicate that the fluid is probably due to ovulation. The open arrow indicates reverberation artifact in the anterior portion of the bladder.

- Color and power Doppler imaging can aid in localization of the ovaries and determining the type of cyst found through the cycle or in early pregnancy
- Volumetric imaging aids diagnosis of normal and abnormal ovarian findings

REFERENCES

1. Standring S. Gray's Anatomy: The Anatomical Basis of Clinical Practice, Expert Consult. Section 8. 40th ed. Philadelphia: Churchill Livingstone; 2008.
2. Moore KL, Dalley AF, Agur AMR. Clinically Oriented Anatomy. Chapter 2. 6th ed. Philadelphia: Wolters Kluwer/Lippincott Williams & Wilkins; 2010.
3. Bonsib SM. Renal anatomy and histology. In: Jennette JC, Olson JL, Schwartz MM, Silva FG, eds. *Heptinstall's Pathology of the Kidney*. 6th ed. Philadelphia: Churchill Livingstone; 2007.
4. Salsgiver TL, Hagan-Ansert S. Normal anatomy and physiology of the female pelvis. In: *Textbook of Diagnostic Medical Ultrasonography*. 6th ed. Volume 2. St. Louis: Mosby; 2006.
5. Sample WF. Gray scale ultrasonography of the normal female pelvis. In: Sanders RC, James AE, eds. *The Principles and Practice of Ultrasonography in Obstetrics and Gynecology*. 2nd ed. New York: Appleton-Century-Crofts; 1980.
6. Levi CS, Lyons EA, Holt SC, et al. Normal anatomy of the female pelvis and transvaginal sonography. In: *Ultrasonography in Obstetrics and Gynecolodgy*. 5th ed. Callen PW, ed. Philadelphia: Saunders Elsevier; 2008.
7. Valentin L, Callen PW. Ultrasound evaluation of the adnexa (ovary and fallopian tubes). In: *Ultrasonography in Obstetrics and Gynecolodgy*. 5th ed. Callen PW, ed. Philadelphia: Saunders Elsevier; 2008.
8. Oike K, Obata S, Takagi K, et al. Observation of endometrial movement with endovaginal ultrasonography (Abstract). *J Ultrasound Med*. 1988;7:S99.
9. Poder L. Ultrasound evaluation of the uterus. In: *Ultrasonography in Obstetrics and Gynecolodgy*. 5th ed. Callen PW, ed. Philadelphia: Saunders Elsevier; 2008.
10. Rumack CM, Wilson SR, Charboneau JW. Gynecologic ultrasound. In: *Diagnostic Ultrasound*. 3rd ed. Volume 1. St. Louis: Elsevier; 2006.
11. Sample WF, Lippe BM, Gyepes MT. Gray-scale ultrasonography of the normal female pelvis. *Radiology*. 1977;125: 477–483.
12. Hagan-Ansert S. Pediatric congenital anomalies of the female pelvis. In: *The Textbook of Diagnostic Ultrasonography*. 6th ed. Volume 1. St. Louis: Mosby Elsevier; 2006.
13. Gibbs RS, Karlan BY, Haney AF, et al., eds. Gynecologic ultrasound. In: *Danforth's Obstetrics & Gynecology*. 10th ed. Philadelphia: Lippincott Williams & Wilkins; 2008.
14. Wallace WH, Kelsey TW. Ovarian reserve and reproductive age may be determined from measurement of ovarian volume by transvaginal sonography. *Hum Reprod*. 2004;19(7): 1612–1617.
15. Valentin L, Callen PW. Ultrasound evaluation of the adnexa (ovary and fallopian tubes). In: *Ultrasonography in Obstetrics and Gynecology*. 5th ed. Philadelphia: Saunders Elsevier; 2008.
16. Blount RF. The digestive system. In: Schaeffer JP, ed. *Morris' Human Anatomy*. 11th ed. New York: McGraw-Hill; 1953.
17. Moore KL, Dalley AF, Agur AMR. Clinically Oriented Anatomy. Chapter 1. 6th ed. Philadelphia: Wolters Kluwer/Lippincott Williams & Wilkins; 2010.
18. Rottem S, Thaler I, Goldstein SR, et al. Endovaginal sonographic technique: Targeted organ scanning without resorting to "planes." *J Clin Ultrasound*. 1990;18:243–247.
19. Fleischer AC, Kepple DM. Normal pelvic anatomy as depicted with endovaginal sonography. In: Fleischer AC, Manning FA, Jeanty P, Romero R, eds. *Sonography in Obstetrics and Gynecology*. 5th ed. Stamford, CT: Appleton & Lange; 1996:43–52.

20. Timor-Tritsch IE. Conducting the gynecologic ultrasound examination. In: Goldstein SR, Timor-Tritsch IE, eds. *Ultrasound in Gynecology*. New York: Churchill Livingstone; 1995:49–54.

21. American College of Radiology. Practical Guideline for the performance of pelvic ultrasound. Revised 2009.

22. Breyer B. Physical principles of the Doppler effect and its application in medicine. In: Kupesic S, ed. *Color Doppler and 3D Ultrasound in Gynecology, Infertility and Obstetrics*. New Delhi: Jaypee Brothers; 2003:1–14.

23. Kurjak A, Kupesic S, Schulman H, et al. Endovaginal color Doppler in the assessment of ovarian and uterine perfusion in infertile women. *Fertil Steril*. 1991;6:870–874.

24. Kupesic S, Kurjak A. Uterine and ovarian perfusion during the periovulatory period assessed by endovaginal color Doppler. *Fertil Steril*. 1993;3:439–443.

25. Kupesic S, Kurjak A, Vujisic S, et al. Luteal phase defect: comparison between Doppler velocimetry, histologic, and hormonal markers. *J Ultrasound Obstet Gynecol*. 1997;9:105–112.

26. Kupesic S, Kurjak A. The assessment of normal and abnormal luteal function by endovaginal color Doppler sonography. *Eur J Obstet Gynecol*. 1997;72:83–87.

27. Zaidi J, Jurkovic D, Campbell S, et al. Description of circadian rhythm in uterine artery blood flow during the peri-ovulatory period. *Hum. Reprod*. 1995;10:1642–1646.

28. Kurjak A, Kupesic S. Clinical Application of 3D Sonography. New York, London: Parthenon Publishing; 2000.

29. Kupesic S, Kurjak A. Diagnosis and treatment outcome of the septate uterus. *Croat Med J*. 1998;39:185–190.

30. Kupesic S, Kurjak A, Skenderovic S, et al. Screening for uterine abnormalities by three-dimensional ultrasound improves perinatal outcome. *J Perinat Med*. 2002;30:9–17.

31. Kupesic S. Three-dimensional ultrasound in reproductive medicine. *Ultrasound Rev Ob Gyn*. 2005;5:304–315.

32. Kupesic S, Kurjak A. Predictors of IVF outcome by three-dimensional ultrasound. *Hum Reprod*. 2002;17:950–955.

33. Kupesic S, Kurjak A, Bjelos D, et al. Three-dimensional ultrasound ovarian measurements and in vitro fertilization outcome are related to age. *Fertil Steril*. 2003;79:190–197.

34. Kupesic S, Kurjak A, Ujevic B. B-mode, color Doppler and three-dimensional ultrasound in the assessment of endometrial lesions. *Ultrasound Rev Obstet Gynecol*. 2001;1:50–71.

35. Kupesic S, Bekavac I, Bjelos D, et al. Assessment of endometrial receptivity by endovaginal color Doppler and three-dimensional power Doppler ultrasonography in patients undergoing in vitro fertilization procedures. *J Ultrasound Med*. 2001;20:125–134.

36. Kupesic S, Plavsic MB. Early ovarian cancer: 3D power Doppler. *Abdominal Imaging*. 2006;31:613–619.

37. Kupesic S, Kurjak A, Hajder E. Ultrasonic assessment of the postmenopausal uterus. *Maturitas*. 2002;41:255–267.

38. Kupfer MC, Ralls PW, Yao SF. Transvaginal sonographic evaluation of multiple peripherally distributed echogenic foci of the ovary: prevalence and histologic correlation. *AJR*. 1998;171(2):483.

39. Muradali D, Colgan T, Hayeems E, et al. Echogenic ovarian foci without shadowing: are they caused by psammomatous calcifications? *Radiology*. 2010;254(2):429–435.

40. Webb JL. I'm seeing spots!: a review of literature regarding echogenic foci of the ovary. *JDMS*. 2002;18:380.

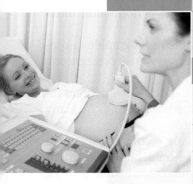

6 Doppler Evaluation of the Pelvis

Michelle Wilson

OBJECTIVES

Summarize changes seen during the female cycle in the flow patterns of the ovaries, uterus, and adnexal vessels

List indications for the Doppler examination of the pelvis

Calculate qualitative measurements to include systolic/diastolic (S/D) ratios, resistance index (RI), and pulsatility index (PI) indices

Describe the importance of low and high resistance flow in pelvic vessels

Identify the correct sampling method for obtaining spectral Doppler tracings

Discuss the flow pattern and formation of a uterine arteriovenous malformation (AVM) and pelvic congestion

Explain ovarian flow patterns in the presence of torsion and neoplastic processes

KEY TERMS

S/D ratio | resistive index | PI | color Doppler | energy or power Doppler impedance indices | pulsed wave Doppler | uterine Doppler study | ovarian Doppler study | pelvic congestion syndrome | arteriovenous malformation of the female pelvis

GLOSSARY

Adnexa Anatomical parts added, attached, or adjunct to another or others

Angiogenesis Physiologic process involving the growth of new blood cells from preexisting vessels

Arcuate vessels Small vascular structures found along the periphery of the uterus

Arteriovenous malformation abnormal connection between veins and arteries

Impedance indices Measurements used to compare the resistance of a medium to the propagation of flow

Ovarian vessels Blood vessels that supply oxygenated blood to and drain deoxygenated blood away from the ovaries

Pourcelot resistive index Doppler measurement that takes the highest systolic peak minus the highest diastolic peak divided by the highest systolic peak

Proliferative phase early Days 5 to 9 of the menstrual cycle

Proliferative phase late Days 10 to 14 of the menstrual cycle

Pulsatility index Doppler measurement that uses peak systole minus peak diastole divided by the mean

S/D ratio Difference between peak systole and end diastole

Secretory phase Days 15 to 28 of the menstrual cycle

Uterine artery Main vessel carrying oxygenated blood toward the uterus

---

Ultrasound has been established and continues to prove itself as an indispensable tool in the evaluation of the female pelvis. Anatomical information is always invaluable in the presence of suspected pathology, and with recent technologic advancements, assessment of physiologic information in both adult and pediatric populations is now routine with sonography. Ultrasound's ease of use, noninvasiveness, and high resolution allow for sonography to be the center of diagnostic imaging for gynecologic concerns.

Doppler techniques allow for a thorough investigation of changes in pelvic structures such as the uterus, ovaries, and adnexa during different phases of the menstrual cycle in the presence of a broad spectrum of pathologies. Sonography is the fundamental diagnostic imaging tool in the determination of the origin, size, location, contour, vascularity, internal consistency, and definition of a pelvic mass, or the presence or absence of ascites in the female pelvis.

Doppler ultrasound is a vital component in the evaluation of pelvic pathology and physiology. As has been well established in the literature, many pathologies elicit an increase in blood flow to the affected pelvic organs. Whether this is attributed to angiogenesis of malignant or benign tumors, hyperemia from inflammatory conditions, or even normal and abnormal physiological blood flow patterns, Doppler studies provide a great deal of information to the investigator. This chapter presents the application of the various modalities of Doppler ultrasound for the investigation of the female pelvis.

PATIENT HISTORY AND PREPARATION

Prior to any sonographic examination, a thorough patient history should be taken to include any pertinent information that might help correlate the sonographic findings with the proper differential diagnosis. This may provide information that will assist in the diagnosis, differential diagnosis, or follow-up of a previously noted pathology.

This patient history includes the patient age, date of the first day of the last menstrual period (LMP), normality or irregularity of the LMP, gravidity, parity, hormone regimen if applicable, and personal history or familial history of cancers. Also document the following: clinical symptoms such as pain or bleeding (and their lengths), any history of pelvic procedures or infections, laboratory data, and any other pertinent medical or surgical history, which should include any biopsies or invasive procedures. After obtaining a thorough patient history, explain the procedure and direct the patient to the examination table.

PERFORMANCE STANDARDS

Multiple major professional organizations have developed recognized statements, recommendations, and standardizations for the use of diagnostic medical sonography in the pelvic examination. These include the Society of Diagnostic Medical Sonography, the American Institute of Ultrasound in Medicine, the American College of Radiology (ACR), and the International Society of Ultrasound in Obstetrics and Gynecology (ISOUG).[1-4] All of these professional foundations have websites full of valuable information, which encourage their use. This chapter will rely on the standards set forth by the ACR, but—as stated on the ACR website— recommendations for clinician requirements, written requests for the examinations, documentation, and quality control vary among these organizations.[1]

The ACR practice guidelines for the ultrasound examination of the female pelvis are briefly summarized by the following:

1. Ultrasound of the female pelvis should be performed only when there is a valid medical reason, in a written or electronic request for the study. This allows for proper exam performance, interpretation, and reimbursement.

2. Use the lowest possible sonographic exposure settings to gain the necessary diagnostic information.

3. Identify all relevant structures through transabdominal (TA) or endovaginal imaging. In many cases, both will be needed.

4. High-quality patient care requires adequate documentation. There should be a permanent record of the ultrasound examination and its interpretation. Record images of all appropriate areas and include both normal and abnormal structures. Include an official interpretation of the ultrasound examination in the patient's medical record.

5. Conduct the sonographic examination of the female pelvis with a real-time scanner. Adjust the transducer to operate at the highest clinically appropriate frequency.

6. Clean all transducers after use according to manufacturer recommendations. Cover vaginal transducers with a protective sheath prior to insertion. Following the examination, dispose of the sheath and clean the transducer in an antimicrobial solution.

The ACR also lists standards for personnel, protocols, quality control, quality improvement, safety, infections control, and patient education concerns as discussed in Chapter 1.

ABDOMINAL AND ENDOVAGINAL IMAGING

The complete ultrasound examination of the female pelvis should utilize both the TA and transvaginal/endovaginal sonography (TV/EVS) approaches, as these methods can complement each other. The TA technique typically provides an opportunity to survey the pelvic anatomy and pathology with a good global overview. The endovaginal approach often provides a more detailed examination of the pelvic organs, but due to its higher frequency and diminished maneuverability of the transducer, is often more limited in its field of view (Table 6-1).

The literature suggests that TA and EVS each have their own limitations and advantages, implying that an optimal gynecologic study of the uterus and adnexa should include both scanning techniques in order to arrive at the proper clinical diagnoses.[5-8] Every lab should have its own written protocols to guide the sonographer/sonologist through the proper methodology in evaluating the female pelvis in its entirety with sonography.

TABLE 6-1		
Benefits and Drawbacks of Transabdominal and Endovaginal Techniques		

Transabdominal Advantages

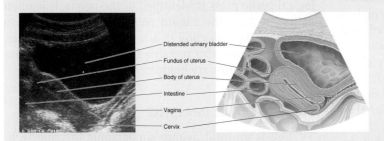

View of entire pelvis
Evaluate large masses
Evaluate small or large masses farther medial or lateral from midline
Can be used on patients with intact hymen
Noninvasive to not cause psychological or emotional harm

Transabdominal Disadvantages

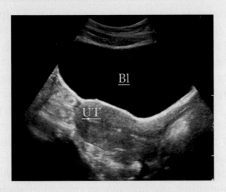

Full bladder must be prepped prior to exam
Full bladder may cause physical pain
Some patients are unable to fill bladder adequately
Retroverted uterus can be difficult to completely visualize
Less detail due to depth and penetration

Endovaginal Advantages

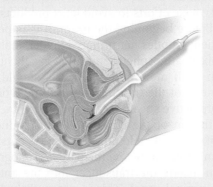

Closer to pelvic organs
Higher frequency transducer/better resolution
Empty bladder/no patient prep
Obese patients with a large panus can be scanned
Abdominal wall scars or openings can be avoided

Endovaginal Disadvantages

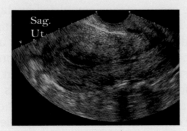

Limited field of view
Large masses can extend past the field of view
Patients with an intact hymen may not be scanned
Physical and emotional limitations not allowing the patient to relax
Small lesions outside of field of view can be missed
Some postmenopausal patients with acute pain cannot tolerate transducer

ABDOMINAL IMAGING

The TA examination is performed from the anterior abdominal wall. The transducer used is based on the fundamental sonographic imaging principle that balances adequate depth penetration while preserving the highest resolution possible. TA transducers used are curvilinear, sector, or linear as required by patient body habitus and certain pathologic presentations. The frequency of the transducer is also adjusted based on patient body habitus, with a higher frequency (5.0 MHz) used for thinner patients and a lower frequency (2.5 MHz) considered for larger patients.

TA pelvic studies are enhanced by a distended urinary bladder, as it generally displaces small bowel and its contained gas from the field of view. For this reason, patients should be instructed to *finish* drinking 32 oz of fluid at least 1 hour prior to their exam. An optimally filled bladder images anterior to the uterus in a midline plane and is noted by its elongated appearance and anechoic lumen, extending from the area of the vaginal canal to the top of the fundus in the normal-sized uterus (Fig. 6-1; Fig. 1-2). Bladder distention was once thought to potentially have an effect on Doppler spectra, producing a notable increase in the impedance indices compared to the Doppler study performed with an empty bladder, but this theory has been disproved.[9] When the urinary bladder is full, the body of the uterus is typically well visualized because of its position; however, the course of the uterine arteries is often less optimal for a Doppler study because of the angle of incidence at which the ultrasound beam intersects the vessels. Also, be aware that an overfilled bladder may displace or push pelvic organs too superiorly or laterally, thereby creating a situation in which they are out of the transducer's plane of view. If this occurs, the study may be enhanced if the patient partially voids.

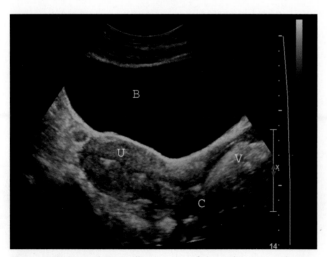

Figure 6-1 Sagittal TA midline image of the pelvic cavity demonstrating the more anterior urinary bladder (B), the uterus (U), the cervix (C), and the vagina (V).

The TA study includes investigation of the uterus, adnexa, and urinary bladder. Identification of the full bladder helps the sonographer to avoid mistaking a cystic mass for the normal pelvic organ. When a pathological cystic mass is identified in the pelvis, it is often helpful to have the patient void and obtain images to document the reduction in size of the urinary bladder. The cystic mass size remains constant if it lacks connection to the urinary bladder.

ENDOVAGINAL IMAGING

TV/EVS is an intracavitary sonographic imaging technique that requires the insertion of an ultrasound transducer into the vaginal canal. EVS provides better anatomic detail when compared to TA imaging, as the transducer can be placed closer to the area of interest and it employs a higher frequency. The course of the uterine artery in a superior to inferior fashion allows for an ideal Doppler angle when obtaining its waveform and indices with this sonographic technique.

The procedure in its entirety must be explained and the intent in performing the study must be conveyed to the patient. Once this is complete, the sonographer must then obtain acceptance of the patient in order to continue on and perform the endovaginal exam. Before beginning any invasive examination such as an EVS, it is imperative that the sonographer/sonologist question the patient about any known latex allergies and, if present, make efforts to avoid latex products.

Before beginning the exam, it is imperative that the patient empties her urinary bladder, making for a more relaxed atmosphere and allowing the uterus to position itself more anteverted. Gel should be applied to the end of the transducer and it must be covered with a protective sheath. Make sure there are no air bubbles at the tip of the cover, as these produce an imaging artifact. Apply additional gel to the outside of the condom or sheath before the patient, sonographer, or clinician inserts the transducer into the anterior fornix of the vaginal canal. This is accomplished by advancing the transducer 3 to 4 inches or 7 to 8 centimeters into the vaginal canal. The sonographic evaluation of the pelvic organs is then completed by directing the sound beam throughout the pelvis, by rotating and angling the transducer from anterior to posterior and right to left.

A common gynecologic examination table that allows for a supine position with heel support or stirrups works well for the endovaginal study. If this type of examination table is not available, the patient can be positioned at the end of the table with her hips elevated by a pillow or foam cushion, allowing for proper movement of the transducer without being impeded by the table. Image the patient in the lithotomy position with a slight reverse Trendelenburg tilt to localize free fluid in the pouch of Douglas. If present, this fluid creates tissue-fluid interfaces, improving the outline of pelvic structures. In some instances, a Trendelenburg position helps to displace bowel from the pelvic structures. When evaluating the adnexa, the transducer can be moved into the lateral fornix for improved visualization.

Use a transducer that employs a frequency of 7.5 MHz or higher to allow for better resolution of the uterine and adnexal morphology. Upon completion of the examination, dispose of the condom or sheath covering the endovaginal transducer. Soak the transducer in an antimicrobial solution, following the manufacturer's directions and soak times.

WAVEFORM ANALYSES

Doppler ultrasound has been used for many years as a noninvasive technique to assess blood flow impedance. When employing pulsed wave Doppler, the sonographer is able to measure the distribution of velocities in the sample volume as well as the changing dynamics noted throughout the cardiac cycle. The Doppler effect and its fundamental principles have been covered in many physics texts; however, a brief explanation of Doppler signal analysis is included in this chapter.

We begin by defining the differences between qualitative and quantitative measurements of Doppler studies. Qualitative Doppler indices offer 'semi-quantitation' of the characteristics of waveforms by demonstrating the direction, breadth, and extent of the individual flow patterns. This type of analyses is better at defining characteristics of the waveforms, which indirectly give an approximation of flow and resistance to flow of the area being interrogated. Qualitative indices use ratios in their formulas or calculations, therefore are not angle dependent, with the three most popular including systolic/diastolic ratios (S/D ratios), resistance index (RI) also called resistive index or Pourcelot's index, and pulsatility index (PI). These measurements are all calculated from the maximum Doppler shift waveform. Quantitative Doppler applications however have proven most useful in noninvasive measurements of estimating absolute blood velocities, assessment of vascular impedances, and quantifying flow disturbances. All of the quantitative indices rely heavily on the correct angle of measurement and the diameter of the vessel being interrogated in order to accurately conclude the correct measurement.[10]

The resistance index was first described by Pourcelot in 1974 as a mathematical derivative of the simple S/D formula or ratio.[12] The resistance index is the difference between systolic and diastolic pressure divided by the systolic pressure See Table 6-2. In 1976, Gosling and King proposed their theory that velocity waveforms are sensitive to changes in the impedance of the vascular bed.[13] They speculated that the difference between peak systolic pressure and end-diastolic pressure divided by the mean maximum frequency over the entire cardiac cycle would evaluate the sensitivity of impedances and arterial resistance. The pulsatility index analyzes diastolic flow differently than the resistive index, by running a cursor along the superior aspect of the mean systolic and diastolic flow, with the mean being calculated by the ultrasound system. Stuart and colleagues first described the S/D ratio in 1980.[14] This is simply the ratio of the peak systolic velocity to the end diastolic velocity. These indices are not dependent on the angle of insonation simply because they use ratios in their calculations, and do not require a measurement of the diameter of the lumen of the vessel, making them easier to obtain than quantitative values. These three indices:

(1) Resistive index (RI)
(2) Pulsatility index
(3) S/D ratio

are widely used in gynecological sonographic studies, and when possible angles of less than 60 degrees between the area being sampled and the ultrasound beam should be implemented, but are not absolute.

Arterial Doppler flow analysis can be categorized into two different types: high-resistance and low resistance. The higher resistance flow pattern demonstrates a high systolic peak and a low diastolic flow. The lower resistance spectral waveform is demonstrated by a sometimes biphasic systolic peak and a relatively high level of diastolic flow, thus demonstrating that a low resistance bed will allow for more blood flow to lapse (Fig. 6-2). Or simply, with a constant perfusion pressure the flow increases as the impedance to flow decreases.[11]

Employing these waveform analysis calculations while using optimal signal recording methods, a sonographer should be able to determine the expected and/or

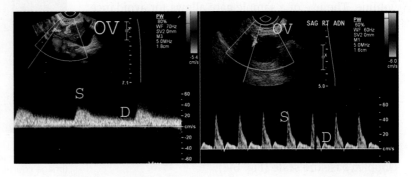

Figure 6-2 This two-image set displays an endovaginal sagittal axis view of the right ovary, with a pulsed wave Doppler waveform of the ovarian artery **(on the left)** demonstrating a low impedance or resistance waveform. Note the higher diastolic flow and slower uptake during systole. The arterial signal of a high impedance **(on the right)** displays a lower diastolic flow pattern and a high uptake with systole. *OV*, ovary; *S*, systole; *D*, diastole.

TABLE	6-2

Procedure for Measuring the Waveform

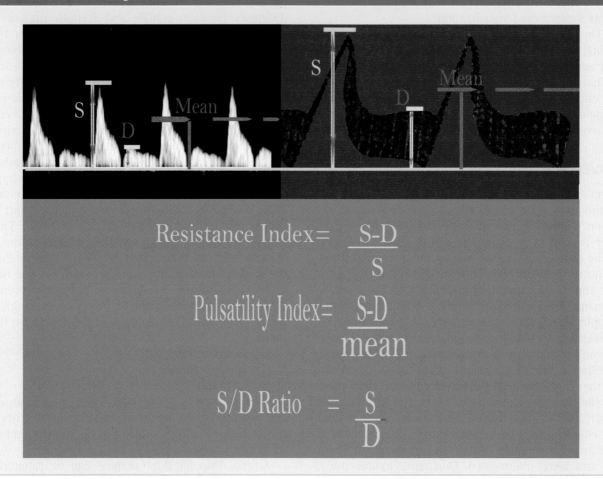

$$\text{Resistance Index} = \frac{S-D}{S}$$

$$\text{Pulsatility Index} = \frac{S-D}{mean}$$

$$\text{S/D Ratio} = \frac{S}{D}$$

the pathologic waveforms in a given area. A high-resistance pattern noted in an area where a low-resistance appearance is typically found raises suspicion of occlusion or compromise. If an area normally expected to be high resistance, like the ovaries during the proliferative phase, is found to have a lower resistance, this could raise the question of neovascularization (Fig. 6-3).

DOPPLER TECHNIQUES

As discussed previously, pulsed Doppler is used to detect the presence of blood flow in a select area or vessel at a known depth, with a given sample gate or sample volume. The use of a sample gate allows for avoidance of proximal vessel movement, allowing for a more concise evaluation of a given vascular structure. When interrogating a vessel with pulsed wave Doppler, note the direction of blood flow as either above or below the baseline. Flow traveling toward the transducer is displayed above the Doppler baseline (unless the scale has been inverted, thus displaying the flow pattern on the opposite side of the baseline), and flow moving away from the transducer is traditionally plotted below the Doppler baseline scale (Fig. 6-4).

If the peak systolic flow and the angle at which the beam intersects the vessel are known, then one can deduce the velocity at which the blood is traveling within the sample gate.[10,11] When attempting to analyze a vascular flow for purposes of determining its velocity by a

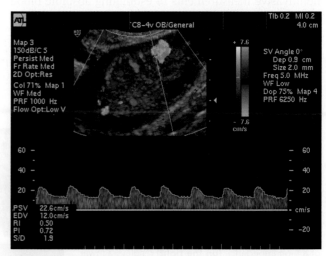

Figure 6-3 This triplex image of ovarian flow utilizes an automatic measuring method which calculates all indices from the waveform. (Image courtesy of Philips Medical Systems, Bothell, WA.)

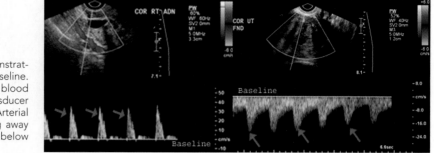

Figure 6-4 Doppler spectral analysis demonstrating arterial flows above and below the baseline. **A:** Arterial Doppler waveform displaying blood flow moving in a direction towards the transducer *(arrows)*, and displayed above the baseline. **B:** Arterial Doppler spectral waveform with flow moving away from the transducer *(arrows)*, being displayed below the baseline.

Doppler shift, a correct angle must be obtained, or the calculation formula used will not allow for the correct velocity. To ensure optimal accuracy when calculating velocities, use angles of less than 60 degrees. The standard measurement used when displaying the spectral waveform is velocity, which is written as meters per second or centimeters per second (m/sec or cm/sec).

FLOW PATTERN

Vascular flow has distinct patterns when analyzed with spectral Doppler methods. Typically, venous vessels have a continuous recurring flow in diastole and systole with a reduced flow signal when compared to arterial signals. Typical arterial flow will have a spectral waveform with an alternating quick uptake systolic peak and a lower diastolic flow level (Fig. 6-5).

Color Doppler is an overlay that assigns different hues to red blood cells traveling through a vessel in a given sample area, based on the degree of the frequency shift, and the direction they are moving, in relation to the transducer. These result in a display of the relative velocity of flow.[15] As with pulsed wave, the fundamental principles of the Doppler equation apply, therefore the displayed results are dependent

on optimization of angles between the flow being interrogated in the region of interest (ROI) and the transducer. This can be achieved by either moving the transducer to the correct location or by manipulating the ROI or color box to coincide with the correct angle desired.

Generally, flow moving toward the transducer displays as red and flow moving away from the transducer displays as blue (Fig. 6-6). To help remember this flow pattern, think BART: blue away, red toward. The color bar, located on the side of the image, should be used to determine flow direction. Different color hues are used to depict the different speeds at which the red blood cells are moving. Traditionally, the faster velocities are brighter and slower velocities are darker; however, color Doppler velocity maps are not standardized, and proprietary colors are programmed into different ultrasound machines. When turbulent flow is detected, one would expect to see a mixture of darker and lighter colors being displayed in the sample area. Today's machines frequently allow users to employ a plethora of color Doppler velocity maps, displaying a variation of colors and hues in vascular structures.

In a normal vessel, it can be assumed that the velocity of blood is highest at the center and is lowest

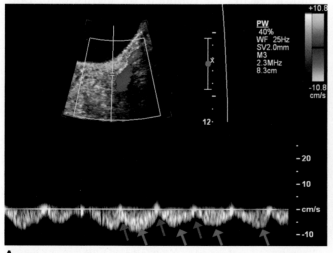

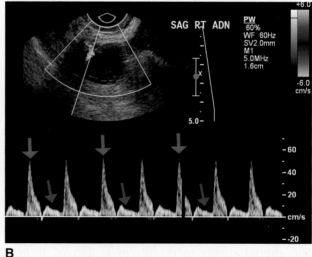

A **B**

Figure 6-5 Venous and arterial waveforms. **A:** Venous waveform with continuous flow during both systole *(red arrows)* and diastole, with the relative reduction in diastolic flow *(blue arrows)*. **B:** Arterial flow is typically distinguishable and distinct, with an alternating quick uptake systolic peak *(red arrows)* and a reduction in flow during diastole *(blue arrows)*.

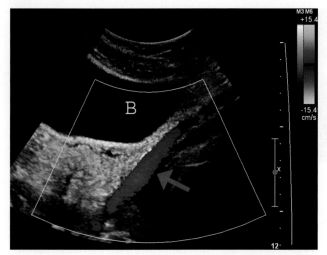

Figure 6-6 TA study of the pelvis displaying the iliac vessels. The lumen of the vessel (red arrow) is filled with a blue color hue, indicating flow moving away from the transducer as referenced from the velocity map located in the upper right of the image. B, bladder.

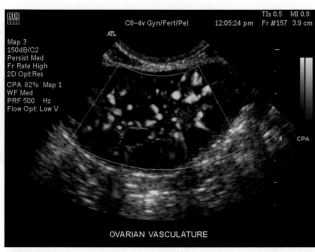

Figure 6-7 Endovaginal sonogram in the coronal plane demonstrating the vascular bed of the ovary, Color Power Angio (CPA). (Image courtesy of Philips Medical Systems, Bothell, WA.)

closer to the wall.[10,11] This principle is termed *laminar flow*. In the presence of an irregularity in the vessel or if the vascular structure is tortuous, the flow can be distorted, causing the greater velocity flow to travel closest to the vessel wall; this is commonly noted in malignant ovarian tumors or prominently vascular pathologies.

Color Doppler and power Doppler allow for the visualization of perfusion within the tissues of the uterus and ovaries. With expected color flow waveforms changing with the fluctuating phases of the menstrual cycle and patient's age, these applications can be used to identify vascular structures for quantitative analysis with pulsed wave Doppler.

Power or energy Doppler displays movement but without the attempt to obtain a frequency shift (Fig. 6-7). Without these stipulations, flow in all directions visualized in the ROI can be noted without the restriction of certain Doppler angles. The application of power Doppler is often implemented when more sensitivity is needed for subtle flow than is otherwise obtained with color Doppler. Power Doppler has also been widely used for the subjective assessment of vascular patterns. When evaluating adnexal lesions with low velocity internal flow, sometimes it is helpful to utilize power Doppler to determine the presence and location of flow, then assess more thoroughly with pulsed wave Doppler. Color Doppler can also be helpful in establishing the solid nature of a hypoechoic solid mass.

NORMAL UTERINE DOPPLER

The arterial supply to the uterus is derived from a complex network of arteries originating from the uterine arteries (Fig. 6-8). The uterine artery receives its vascular supply from the anterior branch of the internal iliac artery. Imaging with either the TA or EV techniques should allow for visualization of the internal iliac vessels, on the lateral aspect of the pelvis, and often can be used as a landmark for the more anterior ovaries (Fig. 6-9). When using color Doppler to identify the iliac vessels, ensure complete color filling of the lumen, and note the artery to be typically anterior to the vein. From its proximal origination on the anterior internal iliac artery, the uterine artery passes medially on the surface of the levator ani muscle, crossing above the ureter and descending to the uterus at the level of the cervix. The uterine artery tends to be tortuous and travels in a spiral fashion on the lateral aspect of the uterus from the level of the cervix in an inferior to superior course within the broad ligament, giving rise to uterine branches throughout its course, until it reaches the cornua of the uterus. Color Doppler helps to demonstrate and interrogate the uterine arteries coursing along the lateral aspects of the body of the uterus; however, the most readily identifiable location for sampling the uterine artery with sonography is at the level of the cervix. Once the uterine artery arrives at the cornua of the uterus, it anastomoses with the ovarian artery (Fig. 6-10).

The main uterine arteries circle the anterior and posterior surfaces of the uterus, forming branches with the arcuate arteries in the myometrium of the uterus.[16] These arcuate arteries are often sonographically identifiable as anechoic tubular structures coursing within the outer portion of the uterus (Fig. 6-11A–D). In the postmenopausal patient, the arcuate arteries may be noted to be calcified, as this occurs normally with age. These calcifications image with sonography as peripheral linear echogenic areas with shadowing (Fig. 6-12).

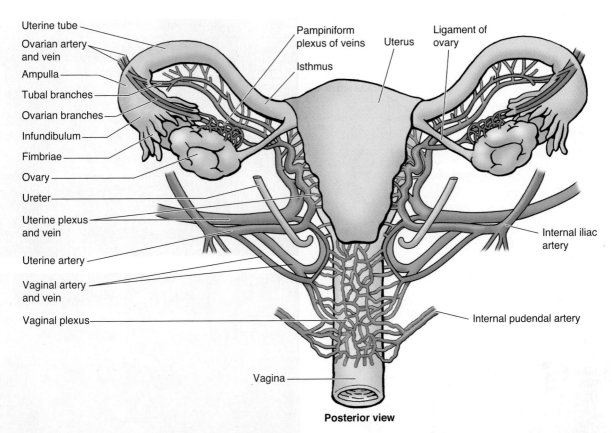

Posterior view

Figure 6-8 Blood supply and venous drainage of the uterus, vagina, and ovaries. The broad ligament of the uterus is removed to show the ovarian artery from the aorta and the uterine artery from the internal iliac artery supplying the ovary, fallopian tube, and uterus. Observe also the anastomosing tubal and ovarian branches within the broad ligament (removed). Examine the pampiniform plexus and ovarian vein and the uterine plexus and vein. (From Moore KL, Dalley AF II. *Clinical Oriented Anatomy.* 4th ed. Baltimore, MD: Lippincott Williams & Wilkins; 1999.)

The radial arteries branch off the arcuate arteries and are directed into the uterine lumen from the myometrium, where the spiral arteries are formed. It is the spiral and radial arteries that supply blood to the functional layer of the endometrium. Color flow and pulsed wave Doppler waveform is typically found only in the periovulatory period in the endometrium or its subendometrial layer (Fig. 6-13). During menses, blood from the spiral arteries is shed as part of the functional layer or zona functionalis of the endometrium.

An increase in uterine volume paralleling the menstrual cycle is heavily dependent on the variance in

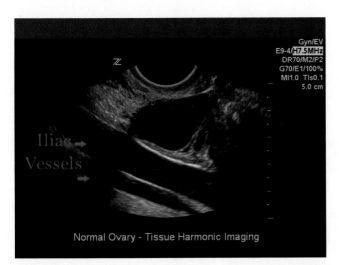

Figure 6-9 Endovaginal image of the right ovary (ovary) in a sagittal plane, and the external iliac artery and vein (iliac vessels).

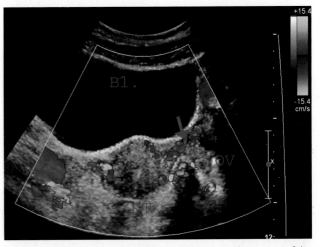

Figure 6-10 TA midline image of the pelvic cavity. The cornua of the uterus is shown with the ovarian arteries anastomosing *(red arrow)* with the uterine arteries. *UT,* uterus; *OV,* ovary; *Bl,* urinary bladder.

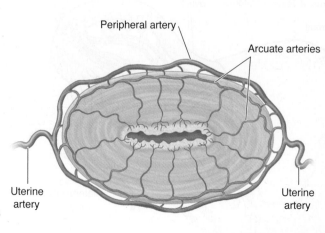

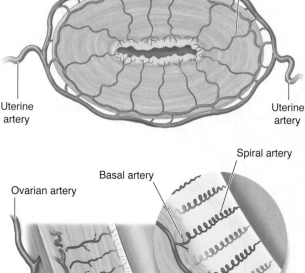

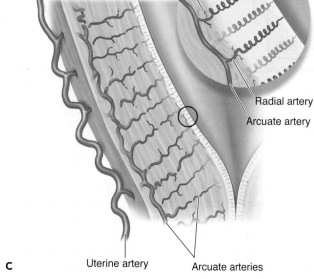

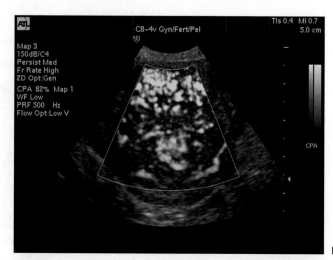

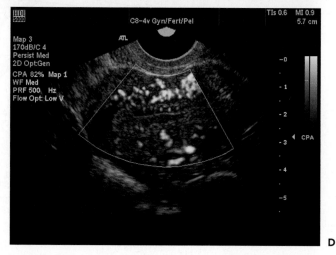

Figure 6-11 Arcuate arteries. **A:** Diagram of the arcuate arteries being supplied by the uterine artery in the transverse plane. The arcuate arteries then continue on to supply the spiral arteries. **B:** Endovaginal coronal view of the mid uterus. Energy Doppler or CPA portrays the course of arcuate arteries within the uterus. **C:** Diagram of the arcuate arteries on the longitudinal plane. **D:** Endovaginal sagittal view of the midline uterus. (Images courtesy of Philips Medical Systems, Bothell, WA.)

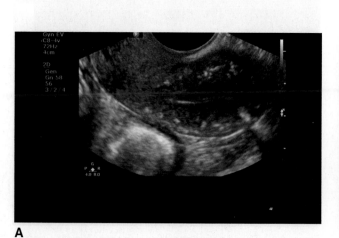

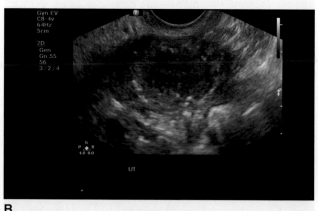

Figure 6-12 A: Sagittal endovaginal image of a uterus with calcified arcuate vessels. **B:** Transverse image of the same uterus. (Images courtesy of Derry Imaging Center, Derry, NH. Robin Davies, Ann Smith, and Denise Raney.)

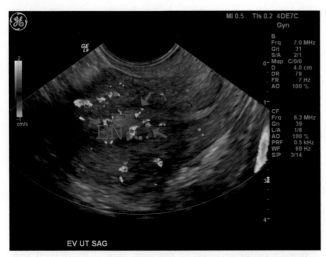

Figure 6-13 Endovaginal sonogram in the sagittal plane with demonstration of spiral arterial flow *(arrows)* within the endometrium. *EN,* endometrium.

vascular supply.[17–21] As with ovarian artery flow, uterine artery velocities vary with the menstrual cycle and dramatically increase with an early pregnancy, while the impedance decreases. The assessment of uterine artery flow by Doppler examination is typically easy to obtain and readily reproducible. Blood flow in the uterine arteries has been shown to be of moderate to high velocity with a high-resistance flow in the nongravid patient. The RI is higher in the proliferative phase of the menstrual cycle (0.88 ± 0.05), then decreases slightly (0.84 ± 0.06) before ovulation and into the luteal phase.[22–24] Cyclical variation in uterine artery flow is well defined and also appears to correlate with fertility.[22–24] Given the variability in menstrual cycles, assessment of reproductive physiology should be based on cyclical changes rather than individual values. It is important to be aware of the fact that mean values for uterine artery flow in postmenopausal patients are similar to those recorded for the midluteal phase in premenopausal patients.[25]

Periuterine veins should course in close proximity with the uterine arterial vessels. They may be prominent but should not distend to measure over 5 mm in the nongravid uterus, and flow velocities should range between 5 and 10 cm/sec[26–28] or suspicion of pelvic congestion syndrome may be raised.

REPRODUCTIVE-AGE FEMALE

OVARIAN ARTERIAL FLOW VARIES WITH MENSTRUAL CYCLE

The ovarian artery originates from the lateral aspect of the aorta at around the level of the lower margin of the renal pelvis. The arteries follow the same inferior course as the ureters over the psoas muscles, crossing the common iliac artery just superior to its bifurcation into the external and internal iliac arteries. The ovarian artery then enters the infundibulopelvic ligament, where it travels to the ovary on the superior aspect to supply the parenchyma. An attempt at a complete or thorough arterial vascular supply is provided to the ovaries by the addition of the ovarian artery forming an anastomoses with the ovarian branches formed from the uterine artery. With two separate arterial supplies to the ovaries, a solid effort is made to provide a well-compensated arterial feed (Fig. 6-14). The ovarian arteries typically follow a tortuous pattern; therefore, it is common to identify only short segments of the artery in any one scan plane.

During the course of the menstrual cycle, the Doppler spectra of the ovarian artery and stromal ovarian flows vary.[29–32] These variations can be attributed to the hemodynamic changes that are involved in the remodeling of ovarian tissue that occurs during the predictable follicular growth, ovulation, and new corpus

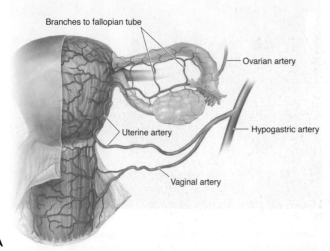

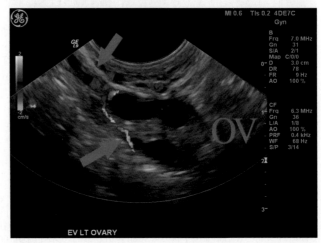

Figure 6-14 A: Diagram of the ovarian and uterine arteries. **B:** Sagittal image of the ovary *(OV)*. Arrows depict the proximal ovarian artery, and the more distal ovarian artery within the ovarian stroma.

luteum development. Intraovarian arterial flow visualizes within the stroma of the ovary using color and power Doppler, with flow being observed more frequently in the luteal phase than in the early follicular or periovulatory phases.

During the follicular phase, before formation of a dominant follicle, normal ovarian artery flow has a low velocity, with a high resistance or impedance pattern. Diastolic flow is low and can be absent, and the mean RI is approximately 0.92 ± 0.08.[32] Irrespective of the side of ovulation, this peak velocity tends to be fairly constant; the impedance, however, has been found to drop dramatically in the ovarian artery on the side with the dominant follicle, especially in the periovulatory period or luteal phase. The RI then rises during the late luteal phase (Fig. 6-15). At the time of ovulation, both the maximal velocity increases and the RI decreases, reaching a low point of 0.44 ± 0.08.

The low impedance of the dominant follicle probably results from neovascularization, as velocities increase hours before follicle rupture and continue to rise until approximately 72 hours after the formation of the corpus hemorrhagicum.[33,34] Similar values for ovarian vascular indices noted in the follicular phase of a premenopausal female have been noted in postmenopausal ovaries but the cyclical variation is lost. Just as with uterine arterial absolute values, cyclic variations and the uniqueness of individuals lend to the conclusion that solitary measurements of ovarian artery impedance is of limited value in the assessment of ovarian function.

In early pregnancy, the corpus luteal cyst helps maintain the pregnancy through secretion of progesterone. Color Doppler studies of the cyst reveal increased vascularity surrounding the cyst. This phenomenon, often called the "ring of fire," supplies blood flow to the cyst

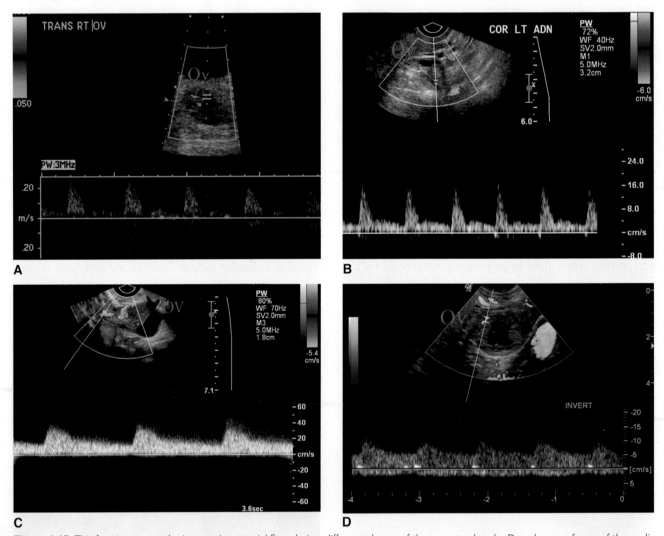

Figure 6-15 This four-image set depicts ovarian arterial flow during different phases of the menstrual cycle. Doppler waveforms of the cyclic changes of the ovarian artery can be seen with these Doppler spectra. **A:** Intraovarian arterial flow during the follicular phase. **B:** Intraovarian arterial flow during the late luteal phase. **C:** Intraovarian arterial flow during the corpus luteal phase. **D:** Intraovarian flow during the corpus hemorrhagicum phase. *OV,* ovary.

wall. Spectral Doppler sampling of these vessels shows prominent diastolic, low-resistance flow.[5,17]

ARTERIOVENOUS MALFORMATION

A vascular plexus of arteries and veins without an intervening capillary network is known as an arteriovenous malformation (AVM). They are rare, occurring anywhere in the body. In the uterus, they typically involve the myometrium, which houses more vessels with lower impedances, but at times may involve the endometrium. As seen with AVMs in other areas of the body, they are acquired through such acute events as trauma or surgery. In the uterus, they have also been reported secondary to gestational trophoblastic disease, with these patients presenting with menorrhagia, which includes hemoglobin-dropping blood loss. In the pelvis, congenital AVMs may also be present, but these occur less frequently than the acquired type.[35-37]

Sonographically, uterine AVMs present with a large variability, ranging in subtleness from minimal findings to the more obvious, as is seen with nonspecific serpiginous, anechoic structures within the pelvis. These findings may be confused with multiloculated ovarian cysts, fluid-filled bowel loops, and hydrosalpinx, giving the use of Doppler studies top priority.

Color Doppler is diagnostic in displaying abundant blood flow within the anechoic structures, so much so that there is often an elaborate color mosaic signal, which is more extensive than the gray-scale abnormality due to the turbulent and chaotic nature of the flow. Spectral Doppler often shows high velocity, low-resistance arterial flow with high-velocity venous flow often being indistinguishable from the arterial signal. Color flow imaging and pulsed wave Doppler are both essential in confirming the vascular nature of an AVM and for distinguishing it from other entities such as a hydrosalpinx, multilocular ovarian cysts, fluid-filled bowel loops, or pelvic varicosities. Typically, treatment includes embolic therapy, with confirmation of a uterine AVM made with angiography[38-41] (Fig. 6-16).

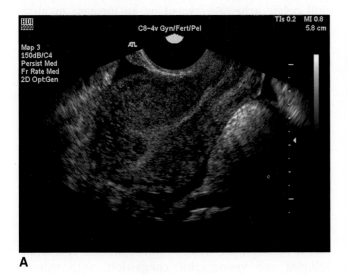

A

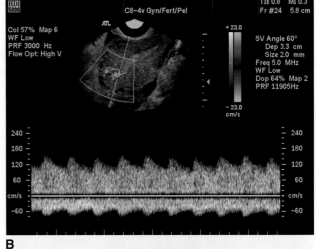

B

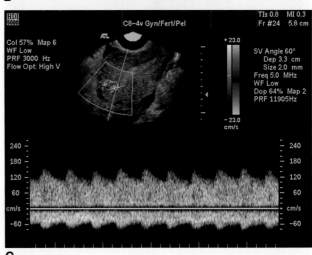

C

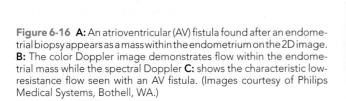

Figure 6-16 A: An atrioventricular (AV) fistula found after an endometrial biopsy appears as a mass within the endometrium on the 2D image. **B:** The color Doppler image demonstrates flow within the endometrial mass while the spectral Doppler **C:** shows the characteristic low-resistance flow seen with an AV fistula. (Images courtesy of Philips Medical Systems, Bothell, WA.)

DOPPLER OF THE OVARIAN VEIN

Venous drainage of the ovaries occurs via the ovarian plexus, which communicates with the uterine plexus in the broad ligament. The ovarian vein arises from the ovarian plexus and ascends superiorly along the psoas major muscle. The ovarian veins course differently on the left and right sides of the pelvis. The left ovarian vein travels superiorly and drains into the left renal vein at a right angle, whereas the right ovarian vein drains directly into the inferior vena cava at an acute angle (Fig. 6-17). They carry blood at lower pressures, so their walls are thinner than those of arteries.

The literature reports a mean ovarian vein diameter in nulliparous women as 2.6 mm as opposed to 3.4 mm in the parous group. The veins are known to enlarge greatly during pregnancy to accommodate the increased blood volume. The ovarian vein Doppler signal displays continual flow throughout the cardiac cycle (Fig. 6-18). Sonography can provide a quick and inexpensive initial examination of venous structures within the pelvis, without risk to the patient. However, exams are frequently limited by overlying bowel gas.

PELVIC CONGESTION

The pathophysiology of pelvic congestion syndrome is not completely understood, but many investigators believe that incompetence of the ovarian veins leads to progressive varicosities in the broad ligament and pampiniform plexus, which are associated with pelvic

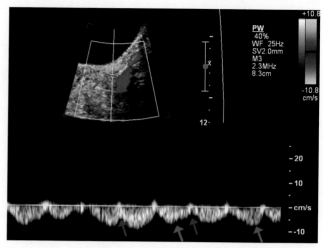

Figure 6-18 TA study of the ovarian vein. This spectral Doppler image displays the ovarian vein with continuous flow throughout the cardiac cycle. The *red arrows* depict systole, and the *blue arrows* depict diastole. *OV,* ovary.

pain. When valves in the veins do not properly close, they allow for retrograde flow and pooling of blood, causing pressure and dilatation in these areas. Patients with pelvic congestion typically complain of a chronic dull pelvic ache, aggravated by an increase in intra-abdominal pressure, such as during bending and lifting, or by walking and prolonged standing.

Patients may complain of premenstrual, menstrual, postcoital, and perineal pain. Pelvic congestion syndrome is often associated with vulvar, perineal, and lower extremity varices. This syndrome is diagnosed most frequently in multiparous women. Therefore, it is suggested that the dilatation of the ovarian veins during pregnancy compensates for the sometimes 60-fold increase in blood flow and is a likely cause of subsequent venous incompetence.[42,43]

The gold standard to diagnosing pelvic congestion is venography, an invasive procedure requiring sedation and irradiation. The literature supports a correlation between the number and diameter of ovarian follicles and venographic congestion, with women having congestion tending to have significantly more and smaller follicles.[44-46] Unfortunately, it has been shown that endovaginal ultrasound measurements of adnexal vasculature, including power Doppler measurements, cannot reliably distinguish between women with pelvic congestion and controls. Ultrasound may remain useful for diagnosis of pelvic congestion, predominantly due to visualizations of larger than expected, multicystic ovaries, and multiple dilated structures lateral to the uterus. Sonographic imaging also helps rule out other pathologies that might contribute to patient symptoms.

When multiple tortuous and dilated venous structures around the uterus and ovaries (larger than 4 to 5 mm in diameter with slow flow velocities [about 3

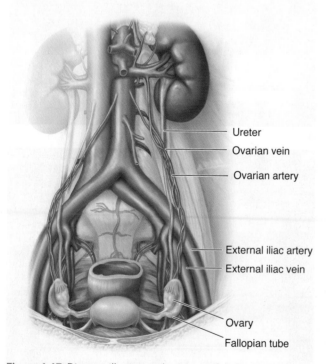

Ureter
Ovarian vein
Ovarian artery

External iliac artery
External iliac vein

Ovary
Fallopian tube

Figure 6-17 Diagram illustrating the course of the ovarian vein and artery coursing anterior to the external iliac vessels.

PATHOLOGY BOX 6-1

Spectral Doppler Waveforms

	Sample Location	Normal cm/sec	Abnormal
Uterine artery	Laterally at the cervical level	Arterial proliferative phase RI = 0.88 ± 0.05 Arterial luteal phase RI = 0.84 ± 0.06	Lack of flow
Uterine vein	Adjacent to the uterine artery	Nulliparous women = 2.6 mm Parous women = 3.4 mm Continuous forward flow	>5 mm in diameter <5 or >10 cm/sec venous flow
Ovarian artery	Within ovary stroma	Arterial follicular phase RI = 0.92 ± 0.08 Arterial luteal phase RI = 0.44 ± 0.08	High diastolic flow
Ovarian neoplasm	Within mass		RI = 0.4 PI = 1.0

cm/sec]) are noted, the suspicion of pelvic congestion syndrome should be raised[47,48] (Fig. 6-19).

OVARIAN TORSION

Ovarian torsion is a differential for patients presenting with localizing pain in the lower pelvis. Torsion is caused by the rotation of the ovary with the vascular pedicle on its axis, resulting in arterial, venous, or lymphatic obstruction. A variety of sonographic ovarian presentations may be found depending on the duration and degree of torsion, including a solid mass, a cystic mass, a solid mass with peripheral follicles, with or without pelvic fluid, thickening of the wall, and cystic hemorrhage. The classic finding of a torsed ovary is one that is enlarged and edematous (hypoechoic), with multiple small peripheral follicles, little to no vascular flow, and free fluid in the pelvis. There is a possibility that an ovary is torsed but still displays blood flow either centrally or peripherally, secondary to torsion that has not yet caused necrosis. In this case, laparoscopic untwisting of the adnexa can be successful in saving the ovary.[26,49]

In the classic case of ovarian torsion, blood flow is absent on the affected side. When this finding is encountered, it is necessary to document blood flow in the contralateral ovary to ensure that Doppler controls are set appropriately and the absence of a waveform is truly due to the absence of blood flow. With the finding of nonexistent vascular flow, open surgery and oophorectomy would be the likely procedure, whereas those with normal flow patterns can be likely managed conservatively.[50]

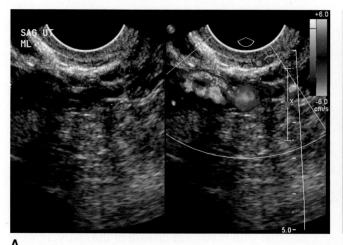

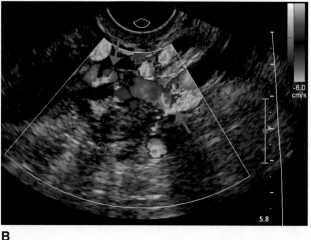

A   **B**

Figure 6-19 Pelvic congestion. **A:** Dual screen image demonstrating multiple anechoic tubular structures measuring greater than 5 mm in size, found adjacent to the lateral aspect of the uterus. When color was applied to these structures, they were characteristic of venous structures. **B:** Dilated venous vessels *(arrows)* adjacent to the ovary *(OV)* in the same patient.

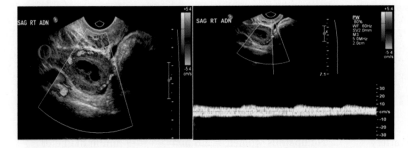

Figure 6-20 Corpus luteal flow. Endovaginal, sagittal image of the right ovary *(OV)* showing color flow around the dominant follicle on the left, and spectral waveform of the low impedance vascular supply to the corpus luteal cyst on the right.

OVARIAN NEOPLASMS

A good deal of literature has been dedicated to the use of Doppler sonography for distinguishing between benign and malignant adnexal masses.[51-53] Because tumor vessels lack a muscular layer, they frequently have a low resistance flow. This resistance is typically obtained and quantified using either the RI or the PI. A RI of 0.4 or less or a PI of 1.0 or less has been associated with malignant disease.[54-57] However, many other physiologic and benign neoplastic lesions can have a low RI. Several scoring systems have been developed to differentiate benign from malignant lesions based on ovarian volume and the complexity of the cyst, including thickness of the cyst wall, number of cysts, papillary projections into the cyst, thickness of septa, surface excrescences, and presence of ascitic fluid.[15,58,59] In many cases, a cyst that has complex features by sonographic standards can be found to be benign, thereby making sonography a less effective diagnostic tool in discriminating benign cysts from malignant cysts.

The corpus luteum typically induces a low resistance flow; therefore, if possible, patients should be scanned in the first 10 days of the cycle to avoid confusion with luteal flow (Fig. 6-20). However, even when physiologic masses are excluded from analysis, the sensitivity and specificity of Doppler RI are not sufficient to replace the morphologic impression of a lesion being benign or malignant; to date, gray-scale morphologic features are more sensitive in this discrimination. However, the emergence of volume imaging has offered many hopeful avenues to help with this controversial diagnostic dilemma.

SUMMARY

- Patient history and examination technique follow the same protocol as a non-Doppler examination.
- Quantitative Doppler results in a numerical value such as a RI, S/D ratios, PI indices, or velocity.
- Quantitative values change as a result of vascular impedance due to physiologic or pathologic processes.
- High resistance flow has a low end-diastolic value with a high peak systolic value. This type of flow images most often in arteries; however, some disease states result in high-resistance venous flow.
- Low-resistance flow has a high end-diastolic and peak systolic velocity. This can be imaged in either veins or arteries.
- The use of a Doppler angle of 60 degrees or less ensures accurate velocity measurements and optimal sensitivity to flow.
- Color and energy/power Doppler are overlays on the gray-scale image.
- In standard color flow imaging, flow toward the transducer (above the baseline) displays red, whereas flow away from the transducer (below the baseline) displays blue.
- The normal vessel has laminar flow.
- Color Doppler displays the Doppler frequency shift as a velocity, whereas energy/power Doppler displays the amount or strength of the blood flow.
- Uterine artery RI is higher in the proliferative phase of the menstrual cycle (0.88 ± 0.05), then decreases slightly (0.84 ± 0.06) before ovulation and into the luteal phase.
- Periuterine vein velocity ranges between 5 and 10 cm/sec, measuring less than 5 mm.
- Follicular phase ovarian RI is approximately 0.92 ± 0.08 due to low to absent diastolic flow. Ovulation RI flow decreases to 0.44 ± 0.08.
- An AVM of the uterus is due to a congenital malformation, some type of trauma such as an endometrial biopsy, or trophoblastic disease.
- The ovarian vein diameter in nulliparous women is 2.6 mm and can be up to 3.4 mm in women who have had children. Dilated venous structures larger than 4 to 5 mm raise suspicion for pelvic congestion.
- Ovarian torsion is the result of twisting of the ovary on its vascular pedicle. Compete torsion results in an absence of flow, whereas partial torsion may demonstrate reduced flow to the ovary.
- A RI of 0.4 or less, or a PI of 1.0 or less, has been associated with malignant disease of the ovary; however, even when physiologic masses are excluded from analysis, the sensitivity and specificity of Doppler RI are not sufficient to replace the morphologic impression of a lesion being benign or malignant.

Critical Thinking Questions

1. A patient presents to the sonography department for an early pregnancy exam. A borderline maternal serum alpha-fetoprotein (MSAFP) level cannot confirm pregnancy. The endovaginal exam reveals a small, round fluid collection without evidence of a yolk sac or embryo. What Doppler measurements help to confirm an early pregnancy?

   ANSWER: As uterine artery flow velocities increase and the presence of a corpus luteal cyst occurs with early pregnancy, a low resistance spectral Doppler pattern will be seen along with an increased in color Doppler surrounding the cystic structure.

2. During an examination of a patient with complaints of irregular bleeding with an endometrial biopsy approximately a month ago. The endovaginal exam shows a complicated mass within the endometrium. Color Doppler displayed a turbulent and chaotic flow pattern within the mass. The spectral tracing showed high-velocity, low-resistance flow that was difficult to differentiate between arterial and venous flow. What would be the differential diagnosis for these patient findings?

   ANSWER: This patient history along with the sonographic findings suggest the presence of an AVM. Without these specific Doppler findings, it would be difficult to differentiate the AVM from a myomatous mass, endometrial polyp, or other invasive uterine or endometrial mass.

3. Determine the differential diagnosis for a patient with the following history and sonographic findings.

History

1. 35 years old

2. Gravida 6 para 5 abortion 1

3. Pain after intercourse

4. Lower extremity sclerosis for various veins

5. Waitressing for the last 10 years

6. General feeling of pelvic pressure after her 10-hour shift

7. Intrauterine contraceptive device (IUCD) placement 3 years ago

Sonographic findings

1. Normal uterus

2. No free fluid

3. T-shaped ICUD in place

4. Muticystic ovaries

5. Multiple dilated structures around the uterus measuring 6 mm in diameter. Color Doppler revealed no detectable flow; power Doppler detected flow; a spectral tracing revealed venous flow of about 2 cm/sec.

   ANSWER: Given the patient's multiparous history, her presenting symptoms of pain after intercourse and pelvic pressure after prolonged periods of standing, and her clinical signs of varicose veins in her lower extremities, attention should be paid for sonographic findings of pelvic congestion. During the sonogram, the normalcy of the uterus, the multicystic ovaries, and the multiple venous structures found proximal to the uterus, should prompt a referral for a pelvic venogram to rule out pelvic congestion.

REFERENCES

1. ACR standard for the performance of ultrasound examination of the female pelvis, ACR Res 23, 2004. http://www.acr.org/SecondaryMainMenuCategories/quality_safety/guidelines/us/us_pelvic.aspx. Accessed July 13, 2009.
2. Society of Diagnostic Medical Sonography. Diagnostic Ultrasound Clinical Practice Standards. http://www.sdms.org/positions/clinicalpractice.asp. Accessed July 13, 2009.
3. American Institute of Ultrasound in Medicine. AIUM Practice Guideline for the Performance of Pelvic Ultrasound Examinations. http://www.aium.org/publications/guidelines/pelvis.pdf.
4. International Society of Ultrasound in Obstetrics and Gynecology. Home Website. http://www.isuog.org/. Accessed July 13, 2009.
5. Hagen-Ansert SL. *Textbook of Diagnostic Ultrasonography.* 6th ed. St. Louis, MO: Mosby Elsevier Health Sciences; 2006.
6. Marveen Crai g. *Essentials of Sonography and Patient Care.* 2nd ed. St. Louis, MO: Saunders Elsevier; 2006.
7. Curry RA, Tempkin BB. Sonography: Introduction to Normal Structure and Function. St. Louis, MO: Elsevier Health Sciences; 2003.
8. Qureshi IA, Ullah H, Akram H, et al. Transvaginal versus transabdominal sonography in the evaluation of pelvic pathology. *J Coll Clinicians Surg Pak.* 2004;14(7):390–393.
9. Steer CV, Williams J, Zaidi J, et al. Diagnostic techniques: intra-observer, interobserver, interultrasound transducer and intercycle variation in colour Doppler assessment of uterine artery impedance. *Hum Reprod.* 1995;10(2):479–481.
10. Kremkau FW. Diagnostic Ultrasound: Principles and Instruments. St. Louis, MO: WB Saunders; 2005.
11. Well PN. Doppler studies of the vascular system. *Eur J Ultrasound.* 1998;7:3–8.
12. Pourcelot L. Application clinques de l'examen Doppler transcutanie. In: Peronneau P, ed. *Velometric Ultrasonor Doppler.* Vol 34. Paris, France: 10 Inserm; 1974:625.
13. Gosling RG, King DH. Ultrasound angiology. In: Marcus AW, Adamson L, eds. *Arteries and Veins.* Edinburgh, United Kingdom: Churchill Livingstone; 1975.

14. Stuart B, Drumm J, Fitzgerald DE, et al. Fetal blood velocity waveforms in normal and complicated pregnancies. *Br J Obstet Gynaecol*. 1980;87:780.

15. Hendrick WR, Hykes DL, Starchman DE. *Ultrasound Physics and Instrumentation*. 4th ed. St. Louis, MO: Mosby; 2004.

16. Dietz HP. *Atlas of Pelvic Floor Ultrasound*. London, United Kingdom: Springer-Verlag; 2008.

17. Dal J, Vural B, Caliskan E, et al. Power Doppler ultrasound studies of ovarian, uterine, and endometrial blood flow in regularly menstruating women with respect to luteal phase defects. *Fertil Steril*. 2005;84(1):224–227.

18. Lyall F, Bulmer JN, Kelly H, et al. Human trophoblast invasion and spiral artery transformation: the role of nitric oxide. *Am J Pathol*. 2001;54(4):1105–1114.

19. Ng EHY, Chan CCW, Tang OS, et al. Relationship between uterine blood flow and endometrial and subendometrial blood flows during stimulated and natural cycles. *Fertil Steril*. 2006;85:721–727.

20. Ziegler WF, Bernstein I, Badger G, et al. Regional hemodynamic adaptation during the menstrual cycle. *Obstet Gynecol*. 1999;94:695–699.

21. Raine-Fenning NJ, Campbell BK, Clewes JS, et al. Quantifying the changes in endometrial vascularity throughout the normal menstrual cycle with three-dimensional power Doppler angiography. *Hum Reprod*. 2004;19:330–338.

22. Carbillon L, Perrot N, Uzan M, et al. Doppler ultrasonography and implantation: a critical review. *Fetal Diagn Ther*. 2001;16:327–332.

23. Bernstein IM, Ziegler WF, Leavitt T, et al. Uterine artery hemodynamic adaptations through the menstrual cycle into early pregnancy. *Obstet Gynecol*. 2002;99:620–624.

24. Jauniaux E, Jhons J, Burton J. The role of ultrasound imaging in diagnosing and investigating early pregnancy failure. *Ultrasound Obstet Gynecol*. 2005;25:613–624.

25. Alcázar JL, Castillo G, Mínguez JA, et al. Endometrial blood flow mapping using transvaginal power Doppler sonography in women with postmenopausal bleeding and thickend endometrium. *Ultrasound Obstet Gynecol*. 2003;21(6):583–588.

26. Allan P, Dubbins P, Pozniak M, et al. *Clinical Doppler Ultrasound*. 2nd ed. China: Churchill Livingstone Elsevier; 2006.

27. Venbrux AC. Ovarian vein and pelvic varices in the female. In: Savader SJ, Trerotola SO, eds. *Venous interventional radiology with clinical perspectives*. New York, NY: Thieme; 1996:159–162.

28. Park SJ. Diagnosis of pelvic congestion syndrome with transabdominal and transvaginal ultrasound. *UMB* 2006;32(5):41.

29. Pan Ha, Wu MH, Cheng YC, et al. Quantification of ovarian stromal Doppler signals in poor responders undergoing in vitro fertilization with three-dimensional power Doppler ultrasonography. *Am J Obstet Gynecol*. 2004;190:338–344.

30. Fleischer AC. New developments in the sonographic assessment of ovarian, uterine, and breast vascularity. *Semin Ultrasound CT MR*. 2001;22:42–49.

31. Nyberg DA, Hill LM, Bohm-Velez M, et al. eds. *Transvaginal ultrasound*. St. Louis, MO: Mosby Year Book; 1992.

32. Wiebe ER, Switzer P. Arteriovenous malformation of uterus associated with medical abortion. *Int J Obstet Gynaecol*. 2000;71:155–158.

33. Renu A, Achla B, Pinkee S, et al. Arteriovenous malformations of the uterus. *N Z Med J* 2004;117:1206.

34. Grivell RM, Reid KM, Mellor A. Uterine arteriovenous malformations: a review of the current literature. *Obstet Gynecol Surv*. 2005;60(11):761–767.

35. Agarwal S, Magu S, Goyal M. Pelvic arteriovenous malformation. An important differential diagnosis of a complex adnexal mass. *J Ultrasound Med*. 2009;28(8):1111–1114.

36. Elia G, Counsell, Singer SJ. Uterine artery malformation as a hidden cause of severe uterine bleeding. A case report. *J Reprod Med*. 2001;46:389–400.

37. Goldberg RP, Flynn MK. Pregnancy after medical management of uterine arteriovenous malformations. A case report. *J Reprod Med*. 2000;45:961–963.

38. Lin AC, Hung YC, Huang LC, et al. Successful treatment of uterine arteriovenous malformation with percutaneous embolization. *Taiwan J Obstet Gynecol*. 2007;46(1):60–63.

39. Halligan S, Campbell D, Bartram C, et al. Transvaginal ultrasound examination of women with and without pelvic venous congestion. *Clin Radiol*. 2000;55(12):954–958.

40. Campbell D, Halligan S, Bartram CI. Transvaginal power doppler ultrasound in pelvic congestion: a prospective comparison with transuterine venography. *Acta Radiologica*. 2003;44(3):269–274.

41. Hobbs JT. The pelvic congestion syndrome. *Br J Hosp Med*. 1990;43:200–206.

42. Mathis BV, Miller JS, Lukens ML, et al. Pelvic congestion syndrome: a new approach to an unusual problem. *Am Surg*. 1995;61:1016–1018.

43. Adams J, Reginald PW, Franks S, et al. Uterine size and thickness and the significance of cystic ovaries in women with pelvic pain due to congestion. *Br J Obstet Gynaecol*. 1990;97:583.

44. Giacchetto C, Catizone F, Cotroneo GB, et al. Radiologic anatomy of the genital venous system in female patients with varicocele. *Surg Gynecol Obstet*. 1989;169:403–407.

45. Alla M, Rozenblit Z, Ricci J, et al. Incompetent and dilated ovarian veins: a common CT finding in asymptomatic parous women. *AJR*. 2001;176:119–122.

46. Willms AB, Schlund JF, Meyer WR. Endovaginal Doppler ultrasound in ovarian torsion: a case series. *Ultrasound Obstet Gynecol*. 1995;5(2):129–132.

47. Smorgick N, Maymon R, Mendelovic S, et al. Torsion of normal adnexa in postmenarcheal women: can ultrasound indicate an ischemic process? *Ultrasound Obstet Gynecol*. 2008;31(3):338–341.

48. Valentin L, Ameye L, Testa A, et al. Ultrasound characteristics of different types of adnexal malignancies. *Gynecol Oncol*. 2006;102(1):41–48.

49. Milad MP, Cohen L. Preoperative ultrasound assessment of adnexal masses in premenopausal women. *Int J Gynecol Obstet*. 1999;66(2):137–141.

50. Kupesic S, Plavsic BM. Early ovarian cancer: 3-D power doppler. *Abdom Imaging*. 2006;31(5):613–619.

51. Fruscella E, Testa AC, Ferrandina G, et al. Ultrasound features of different histopathological subtypes of borderline ovarian tumors. *Ultrasound Obstet Gynecol*. 2005;26:644–650.

52. Emoto M, Udo T, Obama H, et al. The blood flow characteristics in borderline ovarian tumors based on both color Doppler ultrasound and histopathological analysis. *Gynecol Oncol*. 1998;70:351–357.

53. Wu CC, Lee CN, Chen TM, et al. Incremental angiogenesis assessed by color Doppler ultrasound in the tumorogenesis of ovarian neoplasms. *Cancer*. 1994;73:1251–1256.

54. Seidman JD, Soslow RA, Vang R, et al. Borderline ovarian tumors: diverse contemporary viewpoints on terminology and diagnostic criteria with illustrative images. *Hum Pathol*. 2004;35:918–933.

55. Valentin L. Use of morphology to characterize and manage common adnexal masses. *Best Pract Res Clin Obstet Gynaecol*. 2004;18(1):71–89.

56. Varras M. Benefits and limitations of ultrasonographic evaluation of uterine adnexal lesions in early detection of ovarian cancer. *Clin Exp Obstet Gynecol*. 2004; 31(2):85–98.

57. Marret H. Doppler ultrasonography in the diagnosis of ovarian cysts: indications, pertinence and diagnostic criteria. *J Gynecol Obstet Biol Reprod*. 2001;30(1):20–33.

58. Fleischer AC. Recent advances in the sonographic assessment of vascularity and blood flow in gynecologic conditions. *Am J Obstet Gynecol*. 2005;193(1): 294–301.

59. Fleischer AC, Andreotti RF. Color Doppler sonography in obstetrics and gynecology. *Expert Rev Med Devices*. 2005;2(5):605–611.

7 Pediatric Pelvis

Jennifer Martin, Linda Woolpert, and Susan R. Stephenson

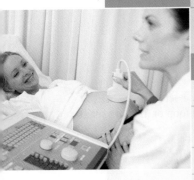

KEY TERMS

hydrocolpos | hematocolpos | hydrometra | hematometra | hydrometrocolpos | hematometrocolpos | rhabdomyosarcoma | pheochromocytoma | dysgerminoma | Rokitansky nodules | germ cell tumors | precocious puberty | gonadal dysgenesis | ambiguous genitalia | ovarian torsion

GLOSSARY

Adrenarche Increase in adrenal gland activity seen at the onset of puberty

Ambiguous genitalia Intersexual genitalia

Café au lait skin pigmentation Irregular flat spots of increased skin pigmentation

Diethylstilbestrol (DES) Synthetic estrogen, used from 1940 to 1971 to aid in pregnancy maintenance, that resulted in a T-shaped uterus in female children

Germ cell tumors Class of tumors that originate in either the egg or sperm

Gonadal dysgenesis Loss of primordial germ cells in the gonads of an embryo

Hermaphrodite Having both male and female sexual characteristics

Pheochromocytoma Vascular tumor of the adrenal gland

Precocious puberty Early onset of puberty, usually before 8 years of age

Pseudohermaphrodite Individual with external genitalia of one sex and the internal organs of another sex

Rhabdomyosarcoma Malignancy derived from striated or skeletal muscle

Rokitansky nodule (a.k.a. dermoid plug) Nodule projecting from a thickened cyst wall, usually ovarian in origin

Thelarche Start of breast development at the onset of puberty

Turner syndrome Genetic syndrome characterized by an X and O chromosome combination resulting in a female with premature ovarian failure and lack of puberty

Ultrasonography has opened new horizons in the field of pediatric gynecologic imaging. Much information about the nature and extent of an abnormality can be collected with little trauma to the child. Because internal pelvic examination of young girls is not generally desirable or possible, ultrasound assumes a role of great importance as a relatively simple and painless method of viewing the internal anatomy. The virginal patient or child prohibits the use of endovaginal ultrasound, which is helpful in the older patient. Transperineal imaging has occasionally proven useful by providing imaging close to the uterus without transducer insertion.

More invasive procedures, such as examination under anesthesia, diagnostic laparoscopy, or exploratory laparotomy, may be avoided or postponed. In recent years, spectral, color flow, and duplex Doppler have added to our ability to examine the child sonographically. Major indications for gynecologic ultrasound examination of young girls include vaginal bleeding or discharge, ambiguous genitalia, pelvic pain, and abdominal masses. Although pregnancy is often found to be the cause of an abdominal mass in older adolescents, because this chapter deals with premenarchal patients, pregnancy is not discussed here.

SONOGRAPHIC EXAMINATION TECHNIQUE AND PROTOCOLS

Taking a few minutes to prepare the child and her parent(s) before beginning the ultrasound exam is highly beneficial. Reduction in the anxiety level of the child creates a culture of trust. The explanation and demonstration should be tailored to the age of the patient. For example, allow the child to touch the transducer "camera," feel the gel, and locate the "TV" where she will "see her belly." Allowing a parent to stay with the child during the examination and discussing ways he or she can support the child reduces the anxiety level of all concerned. A bottle, pacifier, and a key ring for an infant and perhaps a favorite toy for an older child is another method to alleviate patient anxiety. Visual and auditory distractions (including nursery rhymes, songs, bubbles, and toys) can also distract the child's attention from the procedure. Often, a child will cry at the start of the examination despite the examiner's explanations and endeavors; invariably she will stop once she realizes the examination is not painful and that her parents are not going to leave her. Child Life Specialists are often available at freestanding children's hospitals; they may offer education to the patient and family prior to the procedure and can offer distraction techniques during the examinations. A common practice used at the end of pediatric exams is to have either a toy basket or similar small reward such as a lollipop or sticker in recognition of successful completion of the examination.

High-resolution, real-time, and three-dimensional (3D) ultrasound have become vital imaging techniques for the lower abdominal and pelvic structures of infants, children, and adolescents. The distended urinary bladder is used as an acoustic window to evaluate the lower urinary tract, uterus, adnexa, prostate gland, seminal vesicles, pelvic muscles, and vasculature.[1]

The size of the child and area of interest for the ultrasound examination determine the frequency range and type of transducer that is most appropriate. For visualization of the lower urinary tract, uterus, adnexa, and prostate gland, either a phased array or curved linear transducer in the 4-to-10 MHz range is used for infants and small children. These same structures may require a 1-to-5 MHz phased array or curved linear transducer for larger children. To best visualize pelvic muscles, vasculature, superficial structures, and bowel, use a high-frequency linear transducer in the

7-to-15 MHz range. Pediatric sonographic examinations mirror adult exams in scanning planes and exam protocol. Children may move during the exam. To reduce motion on still images, use a lower persistence, and captures from cine loops. If available, 3D data sets containing anatomic sweeps is another method to acquire the needed images.

Preparation for the pelvic exam begins with the older child ingesting and finishing 24 oz of fluid 45 minutes to an hour prior to the exam. An infant can be fed a bottle 30 minutes before the exam.[1,2] If bladder filling cannot be accomplished via fluid ingestion, catheterization may be required. The speed and accuracy of the examination is critical, as it is difficult for the pediatric patients to maintain control of their full urinary bladder. Endovaginal ultrasound in mature, sexually active adolescents helps to delineate the pelvic organs.[1,3]

Transperineal imaging may be particularly helpful in evaluating cases of vaginal pathology or imperforate anus. As in adults, if an abnormality is found in the pelvis, the appropriate upper abdominal organs should be examined to preclude related findings, such as hydronephrosis or metastatic lesions in the lymph nodes or liver.

In recent years, radiation dose concerns have shifted many institutions to utilizing ultrasound as the first line of imaging versus the common practice of using computed tomography (CT) as an imaging modality for children with lower abdominal pain. The performance and interpretation of the sonographic exam by properly trained medical professionals has proven to be the only diagnostic modality required for many pediatric pelvic disorders.[4]

NORMAL ANATOMY

UTERUS

The uterus and ovaries develop in a series of changes in size and configuration during normal growth and development.[5] In the newborn female, the uterus is prominent and thickened with a brightly echogenic endometrial lining caused by in utero hormonal stimulation.[2,3] The spade-shaped uterus length is approximately 3.5 cm, with a fundus-to-cervix ratio of 1:2. At 2 to 3 months of age, the

---

PATHOLOGY BOX 7-1

Methods to Reduce Motion

1. Decrease
   - Focal zone number
   - Sector size
   - Persistence
2. Obtain cine loop or 3D data set
3. Measure organs from cine loop or 3D data set

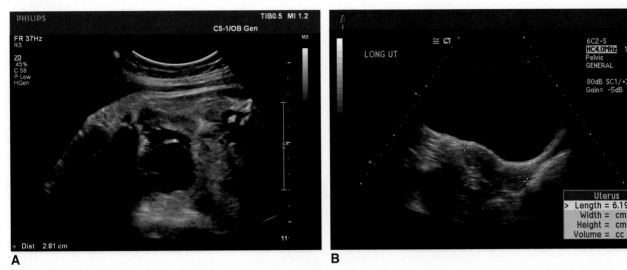

Figure 7-1 A: Normal uterus in a 38-week fetus. **B:** Uterus in a 12-year-old prepubescent girl.

uterus reverts to prepubertal size with a tube-shaped configuration, is 2.5 to 3 cm long, has a fundus-to-cervix ratio of 1:1, and with a nonvisualized endometrial stripe. The uterus remains this size and shape until puberty, when it gradually increases to 5 to 7 cm and the fundus-to-cervix ratio becomes 3:1 (Fig. 7-1).[3,6–8] In the adolescent, the echogenicity and thickness of the endometrial lining varies according to the phase of the menstrual cycle. The right and left uterine arteries, branches of the internal iliac arteries, supply the uterus. Color Doppler modes demonstrate flow in the myometrium with little or no flow in the normal endometrium (see Table 4-11).[3,7]

VAGINA

High-resolution ultrasound offers an alternative to digital and visual examination of the vagina in the pediatric population. In the infant or girl presenting with an interlabial mass, ultrasound in conjunction with other imaging modalities can usually determine the cause.[8] The best method to assess the vagina is in the longitudinal scan plane through the distended urinary bladder. The vagina visualizes as a long tubular structure continuous with the uterine cervix. The opposing mucosal walls of the vagina appear with a bright central echo. The transperineal approach can also be useful in evaluating vaginal pathology.

OVARIES

Ultrasound visualization of the ovaries in children varies greatly dependent upon their location, size, and the patient's age (Fig. 7-2). Neonatal ovaries generally are on a long pedicle within a relatively small pelvis and may locate anywhere between the lower pole of either kidney and the true pelvis. Calculation of the ovarian volume is the best assessment of ovarian size. The simplified prolate ellipse formula can be used to

calculate the volume. The mean ovarian volume from birth to age 5 years is usually less than or equal to 1 cm³.[2,3] The mean ovarian volume in premenarchal girls between ages 6 and 10 years ranges between 1.2 and 2.1 cm³.[2,3] The ovarian volume markedly enlarges postpuberty; therefore, ovarian volumes in menstruating children will be greater than their premenarchal counterparts.

Starting in the neonatal period, the usual appearance of ovaries is heterogeneous secondary to small cysts. Ovarian cysts are extremely common in the pediatric population. Observations of ovarian cysts in children from birth to 2 years found that most had some cysts, with a steady reduction until the age of 12. Large cysts (macrocysts) measuring over 9 mm image in the first year of life more often than in the second. These findings correlate to the higher levels of maternal hormones found in the neonate. Ovarian blood supply is dual: Blood comes from the ovarian artery, which originates at the aorta, and from an adnexal branch of the uterine artery.[2,3,5] The Doppler modes (color, spectral) demonstrate flow in the majority of adolescent ovaries; however, separation of the dual blood supplies is not possible.[2,5]

PATHOLOGY BOX 7-2	
Ovarian Volume[2,3]	
Formula	Length × Depth × Width × 0.523
Size (cm³; ± SD)	
Birth–5 years	≤1
6–10 years	1.2–2.1 (± 0.5)
11–13 years	2.5–4.2 (± 1.3–2.3)
Menstrual	9.8 (± 5.8)

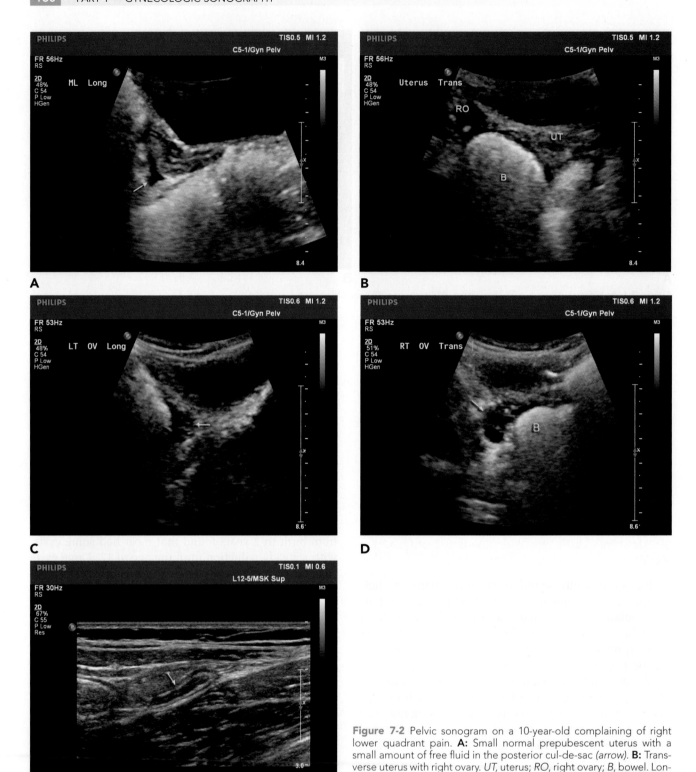

Figure 7-2 Pelvic sonogram on a 10-year-old complaining of right lower quadrant pain. **A:** Small normal prepubescent uterus with a small amount of free fluid in the posterior cul-de-sac *(arrow)*. **B:** Transverse uterus with right ovary. *UT,* uterus; *RO,* right ovary; *B,* bowel. Longitudinal image of the normal left ovary **(C)** and transverse of the right ovary **(D)**. **E:** Exploration of the appendiceal area revealed a tubular structure *(arrow)*. The transverse dual with compression and noncompression views confirm appendicitis *(arrows)*.

PATHOLOGY

Tumors of the genitalia are rare in the pediatric and adolescent populations; but of the tumors that are found, approximately half are malignant or have a malignant potential.[9] Tumors found in the adult population have almost all been found in the pediatric population. The following sections describe the most frequently found malignant and benign tumors in children and adolescents.

LOWER URINARY TRACT

Malignant Lesions

Rhabdomyosarcoma is the tumor found most commonly in the lower urinary tract of the pediatric population.[2] This tumor originates from the genitourinary tract in 21% of cases at the prostate or trigone of the bladder. Less common sites include the seminal vesicles, spermatic cord, vagina, pelvic muscles, uterus, vulva, urachus, and the area surrounding the scrotum.[2] CT and ultrasound imaging of the pelvis help diagnose rhabdomyosarcoma in children.[2,10]

Males have a higher incidence of rhabdomyosarcoma by a 1.6:1 ratio.[2] The age of highest incidence is 3 to 4 years, with the second highest incidence peak seen again in adolescence.[2] The embryonal form of rhabdomyosarcoma is the most common cellular type of this disease; sarcoma botryoides is a subtype of this cellular form. The alveolar cellular form is the next most common type; undifferentiated and pleomorphic are rarely seen. When the tumor originates from the bladder or prostate, patients commonly present with urinary tract obstruction and hematuria. These tumors have been associated with fetal alcohol syndrome, basal cell nevus syndrome, and neurofibromatosis.[2]

The sonographic appearance of rhabdomyosarcoma is a homogeneous, solid mass with similar acoustic characteristic presentation to that of muscle tissue. Necrosis and hemorrhage within the tumor can lead to anechoic foci within the rhabdomyosarcoma. Calculi are rarely seen with this tumor type. Polypoid projections caused by sarcoma botryoides infiltration into the bladder wall can be seen when the tumor originates in the submucosa of the urinary bladder. Prostate origination of the tumor can cause concentric or asymmetric enlargement of the gland, resulting in potential for infiltration of the bladder neck, perirectal region, and posterior urethra. Lymph node metastases in the area of tumor origination and the retroperitoneum are common.[2]

Benign Lesions

Benign lesions of the lower urinary tract in the pediatric population are extremely uncommon. Transitional cell papilloma, leiomyoma, neurofibroma, fibroma, and hemangioma are among these benign tumors of young children and adolescents (Fig. 7-3).[2] *Pheochromocytoma* is a rare tumor that most likely originates in the paraganglia of the autonomic nervous system and may be either in the submucosal layer of either the posterior wall of the bladder close to the trigone or in the dome of the urinary bladder. Of note, in the pediatric population, 2% of bladder pheochromocytomas are malignant.[2] Congenital diseases that may involve pheochromocytomas are neurofibromatosis, tumerous sclerosis, type A multiple endocrine neoplasia (medullary thyroid carcinoma, hyperparathyroidism), Hippel-Lindau disease, Sturge-Weber syndrome, and multiple endocrine neoplasia type IIB (medullary thyroid carcinoma, mucosal neuromas, and pheochromocytoma).

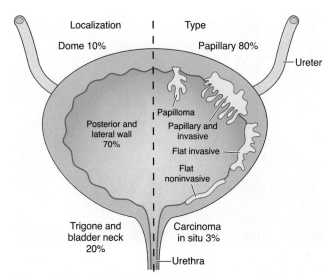

Figure 7-3 Urothelial neoplasms. Most tumors occur in the urinary bladder and are classified histologically as urothelial (transitional cell) carcinomas (TCCs). Ureters and the posterior urethra are also lined by transitional epithelium and can give rise to TCC. TCCs can be flat, papillary, papillary and invasive, or simply invasive. Benign transitional cell papillomas are rare.

Symptoms of pheochromocytomas of the bladder include headache, intermittent high blood pressure (70%), hematuria (6%), blurred vision, diaphoresis, and palpitation.[2]

Urinary obstruction can also be caused by benign polyps in the male urethra. The fundus of the bladder is the most common location for these well-defined, solid, intramural bladder mass.[2]

VAGINA, UTERUS, AND FALLOPIAN TUBES

Tumors originating in the uterus and vagina are rare in the pediatric population. Malignant tumors are more common than benign tumors, and the vagina is involved more often than the uterus.[2] Foreign bodies in the vagina are the most common cause of vaginal bleeding in pediatric patients, toilet paper is the most common source of this material. Premenarchal vaginal bleeding can also be caused by precocious puberty. Vascular malformations and hemangiomas are also potential causes of prepubertal vaginal bleeding.[11] The workup of vaginal bleeding may include measurement of blood estradiol levels, gonadotropin-releasing hormone (GnRH) stimulation test, pelvic sonography and possibly CT or magnetic resonance imaging (MRI) to rule out adrenal or gonadal tumors, and a head CT to rule out central nervous system lesions,[4] particularly in the evaluation of precocious puberty (Fig. 7-4).[12]

Benign Lesions

Although benign solid lesions in the uterus and vagina are rare in the pediatric population, cystic benign vaginal lesions are not uncommon. Examples of these types of masses include Gartner duct cysts and pelvic inflammatory disease. The most common type of cystic

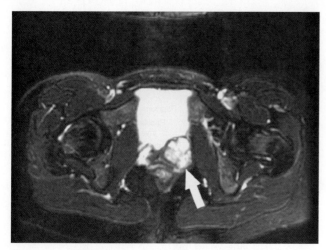

Figure 7-4 Pheochromocytoma of the vagina. Axial fat-suppressed T2-weighted image shows lobulated high signal intensity mass (arrow) in left wall of vagina.

lesion in the vagina is a Gartner duct cyst. These benign cysts are remnants of the distal wolffian or mesonephric duct.[2] There can be multiple cysts or a single cyst and are most commonly located in the anterolateral aspect of the vagina. These cysts look like fluid-filled structures within the vaginal wall on sonographic examination (see Fig. 8-28).

Pelvic inflammatory disease (PID) can occur in sexually active adolescents or in sexually abused pediatric patients. This infection has the potential of affecting the ovaries, uterus, and fallopian tubes. PID can lead to tubo-ovarian abscess, endometritis, salpingitis, oophoritis, and/or pelvic peritonitis, which sequentially leads to chronic pelvic pain, impaired fertility, or ectopic pregnancy.

Malignant Lesions

The most common malignant vaginal and uterine mass in pediatric females is rhabdomyosarcoma. Typical presentation is a cluster of cysts called *sarcoma botryoides* protruding from the vagina or presentation with vaginal bleeding in the 6-to-18-month age group. This tumor typically originates in the vagina and spreads to the uterus, although it may follow the opposite path occasionally (Fig. 7-5).[2]

The sonographic appearance of rhabdomyosarcoma is a homogeneous mass either filling the vaginal cavity or causing an irregular mass effect of the uterus. The size and extension of this tumor can make it difficult to determine the origin of the tumor on the ultrasound exam.[14] Radiation and chemotherapy are used to shrink the mass to a size suitable for conservative excision. Ultrasound, MRI, and CT may be used for serial follow-up examinations.[1,10]

Endodermal sinus or yolk sac tumors have a similar clinical and sonographic presentation as dysgerminoma and rhabdomyosarcomas, although it is much less common.[2]

Various other tumors of the uterus and vagina are rare. Vaginal carcinoma (typically clear cell adenocarcinoma) is found most commonly in teenagers that were exposed to diethylstilbestrol (DES) in utero.[2]

OVARY

Ovarian cysts have been found to be much more common than originally thought since the advent of pediatric pelvic sonography. In the pediatric age group, 60% of ovarian masses are functional cysts and 40% are neoplasms. The most common site of tumors in the pediatric female genital tract is the ovary. Prior to menarche, one-third of these tumors are malignant with two-thirds of these neoplasms benign mature teratomas.[4] Ovarian tumors present with a variety of symptoms including pelvic pain, swelling, and inflammation. Ultrasound is a useful diagnostic tool when used in conjunction with tumor markers. With the exception of ovarian cancer, these tools allow for successful tumor management and ovarian preservation.[15]

Benign Masses

Ovarian cysts in the pediatric and adolescent population are quite common. Follicular retention cysts, corpus luteum cysts, or hemorrhagic cysts are the most commonly seen cysts in this population. Precocious puberty can be precipitated by the secretion of hormones from the lining of these cysts. Aside from hemorrhagic cysts, which have a complex appearance, the remainder of cysts tend to be anechoic. The greatest risk associated with various ovarian cysts is the possibility of ovarian torsion once they attain a certain size. Ovarian cysts

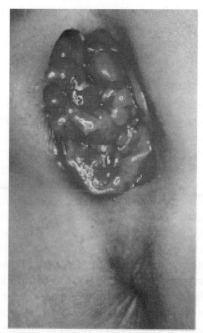

Figure 7-5 Embryonal rhabdomyosarcoma (sarcoma botryoides) of vagina. The grape-like tumor protrudes through the introitus.

in the fetus are related to the secretion of maternal and placental chorionic gonadotropin. Larger ovarian cysts are more common in fetuses of mothers with toxemia, Rh isoimmunization, and diabetes, as these conditions all cause an increase in the release of placental chorionic gonadotropin.[16]

Over time, management of neonatal ovarian cysts has changed. Follow-up sonographic assessment of neonatal ovarian cysts found that many regress on their own during the first few months of life. Monitoring of gonadotropin levels and follow-up ultrasound exams have replaced surgical excision of ovarian cysts or oophorectomy.[17]

Cyst removal is still promoted by some in regard to neonatal cysts that are larger than 5 cm, hemorrhagic cysts that may be caused by torsion or infarction, and even small cysts if they persist longer than 4 months, enlarge, or become symptomatic.[2] It is thought that surgery may avoid the potential morbidity of ovarian autoamputation due to torsion, peritonitis caused by cyst rupture, or intestinal obstruction due to cyst size. The possibility of a potentially lethal cyst rupture, or peritonitis from cyst torsion with infarction, or bowel obstruction is raised when a neonatal cyst has associated ascites.[18]

Color Doppler ultrasound in characterization of ovarian cysts has not proven to increase the specificity of diagnosis, rather it helps to accurately detect the presence or absence of ovarian blood flow, enabling the clinician to either confirm or disregard the diagnosis of ovarian torsion.[7]

The most common tumor during the reproductive years is benign cystic teratoma (BCT, dermoid cyst), but it is relatively uncommon before puberty. It occurs more often on the right side and often presents with abdominal pain secondary to torsion; therefore, it can mimic the symptoms of appendicitis.[2,3] The mass is predominantly cystic in children, with small foci of fat, hair, and calcification.[19] Ovarian teratomas may contain sonographically visible mural nodules (called *Rokitansky nodules*) and exhibit posterior acoustic shadowing.[19] Approximately 10% of these teratomas are present bilaterally.[19]

Rarely seen, benign serous and mucinous cystadenomas occur in prepubertal girls. In children, the benign form occurs more often than the malignant type and is commonly unilateral; they are epithelial in origin.[20] Septa seen within these lesions aids the clinician in providing the differential diagnosis. The combination of ascites, pleural effusion, and a fibroma (Meigs syndrome), which is a rare benign solid connective tissue tumor, can lead to ovarian torsion.[21,22]

Malignant Masses

Germ cell tumors are the most common malignant tumors involving the pediatric genital tract. The counterpart of the testicular mass seminoma is dysgerminoma, which is the most common pediatric ovarian mass.

It is fortunate this tumor has low-grade malignancy and is very radiosensitive, therefore potentially curable. Typical ultrasound presentation is a solid mass ranging in size from a small nodule to one extending from the pelvis into the abdominal cavity. Lobulations, areas of hemorrhagic necrosis and fibrovascular septa may be seen within this mass.[20] Liver metastases, ascites, and retroperitoneal lymphadenopathy may be present in cases of advanced disease (Fig. 7-6).

Color Doppler ultrasound demonstrates prominent arterial flow within the fibrovascular septa of dysgerminoma. Kim and Kang described imaging findings in several cases, including a particular case of a 7-year-old girl. On her MRI evaluation, the septa were hypointense or isointense on T2-weighted images and showed marked enhancement on both contrast-enhanced CT and contrast-enhanced T1-weighted MRI. Tanaka and coworkers also described this unique finding.[20,23]

Lab work is also an essential tool to differentiate this tumor from other diseases with similar sonographic appearance, such as ovarian torsion and appendiceal abscess. Human chorionic gonadotropin (hCG), lactic dehydrogenase (LDH), and alpha-fetoprotein (AFP) may all be elevated with dysgeminoma. In 10% to 15% of cases, these masses occur bilaterally and contain calcifications.[24]

Unilateral tumor localization is sometimes treated with single oophorectomy in conjunction with radiation; however, some advocate total abdominal hysterectomy with postoperative radiation. If the tumor is bilateral, locally extensive, or accompanied by lymphadenopathy and/or ascites, a total abdominal hysterectomy followed by postoperative radiation is the usual treatment.[25]

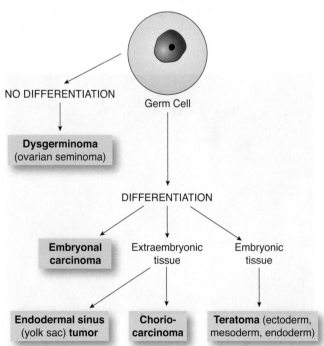

Figure 7-6 Classification of germ cell tumors of the ovary.

Endodermal sinus tumor, malignant teratoma, primary choriocarcinoma of the ovary, and embryonal carcinoma are other germ cell tumors. Growth of endodermal sinus tumor is rapid and unilateral; this is the second most common germ cell tumor.[11] Peak incidence of malignant teratomas is at age 3, and 60% of teratomas show calcification on radiographic examination. This tumor may not be distinguishable from BCT, although it typically contains more solid portions.[20] A highly malignant, unilateral tumor that may lead to precocious puberty is embryonal carcinoma. Another, less common precursor to precocious puberty is non-gestational choriocarcinoma.[2] These tumors range in sonographic presentation from highly echogenic to purely cystic, with cul-de-sac fluid in half of these patients. Liver and nodal metastases, and ascites are common with these tumors (Fig. 7-7).[26]

Granulosa-theca cell and arrhenoblastoma (Sertoli-Leydig cell) tumors of gonadal origin are less often malignant and tend to exert influence on hormones. Precocious puberty can be brought on by granulosa-theca cell tumors that are feminizing tumors and are only found 5% of the time prior to puberty. Less than 5% of these tumors are bilateral. They have a prevalence of late recurrence, requiring that postoperative follow-up surveillance be performed on these patients for the remainder of their lives. Arrhenoblastomas are an example of masculinizing tumors. If these tumors recur, it is within the first 3 years after treatment.[24]

In children, epithelial originating tumors, serous and mucinous cystadeonocarcinoma, are rarer than their benign counterparts. Serous tumor types commonly present with thick septa and solid elements and are multilocular. Serous tumors are twice as common as mucinous tumors.

Metastases can spread to one or both ovaries. Leukemia, lymphoma, Krukenberg tumor, neuroblastoma, and rhabdomyosarcoma have all been shown to have the potential of spreading to involve the ovary.[1,12] Autopsy has shown genital involvement of acute lymphocytic leukemia to be 11.5% to 80% in females. Sonographically, this is represented as solid, hypoechoic ovarian masses. Marrow remission often coincides with gonadal involvement. Recurrence of tumor is likely if the sequestered tumor is not treated adequately (Table 7-1).

GENITAL ANOMALIES, GONADAL DYSGENESIS, AND AMBIGUOUS GENITALIA

Ultrasound can be obtained in cases where congenital uterine anomalies are suspected in infants and young children; however, these can be difficult to detect. Associated anomalies such as absence of the vagina, imperforate anus, or urinary tract abnormalities can lead to clinical suspicion and result in a pelvic sonogram. Potential diagnosis made by pelvic sonography would be either the presence of a smaller than normal uterus or a uterine obstruction, which would suggest a congenital uterine anomaly. Distension of the endometrial cavity and vagina would be suggestive of an imperforate hymen or anomaly of the vagina. Certain syndromes involving müllerian anomalies may reveal agenesis of the uterus, vagina, or kidneys. Mayer-Rokitansky-Küster-Hauser syndrome present with a normal karyotype. These children have normal secondary sexual characteristics but have coexistent renal (50% to 90%) and skeletal anomalies. Sonography helps establish the presence of a vagina, but specific vaginal anomalies are difficult to characterize. Ultrasound aids in surgical planning for corrective surgery in cases of vaginal atresia, stenosis, or hypoplasia by depicting the extent of vaginal presence or absence in the upper one-third of the vagina, the uterus, and the ovaries.[14]

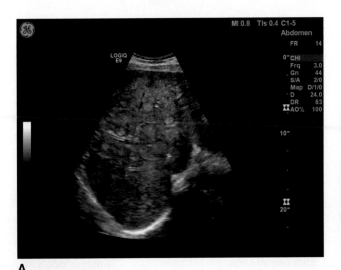

A

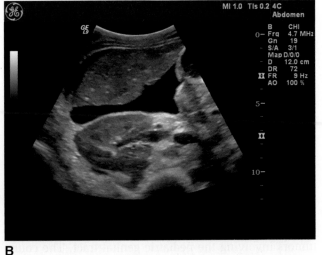

B

Figure 7-7 A: Example of liver metastasis. **B:** Transverse image of ascites in the right upper quadrant in a different patient. (Images courtesy of GE Healthcare, Wauwatosa, WI.)

TABLE 7-1

Differential Diagnoses of the Complex Pediatric Ovarian Mass

Mass	History	Physical Findings	Laboratory Studies	Sonographic Findings
Hemorrhagic ovarian cyst	Lower abdominal pain, occasional nausea	None, or palpable mass; fever with torsion	↑ WBC if torsion	Variable: thick-walled cyst; septated cyst; homogeneous low-level echoes with poor sound attenuation; cyst containing solid components, may have fluid in cul-de-sac; change in appearance in follow-up study
Benign cystic teratoma	Lower abdominal pain, nausea, vomiting; pain increase with torsion	Lower abdominal or pelvic mass; torsion in 25% cases, with associated fever and acute abdomen	↑ WBC if torsion	Complex mass with hyperechoic zones with acoustic shadowing; "tip-of-the-iceberg sign"; solid mass with cystic components with or without scattered internal echoes; fat-fluid level; pelvic radiograph shows calcification in 47% to 54%
Torsion of normal uterine adnexa	Acute abdominal pain; 50% have had similar episodes with spontaneous recovery in past; nausea, vomiting	Small, tender adnexal mass or lower abdominal mass; possible rebound tenderness; fever	↑ WBC	Predominantly solid ovarian mass with good through-transmission; may have fluid in cul-de-sac; solid mass (enlarged ovary) with peripheral cysts; infarction may mimic hemorrhagic cyst
Appendiceal abscess	Right lower quadrant pain, nausea, fever, vomiting	Tender right, lower abdominal mass; may have rebound tenderness; fever	↑ WBC	Nonspecific complex adnexal mass; fecalith with or without shadowing; fluid in cul-de-sac
Tubo-ovarian abscess	Lower abdominal pain, vaginal discharge; history of pelvic inflammatory disease	Tender lower abdominal or adnexal mass; fever; purulent cervical drainage	↑ WBC	Nonspecific complex mass; may simulate hemorrhagic cyst in enlarged adnexa; fluid in cul-de-sac
Malignant neoplasm	May have lower abdominal pain that is acute, subacute, or chronic; nausea, vomiting	Lower abdominal mass; fever with torsion; ascites, lymphadenopathy, metastases	↑ WBC if torsion	Nonspecific complex ovarian mass; central cystic area of necrosis; may be cystic with multiple septations; uterus may not be identifiable; fluid in cul-de-sac in 50%; ascites, liver and peritoneal metastases, and lymphadenopathy may occur

WBC, white blood cell count; ↑, increased

(Adapted from Haller JO, Bass IS, Friedman AP. Pelvic masses in girls: an 8-year retrospective analysis stressing ultrasound as the prime imaging modality. *Pediatr Radiol.* 1984;14:367.)

The occurrence of ovarian agenesis is so rare that it is even thought to be an acquired condition as a result of ovarian torsion and eventual necrosis in utero. Ovarian hypoplasia is commonly associated with endocrine disorders, intersex disorders, and gonadal dysgenesis.[14]

Turner syndrome is the most familiar type of gonadal dysgenesis. Ovarian development in this syndrome ranges from adult to infantile to absent. Turner patients have deficient ovaries and a 45,XO karyotype. Physical characteristics include dwarfism, webbed neck, shield-shaped chest, amenorrhea, and infantile sexual development. Ovaries do not contain follicles and are typically only a fibrous streak. Ultrasound does not commonly demonstrate ovaries in these patients prior to hormone therapy; the uterus is prepubertal in size and shape independent of the patient's age. It is useful to utilize ultrasound for changes in the size and shape of the uterus and ovaries following the administration of hormonal therapy.

In the individual with the abnormal karyotype of 46,XY, testicular feminization occurs due to androgen insensitivity. Physical characteristics include uterine and vaginal anomalies, little or no pubic or axillary hair, and testis within the abdomen or inguinal canal. Although testosterone levels may be normal, the end organs are typically not sensitive.[16] Gonadal dysgenesis patients may have "streak" gonads. They resemble ovaries but contain no germ cells or follicles. The Y chromosome in these children is cause for concern because the child's risk for development of a tumor such as a dysgerminoma or a gonadoblastoma is greater than 30%. Therefore, gonadectomy is recommended for these patients.

One of the main indications for sonography of the neonate is ambiguous genitalia. Serious psychological disturbances can be avoided with early diagnosis. Vaginal atresia, fused labia, clitorimegaly, or cryptorchidism should result in ultrasound investigation in an effort to define the internal anatomy. Careful sonographic surveillance of the retroperitoneum and labia for gonads and the pelvis for müllerian structures provides clinicians with vital information for diagnosis and treatment. Sonographic images should also be obtained of the adrenal glands and kidneys to exclude associated anomalies of adrenal hyperplasia and renal anomalies.[12] Hormonal and chromosomal

studies are typically run in parallel with the ultrasound examination (Fig. 7-8).

Ambiguous genitalia is seen in approximately 1 in 50,000 to 70,000 babies.[12] This is an isolated occurrence of intersex in 1 birth in 1,000 and is much more commonly associated with other anomalies.[14] Definition of the internal anatomy via ultrasound helps accelerate diagnosis and sex assignment of such infants.[3,14] True hermaphrodites have both ovarian and testicular tissue. Ovaries and testes may be separated on either side of the pelvis, or the structures can be joined as ovitestis; presence or absence of the uterus also varies. A chromosomal female (46,XX) is considered a female pseudohermaphrodite because of physical characteristics of the presence of ovaries along with masculinized external genitalia, including prominent fused labia, which may be hyperpigmented secondary to increased adrenocorticotropin levels and enlarged clitoris. The cause of this

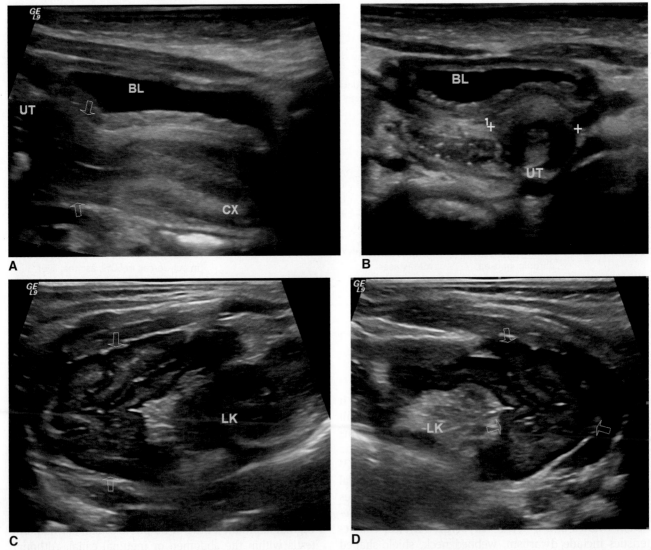

Figure 7-8 Newborn with ambiguous genitalia. **(A)** Longitudinal *(arrows)* and transverse. **(B, calipers)** Images of the pelvis reveal a normal infantile uterus. Longitudinal **(C)** and transverse **(D)** images of the left adrenal gland *(arrows)* reveal an enlarged adrenal gland with convolutions reminiscent of the brain (cerebriform) consistent with CAH. *LK,* left kidney; *BL,* bladder; *UT,* uterus; *BL,* bladder; *CX,* cervix. (Images courtesy of Helen DeVos Children's Hospital, Grand Rapids, MI.)

condition could be increased androgen production due to a virilizing maternal condition where the uterus may or may not be present, or congenital adrenal hyperplasia (CAH); a uterus is always present in this condition. A characteristic of CAH is adrenal gland enlargement with a cerebriform appearance.

A chromosomal male (46,XY) with feminized external genitalia is considered a pseudohermaphrodite. This condition can be due to a decrease in androgens, poor target organs, or an enzyme defect. High serum testosterone to dihydrotestosterone ratios confirm this diagnosis. Ultrasound of the pelvis may demonstrate müllerian structures. Androgen insensitivity commonly leads to inguinal hernias and may contain a testicle. The testicle may be found in the retroperitoneum or labia as well. Patients with this condition may have one or two testicles, or they may have one testicle and one streak gonad.

PRECOCIOUS PUBERTY

The onset of normal physiologic and endocrine processes of puberty in girls before the age of 8 years is the definition of *precocious puberty*. This condition in its true form is idiopathic in most cases and is secondary to activation of the hypothalamus-pituitary-gonadal axis. Laboratory tests reveal pubertal luteinizing hormone (LH) and follicle-stimulating hormone response to GnRH, elevated levels of gonadal sex steroids, and advanced bone age. The sequelae of precocious puberty typically follows the physical developmental sequence seen in normal children at puberty: breast development, pubic and axillary hair appearance, then the commencement of menstruation. The uterus and ovaries will also reach their postpubertal size as in adults, with a corpus-to-cervix ratio of 1:1 (see Fig. 5-40).[3] Central nervous system lesions affecting the hypothalamus can lead to true precocious puberty.

Adrenal or ovarian dysfunction can cause pseudoprecocious or incomplete precocious puberty; this is not dependent on the pituitary gonadotropins. Patients may present with clinical signs that are the same as the true type, but menstruation is typically more irregular. Ovarian-caused cases are accounted for by granulosatheca cell tumors 60% of the time.[26] Pseudoprecocious puberty has been caused by dysgerminoma, choriocarcinoma, arrhenoblastoma, follicular retention cysts, and autonomous function of an ovarian cyst in rare cases. Causes of adrenal origin include congenital hyperplasia, adenoma, and carcinoma. Occasionally, hypothyroidism can cause breast development in prepubertal girls, but this has not been reported to produce menses.[3]

An association exists between patients with *McCune-Albright syndrome*, a condition characterized by fibrous dysplasia of bone associated with café au lait skin pigmentation. Possible endocrine hyperfunction has also been associated with precocious puberty. Sonographic

evaluation of these patients demonstrates their tendency to have the largest ovarian cysts and the largest size discrepancy between the two ovaries.

Sonography can accurately assess the size of the uterus and ovaries. A diagnosis of pituitary axis stimulation can be made when ultrasound reveals a large uterus and symmetric ovarian enlargement. A prepubertal-sized uterus and unilateral ovarian enlargement suggests an ovarian tumor, although primordial cysts may be a normal cause of an enlarged ovary. King and colleagues conducted a study that looked at ovarian cysts in patients with precocious puberty. They found the presence of small (<9 mm) cysts alone could not separate those patients with precocious puberty from normal girls. According to their study, the best predictor of true precocious puberty was bilateral ovarian enlargement, whereas unilateral enlargement associated with macrocysts (>9 mm) was suggestive of pseudoprecocious puberty. Sonographic representation of an infantile uterus and ovaries is suggestive of premature thelarche or adrenarche and does not lead to a diagnosis of precocious puberty. In these cases, careful analysis of the adrenal and hypothalamic regions must also be undertaken before precocious puberty can be attributed to an ovarian cyst.[12] CT and MRI are both superior to sonography in the evaluation of these areas and should be utilized to evaluate these regions.

Sonography is useful as a tool to assess patients with precocious puberty during hormone replacement therapy (LH-releasing factor analog therapy to decrease the pituitary response to GnRH) and to monitor the size and volume changes of the uterus and ovaries.[3] GnRH-a (GnRH agonist) medications are targeted at suppression of the pituitary-gonadal axis and downregulation of pituitary gonadotropin secretion, leading to a return to hypogonadal status as soon as possible. Serial ultrasound exams document regression in response to therapy (Fig. 7-9).

HYDROCOLPOS, HEMATOCOLPOS, HYDROMETRA, HEMATOMETRA, HYDROMETROCOLPOS, AND HEMATOMETROCOLPOS

Hydrocolpos is fluid in the vagina; *hematocolpos* is blood in the vagina; *hydrometra* is fluid in the uterus; *hematometra* is blood in the uterus; *hydrometrocolpos* is fluid in both; and *hematometrocolpos* is blood in both. Imperforate hymen, vaginal septum, duplication anomalies with unilateral obstruction, or acquired obstructing lesions are the most common causes.[2,14,21,26] The cervix may also distend with blood. Causes include atresia or stenosis which may occur in association with vaginal atresia (Fig. 7-10).[2,3] These conditions may present in the neonatal period as an abdominal mass or bulging hymen; typically, they are not detected until menarche.

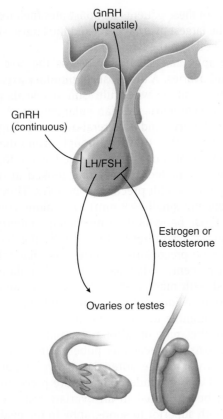

Figure 7-9 Effects of GnRH on the hypothalamic-pituitary and reproductive axis. GnRH is secreted by the hypothalamus in a pulsatile fashion, stimulating gonadotroph cells of the anterior pituitary gland to secrete LH and follicle-stimulating hormone (FSH). LH and FSH stimulate the ovaries or testes to produce the sex hormones estrogen or testosterone, respectively, which inhibit further release of LH and FSH. Exogenous pulsatile GnRH is used to induce ovulation in women with infertility of hypothalamic origin. Conversely, continuous administration of GnRH suppresses gonadotroph response to endogenous GnRH, and thereby causes decreased production of sex hormones. Analogues of GnRH with increased metabolic stability and prolonged half-lives take advantage of this effect and are used to suppress sex hormone production in clinical conditions such as precocious puberty and prostate cancer.

visualization of low-lying obstruction and determination of the thickness of an obstructing vaginal septum. Scanlan and associates reported this technique.

Hydronephrosis and obstruction of venous and lymphatic channels of the lower extremity can be caused by severe distention.[3] In utero presentation can lead to urinary tract obstruction associated with fetal anuria, oligohydramnios, and pulmonary hypoplasia (Fig. 7-12).[2]

With the exception of pure imperforate hymen, hydrocolpos is often accompanied by other congenital malformations such as imperforate anus and urinary tract anomalies, as well as genital, cardiac, and skeletal anomalies.[2] Associated anomalies such as unilateral renal agenesis or hypoplasia are possible, and a thorough examination of the kidneys should be made to either identify or eliminate these diagnoses. In females with renal abnormalities, uterine anomalies are present 48% to 70% of the time; but in all females, the incidence of uterine anomalies is only 0.1% to 0.5%. Therefore, findings of renal anomalies in females should prompt investigation of the uterus.[2,3,5] Early diagnosis of a double uterus with an obstructed hemivagina—where the septum must be resected surgically to avoid the possibility of pyocolpos due to closure spontaneously after drainage—can lead to conservative treatment, thus preserving the maximum reproductive capability of these patients (Table 7-2).

OVARIAN TORSION

An infrequent yet important cause of abdominal pain is torsion of a normal or an abnormal ovary.[2] Rotation of the ovary about the ovarian pedicle causes sequential obstruction to the lymphatic and venous outflow and eventually arterial inflow. Torsion of the ovary has a right-sided predominance ratio of 3:2 potentially due

This condition represents 15% of abdominal masses in newborn females, surpassing the incidence of ovarian cysts by a small amount.[12] Newborn females' uterine secretions may be increased by maternal hormones that can lead to distention of the uterus or vagina proximal to the point of obstruction.

Sonographic appearance of hydrocolpos is a cystic, pear-shaped mass in the midline arising from the pelvis between the bladder and rectum. The mass may contain internal echoes resulting from cellular debris or blood; a fluid–fluid level may be present. A normal uterus can be identified at the superior aspect of an isolated distended vagina.[1,26] The urinary bladder needs to be distended in order to distinguish the mass from the bladder (Fig. 7-11).

Vaginal reconstruction planning may be aided by transperineal sonography to visualize the entire length of the vagina. Sagittal and coronal scans allow

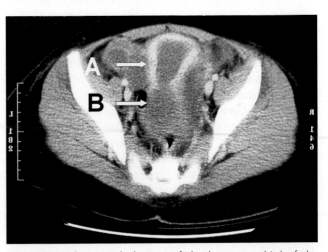

Figure 7-10 Congenital absence of the lower one-third of the vagina. MRI demonstrates that a uterus is present (A) as well as an upper vaginal pouch (B). The upper vagina has formed a hematocolpos which began soon after menarche and presented as a pelvic mass.

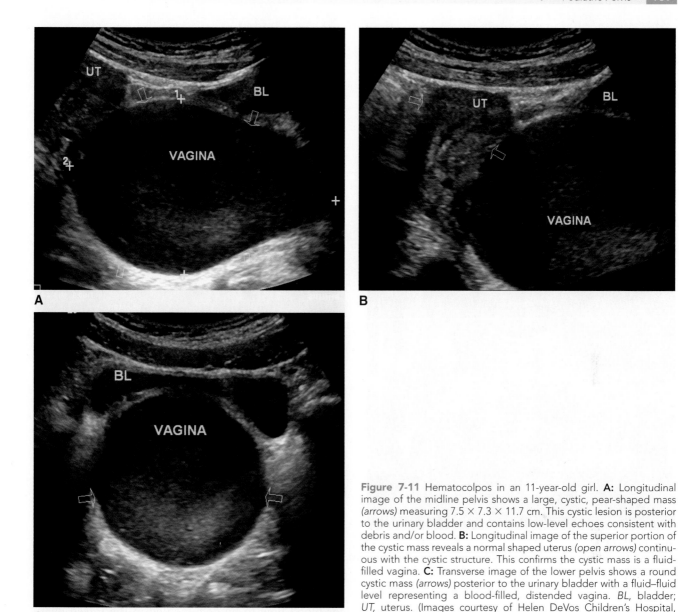

Figure 7-11 Hematocolpos in an 11-year-old girl. **A:** Longitudinal image of the midline pelvis shows a large, cystic, pear-shaped mass *(arrows)* measuring 7.5 × 7.3 × 11.7 cm. This cystic lesion is posterior to the urinary bladder and contains low-level echoes consistent with debris and/or blood. **B:** Longitudinal image of the superior portion of the cystic mass reveals a normal shaped uterus *(open arrows)* continuous with the cystic structure. This confirms the cystic mass is a fluid-filled vagina. **C:** Transverse image of the lower pelvis shows a round cystic mass *(arrows)* posterior to the urinary bladder with a fluid–fluid level representing a blood-filled, distended vagina. *BL,* bladder; *UT,* uterus. (Images courtesy of Helen DeVos Children's Hospital, Grand Rapids, MI.)

to partial immobilization of the left adnexa by its proximity to the sigmoid mesentery. The first decade of life is the most common time for torsion of the normal adnexa, which is not as common as torsion of an ovary containing a mass (i.e., BCT or dysgerminoma). Mobility of the pediatric adnexa, which allows twisting at the mesosalpinx as a result of changes in intra-abdominal pressure or in body position, is thought to be the cause of this prevalence. An extrapelvic location of the twisted ovary is more common in prepubertal females. Torsion may involve the tube, the ovary, or both. For preservation of the ovary, surgical treatment must be carried out promptly.[12]

Clinical symptoms of torsion include lower abdominal pain, usually of more than 48 hours, fever, lack of appetite, nausea, and vomiting. It is typical for the pain to be acute in onset, sharp, and radiate to the groin or flank. Fever and increased white blood cell count usually indicates that necrosis or abscess formation has begun. Half of patients with a history of pain have spontaneous recovery.[2,3] This can lead to diagnostic confusion, especially in the case of pediatric patients, whose symptoms may be attributed to such entities as appendicitis, gastroenteritis, pyelonephritis, intussusception, or Meckel's diverticulitis. Pelvic ultrasound can be used to exclude these other causes of acute pelvic pain.

The sonographic appearance of ovarian torsion is varied, may be nonspecific, and includes a markedly enlarged ovary (mean volume may be 28 times normal), cul-de-sac fluid, peripheral structures most likely representing follicles, and other adnexal lesions such as a cyst or tumor.[2,3] When cul-de-sac fluid is caused exclusively by ovarian torsion, it is usually a

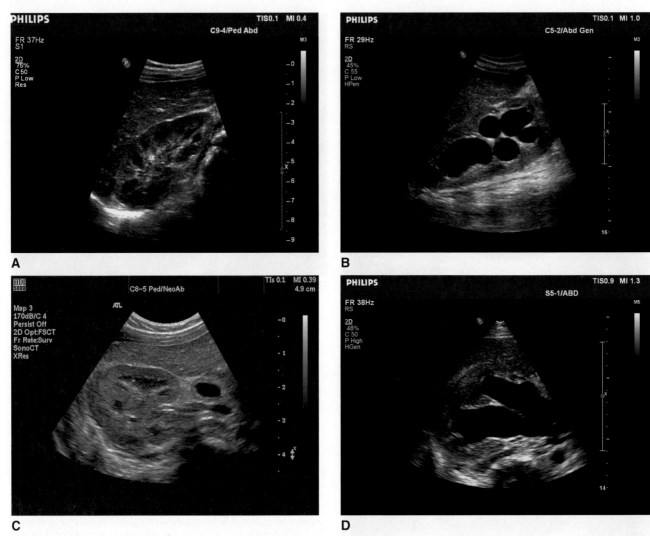

Figure 7-12 Normal sagittal neonatal kidney with fetal lobulations **(A)** and hydronephrosis **(B)**. Normal transverse kidney **(C)** and hydronephrosis **(D)**. (Images courtesy of Philips Medical Systems, Bothell, WA.)

late manifestation and associated with hemorrhagic, necrotic ovarian tissue.[2,3] Vascular congestion in the mass causes good sound transmission and numerous internal echoes. The appearance of a solid mass can be caused by abnormal venous and lymphatic drainage, leading to marked ovarian enlargement caused by incomplete torsion. The sonographic appearance of massive ovarian edema caused by either partial or intermittent torsion varies from solid to multicystic to complex. It is unclear whether the torsion is the primary event or the result of the enlarged size of the ovary.[2,7] When torsion is found in conjunction with an intraovarian mass, a complex pelvoabdominal mass is usually identified.

The diagnosis of ovarian torsion may be aided by spectral and color flow Doppler.[2,3,7] First, image the normal ovary to establish the proper technical factors. Next, examine the abnormal side for the presence or absence of flow.[2,7] Venous flow is absent although arterial perfusion may be variable depending on the degree of vascular compromise; therefore, it is possible

for blood flow to be documented in the torsed ovary (Fig. 7-13).

Differential sonographic diagnosis includes ovarian neoplasm, ectopic pregnancy, hemorrhagic cyst, PID,

TABLE	7-2	
Differential Diagnoses of Cystic and Solid Gynecologic Masses or Their Simulators in Children		

Cystic	Solid
Anterior meningocele	Chordoma neuroblastoma
Neurenteric cysts	Ganglioneuroma
Retrorectal cysts	Neurofibroma
Ectopic kidney (hydronephrotic)	Sacral bone tumors
Massive hydroureter	Retroperitonealsarcomas
Bladder diverticulum	Lymphosarcoma
Hydrosalpinx	Rhabdomyosarcoma
Ovarian cyst	Yolk sac carcinoma
Hydrometrocolpos	Intussusception

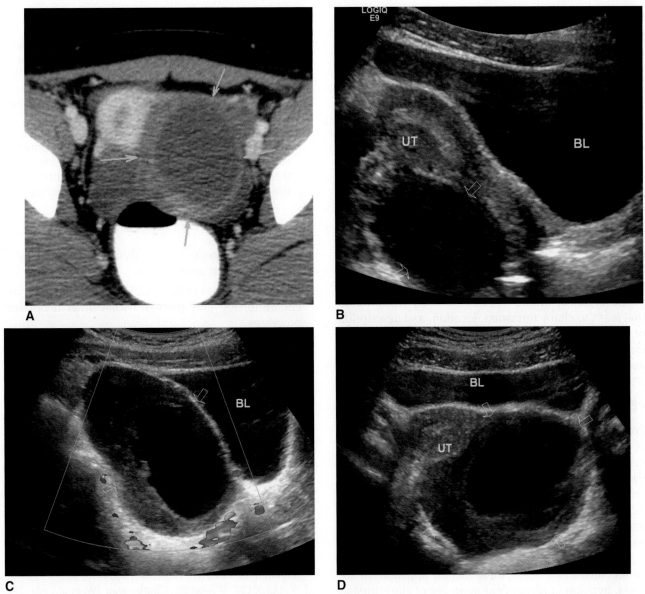

Figure 7-13 13-year-old with pelvic pain. **A:** Contrast-enhanced axial CT image shows a complex 10-cm ovarian mass (*arrows*) posterior to the uterus and displacing the uterus to the right. There is mild peripheral enhancement of the lesion. The uterus and left ovary appear normal. **B:** Sagittal midline ultrasound image of the pelvis shows a normal uterus and endometrium with an oval, cystic mass seen posterior to the uterus (*arrows*). **C:** Sagittal image of the pelvic mass shows a large anechoic cyst surrounded by ovarian tissue measuring 10.1 × 5.5 × 9.1 cm (*arrows*). Color Doppler imaging using the same imaging parameters used on the contralateral ovary demonstrate a lack of vascularity within the mass. **D:** Transverse image of the pelvis corresponding to the CT exam performed 1 week prior. A large mass containing a cystic structure is seen in the posterior, left pelvis (*arrows*) resulting in deviation of the uterus anterior and to the right. A normal right ovary was not identified; therefore, this mass most likely represents a torsed right ovary. At surgery, the ovary was black, necrotic, and torsed. *BL*, bladder; *UT*, uterus. (Images courtesy of Helen DeVos Children's Hospital, Grand Rapids, MI.)

and periappendiceal abscess. Thorough clinical history coupled with a proper index of suspicion in the face of a clinical history that is atypical for these diagnoses may lead to early diagnosis of torsion and preservation of the ovary.[2,3]

Some authors have been advocates for oophoropexy on the noninvolved side, tacking the ovary to the broad ligament or pelvic sidewall to prevent ovarian torsion. The thought process behind this decision is that subsequent torsion of the ovary in a female with prior oophorectomy prevents both emotional and reproductive concerns in this population.

PATHOLOGY DIAGNOSTIC CRITERIA

Sonographic diagnostic criteria are in general described the same for pediatric pelvic examinations as they are for the adult population. Terminology for masses is either cystic, solid, or complex. Ascites, irregular borders, or papillary projections with thickened septa in a

Critical Thinking Questions

A premenstrual 11-year-old girl presents to the department with complaints of right lower quadrant pain, fever, nausea, and vomiting for the last 2 days. Laboratory findings include an increased white blood count. The sonographic examination shows a normal uterus and left ovary. There is fluid in the posterior cul-de-sac and a complex, cylindrical right-sided mass. On color Doppler, this mass has a hyperemic appearance. Discuss differential diagnoses for this clinical scenario.

ANSWER: At first glance, this would appear to be non-specific to ovarian torsion, appendicitis, hemorrhagic cyst, pelvic inflammatory disease, or ovarian neoplasm. As the patient is virginal and not sexually active, it is unlikely that there would be an ectopic pregnancy. PID can image as a tubular structure lateral to the uterus; however, in this patient, this diagnosis is unlikely. The symptoms include right lower quadrant (RLQ) pain, fever, nausea and vomiting, and the increased white blood count. The finding of hyperemia of the right-sided mass gives us our best clue. In the case of torsion, there would be lack of flow. The most likely cause for this patient's symptomology is a case of appendicitis.

mass favors, but is not diagnostic of, malignancy. Any abnormality requires identification in relation to normal anatomical landmarks, and this many times leads to the organ of origin. Ultrasound is an examination that leads to characterization, location, and description of anatomy; it is used in conjunction with clinical history and physical examination and both radiographic and laboratory tests to arrive at a differential diagnosis.

PELVIS MASS DIFFERENTIAL DIAGNOSIS

Pediatric gynecologic disorders range across a variety of differential diagnoses. Masses composed of cystic material may be of gynecologic origin (e.g., ovarian cyst, hydrosalpinx, hydrocolpos) or they may arise from the urinary tract (e.g., bladder diverticulum, hydroureter). Additionally, such conditions as mesenteric cyst, gastrointestinal (GI) duplication cyst, pseudocyst, and presacral meningocele are also potential differential diagnoses.

Masses that are complex in nature could potentially be secondary to abscess; these include appendiceal abscess, hematoma (dependent upon age of clot), torsion of a mass, or an ectopic pregnancy.

Masses composed of solid material may represent gynecological tumors, presacral neural tumors, intussusception, lymph nodes, and sarcomas originating in the pelvic bones.

To reach a most likely diagnosis, all information is needed, including the clinical history, laboratory test results, sonographic impressions, and hormone levels.

SUMMARY

- Ovarian cysts are a common finding in the pediatric population.
- Most urinary tract neoplasms originate in the bladder.
- The ovary is the most common site for pelvic neoplasms in the child.
- Functional ovarian neoplasms, adrenal hyperplasia, and endocrine processes can result in precocious puberty.
- Fibrovascular septi of the dysgerminoma demonstrate prominent arterial flow.
- Laboratory values of hCG, LDH, and AFP help differentiate torsion and abscesses from other neoplastic processes.
- In the child with ambiguous genitalia, sonography aids in gender determination through visualization of the uterus, ovaries, and/or testicles.
- Hydrocolpos, hematocolpos, hydrometra, hematometra, hydrometrocolpos, and hematometrocolpos are all variations of fluid or blood within the uterus and vagina due to some type of obstruction.
- Congenital and mechanical uterine, ovarian, and renal anomalies often coexist.
- Ovarian torsion occurs more often on the right side.

REFERENCES

1. Atra A, Ward HC, Aitken K, et al. Conservative surgery in multimodal therapy for pelvic rhabdomyosarcoma in children. *Br J Cancer.* 1994;70(5):1004–1008.
2. Rumack CM, Wilson SR, Charboneau JW, et al., eds. *The Pediatric Pelvis. Diagnostic Ultrasound.* 4th ed. St. Louis, MO: Mosby; 2010.
3. Hagan-Ansert S. Pediatric congenital anomalies of the female pelvis. In: Hagan-Ansert SL, ed. *Textbook of Diagnostic Ultrasonography.* 6th ed. St. Louis, MO: Mosby Elsevier; 2006.
4. Coley BD, Kane RA, Kruskal JB, eds. *Ultrasound Clinics. Pediatric Ultrasound/Intraoperative Ultrasonography of the Abdomen.* Vol. 1, issue 3. Philadelphia, PA: Elsevier Saunders; 2006:471.
5. Moore KL, Persaud TVN. *The Developing Human: Clinically Oriented Embryology.* 8th ed. Philadelphia, PA: Saunders; 2007. Hagan-Ansert SL, ed. *Textbook of Diagnostic Ultrasonography.* 6th ed. St. Louis, MO: Mosby Elsevier; 2006.
6. Khadilkar VV, Khadilkar AV, Kinare AS, et al. Ovarian and uterine ultrasonography in healthy girls between birth to 18 years. *Indian Pediatr.* 2006;43(7):625–630.
7. Dubbins, PA. Doppler ultrasound of the female pelvis. In: Allen PL, Dubbins PA, Pozniak MA, et al., eds. *Clinical Doppler Ultrasound.* 2nd ed. Philadelphia, PA: Churchill Livingstone Elsevier; 2006.

8. Nussbaum AR, Lebowitz RI. Interlabial masses in little girls: review and imaging recommendations. *AJR*. 1983;141:65–71.

9. Foster CM, Feuillan R, Padmanabhan V, et al. Ovarian function in girls with Mccune-Albright syndrome. *Pediatr Res*. 1986;20:859–863.

10. Park K, van Rijn R, McHugh K. The role of radiology in paediatric soft tissue sarcomas. *Cancer Imaging*. 2008;8:102–115.

11. Garel L, Dubois J, Grignon A, et al. US of the pediatric female pelvis: a clinical perspective. *RadioGraphics*. 2001;21:1393–1407.

12. Haller JO, Fellows RA. The pelvis. In: Haller JO, Shkolnik A, eds. *Ultrasound in Pediatrics Clinics in Diagnostic Ultrasound*. Vol. 8. New York, NY: Churchill Livingstone; 1981.

13. Bulas DI, Ahlstrom PA, Sivit CJ, et al. Pelvic inflammatory disease in the adolescent: comparison of transabdominal and transvaginal sonographic evaluation. *Radiology*. 1992;183:435–439.

14. Haller JO, Bass IS, Friedman AP. Pelvic masses in girls: an 8-year retrospective analysis stressing ultrasound as the prime imaging modality. *Pediatr Radiol*. 1984;14:363–368.

15. Laufer MC. Ovarian cysts and neoplasms in infants, children, and adolescents. *J Reprod Med*. 2004;49:329.

16. Nussbaum AR, Sanders RC, Hartman DS, et al. Neonatal ovarian cysts: sonographic-pathologic correlation. *Pediatr Radiol*. 1988;168:817–821.

17. Widdowson DJ, Pilling DW, Cook RCM. Neonatal ovarian cysts: therapeutic dilemma. *Arch Dis Child*. 1988;63:737–742.

18. Nussbaum AR, Sanders RC, Hartman DS, et al. Neonatal ovarian cysts: sonographic-pathologic correlation. *Pediatr Radiol*. 1988;168:817–821.

19. Valentin L, Callen PW. Ultrasound evaluation of the adnexa (ovary and fallopian tubes). In: Callen PW, ed. *Ultrasonography in Obstetrics and Gynecology*. 5th ed. Philadelphia, PA: Saunders Elsevier; 2000.

20. Kim SH, Kang SB. Ovarian dysgerminoma: color doppler ultrasonographic findings and comparison with CT and MR imaging findings. *J Ultrasound Med*. 1995;14:843–848.

21. Vander Werff BJ, Hagen-Ansert S. Pathology of the ovaries. In: Callen P, ed. *Ultrasonography in Obstetrics and Gynecology*. 5th ed. Philadelphia, PA: Elsevier; 2008.

22. Vijayaraghavan GR, Levine D. Case 109: Meigs syndrome. *Radiology*. 2007;242(3):940–944.

23. Tanaka YO, Kurosaka Y, Nishida M, et al. Ovarian dysgerminoma: MR and CT appearance. *J Comput Assist Tomogr*. 1994;18:443–448.

24. Foster CM, Feuillan R, Padmanabhan V, et al. Ovarian function in girls with Mccune-Albright syndrome. *Pediatr Res*. 1986;20:859–863.

25. Salardi S, Orsini LF, Cacciari E, et al. Pelvic ultrasonography in premenarchal girls: relation to puberty and sex hormone concentrations. *Arch Dis Child*. 1985;60:120–125.

26. Schaffer RM, Haller JO, Friedman AP, et al. Sonographic diagnosis of ovarian dysgerminoma in children. *Medical Ultrasound*. 1982;6:118–119.

27. Fleischer AC, Entmann SS. Sonographic evaluation of the ovary and related disorders. In: Sabbagha RE, ed. *Diagnostic Ultrasound Applied to Obstetrics and Gynecology*. 3rd ed. Philadelphia, PA: JB Lippincott; 1994.

28. Bicker GH, Siebert JJ, Anderson JC, et al. Sonography of ovarian involvement in childhood acute lymphocytic leukemia. *Am J Roentgenol*. 1981;137:399–401.

29. Pal R, Manglik A, Sinha N. A case of Mayer-Rokitansky-Küster-Hayser syndrome with absence of the right thumb. *Saudi J Kidney Dis Transpl*. 2008;19:236–240.

30. Acién P, Galán F, Manchón I, et al. Hereditary renal adysplasia, pulmonary hypoplasia, and Mayer-Rokitansky-Küster-Hauser (MRKH) syndrome: a case report. *Orphanet J Rare Dis*. 2010;14:5–6.

31. Westphalen AC, Qayyum Aliya. The role of magnetic resonance imaging in the evaluation of gynecologic disease. In: Callen PW, ed. *Ultrasonography in Obstetrics and Gynecology*. 5th ed. Philadelphia, PA: Elsevier; 2000.

32. Ramos ES. Turner syndrome: counseling prior to oocyte donation. *Sao Paulao Med J*. 2007;125(2):112–114.

33. Oakes MB, Eyvazzadeh AD, Quint E, et al. Complete androgen insensitivity syndrome—a review. *J Pediatr Adolesc Gynecol*. 2008;21(6):305–310.

34. Ambrosino MM, Hernanz-Schulman M, Genieser NB, et al. Monitoring of girls undergoing medical therapy for isosexual precocious puberty. *J Ultrasound Med*. 1994;13:501–508.

35. Midyett LK, Moore WV, Jacobson JD. Are pubertal changes in girls before age 8 benign? *Pediatrics*. 2003;111(1):47–51.

36. King LR, Siegel MJ, Solomon AL. Usefulness of ovarian volume and cysts in female isosexual precocious puberty. *J Ultrasound Med*. 1993;12:577–581.

37. Matarazzo P, Lala R, Andreo M, et al. McCune-Albright syndrome: persistence of autonomous ovarian hyperfunction during adolescence and early adult age. *J Pediatr Endocrinol Metab*. 2006;19(suppl 2):607–617.

38. Ben-Haroush A, Goldberg-Stern H, Phillip M, et al. GnRH agonist treatment in girls with precocious puberty does not compromise post-pubertal uterine size. *Hum Reprod*. 2007;22(3):895–900.

39. Geipel A, Berg C, Germer U, et al. Diagnostic and therapeutic problems in a case of prenatally detected fetal hydrocolpos. *Ultrasound Obstet Gynecol*. 2001;18(2):169–172.

40. Scanlan KA, Pozniak MA, Fagerholm M, et al. Value of transperineal sonography in the assessment of vaginal atresia. *Am J Roentgenol*. 1990;154:545–548.

41. Donnez O, Jadoul P, Squifflet J, et al. Didelphic uterus and obstructed hemivagina: recurrent hematometra in spite of appropriate classic surgical treatment. *Gynecol Obstet Invest*. 2007;63(2):98–101.

42. Chang HC, Bhatt S, Dogra VS. Pearls and pitfalls of diagnosis of ovarian torsion. *Radiographics*. 2008;28(5):1355–1368.

43. Moore KL, Dalley AF, Agur AMR, eds. *Clinically Oriented Anatomy*. 6th ed. Baltimore, MD: Wolters Kluwer | Lippincott Williams & Wilkins; 2010.

44. Davis AJ, Feins NR. Subsequent asynchronous torsion of normal adnexa in children. *J Pediatr Surg*. 1990;25:687–689.

45. Abu-Rustum RS, Chaaban M. Is 3-dimensional sonography useful in the prenatal diagnosis of ambiguous genitalia? *J Ultrasound Med*. 2009;28:95–97.

46. de Sousa G, Wunsch R, Andler W. Precocious pseudopuberty due to autonomous ovarian cysts: a report of ten cases and long-term follow-up. *Hormones*. 2008;7(2):170–174.

8 Benign Disease of the Female Pelvis

Susan Raatz Stephenson

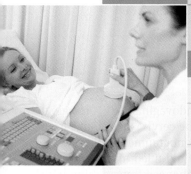

OBJECTIVES

List benign neoplasms of the vagina, cervix, uterus, and ovaries

Describe the sonographic and complementary imaging appearance of benign neoplasms of the female reproductive organs

Summarize the results of surgery and trauma to the uterus (i.e., synechiae, uterine, and dehiscence)

Distinguish extrauterine masses such as abscesses, hematomas, lymphoceles, and appendicitis from uterine masses

List types of ovarian cysts as well as their cause and their sonographic appearance

Explain the results and imaging appearance of ovarian torsion

KEY TERMS

nabothian cysts | endometrial hyperplasia | Asherman's syndrome | synechiae | uterine dehiscence | leiomyoma | abscess | hematoma | lymphocele | appendicitis | hydrosalpinx | functional cyst | follicular cyst | corpus luteum cyst | theca lutein cysts | hemorrhagic cyst | torsion | polycystic ovary syndrome (PCOS) | cystic teratomas | dermoid | mucinous cystadenoma | serous cystadenoma | Brenner tumor | thecoma-fibroma | granulosa stromal tumor | gonadoblastoma | Sertoli-Leydig cell tumor | Meigs' syndrome

GLOSSARY

Adhesiolysis Surgical removal of adhesions (scar tissue)

Anovulation Failure to ovulate

Chorioadenoma destruens Form of carcinoma that grows into the uterine musculature

Crohn's disease Inflammation of the bowel

Electrosurgery Surgery performed with an electrical device such as an electrocautery

Endometrioma Blood-filled ovarian cyst resultant from endometriosis implants

Follicle-stimulating hormone (FSH) Hormone produced by the anterior pituitary gland that stimulates growth of the Graafian follicle

Hirsutism Excessive hair on a woman

Hydatidiform mole Genetically abnormal pregnancy that develops into a grape-like mass with the uterus

Hyperandrogenemia Increased testosterone levels associated with polycystic ovary syndrome (PCOS)

Hyperandrogenism Excessive production/secretion of androgens

Hysteroplasty Reconstructive surgery of the uterus

Hysteroscope Instrument allowing visualization of the uterus

Involute Collapsing and rolling inward

Luteinizing hormone (LH) Hormone produced by the anterior pituitary gland that stimulates ovulation

Lysis Breaking up of tissue

Menorrhagia Abnormally heavy or prolonged menses

Oligoanovulation Infrequent ovulation

Oligomenorrhea Infrequent menses

Omentum Peritoneal fold supporting the abdominal viscera

Placenta accrete Growth of the placenta into the myometrium

Placenta previa Implantation of the placenta in the lower uterine segment or on the cervix

Psammoma bodies Microscopic collection of calcium associated with specific tumor types

Radiodense (radiopaque) Tissue that absorbs X-rays appearing white on the resulting radiograph

Red degeneration Hemorrhage into a leiomyoma that has outgrown its blood supply

Tamoxifen Anti-estrogenic drug used to decrease the occurrence of certain estrogen-sensitive breast cancers

Uterine dehiscence Partial separation of the myometrium at the location of uterine scar

The diagnostic ultrasound examination has become the modality of choice to evaluate the organs of the female pelvis because of the ease of imaging the female reproductive system. Pathology found during the sonographic examination often shares features of malignant and benign disease, requiring correlation with clinical, laboratory, and pathologic findings. This chapter focuses on benign disease of the female pelvis ranging from leiomyomas found in the uterus to ovarian findings of physiologic cysts and multistructure processes such as a tubo-ovarian abscess or neoplasm.

THE UTERUS

THE CERVIX

Anomalies of uterine development are relatively frequent. They can be divided into those caused by abnormal uterine fusion (see Chaps. 2 and 3), those caused by abnormal cervical function (incompetent cervix), and those produced by maternal exposure to diethylstilbestrol (DES). Benign conditions that may produce an enlarged cervix include cervical leiomyoma, nabothian cysts, and cervical polyps (Table 8-1).

Nabothian Cysts/Inclusion Cysts

Nabothian or inclusion cysts are located within the cervix at the opening of a nabothian duct. The cyst forms due to retention of nabothian gland secretions.[1,2] This normal asymptomatic variation is a common finding in the adult cervix and is often noted after pregnancy or chronic cervicitis (Fig. 8-1).[3]

Imaging Findings
Sonography

Sonography, particularly endovaginal (EV) imaging, helps cyst detection within the cervix. Sizes range from as small as 3 mm to 3 cm. Sonographically, these cysts image as smooth bordered, fluid-filled masses. A common finding of artifactual enhanced transmission with refractive edge shadowing (Fig. 8-2) may be eliminated through technique adjustments. Proper imaging techniques help the sonographer avoid confusing the nabothian cyst with developing ovarian follicles or loculated pelvic fluid.

Magnetic Resonance Imaging

Nabothian cysts image easily on the magnetic resonance imaging (MRI) examination. These incidental findings display as an intermediate to high intensity signal on the T2-weighted image. The difficulty with the finding of the inclusion cyst is that it often mimics malignant pathology of the cervix (Fig. 8-3).[4]

Treatment

Nabothian cysts are not usually treated if they are small and asymptomatic. If malignancy cannot be ruled out or they become large, drainage may be necessary.[5]

Polyps

Cervical polyps are the most common benign neoplasms of the cervix. Found in at least 4% of women, they most often occur in multigravidas in the perimenopausal and postmenopausal years. Usually asymptomatic, cervical polyps may be a cause for profuse bleeding or

TABLE	8-1

Benign Lesions of the Vagina, Cervix, and Uterus

Lesion	Ages Affected	Sonographic Characteristics
Gartner's duct cyst	Reproductive years	Anechoic fluid-filled mass with well-defined margins and good through-transmission. Located in the anterolateral wall of the vagina.
Nabothian cyst	Usually seen after pregnancy	Fluid-filled mass located in the cervical canal, often with refractive edge shadowing.
Polyps (endometrial)	Peri menopausal and postmenopausal	Appear increased in echogenicity when compared to the surrounding endometrium. May be focal or diffuse.
Leiomyoma (myoma, fibroids)	Reproductive years	May be increased, decreased, or same echogenicity as myometrium. Hyaline degeneration; anechoic mass with poor sound transmission. Cystic degeneration: anechoic mass with good sound transmission. Calcific degeneration: echogenic focal areas with distal acoustic shadowing.

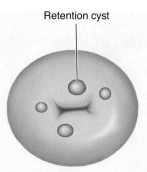

Retention cyst

Figure 8-1 Variations in the cervical surface. Two kinds of epithelia may cover the cervix: (1) shiny pink squamous epithelium, which resembles the vaginal epithelium, and (2) deep red, plushy columnar epithelium, which is continuous with the endocervical lining. These two meet at the squamocolumnar junction. When this junction is at or inside the cervical os, only squamous epithelium is seen. A ring of columnar epithelium is often visible to a varying extent around the os—the result of a normal process that accompanies fetal development, menarche, and the first pregnancy. With increasing estrogen stimulation during adolescence, all or part of this columnar epithelium is transformed into squamous epithelium by a process termed metaplasia. This change may block the secretions of columnar epithelium and cause retention cysts (sometimes called nabothian cysts). These appear as one or more translucent nodules on the cervical surface and have no pathologic significance.

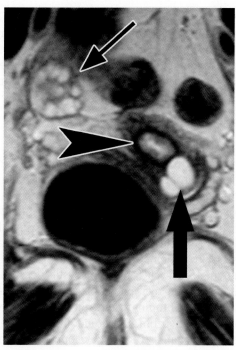

Figure 8-3 Nabothian cyst seen on a high-resolution T2-weighted MRI image performed axial with respect to cervix shows two small nabothian cysts *(arrow)*. Note zonal anatomy of cervix *(arrowhead)* and normal right ovary with follicles *(thin arrow)*.

discharge.[3] Polyps are usually attached to the cervical wall by a pedicle and may reach a size of several centimeters.[3] Although it is easier to identify small polyps with the EV approach than transabdominally, they may be difficult to identify sonographically because of their size. Occasionally, a pedunculated intracavity or cervical leiomyoma protrudes through the os, mimicking the polyp (Fig. 8-4).[3,4]

Treatment

Asymptomatic polyps do not need removal. If they begin to bleed, grow large, or have an unusual appearance on visual examination, removal becomes warranted. Removal of a cervical polyp is achieved through twisting or use of forceps.[6]

Myomas

Cervical myomas share similar histology to myomas (leiomyomas) of the uterine corpus. Most of the small, asymptomatic cervical myomas comprise from 3% to 8% percent of these types of neoplasms. If symptoms do occur, they may include dyspareunia, dysuria, urgency, genitourinary obstruction, cervical obstruction, prolapse, bleeding, and obstructed labor. Depending on the age and reproductive plans of the patient, the clinician may choose to resect symptomatic lesions or perform a hysterectomy.[7] Sonographically, cervical myomas may distort the cervix and present a sonographic pattern similar to that of corpus myomas. Serial sonographic examinations aid in observation of growth of the asymptomatic tumors.

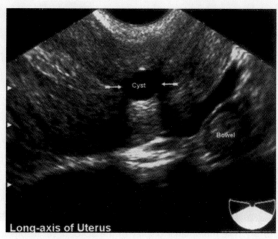

Long-axis of Uterus

Figure 8-2 Long-axis EV image of the cervix in an anteverted uterus. A rounded, fluid-filled mass *(arrows)* demonstrates posterior enhancement and refractive edge artifacts consistent with a nabothian cyst.

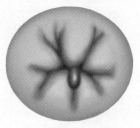

Figure 8-4 A cervical polyp usually arises from the endocervical canal, becoming visible when it protrudes through the cervical os. It is bright red, soft, and rather fragile. When only the tip is seen, it cannot be differentiated clinically from a polyp originating in the endometrium. Polyps are benign but may bleed.

Treatment

Asymptomatic cervical myomas require no treatment. If symptoms become present with a small to medium leiomyoma, a myomectomy allows for removal of the mass; very large myomas may require a total hysterectomy.[8]

THE ENDOMETRIUM

Endometrial Hyperplasia

Excessive growth of the endometrium is a condition called endometrial hyperplasia. High hormone levels cause the endometrium to thicken due to high levels of estrogen (i.e., as a result of fertility treatments, hormone replacement therapy [HRT], or tamoxifen therapy [Fig. 8-5]). Hyperplasia of the endometrium has also been seen in patients with diabetes, obesity, persistent anovulatory cycles, and polycystic ovary disease. Estrogen-producing ovarian neoplasms such as the theca and granulosa cell tumor also result in the development of a thick endometrium. Since endometrial hyperplasia increases a woman's risk for development of endometrial cancer, close monitoring becomes important.[9,10]

Hyperplasia is the most common cause of abnormal uterine bleeding in women, with the upper limit endometrial thickness of 14 mm[3] in premenopausal woman, 10 mm[11] in women on tamoxifen, and 8 mm[3] in postmenopausal women. All measurements include the anterior and posterior layer of the endometrium.

Imaging Findings

Sonography

The main sonographic finding is one of a thickened endometrium (Fig. 8-6). The homogeneous, heterogenic endometrium with small cystic areas—which represent dilated cystic glands, cystic atrophy, or endometrial polyps—indicate a benign process.[12] Because of the

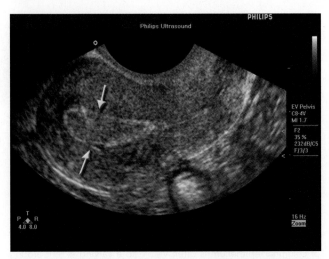

Figure 8-6 This EV image demonstrates a thickened endometrium (*arrows*) seen with endometrial hyperplasia. (Image courtesy of Philips Medical Systems, Bothell, WA.)

nonspecificity of the sonographic findings, a biopsy becomes necessary to confirm diagnosis.[10]

The three-dimensional (3D) examination of the patient with endometrial hyperplasia has the added benefit of imaging anatomy on planes absent on two-dimensional (2D) imaging. The coronal plane, only seen with the multiplanar reconstructions done with the 3D data set, allow for further evaluation of the uterine lining (Fig. 8-7). The superimposition of color Doppler information onto the reconstructed 3D image helps to distinguish a benign from a malignant process. A study done by Hosny et al. confirmed the peripheral location of regularly separated vessels with the hyperplastic endometrium. Couple the color finding with a resistive index (RI) of greater than 0.5 in the endometrium and 0.85 ± 0.08, and the probability of a benign process increases.[12]

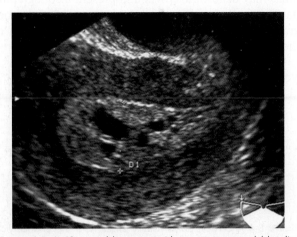

Figure 8-5 A 62-year-old woman with postmenopausal bleeding undergoing tamoxifen therapy. EV long-axis view of the uterus reveals a thickened endometrial lining (19 mm) with cystic changes. A polyp was confirmed.

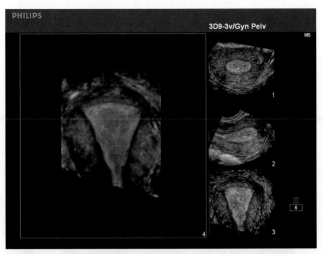

Figure 8-7 The multiplanar display of the 3D data set results in an image of the coronal plane. The coronal image, displayed as *frame 3*, has been reconstructed in *frame 4* as the volume. (Image courtesy of Philips Medical Systems, Bothell, WA.)

Treatment

The American Congress of Obstetricians and Gynecologists (ACOG) suggests hysteroscopy and dilation and curettage (D&C) for use in patients with endometrial hyperplasia.[13] Other treatments, depending on the type of hyperplasia present and the fertility status of the patient, include progesterone treatment using an oral medication, or an intrauterine contraceptive device (IUCD) delivery method.[14] In extreme cases, a hysterectomy may also be recommended.[14]

Asherman's Syndrome/Synechiae

Adhesions of the endometrium develop as a result of trauma to the uterine lining. This includes a history of cesarean section (C/S) and the D&C often performed during an elective abortion or as a result of a pregnancy failure. The D&C performed for placental fragment retention also increases the risk of developing synechiae. After the procedure, the damaged endometrial surfaces heal into the adhesion. As a result, the patient may experience fertility problems or recurrent pregnancy loss.

Imaging Findings

Sonography

Hysterosonography, hysterosonosalpingography, and sonohysterography are similar terms describing the saline injection procedure performed with ultrasound guidance. Chapter 31 provides a detailed description of this procedure (Fig. 8-8).

Lysis (hysteroplasty) of the uterine synechiae with a hysteroscope allows for direct treatment of the adhesion. A laparoscope, in conjunction with the hysteroscope, may be used for complicated cases to perform adhesiolysis.[10,15,16]

Hysterosalpingography

Hysterosalpingography (HSG) has been the gold standard in diagnosing pathology of the uterine cavity and tubes. This procedure occurs through the use of radiographic fluoroscopy and the injection of contrast material through the cervix into the uterus. To prevent radiation exposure to an early pregnancy, this procedure occurs during the first portion (day 7 to 12) of the woman's cycle.[17,18] Complications of this procedure include bleeding, infection, contrast reaction, perforation of the uterus, and radiation exposure of an early pregnancy.

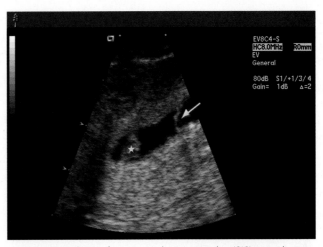

Figure 8-8 Saline infusion sonohysterography (SIS) revealing an intrauterine synechiae *(star)* and an adhesion *(arrow)*. Note the decrease in sector size (increasing the line density within the sector) and depth to increase the image detail.

During the hysterosalpingogram, a radiographic procedure, synechiae appear as filling defects within the uterine cavity. These areas display as darker than the surrounding contrast material and can be followed to the uterine wall. Care must be taken to differentiate uterine folds, which appear as linear filling defects parallel to the uterine walls from adhesions (Fig. 8-9).[18]

Treatment

Removal or rupture of the intrauterine adhesions is under direct visualization through a hysteroscope. This procedure takes the form of adhesion rupture, cutting of adhesions with scissors, *and excision through* electrosurgery *or using* via a laser.[15]

THE MYOMETRIUM

Uterine Dehiscence

C/S is a common procedure performed in developed countries. The safety of this procedure has become an assumption; however, any surgery raises the risk for development of pelvic adhesions, uterine dehiscence (scar rupture), and future placental implantation complications (placenta previa and accreta).[19] Other causes for uterine scarring include myomectomies and instrument perforation.[20,21] Though a rare complication,

---

PATHOLOGY BOX 8-1

Asherman's Syndrome[10,17]

Signs and Symptoms	Diagnosis	Endometrial Sonographic Appearance
• Normal to absent menses • Recurrent miscarriage • Infertility	• Hysteroscope • HSG • Sonohysterography (SHG)	• 2D imaging: normal or hypoechoic bridgelike bands • Sonohystogram: bridging tissue bands; cavity distortion; thin, free-floating membranes; lack of distention in the presence of thick membranes

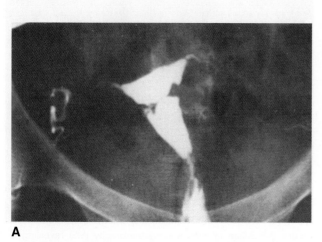

A

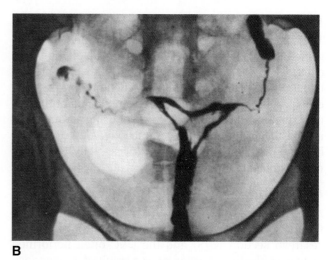

B

Figure 8-9 A: Filling defect typical of a marginal synechiae. In this case, the adhesion is circular and is visible on both lateral contours of the hysterogram. **B:** Intrauterine adhesions showing a persistent filling defect with hourglass appearance (i.e., column-shaped adhesion stretching between anterior and posterior walls of the uterus).

uterine scar dehiscence becomes an acute event during pregnancy often resulting in maternal and fetal morbidity.[19] This condition is the separation of the uterine myometrium with an intact peritoneum. In the case of a gravid uterus, the fetal membranes remain intact.[20] This section focuses on scar rupture in the nongravid uterus.

Imaging Findings

Sonography

The best method to identify the C/S scar in the uterus is to image the lower uterine segment (LUS) with an EV transducer.[20,22] The majority of cesarean deliveries use a transverse segmental uterine incision just superior to the bladder. This results in uterine scarring on the anterior section of the uterus at the internal os of the cervix.[22] A study by Ofili-Yebovi et al. confirmed previous findings of the ability to identify 95% or more of C/S scarring with EV imaging. The majority were in a location close to the internal os.[19]

The LUS consists of the uterine muscularis and bladder mucosa to include the visceral–parietal peritoneum. This section of the uterus images as two echogenic layers, which contrasts to the hypoechoic myometrium.[23] Identification of the scar occurs through the location of linear or triangular hypoechoic areas in the LUS and thinning of the endometrium and myometrium (Fig. 8-10). The retroflexed LUS had a 50% increase in scarring possibly due to tension on the healing wound.

MRI

MRI may be used in addition to ultrasound to confirm the extent of myometrial separation, especially in the case of suboptimal or confusing sonographic findings.[20] The ability to obtain images without the use of contrast or radiation has led to the use of MRI in fetal imaging. In the case of uterine rupture, MRI detail allows imaging of the separate uterine muscle layers (Fig. 8-11).[24]

Treatment

Defect closure at the C/S location include hysteroscopy, laparoscope-vaginal combinations, and laparotomy.[25] Severe cases may require a hysterectomy.

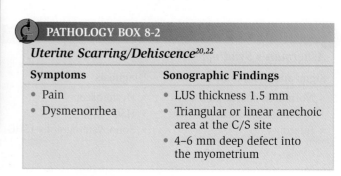

Figure 8-10 C/S scar rupture. Note the thinning and hypoechoic area extending from the internal os into the cervical tissue *(arrow)*. (Image courtesy of Philips Medical Systems, Bothell, WA.)

PATHOLOGY BOX 8-2

Uterine Scarring/Dehiscence[20,22]

Symptoms	Sonographic Findings
• Pain	• LUS thickness 1.5 mm
• Dysmenorrhea	• Triangular or linear anechoic area at the C/S site
	• 4–6 mm deep defect into the myometrium

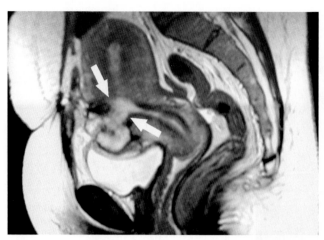

Figure 8-11 Uterine dehiscence following C/S. Sagittal T2-weighted image of uterus in patient with pain and bleeding after C/S. Note disruption of myometrium at the incision site *(arrows)*.

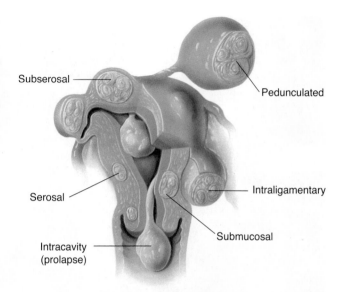

Figure 8-12 Possible locations of myomas. This schematic diagram illustrates the many locations at which myomas may develop. Symptoms related to heavy vaginal bleeding are generally greater when the myoma is in close proximity to the endometrial cavity, with serosal tumors able to attain large size with virtually no change in menstrual bleeding. Fibroids can develop anywhere in the uterus, with the cervix having proportionally fewer because of its lower complement of myometrial cells.

Leiomyoma

Leiomyomas are the most common tumor of the female pelvis. They have been estimated to occur in 20% to 30% of women of reproductive age.[24] The rate of occurrence is markedly greater in African Americans than Whites,[3,26] and there is a familial pattern to development of these benign tumors. A woman with a mother or sister with myomas has a 40% chance of developing myomas in her lifetime.[26] The cause of leiomyoma is unknown; however, they typically arise after menarche and regress after menopause, implicating estrogen as a promoter of growth.[10,24] Patients on tamoxifen treatment may see an increase in leiomyoma growth.[10]

Uterine leiomyomas are benign tumors of smooth muscle cells and fibrous connective tissue arising from uterine smooth muscle. Other frequently used descriptive terms include leiomyoma, myoma, leiomyomata, and fibromyoma. They may be single or multiple and variable in size, and they are surrounded by a pseudocapsule of compressed muscle fibers.[3,24,27] Leiomyomas affect any area of the uterus and are described by their relation to the uterine cavity. Those located within the myometrium are termed intramural, whereas the submucous forms lie beneath the endometrium and often protrude and distort the endometrial cavity. Subserosal or serosal myomas are at the serosal surface of the uterus, projecting into the peritoneal cavity. This classification often includes pedunculated myomas that image as an extrauterine neoplasm (Fig. 8-12). Five to 10 percent of myomas are submucosal, and these are the most symptomatic.[3] Subserosal myomas may become pedunculated at times and are the most difficult to assess sonographically. The term *parasitic myoma* is used when the blood supply of a leiomyoma is from other organs (Fig. 8-13). These myomas may be attached to the omentum or intestine or may grow laterally into the broad ligament.[3]

Degenerative Changes

Degeneration occurs when myomas outgrow their blood supply. The extent of degeneration depends on the severity of the discrepancy between the leiomyoma's growth and its blood supply,[26] with up to two-thirds of all myomas demonstrating some form of degeneration. The signs and symptoms of degeneration depend on the size and location of the leiomyoma. Various types of degeneration can occur, including hyaline, myxomatous, cystic, calcific, fatty, red degeneration (hemorrhagic), and necrosis.[26–28] Pain may indicate some form of a degenerative process or may be the result of torsion of a pedunculated leiomyoma or large tumor pressing on pelvic nerve roots.

In hyaline degeneration, smooth muscle cells are replaced by fibrous tissue. In cystic degeneration (4%), degeneration of hyaline tissue occurs, which leads to liquefaction necrosis. Calcific degeneration occurs most often after menopause[29] and is easily recognized sonographically (Fig. 8-14). Red degeneration is an acute form resulting from muscle infarction and occurs more commonly during pregnancy.[27] This may cause acute pain requiring surgical treatment. If laparotomy or myomectomy is necessary in the pregnant patient, there is usually a favorable maternal and fetal outcome.[27]

Signs and Symptoms

The size and location of myomas determine the symptomatology; however, many women with myomas have no symptoms. Submucous and intramural myomas that distort or deviate the endometrial cavity often result in

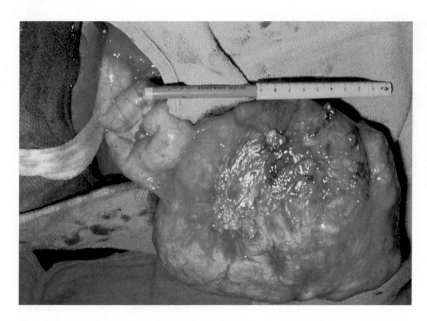

Figure 8-13 A parasitic myoma. A large tumor has become parasitic to a loop of small bowel, deriving its blood supply from the new vascular source. This typically only happens with large posterior or fundal tumors and is more common when they are pedunculated. The mechanism is felt to be pressure necrosis and revascularization during healing of the necrosis of the bowel wall.

abnormal bleeding that presents clinically as menorrhagia, but intermenstrual spotting and irregular periods may also occur. A very large myomatous tumor may result in increasing abdominal girth with or without associated pain.[15,28] A leiomyoma pressing on the bladder anteriorly often produces urinary frequency and urgency exaggerated perimenstrually.[26] A posterior leiomyoma may produce rectal pressure, causing constipation or lower back and leg discomfort and swelling.[3]

Imaging Findings

Imaging the leiomyoma becomes important, as large myomas can disrupt uterine contour more than smaller ones. Multiple large subserosal myomas may result in an enlarged uterus with a lobulated contour; large intramural and submucous myomas may distend the uterine cavity and distort the endometrial lining. It is important to indicate the location of myomas, whether subserosal, intramural, and/or submucosal, and whether distortion of the endometrial lining is present. Different surgical approaches may be used depending on the position and size of the myomas.

Because leiomyomas can enlarge the uterus considerably and may present outside the uterus in a pedunculated form, care must be taken to demonstrate the entire pelvic area to document both uterine and extrauterine myomas. A pedunculated leiomyoma can be mistaken for a number of conditions, including bicornuate uterus, blind uterine horn, ovarian mass, hydatidiform mole, and ectopic pregnancy (Fig. 8-15).[26] The use of complementary imaging modalities, such as sonography, radiography, MRI, and contrast studies, may be necessary to confirm diagnosis.

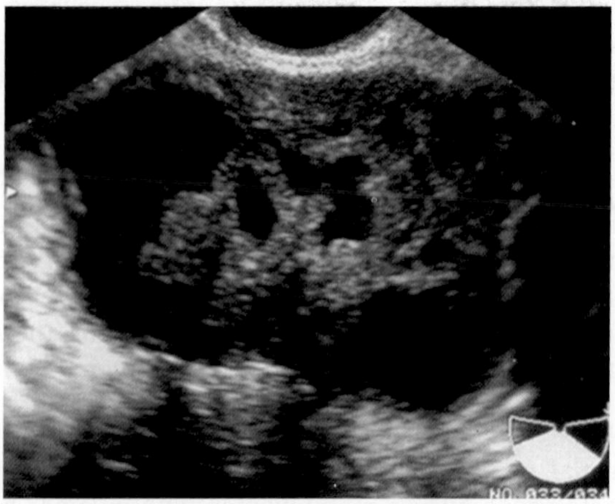

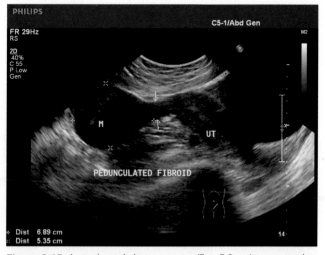

Figure 8-15 A moderately large myoma (7 × 5.3 cm) connected to the fundus of the uterus by a thin stalk (peduncle). A push–pull technique (sliding the scanning hand back and forth so that the transducer is in the proximal and distal portion of the vagina) with the vaginal transducer can often help identify the stalk of the myoma and its movement. (Image courtesy of Joe Antony, MD, Cochin, India. From the website at: http://www.ultrasound-images.com/fetus-general.htm.)

Figure 8-14 This large, complex mass with cystic degeneration was located anterior to the uterus and proved to be a degenerating pedunculated myoma.

Sonography

Routine sonography for imaging of myomas allows for assessment of dimensions, number, and location of tumors.[2] As with all imaging modalities, the leiomyoma measurement includes three dimensions: length, width, and height. Frequently, the sonographer may need to use the lowest-frequency transducer possible, increase the overall and time gain compensation (TGC), and increase the output power because myomas tend to attenuate the sound beam, which in turn makes it difficult to define the posterior wall of the tumor. Serial examinations help monitor and document interval growth. The enlarged uterus compromises the physical assessment completed by the clinician of the adnexa. In these instances, sonography is an excellent modality to evaluate the ovaries. Frequently, with a large myomatous uterus, the ovaries are low in the pelvis, requiring EV evaluation. The extremely high ovary images better with a transabdominal approach. The enlarged uterus often obstructs the ureters, resulting in hydronephrosis and underscoring the importance of imaging the kidneys.

A wide range of sonographic findings is associated with myomas.[9,30] The sonographic appearance of myomas depends on their size, location, and whether degeneration exists. Small myomas appear as subtle changes in myometrial echogenicity and may displace the endometrial cavity echo (Fig. 8-16). Degeneration may be present and can range from hypoechoic to echogenic. Cystic degeneration can cause hypoechoic areas within the leiomyoma. A whorled internal architecture may be seen when bundles of smooth muscle and fibrous tissue are arranged concentrically within a leiomyoma. Red degeneration can present as medium echoes with good through-transmission.[31]

Calcific degeneration is commonly seen and sonographically is recognized as clusters of bright reflectors

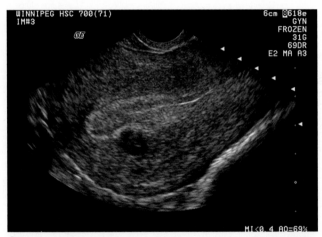

A

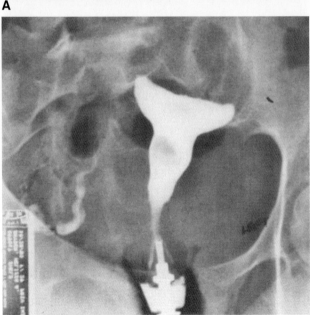

C

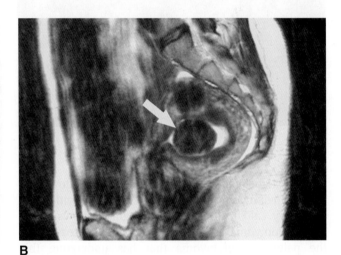

B

Figure 8-16 A: Submucosal myoma on a longitudinal EV image appears as a hypoechoic mass distorting the endometrial echo. **B:** Sagittal T2-weighted MRI image shows a submucosal myoma *(arrow)* centered in the endometrial cavity. **C:** Radiographic view of submucosal myoma, which images as a darker filling defect within the uterine cavity. (Sonographic image courtesy of GE Healthcare, Wauwatosa, WI.)

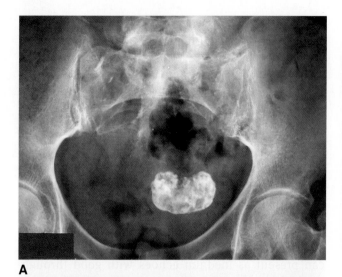

A

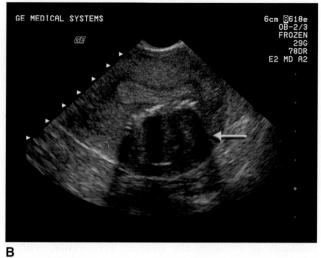

B

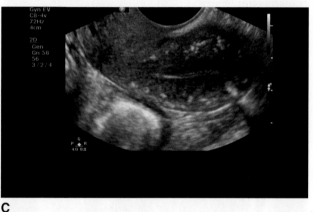

C

Figure 8-17 A: Pelvic radiograph shows a calcified mass just to the left of midline. Calcifications in fibroids often look like popcorn. **B:** An ultrasound image on a different patient demonstrates the appearance of a calcified, echogenic myoma *(arrow)*. (Sonographic image courtesy of GE Healthcare, Wauwatosa, WI.) **C:** Arcuate artery calcifications of the uterus image as echogenic foci in the periphery. (Image courtesy of Philips Medical Systems, Bothell, WA.)

that are associated with a distal acoustic shadow. The calcified leiomyoma should not be confused with arcuate artery calcifications. The radiograph shows a calcified leiomyoma as a radiodense (white) area within the pelvis. A leiomyoma that has undergone this type of degeneration usually images as a larger mass with posterior shadowing on the sonographic image. Calcifications of the arcuate arteries of the uterus image as bright echoes in the periphery of the uterus. Both types of calcifications are considered benign processes (Fig. 8-17).

Large myomas in the anterior and posterior uterine musculature can cause extrinsic compression of the urinary bladder and rectum that appears sonographically to indent the usually smooth uterus-bladder and rectum interface. See Figures 8-18, 8-19, 8-20, and 8-21 for examples of myomas.

MRI

Studies indicate that MRI may, in some instances, visualize leiomyomas better than ultrasound.[25,32] MRI evaluation may be recommended to locate myomas before surgery,[25] but this diagnostic examination is much more expensive than an ultrasound examination (Figs. 8-16B and 8-21A).

Hysterosalpingogram and Sonohysterography

Both HSG and SHG provide information on myomatous extension onto the endometrium through the visualization of filling defects. Both invasive procedures

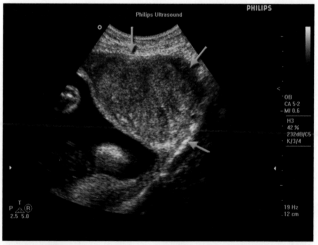

Figure 8-18 Transverse sonogram in a pregnant patient demonstrating a myoma *(arrows)*. A color overlay, called *chroma*, results in the gold hue seen on this image. (Image courtesy of Philips Medical Systems, Bothell, WA.)

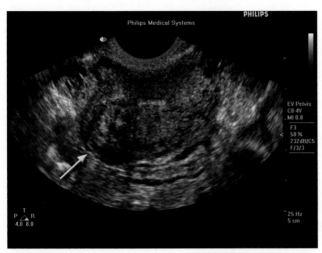

Figure 8-19 Subserosal myoma *(arrow)* imaged on the transverse EV exam. (Image courtesy of Philips Medical Systems, Bothell, WA.)

<table>
<tr><td colspan="2">

PATHOLOGY BOX 8-3

Leiomyoma

Symptoms	Sonographic Findings
• Symptomatic • Menorrhagia • Spotting • Increased abdominal girth • Pain • Urinary frequency/urgency • Lower back pain • Leg discomfort/swelling	• Heterogeneous myometrium • Irregular endometrial stripe • Hypoechoic areas within the myometrium • Whorled internal architecture of a mass • Calcifications • Posterior bladder contour changes
</td></tr>
</table>

come with risks of infection and bleeding and are often quite uncomfortable for the patient. HSG, since it is a radiographic procedure, has the added factor of radiation exposure. Since these procedures essentially only provide information on submucosal myomas, other diagnostic methods would be used (Figs. 8-16C and 8-21B,C).

Treatment

Treatment is as varied as the patients that present with a large uterus due to myomas. Asymptomatic women require only routine follow-up. The use of a prostaglandin or oral contraceptive may reduce or eliminate symptoms.[26] In the case of a patient with large myomas and a desire to become pregnant, a myomectomy would be appropriate. If the tumors obstruct the kidneys, removal becomes critical due

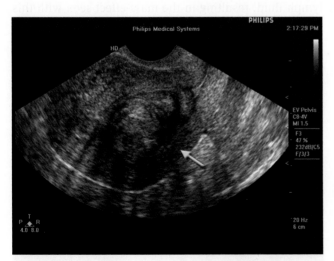

Figure 8-20 Myoma location may be difficult to determine. In this case, it is probably an intramural myoma *(arrow)*; however, distortion of the endometrium could result in categorization as a submucosal. (Image courtesy of Philips Medical Systems, Bothell, WA.)

to renal function impairment.[26] Each case differs and the clinician must determine the appropriateness of hormone therapy,[26] hysterectomy,[26] hysteroscopic myomectomy,[15,26] abdominal myomectomy,[26,33] or laser[1] or uterine artery embolization[34] in treatment of the benign fibroid.

EXTRAUTERINE PELVIC MASSES

ABSCESS

Abscess formation within the pelvis may be due to an infectious process involving the tubes, ovaries, appendix, bowel, peritoneum,[10,21] or bowel perforation.[30] This process is due to necrosis of the tissue or the development of purulent material. Peritonitis (infection of the serous membrane lining of the abdomen) is a complication of surgery. Bowel perforation, appendicitis, or tubo-ovarian abscess spread are also causes of a pelvic abscess.[35]

Patients with suspected abscess present postoperatively with fever, tenderness or pain, and swelling at the surgery site. Chills, general malaise, and weakness may also accompany this process. These patients also present with laboratory findings of an increased white blood count (WBC), sepsis, and possibly positive bacterial cultures.[35,36]

Imaging Findings
Sonography

Sonographically, this process may be difficult to image because of the formation of gas bubbles. Areas of infection may be loculated and located within the pelvis, paracolic gutters, or extend out of the pelvis. The complex or clear fluid has the tendency to collect in both the left upper and right upper quadrants surrounding the kidneys. Debris settling may result in fluid levels within the mass. Careful monitoring of the suspected mass for peristalsis helps differentiate the area from the bowel (Fig. 8-22).[35,36]

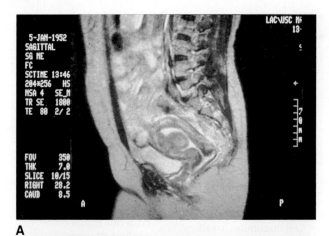

A

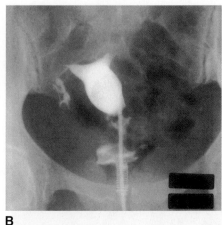

B

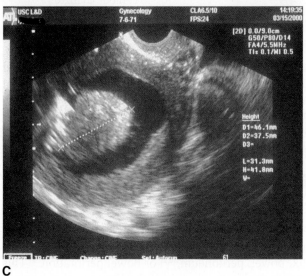

C

Figure 8-21 **A:** MRI of a submucous myoma. **B:** HSG of same myoma. **C:** Saline infusion sonogram of same myoma.

Computed Tomography

Computed tomography (CT) is a highly accurate method to diagnose infectious disease within the pelvis. Abscesses have a characteristic appearance on CT as a localized, loculated fluid collection. A mass effect may occur on surrounding structures (Fig. 8-23).[37]

HEMATOMA

The hematoma is any collection of blood, due to trauma or a disease process, within an organ or potential space. The patient with internal bleeding presents with a decreased hematocrit level, possibly a palpable mass, hypertension, and a decreased renal function.[36] Causes of the pelvic hematoma include an ectopic pregnancy or cyst rupture, postoperative bleeding due to a renal transplant, surgery, or trauma.

During the ultrasound examination, the sonographer may find a well-defined, walled-off mass. This area may have a complex appearance, ranging from swirling mobile mass contents to partially solid and anechoic to totally anechoic. The appearance depends on the age of the hematoma.[10,36]

LYMPHOCELE

The lymphocele is a pocket of lymph fluid resulting from some type of trauma to the lymph vessels within the pelvis. A fibrous reaction occurs to this leaking lymph fluid, resulting in the mass-effect seen with this

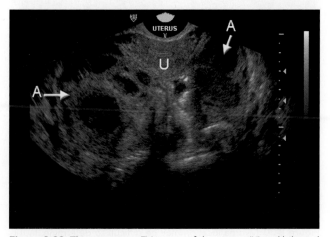

Figure 8-22 This transverse EV image of the uterus (*U*) and bilateral abscesses (*A*) demonstrates the complex appearance seen with this infectious process. (Images courtesy of Philips Medical Systems, Bothell, WA.)

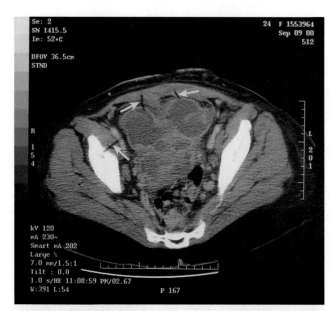

Figure 8-23 Postcesarean delivery abscess. CT scan showing multi-loculated abscesses anteriorly and low in the pelvis in the region of uterine incision.

process. This common complication of renal transplantation occurs in about 12%[36] of cases.

The sonographic appearance of the lymphocele mimics other pelvic masses with its septated, well-defined appearance. Differential diagnosis for the mass, which indents the bladder, include a uroma, hematoma, or abscess (Fig. 8-24). Many different masses share sonographic appearances, as demonstrated by Figure 8-25.

Treatment

To relieve symptoms of a large lymphocele, the clinician may drain it via surgery or an abdominal puncture (percutaneous) or perform a marsupialization procedure.[38]

APPENDICITIS

Appendicitis in both its forms, acute and chronic, may result in an abscess. Usually because of fecolith obstruction of the lumen or lymphoid hypertrophy, this process may also mimic cecal cancer,[30,39] ovarian masses, Crohn's disease, or diverticulitis.[40] This common inflammatory process becomes difficult to diagnose because of the lack of specific physical and laboratory findings. The most common finding is right lower quadrant pain at McBurney's point. To find this area, simply draw a line between the umbilicus and the anterior superior iliac spine (ASIS) and locate McBurney's point 5 cm (2 in) back toward the umbilicus.[36] This is also the area to check for rebound tenderness.

Imaging Findings

Sonography

Sonographic imaging of the appendix has a characteristic appearance of bowel. The three layers of bowel image well, especially in the infected appendix. To image

the appendix, begin by selecting the lowest frequency that allows visualization, usually a 5 to 12 MHz transducer with the focal zone at the appendix depth.[36,40] Pressure applied abdominally (graded compression) during the exam allows for localization of the pain and moves bowel out of the field of interest. When imaged, the appendix appears as a bull's-eye structure on the transverse plane lateral to the iliac vessels and anterior/medial to the psoas muscle.

It is often difficult to image the normal appendix with sonography due to patient habitus, bowel gas, or the location of the appendix. If seen, the appendix collapses with compression due to the normal wall thickness. The inflamed appendix has thick walls, often imaged as hypoechoic, due to edema, preventing collapse. Measurements of the appendix add to the diagnosis of inflammation. The normal appendix measures less than 6 mm from outer edge to outer edge.[36,40] Increased color or power Doppler indicates the characteristic hyperemia seen with an infectious process.[36,40] If the appendix ruptures, the only finding may be thickened bowel, loculations, abscess, phlegmon, fluid, and prominent fat surrounding the cecum and appendix (Fig. 8-26).[40]

Radiography

Radiographs demonstrate ureteral displacement changes in the psoas muscle margin, abnormal masses, air within the abdomen, and a nonfilling appendix during the barium enema examination.[30]

Computed Tomography

CT is another method to diagnose appendicitis and the resultant abscess.[30] The gravid patient presenting with complaints of right lower quadrant pain presents a challenge for the sonographer. The growing uterus displaces the appendix out of the pelvis, making the determination of location—much less diagnosis—difficult

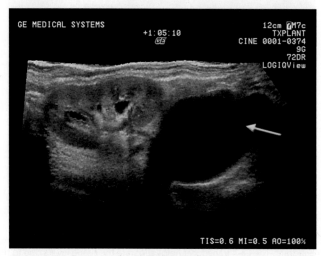

Figure 8-24 Posttransplant lymphocele formation results in an anechoic mass (*arrow*) extending into the pelvis. (Sonographic image courtesy of GE Healthcare, Wauwatosa, WI.)

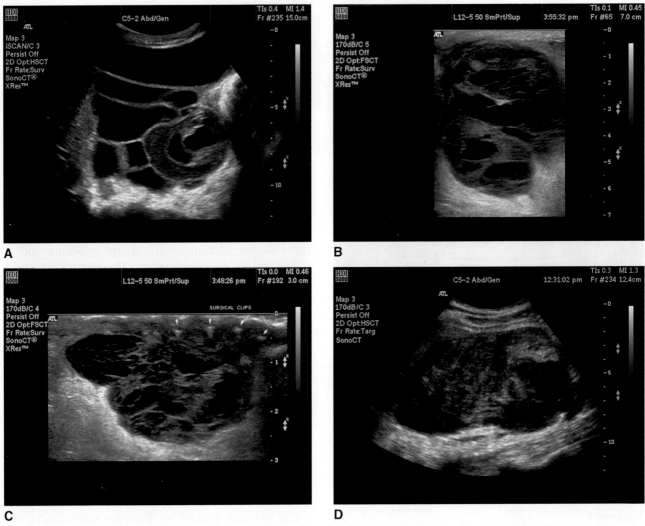

Figure 8-25 A: This image demonstrates the appearance of loculated complex ascites. **B:** An abscess found at an incision site. **C:** Postsurgical seroma. **D:** An abdominal wall sarcoma. (Images courtesy of Philips Medical Systems, Bothell, WA.)

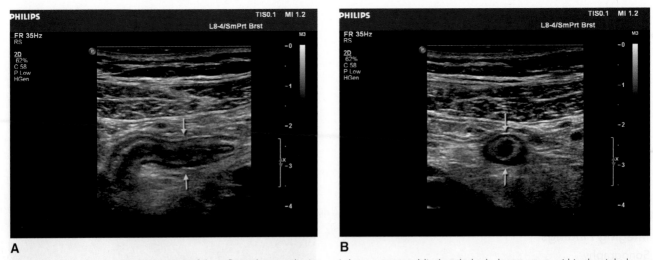

Figure 8-26 A: The longitudinal image of the inflamed appendix *(arrows)* demonstrates a blind-ended tubular structure within the right lower quadrant. The L8-4 transducer helps separate the tissue layers due to the increased image detail found with the higher frequency transducer. This increase in quality had to be balanced with the decrease in penetration seen at this frequency. **B:** This transverse image of the same appendix illustrates the characteristic "bull's-eye" appearance of inflamed bowel. (Images courtesy of Philips Medical Systems, Bothell, WA.)

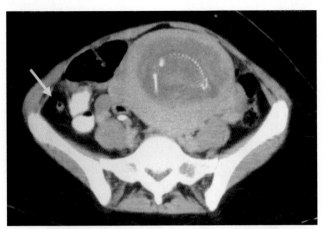

Figure 8-27 CT scan of a woman in the 18th week of gestation presenting with a 12-hour history of right-sided abdominal pain. Abdominal examination on presentation revealed significant tenderness and, after a nondiagnostic ultrasound, a laparotomy is considered for presumed appendicitis. A CT scan is obtained instead, revealing a normal, air-filled appendix with no sign of periappendiceal inflammation (arrow). The laparotomy was postponed, and 12 hours later, the patient aborted a septic fetus. An unnecessary laparotomy for an atypical presentation of chorioamnionitis was avoided by the judicious use of the CT scan. (Courtesy of Dr. David Weiss, Chestnut Hill Hospital, University of Pennsylvania Health System, Chestnut Hill, PA.)

with ultrasound.[41,42] In the case of nonvisualization by sonography, CT becomes the modality of choice because of the high incidence of perforation, preterm labor, and fetal loss in this patient population.[42] The cecum demonstrates a focal mass indention (Fig. 8-27).[41]

Treatment

Surgery is the treatment of choice.

THE VAGINA

GARTNER'S DUCT CYST

Gartner's duct cysts are usually asymptomatic and are most commonly discovered on routine pelvic examinations. These cysts may be single or multiple and are a common lesion of the vagina. They are a remnant of the mesonephric duct, an embryonic urogenital structure.[43] They rarely cause symptoms but, if large, they may cause pressure symptoms and dyspareunia. When symptomatic, they often originate high in the vagina adjacent to the cervix and extend into the labia at the vaginal opening.

Imaging Findings

Sonography

Sonography is helpful in delineating the location of the cyst in the anterolateral vaginal wall. The lesion appears as an anechoic or complex mass, with well-defined margins and good sound transmission (Fig. 8-28).

Computed Tomography

CT, like ultrasound, shows a thin-walled cyst with defined borders that does not enhance. MRI helps with diagnosis through the location and cystic appearance

---

PATHOLOGY BOX 8-4

Extrauterine Pelvic Masses[10,35,36,39,40]

Mass	Cause	Sonographic Appearance
Abscess	Infectious process	Complex mass, dirty shadowing due to gas bubbles, loculations, fluid in pericolic gutters
Hematoma	Surgery, trauma	Varies on age of hematoma. Initial stages complex with mobile particles, solid as the blood consolidates, returning to complex with solid/anechoic areas
Lymphocele	Renal transplant, trauma, lymph node dissection	Septate, well-defined mass, may appear complex, located lateral to the bladder
Urinoma	Renal transplant, trauma, obstructing lesion	Anechoic cyst located in close proximity of the transplanted kidney, consisting of urine encapsulated by a fibrous capsule. Displacement of pelvic organs
Seroma	Surgery, trauma	Complex mass at the surgical site
Appendicitis	Fecolith, obstruction, bacterial infection, pelvic abscess	Noncompressible bull's-eye structure on the transverse plane at McBurney's point, blind-ended tubular structure greater than 6 mm, free fluid
Bowel neoplasm	Infectious process (Crohn's disease), cancer, obstruction	Mimics complex adnexal mass, target sign of bowel, echogenic central echo due to gas, hypoechoic wall
Pelvic kidney	Renal failure	Similar appearance to the native kidney usually located in the left iliac fossa.
Diverticula of the bladder	Congenital or acquired	Anechoic outpouching of the bladder wall, may image the connecting neck, may mimic an ovarian cyst, changes shape/size with voiding
Ureteral dilatation	Obstruction	Mimic ovarian cyst on transverse view; however, rotation elongates the ureter

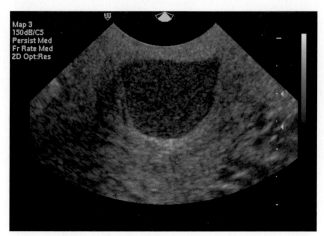

Figure 8-28 This EV image demonstrates a Gartner's duct cyst. The complex appearance is most likely due to protein in the fluid. (Image courtesy of Philips Medical Systems, Bothell, WA.)

of the vaginal mass. The Gartner's duct cyst displays a high signal intensity because of the protein found within the cyst fluid (Fig. 8-29).[44]

Treatment

Asymptomatic Gartner's duct cysts require no follow-up. If they become symptomatic, drainage or removal relieves symptoms.[44]

IMAGING THE VAGINAL CUFF POSTHYSTERECTOMY

The pelvic examination in posthysterectomy patients demonstrates the vaginal cuff. Anterior-to-posterior (AP) measurements of the vaginal cuff should not exceed 2.1 cm.[3] Enlargement may be due to a mass, cancer, or radiation induced fibrosis. The vaginal length varies depending on which level the surgeon uses during the hysterectomy (Fig. 8-30).[45]

THE FALLOPIAN TUBES

The normal fallopian tubes are narrow and are not routinely seen with the transabdominal approach unless surrounded by fluid.[46] Endovaginally, a combination of the fallopian tube and the suspensory ligament may be seen in a short-axis view and frequently may assist in locating the ovary. This normal structure is easier to see with EV sonography when surrounded by fluid. Benign disease of the fallopian tubes is restricted to pelvic inflammatory processes.

INFLAMMATORY PROCESSES

Inflammatory processes in the pelvis include pelvic inflammatory disease (PID; pyosalpinx and tubo-ovarian abscess) and nongynecologic abscesses. PID is associated primarily with gynecologic infections

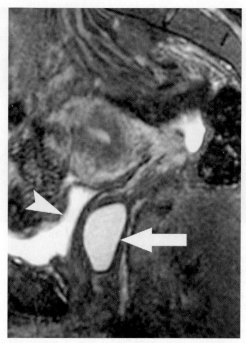

Figure 8-29 Gartner's duct cyst. Midline sagittal fat-suppressed T2-weighted image of female pelvis shows high-signal intensity simple cystic lesion *(arrow)* posterior to bladder *(arrowhead)*. (Courtesy of Timothy G. Sanders, MD.)

and intrauterine contraceptive devices. A complete discussion of PID is presented in Chapter 11. Patients with pelvic abscesses present with fever, pain, and elevated WBC count.

A variety of sonographic patterns can be displayed by pelvic abscesses. Such collections usually demonstrate good through-transmission and may have irregular borders, internal septa, debris levels, and air. Gas within an abscess produces bright echoes and may shadow.

Pyosalpinx may appear sonographically similar to hydrosalpinx, but usually, there are low-level internal echoes representing pus. Visualization of the

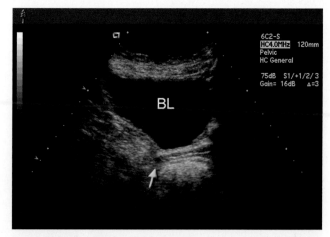

Figure 8-30 Transabdominal image of a posthysterectomy patient. The vaginal cuff *(arrow)* images posterior to the bladder *(BL)*.

ovary at one wall of the abscess raises suspicion for a tubo-ovarian abscess.

The differential diagnosis for a pelvic abscess includes hematoma, endometrioma, ectopic pregnancy, necrotic gynecologic tumor, and abscess of nongynecologic origin (e.g., diverticular abscess, periappendiceal abscess, Crohn's disease, psoas abscess, postsurgical abscess). Because many of these entities have similar sonographic patterns, a complete patient history is critical for distinguishing which disease process has most likely been demonstrated.[35]

HYDROSALPINX

Hydrosalpinx is a fluid collection in a scarred or blocked fallopian tube. Usually secondary to pyosalpinx, it evolves when the purulent material is replaced by serous fluid. This appearance suggests a chronic or old infection.[47] Frequently, patients have no acute symptoms and the hydrosalpinx is discovered endovaginally as an incidental finding.

Sonographically, hydrosalpinx appears as a tubular, tortuous, fluid-filled mass with smooth, well-defined walls.[10] Hydrosalpinx can be unilateral or bilateral, and the tube may become quite large. The distinguishing sonographic characteristic of a hydrosalpinx is that the proximal end of the fusiform fluid-filled structure tapers as the tube enters the cornual region of the uterus. This fluid collection may mimic sonographically an adnexal cyst or surrounding bowel. However, the lack of peristalsis helps to differentiate this entity from bowel. Bladder diverticulum, urachal cyst, and mesenteric cyst are some of the nongynecologic entities that can also appear as fluid-filled pelvic masses (Fig. 8-31).

THE OVARIES

BENIGN CYSTS

Most fluid-filled pelvic masses originate in the ovary. The sonographic criteria for simple cysts are (1) smooth, well-defined borders, (2) absence of internal echoes, and (3) increased posterior acoustic enhancement (Fig. 8-32).[10] Thick, irregular walls or thick septations (>3 mm) may be associated with inflammation, endometriosis, or malignancy. Adnexal masses containing extremely echogenic foci may be benign cystic teratomas. Adnexal masses that are of homogeneously increased echogenicity tend to be solid masses, hemorrhage, or endometriomas. A list of benign cystic masses of the adnexa is presented in Table 8-2.

Ovarian cysts may be visualized sonographically in women of all reproductive stages, including pregnancy. Cysts measuring less than 3 cm in greatest diameter usually regress spontaneously and represent follicles and physiologically normal functioning of the ovary.[48] Careful sonographic evaluation to detect septa or solid components is recommended for any ovarian cyst, especially those measuring more than 5 cm in greatest dimension. Up to 60% of cysts with thin septa and no solid components have been reported to regress spontaneously, usually within 3 months. Even cysts that appear simple by sonographic criteria rarely resolve if they measure more than 10 cm in greatest diameter. Cysts of this size have a greater potential to be malignant or invasive, and thus are usually removed. Cysts detected during pregnancy that measure more than 8 cm in diameter traditionally have been removed during the second trimester because of the risk of increased complications during pregnancy or delivery and may represent a malignancy.

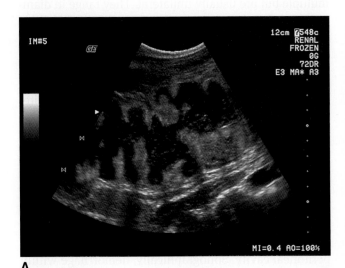

A

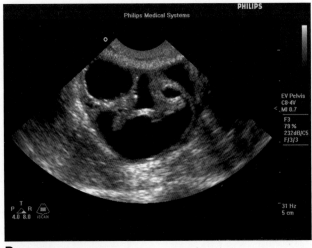

B

Figure 8-31 Inflamed large bowel due to colitis **(A)** could be mistaken for hydrosalpinx **(B)**; however, the bowel demonstrates peristalsis and internal rugae that are not seen in the fallopian tube. (Image **A** courtesy of GE Healthcare, Wauwatosa, WI. Image **B** courtesy of Philips Medical Systems, Bothell, WA.)

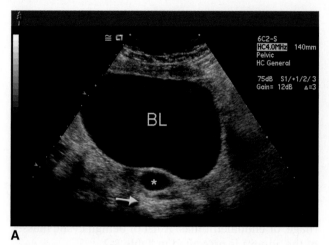
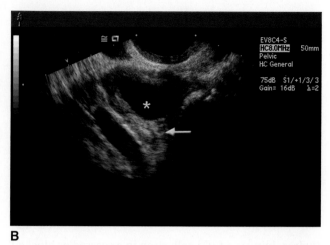

A   B

Figure 8-32 A: A transabdominal sagittal image of a follicular cyst *(star)* posterior to the full bladder *(BL)*. Notice the posterior enhancement *(arrow)*. **B:** EV image of the same patient with the follicular cyst *(star)* and minimal posterior enhancement *(arrow)*.

FUNCTIONAL CYSTS

Functional or physiologic cysts of the ovary include ovarian follicles, follicular cysts, corpus luteum cysts, and theca lutein cysts.[10] Ovarian follicles are visualized as anechoic structures in the ovary. Ultrasound images follicles as small as 5 mm. Approximately 10 days before ovulation, the ovaries contain many small follicles. Not all of the follicles mature to the point of ovulation. A single follicle usually becomes dominant, measuring 2 to 2.5 cm in greatest dimension.[10] During the mid-portion of the menstrual cycle, a release of luteinizing hormone (LH) leads to ovulation with follicular rupture and conversion into a corpus luteum.[10] If conception occurs, the corpus luteum continues to produce progesterone until approximately the 11th or 12th week of pregnancy, when the placenta takes over production of progesterone. If conception does not occur, the corpus luteum usually regresses within 2 weeks of ovulation.

Complementary imaging modalities, such as CT and MRI, often image normal physiologic changes in the female pelvis. Sonographers often are asked to confirm a functional cyst seen on these modalities (Fig. 8-33). Often, as in the case of the functional cyst, this finding often resolves by the time a sonographic examination occurs.

Follicular Cysts

Follicular cysts result from either nonrupture of the dominant mature follicle or failure of an immature follicle to undergo the normal process of atresia, with absence of follicular fluid reabsorption. They may be multiple but are usually unilateral. They range in diameter from 3 to 10 cm, averaging 2 cm.[49] Solitary follicular cysts are common and may occur from fetal life to menopause. Most patients with physiologic cysts experience no symptoms because these cysts usually regress spontaneously.

Sonographically, follicular cysts meet the criteria for a simple cyst, as described earlier. In general, any simple ovarian cyst measuring less than 5 cm in greatest dimension in an ovulating woman should be reevaluated sonographically, 6 to 8 weeks later. A change in the size or appearance or complete resolution of the cyst usually is seen. In some cases, patients with follicular cysts present with mild to severe pelvic pain. The cyst may become symptomatic, with the occurrence of hemorrhage, torsion, or rupture into the peritoneal cavity. Sonographically, hemorrhage within the cyst will appear variable in its echo pattern. In the case of a ruptured cyst, changes in the appearance of the cyst may be associated with free fluid in the cul-de-sac.

TABLE 8-2
Benign Cystic Masses of the Adnexa

Physiologic or Functional
Ovarian follicles
Follicular cysts
Corpus luteum cysts
Theca lutein cysts (hyperreactio luteinalis)
Surface inclusion cysts
Miscellaneous
Paraovarian cysts
Peritoneal inclusion cysts
Hemorrhagic cysts
Endometriomas
Hydrosalpinx
Paratubal cysts
Polycystic ovary
Inflammatory processes

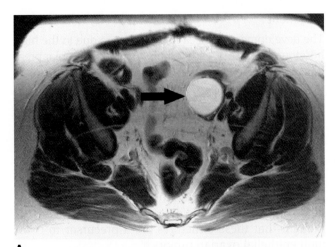

A

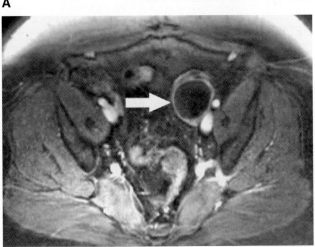

B

Figure 8-33 Functional ovarian cyst. **A:** Axial T2-weighted image of female pelvis shows simple-appearing left ovarian cyst *(arrow)*. **B:** No internal enhancement of cyst *(arrow)* is present on fat-suppressed T1-weighted image.

Corpus Luteum Cysts

Failure of absorption of the follicular cyst often results in a corpus luteum cysts.[48] The corpora lutea forms from the graafian follicle within hours of ovulation. As the dominant follicle ruptures, the corpora lutea develops. The corpora lutea measures 1.5 to 2.5 cm and may appear hypoechoic and possess irregular or thick borders around a central anechoic area. Because of their variable appearance, these cysts have been called "the great pretender." These cysts are routinely visualized with the EV approach but frequently are not seen with the transabdominal approach. Corpora lutea are not considered to be corpus

PATHOLOGY BOX 8-5

Functional Cyst Sonographic Appearance

- Anechoic
- Thin-walled
- Posterior enhancement

luteum cysts unless their size is at least 3 cm in diameter. This cyst results from intracystic hemorrhage[48] resulting in the sonographic appearance of low-level echoes or a fluid-debris level within the cyst. Most patients present with acute pain of less than 24 hours' duration, though one-fourth of patients have pain for a duration of 1 to 7 days. Corpus luteum cysts usually are unilocular and unilateral and measure 6 to 8 cm, with an average diameter of 4 cm. Unless torsion occurs, no treatment is required,[49] and regression occurs after two to three menstrual cycles. Rupture results in fluid in the cul-de-sac and elsewhere in the abdomen. Hemorrhage and rupture frequently cause increased symptoms.

Should fertilization take place, a corpus luteum cyst of pregnancy may result. In Figure 8-39, a corpus luteum cyst of pregnancy and a gravid uterus are demonstrated on a single sonographic image. During pregnancy, corpus luteum cysts typically reach a maximum size of 3 cm, but can enlarge up to 5 to 10 cm. They usually resolve by the 16th week of gestation. At any point during this time, hemorrhage or rupture can occur, causing pelvic pain and posing a threat to both mother and fetus.

Color or power Doppler imaging of the cyst demonstrates flow in the periphery of the cyst often called the "ring of fire." Spectral Doppler tracings show a low resistance flow pattern with prominent diastolic flow (Fig. 8-34).[48]

Treatment

Corpus luteal cysts require no treatment.

Theca Lutein Cysts

Theca lutein cysts (a.k.a., *hyperreactio luteinalis*) are the largest of the functional cysts and may range in size from 3 to 20 cm. Theca lutein cysts represent an exaggerated corpus luteum response in patients with high levels of human chorionic gonadotropin (hCG), the hormone produced during pregnancy.[10,48] Theca lutein cysts are associated with gestational trophoblastic

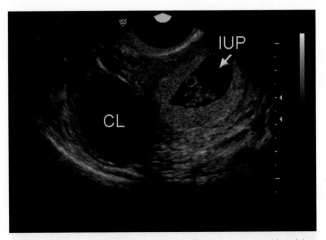

Figure 8-34 Corpus luteum cyst *(CL)* of pregnancy visualized lateral to the uterus containing an intrauterine pregnancy *(IUP)*. (Image courtesy of Philips Medical Systems, Bothell, WA.)

PATHOLOGY BOX 8-6

Corpus Luteum Cyst

Signs and Symptoms	Sonographic Appearance
Pain Nausea Vomiting Enlarged tender ovary	Complex appearance if hemorrhage present Gravid patient • Thin-walled • Unilateral • Possible posterior cul-de-sac fluid with rupture

diseases such as hydatidiform mole, chorioadenoma destruens, and choriocarcinoma. Theca lutein cysts may also be seen with ovarian hyperstimulation syndrome, a complication of infertility drug therapy.[10] In rare instances, theca lutein cysts are seen with a normal singleton or multiple gestations.

Theca lutein cysts are usually treated conservatively because they involute when the source of gonadotropin is removed, though they may persist for several months after trophoblastic evacuation. In some patients, the cysts persist long after the hCG levels are no longer detectable. On occasion, theca lutein cysts, like other functional cysts, may undergo hemorrhage, torsion, or rupture, causing the patient pain.[10,48] Surgery may be necessary if they become very large or in the event of intraperitoneal rupture or hemorrhage.

Sonographically, theca lutein cysts are multilocular, thin-walled, large, bilateral, fluid-filled masses (Fig. 8-35).[10,48] Bilateral development is thought to be a response to hormonal stimulation. Because of their association with gestational trophoblastic disease, it is important to evaluate the uterus carefully when theca lutein cysts are seen. A good patient history also is helpful in evaluating the cause of theca lutein cysts.

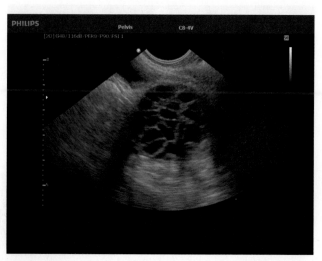

Figure 8-35 The hyperstimulated ovary contains multiple theca lutein cysts. (Image courtesy of Philips Medical Systems, Bothell, WA.)

Treatment

The development of theca-luteal cysts are due to the high hormone levels seen with fertility treatment or molar pregnancies. Once levels return to normal, these cysts resolve.

Surface Epithelial Inclusion Cysts

The peripherally located surface epithelial inclusion cyst occurs most often in postmenopausal women; however, these occur at any age.[10] These structures, which occur on the periphery of the ovary, are due to cortical invaginations of the surface epithelium.[10,50] Diagnosis of these tiny, unilocular, thin-walled cysts is made through the detection of psammoma bodies. It is thought that these structures are a precursor to common epithelial ovarian tumors.[50]

HEMORRHAGIC CYSTS

Bleeding into a cyst, whether functional or corpus luteal, results in an acute case of pelvic pain.[10] Sonographically, fresh blood appears anechoic, progresses subacutely to a mixed echogenicity, and finally becomes anechoic again. In the late acute phase, the cyst appears hyperechoic because of the hemorrhage mimicking a solid mass. Differentiators from an ovarian mass include posterior enhancement, a smooth posterior wall, and lack of color flow within the area.[10,48] Debris may be seen in the posterior portion of a hemorrhagic cyst. Follow-up ultrasound examinations often allow monitoring of clot lysis and forming septations. As the clot retracts, a solid fluid level or fluid mass complex often images. Care must be taken, as a hemorrhagic cyst has similar sonographic features to an ectopic pregnancy or a tubal infection (Fig. 8-36).[10,48,49]

Treatment

Cysts with suspected hemorrhage can be followed to ensure resolution. If the mass fails to resolve or decrease in size, other neoplastic processes become suspect. These complex masses may result in torsion and treatment because of the vascular occlusion. These complex masses may result in torsion and **require** treatment due to the vascular occlusion.

TORSION

Partial or complete rotation of the ovary with an adnexal cyst or mass at the ovarian pedicle results in the sudden onset of pain.[10,46] Although torsion may occur with normal ovaries, most reported cases have involved children with ovarian masses or women younger than 30 years of age.[10,46] The hyperstimulated ovary,[46] and those patients with congenital anomalies of the tube or mesosalpinx,[51] have an increased risk of twisting. There is also an increased incidence of torsion with a previous history.[48] Although there is an increased incidence in pregnant patients[10]; in a nonpregnant patient with an acute onset of pelvic pain, with or without a mass on the physical exam,

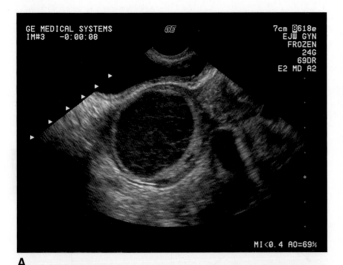

A

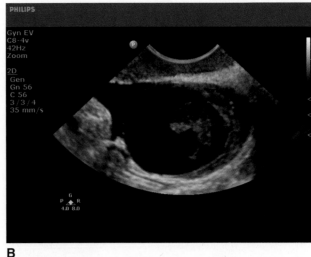

B

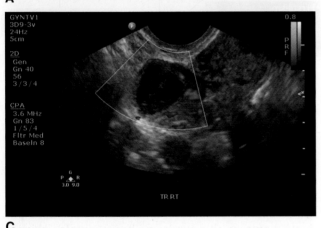

C

Figure 8-36 A: Organized hemorrhagic cyst within the right ovary. **B:** As the cyst ages, the hemorrhage begins to liquefy. **C:** Color power angio confirms the lack of flow within this hemorrhagic cyst. (Image **A** courtesy of GE Healthcare, Wauwatosa, WI. Images **B** and **C** courtesy of Philips Medical Systems, Bothell, WA.)

the primary diagnosis includes hemorrhage and torsion.

Torsion of the adnexa is usually unilateral; however, there is a slightly higher incidence of right-sided occurrence, which is thought to be due to the space occupied by the bowel.[10,48,51] The clinical presentation is recurrent or acute onset of localized pain and tenderness, nausea, vomiting, and a palpable pelvic mass.[10] Because of this occlusive process, varying degrees of circulatory obstruction, to include the lymphatics, occur.[46] The result is edema and infarction and, in the worst case, development of gangrene, explaining the imaging findings.

Imaging Findings
Sonography

Nonspecific findings (cystic, solid, or complex mass with or without pelvic fluid, thickening of the cyst wall, hemorrhage) on ultrasound make a diagnosis of ovarian torsion difficult. Even with this difficulty, ultrasound is the primary diagnostic tool for ovarian torsion.[52,53] If the torsion is incomplete and intermittent, the ovary may enlarge with edema to greater than 4 cm.[48] The most characteristic finding is a large ovary[52] that loses the characteristic almond shape, becoming round or globular.[46] Areas of decreased and increased echogenicity,

representing hemorrhage, infarct, or necrosis, image on the ovary.[48] The torsed ovary of the adolescent woman results in unilateral enlargement and multiple peripherally located cystic structures.[46] Multifollicular enlargement is thought to result from fluid transudation into follicles because of the ovarian congestion caused by circulatory impairment.[10] Intraperitoneal fluid may be present secondary to obstruction of venous and lymphatic return, resulting in a transudate from the capsule of the ovary.[10] If the whole vascular pedicle twists, a hypoechoic round structure with concentric hypoechoic stripes images, referred to as the target appearance. The development of an ellipsoid or tubular structure with heterogeneous internal echo pattern may also image.[10]

Doppler flow studies (spectral, color, and power) may help in diagnosis of torsion, as three-quarters of cases result in the absence of arterial flow and, in over 90% of cases, there is either a decrease or absence of venous flow.[52] Ovarian torsion results in the partial or complete obstruction of blood flow because of this twisting.[10,48] The absence of flow within one ovary, and the confirmation of flow in the contralateral, raises suspicion for this mechanical process. In the case of intermittent torsion and collateral flow from the uterine artery branches, Doppler studies may not be helpful.[53] Doppler evaluation may be useful in determining whether the ovary is

PATHOLOGY BOX 8-7

Ovarian Torsion

Signs and Symptoms	Sonographic Appearance
Sudden onset of severe pelvic pain	Ovarian enlargement
	Loss of normal ovarian shape
Nausea	Hyperechoic ovary
Vomiting	Heterogeneous texture
Palpable adnexal mass	Dilated vessels on the periphery of the ovary
	Doppler may demonstrate absence or decreased blood flow
	Posterior cul-de-sac fluid

receiving blood, because torsion initially involves the ovarian vein, but it may progress to involve the ovarian artery as well.[10,48] It is important to note if the flow has a central or peripheral pattern, as ovarian viability increases with central flow.[52] The presence of coiled, twisted, or circular vessels (whirlpool sign) within the affected adnexa is another sonographic sign of torsion.[10,31,48]

Computed Tomography and MRI

CT and MRI share imaging features of ovarian torsion. These mimic the sonographic findings of a large ovary, fallopian tube thickening, peripheral cystic structures, and free fluid. Because of the global nature of these imaging modalities, a global view of the pelvis allows for detection of uterine deviation toward the affected side.[52,53]

Treatment

The usual course of treatment is an adnexectomy; however, there has been some success with untwisting the vascular pedicle restoring flow to the affected ovary.[52] In postmenopausal women, an oophorectomy is the treatment of choice.[52]

POLYCYSTIC OVARY SYNDROME

Polycystic ovary syndrome (PCOS) is the most common androgen disorder and is associated with obesity, amenorrhea, anovulation, hirsutism, and infertility.[54,55] Originally described by Stein and Leventhal—hence the name, Stein-Leventhal syndrome—the disorder is characterized by four criteria: infertility, obesity, oligomenorrhea, and hirsutism.[48] The problem with the initial classification is the wide variety of findings—both physical and metabolic—that women with this syndrome exhibit. The Rotterdam criteria established in 2003 uses the trilogy of oligoanovulation, hyperandrogenism and/or hyperandrogenemia, and the exclusion of related disorders as a diagnostic criteria for PCOS.[54,55]

Anovulation is thought to result from the unusually thick pseudocapsule surrounding the ovaries[56] and

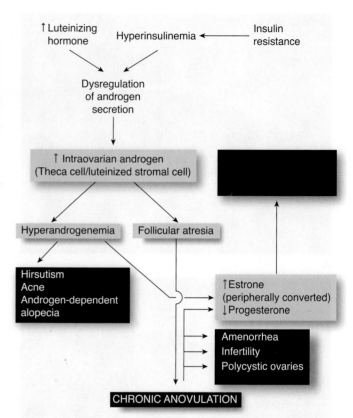

Figure 8-37 Pathogenesis of the PCOS.

the associated endocrine abnormalities in these patients; however, this syndrome has a complex physiologic process (Fig. 8-37). The abnormal estrogen and androgen production results in an imbalance between LH and follicle-stimulating hormone (FSH) blood serum levels.[10,48,56] In PCOS, the low FSH and high LH results in an elevated LH/FSH ratio.[10,48,55] The result of the chronic stimulation of the ovarian stroma is an increase in the production of androgens, which converts into estrogens.[56] The estrogen increases the LH while depressing the FSH secretion.[56] This type of hormone cycle results in an anovulatory cycle with the outcome of endometrial hyperplasia and infertility problems.[56]

The clinical presentation varies greatly with the degree and duration of the hormone imbalance and any coexisting syndromes or diseases (Table 8-3).[48] The most common clinical and imaging finding is that of bilateral large ovaries (Fig. 8-38). Because certain adrenal tumors can also cause oligomenorrhea or amenorrhea and infertility, adrenal tumor should be considered in the clinical differential diagnosis of these patients.

Imaging Findings

Sonography

The sonographic appearance of the ovaries in patients with polycystic ovary disease varies widely and is considered the gold standard for diagnosis of PCOS.[54] In

TABLE 8-3		
Syndromes or Disease Entities that Have Been Associated with Polycystic Ovaries		
HYPERANDROGENISM WITHOUT INSULIN RESISTANCE		
Steroidogenic enzyme deficiencies		
Congenital adrenal hyperplasia		
Aromatase deficiency		
Androgen-secreting tumors		
Ovarian		
Adrenal		
Exogenous androgens		
Anabolic steroids		
Transsexual hormone replacement		
Other		
Acne		
Idiopathic hirsutism		
HYPERANDROGENISM AND INSULIN RESISTANCE		
Congenital		
Type A syndrome		
Type B syndrome		
Leprechaunism		
Lipoatrophic diabetes		
Rabson-Mendenhall syndrome		
PCOS		
Acquired		
Cushing's syndrome		
INSULIN RESISTANCE		
Glycogen storage disease		
Type 2 diabetes mellitus		
OTHER		
Central nervous system lesions		
Trauma/lesions		
Hyperprolactinemia		
Nonhormonal medications		
Valproate		
Hereditary angioedema		
Bulimia		
Idiopathic (includes normoandrogenic women with cyclic menses)		

From: Legro RS, Azziz R. Androgen Excess Disorders. In: *Danforth's Obstetrics and Gynecology.* 10th ed. Philadelphia, PA: Lippincott Williams & Wilkins; 2003.

classic cases, the ovaries are enlarged bilaterally and contain multiple, small peripheral cysts sometimes referred to as a "string of pearls"[54] or "black pearl necklace"[55] sign (Fig. 8-39). The cysts (12 or more) may range in diameter from 2 to 9 mm, resulting in an

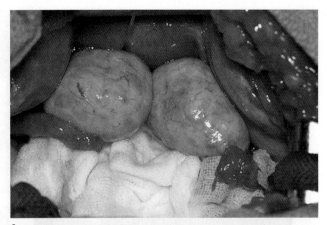

A

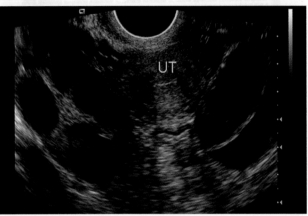

B

Figure 8-38 A: The ovaries in a woman with PCOS at laparotomy. Note the large size of the ovaries relative to the uterus, with a smooth ovarian capsule without evidence of ovulatory events. **B:** Transverse EV image of bilateral polycystic ovaries. *UT*, uterus. (Image courtesy of Siemens Healthcare, Mountain View, CA.)

ovarian volume of greater than 10 cm.[3,54] Because they can be quite small, often only the echogenic linear wall may be visualized. The cysts may be subcapsular or randomly distributed throughout the parenchyma of the ovary. Up to a third of pelvic sonograms performed on patients with the clinical findings of PCOS reveal sonographically normal ovaries.[10] Bright stromal echogenicity is the most common finding with PCOS.[48,54]

3D ultrasound may become helpful in the diagnosis of PCOS because of the ability to perform volumes. The ability to display the ovary on three planes, performing the volume from this display, allows for increased accuracy of the volume measurement.[57]

Studies performed to determine the use of color and spectral Doppler measurements found that the uterine artery had a higher pulsatility index (PI) in patients with PCOS. The resistance index (RI) suggested increased resistance with a lower value.[57]

Women with true polycystic ovary disease may have no clinical manifestations; however, the cysts

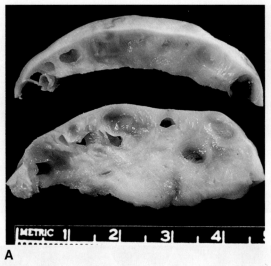
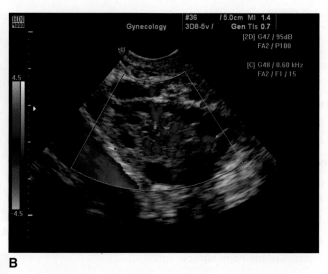

A B

Figure 8-39 A: Cut sections of an ovary show numerous cysts embedded in a sclerotic stroma. **B:** A sonographic image demonstrating the peripherally located cysts with color flow Doppler active. (Image courtesy of Philips Medical Systems, Bothell, WA.)

are always bilateral. The sonographic appearance of polycystic ovaries may also be seen in women being treated with FSHs or in newborn girls whose ovaries are responding to maternal hormones.[44] A history of PCOS increases the risk of cardiovascular disease[57] and endometrial and breast cancers because of the high levels of estrogen levels found with this syndrome.[10,48]

MRI

MRI becomes helpful in patients that have biochemical markers for PCOS that do not demonstrate the typical cystic/stromal ovarian pattern on the sonographic examination.[58] MRI of the patient with PCOS reveals slightly enlarged ovaries with small peripherally located cysts and a central area of low signal intensity.[56,59] Hypertrophy of the ovarian stroma results in the low signal intensity seen in the central portion of the ovary.[58] The use of the contrast agent gadolinium results in stromal enhancement, confirming increased vascularization of the ovary.[57] As with sonography, MRI findings alone are nonspecific to PCOS and must be viewed as part of the diagnostic workup.[56,57]

PATHOLOGY BOX 8-8

Polycystic Ovary Syndrome

Signs and Symptoms	Sonographic Appearance
Amenorrhea	Bilateral ovarian enlargement
Hirsutism	Multiple, small peripheral cysts
Infertility	
Oligoanovulation	Ovarian volume of greater than 10 cm³
Hyperandrogenism	
Hyperandrogenemia	

Treatment

The regulation of the complex androgenic imbalance is the first step in resolving PCOS. In the patient wishing to become pregnant, ovarian ablation treatments such as surgical destruction of the ovarian stroma through the use of ovarian drilling or resection has shown some promise.[55]

BENIGN NEOPLASMS

Eighty percent of all ovarian tumors are benign. Benign ovarian neoplasms may be categorized as germ cell tumors, epithelial tumors, or stromal tumors, depending on the ovarian tissue elements and derivation of these tumors. The most common benign adnexal neoplasms are benign cystic teratomas (germ cell tumor) and cystadenomas (epithelial tumors). Stromal tumors include fibroma and theca. Benign neoplasms are summarized in Table 8-4.

Koonings and associates performed a retrospective study spanning 10 years (encompassing real-time sonography) evaluating 861 surgically confirmed cases of ovarian neoplasm.[49] In their series, cystic teratoma was the most prevalent neoplasm, accounting for 44% of all ovarian tumors (Table 8-5). Twenty-eight percent of the neoplasms measured less than 6 cm, 53% ranged from 6 to 11 cm, whereas 19% were larger than 11 cm. In premenopausal women, 75% of the tumors were benign, whereas 25% were benign in postmenopausal women (Table 8-6).

BENIGN CYSTIC TERATOMA

Benign cystic teratomas are the most common germ cell tumor of the pelvis.[10,48,60] They are also the most frequently seen ovarian tumor in women younger than age 20 years arising from germ cells found in the

TABLE 8-4

Benign Ovarian Neoplasms

Lesions	Ages Affected	Signs and Symptoms	Laterality	Sonographic Characteristics
GERM CELL TUMORS				
Mature (Cystic) Teratoma (Dermoid)	Any age; usually reproductive or younger	Mild to acute abdominal pain Palpable adnexal mass/fullness Pressure on bladder and/or bowel	15% Bilateral	Cystic to complex Fluid/solid or fluid/fat levels Calcification with shadowing Echogenic foci Floating hair strands
EPITHELIAL TUMORS				
Serous cystadenoma	20s to 50s	Pelvic pressure, bloating, acute onset of pain, palpable pelvic mass	25% Bilateral	Unilocular or multilocular Cystic with low-level debris Thin smooth walled Possible septae and papillary projections
Mucinous cystadenoma	20s to 50s	Same as serous cystadenoma	5% Bilateral	Multiseptate tumor Large Variable fluid echogenicity Regular wall thickness and appearance Ascites Fixation to surrounding structures
Brenner tumor	Any age, usually around 50 y	Usually asymptomatic	6.5% Bilateral	Solid; hypoechoic, may exhibit acoustic enhancement; ranges in size from microscopic to 8 cm in diameter
STROMAL TUMORS				
Theca cell tumor a.k.a. theca, fibrothecoma	Common among menopausal or postmenopausal women, but age distribution ranges from 15 to 86 y	Similar to GCT if hormonally active	Usually unilateral, but multiple in 10% of cases	Hypoechoic; attenuates sound, which can produce distal acoustic shadow; measures 5–16 cm in diameter, Meigs' syndrome, Large ovaries Calcifications Cystic degeneration
Granulosa cell tumors (GCTs)	Any age	Prepubertal: precocious pseudopuberty Premenopausal: oligomenorrhea, menorrhagia, increasing abdominal girth Post menopausal: bleeding, breast tenderness	Unilateral	Up to 12 cm, solid to complex, isoechoic to slightly hypoechoic and heterogeneous, low-level internal echoes, multiloculated if torsed
Gonadoblastoma	20s	Primary amenorrhea, virilization, abnormal development of genitalia	33% Bilateral	Soft tissue density, calcifications
Sertoli-Leydig cell tumor	30 y	Masculinization Cushing's syndrome, oligomenorrhea followed by amenorrhea, acne, breast atrophy, hirsutism, voice deepening, temporal balding, clitoral enlargement, abdominal swelling, pain	Unilateral	Echogenic mass or hypoechoic mass

TABLE 8-5

Incidence of Benign Ovarian Neoplasms

Type	Occurrence
Cystic teratoma	58%
Serous cystadenoma	25%
Mucinous cystadenoma	12%
Benign stromal	4%
Brenner tumor	1%

(Modified from Koonings PP, Campbell K, Mishell DR, et al. Relative frequency of primary ovarian neoplasms: a 10-year review. *Obstet Gynecol.* 1989;84:921. Reprinted with permission from The American College of Obstetricians and Gynecologists.)

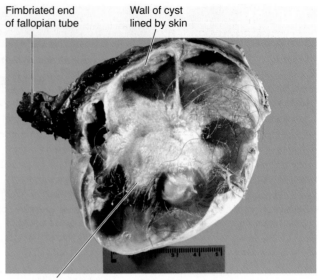

Fimbriated end of fallopian tube

Wall of cyst lined by skin

Mass of hair and sebaceous material

Figure 8-40 Benign ovarian cystic teratoma (teratoma cyst). Note hair and sebaceous material.

embryonic yolk sac.[60] Although teratomas may occur in any age group, they are most often seen during the second to fourth decades.[54,60] The terms "dermoid tumor" and "teratoma" are often used interchangeably, though teratomas contain tissue of all three germ layers (ectoderm, mesoderm, endoderm),[48] whereas dermoids are composed of ectodermal tissue only.[10] Pathology specimens of teratomas include teeth, hair, and glandular tissues (sweat, apocrine, sebaceous). Neural and thyroid tissue (stroma ovarii)[48,54] have also been seen on histopathologic examination (Fig. 8-40). The malignant potential of a teratoma is related inversely to its tissue maturity, but malignant change rarely occurs (~1%) in benign cystic teratomas.[10,48]

Although patients with teratomas usually have no symptoms, they may present with pain, pelvic pressure, or a palpable mass.[10] Teratoma pedicles may twist, but they rarely rupture, because of their thick capsules. Teratomas are often first detected with a bimanual pelvic examination. Teratomas containing high fat content may cause the ovary to be located superior to the uterine fundus. They are bilateral in approximately 10% to 15% of patients.[48] Benign cystic teratomas are associated with torsion[10,52,53] because of the mobility of the tumor,[60] which may result in rupture and the development of peritonitis.[61]

TABLE 8-6

Ovarian Neoplasms (861 Cases)

Type	Occurrence
Premenopausal	85% (13% malignant)
Postmenopausal	25% (45% malignant)
Benign	85%
Malignant	21%
Low malignant potential	4%

(Modified from Koonings PP, Campbell K, Mishell DR, et al. Relative frequency of primary ovarian neoplasms: a 10-year review. *Obstet Gynecol.* 1989;84:921. Reprinted with permission from The American College of Obstetricians and Gynecologists.)

Two processes, the mature and immature cystic teratomas, share some findings and symptomology; however, they are different types of masses. First, the mature teratoma is a benign process, whereas the immature teratomas is a malignancy. The immature teratoma contains the same three germinal layers in addition to embryonic tissue. This is the most common malignant tumor occurring in women before the age of 30,[60] with half demonstrating an elevated alpha fetoprotein.[48] Histology shows both mature and immature components within some teratomas, requiring grading of the tumor by the amount of each type of tissue.[60] A third type of dermoid, the monodermal teratomas, consists of one type of tissue. This is the case with struma ovarii, which is a mass which consists of thyroid tissue.[52,54]

Imaging Findings

Sonography

There is a wide spectrum of sonographic appearances to teratomas, including a predominantly cystic mass, a complex mass with calcifications, fat-fluid level within a complex mass, and a diffusely echogenic mass without shadowing.[10] Most commonly, teratomas appear sonographically as complex masses that are predominantly solid, containing echogenic foci that represent calcium or fat with or without acoustic shadowing. This type of teratoma is the most difficult to detect because the sonographic appearance mimics that of bowel gas. An echogenic nodule within a cystic mass is called a *dermoid plug*[10,48] or *Rokitansky nodule*,[54] which may contain teeth, hair, or fat. Occasionally, the "tip of the iceberg" sign is demonstrated; this refers to a very echogenic anterior component with a posterior shadow, which prevents visualization of the more posterior aspect of the mass.[10,48] When a fat-fluid level is identified, the fluid component is seen in the more dependent position,

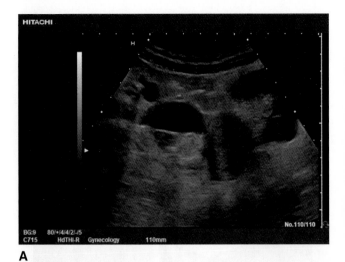

A

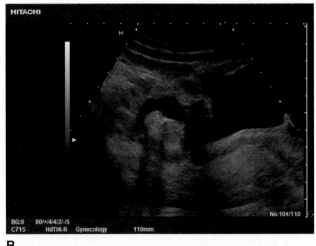

B

Figure 8-41 A: This image demonstrates the fluid/solid level commonly imaged with a teratomas. **B:** Posterior shadowing within the mass indicates areas of increased density within the mass. (Image courtesy of Hitachi.)

whereas the echodense fat floats on top of the fluid. The sonographic appearance of a teratoma varies according to its elemental components—skin, hair, teeth, bone, fat. Strands of hair may be seen floating in fluid and is a specific sign of the teratomas called the *dermoid mesh*.[10] With the presence of significant bone and teeth components, echogenic foci with distal shadowing should be demonstrated on ultrasound examination (Fig. 8-41).

Care while imaging the suspected teratomas must be taken, as other processes mimic this pathology. The resolving hemorrhagic cyst[10] or endometrioma[48,54] may have mural nodules during resolution; however, the posterior enhancement differentiates this mass from the shadowing teratomas. The pedunculated leiomyoma and perforated appendiceal feoclith has a simular sonographic appearance to the teratoma.[10,48] Nonperistalsing bowel may also mimic the teratoma.[54]

Sonographic Imaging Tips

Decubitus positioning during transabdominal imaging may aid in demonstrating fat-fluid or fluid-debris levels, because shifting should occur when different parts of the mass are dependent. Palpating the mass with the free hand may also produce movement at the fat-fluid interface. Water enemas may help differentiate a teratoma from bowel due to microbubbles, providing a sonographic contrast that helps to distinguish rectum from pelvic masses.

Radiography

A pelvic radiograph may show fat, teeth, or bony components of teratomas. Before the advent of EV imaging, diagnosis of a teratoma was made through radiographic findings. The patient presenting with acute abdominal pain with findings of osseous masses or teeth within the pelvis raised suspicion for a teratoma (Figs. 8-42A and 8-43).[60]

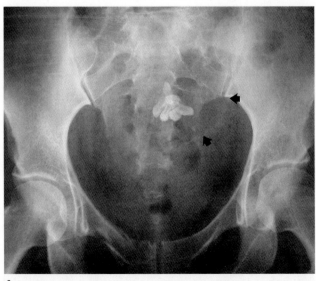

A

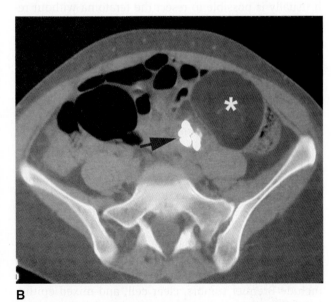

B

Figure 8-42 Ovarian teratoma tumor (teratoma). **A:** Detailed view of the pelvis shows a lucent mass *(arrows)* on the left containing malformed teeth. **B:** CT image shows the tumor with varying fatty *(star)* and dental *(arrow)* components.

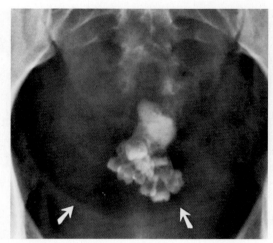

Figure 8-43 Teratoma cyst containing multiple well-formed teeth. Note the relative lucency of the mass (*arrows*), which is composed largely of fatty tissue.

Computed Tomography and MRI

CT and MRI also display some characteristic findings of benign cystic teratoma. Fat has a characteristic appearance on CT, and CT can demonstrate fat-fluid or fluid-debris levels in these tumors.[62] CT of the cystic mass with a dermoid plug identifies the sonographically anechoic sebum that fills the mass (Fig. 8-42B).[10]

Benign cystic teratomas with high fat content have been demonstrated with MRI: the fat component in the tumors gives very high signal intensity on T1-weighted images. MRI becomes especially helpful in the pregnant patient or with an uncertain diagnosis with other complementary imaging modalities (Fig. 8-44).[60]

Treatment

Surgical removal of benign cystic teratomas is usually indicated. In the younger patient, an ovarian cystectomy helps preserve unaffected ovarian tissue and fertility.[60] It usually is possible to resect the teratoma without removing the entire ovary through the performance of a laparotomy procedure (Fig. 8-45).[60]

EPITHELIAL TUMORS

The membranous epithelium is a tissue layer that covers the external portions of organs and the body cavities. Epithelial neoplasms occur in multiple locations to include the liver, lung, salivary glands, fallopian tubes, and the ovary. The common finding with these tumors is the histologic features of the spindle-shaped columnar cells.[63] This section focuses on the benign ovarian form of serous cystadenoma and mucinous cystadenoma that arise from the surface epithelium of the ovary.[10] Their malignant counterparts are serous cystadenocarcinoma and mucinous cystadenocarcinoma. Less common benign epithelial tumors include Brenner tumors, clear cell, and mixed epithelial tumors.[10]

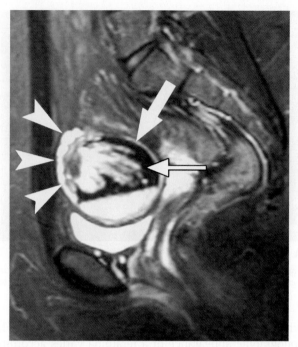

Figure 8-44 Mature cystic teratoma. Sagittal fat-suppressed T2-weighted image of female pelvis demonstrates heterogeneous mass (*arrow*) with high signal intensity follicles (*arrowheads*) draped around it, confirming ovarian origin of mass. Low signal component of mass (*thin arrow*) represents fatty component on this fat-suppressed sequence.

Cystadenomas

A cystadenoma is a benign tumor originating in glandular tissue. Secretions from these epithelial-lined tumors are either serous or mucinous and occur in the salivary gland, pancreas, or the ovaries. The most common type of benign cystic ovarian tumor is a cystadenoma, representing approximately a quarter of all ovarian neoplasms.[10,54] In general, cystadenomas may grow very large[48] and are seen in postmenopausal women, though they are occasionally encountered in women of childbearing ages.[10] As their names suggest,

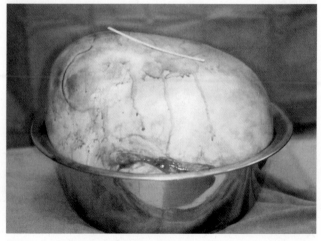

Figure 8-45 Removal of a large cystic teratoma.

serous cystadenomas contain thin, serous fluid and mucinous cystadenomas contain thicker mucin. Serous cystadenomas are more common than mucinous cystadenomas and more frequently malignant. They are usually unilocular and may be bilateral in 25% of cases.[48,54] Serous cystadenomas, the malignant counterpart to the serous cystadenoma, may contain very thin septations, and, on occasion, papillary projections (Fig. 8-46).

Mucinous cystadenomas, the largest of the ovarian cysts, are bilateral less than 5%[10,54] of the time and grow larger than the serous cystadenoma (up to 50 cm),[10,54] with multiple prominent septations and debris.[4,37] The age of occurrence ranges from the second to fifth decades.[54] It may be possible to differentiate serous from mucinous cystadenomas based on the echogenicity of fluid. It is difficult to differentiate sonographically between benign and malignant forms of cystadenoma, so it is important to look for secondary signs of malignancy, such as ascites or fixation of the mass. Histopathologic analysis is required for a definitive diagnosis (Fig. 8-47).

Patients with either a serous or mucinous cystadenoma complain of pelvic pressure, bloating, and possibly an acute onset of pain upon rupture.[48] Because of the large size of these tumors, the clinical exam may reveal a palpable pelvic mass.[54]

Imaging Findings

Sonography

The serous cystadenoma has a unilocular or multilocular appearance during the sonographic examination.[10] Though the neoplasm is usually unilateral, they can occur bilaterally.[48] This mass, which ranges from 5 to 15 cm may exhibit papillary projections from the cyst wall (Fig. 8-48).[10,48,54]

The mucinous cystadenoma is usually a unilateral neoplasm, which upon rupture results in abdominal ascites called *pseudomyxoma peritonei*.[10] This fluid images with bright pinpoint echoes, whereas the mass itself has thick, irregular walls and septations.[48] Because of the common sonographic findings between these neoplasms, it is difficult, if not impossible, to render a diagnosis from images (Fig. 8-49).[45]

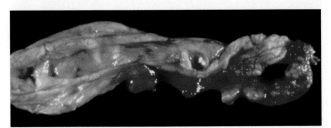

Figure 8-46 Serous cystadenoma of the ovary. This unilocular cyst has a smooth lining, microscopically resembling the fallopian tube epithelium.

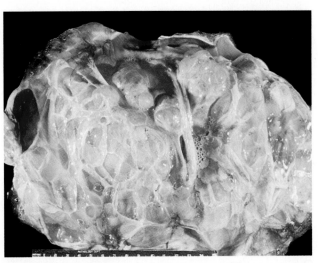

Figure 8-47 Mucinous cystadenoma of the ovary. The tumor is characterized by numerous cysts filled with thick, viscous fluid.

Computed Tomography and MRI

The CT and MRI examinations of a cystadenoma have similar findings as the sonographic exam. The cyst may appear large (macrocystic) or very small (microcystic) resulting in a characteristic honeycomb appearance.[64] The thin walls may or may not contain punctuate intracystic calcifications.[64,65] Cyst walls are thin, with some lobulations commonly without mural nodules.[64] Another feature, the *central scar*, is an area of fibrous scarring surrounded by cysts[66] that is found in up to half of masses (Figs. 8-48C and 8-50).[67]

Treatment

In the patient of childbearing age, an ovarian cystectomy is the best choice, whereas the postmenopausal patient would have a unilateral salpingo-oophorectomy.[54] If the tumors are bilateral, a total hysterectomy is a consideration.[54] In the case of a confirmed mucinous cystadenoma of the ovary, there is an increased risk of an appendiceal mucinous tumor.[54] This often results in the concurrent removal of the appendix.[54]

Brenner Tumors

The transitional cell is a type of epithelial tissue that stretches, such as in the cyst wall, changing shape from cuboidal to squamous with distention. These cells are found not only in the ovary but in the bladder, ureters, and the prostate. In the ovary, the Brenner or transitional cell tumors are an uncommon solid tumor arising from the ovarian surface epithelium.[10] They account for approximately 2%[10,48,54] of all ovarian neoplasms. Brenner tumors can be seen in any age group but usually are found in women in the fifth to seventh decades of life[48,54] who are asymptomatic or present with a palpable pelvic mass, pain, and abnormal uterine bleeding.[54] The tumors are bilateral in 6.5%[48] of cases and range in size from microscopic to 30 cm[54] in diameter. Brenner

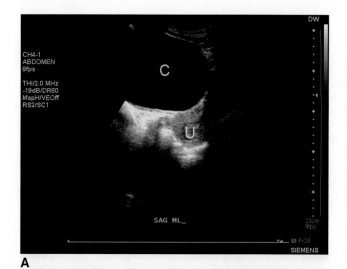

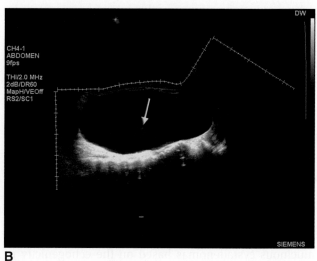

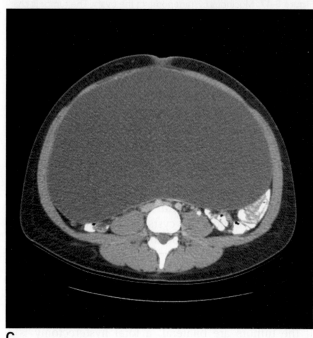

Figure 8-48 A: A large serous cystadenoma extends out of the pelvis. *C*, cyst; *U*, uterus. **B:** Panoramic image of the same cyst. Note the artifact *(arrow)* seen in the central portion of the cystic structure. **C:** Axial CT image of the same structure. (Images courtesy of Derry Imaging Center, Derry, NH. Robin Davies, Ann Smith, and Denise Raney.)

tumors often are diagnosed histopathologically as incidental findings in specimens removed for associated pelvic disease, usually a serous or mucinous cystadenoma (Fig. 8-51).[10,54] Malignant changes in Brenner tumors are rare. Malignant forms of this tumor usually are large, fluid-filled masses.

Imaging Findings

Sonography

The usual sonographic presentation is a solid[54] hypoechoic[10] mass that may contain wall calcifications.[10,48] Contours of the mass may show a slightly lobulated appearance.[54] Imaging of small cystic spaces increases suspicion of a coexisting cystadenoma.[10] Because of the fibrous stroma composition, a Brenner tumor images similar to a leiomyoma, fibroma, or theca, both sonographically[10,46,48] and hystologically.[10]

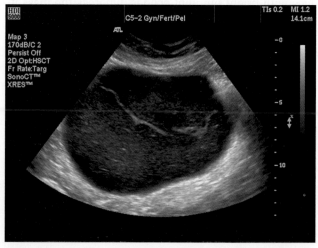

Figure 8-49 This transabdomal image acquired with a C5-2 transducer demonstrates characteristics of a mucinous cystadenoma. (Image courtesy of Philips Medical Systems, Bothell, WA.)

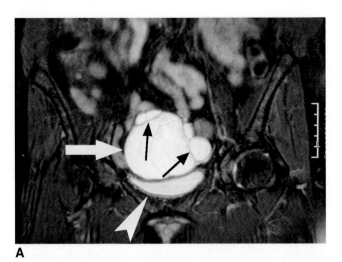

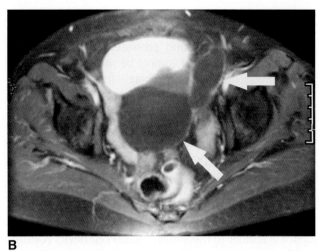

Figure 8-50 Serous ovarian cystadenoma. **A:** Coronal fat-suppressed T2-weighted image shows cystic mass *(arrow)* superior to bladder *(arrowhead)*. A few septa are present *(thin arrows)*. **B:** Axial fat-suppressed, gadolinium-enhanced T1-weighted image demonstrates walls of mass *(arrows)* to be thin and without enhancing nodules. Mass was benign at surgery.

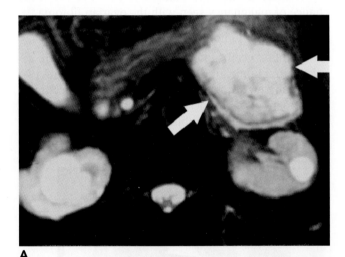

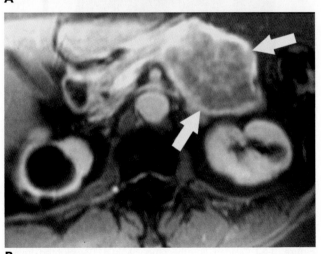

Figure 8-51 Mucinous cystadenoma. **A:** Axial, heavily T2-weighted, fat-suppressed image demonstrates a complex cystic mass *(arrows)* in tail of pancreas. **B:** Fat-suppressed, gadolinium-enhanced gradient echo image shows faint enhancement of internal architecture of mass *(arrows)*.

Computed Tomography and MRI

As with ultrasound, CT and MRI findings are relatively nonspecific. The modalities demonstrate solid masses. CT detects possible calcifications found in the mass, whereas the low-signal T2-weighted MRI results in a mass finding with a low signal intensity similar to the ovarian fibroma.

Treatment

Resection of the tumor, which may involve a partial or total hysterectomy, is the usual treatment for the Brenner tumor.[54]

Ovarian Sex Cord-Stromal Tumors

The World Health Organization (WHO) classifies the granulosa cell and the thecoma-fibroma tumor as a granulosa stromal cell tumor. These tumors arise for the embryonic gonad or ovarian stroma.[10] Classification of these benign stromal tumors, as well as Sertoli-Leydig cell tumors (also referred to as androblastomas and arrhenoblastomas), is achieved through the use of cellular typing, as they often share symptomology and physical and imaging findings. For example, fibromas, thecomas, Sertoli-Leydig cell tumors, and Brenner tumors are all sonographically hypoechoic or echogenic adnexal masses individually indistinguishable from benign or malignant tumors of the ovary.[46,60,68] Differential diagnosis between these ovarian tumors and uterine myomas may be made by establishing, if possible, the ovarian origin of the mass.[60]

Granulosa Stromal Cell Tumors

Theca Cell Tumor/Thecomas

Thecomas, sometimes called fibrothecomas, are estrogen-producing, solid ovarian masses that account for 1% to 2%[10,60] of ovarian tumors that arise from the ovarian stroma.[10] Estrogen production is responsible for the presenting complaint of abnormal uterine bleeding, pelvic pain, abdominal distention, and pressure.[60] Adenocarcinoma often accompanies these tumors because of the high estrogen production.[60] Thecomas are usually unilateral and may measure up to 20 cm in diameter.[60] They occur most frequently in menopausal, postmenopausal[10] and, rarely, in women younger than 35 years.[60] Although they are not considered malignant, they may become invasive. Increased estrogen production may place the patient at greater risk for endometrial cancer.[60]

A fibroma is very similar to the theca; however, it differs in that there is no hormone production.[60] Meigs' syndrome (see subsequently), size, treatment, and incidence is similar to thecomas.[60] Basal cell nevus (Gorlin) syndrome patients have a higher incidence of fibroma development, resulting in bilateral, calcified ovarian neoplasms developing in the third decade.[10,60,68]

Imaging Findings

Sonography

The theca images as a solid, hypoechoic mass, possibly with cystic changes and calcifications.[10,60,68] This smooth-contoured mass demonstrates posterior shadowing because of attenuation by the dense fibrous tissue composing the neoplasm.[10,48,68] Occasionally, the large ovary may appear edematous as a result of torsion of the pedicle due to the weight of the theca.[10,48] The theca becomes indistinguishable from a pedunculated leiomyoma because of the similar appearance of a solid, round or oval, smooth contoured mass with regular echogenicity.[46]

Computed Tomography and MRI

The CT appearance of the theca becomes dependent on the presence or absence of torsion. In the contrast study, the theca images as a well-defined solid homogeneous or heterogeneous mass with delayed enhancement.[68,69] The degree of enhancement varies dependent on the tumor composition with the homogeneous tumor enhancing more than the heterogeneous tumor.[69]

During the MRI exam, delayed weak enhancement occurs in the normal ovary because of the highly vascularized theca cells. As the fibrotic tissue content varies in the theca, so does the degree of enhancement seen during the MRI exam.[70] Imaging of the smaller homogeneous solid fibroma results in a low-intensity T1 and T2 signal. This signal intensity is due to the fibrous tissue found in the smaller fibroma.[68,70] Large fibromas display a high signal intensity because of edema or cystic degeneration of the mass (Fig. 8-52).[70,71]

Treatment

Age is the main determination for patient treatment with a total hysterectomy and bilateral oophorectomy in the menopausal or postmenopausal patient. For the patient wishing to retain fertility, ovarian cystectomy or salpingo-oophorectomy are the procedures of choice.[60,68] Removal

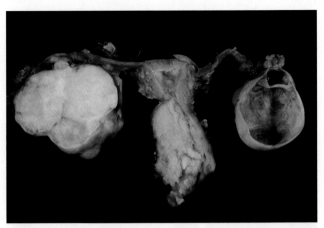

Figure 8-52 This TAH-BSO specimen is demonstrated in standard anatomic position, with the right adnexa on the left side of the image. The right ovary is replaced by a Brenner tumor, the left ovary by a mucinous cystadenoma. The cervical tumor is a nonkeratinizing squamous carcinoma.

of the mass is the only method to rule out the small chance of malignancy seen with the ovarian fibroma.[68]

Granulosa Cell Tumors

All granulosa cell tumors (GCTs) secrete estrogen, resulting in feminization of the patient.[48,70] There are two types, adult and juvenile type, with most occurring in women of reproductive or postmenopausal age.[10] Composed of cells resembling the graafian follicle, half

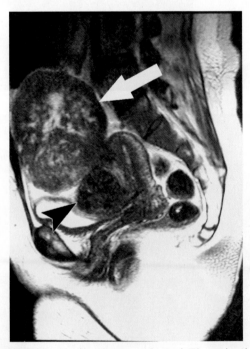

Figure 8-53 Ovarian fibrothecoma. Sagittal T2-weighted image through the pelvis of a perimenopausal woman shows a large, predominately low signal–intensity mass (arrow) adjacent to the uterus with some internal areas of high signal intensity. The ovaries could not be identified. Uterine fibroids were also present (arrowhead). This mass was initially mistaken for a subserosal leiomyoma.

of all cases are found in menopausal women, with the other half found in reproductive (45%) and adolescent women.[48] This low malignancy potential tumor makes up 1% to 2% of ovarian neoplasms[11,46]; however, up to 15% of patients develop endometrial carcinoma because of the high estrogen levels.[10]

Juvenile GCTs occur in women up to 30 years of age. This ovarian neoplasm has associations with Ollier's disease, Maffucci's syndrome, and abnormal karyotypes in the younger patient.[60]

Symptoms depend on the age of onset, with the younger patient presenting with isosexual precocious puberty, pain, increasing abdominal girth, and the older woman with tender breasts and abnormal vaginal bleeding.[10,48,60,70] As with any solid tumor, torsion results in pain and rupture of the tumor. Pseudo-Meigs' syndrome may also occur.[48]

Imaging Findings

Sonography

In the adult, these unilateral tumors can become quite large (average 10 to 12 cm[48,60]) and vary in appearance. Smaller masses appear solid to complex because of hemorrhage or fibrosis.[10,48] The tumors vary in presentation from isoechoic to slightly hypoechoic and heterogeneous.[72] Low-level internal echoes image similar to an endometrioma or cystadenoma.[48] In the presence of torsion, the mass becomes multiloculated with blood or fluid contents.[48] Endometrial hyperplasia or polyps occur because of the high estrogen levels.[48,60,71]

In a small study, color flow Doppler was found to be consistent with benign findings of peripheral flow indicative of a borderline malignant mass.[72] Cystic liver masses may be an indication of liver metastasis from a malignant form of the GCT.[10]

Computed Tomography and MRI

Imaging features of the germ cell tumor correlate well between CT, MRI, and sonography.[72] CT demonstrate multiloculated cystic lesions with fibrotic, infarct, necrosis, and hemorrhagic changes.[71,72] One benefit of CT or MRI over sonography is the ability to image any peritoneal seeding or hemoperitoneum.[71] MRI has the added benefit of imaging any endometrial or uterine enlargement that is the result of the high estrogen levels.[72,73]

Treatment

Treatment of young women for this type of tumor includes removal of the affected ovary and tube. Staging of the tumor determines any potential for malignancy. A bilateral salpingo-oophorectomy with a hysterectomy in the postmenopausal patient eliminates late malignant behavior in the following 10 to 20 years.[60] Patients wishing to preserve fertility may undergo removal of the ovary or tumor. Adjunct chemotherapy is another step that helps prevent the chance of malignant spread.[60]

Gonadoblastoma

The gonadoblastoma is a rare tumor found in either males or females and is composed of sex cord cells and stromal elements arising from dysplastic gonads. The karyotypes that result in a male pseudohermaphrodite have the highest incidence of this tumor with a four to one ratio between the male and female phenotypes.[60] Approximately half contain dysgerminoma cellular patterns and about a third of cases are bilateral.[60,74] Other tumors associated with the gonadoblastoma include the yolk sac tumor, embryonal carcinoma, and choriocarcinoma.[60]

Symptoms in these patients include primary amenorrhea, virilization, and abnormal development of genitalia. Gonadoblastoma is frequently detected in the second decade of life.[60]

Imaging Findings

The sonographic examination reveals a soft tissue density and the diagnosis is made through histologic analysis[75] Size ranges up to 8 cm in size demonstrating areas of calcification.[60] Radiography may image any calcifications. The larger field of view seen with an MRI exam allows for tumor localization in the patient with gonadal dysgenesis and dysmorphic gonads.[75]

Treatment

Bilateral gonadectomy is the treatment of choice with gonadal dysgenesis because of the increased risk of developing a gonadoblastoma.[60] Prognosis and treatment upon development of this tumor depends on the presence of any associated tumors, such as embryonal carcinoma or choriocarcinoma.[60]

Sertoli-Leydig Cell Tumors

These unilateral tumors have several names: the Sertoli-Leydig cell tumor, Sertoli-stromal cell tumors, arrhenoblastoma, or androblastoma.[34,48,60,71] These account for less than 0.5% of tumors. Patients present with pain or abdominal swelling, and one-third suffer masculinization effects from elevated androgen levels.[34,48] This tumor is also associated with Cushing's syndrome.[71] Most cases occur in women approximately 30 years of age.[34,48,60] Occasionally, these tumors relate to increased estrogen production and may be malignant in up to 20% of patients.[10,60]

Patients present with oligomenorrhea followed by amenorrhea, acne, atrophy of the breasts, hirsutism, voice deepening, temporal balding, and clitoral enlargement. Abdominal swelling and pain in patients without the endocrine symptoms occur in some patients partially due to the large size (12 to 15 cm) of the mass.[60]

Imaging Findings

These nonspecific solid ovarian neoplasms image on the sonogram as echogenic or hypoechoic masses.[48] Areas of necrosis or hemorrhage may image.[60] On the

MRI exam, the tumor images as a hyperintense mass on the T1-weighted image.[71]

Treatment

Treatment for these tumors, as with any other, becomes dependent on the composition. The patient with a tumor limited to the affected ovary who wishes to preserve fertility could do well with removal of the affected tube and ovary. In the postmenopausal patient, a total hysterectomy and bilateral salpingo-oophorectomy is the procedure of choice.[60]

A Note about Meigs' Syndrome

The triad of ascites, pleural effusion, and an ovarian neoplasm often is referred to as Meigs' syndrome.[76,77] This mass may be a fibroma, theca, or granulosa tumor.[76] This rare clinical sequelae has several iterations dependent on the disease process. Pseudo-Meigs' syndrome has the same clinical findings; however, the cell types originally described by Meigs' are absent. Ovarian tumors found with pseudo-Meigs' include fallopian tube, uterine, mature teratomas, struma ovarii, and ovarian leiomyomas.[76-78] Upon removal of the tumor, the pleural effusion and ascites resolve.[76]

Yet another variation, pseudo-pseudo Meigs' syndrome, is the result of enlarged ovaries, ascites, and pleural effusion in a patient with systemic lupus erythematosus. Ovaries in this patient population measure large without the accompanying masses seen with either Meigs' or pseudo-Meigs' syndromes.[76]

OVARIAN REMNANT SYNDROME

A complication of prior bilateral salpingo-oophorectomy is the ovarian remnant syndrome. In this syndrome, postoperative remnants of ovarian tissue become functional.[10] Women can present with chronic pelvic pain, a mass, or both.[10,32] This occurs most frequently in patients who have undergone pelvic exploration because of severe endometriosis.[32] Ovarian remnant syndrome can also develop in patients who had severe adhesions where dissection of the ovary may have been difficult. Sonographically, solid tissue similar in echogenicity to ovarian tissue visualizes with or without accompanying cysts.[10,48]

MISCELLANEOUS

Paraovarian and Paratubal Cysts

Paraovarian or paratubal cysts develop from vestigial wolffian duct structures or arise from the tubal epithelium. The paraovarium is located in the mesosalpinx, the portion of broad ligament between the fallopian tube and the hilum of the ovary.[46] These cysts represent 10% of all adnexal masses and occur over a wide range of ages.[48] They are seen most commonly in the third and fourth decades of life and range in size from 1.5 to 19 cm. Paraovarian cysts are difficult to distinguish from other ovarian lesions by physical or ultrasound examination. Most symptomatic patients present with menstrual irregularities, increased lower abdominal girth, and pain if the cyst is large. Some small cysts remain asymptomatic and are found incidentally on ultrasound examination or at surgery.

Sonographically, paraovarian cysts appear thin walled, unilocular, and free of internal echoes. They arise from the adnexa and not the ovary, but this may not be a simple ultrasound diagnosis.[46] Because they do not respond to cyclic changes, their size does not change in relation to the menstrual cycle.[48] On occasion, a paraovarian cyst may be recognized when a cyst is noted to be separate from an intact ovary and the fallopian tube is draped or stretched over the cyst. With the EV technique, the sonographer may be able more easily to establish the separation of the paratubal mass from the ovary. As with other cystic masses, hemorrhage, torsion, and rupture alter the sonographic appearance.

Peritoneal Inclusion Cysts

Fluid-filled masses resulting from accumulations of serous fluid between adhesions or layers of peritoneum may be seen sonographically, usually in patients with a history of pelvic adhesions or surgery.[48] These collections are referred to as *peritoneal inclusion cysts*. Noted almost exclusively in premenopausal women, affected patients present with pelvic pain or mass.[48] The patient histories includes previous surgery (frequently multiple operations), endometriosis, or a history of PID.[48]

Peritoneal inclusion cysts are usually contiguous with the adnexa and may distort the appearance of the ovaries by displacing them. EV sonography often reveals multiple septations within fluid surrounding an intact ovary, reminiscent of "a spider in a web." When large, these inclusion cysts may be better evaluated with the transabdominal approach. Sohaey and colleagues used color Doppler and pulsed Doppler to reveal relatively low resistive flow in the septations of peritoneal inclusion cysts.

Differential Diagnosis

In the proper clinical setting, it is imperative that ectopic pregnancy and endometriosis be included in the differential diagnosis of the pelvic mass. The sonographic presentation of ectopic pregnancy and endometriosis ranges from predominantly cystic to complex pelvic masses. These entities are discussed in detail in Chapters 11 and 15.

The differential diagnoses for benign cystic and solid ovarian masses are presented in Table 8-7.

TABLE	8-7

Differential Diagnosis for Benign Adnexal Masses

CYSTIC ADNEXAL MASSES
Follicular cyst
Corpus luteum cyst
Paraovarian cyst
Peritoneal inclusion cyst
Hemorrhagic cyst
Hydrosalpinx
Endometrioma
Benign cystic teratoma

PREDOMINANTLY CYSTIC ADNEXAL MASS WITH SEPTATIONS OR DEBRIS
Theca lutein cyst
Hemorrhagic cyst
Cystadenoma
Tubo-ovarian abscess
Ectopic pregnancy
Cystic adnexal mass

SOLID ADNEXAL MASS
Endometrioma
Hemorrhagic cyst
Brenner tumor
Theca
Fibroma

Fluid-filled bowel or abnormal bowel may mimic cystic, complex, or solid adnexal masses. Sonography cannot differentiate between benign and malignant masses, but it can identify tissue characteristics suggestive of benignity or malignancy. Solid adnexal tumors tend to be more malignant, as do cysts with multiple septations or solid mural nodules. Associated ascites, peritoneal implants, or visceral metastases also favor malignancy.

SUMMARY

- Nabothian cysts are a common finding in gynecologic imaging, appearing as a hypoechoic cystic area within the cervix.
- Diagnosis of endometrial hyperplasia is made through measurement of two layers of endometrium equaling 14 mm in premenopausal women, 10 mm in women on tamoxifen, and 8 mm in postmenopausal women.
- Asherman's syndrome images as hyperechoic bands within the uterine cavity and is due to scar development after surgical procedures.

- Rupture of a uterine scar (dehiscence) is a complication occurring in pregnancy after a C/S, myomectomy, or instrument perforation.
- Leiomyomas occur in any area of the cervix or uterus.
- Degenerated leiomyomas may mimic ovarian or uterine pathology.
- Extrauterine infectious process often image similarly to a neoplasm; however, they have additional symptoms of fever, chills, increased WBC, and possible positive bacterial cultures.
- Hematomas and lymphocele can be due to surgical processes such as renal transplants.
- The abnormal appendix measures greater than 6 mm, demonstrates hyperemia with color modes, and may mimic or cause tubo-ovarian abscesses.
- Physiologic ovarian cysts include functional, follicular, corpus luteal, and theca lutein cysts.
- Hemorrhagic cysts have a variable appearance dependent on the stage of resolution.
- Ovarian torsion can result due to a functional cyst, hyperstimulation, or a neoplasm. The sonographic appearance varies on the amount of time the ovary has been torsed.
- PCOS is a complex, androgen-dependent process often resulting in sonographically large ovaries with multiple small cysts located in the periphery of the ovary.
- Tumors containing teeth, hair, glandular tissues, and possibly neural or thyroid tissue are teratomas or dermoid tumors.
- Serous or mucinous material fills the cystadenoma, resulting in low-level pinpoint internal echoes in the large mass during the sonographic exam.
- Brenner tumors image similar to leiomyoma, fibroma, or theca tumors.
- Theca cell tumors, thecomas, and GCT have similar composition with determination of the type through the predominance of the cell type and hormone production of the tumors.
- Gonadoblastomas occur in a karyotypical male pseudohermaphrodite with a female phenotype.
- Sertoli-Leydig cell tumors result in high androgen levels presenting with nonspecific ovarian findings on imaging studies.
- Meigs' syndrome is the triad of an ovarian neoplasm, ascites, and pleural effusion. Originally used to describe findings with a fibroma, additional academic-based categories of pseudo-Meigs' and pseudo-pseudo Meigs' are in use.
- Additional causes of cystic pelvic masses include ovarian remnant syndrome, paraovarian, paratubal, and peritoneal inclusion cysts.

Critical Thinking Questions

1. Sue is a 26-year-old complaining of few and light periods. She has been trying to conceive without success for the last year and has begun a workup for infertility. Initial laboratory findings include an LH/FSH ratio.

   SONOGRAPHIC FINDINGS: Thick endometrium measuring 15 mm on the AP dimension. Bilateral large ovaries demonstrating multiple small peripheral cysts with echogenic central ovarian tissue. The cervix contains two anechoic, smooth-walled areas.

   What do the sonographic findings indicate? Explain the primary cause of the findings.

   ANSWER: Endometrial hyperplasia due to PCOS. The hormone imbalance accompanying PCOS results in the lack of ovulation and thus the development of the characteristic ovarian appearance. This lack of menses also results in the thickened endometrium. Nabothian cysts within the cervix are an incidental finding and of no consequence if the patient is asymptomatic.

2. A 30-year-old patient presents to the sonography department with complaints of intermittent right lower quadrant pain. She has been using over-the-counter pain medication and currently has a pain score of 6. Her clinician found no fever, normal WBC, negative pregnancy test, and a large palpable right ovary. She is G4P3A0 with an LMP 3 weeks ago.

   SONOGRAPHIC FINDINGS: Normal uterus with a secretive phase endometrium. The left ovary is normal in size with a 2-cm hypoechoic area with irregular borders containing low-level echoes. The right adnexa demonstrates a 4-cm cystic mass with an echogenic nodule with posterior shadowing. A structure identified as the right ovary imaged as a hypoechoic structure with striations. The mass and ovary remained connected with patient position, transducer, and external manipulation. Color Doppler imaging of the left ovary demonstrates increased flow in the periphery of the left hypoechoic area. Color and power Doppler of the right adnexa demonstrated a lack of flow in the cystic mass and the ovary.

   Summarize the pertinent clinical and imaging findings, relating them to probable disease differentials. Explain the difference between this case and one with an infectious process.

   ANSWER: The left ovary contains a resolving corpus luteum cyst, which correlates to the secretory phase of the patient's cycle. These findings correlate to the presence of a dermoid/teratoma on the right ovary with intermittent torsion.

   This would not be an infectious process such as appendicitis or PID because of the lack of correlating symptoms such as a fever or an increased WBC. An ectopic pregnancy would also be unlikely, as the pregnancy test is negative.

   To gauge a patient's pain, we use a scale from 1 to 10 with 10 the worst and 1 the least. Though subjective, it is one method to gauge the intensity of pain experienced.

REFERENCES

1. Nabothian follicles. Merck Source Web site. http://www.merncksource.com/pp/us/cns/cns_hl_dorlands_split.jsp?pg=/ppdocs/us/common/dorlands/dorland/three/000041439.htm#000041439. Accessed March 30, 2010.

2. Nabothian cyst. MedlinePlus Web site. http://www.nlm.nih.gov/medlineplus/ency/article/001514.htm. Accessed March 30, 2010.

3. Vander Werff BJ, Hagen Ansert S. Pathology of the uterus. In: *Textbook of Diagnostic Medical Ultrasonography*. Vol 2. 6th ed. St. Louis, MO: Mosby; 2006.

4. Okamoto Y, Tanaka YO, Nishida M, et al. MR imaging of the uterine cervix: imaging-pathologic correlation. *Radiographics*. 2003;23:425–445.

5. Sosnovski V, Barenboim R, Cohen HI, et al. Complex nabothian cysts: a diagnostic dilemma. *Arch Gynecol Obstet*. 2009;279:759–761.

6. Cervical polyps. WebMD Web site. http://women.webmd.com/tc/cervical-polyps-topic-overview. Accessed April, 2010

7. Katz VL, Lentz G, Lobo RA, et al. *Comprehensive Gynecology*. 5th ed. St. Louis, MO: Mosby; 2007.

8. Cervical myomas. Merck Web site. http://www.merck.com/mmhe/sec22/ch262666/ch262666c.html. Accessed April 2010

9. The American Congress of Obstetricians and Gynecologists. Endometrial hyperplasia patient education pamphlet. http://www.acog.org/publications/patient_education/bp147.cfm. Accessed March 30, 2010.

10. Salem S, Wilson SR. Gynecologic ultrasound. In: *Diagnostic Ultrasound*. Vol 1. 3rd ed. St. Louis, MO: Elsevier Mosby; 2005.

11. Weaver J, McHugo JM, Clark TJ. Accuracy of transvaginal ultrasound in diagnosing endometrial pathology in women with post-menopausal bleeding on tamoxifen. *Br J Radiol*. 2005;78(929):394–397.

12. Hosny IA, Elghawabit HS, Mosaad MM. The role of 2D, 3D ultrasound and color Doppler in the diagnosis of benign and malignant endometrial lesions. *J Egypt Natl Canc Inst*. 2007;19(4):275–281.

13. The American Congress of Obstetricians and Gynecologists (ACOG). Endometrial hyperplasia. Patient Education Pamplet Web site. http://www.acog.org/publications/patient_education/bp147.cfm . Accessed April 2010.

14. Chundnoff SG. Endometrial hyperplasia. *Medscape Ob/Gyn & Women's Health*. 2005;10(1). http://www.medscape.com/viewarticle/507187?rss. Accessed April 2010.

15. Williams RS. Hysteroscopic surgery. In: *Danforth's Obstetrics and Gynecology*. 10th ed. Philadelphia, PA: Lippincott Williams & Wilkins; 2003.

16. Yasmin H, Nasir A, Noorani KJ. Hystroscopic management of Ashermans syndrome. *J Pak Med Assoc.* 2007;57(11): 553–555.

17. Baramki TA. Hysterosalpingography. *Fertil Steril.* 2005;83 (6):1595–1606.

18. Simpson WL, Beitia LG, Mester J. Hysterosalpingography: a reemerging study. *Radiographics.* 2006;26:419–431.

19. Ofili-Yebovi D, Ben-Nagi J, Sawyer E, et al. Deficient lower-segment Cesarean section scars: prevalence and risk factors. *Ultrasound Obstet Gynecol.* 2008;31:72–77.

20. Hunter TJ, Maouris P, Dickinson JE. Prenatal detection and conservative management of a partial fundal uterine dehiscence. *Fetal Diagn Ther.* 2009;25: 123–126.

21. Hasbargen U, Summerer-Moustaki M, Hillemanns P, et al. Uterine dehiscence in a nullipara, diagnosed by MRI, following use of unipolar electrocautery during laparoscopic myomectomy: case report. *Human Reproduction.* 2002;17(8):2180–2182.

22. Koskas M, Nizard J, Salmon LJ, et al. Abdominal and pelvic ultrasound findings within 24 hours following uneventful Cesarean section. *Ultrasound Obstet Gynecol.* 2008;32:520–526.

23. Cheung V. Sonographic measurement of the lower uterine segment thickness in women with previous caesarean section. *J Obstet Gynaecol Can.* 2005;27(7): 674–681.

24. Leyendecker JR, Gorengaut V, Brown JJ. MR imaging of maternal diseases of the abdomen and pelvis during pregnancy and the immediate postpartum period. *Radiographics.* 2004;24:1301–1316.

25. Donnez O, Jadoul P, Squifflet J, et al. Laparoscopic repair of wide and deep uterine scar dehiscence after cesarean section. *Fertil Steril.* 2008;89(4):974–980.

26. Haney AF. Leiomyomata. In: *Danforth's Obstetrics and Gynecology.* 10th ed. Philadelphia, PA: Lippincott Williams & Wilkins; 2003.

27. Mason TC. Red degeneration of a leiomyoma masquerading as retained products of conception. *J Natl Med Assoc.* 2002;94(2):124–126.

28. Poder L. Ultrasound evaluation of the uterus. In: *Ultrasonography in Obstetrics and Gynecology.* 5th ed. Philadelphia, PA: Elsevier; 2008.

29. Novak ER, Woodruff JD, eds. Novak's gynecologic and obstetric pathology. 8th ed. Philadelphia, PA: WB Saunders; 1979.

30. Okita A, Kubo Y, Tanada M, et al. Unusual abscesses associated with colon cancer: report of three cases. *Acta Med Okayama.* 2007;61(2):107–113.

31. Vijayaraghavan SB. Sonographic whirlpool sign in ovarian torsion. *J Ultrasound Med.* 2004;23(12):1643–1649.

32. Sharp HT. Chronic pelvic pain. In: *Danforth's Obstetrics and Gynecology.* 10th ed. Philadelphia, PA: Lippincott Williams & Wilkins: 2003.

33. Tucker RD, Baggish MS. Lasers and electrosurgery in hysteroscopy. In: *Hysteroscopy: Visual Perspectives of Uterine Anatomy, Physiology and Pathology.* 3rd ed. Philadelphia, PA: Lippincott Williams & Wilkins; 2003.

34. Westphalen AC, Qayyum A. The role of magnetic resonance imaging in the evaluation of gynecologic disease. In: *Ultrasonography in Obstetrics and Gynecology.* 5th ed. Philadelphia, PA: Elsevier; 2008.

35. Vander Werff BJ, Hagen-Ansert S. Pathology of the adnexa. In: *Ultrasonography in Obstetrics and Gynecology.* 5th ed. Philadelphia, PA: Elsevier; 2008.

36. Hagan-Ansert S. The peritoneal cavity and abdominal wall. In: *Textbook of Diagnostic Medical Ultrasonography.* Vol 2. 6th ed. St. Louis, MO: Mosby; 2006.

37. Pinto LN, Pereira JM, Cunha R, et al. CT evaluation of appendicitis and its complications: imaging techniques and key diagnostic findings. *AJR Am J Roentgenol.* 2005;185(2):406–417.

38. Muradali D, Wilson S. Organ transplantation. In: *Diagnostic Ultrasound.* Vol 1. 3rd ed. St. Louis, MO: Elsevier Mosby; 2005.

39. Downey DB. The retorperitoneum and great vessels. In: *Diagnostic Ultrasound.* Vol 1. 3rd ed. St. Louis, MO: Elsevier Mosby; 2005.

40. Wilson SR. The gastrointestinal tract. In: *Diagnostic Ultrasound.* Vol 1. 3rd ed. St. Louis, MO: Elsevier Mosby; 2005.

41. Levine D. The role of computed tomography and magnetic resonance imaging in obstetrics. In: *Textbook of Diagnostic Medical Ultrasonography.* Vol 2. 6th ed. St. Louis, MO: Mosby; 2006.

42. Krakow D. Medical and surgical complications of pregnancy. In: *Danforth's Obstetrics and Gynecology.* 10th ed. Philadelphia, PA: Lippincott Williams & Wilkins; 2003.

43. Rosenberg HK. Pediatric pelvic sonography. In: *Diagnostic Ultrasound.* Vol 2. 3rd ed. St. Louis, MO: Elsevier Mosby; 2005.

44. Gartner's duct cyst. Medcyclopaedia. http://www.medcyclopaedia.com/library/topics/volume_iv_2/g/gartners_duct_cyst.aspx. Accessed March 27, 2010.

45. DeLancy JOL. Epidemiology, pathophysiology, and evaluation of pelvic organ support. In: *Danforth's Obstetrics and Gynecology.* 10th ed. Philadelphia, PA: Lippincott Williams & Wilkins; 2003.

46. Valentin L, Callen PW. Ultrasound evaluation of the adnexa (ovary and fallopian tubes). In: *Ultrasonography in Obstetrics and Gynecology.* 5th ed. Philadelphia, PA: Sanders Elsevier; 2008.

47. Eschenbach DA. Pelvic and sexually transmitted infections. In: *Danforth's Obstetrics and Gynecology.* 10th ed. Philadelphia, PA: Lippincott Williams & Wilkins; 2003.

48. Vander Werff BJ, Hagen-Ansert S. Pathology of the ovaries. In: *Ultrasonography in Obstetrics and Gynecology.* 5th ed. Philadelphia, PA: Elsevier; 2008.

49. Davidson SA. Management of the adnexal mass. In: *Danforth's Obstetrics and Gynecology.* 10th ed. Philadelphia, PA: Lippincott Williams & Wilkins; 2003.

50. Survace epithelial inclusion cysts. Medcyclopaedia. http://www.medcyclopaedia.com/library/topics/volume_iv_2/s/surface_epithelial_inclusion_cyst_ovarian.aspx. Accessed March 27, 2010.

51. Lin CK, Chu TW, Yu MH. Painless ovarian torsion mimicking a uterine myoma. *Taiwan J Obstet Gynecol.* 2006;45(4):340–342.

52. Chang HC, Bhatt S, Dogra VS. Pearls and pitfalls in diagnosis of ovarian torsion. *Radiographics.* 2008;28(5): 1355–1368.

53. Singh A, Danrad R, Hahn PF, et al. MR imaging of the acute abdomen and pelvis: acute appendicitis and beyond. *Radiographics.* 2007;27(5):1419–1431.

54. Pierson RA. Ultrasonic imaging in infertility. In: *Ultrasonography in Obstetrics and Gynecology*. 5th ed. Philadelphia, PA: Sanders Elsevier; 2008.

55. Legro RS, Azziz R. Androgen excess disorders. In: *Danforth's Obstetrics and Gynecology*. 10th ed. Philadelphia, PA: Lippincott Williams & Wilkins: 2003.

56. Mitchell DG, Gefter WB, Spritzer CE, et al. Polycystic ovaries: MR imaging. *Radiology*. 1986;160:425–429.

57. Lakhani K, Seifalian AM, Atiomo WU, et al. Polycystic ovaries. *Br J Radio*. 2002;75(889):9–16.

58. Faure N, Prat X, Bastide A, et al. Assessment of ovaries by magnetic resonance imaging in patients presenting with polycystic ovarian syndrome. *Human Reproduction*. 1989;4(4):468–472.

59. Tanaka YO, Tsunoda H, Kitagawa Y, et al. Functioning ovarian tumors: direct and indirect findings at MR imaging. *Radiographics*. 2004;24 (suppl 1):S147–S166.

60. Cass I, Karlan B. Ovarian and tubal cancers. In: *Danforth's Obstetrics and Gynecology*. 10th ed. Philadelphia, PA; Lippincott Williams & Wilkins: 2003.

61. Chang YT, Lin JY. Intraperitoneal rupture of mature cystic ovarian teratoma secondary to sit-ups. *J Formos Med Assoc*. 2009;108(2):173–175.

62. Okada S, Ohaki Y, Inoue K, et al. A case of dermoid cyst of the ovary with malignant transformation complicated with small intestinal fistula formation. *Radiat Med*. 2005;23(6):443–446.

63. Metaxas G, Tangalos A, Pappa P, et al. Mucinous cystic neoplasms of the mesentery: a case report and review of the literature. *World J Surg Oncol*. 2009;7:47.

64. Shah AA, Sainani NI, Kambadakone AR, et al. Predictive value of multi-detector computed tomography for accurate diagnosis of serous cystadenoma: radiologic-pathologic correlation. *World J Gastroenterol*. 2009;15(22):2739–2747.

65. Okada S, Ohaki Y, Inoue K, et al. Calcifications in mucinous and serous cystic ovarian tumors. *J Nippon Med Sch*. 2005;72(1):29–33.

66. Jacob S, Rawat P, Mark RP. Serous microcystic adenoma (glycogen rich cystadenoma) of the pancreas. *Indian J Pathol Microbiol* [serial online] 2010 [cited 2010 Apr 7];53:106–8. http://www.ijpmonline.org/text .asp?2010/53/1/106/59195

67. Hong SG, Kim JS, Joo MK, et al. Pancreatic tuberculosis masquerading as pancreatic serous cystadenoma. *World J Gastroenterol*. 2009;15(8):1010–1013.

68. Ovarian Fibroma. Medcyclopaedia Web site. Accessed April 2010.

69. Mak CW, Tzeng WS, Chen CY. Computed tomography appearance of ovarian fibrothecomas with and without torsion. *Acta Radiol*. 2009;50(5):570–575.

70. Tanaka YO, Tsunoda H, Kitagawa Y, et al. Functioning ovarian tumors: direct and indirect findings at MR imaging. *Radiographics*. 2004;24:S147–S166.

71. Jung SE, Rha SE, Lee JM, et al. CT and MRI findings of sex cord-stromal tumor of the ovary. *AJR*. 2005;185(1):207–215.

72. Ko SF, Wan YL, Ng SH, et al. Adult ovarian granulosa cell tumors: spectrum of sonographic and CT findings with pathologic correlation. *AJR*. 1999;172(5):1227–1233.

73. Jung SE, Lee JM, Rha SE, et al. CT and MR imaging of ovarian tumors with emphasis on differential diagnosis. *Radiographics*. 2002;22(6):1305–1325.

74. Rosenberg HK. Pediatric pelvic sonography. In: *Diagnostic Ultrasound*. Vol 2. 3rd ed. St. Louis, MO: Elsevier Mosby; 2005.

75. Gonadoblastoma, ovarian. Medcyclopaedia Web site. Accessed April 16, 2010.

76. Cheng MH, Yen MS, Chao KC, et al. Differential diagnosis of gynecologic organ-related diseases in women presenting with ascites. *Taiwan J Obstet Gynecol*. 2008;47(4):384–390.

77. Vijayaraghavan GR, Levine D. Case 109: Meigs' syndrome. *Radiology*. 2007;242(3):940–944.

78. Uehara T, Sawada M. Struma ovarii associated with Meigs' syndrome. *Jpn J Clin Oncol*. 2007;37(1):73.

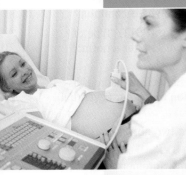

9

Malignant Disease of the Uterus and Cervix

Faith Hutson

OBJECTIVES

Associate endometrial carcinoma with its risk factors, imaging appearance, and prognosis

Distinguish the difference between a leiomyoma and leiomyosarcoma

Identify fallopian tube carcinoma risk factors, imaging characteristics, and long-term prognosis

List the disease process and imaging characteristics for cervical carcinoma

Summarize the genetic makeup of persistent trophoblastic neoplasia

KEY TERMS

adenocarcinoma | cervical carcinoma | cervical polyp | choriocarcinoma | endometrial carcinoma | endometrial hyperplasia | endometrial polyp | epithelioid trophoblastic tumor | fallopian tube carcinoma | hereditary nonpolyposis colon cancer (HNPCC) | human papillomavirus (HPV) | hydrops tubae profluens | invasive mole | leiomyosarcoma | Papanicolaou (Pap) smear | persistent trophoblastic neoplasia (PTN) | placental site trophoblastic tumor (PSTT) | sonohysterography, squamous cell carcinoma | tamoxifen

GLOSSARY

Adenocarcinoma Malignant tumor arising from any glandular organ

Adenosis Any disease of a gland or of glandular tissue

Androstenedione Pivotal adrenal steroid that is a precursor to testosterone and other androgens

Antiestrogen Any substance that blocks or modifies the action of estrogen

Antineoplastic Prevents the development, growth, or proliferation of malignant cells

Cervical polyp Hyperplastic growth that protrudes from the epithelium of the cervix; may be broad based or pedunculated

Cervical stenosis Narrowing or obstruction of the cervical canal caused by an acquired condition

Choriocarcinoma Metastatic type of persistent trophoblastic neoplasia that can result from any type of pregnancy but most often occurs with a molar pregnancy

Endometrial carcinoma Malignant condition that presents with abnormal thickening of the endometrial cavity and irregular bleeding in perimenopausal and postmenopausal women

Endometrial hyperplasia Condition that results from estrogen stimulation to the endometrium without the influence of progestin; frequent cause of bleeding, especially in postmenopausal women

Endometrial polyp Pedunculated or sessile mass attached to the endometrial cavity

Endometrioid Presence of endometrial tissue of varying differentiation

Epithelioid trophoblastic tumor Variant of placental site trophoblastic tumor

Fallopian tube carcinoma Very rare gynecologic malignancy occurring most often in postmenopausal patients in the sixth decade; adenocarcinoma is the most common histologic type

Gadolinium Rare earth metallic element possessing paramagnetic properties that are used in contrast media for magnetic resonance imaging (MRI)

Gestational trophoblastic neoplasia (GTN) Trophoblastic tissue that has overtaken the pregnancy and propagated throughout the uterine cavity; these tumors arise from the placental chorionic villi

Granulosa cell tumor Fleshy ovarian tumor with yellow streaks that originates in cells of the primordial membrana granulosa and may grow to an extremely large size

Human chorionic gonadotropin (hCG) Hormone secreted by the placental trophoblastic cells; it is found in the urine and blood of pregnant women; elevated levels are found with GTN

Human papillomavirus (HPV) Virus that is transmitted through sexual contact and produces lesions on the mucous membranes; considered a causative factor in cervical carcinoma

Hydrops tubae profluens Watery discharge sometimes present with fallopian tube carcinoma

Invasive mole Tumor penetrating into and possibly through the uterine wall

Leiomyoma Benign tumor composed of smooth muscle cells and fibrous connective tissue that occurs in the uterus

Leiomyosarcoma Malignant uterine tumor composed of smooth muscle cells and fibrous connective tissue; sonographically, it appears like a benign leiomyoma

Metastases Spread of bacteria or body cells, especially of cancer cells, from one part of the body to another

Methotrexate Drug prescribed in the treatment of severe psoriasis and a variety of malignant neoplastic diseases

Papanicolaou (Pap) smear Cytological study (developed by George Nicholas Papanicolaou) used to detect cancer in cells that an organ has shed; used most often in the diagnosis and prevention of cervical cancer and also valuable in the detection of pleural or peritoneal malignancies

Pelvic inflammatory disease Infection of the uterus, fallopian tubes, and adjacent pelvic structures; usually caused by an ascending infection in which disease-producing germs spread from the vagina and cervix to the upper portions of the female reproductive tract

Persistent trophoblastic neoplasia (PTN) Malignant end of the GTN spectrum; this group of life-threatening diseases persists most often from a molar pregnancy

Peutz-Jeghers syndrome Inherited disorder characterized by the presence of polyps of the small intestine and melanin pigmentation of the lips, mucosa, fingers, and toes; anemia from the intestinal polyps is common

Placental site trophoblastic tumor (PSTT) Type of PTN that usually occurs several years after a normal term pregnancy

Polycystic ovarian syndrome Endocrine disorder associated with chronic anovulation and Stein-Leventhal syndrome

Polypoid Containing more than two normal sets of chromosomes

Pulsatility index (PI) Doppler measurement that uses peak systole minus peak diastole divided by the mean

Radiation therapy Treatment of neoplastic disease by using X-rays or gamma rays; deters the proliferation of malignant cells by decreasing mitosis or by impairing DNA synthesis

Resistive index (RI) Peak systole minus peak diastole divided by peak systole; an RI 0.7 or lower indicates good perfusion of an organ, whereas an RI greater than 0.7 indicates decreased perfusion

Salpingo-oophorectomy Surgical removal of the fallopian tubes and ovaries

Sonohysterography Injection of sterile saline into the endometrial canal under ultrasound guidance; this procedure allows for good visualization of the endometrial borders to rule out pathology

Squamous cell carcinoma Slow-growing malignant tumor composed of squamous epithelium; most common type of cervical cancer

Submucosal leiomyoma Type of leiomyoma that deforms the endometrial cavity and can cause heavy or irregular menses

Tamoxifen Nonsteroidal antiestrogen compound that is currently the most widely prescribed drug for the treatment of breast cancer

Teratogenic Causing congenital anomalies or birth defects

Sonography is a relatively inexpensive and noninvasive tool for detecting and evaluating female pelvic pathology. Its ability to visualize characteristics, morphology, size, and location of a mass makes sonography useful in imaging pelvic pathology. Intracavitary transducers, both endovaginal and endorectal, give improved visualization of the regional anatomy, providing information that can aid in staging of uterine and cervical malignancies. Three-dimensional (3D) ultrasound simultaneously displays sagittal, transverse, and coronal planes. By creating a voxel of stored information, the rendered images can be manipulated to evaluate pelvic structures in different planes. Additionally, 3D ultrasound provides more specific information by reconstructing organ volume that can be indicative of pathology. Sonohysterography and particularly 3D sonohysterography can elucidate the etiology of endometrial thickening and the exact location of intrauterine pathology. Color and spectral Doppler evaluation of uterine endometrial and myometrial blood flow is a helpful adjunct to facilitate treatment of pelvic carcinomas. Sonography is also valuable in guiding biopsies and other interventional procedures. Magnetic resonance imaging (MRI) and computed tomography (CT) are two other imaging methods. MRI is used for tissue characterization and staging of malignancies. CT has a more limited role but is used for determining metastatic spread or tumor recurrence.

ENDOMETRIAL CARCINOMA

CLINICAL INFORMATION

Epidemiology and Risk Factors

In developed countries such as the Unites States, endometrial carcinoma is the most common gynecological malignancy; by contrast, in developing countries, carcinoma of the cervix is more common. In 2007, approximately 39,000 cases of endometrial carcinoma were predicted to occur in the United States; 7,400 of these patients will die.[1] Fortunately, despite the increased incidence, endometrial carcinoma has the best prognosis when diagnosed early compared to other gynecological carcinomas.

Multiple risk factors are associated with the development of endometrial carcinoma. Obese patients have a higher risk because fat is responsible for the conversion of androstenedione to estrogen compounds at a much higher rate than if fat is not present. Current data indicate that women who are 50 lb heavier than their ideal weight have a twofold to threefold increased risk of developing endometrial cancer. Nulliparity also increases the risk twofold to threefold when compared with parity.

Late menopause (after 52 years old) also seems to be a risk factor. Also, a higher incidence is associated with adenomatous polyps, family history of endometrial carcinoma, and the use of unopposed estrogen, either as replacement therapy or endogenously produced, including polycystic ovarian syndrome or granulosa cell tumors.[1] Estrogen has a proliferative effect on the endometrium; approximately 25% of patients with atypical endometrial hyperplasia develop endometrial carcinoma.[2,3]

Several other medical conditions predispose women to endometrial cancer. Patients who have hereditary nonpolyposis colon cancer (HNPCC) and those who have had breast cancer have a twofold to threefold increase.[1,4] Tamoxifen, a nonsteroidal antiestrogen compound, is currently the most widely prescribed antineoplastic drug in the world for the treatment of breast cancer. Tamoxifen is effective because it competes with estrogen for estrogen receptors. In premenopausal women, it has an antiestrogen effect; however, in postmenopausal women, it may have estrogenic effects. An increased risk of endometrial carcinoma, endometrial hyperplasia, and polyps has been reported in patients on tamoxifen

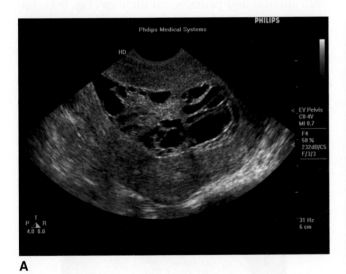

A

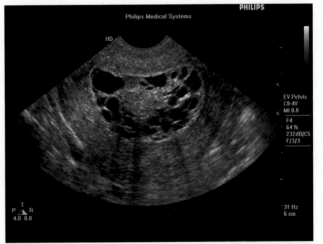

B

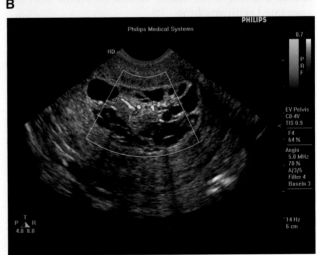

C

Figure 9-1 A: This sagittal, endovaginal image demonstrates the typical appearance of an endometrium in a patient undergoing tamoxifen therapy. **B:** A transverse image of the same endometrium. **C:** A Color power angio image of the endometrium demonstrates flow in the central portion of the complex mass. (Images courtesy of Philips Medical Systems, Bothell, WA.)

PATHOLOGY BOX 9-1

Endometrial Cancer

Risk Factors	Signs/Symptoms	Sonographic Findings
Obesity	Uterine bleeding	Heterogeneous endometrium
Nulliparity	Pain	Irregular or poorly defined endometrial margins
Menopause after age 52		Cystic changes
Adenomatous polyps		Hydrometra or hematometra
Family history of endometrial cancer		Enlarged uterus
Use of unopposed estrogen		Lobular uterine contour
PCOD		
Granulosa cell tumors		
Endometrial hyperplasia		
HNPCC		
Tamoxifen use		

therapy (Fig. 9-1).[5] According to Callen,[3] data point to high-risk and low-risk groups that can be identified prior to tamoxifen treatment. Patients are screened with endovaginal sonography, and those with no uterine abnormalities appear to be at a very low risk for developing atypical hyperplasia. Patients with any uterine lesion seem to have an 18-fold increased risk and, even if asymptomatic, may be candidates for serial surveillance.[6]

Recent studies show that, in contrast with tamoxifen, the use of combination oral contraceptives (OCs) decreases the risk of developing carcinoma of the endometrium. Women who have been on an OC for at least 12 months are protected for approximately 10 years after OC use. This protection is most notable for nulliparous women.[1]

Smoking also appears to decrease the risk of endometrial carcinoma because it decreases body weight, with obese smokers having the greatest risk reduction. Additionally, smokers undergo menopause approximately 1 to 2 years earlier than nonsmokers. Unfortunately, these benefits are offset by the huge risk of lung cancer and the other major health problems that are associated with smoking.[1]

Pathophysiology

Histologically, over 80% of endometrial carcinomas are of the endometrioid type. *Endometrioid* simply refers to the presence of endometrial tissue of varying differentiation and can be subdivided into two groups: type 1 (low grade) and type 2 (high grade). Type 1 carcinomas are connected to long-term unopposed estrogen therapy; they progress from endometrial hyperplasia and have a good prognosis. Type 2 carcinomas, which are less common (approximately 10% of cases), are most often associated with an atrophic endometrium and have a much poorer prognosis. About 8% of patients with endometrial carcinoma also present with histologically similar ovarian carcinoma (Fig. 9-2).[6]

Endometrial carcinoma is also classified into grades 1 through 3, depending on the histopathology and degree of tumor differentiation. This classification is different than the staging of the disease, which is based on the extent of tumor spread. Current International Federation of Gynecologists and Obstetricians (FIGO) staging for endometrial carcinoma is based on both surgical and pathological findings (Fig. 9-3). Important diagnostic features in staging the disease include the depth of myometrial invasion; involvement of the cervix; extension to the tubes, ovaries, or pelvic lymph nodes; and distant metastases to lungs or other organs.

Clinical Diagnosis

Carcinoma of the endometrium is usually diagnosed in the sixth or seventh decade. There is a higher rate of

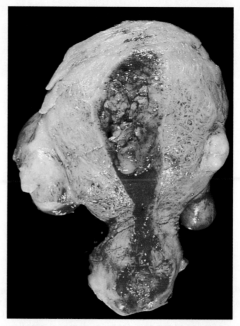

Figure 9-2 Adenocarcinoma of the endometrium. The uterus has been opened to reveal a partially necrotic, polypoid endometrial cancer. (Image from Rubin E, Farber JL. *Pathology.* 3rd ed. Philadelphia, PA: Lippincott Williams & Wilkins; 1999.)

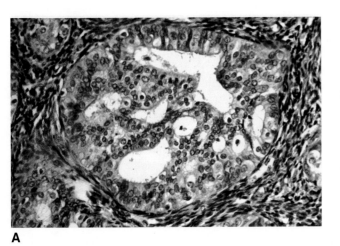

A

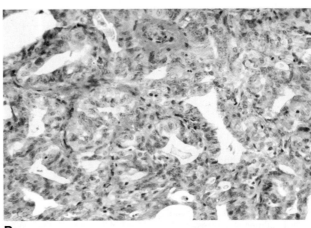

B

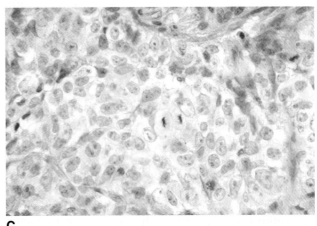

C

Figure 9-3 A: Adenocarcinoma of the endometrium (FIGO grades 1 to 3). Grade 1: The tumor is well differentiated and composed entirely of glands. **B:** Adenocarcinoma of the endometrium (FIGO grades 1 to 3). Grade 2: The cancer is moderately differentiated and shows both glands and solid sheets of cells. **C:** Adenocarcinoma of the endometrium (FIGO grades 1 to 3). Grade 3: The tumor is poorly differentiated and is composed entirely of sheets of cells. Numerous mitoses are present. (Image from Rubin E, Farber JL. *Pathology.* 3rd ed. Philadelphia, PA: Lippincott Williams & Wilkins; 1999.)

occurrence among white women compared with black women: 26.1 cases per 100,000 compared to 19.6 cases per 100,000, respectively. However, there is a higher rate of mortality among black women compared to white women: 7.1 deaths per 100,000 versus 3.9 deaths per 100,000.[10]

The most common clinical presentation is uterine bleeding, although only 10% of patients with postmenopausal bleeding actually have endometrial carcinoma.[11] Pain may also occur because of uterine distention resulting from intracavitary bleeding associated with cervical stenosis. Symptoms of postmenopausal pelvic

---

PATHOLOGY BOX 9-2

Surgical-Pathologic Staging of Endometrial Carcinoma

Stage	Characteristics
Stage I	A: Tumor limited to endometrium
	B: Invasion to less than one-half the myometrium
	C: Invasion to more than one-half the myometrium
Stage II[a]	A: Endocervical glandular involvement only
	B: Cervical stromal invasion
Stage III[a]	A: Tumor invades serosa or adnexa and/or positive peritoneal cytology
	B: Vaginal metastases
	C: Metastases to pelvic and/or para-aortic lymph nodes
Stage IV[a]	A: Tumor invades of the bladder and/or bowel mucosa
	B: Distant metastases including intra-abdominal and/or inguinal lymph nodes
[a]Pathologic stages	G1: Highly differentiated adenomatous carcinomas
	G2: Differentiated adenomatous carcinomas with partly solid areas
	G3: Predominantly solid or entirely undifferentiated carcinomas

Adapted from the International Federation of Gynecologists and Obstetricians [FIGO] Cancer Committee Report. Rio de Janeiro, Brazil, October 1989.

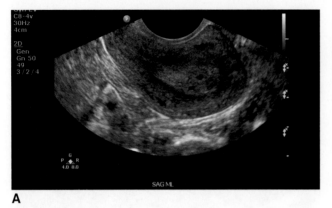

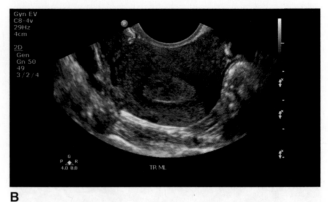

A   **B**

Figure 9-4 A: Sagittal endovaginal image of an endometrium demonstrating cystic changes. **B:** Transverse view of the thickened, cystic endometrium. (Images courtesy of Philips Medical Systems, Bothell, WA.)

inflammatory disease may be present secondary to tumor necrosis and infection. Dilation and curettage and endometrial biopsy provide the tissue necessary to confirm the diagnosis.

Treatment

Treatment includes a total hysterectomy, bilateral salpingo-oophorectomy, and peritoneal fluid aspiration and washings. Depending on tumor stage and grade, selective pelvic and para-aortic lymphadenectomy is performed. Radiation therapy is usually prescribed as an adjunctive treatment; sometimes chemotherapy (cisplatin) is used even though it has a greater toxicity.

SONOGRAPHIC IMAGING

Diagnostic Features

For patients with abnormal uterine bleeding, pelvic ultrasound is initially the modality of choice. Endovaginal scanning facilitates a detailed study of endometrial and myometrial texture. If the endometrium has a heterogeneous echotexture with irregular or poorly defined margins, cancer is more likely. Cystic changes

(Fig. 9-4) within the endometrium are more likely to be the result of endometrial atrophy, hyperplasia, or polyps but can also be seen with cancer. Endometrial carcinoma is also likely to obstruct the endometrial canal and cause hydrometra or hematometra (Fig. 9-5). Enlargement with lobular contour of the uterus and mixed echogenicity is more indicative of an advanced disease stage.

A detailed analysis of the endometrial lining and the subendometrial hypoechoic halo, which corresponds to the compact vascular inner myometrial segment, may provide a clue to the presence or extent of myometrial invasion. It has been suggested that an intact subendometrial halo in the presence of endometrial carcinoma would imply superficial involvement only and that disruption or obliteration of the halo would indicate deep myometrial invasion.[12] Deep myometrial invasion (stage IC) constitutes more than 50% extension into the myometrial thickness with an intact outer rim.[6]

Ultrasound can be helpful in distinguishing stage I or II carcinoma (carcinoma confined to the uterus) from stage III or IV (carcinoma extending beyond the uterus). By using simultaneous display of the transverse

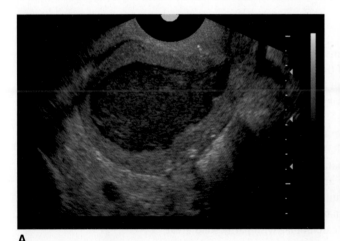

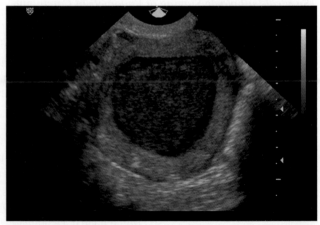

A   **B**

Figure 9-5 Sagittal **(A)** and transverse **(B)** endovaginal images of hematometra demonstrating the characteristic complex appearance of blood within the endometrium. (Images courtesy of Philips Medical Systems, Bothell, WA.)

plane with 3D ultrasound, it is possible to detect infiltration of endometrial or cervical carcinoma into the bladder or rectum. Presence of a mass adjacent to the uterus may represent direct extension, metastases to the ovary, lymph node enlargement, or a coincidental ovarian mass. If the urinary bladder is involved, ureteral obstruction is likely to be present and the kidneys should be scanned for evidence of hydronephrosis.

Because of tumor angiogenesis, color and pulsed Doppler can give accurate information for the diagnoses of endometrial carcinoma. Endometrial blood flow is usually not seen in the normal or atrophic endometrium nor in most cases of endometrial hyperplasia. According to Kupesic et al.,[5] in 91% of their cases, neovascularization was demonstrated. Intratumoral flow indicates low vascular resistance, *resistive index* (RI) = 0.42 ± 0.02. Invasion of the myometrial vessels is suspected if there is an increase in flow signals surrounding a lesion; this is due to an absent or incomplete myometrial membrane.

Technique and Protocol

It is important to identify the endometrial lining, which represents the endometrial canal. Endometrial lining thickness is measured from the reflective interface of the basalis layer of the endometrium, anterior to posterior. The hypoechoic myometrial layer should not be included. Also, any fluid present within the endometrial canal should be excluded from the measurement.

There are disadvantages in distinguishing benign from malignant pathology when using conventional two-dimensional (2D) ultrasound to measure endometrial thickness. In itself, a prominent endometrium is not a specific sign of endometrial carcinoma. Endometrial thickness varies considerably with different factors. These include whether the patient is obese or diabetic, whether she is perimenopausal or postmenopausal and for how long, and whether the patient is taking hormone replacement therapy, either estrogen alone or a combination of estrogen and progesterone.[1] 3D sonography assesses endometrial volume, which is superior in distinguishing carcinoma from benign pathology. Studies have found that the endometrial volume was markedly higher in patients with carcinoma than in those with benign changes. In symptomatic postmenopausal patients, the endometrial volume measurements were superior to endometrial thickness measurements as a diagnostic test for the detection of carcinoma. Increasing endometrial volume is related to an increased severity or higher grade of endometrial cancer and myometrial invasion.[5] In addition to endometrial volume, Kupesic et al. used other 3D sonographic and power Doppler criteria to diagnose endometrial carcinoma. These criteria include subendometrial halo irregularity, presence of endometrial fluid, vessel architecture, and vessel branching pattern.[5]

Any changes in size and echogenicity of either the uterus or cervix should be noted and the adnexal region imaged to identify the ovaries and any adnexal masses. Also note the presence of pelvic or abdominal ascites. If the sonographic findings in the pelvis suggest a neoplasm, extend the examination to include the liver and abdominal viscera to search for possible metastases. Image the kidneys to document the presence or absence of hydronephrosis and scan the para-aortic and para-caval areas for adenopathy.

OTHER IMAGING MODALITIES

Both MRI and CT are useful in determining lymphadenopathy and distal metastatic disease (stages III and IV). In addition, CT is commonly used to determine recurrent disease because it affords great definition of pelvic sidewalls and retroperitoneal anatomy.

PATHOLOGY BOX 9-3

Three-Dimensional Sonographic and Power Doppler Criteria for the Diagnosis of Endometrial Malignancy

3D Sonographic and Power Doppler Criteria	Score
Endometrial volume	<13 mL score 0
	≥13 mL score 2
Subendometrial halo	Regular score 0
	Disturbed score 2
Intracavitary fluid	Absent score 0
	Present score 2
Vessel's architecture	Linear vessel arrangement score 0
	Chaotic vessel arrangement score 2
Branching pattern	Simple score 0
	Complex score 2

TOTAL SCORE
Total score = sum of individual scores

Cut off score = greater or equal to 4 is associated with a high risk of endometrial malignancy. Reprinted with permission from Kupesic S. Color Doppler and 3D Ultrasound in Gynecology, Infertility and Obstetrics 1st ed. New Delhi: Jaypee Brothers Medical Publishers (P) Ltd, 2003.

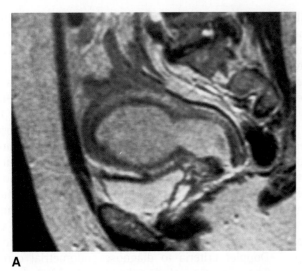
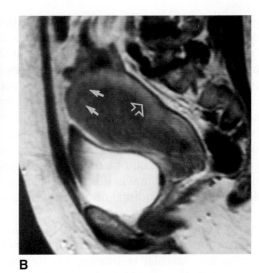

A   **B**

Figure 9-6 Endometrial carcinoma (value of gadolinium). **A:** Sagittal T2-weighted image shows a markedly enlarged endometrial cavity with intact junctional zone (suggesting a stage IA tumor confined to the myometrium). **B:** Sagittal gadolinium-enhanced T1-weighted scan at the same level (bladder contains more urine) shows intermediate-intensity tumor invading the junctional zone and myometrium of the fundus *(solid arrows),* which was proved at surgery to represent stage IC tumor (invasion to more than 50% of the endometrium). Note the normal high-intensity enhancement of the posterior myometrium *(open arrow).*

The overall accuracy of MRI in the staging of endometrial carcinoma is approximately 85%; the use of gadolinium increases this accuracy even further. The reported accuracy in the identification of deep myometrial invasion varies from 74% to 95%, compared with 68% to 73% for endovaginal sonography. However, if the cancer stretches and thins the myometrium, the amount of malignant invasion can be overestimated by MRI (Fig. 9-6).[6,7]

DIFFERENTIAL DIAGNOSIS

The differential diagnosis for endometrial carcinoma includes endometrial hyperplasia, which in some cases can be a precursor to endometrial carcinoma (Fig. 9-7). Endometrial polyps can appear as nonspecific echogenic endometrial thickness, which may be diffuse or focal

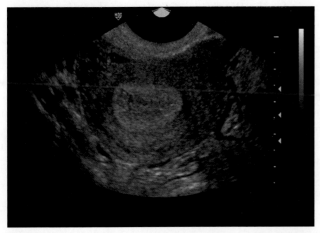

Figure 9-7 This endovaginal image demonstrates hyperplasia of the endometrium. (Image courtesy of Philips Medical Systems, Bothell, WA.)

(Fig. 9-8). Enlarged, bulbous, or lobulated uterus may be due to leiomyomas and associated with abnormal bleeding. Myomas can also distort the endometrial lining, giving the appearance of endometrial thickening. Cervical carcinoma invasion into the uterus can also give the endometrium a thickened appearance.

LEIOMYOSARCOMA

CLINICAL INFORMATION

Epidemiology and Risk Factors

Leiomyosarcoma is a rare, fast-growing malignancy, accounting for only 3% of uterine tumors. These lesions are derived from smooth muscle in the wall of the uterus and are notorious for their aggressive nature and poor prognosis. Because of its aggressive nature, local pelvic recurrence and metastasis are common. The lung is a common site of metastasis; other sites include the bone, brain, and abdomen.[1] Risk factors for the development of uterine sarcomas including leiomyosarcomas are nulliparity, increasing age (perimenopausal and postmenopausal women in the fifth decade of life), obesity, history of pelvic radiation, and exposure to tamoxifen.[2]

Pathophysiology

It was previously thought that leiomyosarcomas of the uterus arose from existing leiomyomas. Although this is possible, genetic studies suggest that they are two different entities arising from separate pathways.[6] Leiomyosarcomas tend to be intramural but may be found anywhere within the uterus. Their gross appearance is fleshy, hemorrhagic, and necrotic, without the typical whorl-like appearance seen in benign leiomyomas. The

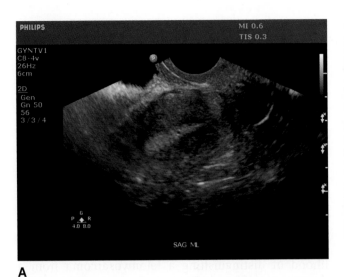

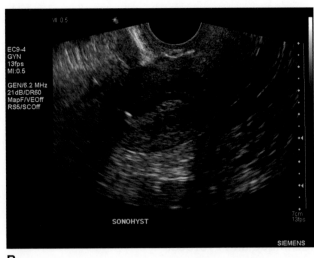

Figure 9-8 **A:** Thickened, echogenic endometrium. **B:** The sonohystogram image demonstrating endometrial polyps. (Images courtesy of Derry Imaging Center, Derry NH Robin Davies, Ann Smith, and Denise Raney.)

borders of these masses are infiltrative rather than well circumscribed.[22]

Clinical Diagnosis

Abnormal vaginal bleeding and pelvic or abdominal pain are the most common presenting symptoms. Since these are the same symptoms that typically present with benign leiomyomas, an accurate diagnosis of malignancy is rarely made. With the increasing use of nonsurgical conservative techniques for treating benign uterine fibroids, the likelihood of a delay in diagnosis or of a misdiagnosis of a sarcoma is a disturbing reality.[2] Some authors suggest using a transcervical needle biopsy combined with MRI to differentiate between a leiomyosarcoma and a benign myoma.[2] Clinically, a rapid increase in the size of a uterine tumor after menopause should arouse suspicion of sarcoma.

Treatment

Universally, surgery is the primary treatment for any leiomyosarcoma. Total hysterectomy and bilateral salpingo-oophorectomy are standard, along with peritoneal washings and sampling of any suspicious nodules.

Because uterine leiomyosarcomas are extremely aggressive, prognosis depends on tumor stage and grade at the time of surgery. The FIGO criteria used for staging endometrial carcinoma are also used to stage uterine leiomyosarcomas. Survival is also greater in premenopausal women and in women with tumors that are less than five centimeters. Tumors with vascular invasion or extrauterine spread have a very grave prognosis.[1] The use of adjuvant radiotherapy has not proven to be very useful, but adjuvant anthracycline-based chemotherapy may have a role in management; however, more studies are needed.

SONOGRAPHIC IMAGING

Diagnostic Features

The sonographic appearance of this type of sarcoma is a rapidly growing, heterogeneous uterine mass very similar to a leiomyoma undergoing degenerative changes. In many cases, the leiomyosarcoma is single and very large. More than 90% have a mean diameter of 10 cm³ and show pronounced acoustic enhancement due to increased vascularity and areas of liquefaction.

PATHOLOGY BOX 9-4

Uterine Sarcomas and Leiomyosarcomas

Risk Factors	Signs/Symptoms	Sonographic Findings
Nulliparity	Vaginal bleeding	Rapidly growing heterogeneous mass
Increasing age (perimenopausal and postmenopausal women in the fifth decade of life)	Abdominal pain	Usually single
	Rapid increase in uterine mass size	Large mass
Obesity		Acoustic enhancement
History of pelvic radiation		Anechoic or complex areas due to tumor liquefaction
Tamoxifen exposure		

Because of its invasive nature, myometrial involvement may also be seen. Doppler has been used to assess increased intratumoral flow, but this has had little effect in differentiating benign from malignant masses. Szabo et al. used color and pulsed Doppler to determine if blood flow analysis could differentiate between uterine leiomyomas and sarcomas. They discovered that the mean intratumoral RI and pulsatility index (PI) were significantly lower and the peak systolic velocity (PSV) was significantly higher in patients with leiomyosarcomas; however, there was a significant reduction of RI and PI and increased PSV with leiomyomas that were very large and had necrotic and/or degenerative and inflammatory changes.[5]

Technique and Protocol

In general, both a transabdominal and an endovaginal technique should be used. Give particular attention to the size and echotexture of the uterus and the adnexa for extrapelvic masses and free fluid. In the presence of a neoplasm, extend the sonographic examination to the liver and other abdominal visceral organs for possible metastases. Additionally, scan the para-aortic and para-caval areas to search for adenopathy.

OTHER IMAGING MODALITIES

Both CT and conventional MRI give useful information about the number of uterine tumors, as well as their size, exact location, and extent of degeneration; both are limited in their ability to distinguish benign from malignant neoplasms. Using MRI with a gadolinium-based contrast agent increases the likelihood of distinguishing a leiomyosarcoma from a degenerative fibroid. Goto et al. showed that specificity, positive predictive value, negative predictive value, and diagnostic accuracy of conventional MRI are 93%, 53%, 100%, and 93%, respectively; however, with gadolinium-based contrast MRI, this increases to 93%, 83%, 100%, and 95%, respectively.[2] Fluorodeoxyglucose-positron emission tomography (FDG-PET) has also been somewhat useful in the differentiation of leiomyosarcomas from other uterine masses (Fig. 9-9).[2]

DIFFERENTIAL DIAGNOSIS

The differential diagnosis includes degenerating leiomyomas (Fig. 9-10), other types of uterine sarcomas, endometrial adenocarcinoma, adenomyomas, or gastrointestinal and bladder carcinomas. Many times, the diagnosis of leiomyosarcoma is not made until surgery is performed; approximately 0.5% of women who have had routine hysterectomies for uterine fibroids actually have leiomyosarcomas.[3]

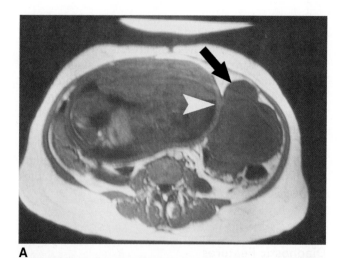

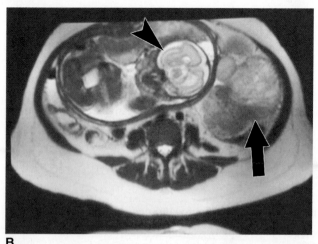

B

Figure 9-9 Myxoid leiomyosarcoma. **A:** T1-weighted axial image of pregnant patient with size greater than dates shows a lobulated intermediate signal intensity mass *(arrow)* adjacent to the uterus *(arrowhead)*. **B:** T2-weighted axial image shows mass *(arrow)* to have areas of high signal intensity. *Arrowhead* denotes fetal head. Resected specimen demonstrated invasion of surrounding fat by tumor.

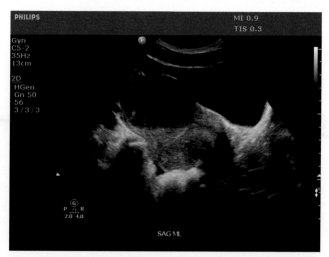

Figure 9-10 Degenerating leiomyoma. (Image courtesy of Derry Imaging Center, Derry NH Robin Davies, Ann Smith, and Denise Raney.)

FALLOPIAN TUBE CARCINOMA

CLINICAL INFORMATION

Epidemiology and Risk Factors

Fallopian tube carcinoma comprises less than 1% of all gynecologic malignancies. It is an aggressive tumor occurring most often in postmenopausal patients in the sixth decade. Of the fallopian tube carcinomas, metastatic tumors account for 85%, with the primary sites being the ovary, uterus, or gastrointestinal tract.[8,9] Other risk factors include infertility, nulliparity, low parity, pelvic inflammatory disease, and a family history of ovarian carcinoma.

Pathophysiology

Adenocarcinoma is the most common histologic type of primary fallopian tube carcinoma. An elevated CA-125 can be suggestive of a malignancy; however, an abnormal level can also be caused by myomas, endometriosis, adenomyosis, pregnancy, and pelvic inflammatory disease.[9]

Clinical Diagnosis

Clinical symptoms range from asymptomatic to abdominal pain and increased abdominal girth, abnormal vaginal bleeding, and a palpable pelvic mass; these tumors are usually small and hard to detect on a pelvic exam. A small percentage of women have a profuse watery discharge known as *hydrops tubae profluens*.[8] The tumor can involve the entire length of the tube; however, it is usually located in the distal wall or within the lumen. These tumors may also become pedunculated (Fig. 9-11).

Treatment

Surgical staging plus a total hysterectomy and bilateral salpingo-oophorectomy are the standard treatments, along with peritoneal biopsies and lymph node sampling. Radiation therapy and chemotherapy are also usually prescribed.

SONOGRAPHIC IMAGING

Diagnostic Features

High-frequency endovaginal sonography is valuable in evaluating abnormal adnexal masses. In the presence of an adnexal mass with solid or cystic components, suspicion should be raised for a potential malignancy, especially in postmenopausal women. The sonographic appearance of fallopian tube carcinoma is limited because of its rarity; however, this type of cancer can appear as an ill-defined or sausage-shaped adnexal mass with papillary projections. Sometimes, hydrosalpinx may be visualized because of tubal blockage (Fig. 9-12).

Technique and Protocol

A systematic sonographic examination of the pelvis should be performed, with special attention to the adnexa and uterus since this is the primary location of metastasis to the fallopian tubes. Endovaginal sonography

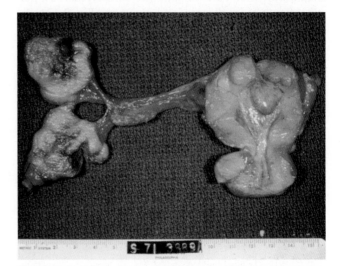

Figure 9-11 Fallopian tube carcinoma. The fallopian tube lumen and its wall have been replaced by tumor. (Scott JR, Gibbs RS, Karlan BY, et al. eds. *Danforth's Obstetrics and Gynecology*. 9th ed. Philadelphia, PA: Lippincott Williams & Wilkins; 2003.)

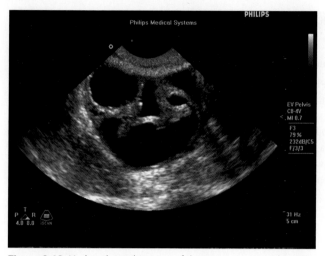

Figure 9-12 Hydrosalpinx, because of the many curves and turns in the fallopian tube, often images as a complex cystic mass. (Images courtesy of Philips Medical Systems, Bothell, WA.)

is excellent for showing tumor location and mass detail. If the sonographic findings in the pelvis suggest a neoplasm, the examination should be extended to the kidneys, liver, and other abdominal viscera for possible distal metastases. Document the presence of abdominal and pelvic ascites, hydronephrosis, and lymphadenopathy.

OTHER IMAGING MODALITIES

Since nearly 90% of fallopian tube carcinoma is metastatic, CT is useful in imaging the primary malignancy location and determining metastatic spread.

DIFFERENTIAL DIAGNOSIS

The differential diagnosis for this particular pathology includes ovarian carcinoma, other adnexal masses, pelvic inflammatory disease, and myomas. (Fig. 9-13)

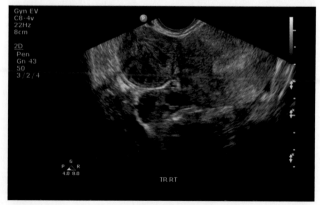

Figure 9-13 A pedunculated myoma anterior to the cystic ovary presents the appearance of a complex adnexal mass. (Image courtesy of Derry Imaging Center, Derry NH Robin Davies, Ann Smith, and Denise Raney.)

CARCINOMA OF THE CERVIX

CLINICAL INFORMATION

Epidemiology and Risk Factors

Cervical carcinoma is the second most common gynecologic malignancy in the United States and typically presents between the third and fourth decades. It is estimated that more than 11,150 women were diagnosed with this carcinoma in 2007, and approximately 3,670 women died from this disease.[4] The majority of noninvasive cervical cancers are asymptomatic and detected only by Pap smear. With invasive cancer, patients may also be asymptomatic but in general have a history of instrumental or postcoital bleeding.

The greatest risk factor for the development of cervical carcinoma is infection by human papillomavirus (HPV). There is evidence that infection by HPV has causal effect.[6] Other risk factors include early sexual activity, multiple sexual partners, low socioeconomic status, smoking, use of OCs, and a weakened immune system.[3] It is unclear if these other risk factors are independent or related to the HPV infection.[6] Cancer of the cervix develops at an earlier age in India, where early marriages are customary. Conversely, the disease is unknown among celibate women. In the United States, the disease is more prevalent among the Puerto Rican and African American populations and least common among Jewish women. This ethnic variation has led some authors to speculate on the possible significance of coitus with uncircumcised men. It has been suggested that secretions contained in the smegma of uncircumcised men constitute an irritant to the cervical mucosa that promotes cancer in susceptible women.[3]

Since the cervix is easily accessible to visual inspection and palpation during a gynecologic examination, there has been an increase in the diagnosis of carcinoma in situ. The availability of cytologic screening has also led to a reduction in mortality.

Women who were exposed to diethylstilbestrol in utero have a higher incidence of adenocarcinoma of the cervix and vagina. This drug was used during the 1940s and 1950s to support pregnancy for habitual aborters.

Pathophysiology

The cervical lining is composed of two types of cells. The lower cervix is covered with squamous epithelium, which gives rise to squamous cell carcinoma and accounts for 85% to 90% of lesions. The endocervix or cervical canal is lined with columnar epithelium, which gives rise to adenocarcinoma (10% to 15%). The junction between the two types of epithelium is called the *squamocolumnar junction*. Because this junction is the site of active mitotic activity, cervical cancer invariably arises here, initially as carcinoma in situ. The concept that has been proposed is that this site of mitotic activity is subject to transformation into

PATHOLOGY BOX 9-6

Cervical Cancer

Risk Factors	Signs/Symptoms	Sonographic Findings
Infection by HPV	Asymptomatic	Normal appearance in stage I and II
Early sexual activity	Postcoital bleeding	Hematometra with cervical stenosis
Multiple sexual partners	Superficial ulcerating mass on the cervix	Multiple cystic areas within a solid cervical mass
Low socioeconomic status		Bulky cervix
Smoking	Copious watery vaginal discharge	Irregular cervical borders
Use of OCs	Back pain	Mass extending from the cervix to pelvic sidewall
Weakened immune system	Bladder irritability	Tumor invasion of the bladder
Indian, Puerto Rican, or African descent	Ureteral obstruction	Hydronephrosis
	Uremia	Liver metastasis
Diethylstilbestrol in utero		Para-aortic nodes

neoplastic growth by exposure to external carcinogens. (Fig. 9-14)

Initially, the tumor is confined to the cervix and may form a superficial ulcerating mass with bulky expansion of the cervix. If untreated, the lesion spreads locally to the vagina, upper cervix, and parametrium, and may spread to neighboring structures such as the bladder and rectum.

Adenoma malignum is an extremely rare (3%) form of cervical adenocarcinoma. Also called *minimal deviation adenocarcinoma*, it is often associated with Peutz-Jeghers syndrome.[11] Multiple cystic areas are seen within a solid cervical mass. Copious watery vaginal discharge is associated with this pathology, and it is diagnosed only with deep biopsies of the cervix.

Even though histologically it is a well-differentiated lesion, it has very poor prognosis and response to therapy (Fig. 9-15).

Clinical Diagnosis

Cervical cancer occurs at a younger age than carcinoma of the endometrium. Carcinoma in situ is often diagnosed between the ages of 25 and 40 years. Typical presenting symptoms include abnormal vaginal discharge and bleeding, particularly after intercourse. Frequently, patients delay seeking medical attention after the onset of symptoms. In more advanced stages, symptoms include bladder irritability, low back pain from lumbosacral root involvement, and parametrial involvement. Unilateral or bilateral ureteral obstruction is invariably

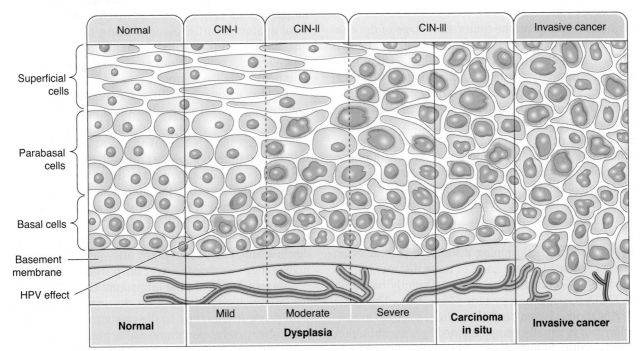

Figure 9-14 Development of dysplasia and carcinoma of the cervix. Repeated HPV infections convert normal epithelium **(left)** into increasingly severe dysplasia until malignant epithelium breaks through the basement membrane to become invasive cancer, capable of metastasis by invasion of blood vessels and lymphatics.

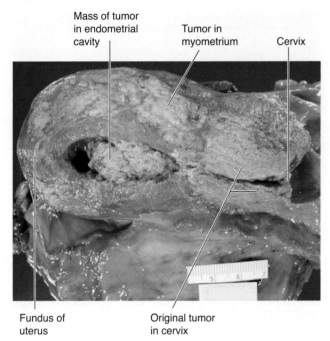

Mass of tumor in endometrial cavity

Tumor in myometrium

Cervix

Fundus of uterus

Original tumor in cervix

Figure 9-15 Invasive carcinoma of the cervix. Extensive involvement of the cervix, endometrium, and uterus is evident.

present in advanced disease, and the resultant uremia has been the most common cause of death from cervical carcinoma. Diagnosis in most of these cases is established through Pap smear or by cervical biopsy. The effective use of screening has caused a decline in incidence and mortality from invasive squamous cell carcinoma; however, there has been an increase in the incidence of adenocarcinoma.[6]

Treatment

Prognosis depends on the tumor size, stage of the cancer, and the patient's age. The type of treatment used is determined by the stage of disease. When fertility preservation is desired, patients with microinvasive cervical cancer can be treated with cone biopsy. Primary radiotherapy is another alternative for early macroinvasive disease. For patients whose disease involves the parametrium and pelvic lymph nodes, treatment is usually a combination of surgery, radiotherapy, and chemotherapy. Intracavitary radiotherapy involves placing radioactive material into the uterus and the vaginal fornices to deliver high-intensity focal radiation. Knowledge of the distance from the radiation source to sensitive adjacent organs such as the bladder is imperative, and sonography is useful in determining distances. The radiation dose is calculated on the basis of these distances.

Staging of cervical carcinoma is currently based on the FIGO classification system (Table 9-1). The FIGO classification is based on findings from physical examination and is usually complemented by a combination of colposcopy, biopsy, chest radiography, intravenous excretory urography, barium enema, cystoscopy, or proctosigmoidoscopy. Although studies have shown the value of cross-sectional imaging, it has not yet been included in the FIGO staging system. The FIGO staging system is being used to predict patient survival, but it has limitations. Studies have indicated a poor correlation between the clinical stage and surgical-pathologic findings. Errors in staging have been reported to be 30% for stage I tumors, 50% for stage II, and 75% for stage III. Part of the reason for these limitations is a failure to accurately estimate the tumor size and a failure to detect parametrial, pelvic sidewall, and bladder and rectal wall invasion, as well as other organ metastasis.[6]

SONOGRAPHIC IMAGING

Diagnostic Features

The cervix is typically of normal size and echogenicity in stage I and II of cervical carcinoma. Ultrasound may offer very little diagnostic information; however, if there is a cervical stenosis, hematometra may be noted. In more advanced stages of disease, endovaginal sonography may show a bulky cervix with irregular borders, possible extension into the vagina or peritoneum, a mass that extends from the cervix to pelvic sidewall, invasion of the bladder, hydronephrosis due to ureteral obstruction, metastasis to the liver, and para-aortic node formation (Fig. 9-16).[9] Sonography is very reliable in determining the size, shape, vascularity, and echotexture of the tumor.

Technique and Protocol

Translabial or transperineal sonography can be used along with an endovaginal approach to define the cervical anatomy. Partial bladder filling can also assist in visualization of the cervix. Positioning the patient with hips elevated helps to displace rectal gas and should also help visualize anatomy.

Bladder involvement in stage IV disease may be readily appreciated with ultrasound since fluid in the bladder provides a natural contrast. It is more difficult to determine rectal involvement and parametrial infiltration unless a bulky adnexal mass is present. Obstruction and dilatation of the distal ureter may mimic an ovarian cyst, but the identification of ipsilateral hydronephrosis will clarify this. Image the kidneys to exclude obstructive hydronephrosis, which would indicate stage III disease. Survey the retroperitoneal area to disclose any lymphadenopathy and—as with any pelvic malignancy—survey the liver for possible metastases.

Conventional real-time ultrasound is used as a guide for interventional procedures in managing patients with pelvic malignancy. In the presence of bilateral ureteral obstruction, percutaneous nephrostomy is often performed using ultrasound guidance. Cervical biopsies are also performed with ultrasound guidance.

TABLE 9-1

Summary of International Federation of Gynecology and Obstetrics (FIGO) Cervical Cancer Staging/Clinical Findings

Stage	Characteristics	
Stage 0 carcinoma in situ	*Confined to the cervix*	
Stage I confined to cervix	A: <5 mm invasion depth B: All other stage I	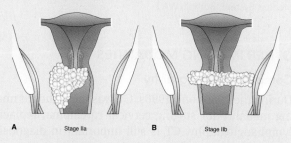
Stage II extends beyond cervix: upper two-thirds of vagina or parametrial tissue	A: No parametrial involvement B: Parametrial involvement	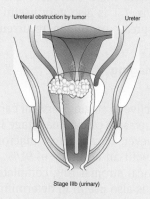
Stage III extends to pelvic wall or lower third of vagina or causes ureteral obstruction	A: No pelvic wall involvement B: Pelvic wall involvement or ureteral obstruction	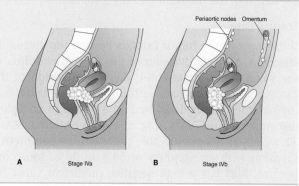
Stage IV extends beyond true pelvis or involves bladder or rectal mucosa	A: Spread to adjacent organs B: Spread outside pelvis	

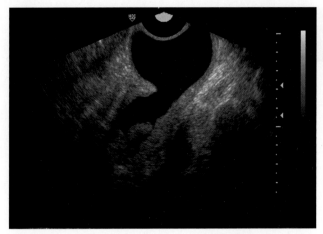

Figure 9-16 A complex-appearing cervical polyp raises the possibility of hematometra due to cervical cancer. (Image courtesy of Philips Medical System, Bothell, WA.)

OTHER IMAGING MODALITIES

Computed Tomography

During the 1980s and 1990s, CT was the standard imaging modality for staging cervical carcinoma, replacing lymphangiography. CT is still important in diagnosing when the size of the cervical mass exceeds 4 cm or is located in the endocervix. CT is also very useful in determining metastatic spread or tumor recurrence (Fig. 9-17).

Magnetic Resonance Imaging

Early Stage Disease

Overall, MRI is highly effective in staging cervical carcinoma. Detection of microinvasive carcinoma (stage IA) with MRI is limited; however, it can detect macroinvasive disease (stage IB) with an accuracy of 91%. In stage IB disease, the cervical stromal ring completely surrounds the tumor. MRI is also useful in determining the depth of the invasion into the stroma.[6]

Stage II Disease

With stage II, the tumor extends beyond the uterus. In stage IIA, there is invasion of the upper two-thirds of the vagina, and in stage IIB, there is extension of the carcinoma into the parametrium. This extension into the parametrium is diagnosed by a partial or complete disruption of the dark ring of cervical stroma. Axial T2-weighted images are able to determine parametrial invasion with an accuracy of 68% to 96%. More important, MRI has a high negative predictive value for parametrial invasion, ranging from 79% to 100%.[6]

Stage III Disease

Stage III is an invasion of the lower third of the vagina and pelvic sidewall. An important indicator of pelvic sidewall invasion is the presence of hydronephrosis. MRI's accuracy is approximately 95% in diagnosing stage III disease.[6]

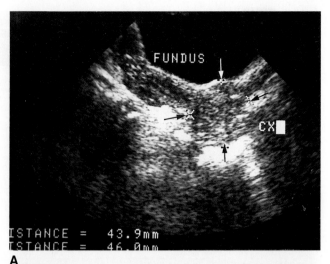

A

B

Figure 9-17 Cervical carcinoma. **A:** Longitudinal scan shows enlargement of the underlying cervix *(arrows)*. **B:** CT image shows the mass immediately behind the bladder *(large arrow)*. A small amount of gas is present within the mass *(small arrow)* secondary to necrosis. *CX*, cervix.

Stage IV Disease

Bladder and rectal invasion is an indication of stage IV cervical carcinoma. MRI is 96% accurate in making this diagnosis.[6] Tumor size has been shown to be significant in the patient's prognosis, and several studies have demonstrated that MRI is very accurate in assessing tumor size. MRI measurements are within 0.5 cm of surgical measurements in 70% to 90% of the cases (Fig. 9-18).[6]

DIFFERENTIAL DIAGNOSIS

When a bulky cervix is present on ultrasound, the main consideration is a leiomyoma involving the lower uterine segment. Sometimes, benign endometrial polyps can enlarge and prolapse into the cervical canal; this causes expansion of the cervix and changes in its acoustic texture. Occasionally, cancer of the endometrium may involve the cervix, causing bulky expansion.

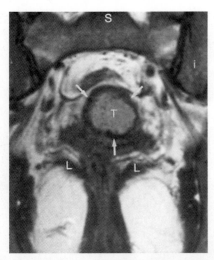

Figure 9-18 Cervical carcinoma without full-depth stromal invasion. Coronal T2-weighted image through the cervix demonstrates a thin, intact, low-signal-intensity rim *(arrows)*, representing residual cervical stroma surrounding the medium-signal-intensity tumor *(T)*, which expands the cervix. Identification of this intact rim has high predictive value for excluding invasion into the parametrial and paracervical areas. The sacrum *(S)*, iliac bones *(i)*, and levator ani muscles *(L)* are labeled for orientation.

GESTATIONAL TROPHOBLASTIC NEOPLASIA

CLINICAL INFORMATION

Epidemiology and Risk Factors

The term *gestational trophoblastic neoplasia* (GTN) is used to describe a group of uterine neoplasms that occur as a complication of pregnancy. These lesions include benign hydatidiform mole, invasive mole, choriocarcinoma, and placental site trophoblastic tumor (PSTT). This chapter focuses on the malignant end of the spectrum of GTN. This group of life-threatening diseases—termed *persistent trophoblastic neoplasia* (PTN)—includes invasive mole, choriocarcinoma, PSTT, and epithelioid trophoblastic tumor (a variant of PSTT).

PTN occurs most often with molar pregnancies. One-half of all complete molar pregnancies with very severe trophoblastic proliferation develop into persistent disease. The statistics are the same for complete mole with a coexisting fetus, since the diagnosis is probably delayed. Approximately 5% of cases of partial molar pregnancies turn into persistent disease. There have also been infrequent reports of PTN developing from a normal term delivery, spontaneous abortion, or ectopic pregnancy (Fig. 9-19).[6]

The normal genetic makeup of a fertilized ovum has 46 chromosomes, with 44 autosomes and two sex chromosomes. In the complete mole, the resulting karyotype is a 46,XX, which is derived through an abnormal sperm chromosome type. In effect, the sperm duplicates without the usual cell division in an ovum with either inactive or absent maternal chromosome material. This chromosomal makeup is considered a diploid karyotype and only occurs with 46,XX, as the 46,XY inheritance is incompatible with life. In a partial mole, the resulting karyotype is called a *triploid* because of the 69,XXX, 69,XYY, or 69,XXY pattern. This conceptus is the result of fertilization by more than one sperm. There is no association of the complete mole with triploidy as a result of maternal chromosomes (Fig. 9-20).[3]

Pathophysiology of Persistent Trophoblastic Neoplasia

Invasive Mole

Because the mechanisms that normally control trophoblastic tissue in a pregnancy are lost, there is extensive proliferation of trophoblastic tissue resulting in GTN. Invasive mole contains chorionic villi from a complete or partial mole that persists following uterine evacuation. This disease becomes clinically apparent with elevated human chorionic gonadotropin (hCG) and persistent heavy vaginal bleeding. Invasive mole is the most common form of PTN, accounting for approximately 80% to 95% of cases.[6] Located in the endometrium and myometrium, this focal invasion can, on rare occasions, penetrate through the myometrium and blood vessels, causing uterine rupture and potential death from severe intraperitoneal hemorrhage.

Choriocarcinoma

In contrast to invasive mole, choriocarcinoma has an absence of chorionic villi, possibly because of their rapid destruction by the malignant tissue. This type of PTN can occur after complete mole, partial mole, normal pregnancy, stillbirth, spontaneous abortion, or ectopic pregnancy. The occurrence of choriocarcinoma is 1,000-fold greater after a complete molar versus nonmolar pregnancy.[6] Choriocarcinoma metastasizes early, and nodules may be seen in the cervix and vagina. Invasion of blood vessels and embolization of trophoblastic tissue to the lungs may occur, which can obstruct the pulmonary venous circulation, causing right-sided heart failure or spread of tumor into the pulmonary arterial system (cor pulmonale). Embolization to the systemic circulation is not uncommon, accounting for tumor implants in brain, liver, and other organs. Therefore, women of reproductive age with unexplained acute cor pulmonale or intracerebral hemorrhage should raise suspicion of choriocarcinoma (Fig. 9-21).[6]

Placental Site Trophoblastic Tumor

PSTT differs from the other forms of PTN in several areas. First, it arises from nonvillus, "intermediate" trophoblast, which infiltrates the decidua, myometrium, and spiral arteries at the placental site. Second, the hCG level elevates mildly, making it an unreliable marker. Third, although it can occur with any type of gestation, it usually presents months or years after a term delivery. Though a less common occurrence

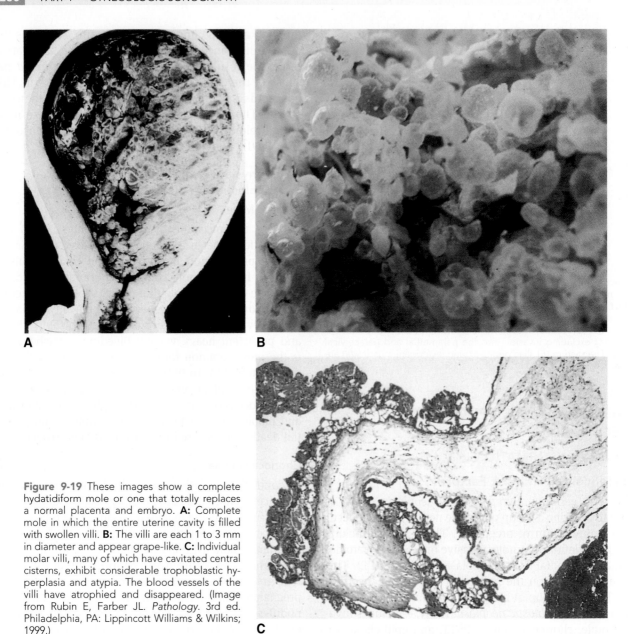

A

B

C

Figure 9-19 These images show a complete hydatidiform mole or one that totally replaces a normal placenta and embryo. **A:** Complete mole in which the entire uterine cavity is filled with swollen villi. **B:** The villi are each 1 to 3 mm in diameter and appear grape-like. **C:** Individual molar villi, many of which have cavitated central cisterns, exhibit considerable trophoblastic hyperplasia and atypia. The blood vessels of the villi have atrophied and disappeared. (Image from Rubin E, Farber JL. *Pathology*. 3rd ed. Philadelphia, PA: Lippincott Williams & Wilkins; 1999.)

than with choriocarcinoma, PSTT can metastasize to the ovary, perimetrium, rectum or bladder, and distal organs.

Epithelioid Trophoblastic Tumor

This is the most recently described and rarest type of PTN and is actually a variant of PSTT. It presents much later than other PTN, usually 6 to 7 years after the last term pregnancy.[6]

Effects on the Ovary

Theca-lutein cysts involving one or both ovaries are frequently observed with gestational trophoblastic disease. It has been suggested that these cysts may be the result of the high levels of the β subunit of human chorionic gonadotropin (β-hCG), a hormone similar to luteinizing hormone produced by the pituitary. Theca-lutein cysts may be seen in 25% of cases of trophoblastic disease. When they are present, they constitute an additional risk factor for the presence or development of postmolar trophoblastic disease.[3]

Clinical Diagnosis

Invasive mole is usually diagnosed after previous evacuation of a hydatidiform mole based on persistent vaginal bleeding and elevation of beta-hCG titers. If uterine perforation or intrauterine hemorrhage occur, the patient is likely to react with shock.

As with invasive mole, abnormal vaginal bleeding in conjunction with evacuated molar pregnancy is a common presenting symptom of choriocarcinoma. Other presenting symptoms include cough, hemoptysis,

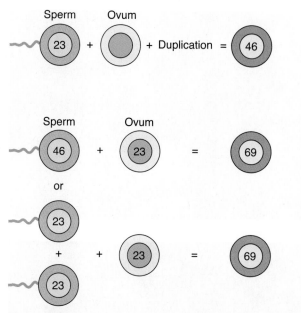

Figure 9-20 Chromosomal formation of gestational trophoblastic disease. **A:** Complete mole. **B:** Partial mole. (From Pillitteri A. *Maternal and Child Nursing.* 4th ed. Philadelphia, PA: Lippincott Williams & Wilkins; 2003.)

neurologic disturbances, or cerebral hemorrhage, which may be related to metastatic disease.

Patients with PSTT usually present with amenorrhea or irregular vaginal bleeding months or years after the last pregnancy. An enlarged uterus and mildly elevated hCG are also clinical symptoms. The clinical presentation of epithelioid trophoblastic tumor is similar to PSTT but occurs even later. In all of these pathologies, an enlarged uterus is present on pelvic examination.

Treatment

With low-risk patients, treatment is usually single-agent chemotherapy such as methotrexate with or without folinic acid. The overall survival rate with this treatment is nearly 100%. The cure rate for just methotrexate alone is approximately 70%; the remaining 30% who are resistant to methotrexate are treated with an additional second-agent or multiagent chemotherapy.

High-risk patients with PTN are treated with a multidrug chemotherapy that is administered around weekly EMA-CO (etoposide + methotrexate + actinomycin D + cyclophosphamide + ocovin) protocols.

In the past, there were various prognostic scoring systems for patients with GTN. In 2000, a more unified worldwide system was agreed upon. According to FIGO, the modified prognostic scoring system is expressed as a risk score. A number is assigned to each prognostic variable, and the risk score is expressed as a sum of these values. The low-risk score is 0 to 6, whereas the high-risk score is 7 and over. This score correlates with the risk of the tumor becoming resistant to single-agent chemotherapy.[13] Surgery is not typically used in the initial management of most PTN cases; however,

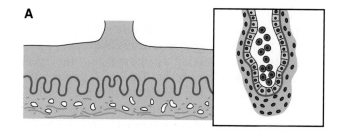

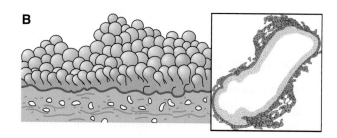

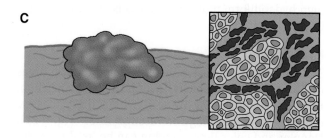

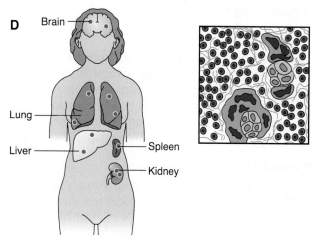

Figure 9-21 Proliferative disorders of the trophoblast. **A:** Normal chorionic villus of 8-week fetus, with blood vessel containing nucleated red blood cells. **B:** Complete hydatidiform mole with hydropic villi. The villi are enlarged by an edematous stroma devoid of blood vessels. The trophoblastic epithelium is hyperplastic and exhibits variable atypia. **C:** Choriocarcinoma, which has arisen in a molar pregnancy, invades the myometrium and consists of admixed syncytiotrophoblastic and cytotrophoblastic elements. **D:** Common sites of metastasis from choriocarcinoma. (Image from Rubin E, Farber JL. *Pathology.* 3rd ed. Philadelphia, PA: Lippincott Williams & Wilkins; 1999.)

it is the treatment of choice with PSTT and epithelioid trophoblastic tumors, which are very chemoresistant. For these patients, surgery is usually curative.

Patients are counseled to avoid pregnancy for 1 year after completion of treatment. This is to prevent the teratogenic risk from the chemotherapy and to eliminate confusion between recurrence of the disease and a new pregnancy. The risk of relapse is around 3% and is most likely to occur during the first year. At some treatment centers, life-long monitoring of hCG is done since it is unclear at this point when it is safe to stop surveillance.[13]

SONOGRAPHIC IMAGING

Diagnostic Features

Sonography is still the best imaging modality for assessing PTN since it is less expensive, well tolerated by patients, and reproducible with serial examinations. The ultrasound appearance of invasive mole or choriocarcinoma may be indistinguishable from that of benign hydatidiform mole. The uterus is usually enlarged in both conditions.

Invasive Mole

Sonographically, invasive mole appears as focal areas of increased echogenicity within the myometrium. Hypoechoic areas may be seen within these masses, representing hemorrhage or vascular lakes (Fig. 9-22). Doppler and color flow mapping can be used to evaluate the extent of the tumor and, therefore, its response to chemotherapy.

Choriocarcinoma

If confined to the uterus, the tumor appears as a focal, hemorrhagic nodule within the myometrium and possibly the endometrium. Since choriocarcinoma metastasizes quickly, secondary masses may be seen in the cervix or vagina. The liver is a common site of metastases, and it should be included in the sonographic evaluation.

Placental Site Trophoblastic Tumor

There are no specific distinguishing features to identify PSTT, but an irregular usually localized uterine mass in conjunction with the patient's clinical history can help with the diagnosis. If the tumor replaces the entire myometrium, it will appear as bulky uterine enlargement. The myometrium will have a heterogeneous, lobulated appearance. There may also be extension into the parametrium, pelvic sidewall, and adjacent organs.

There is marked hypervascularity associated with PTN because the uterine spiral arteries feed into prominent vascular spaces that communicate with draining veins. Abnormal blood flow demonstrates high PSV and low RI, indicating increased perfusion with low impedance to blood flow. PSV is greater than 50 cm/sec and many times is over 100 cm/sec. RI is typically less than

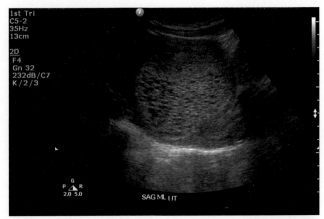

A

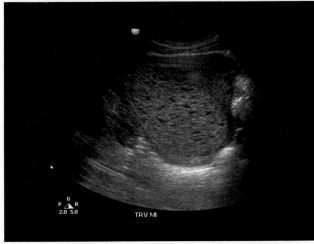

B

Figure 9-22 A: Sagittal endovaginal image of the uterus demonstrating the bulky uterus seen with an invasive mole. There is no evidence of an endometrial canal. **B:** Transverse view illustrates the cystic spaces filling the echogenic endometrium. (Images courtesy of Derry Imaging Center, Derry NH Robin Davies, Ann Smith, and Denise Raney.)

0.50 and many times is below 0.40. Normal myometrial flow, by contrast, has a PSV of less than 50 cm/sec and an RI in the range of 0.70.[2,3,5,12]

Color Doppler typical of PTN shows extensive color aliasing, admixture of color signals, loss of vessel discretion, and chaotic vessels patterns (Table 9-2).

Technique and Protocol

Endovaginal imaging is excellent for recording the small myometrial lesions typical with these disorders. A thorough examination to include the uterus and adjacent pelvic organs helps avoid a misdiagnosis. Power Doppler demonstrates PSV and RI.

OTHER IMAGING MODALITIES

MRI of the brain and pelvis, and CT of the chest and abdomen, are commonly used in patients that have been diagnosed with choriocarcinoma and PSTT, as well as in relapsed or drug-resistant cases (Fig. 9-23).

TABLE 9-2	
Sonographic Signs of Trophoblastic Disease	
Type	**Sonographic Appearance**
Invasive mole	Enlarged uterus
	Increased echogenicity within the endometrium
	Hypoechoic areas
	Presence of color/spectral Doppler
Choriocarcinoma	Enlarged uterus
	Focal, hemorrhagic nodule within the myometrium
	Masses in the cervix or vagina
	Liver metastases
PSTT	Few distinguishing features
	Irregular localized uterine mass
	Enlarged uterus
	Parametrium, pelvic sidewall, and adjacent organ extension hypervascularity

DIFFERENTIAL DIAGNOSIS

Sonographically, an early failed pregnancy with incomplete abortion and hydropic degeneration of the placenta could be mistaken for trophoblastic disease; however, in this condition, the β-hCG titer is likely to be low because there is an absence of trophoblastic proliferation and the function of this tissue is decreased or diminished. Retained products of conception or a degenerating uterine fibroid with areas of hemorrhage may also appear as numerous small cysts within an expanded uterine outline. Intramural fibroids undergoing degeneration may resemble

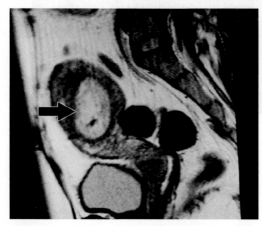

Figure 9-23 Gestational trophoblastic disease. Sagittal T2-weighted fast spin echo image through uterus in patient with abnormally elevated hCG level and abnormal endovaginal ultrasound. Nonspecific thickening of the endometrium is seen *(arrow)* without evidence of fetal development or gestational sac. Dilatation and curettage revealed complete molar pregnancy.

invasive molar tissue. The sonographic appearance of adenomyosis is also very similar to PTN. Certain ovarian tumors such as dermoids and cystic papillary adenomas may have a morphologic similarity to molar tissue; this source of confusion can be minimized if the uterus is identified. One of the strengths of endovaginal scanning is its ability to separate uterine from adnexal structures, thereby enhancing the value of the ultrasound examination.

SUMMARY

- Endometrial cancer is the most common gynecologic malignancy in developed countries.
- Risk factors for endometrial cancer include obesity, nulliparity, late menopause, adenomatous polyps, family history, race, age (60 to 70 years), the use of unopposed estrogen, HNPCC, breast cancer, and tamoxifen therapy.
- Sonographic signs for endometrial cancer include endometrial cysts, hydrometra or hematometra, uterine enlargement with lobular contour, mixed echogenicity in advanced disease stages, and increased vascularity of the endometrium.
- Leiomyosarcoma is a smooth muscle aggressive tumor of the uterus.
- The infiltrative leiomyosarcoma may or may not arise from a leiomyoma.
- Sonographic signs of a leiomyosarcoma include rapidly growing heterogeneous mass, possibly with degenerative changes, and posterior enhancement.
- Clinical signs for endometrial cancer and leiomyosarcomas are nonspecific, with the most common presentation being uterine bleeding, possibly with pain.
- Fallopian tube carcinoma clinical symptoms may be nonexistent or include abdominal pain, vaginal bleeding, and hydrops tubae profluens.
- Sonographic signs of fallopian tube carcinoma include an ill-defined solid or cystic sausage-shaped adnexal mass with possible hydrosalpinx.
- Treatment for endometrial cancer, leiomyosarcoma, or fallopian tube carcinoma is a total hysterectomy.
- Cervical cancer is the second most common gynecologic malignancy occurring in women aged 30 to 40 years.
- Risk factors for developing cervical cancer include HPV infection, early sexual activity, multiple sexual partners, low socioeconomic status, smoking, use of OCs, ethnicity, diethylstilbestrol exposure, and a weakened immune system.
- Clinical symptoms of cervical cancer include vaginal discharge, postcoital bleeding, bladder irritability, and low back pain.

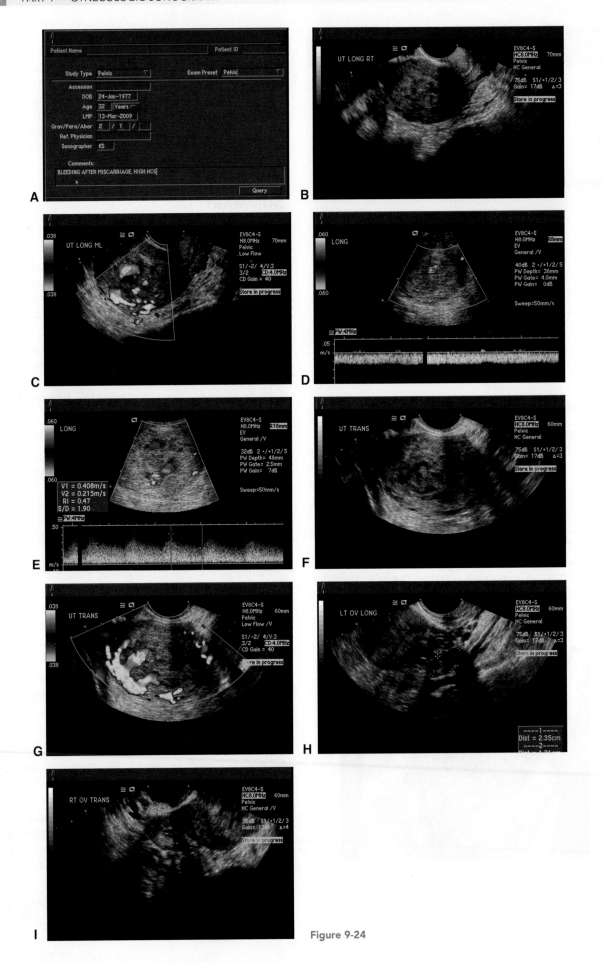

Figure 9-24

Critical Thinking Questions

Figure 9-24

1. After viewing the images, what is the probable differential diagnosis for the findings?

2. What transducer was used to image this patient?

3. How would the differential change if the patient was a 60-year-old postmenopausal woman with bleeding?

4. Contrast this endometrial pattern with findings seen in patients on tamoxifen therapy.

ANSWER 1: The patient history and images would raise suspicion for a molar pregnancy.

ANSWER 2: The transducer used to image this patient was an EV8C4-S, which is listed in the upper right of each image.

ANSWER 3: The differential would change to endometrial carcinoma.

ANSWER 4: Endometrial changes due to tamoxifen have a more cystic appearance; however, the molar pregnancy would share some common sonographic appearance. This is an example of the importance of a good patient history.

- Sonographic signs of cervical cancer in the early stages are nonspecific unless there is cervical stenosis, which results in hematometra. Advanced cancer images with a large cervix with irregular borders, possible extension into the vagina or peritoneum, mass extension from the cervix to pelvic sidewall, invasion of the bladder, hydronephrosis, liver metastasis, and para-aortic nodes.

- Treatment for cervical cancer depends on the stage and tumor size.

- GTN is a group of uterine neoplasms that occur as a complication of pregnancy and include benign hydatidiform mole, invasive mole, choriocarcinoma, and PSTT.

- Due to fertilization by more than one sperm, the triploid molar karyotype has a 69,XXX, 69,XYY, or 69,XXY chromosomal pattern.

- Invasive mole contains chorionic villi from a complete or partial mole that persists following uterine evacuation, whereas choriocarcinoma has an absence of chorionic villi, possibly because of their rapid destruction by the malignant tissue. In PSTT, the formation occurs via the nonvillous trophoblast infiltrating the decidua, myometrium, and spiral arteries. PTN is the late (6 to 7 years) development of trophoblastic disease.

- The invasive mole and choriocarcinoma present with a high hCG, but PSTT shows only a mild elevation.

- Theca-luteal cysts of the ovaries develop in 25% of the cases because of the high levels of β-hCG.

REFERENCES

1. Creasman W. Endometrial carcinoma. *eMedicine Web site.* http://emedicine.medscape.com/article/254083. Accessed: July 9, 2007.

2. Rumack C, Wilson S, Charboneau JW. *Diagnostic Ultrasound.* Vol 1. 3rd ed. St. Louis, MO: Mosby; 2005.

3. Callen P. *Ultrasonography in Obstetrics and Gynecology.* 5th ed. Philadelphia, PA: Saunders Elsevier; 2008.

4. Horner MJ, Ries LAG, Krapcho M, et al. *SEER Cancer Statistics Review, 1975–2006.* Bethesda, MD: National Cancer Institute. http://seer.cancer.gov/csr/1975_2006/. Based on November 2008 SEER data submission, posted to the SEER Web site, 2009.

5. Kupesic S. *Color Doppler and 3D Ultrasound in Gynecology, Infertility and Obstetrics.* 1st ed. New Delhi, India: Jaypee Brothers Medical Publishers (P) Ltd; 2003.

6. Reif, P. Uterine leiomyosarcoma mimicking benign submucosal leiomyoma. *J Diagn Med Sonogr.* 2007;23:368.

7. Harry VN, Narayansingh GV, Parkin DE. Uterine leiomyosarcomas: a review of the diagnostic and therapeutic pitfalls. *Obstet Gynaecol.* 2007;9:88–94.

8. Johnson, J. Fallopian tube cancer. *J Diagn Med Sonogr.* 2003;19:252.

9. Hagen-Ansert S. *Textbook of Diagnostic Ultrasonography.* Vol 2. 6th ed. St. Louis, MO: Mosby; 2006.

10. Shenavai F. Cervical carcinoma. *J Diagn Sonogr.* 2008;24:317–320.

11. Jones HW, Jones GS. *Novak's Textbook of Gynecology.* 11th ed. Baltimore, MD: Williams & Wilkins; 1988.

12. Sanders R, Winter T. *Clinical Sonography: A Practical Guide.* 4th ed. Baltimore, MD: Lippincott Williams & Wilkins; 2007.

13. Ngan S, Seckl M. Gestational trophoblastic neoplasia management: an update. *Curr Opin Oncol.* 2007;19:486–491.

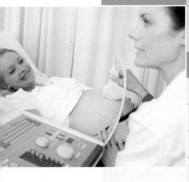

10 Malignant Diseases of the Ovary

Danielle M. Bolger

OBJECTIVES

Relate clinical signs, symptoms, and laboratory tests specific to ovarian cancer

Summarize diagnostic imaging diagnosis of ovarian malignancies

List the forms of ovarian carcinoma

Identify common risk factors for ovarian cancer

Describe the treatment and prognosis of ovarian cancer

KEY TERMS

serous/mucinous cystadenocarcinoma | serous carcinoma | mucinous cystadenoma | Krukenberg tumor | CA 125 | epithelial ovarian cancer | dysgerminoma | yolk cell tumor/endodermal sinus tumor | teratoma | endodermal sinus tumor | struma ovarii | clear cell adenocarcinoma | sex cord stromal tumors | Sertoli-Leydig cell tumors/androblastoma

GLOSSARY

Alpha fetoprotein (AFP) Used as a tumor marker for carcinomas of embryonic origin

BRCA1/BRCA2 Inherited gene mutation associated with a significant increase of breast and ovarian cancer risk

CA 125 Protein found in tumor cells that results in an elevation of blood levels

Carcinoembryonic antigen (CEA) Tumor marker for colon, stomach, breast, lung, some thyroid, and ovarian cancers

Clear cell adenocarcinoma Neoplasm involving the surface epithelium of the female reproductive organs (ovary), which involves cells with a clear appearance on microscopic examination

Dysgerminoma Malignant tumor of the ovary arising from undifferentiated germ cells of the embryonic gonad; histologically identical to seminoma found in the testicle

Endometrioid tumor Tumor of the ovary containing epithelial or stromal elements resembling endometrial tissue; typically arises from endometriosis; a large percentage are malignant

Epithelial ovarian cancer Neoplasm involving the surface epithelium of the ovary

HER2/neu Gene that produces a protein that rebulates normal cell growth found in breast and ovarian cancer cells; identification of this protein enables determination of treatment options

Krukenberg tumor Carcinoma of the ovary, usually metastatic from gastrointestinal cancer, marked by

areas of mucoid degeneration and by the presence of signet-ring cells

Lactate dehydrogenase (LDH) Enzyme involved in production of energy of the cells; elevated levels in the blood indicates tissue damage, cancers, or other diseases

Laparotomy Surgical incision into the abdomen usually performed to evaluate the organs

Meigs' syndrome Finding of pleural effusion, ascites, and an ovarian mass

Mucinous cystadenoma Cystic mass filled with thick gelatinous cystic fluid

Mucinous cystadenocarcinoma Large cystic ovarian mass with thick-walled septations; may have internal debris-layering components

Pseudomyxoma peritonei Accumulation of mucinous material in the peritoneal cavity, either because of rupture of a benign or malignant cystic neoplasm of the ovary or mucocele rupture of the appendix

Salpingo-oophorectomy Surgical removal of the ovary and fallopian tube

Serous carcinoma Type of epithelial ovarian cancer, which presents as a partially cystic mass with solid components

Serous cystadenocarcinoma Large multilocular ovarian neoplasm with papillary projections

Sertoli-Leydig cell tumors/androblastoma Related to the sex-cord (cordlike masses of gonadal epithelial tissue) stromal tumors seen in ovaries, mostly in young adults

Sex cord stromal tumors Solid ovarian mass originating from the embryonic gonadal ridges and Sertoli cells

Struma ovarii Extremely rare neoplasm of the ovary containing thyroid tissue

Teratoma/teratocarcinoma Rare malignant form of a common germ cell tumor found in young adults; contains fat, bone, hair, skin, and/or teeth

Yolk cell tumor/endodermal sinus tumor Neoplasm originating in the germ cells (ovum)

The sonographic examination has maintained an important role in the imaging of ovarian malignancy because of its utility in evaluating patients with a suspected pelvic mass. In a patient with a diagnosis of ovarian carcinoma, sonography helps determine the presence of recurrent or persistent disease after surgery and chemotherapy. Sonography, as a routine screening modality for the diagnosis of ovarian cancer in the general population, has not been successful or cost effective. The combination of sonographic screening in patients with elevated tumor markers or with a hereditary propensity for ovarian carcinoma is under active investigation and is proving to be of value.[1,2]

INCIDENCE AND PROGNOSIS

Ovarian malignancy is a disease of low prevalence, accounting for only 5% of all cancers in women.[3] However, it causes more deaths than any other cancer of the female reproductive system and is the fifth leading cause of cancer deaths among women, trailing cancer of the lung, breast, colon, and pancreas. The relatively high mortality of ovarian malignancy is a reflection of its low cure rate and late diagnosis. The American Cancer Society estimates that approximately 21,550 new cases are diagnosed each year in the United States.[3] Although mortality rates from other gynecologic malignancies are declining, there is evidence to suggest an increase in both the incidence and mortality rate of ovarian cancer.[4-9] Scandinavian countries and the United States have more cases of ovarian cancer than are reported in India and Japan.[6-8]

The poor prognosis of ovarian malignancy is in great measure related to late-stage diagnosis of the disease. In such cases, the overall 5-year survival rates are around 30% to 50%. The majority of ovarian cancer cases spread well beyond the ovaries before diagnosis occurs.

Stage I (confined to the ovary) ovarian cancer has few symptoms; however, the survival rate is over 90% with early detection.[3] Factors that determine the prognosis are (1) stage or extent of the disease when it is first diagnosed; (2) tumor grade (the histopathologic classification or the degree of cellular differentiation); (3) extent of residual disease after initial surgical excision; and (4) tumor response to types of treatment given.

Early detection of ovarian malignancy offers the most effective means of reducing the current high mortality rate. Research in a number of medical disciplines, including epidemiology, gynecologic oncology, and diagnostic imaging, has been directed toward this goal. Extensive epidemiologic studies have helped to define the population at risk.[3,11] Possibly, this data will help direct screening, making it economically feasible to target the at-risk populations despite the low prevalence of ovarian malignancy. Biochemical research has tried to develop immunologic studies to detect even a small population of malignant cells by means of tumor markers.[9,11-13] Finally, the ongoing improvement in imaging techniques has enabled the visualization of even minimal ovarian enlargement.

EPIDEMIOLOGY AND RISK FACTORS

Several studies in the epidemiology of ovarian cancer have shed some light on risk factors for this disease. Age is the major risk factor of incidence and mortality for the most common ovarian malignancies. Over 90% of sporadic ovarian cancer cases occur in women over 50.[14] Other risk factors include nulliparity or low parity, delayed childbearing, early onset of menses, late menopause, postmenopausal estrogen use for more than 10 years, and family history of ovarian or breast cancer.[15] A direct relationship has been observed between the number of years of ovulatory activity and the risk for development of epithelial ovarian cancer, the most common type. A woman whose ovulatory activity extends for more than 40 years is considered at high risk.[11] A reduction of ovulatory activity appears to be a protective influence against ovarian cancer development due to a decrease of the surface repeated trauma to the ovarian epithelium.[17] For example, oral contraceptives have been shown to reduce the risk of ovarian cancer.[10]

Ovarian cancer is similar to breast cancer in the fact that a strong family history (maternal or sibling) places a woman at a significantly higher risk, making genetics a criterion for screening studies.[2,9,18] The American College of Radiology (ACR) recommends that women in their early 20s with a positive family history for ovarian cancer consult specialists about their individual risk.[16] Also, several chromosomal deletions have been identified in patients with ovarian malignancy. For example, in carriers of a BRCA1 or BRCA2 gene mutation and a family history of breast or ovarian cancer, prophylactic bilateral oophorectomy by the age of 35 significantly reduces the patient cancer risk.[15] HER2/neu is another identified gene that regulates how cells reproduce and repair themselves. Though HER2/neu was initially linked to breast cancer, there is also an increased risk of developing ovarian cancers in individuals with this gene. This acquired mutation is due to errors in the replication process resulting in excess copies of the gene (overexpression). Uncontrolled division of cells results in development of a cancerous neoplasm.[61] Testing for HER2/neu is achieved through tissue sampling; the higher the levels, the greater the chance of spread.[62]

Numerous hereditary family cancer syndromes involve ovarian neoplasms (Table 10-1). Unaffected family members with hereditary breast/ovarian cancer syndrome have a risk factor of 82% by 70 years of age. Fortunately, only 3% to 7% of the population has a familial syndrome.[16]

Certain environmental factors have been linked to ovarian cancer risk. A three- to five-fold higher incidence of ovarian cancer and mortality has been observed in industrialized countries compared to developing nations.[5,11] Global variations have led epidemiologists to postulate that carcinogens in the air, water, or diet of industrialized communities play a role in the higher incidence of this disease.[8]

PATHOLOGY

HISTOLOGIC CLASSIFICATION

The pathology and pathophysiology of ovarian malignancy are extremely complex. The ovary has both endocrine and reproductive functions and is composed of at least four different cell populations, each of which may undergo malignant transformation. The World Health Organization (WHO) proposed a classification of ovarian tumors with nine broad categories of tumors based on the cell of origin.[56] Each of these categories divides histologically distinguishable lesions

TABLE 10-1	
Ovarian Neoplastic Syndromes[2,35,45,47,56–60]	
Syndrome	**Associated Neoplasms**
Gonadal dysgenesis (Kleinfelter/Turner)	Gonadoblastoma, dysgerminoma
Multiple nevoid basal cell carcinoma (NBCCS)	Ovarian fibroma
Peutz-Jeghers	Granulosa-theca cell tumor, breast, uterine
Hereditary site-specific ovarian cancer	Epithelial ovarian cancer
Hereditary breast/ovarian cancer	Breast and epithelial ovarian cancer
Lynch II (hereditary nonpolyposis colorectal cancer)	Colorectal, stomach, hetaptobiliary, urinary tract, brain, skin, endometrial, breast, and epithelial ovarian cancer

that may be benign, borderline malignant, or frankly malignant into numerical classifications. Different sections of one lesion may contain varying degrees of histologic differentiation. Whereas the most differentiated area of the lesion determines the cell type, the least differentiated portion determines its malignant potential. Tumor grading depends on the degree of cellular differentiation and represents an important criterion in assessing the severity of the disease and therefore its prognosis. Poorly differentiated cancers have a higher likelihood of aggressive growth, and occult metastases may be present even with a small primary lesion.

Tumors originating from the epithelium covering the ovaries and the serous, as well as mucinous cystadenocarcinomas, account for greater than 80% of ovarian malignancies. A much less common group of lesions are the gonadal stromal, or sex cord, neoplasms, some of which may be endocrinologically active and therefore may be diagnosed when smaller. The least common group is the germ cell neoplasms. Metastases to the ovary account for less than 10% of ovarian malignancies. Although the sonographic specificity for a particular histologic type of ovarian malignancy is poor, correlation of the clinical features and the sonographic appearance of the ovarian masses may lead to a more accurate diagnosis. Table 10-2 summarizes the pathologic, clinical, and sonographic features of the most common ovarian malignancies.

PATHOPHYSIOLOGY

A characteristic feature of most epithelial cancers is the tendency to form cystic masses with multiple septa (Fig. 10-1). The masses can be enormous, reaching 30 to 40 centimeters (cm) in diameter, weighing 10 to 15 kilograms (kg), and extending into the abdomen (Fig. 10-2). The cysts contain serous or mucinous fluid. Nodular or papillary growths may project into the cystic fluid or outward on the external surface of the cyst (Fig. 10-3). The tissue is typically friable, and thin-walled blood vessels of the lesion are predisposed to intracystic bleeding. Color Doppler analysis would help demonstrate prominent blood flow in the septations or solid tissue components with elevated diastolic flow

TABLE 10-2

Most Common Malignant Ovarian Neoplasms: Correlation of Clinical and Sonographic Findings[38,45,47,56–60]

Pathology (Frequency)	Clinical Features	Sonographic Findings
Epithelial (65–75%)		
Cystadenocarcinoma, serous (more common) or mucinous	Peri- and postmenopausal; abdominal pain; distention; gastrointestinal symptoms; increased abdominal girth, pelvic pressure	Large (10 to 30 cm), complex cysts with clear or echogenic fluid; multiple septa and papillations; unilocular or multiloculated; 25–60% are bilateral; ascites, tumor fixation, peritoneal implants; pseudomyxoma peritonei
Undifferentiated adenocarcinoma		Fixation; ascites common; echogenic ascites suggests pseudomyxoma peritonei
Endometrioid	May be associated with benign endometriosis and endometrial cancer	Mixed cystic and solid pattern due to hemorrhage or necrosis; 30% are bilateral; may be seen associated with endometrial echo abnormality; papillary projections
Clear cell carcinoma (CCC)	Variant of endometrioid; occurs after age 50; endometriosis	Bilateral; complex predominately cystic mass
Brenner's tumor	Rare; asymptomatic; associated with cystic neoplasm; paraendocrine hypercalcemia	~10% bilateral; hypoechoic; solid; wall calcifications
Germ Cell Neoplasms (15–20%)[a]		
Dysgerminoma	Often seen in adolescence; radiosensitive; may be cause of primary amenorrhea; elevated LDH, possible CA 125 elevation	Usually solid; homogeneous; variable in size; 10%–20% are bilateral; hyperechoic; may have cystic degeneration areas of necrosis and hemorrhage; irregular boundaries; color Doppler demonstrates fibrovascular septa with arterial flow
Immature and mature teratoma	Often seen in adolescence; possible AFP; CA 125, CEA, hCG, and LDH elevation	Solid mass with multiple small cysts; calcifications; unilateral; usually small; well-defined; variable echogenicity; may have cystic degeneration; may result in torsion
Struma ovarii	Teratoma composed of thyroid tissue; increased thyroid hormone levels without thyroid disease; age 50	Centralized flow with color Doppler imaging; solid; ascites
Choriocarcinoma	May cause precocious puberty; aggressive growth; elevated hCG; abdominal enlargement; pain; may develop hemoperitoneum; menstrual abnormalities	Variable consistency; large; unilateral
Teratocarcinoma	Rare tumor; often seen in young adulthood	Variable appearance with cystic and highly echogenic areas with acoustic shadow
Endodermal sinus tumor (Yolk sac tumor)	Often seen in adolescence; radiosensitive; may be cause of primary amenorrhea; AFP elevated; abdominal pain	Predominantly rapidly growing solid mass with areas of necrosis; unilateral; large (3–30 cm); lymphadenopathy
Metastases to Ovary (5–10%)		
Krukenberg tumor	Primary in gastrointestinal tract or from other sites: breast, lung, pancreas, lymphoma; pre- and postmenopausal; may be first manifestation of extraovarian malignant disease; search for gastrointestinal primary	Large masses; usually complex texture and bilateral; more common on right if unilateral; often indistinguishable from ovarian primary malignancy; ascites
Lymphoma		Bilateral; solid; hypoechoic
Sex Cord Stromal Tumors (5–10%)		
Granulosa-theca cell tumor	Wide age range; associated with hyperestrinism; vaginal bleeding due to endometrial hyperplasia or carcinoma; breast tenderness; precocious puberty; pain due to torsion; associated with endometrial and breast carcinoma; abdominal pain; hemoperitoneum due to rupture	Predominantly solid; unilateral; homogenous; may see endometrial thickening; size up to 40 cm; peritoneal metastasis common; Meigs' syndrome; cystic liver masses

TABLE 10-2 (continued)		
Most Common Malignant Ovarian Neoplasms: Correlation of Clinical and Sonographic Findings[38,45,47,56–60]		
Pathology (Frequency)	**Clinical Features**	**Sonographic Findings**
Androblastoma (Sertoli-Leydig cell tumor)	Common in adolescence; may have masculinizing effect; may have elevated AFP	Usually solid; unilateral; hypoechoic; small
Arrhenoblastoma	Infertility; amenorrhea; may have masculinizing effect; ache; hirsutism; high serum testosterone levels	Solid; cystic areas; lobulated; unilateral; well encapsulated; size up to 30 cm

[a]Includes transdermal sinus tumor, malignant mixed germ cell tumor, choriocarcinoma, and embryonal carcinoma.
AFP, alpha fetoprotein; CEA, carcionoembryonic antigen; hCG, human chorionic gonadotropin; LDH, lactate dehydrogenase

(Fig. 10-4). Areas of the lesion lacking adequate blood supply may suffer necrosis. Bleeding and necrosis add to the fluid content of the lesion, therefore increasing the ultrasound echogenicity of the fluid. Dystrophic calcification often occurs within areas of cellular degeneration. Radiographs demonstrate these microcrystals, or psammoma bodies. The epithelial tumors that do not secrete fluid are usually smaller but may still have irregular fluid collections within them secondary to hemorrhage and necrosis.

Associated ascites often occurs with ovarian malignancy. Sixty to seventy percent of postmortem examinations find the typically high protein ascetic fluid in the abdomen. Protein-rich fluid exudes from the tumor-bearing surfaces of the peritoneum because the vessels are more permeable to protein.[20] Fluid accumulates first in the dependent portion of the peritoneal cavity, such as the pelvic cul-de-sac. Subsequently, the fluid ascends into both paracolic gutters but predominantly on the right side because this space is broader and forms a better communication between the right upper quadrant and the pelvis (Fig. 10-5).

When spontaneous leakage or rupture of a mucinous cystadenocarcinoma occurs, the peritoneal cavity is flooded with sticky, gelatinous fluid, leading to massive abdominal distention, a condition known as pseudomyxoma peritonei. Rupture of a mucinous neoplasm of the appendix (most often malignant) is also a cause of this condition.

SPREAD AND STAGING OF OVARIAN MALIGNANCY

The major patterns of spread of ovarian malignancy are direct extension to involve neighboring organs in the pelvis, peritoneal seeding, and lymphatic spread. Ovarian cancer is the most common tumor responsible for peritoneal malignancy in women. Intraperitoneal dissemination occurs when tumor cells are shed from the lesion and establish growth on peritoneal surfaces within the abdomen, particularly the diaphragmatic leaflets, liver capsule, bowel serosa, and omentum. This occurs relatively early in the disease and is often, but not always, associated with ascites. There are several pathways for the lymphatic spread of tumor cells: peritoneal lymphatics draining toward the diaphragm and pelvic lymphatics draining to the retroperitoneum. The pattern of spread of ovarian tumor is not predictable. Because

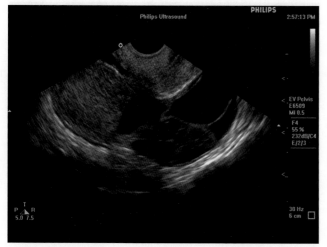

Figure 10-1 This endovaginal image demonstrates the multiple septations seen with ovarian malignancy. (Image courtesy of Philips Medical Systems, Bothell, WA.)

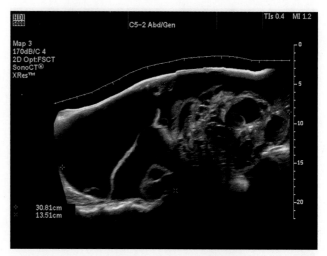

Figure 10-2 Imaging of a large, in this case a 30 × 13 cm, complex mass extending out of the pelvis, probably of ovarian origin. (Image courtesy of Philips Medical Systems, Bothell, WA.)

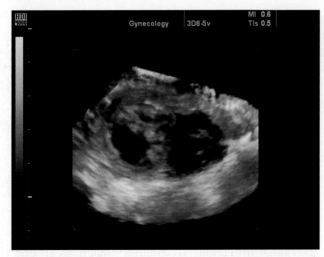

Figure 10-3 This 3D reconstruction of the internal architecture of the ovarian cyst reveals growth of internal projections extending from the cyst wall. (Image courtesy of Philips Medical Systems, Bothell, WA.)

the diaphragmatic lymphatics are the major pathways of peritoneal fluid drainage, blockage of this pathway by tumor may also produce ascites. The diaphragmatic lymphatics that drain to the retrosternal and mediastinal nodes constitute a major avenue for spread of the disease to the chest.

Positive vaginal cytology is due to advanced cases of ovarian malignancy, antegrade spread, or distal migration of tumor cells to the uterus. Frequently, distant metastases occur in the liver (Fig. 10-6). Sonographically, these lesions may have a complex cystic appearance, reflecting the presence of fluid and mucin within them.

The extent of tumor spread or stage of disease at time of diagnosis is an important parameter in determining the patient's clinical course. Staging schemes proposed by the International Federation of Gynecologists and Obstetricians (FIGO) and the American Joint

Committee on Cancer (AJCC) are widely accepted (Table 10-3). The stage of disease is determined at the time of laparotomy. Imaging techniques such as computed tomography (CT), magnetic resonance imaging (MRI), and ultrasound add further information to increase the accuracy of staging (Fig. 10-7).[21-25]

CLINICAL CONSIDERATIONS

SYMPTOMS

Ovarian carcinoma is mainly a disease of perimenopausal and postmenopausal women; mean age at diagnosis is 52 years. The often insidious or vague symptoms of ovarian cancer contribute to delays in diagnosis. Patient complaints of pressure from an enlarging pelvic mass or from accumulation of ascites result in any related symptoms. Less frequently, manifestation of hormone activity (feminizing or masculinizing symptoms) provides clues to the presence of a lesion. Rarely, the diagnosis is made only when the tumor undergoes torsion and the patient presents with an acute abdomen, requiring surgical intervention.

An analysis of clinical studies from the literature disclosed that 95% of women with ovarian cancer reported symptoms prior to diagnosis, the most common being abdominal bloating (77%), followed by complaints of abdominal pain (58%).[26] The mass may produce backache, pelvic pressure, or simply a vague feeling of pelvic discomfort. The pressure from mass and ascites accounts for the urinary symptoms of urgency and frequency seen in 34% of patients. Despite increases in abdominal girth, some patients may experience true weight loss. Such complaints are often treated symptomatically, diverting attention from the pelvis and delaying diagnosis. Undiagnosed, persistent gastrointestinal symptoms in women older than 40 years of age should prompt a search for an ovarian lesion.

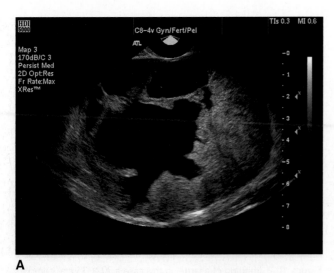

A

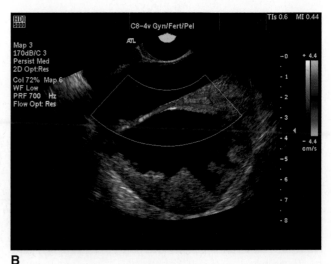

B

Figure 10-4 A: A multiseptated cyst with projections into complex-appearing fluid is a sign of an ovarian malignancy. **B:** Color Doppler imaging reveals flow in the membrane separating the complex cystic areas. (Images courtesy of Philips Medical Systems, Bothell, WA.)

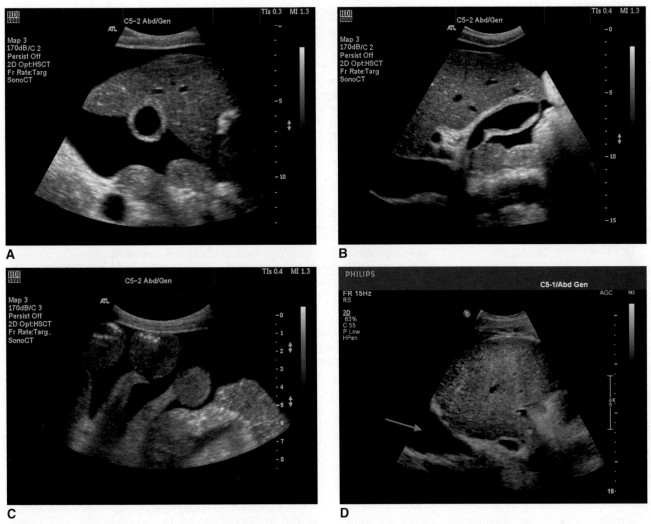

Figure 10-5 Meigs' syndrome is the combination of ascites, pleural effusion, and an ovarian neoplasm. A transverse **(A)** and longitudinal **(B)** image of the right upper quadrant demonstrates the typical appearance of ascites. Bowel floats within the ascetic fluid **(C)** and should not be mistaken for abdominal wall seeding of malignancy. **D:** Pleural fluid *(arrow)*. (Images courtesy of Philips Medical Systems, Bothell, WA.)

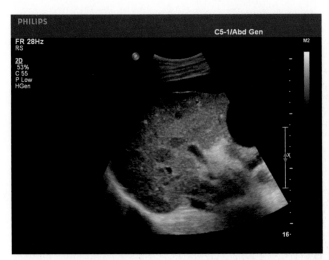

Figure 10-6 This image of the liver demonstrates the typical hypoechoic appearance of metastasis. Note the anechoic ascites seen in the anterior portion of the image. (Image courtesy of Philips Medical Systems, Bothell, WA.)

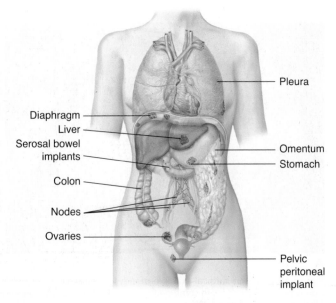

Figure 10-7 Likely metastatic sites for ovarian cancer.

TABLE 10-3		
Staging System for Ovarian Cancer[35, 36, 63]		
FIGO Stage	**TNM Stage**	**Extent of Disease**
	TX	Unable to assess primary tumor
	T0	Primary tumor not seen
I	T1	Growth limited to the ovaries
IA	T1a, N0, M0	Limited to one ovary, capsule intact and free of tumor, no ascites, negative peritoneal cytology
IB	T1b, N0, M0	Neoplasms found in both ovaries, capsule intact and free of tumor, no ascites, negative peritoneal cytology
IC	T1c, N0, M0	Masses are either IA or IB; however the tumor extends outside the ovarian capsule to the surface, ascites, positive peritoneal cytology
II	T2	Growth beyond ovaries but limited to the pelvis
IIA	T2a, N0, M0	Extension or implants to uterus/tubes, no ascites, negative peritoneal cytology
IIB	T2b, N0, M0	Extension to other pelvic structures, including uterus, no ascites, negative peritoneal cytology
IIC	T2c, N0, M0	Pelvic extension or implants similar to IIA or IIB, ascites, positive peritoneal cytology
III	T3	Growth beyond the pelvis; retroperitoneal or inguinal nodes or intraperitoneal omental implants; superficial liver metastases
IIIA	T3a, N0, M0	Negative nodes, histologically confirmed microscopic seeding of abdominal peritoneal surfaces
IIIB	T3b, N0, M0	Same as IIIA with abdominal peritoneal implants <2 cm diameter, negative nodes
IIIC	T3c, N0, M0 or T3c, N1, M0	Same as IIIA with abdominal peritoneal implants >2 cm diameter or positive pelvic, retroperitoneal, or inguinal nodes
IV	T(any), N(any), M1	Distant metastases or pleural involvement; liver parenchymal metastases

T, tumor size; N, spread to nodes; M, metastasis

A significant number of patients with ovarian malignancy present with or develop vaginal bleeding. Bleeding may be secondary to estrogen secretion by the lesion, concurrent endometrial and ovarian carcinoma, or, rarely, direct spread of the lesion to the endometrium. Frequently, the cause of bleeding is undetermined.

Symptoms of abnormal endocrine activity are sometimes a clue to the presence of an ovarian malignancy that is hormonally active or stimulates the normal ovarian tissue to increased hormone production. Feminizing effects due to overproduction of estrogen by a granulosa cell tumor are often associated with vaginal bleeding in the postmenopausal patient. In young girls, a rare cause of primary amenorrhea is dysgerminoma, which is the counterpart of, and histopathologically resembles, the seminoma of the testis (Fig. 10-8). A lesion that often produces defeminizing or masculinizing effects is the arrhenoblastoma or Sertoli-Leydig cell tumor. This lesion occurs in adolescents or young women and is often solid. Other endocrine-like effects, such as Cushing's syndrome, hypoglycemia, hypercalcemia, and hyperthyroidism, may present in association with

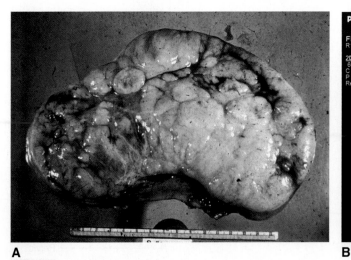

A

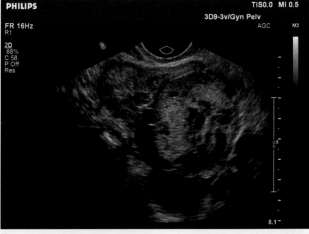

B

Figure 10-8 A: This surgical example of a dysgerminoma shows that it is a solid tumor with a gray, fleshy, and lobulated cut surface. The lesion is principally solid with some cystic areas. **B:** The possible sonographic appearance of the same type of mass. (Image courtesy of Philips Medical Systems, Bothell, WA.)

ovarian malignancy. One consequence of hormonal activity by the ovarian lesion is the possibility of earlier diagnosis. Abnormal hormonal activity is nondiagnostic of ovarian malignancy, as a variety of benign ovarian neoplasms manifest similar abnormalities.

Any mass may undergo sudden compromise of its blood supply as a result of torsion or incarceration. Such an event is likely to produce acute abdominal symptoms that mimic inflammatory disease. In the pediatric age group, ovarian malignancy is likely to present as a pelvic or abdominal mass, with or without torsion. Torsion of any ovarian mass is also more likely to occur in the second or third trimester of pregnancy because of uterine enlargement and the change in position of the ovarian pedicle.[11]

TREATMENT

Early detection of ovarian cancer results in a cure rate of more than 90% with conventional treatment. However, only 25% of ovarian cancers are diagnosed in stage I.[27] Treatment options include surgery, radiation therapy, and chemotherapy.[28] Surgical planning and management begins with appropriate surgical staging and histologic confirmation of the specimen. An attempt to remove the bulk of the tumor (debulking) helps to minimize residual disease and enhance the effectiveness of radiation and chemotherapy. Surgical treatment usually includes bilateral salpingo-oophorectomy, total hysterectomy, and omentectomy. In young women with stage I disease, removal of the involved ovary helps preserve fertility. The diagnosis of stage II or stage IV results in a cyclic course of chemotherapy often paired with radiation therapy. To determine the presence or absence of residual disease and to plan possible further treatment, the clinician may recommend a repeat laparotomy.

LABORATORY TESTS

Laboratory detection of malignancies, including ovarian carcinoma, searches for telltale substances in the serum or plasma of patients who harbor a malignancy.[11] Cancer cells, or the patient's immune system, produces substances, which may be proteins, hormones, or enzymes. These substances have been termed "tumor markers."

Ovarian carcinoma results in significant elevations of certain tumor markers; however, none is unique to the ovary or sensitive enough for use as a screening test. However, in a patient with a known pelvic mass, certain laboratory tests may be helpful in the diagnosis. For example, some assays, such as CA 125 tumor-associated antigen, utilized clinically as a marker of disease status, help in the diagnosis of recurrent ovarian cancer through periodic monitoring.[29] A decreasing level indicates effective therapy, whereas an increasing level indicates tumor recurrence. CA 125 is a cell surface glycoprotein present in 80% of ovarian epithelial cancers.[36] It can be used in combination with two other newly identified markers, CA 72-4 and CA 15-3. A simultaneous elevated level of these antigens is predictive of malignant disease in a majority of cases.[11,12] However, as a screening tool, the sensitivity of CA 125 in detection of early ovarian cancer is low, and a normal antigen level (<35 U/ml) does not necessarily exclude the presence of disease.[16,29,36,41]

Epithelial ovarian cancer results in an elevated CA 125; however, benign processes such as endometriosis, fibroids, and even pancreatitis also result in an increase.[36,38,47,60] Due to this lack of specificity, other values help in diagnosing an ovarian neoplasm, such as an alpha fetoprotein (AFP), carcinoembryonic antigen (CEA), human chorionic gonadotropin (hCG), and lactate dehydrogenase (LDH). Used in conjunction with the CA 125, gray-scale and color Doppler sonography lesion diagnosis and specificity increase.[35,36,38,41,47,58] In addition to helping in diagnosis, serial monitoring after intervention provides an indication of tumor resolution and reoccurrence.[38,57] Table 10-2 outlines which lab values elevate with each ovarian neoplasm.

IMAGING DIAGNOSIS

CONVENTIONAL RADIOLOGY

A plain radiograph of the pelvis often provides important information about the abdomen contents, as does a barium enema study. The principal value of a radiograph of the abdomen, the simplest and least expensive radiographic examination, is that it detects calcifications and abnormal soft tissue masses in patients with abdominal distention. The most common ovarian lesion, serous cystadenoma, and its malignant counterpart, cystadenocarcinoma, may contain fine, granular calcifications that may coalesce to form cloud-like aggregates. The primary lesions, as well as their metastatic deposits, of the cystadenoma or cystadenocarcinoma demonstrate calcifications in approximately 12% of cases (Fig. 10-9). Mucinous cystadenocarcinoma and pseudomyxoma peritonei may develop curvilinear calcifications (Fig. 10-10). A wide range of plain film densities, sometimes quite specific, may be present in cystic teratomas, including their far less common malignant counterpart, the teratocarcinoma. These include teeth, bone, and fat. Malignant teratomas in adolescents or very elderly patients may contain areas of coarse calcification (Fig. 10-11).

A chest radiograph, used routinely to screen for pulmonary metastases, and barium enemas maintain a significant role in patients with suspected ovarian malignancy (Fig. 10-12). Images demonstrate extrinsic displacement or encasement of the colon, or abnormalities of contour, that raise the suspicion of serosal

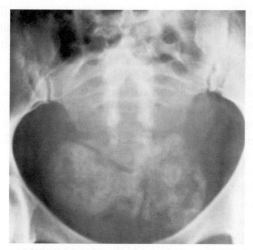

Figure 10-9 Calcified cystadenocarcinoma of the ovary images as a diffuse, ill-defined collection of granular amorphous calcification on this pelvic radiograph.

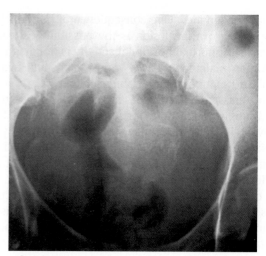

Figure 10-10 One complication of spontaneous rupture of pseudomucinous carcinoma of the ovary is the development of pseudomyxoma peritonei as seen on this pelvic radiograph.

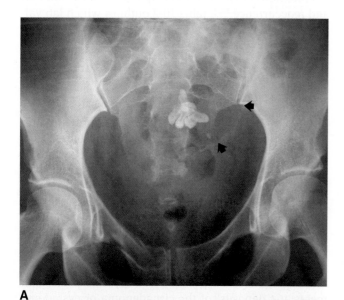

A

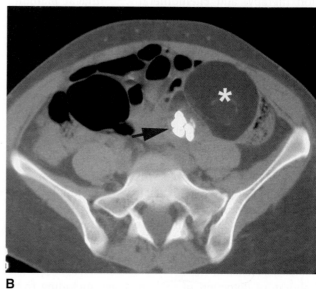

B

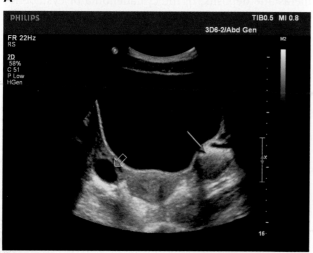

C

Figure 10-11 A: Radiographic detail view of the pelvis showing a lucent mass *(arrows)* on the left containing malformed teeth often imaged with an ovarian teratoma (dermoid). **B:** CT image shows the tumor with varying fatty *(star)* and dental *(arrow)* components. **C:** A transabdominal transverse sonogram of the pelvis. Compare the right-sided simple cyst *(open arrow)* to the dermoid *(arrow)* on the left.

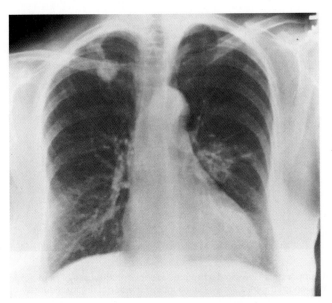

Figure 10-12 This chest radiograph demonstrates the typical appearance of a patient with metastasis from a pelvic cancer. In this case, the bilateral metastasis is from endometrial carcinoma. The well-circumscribed mass in the right upper lobe has the expected radiographic appearance of a metastasis.

involvement. In addition, the barium enema may demonstrate a primary colonic malignancy, which may be coincidental to the ovarian primary or the source from which metastases to the ovary have spread.

COMPUTED TOMOGRAPHY

Specific strengths of the CT examination include the demonstration of pelvic sidewall masses, lymph node enlargement in the retroperitoneum, liver metastases, and calcifications (Fig. 10-13 and 10-14).[30,36] It is not usually indicated in the evaluation of adnexal masses because of poor soft tissue discrimination and the hazards of ionizing radiation.[16]

When intravenous and oral contrast are given, the CT examination provides accurate anatomic information about the urinary tract, the opacified portions of the gastrointestinal tract, and the presence of ascites, in addition to demonstrating the location of the actual mass. CT allows visualization of deep and subcapsular liver metastases that may be difficult or impossible to detect at surgery. Although an exploratory laparotomy remains the gold standard, a CT scan is most helpful as a means of staging the disease. CT may also be useful in determining initial operability.[31,32,36] The scan may show extensive unresectable tumor, thereby preventing unnecessary surgery.[33,36] CT allows for postoperative evaluation for residual disease; after chemotherapy, it is a valuable resource to assess for the response to treatment.

MAGNETIC RESONANCE IMAGING

MRI of adnexal masses offers refinements in tissue characterization over CT and ultrasound.[24,34] Using various parameters, signal intensities can be noted, suggesting fat or blood aiding in the characterization of complex adnexal masses. The addition of intravenous gadolinium to enhance areas of pathology improves the accuracy of diagnosis as well.

Although it is more expensive, MRI has the capability of multiplanar imaging and, together with the good spatial resolution of pelvic anatomy, makes this a choice method for determining the origin of a pelvic mass, regarding its extent and relationship to adjacent structures. MRI with fat-saturation technique is the next step in the imaging workup of any endovaginal sonographic results suspicious of malignancy. The MRI findings most predictive of malignancy are papillary

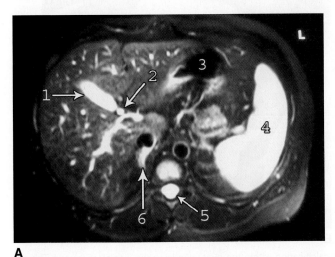

A

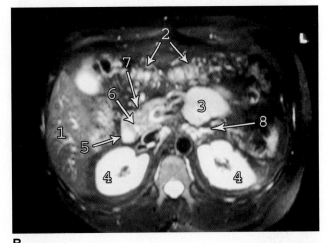

B

Figure 10-13 Axial fat-suppressed T2-weighted anatomy of abdomen. **A:** *1*, gallbladder; *2*, common hepatic duct; *3*, stomach; *4*, spleen; *5*, spinal canal; *6*, right adrenal gland. **B:** *1*, caudal right lobe liver; *2*, transverse colon; *3*, small bowel; *4*, kidneys; *5*, duodenum; *6*, common bile duct; *7*, pancreas; *8*, left adrenal gland. *(continued)*

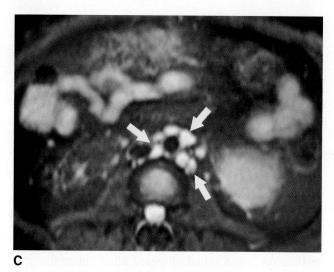

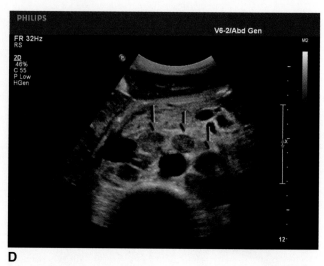

Figure 10-13 *(contniued)* **C:** Lymph nodes are typically very bright on fat-suppressed T2-weighted images as shown in this case of para-aortic lymphadenopathy *(arrows)*. **D:** A transverse sonographic image of lymphadenopathy *(red arrows)* surrounding the aorta. (Image courtesy of Philips Medical Systems, Bothell, WA.)

projections protruding in a cystic tumor and necrosis in a solid tumor (Fig. 10-15).[16] If MRI findings confirm a cystic teratoma or endometrial cyst, further diagnostic procedures may be unnecessary. In all other cases, surgical intervention, such as a laparoscopy, must be considered.[29]

POSITRON EMISSION TOMOGRAPHY

Positron emission tomography (PET) is a tagged radionuclide study used primarily to detect occult or recurrent ovarian malignancy. Some results have been promising, suggesting that it is more sensitive than either CA 125 assay or CT scan in diagnosing recurrence.[35,36] PET

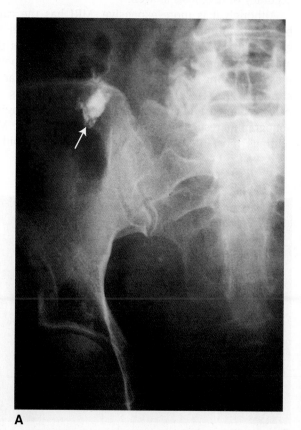

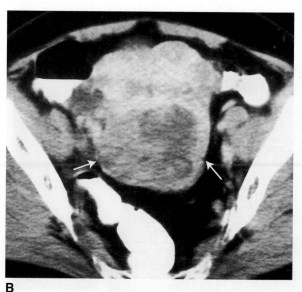

Figure 10-14 Carcinoma of the ovary. **A:** AP pelvis. Note the irregular calcification within the ovary overlying the iliac crest *(arrow)*. The absence of bowel gas centrally overlying the sacrum is caused by a soft tissue mass displacing the gas superiorly. **B:** Axial abdominal CT *(arrows)*. COMMENT: Ultrasound is the modality of choice for the early detection of ovarian masses. CT studies are usually reserved for staging and assessing the therapeutic progress.

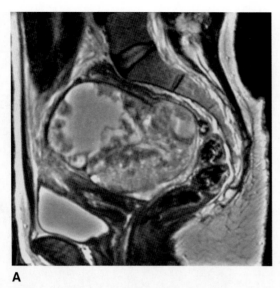
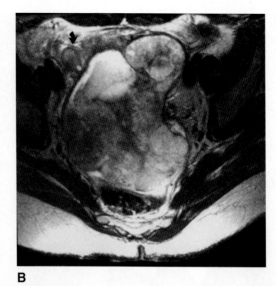

A   B

Figure 10-15 Carcinoma of the ovary. **A:** Sagittal T2-weighted image shows a large cystic and solid mass located above the uterus and anterior to the rectum. Note that the mass does not seem to be arising from either of these structures. **B:** T2-weighted axial image demonstrates the extensive solid components of the mass. Again, the mass does not appear to arise from the rectum and it obliterates the left ovary. Note that the right ovary shows no evidence of tumor (arrow).

scans have shown a diagnostic accuracy of 76%. Because an onsite cyclotron is required for tagging, cost currently precludes its routine use. In addition, physiologic bowel activity may be associated with increased uptake, making it difficult to differentiate bowel loops from adnexal structures. Thus, the usefulness of a PET scan in the preoperative determination of an ovarian lesion's potential for malignancy is limited and appears unsuitable as a routine diagnostic procedure. It should only be used in a select group of patients in whom both ultrasound and MRI have failed to yield unequivocal results (Fig. 10-16).[29]

SONOGRAPHY

Screening for Ovarian Malignancy

Utilization of gray-scale sonography is the most common imaging modality used to separate benign from malignant ovarian disease.[36] Endovaginal sonography is able to image regression in ovarian size, as well as changes in texture and surface characteristics occurring in the premenopausal period. Ovarian dimensions change from approximately 3.5 × 2 × 1.5 cm to 2 × 1 × 0.5 cm, making the ovary impalpable during a pelvic exam in 70% of women.[23] Diminished blood supply and absence of folliculogenesis produce a wrinkled surface and a change in texture. Absence of this normal regression 3 to 5 years after menopause may be considered pathologic and requires prompt investigation. Only women supplementing with hormone replacement therapy (HRT) continue to have normal-sized ovaries. The most promising means of influencing the prognosis of ovarian cancer patients is via endovaginal ultrasound in early detection of adnexal masses.

Endovaginal sonography remains the diagnostic method of choice as a screening technique for ovarian processes. Ultrasound is a safe, well-tolerated examination and can help narrow the differential diagnosis, although it cannot always distinguish a malignant from a benign process.

Ultrasound screening of the normal population of postmenopausal women for ovarian carcinoma has not developed into a successful or cost-effective undertaking, even though a sonogram is a more sensitive tool than the physical examination in measuring ovarian volume and size.[36,40,45] In a genetically high-risk population, an approach that combines tumor markers (i.e., CA 125) with a pelvic ultrasound, including color flow Doppler analysis, and the physical examination is being investigated in numerous studies to see if it improves detection of early malignancy.[20,21,33,36–38]

When screening patients for ovarian malignancy, size as well as sonographic texture are important features to note. To date, ultrasound studies of ovarian volume in postmenopausal women without HRT have suggested a range of 2.5 to 3.7 cm^3 as the upper limit of normal.[6,39,40,64] Significant size discrepancies when comparing both ovaries is another criterion for ovarian enlargement. It has been suggested that one ovary should not be more than twice the size of the contralateral one,[40] but in postmenopausal women, less dramatic size inconsistencies should raise suspicion. Transabdominal sonography has a sensitivity of 83% in detecting postmenopausal ovaries, an improvement over the 67% sensitivity of physical palpation.[23] Transabdominal sonography depicts a global view of the pelvic viscera, permits inspection of the abdomen and retroperitoneum, and can readily demonstrate ascites. A predominantly solid or complex mass is more suspect

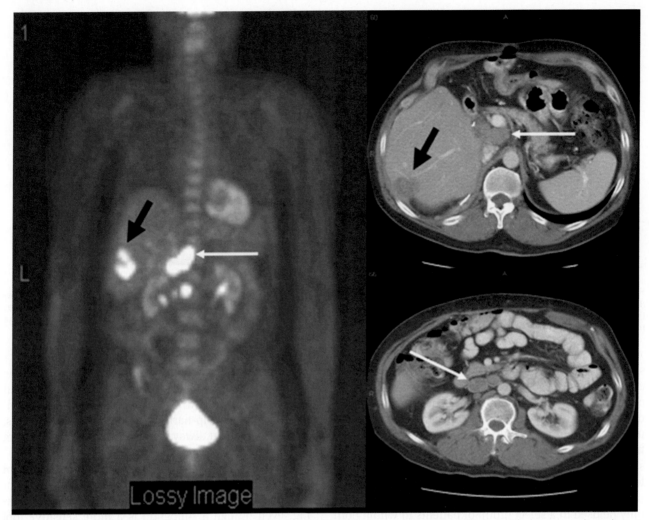

Figure 10-16 PET scan confirming hypermetabolic activity of lesions identified on corresponding CT scans. *Black arrows* indicate hepatic metastases, and the *white arrows* demonstrate portal and para-aortic lymph node metastases. The lossy notation on the PET image indicates the type of compression used on the image.

than a purely cystic mass. Endovaginal ultrasound allows distinctions in tissue texture to be made with greater confidence and provides further refinements in the assessment of ovarian size. The addition of color flow Doppler and spectral analysis permits added information regarding regional blood flow. The best approach to ultrasound imaging of the postmenopausal ovary combines information from both transabdominal and endovaginal studies.[6]

A significant limitation in the ultrasound study of postmenopausal patients is the difficulty in identifying normal postmenopausal ovaries, which are deficient of follicles, a characteristic feature that aids ovarian identification in premenopausal women. It is important to recognize that when ovaries are not visualized sonographically, they cannot be classified as normal.[33,41] Greater experience, careful scanning technique, and endovaginal scanning overcome some of the difficulty.

Doppler of the Ovary

Several studies suggest that both color flow Doppler and spectral analysis may provide clinically useful information in differentiating benign from malignant ovarian neoplasms. The distribution of vascularity is typically peripheral and orderly in benign lesions, but central and haphazard in malignancy.[23,42–47] An overall elevated peak systolic velocity due to neovascularity and arteriovenous shunting has been noted by some authors. A decrease in vascular impedance due to lack of intimal smooth muscle in tumor vessel walls has been

---

PATHOLOGY BOX 10-2

Ovarian volume[6,39,40,45,47,58,64]

Life Stage	Volume
Premenarchal	3.0 cm³ (±2.3)
Menstrual	9.8 cm³ (±5.8)
Postmenopausal*	5.8 cm³ (±3.6)

Ovarian volume in cubic centimeters = length × height (AP thickness) × width × 0.523

*Without hormone replacement

described in several series. A resistive index (RI) less than 0.4 and a pulsatility index (PI) less than 1.0 have been used as measurements denoting malignancy.[36] It has been documented that resistance to flow is lower in vessels supplying ovarian cancers than in those supplying benign ovarian tumors.[48] Other abnormalities may present with similar blood flow patterns. These include inflammatory processes, ectopic pregnancies, and corpus luteal cysts. Current practice is to use the Doppler information as an adjunct to the transabdominal and endovaginal imaging evaluation.

Recently, there have been rapid technological advances in ultrasonography, including the development of three-dimensional (3D) endovaginal power Doppler imaging and 3D volume acquisition. Initial studies suggest an improvement of diagnostic accuracy in the differentiation between benign and malignant adnexal pathology with use of this technology. It allows for thorough evaluation of the lesion's vascularity in three distinct planes and can better assess for internal blood flow in septations and solid papillary projections. Also, there are reported advantages of 3D sonography using surface rendering to improve visualization of the internal architecture of adnexal masses containing cystic and solid components not otherwise appreciated by two-dimensional (2D) technology (Fig. 10-17).[49,50] For detailed information on ovarian Doppler, refer to Chapter 6.

Sonographic Diagnosis

A sonogram is often the initial imaging study for patients with ovarian malignancy. The object of the ultrasound examination is to characterize the mass, define its contours, and obtain measurements. The gross anatomy of the most common form of ovarian malignancy, cystadenocarcinoma, lends itself well to ultrasound depiction because of the propensity of the lesion to form cystic masses with internal septa and soft tissue protrusions. Diffuse, low-amplitude signals within the cystic mass suggest the presence of mucin, as is seen in mucinous cystadenoma and cystadenocarcinoma. However, this finding is nonspecific for mucin, because it may be seen with fresh blood or purulent material. High-amplitude reflections associated with acoustic shadowing are often a clue to the presence of calcifications within the mass.

The ultrasound examination does not have the specificity to distinguish between benign and malignant disease, but a number of sonographic features, if present, favor the diagnosis of ovarian malignancy. As the proportion of solid components of the lesion increases, so does the likelihood of malignancy. Solid portions of the lesion consist of irregular septations, 2 mm thick or greater, and papillary growths.[51] Using endovaginal sonography, a morphologic scoring system has been devised, based on ovarian volume, cyst wall thickness, the presence of septations or papillary growths, and extratumoral fluid. This helps to quantify findings and assign a risk of malignancy.[52] Not infrequently, an ovarian malignancy has a predominantly or completely solid texture. Generally, the likelihood of malignancy is increased by the greater amount of solid tissue in a complex mass and when the volume exceeds 10 cm^3 in postmenopausal women and 20 cm^3 in premenopausal women (Fig. 10-18).[16,48] Nodularity and poor definition of the outer margin of the mass also favors malignancy. Immobility or noncompressibility imply fixation of a mass and suggest malignancy. In addition, bilateral disease can also imply malignancy. This finding is often difficult to ascertain. If the bilateral lesions are large, they may coalesce in the cul-de-sac to form one large mass. In some cases, ascites may be the only clue to the presence of ovarian malignancy, and the ovarian lesion

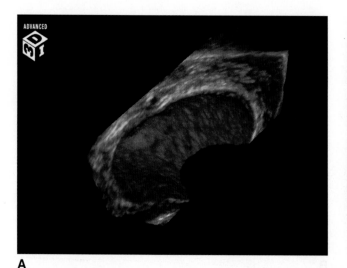

A

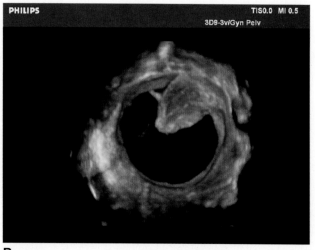

B

Figure 10-17 **A:** Surface rendering of the internal architecture of a simple cyst demonstrates a smooth regular wall. **B:** In contrast, the surface rendering of this cyst clearly shows internal wall projections into an ovarian cyst. (Images courtesy of Philips Medical Systems, Bothell, WA.)

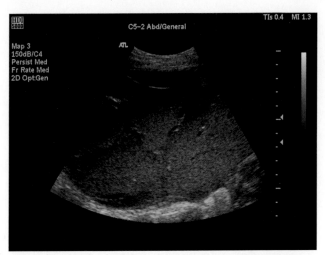

Figure 10-18 This case of ovarian cancer demonstrates a predominately solid mass with a heterogeneous internal echo texture complete with septations. (Image courtesy of Philips Medical Systems, Bothell, WA.)

itself may not be visualized. In such cases, use of an endovaginal transducer would help identify the ovarian mass and be of diagnostic value. The presence of ascites together with a cystic pelvic mass definitely raises the suspicion of malignancy.[53] The ultrasound appearance of the ascitic fluid in pseudomyxoma peritonei is usually echogenic because of the thick globular consistency of the fluid.

Metastasis to the ovary is common and is an important component of treatment failure in female patients with a malignancy. It commonly arises from breast or colon cancer, but also from other affected pelvic organs by direct extension or lymphatic spread. Krukenberg tumors are characterized by the presence of signet ring cells and are marked by areas of mucoid degeneration (Fig. 10-19).[16] They are usually bilateral and solid in appearance, and prognosis is poor.

Ultrasound imaging also has its limitations. There is the difficulty in detecting small-volume disease involving retroperitoneal nodes, peritoneal surfaces, and omentum.[22,54] Lesions situated high in the pelvis may be entirely outside the field of view of the endovaginal transducer. Despite these limitations, ultrasound provides reasonably accurate information for initial staging as well as evaluation for recurrent disease, with a reported accuracy of 90%.[25,54]

Sonographic Monitoring

Ultrasound is often used to monitor patients for persistent or recurrent disease after surgery and during treatment. An exam shortly after surgery may serve as a baseline study. In scanning the patient after a total hysterectomy, it is important to adjust the gain settings so that the increased sound transmission through the urinary bladder does not obscure a small pelvic mass. Endovaginal scanning should clarify any question with regard to the presence of a mass in the true pelvis or involving the vaginal cuff. Survey of the liver and retroperitoneal areas may be part of the postoperative examination as well. If pelvic masses, peritoneal nodules, or loculated areas of ascites are observed, ultrasound may be used to guide for needle aspiration.

Ultrasound Scanning Protocol

The examination consists of a systematic survey of the pelvis in the sagittal and transverse planes with identification of the bladder, uterus, and adnexal and cul-de-sac areas (Table 10-4). During the ultrasound exam, time gain compensation (TGC), focal zone position and number, plus the depth need adjustment to optimized the image and demonstrate posterior transmission patterns.

Often it is not possible to perform the ideal pelvic sonographic examination in the presence of a large mass because it is difficult for the patient to maintain a full

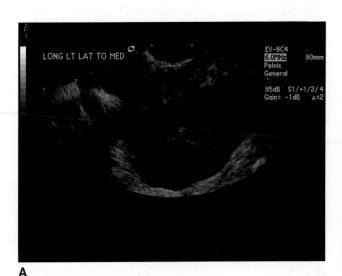

A

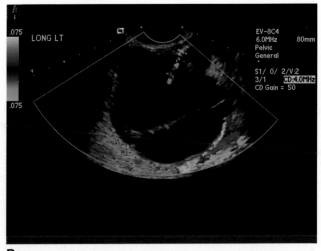

B

Figure 10-19 A: Krukenberg tumor. Endovaginal sagittal images showing a large complex mass with many irregular septations and solid intraluminal nodules. **B:** Sagittal endovaginal image shows hypervascularity of the septations during color Doppler interrogation.

TABLE 10-4	
Summary of Ultrasound Protocol for Ovarian Malignancy	
Purpose	**Sonography Checklist**
Screening	Note any ovarian enlargement. In pre- and postmenopausal women, ovarian linear dimension should not exceed 3 cm in length and 1.5 cm in thickness. Note significant asymmetry in ovarian size.
Diagnosis	Observe texture, contour, size, and sound transmission of mass. Determine whether it is unilateral or bilateral. Note uterine contours and endometrial reflection. Check for ascites. Identify liver, retroperitoneal, or omental masses. Check kidneys for hydronephrosis.
Monitoring	Compare to baseline study to exclude new masses. Check for ascites, retroperitoneal nodes, and liver masses. Survey pelvis, abdomen, and retroperitoneum before second-look operation.

bladder. It is important, however, to have enough fluid in the bladder for identification and use as a landmark and not mistaken for the cystic mass. In some cases, instillation into the bladder of 300 to 500 ml of normal saline with a Foley catheter may be required. An endovaginal exam is a very important adjunct to the examination, especially when an adequate transabdominal scan is not possible. Endovaginal sonography improves the delineation of adnexal masses and increased definition of uterine texture and contour. Thickening and other abnormalities of the endometrium suggest hyperplasia or endometrial carcinoma. Familiarity with Doppler techniques using color flow and spectral analysis is essential for obtaining additional information regarding blood flow to and within the lesion.

When ovarian malignancy is suspected based on the sonographic appearance of the mass, a complete pelvic and abdominal study can be done to provide information for staging (see Table 10-3). Search for ascites is directed to the cul-de-sac, paracolic gutters, especially on the right, and around the liver edge (Fig. 10-20). The inferior surfaces of the diaphragmatic leaflets may be visualized in the presence of moderate ascites. This enables the sonographer to demonstrate nodules on the liver capsule or on the diaphragmatic surface, which would suggest stage IV disease. Attention should be directed to the peritoneal surfaces to detect tumor implants. Observation of peristalsis is an important aspect of real-time scanning and may avoid confusion between tumor nodules and loops of bowel. The sonographer also has the opportunity to perform a "hands-on" maneuver by exerting gentle pressure on the cystic mass (if it is superficially located) to assess

it for compressibility. This is a feature of bowel and is usually not found with cystic malignant lesions. Evaluation of liver parenchyma is an integral part of the ultrasound study in the search for metastases. The costophrenic angles are also evaluated for the presence of pleural effusion. Both kidneys should be studied to assess the presence or absence of hydronephrosis. In the incidence of massive ascites, it may be difficult to image the para-aortic area to demonstrate retroperitoneal adenopathy. In such cases, oblique and coronal scanning should be attempted.

Differential Diagnosis

The differential diagnosis of ovarian malignancies includes a variety of benign ovarian neoplasms. No imaging modality has yet been able to provide the tissue specificity necessary to distinguish between benign and malignant lesions. Most ovarian neoplasms are benign, and their gross pathologic appearance is often indistinguishable from that of their malignant counterparts. In the menstruating woman, nonneoplastic cystic lesions of the ovaries such as large follicular cysts, corpus luteum, and theca-lutein cysts should also be considered in the differential diagnosis. These lesions have a mixed echogenic pattern, particularly when intracystic hemorrhage occurs. Inclusion or paraovarian cysts are nonneoplastic cystic masses of the ovary, but when found in the postmenopausal age group, may resemble neoplasms.

A pedunculated leiomyoma may mimic an ovarian neoplasm, particularly when degeneration due to

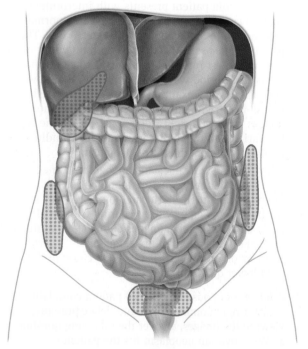

Figure 10-20 Diagrammatic view of the peritoneal cavity. Dotted areas represent the most common sites of ascites fluid collection.

vascular compromise results in the formation of cystic spaces.[55]

Neoplasms of the fallopian tube are exceedingly rare and often malignant. These lesions are sometimes mistaken for ovarian malignancies.

Tumor-like conditions that are morphologically similar to ovarian neoplasms include endometriosis and pelvic inflammatory disease. Furthermore, an ectopic pregnancy should always be considered as a potential cause for a mass in menstruating women. Diverticulitis and colitis, as well as other gastrointestinal diseases, often produce inflammatory masses and fluid collections in the pelvis and should be considered, particularly in postmenopausal patients.

Distended, fluid- and stool-filled loops of bowel imaged in the pelvis may appear tumor-like. Although the observation of peristalsis identifies them as bowel, absence of peristalsis need not exclude this possibility. Ischemic disease of the bowel may be associated with a dynamic ileus and a small amount of ascites.

The examiner faces a number of diagnostic challenges in the presence of a pelvic mass. The first is to determine the origin of the mass: is it ovarian, uterine, or nongynecologic? The second is to identify characteristics that are consistent with benign or malignant neoplasms. Awareness of differential diagnostic possibilities is important because of the morphologic similarity among many masses and disorders in the pelvic area.

SUMMARY

- Ovarian cancer is one of the most lethal forms of cancer due to late diagnosis
- Early treatment of ovarian cancers (Stage I) results in a 90% 5-year survival rate
- Eighty percent of ovarian carcinomas originate in the epithelium of the ovaries
- Epithelial cancers form large cystic masses with nodular papillary growths projecting into the interior
- Color Doppler of the epithelial cancer demonstrates prominent flow in the septations
- Rupture of the mucinous cystadenocarcinoma results in pseudomyxoma peritonei
- The combination of ascites, pleural fluid, and a solid ovarian mass is called Meig's syndrome
- Lymphatic spread and intraperitoneal seeding of tumor cells occurs with ovarian cancer spread
- Staging of ovarian malignancies is through the FIGO and TMN classification systems used at the time of laparotomy
- Vague clinical symptoms, often shared by other disease processes, often result in the late diagnosis of ovarian cancers
- Ovarian masses, whether malignant or benign, can result in torsion of the ovary

Critical Thinking Questions

1. A 18-year-old patient presents with intermittent right lower quadrant pain. Labs revealed normal red and white blood counts (RBC and WBC). The patient denies sexual activity even though her urine pregnancy test returned positive. Her last normal menstrual period was about 2 months ago; however, the clinical exam revealed a normal sized uterus with right-sided fullness. The sonographic images confirm a right-sided mass. Select one type of ovarian pathology that presents these findings. Explain why you chose this neoplasm.

   ANSWER: The lab values and sonographic images fit with an immature or mature teratoma. Possible differentials include a choriocarcinoma. The key lab is the positive pregnancy test occuring with an elevated hCG. The sonographic images demonstrate a unilateral solid mass with multiple small cysts. Intermittent torsion of the mass is likely the cause of the right lower quadrant pain.

2. A 60-year-old postmenopausal patient complains of heartburn, abdominal pain, and pelvic pressure. After viewing the images, answer the following questions:
   a. What ovarian neoplasm fits the patient's symptoms and the sonographic findings?

   b. There are no measurements on the image of the pelvic mass. How would you estimate the size?
   c. From these images, how would you grade this tumor? What image findings did you use to classify the neoplasm?

   ANSWER: This is probably a serous or mucinous cystadenocarcinoma. In the FIGO staging system, this would be classified as a stage IV. TMN. staging would classify this mass as a T3c, N1, M1 because of the positive retroperitoneal nodes, liver metastasis, and ascites.

   These longitudinal and transverse images demonstrate lymphadenopathy (stars).

   This image of the liver demonstrates the heterogeneous appearance of liver metastasis. A small amount of ascites (arrow) is just inferior to the diaphragm.

   An endovaginal image of the pelvic mass reveals a 10 cm mass. The size estimate would be approximately 10 cm, as indicated by the measurement bar located to the right of the image. Complex fluid along with the papillations (solid yellow arrow) suggest that this is a cystadenocarcinoma. The open arrow indicates a side lobe artifact.

- Eighty percent of ovarian epithelial cancers result in an elevated CA 125; however, many benign processes result in increased blood levels
- Adjunct lab tests include CA 72-4, CA 15-3, AFP, CEA, hCG, and LDH; these are also used in post treatment monitoring
- The upper limit of the normal ovarian volume in a postmenopausal woman is 2.5 to 3.7 cm^3
- Ovarian volume discordance raises suspicion for malignancy
- Spectral Doppler RI less than 0.4 and PI less than 1.0 have been used as measurements denoting malignancy
- Color Doppler demonstrates a disorganized central vascularity pattern in malignant lesions
- 3D surface rendering of the internal architecture of a cystic ovarian structure aids in imaging papillary projections
- Sonographic imaging lacks specificity in diagnosis of ovarian masses
- Breast, colon, or other pelvic malignancies often metastasize to the ovary, resulting in Krukenberg tumors

REFERENCES

1. Terplan M, Temkin S, Tergas A, et al. Does equal treatment yield equal outcomes? The impact of race on survival in epithelial ovarian cancer. *Gynecol Oncol.* 2008;111(2):173–178.
2. Garber JE, Offit K. Hereditary cancer predisposition syndromes. *J Clin Oncol.* 2005;23(2):276–292.
3. American Cancer Society. *Cancer statistics, 2009. CA Cancer J Clin.* 2009;59(4):225–249.
4. Aletti GD, Gallenberg MM, Cliby WA, et al. Current management strategies for ovarian cancer. *Mayo Clin Proc.* 2007;82(6):751–770.
5. Cooper N, Quinn MJ, Rachet B, et al. Survival from cancer of the ovary in England and Wales up to 2001. *Br J Cancer.* 2008;99(Suppl 1):S70–S72.
6. Alston RD, Geraci M, Eden TOB, et al. Changes in cancer incidence in teenagers and young adults (ages 13 to 24 years) in England 1979–2003. *Cancer.* 2008;113(10):2807–2815.
7. Jensen KE, Hannibal CG, Nielsen A, et al. Social inequality and incidence of and survival from cancer of the female genital organs in a population-based study in Denmark, 1994–2003. *Eur J Cancer.* 2008;44(14):2003–2017.
8. Chung HH, Hwang SY, Jung KW, et al. Ovarian cancer incidence and survival in Korea: 1993–2002. *Int J Gynecol Cancer.* 2007;17(3):595–600.
9. Rosenthal AN, Menon U, Jacobs IJ. Screening for ovarian cancer. *Clin Obstet Gynecol.* 2006;49(3):433–447.
10. Tworoger SS, Fairfield KM, Colditz GA, et al. Association of oral contraceptive use, other contraceptive methods, and infertility with ovarian cancer risk. *Am J Epidemiol.* 2007;166(8):894–901.
11. Hamilton W, Peters TJ, Bankhead C, et al. Risk of ovarian cancer in women with symptoms in primary care: population based case-control study. *BMJ.* 2009;339:b2998. doi: 10.1136/bmj.b2998

12. Schutter EM, Davelaar EM, Van Kamp GJ, et al. The differential diagnostic potential of a panel of tumor markers in patients with a pelvic mass. *Am J Obstet Gynecol.* 2002;187(2):385–392.
13. Köbel M, Kalloger SE, Boyd N, et al. Ovarian carcinoma subtypes are different diseases: implications for biomarker studies. *PLoS Med.* 2008;5(12):e232.
14. Jacobs IJ, Menon U. Progress and challenges in screening for early detection of ovarian cancer. *Mol Cell Proteomics.* 2004;3(4):355–366.
15. Berkelmans CT. Risk factors and risk reduction of breast and ovarian cancer. *Curr Opin Obstet Gynecol.* 2003;15(1):63–68.
16. Togashi K. Ovarian cancer: the clinical role of US, CT, and MRI. *Eur Radiol.* 2003;13(Suppl 4):L87–L104.
17. Smith ER, Xu XX. Ovarian ageing, follicle depletion, and cancer: a hypothesis for the aetiology of epithelial ovarian cancer involving follicle depletion. *Lancet Oncol.* 2008;9(11):1108–1111.
18. Tchagang AB, Tewfik AH, DeRycke MS, et al. Early detection of ovarian cancer using group biomarkers. *Mol Cancer Ther.* 2008;7(1):27–37.
19. Aebi S, Castiglione M. Epithelial ovarian carcinoma: ESMO clinical recommendations for diagnosis, treatment, and follow-up. *Ann Oncol.* 2008;19(Suppl 2):ii14–ii16.
20. Wang E, Ngalame Y, Panelli MC, et al. Peritoneal and subperitoneal stroma may facilitate regional spread of ovarian cancer. *Clin Cancer Res.* 2005;11(1):113–122.
21. deSouza NM, O'Neill R, McIndoe GA, et al. Borderline tumors of the ovary: CT and MRI features and tumor markers in differentiation from stage I disease. *AJR Am J Roentgenol.* 2005;184(3):999–1003.
22. van Nagell JR Jr, DePriest PD, Reedy MB, et al. The efficacy of endovaginal sonographic screening in asymptomatic women at risk for ovarian cancer. *Gynecol Oncol.* 2000;77(3):350–356.
23. Spencer JA. A multidisciplinary approach to ovarian cancer at diagnosis. *Br J Radiol.* 2005;78(Spec No 2):S94–S102.
24. Outwater E, Dressel HY. Evaluation of gynecologic malignancy by magnetic resonance imaging. *Radiol Clin North Am.* 1992;30(4):789–806.
25. Sanders RC, McNeil BJ, Finberg HJ, et al. A prospective study of CT and US in the detection and staging of pelvic masses. *Radiology.* 1983;146(2):439–442.
26. Goff BA, Mandel LS, Melancon CH, et al. Frequency of symptoms of ovarian cancer in women presenting to primary care clinics. *JAMA.* 2004;291(22):2705–2712.
27. Bast RC. Status of tumor markers in ovarian cancer screening. *J Clin Oncol.* 2003;21(10 Suppl):200s–205s.
28. Morrow CP. Malignant and borderline epithelial tumors of ovary: clinical features staging diagnosis. Intraoperative assessment and review of management. In: Coppleson M, ed. *Gynecologic Oncology: Fundamental Principles and Clinical Practice.* (Vol. 2). New York: Churchill Livingstone; 1981:655–679.
29. Rieber A, Nussle K, Stohr I, et al. Preoperative diagnosis of ovarian tumors with MR imaging. *Am J Roentgenol.* 2001;177(1):123–129.
30. Mitchell DG, Hill MC, Hill S, et al. Serous carcinoma of the ovary: CT identification of metastatic calcified implants. *Radiology.* 1986;158(3):649–652.

31. Nelson BE, Rosenfield AT, Schwartz PE. Preoperative abdominopelvic computed tomographic prediction of optimal cytoreduction in epithelial ovarian carcinoma. *J Clin Oncol*. 1993;11(1):166–172.

32. Akin, O, Sala, E, Moskowitz CS, et al. Perihepatic metastases from ovarian cancer: sensitivity and specificity of CT for the detection of metastases with and those without liver parenchymal invasion. *Radiology*. 2008;248(2): 511–517.

33. Kushtagi P, Kulkarni KK. Significance of the 'ovarian crescent sign' in the evaluation of adnexal masses. *Singapore Med J*. 2008;49(12):1017–1020.

34. Sohaib SA, Reznek RH. MR imaging in ovarian cancer. *Cancer Imaging*. 2007;7(Spec No A):S119–S129.

35. Iyer RB, Balachandran A, Devine CE. PET/CT and cross sectional imaging of gynecologic malignancy. *Cancer Imaging*. 2007;7(Spec No A):S130–S138.

36. Myers ER, Bastian LA, Havrilesky LJ, et al. Management of adnexal mass. *Evid Rep Technol Assess (Full Rep)*. 2006;(130):1–145.

37. Liu J, Xu Y, Wang J. Ultrasonography, computed tomography, and magnetic resonance imaging for diagnosis of ovarian carcinoma. *Eur J Radiol*. 2007;62(3):328–334.

38. Neesham D. Ovarian cancer screening. *Aust Fam Physician*. 2007;36(3):126–128.

39. Healy DL, Bell R, Robertson DM, et al. Ovarian status in healthy postmenopausal women. *Menopause*. 2008;15(6): 1109–1114.

40. Sherman ME, Lacey JV, Buys SS, et al. Ovarian volume: determinants and associations with cancer among postmenopausal women. *Cancer Epidemiol Biomarkers Prev*. 2006;15(8):1550–1554.

41. Van Calster B, Timmerman D, Bourne T, et al. Discrimination between benign and malignant adnexal masses by specialist ultrasound examination versus serum CA-125. *J Natl Cancer Inst*. 2007;99(22):1706–1714. Epub 2007 Nov 13.

42. Kurjak A, Prka M, Arenas JM, et al. Three-dimensional ultrasonography and power Doppler in ovarian cancer screening of asymptomatic peri- and postmenopausal women. *Croat Med J*. 2005;46(5):757–764.

43. Alcázar JL. Tumor angiogenesis assessed by three-dimensional power Doppler ultrasound in early, advanced, and metastatic ovarian cancer: a preliminary study. *Ultrasound Obstet Gynecol*. 2006;28(3):325–329.

44. Shwayder JM. Pelvic pain, adnexal masses, and ultrasound. *Semin Reprod Med*. 2008;26(3):252–265.

45. Hagan-Ansert S. The sonographic and Doppler evaluation of the female pelvis. In: *Textbook of Diagnostic Medical Ultrasonography*. 6th ed. Volume 2. St. Louis: Mosby; 2006:873–897.

46. Van Holsbeke C, Domali E, Holland TK, et al. Imaging of gynecological disease (3): clinical and ultrasound characteristics of granulosa cell tumors of the ovary. *Ultrasound Obstet Gynecol*. 2008;31(4):450–456.

47. Rumack CM, Wilson SR, Charboneau JW. Gynecologic ultrasound. In: *Diagnostic Ultrasound*. 3rd ed. Volume 1. St. Louis: Elsevier; 2006.

48. Ueland FR, DePriest PD, Pavlik EJ, et al. Preoperative differentiation of malignant from benign ovarian tumors: the efficacy of morphology indexing and Doppler flow sonography. *Gynecol Onc*. 2003;91(1):46–50.

49. Cohen LS, Escobar PF, Scharm C, et al. Three-dimensional power Doppler ultrasound improves the diagnostic accuracy for ovarian cancer prediction. *Gynecol Onc*. 2001; 82(1):40–48.

50. Kurjak A, Kupesic S, Sparac V, et al. The detection of stage I ovarian cancer by three-dimensional sonography and power Doppler. *Gynecol Onc*. 2003;90(2):258–264.

51. Moyle JW, Rochester D, Sider L, et al. Sonography of ovarian tumors: predictability of tumor type. *Am J Roentgenol*. 1983;141(5):985–991.

52. Sassone AM, Timor-Tritsch IE, Artner A, et al. Endovaginal sonographic characterization of ovarian disease: evaluation of a new scoring system to predict ovarian malignancy. *Obstet Gynecol*. 1991;78(1):70–76.

53. Requard CK, Mettler FA Jr, Wicks JD. Preoperative sonography of malignant ovarian neoplasms. *Am J Roentgenol*. 1981;137(1):79–82.

54. Khan O, Wiltshaw E, McGready VR, et al. Role of US in the management of ovarian carcinoma. *J Royal Soc Med*. 1983;76(10):821–827.

55. Nocera RM, Fagan CJ, Hernandez JC. Cystic parametrial fibroid mimicking ovarian cystadenoma. *J Ultrasound Med*. 1984;3(4):183–187.

56. World Health Organization. Classification of human ovarian tumors. *Environ Health Perspect*. 1987;73:15–25.

57. Gibbs RS, Karlan BY, Haney AF, et al, eds. Gynecologic ultrasound. In: *Danforth's Obstetrics & Gynecology*. 10th ed. Philadelphia: Lippincott Williams & Wilkins; 2008.

58. Valentin L, Callen PW. Ultrasound evaluation of the adnexa (Ovary and Fallopian Tubes). In: *Ultrasonography in Obstetrics and Gynecology*. 5th ed. Philadelphia: Saunders Elsevier; 2008.

59. Kumar V, Abbas AK, Fausto N, et al. *Robbins Basic Pathology*. 8th ed. Philadelphia: Saunders; 2007.

60. Mills SE. *Sternberg's Diagnostic Surgical Pathology*. 5th ed. Volume II chapters 54 and 55. Baltimore: Lippincott Williams & Wilkins; 2010.

61. Genetics Home Reference. Retrieved from http://ghr.nlm.nih.gov/ Accessed: 1/2010.

62. Tuefferd M, Couturier J, Penault-Llorca F, et. al. HER2 status in ovarian carcinomas: a multicenter GINECO study of 320 patients. *PLoS ONE*. 2007;2(11):e1138.

63. American Joint Committee on Cancer. *AJCC Cancer Staging Manual*. 7th ed. New York: Springer; 2009.

64. Wallace WH, Kelsey TW. Ovarian reserve and reproductive age may be determined from measurement of ovarian volume by transvaginal sonography. *Human Reprod*. 2004;19(7):1612–1617.

11 Pelvic Inflammatory Disease and Endometriosis

Allison A. Cowett

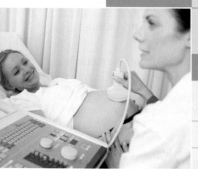

OBJECTIVES

Describe the etiology, clinical presentation, and management of pelvic inflammatory disease (PID) and endometriosis

Discuss the role of ultrasound in diagnosis and management of PID and endometriosis

Classify the severity of PID and endometriosis using current staging categories

Summarize the differences between endometriosis and adenomyosis

KEY TERMS

pelvic inflammatory disease | adenomyosis | endometriosis

GLOSSARY

Adenomyosis Presence of endometrial glands and tissues found in the uterine wall

Dysmenorrhea Painful menstruation

Dyspareunia Painful intercourse

Endometriosis Implants of endometrial tissue outside the uterus

Endometrioma Blood-filled cyst located on the ovary that is the result of endometriosis

Endometritis Bacterial infection of the endometrium with potential extension into the surrounding (parametrial) tissues

Fitz-Hugh-Curtis syndrome (aka perihepatitis) Rare complication of PID resulting in the development of liver adhesions due to the inflammatory exudates

Myometritis Myometrial inflammation

Oophoritis Infection of the ovaries

Parametritis Infection of the connective tissue surrounding the uterus

Pelvic inflammatory disease (PID) Infection of the female reproductive tract

Pyosalpinx Pus within the fallopian tube

Peritonitis Infection of the peritoneum

Salpingitis Infection of the fallopian tube

Tubo-ovarian abscess (TOA) Infection found in the late stages of PID resulting in the inability to differentiate tubal and ovarian structures

Tubo-ovarian complex Ability to identify the ovary and tube in the presence of adhesions or infection

Pelvic inflammatory disease (PID) and endometriosis are disease processes of the female pelvis that cause diffuse morphologic and vascular changes. Both display a varied pattern of tissue involvement and clinical findings. Clinical presentation in the early stages of both disease entities may be nonspecific. Endometriosis often mimics functional bowel disease, and PID often mimics ectopic pregnancy or appendicitis. While these two disease processes are physiologically distinct, they exhibit similar sonographic findings. Attention to the details of the patient history and clinical findings in correlation with pelvic ultrasound findings allow the careful clinician to distinguish between PID and endometriosis. In this chapter, we consider PID and endometriosis separately in terms of etiology, clinical presentation, management,

and sonographic findings. Table 11-1 summarizes the differences and similarities of these two distinct disease processes in relation to etiology, clinical presentation, disease progression, treatment, and sequelae.

PELVIC INFLAMMATORY DISEASE

The term pelvic inflammatory disease or PID refers to the clinical entity of diffuse inflammation of the upper female genital tract resulting from infection. Locations affected by PID include the endometrium (endometritis), the uterine wall (myometritis), the uterine serosa and broad ligaments (parametritis), and the ovary (oophoritis). The most common location of infection is the oviducts or fallopian tubes (salpingitis).

TABLE 11-1

Characteristics of Pelvic Inflammatory Disease (PID) and Endometriosis Compared

	PID	Endometriosis
Definition	Diffuse inflammation of the upper genital tract resulting from infection	Presence of ectopic endometrial tissue located outside the uterus
Etiology	Ascending infection from vaginal and cervical flora	Retrograde menstruation, coelomic metaplasia, hematologic or lymphatic spread
Clinical presentation	Lower abdominal and/or pelvic pain, uterine, adnexal or cervical motion tenderness	Dysmenorrhea, dyspareunia, dysuria, pain on defecation, chronic pelvic pain, infertility
Clinical progression	**Stage 1** Endometritis **Stage 2** Salpingitis **Stage 3** Tubo-ovarian complex or tubo-ovarian abscess (TOA) **Chronic disease**	**Stage 1** Minimal **Stage 2** Mild **Stage 3** Moderate **Stage 4** Severe
Treatment	Broad-spectrum antibiotics, surgical drainage of TOA	Analgesics, hormonal medical management, surgical excision, oophorectomy
Sequelae	Chronic pelvic pain, ectopic pregnancy, infertility	Chronic cyclic pelvic pain, infertility

PID has a significant immediate economic impact as well as costly long-term sequelae. There are currently an estimated 1.5 million cases of PID diagnosed per year in the United States, associated with an estimated cost of $1.88 billion for diagnosis and management of PID and its three major sequelae, chronic pelvic pain, ectopic pregnancy, and infertility.[1] Following a single episode of PID, the risks of tubal factor infertility and ectopic pregnancy, increase sixfold. The second episode increases these risks up to 17 times that of a woman who has never had PID.[2] In addition, chronic pelvic pain and tubo-ovarian abscess (TOA) are common sequelae of salpingitis. The burden of this disease falls disproportionately on younger women, with the prevalence of PID in sexually active adolescents estimated as one in eight as compared to a rate of one in eighty in the 25–29 age group.[3]

ETIOLOGY

The cause of PID is almost invariably (99%) polymicrobial, resulting from the invasion of pathogens ascending from the mixed flora of the vagina and cervix into the upper genital tract. A number of organisms have been implicated in PID, and the rates of infection with the individual entities vary by community. The sexually transmitted infections *Chlamydia trachomatis* and *Neisseria gonorrhoeae* are commonly implicated in PID, and all women diagnosed with PID should be tested for these organisms. PID can also result from infection of the upper tract with endogenous vaginal flora such as anaerobes and aerobes (*Haemophilus influenzae*, enteric gram-negative rods, and *Streptococcus agalactiae*). *Mycobacterium tuberculosis*, cytomegalovirus, *M. hominis, U. urealyticum,* and *M. genitalium* have also been implicated.[2,4,5] Bacterial vaginosis (BV) is

the most common infection of the lower genital tract in reproductive-age women, and the causal association between BV and upper genital tract infection remains controversial.[4]

The majority of patients who develop PID become infected through sexual transmission; therefore, risk factors for PID are similar to those associated with STD acquisition These include early age at first intercourse, young age, increased number of sexual partners with frequent change in partners, amd frequent sexual intercourse.[4] Inconsistent condom use has also been associated with upper genital tract infection.[6] The connection between nonbarrier contraceptive use and PID has also been extensively examined. The use of combined oral contraceptive pills may be associated with reduced clinical severity of PID. The use of an intrauterine device (IUD) confers an increased risk of PID at the time of device insertion and for 3 weeks following insertion, likely secondary to iatrogenic introduction of cervical or vaginal pathogens into the upper genital tract.[7] Following this initial period of increased risk, the risk of PID in IUD users appears to return to equal that of women who do not have an IUD in place.[8] These findings have led to recommendations for STD screening and treatment in high-risk populations prior to IUD insertion.[4,8]

Tobacco use and engaging in vaginal intercourse while menstruating have also been associated with increased risk of PID. Studies evaluating the relationship between vaginal douching and PID have been inconclusive.[4] Additionally, organisms from the lower genital tract may be introduced into the upper genital tract following invasive gynecologic procedures such as endometrial biopsy, dilation and curettage, hysteroscopy, hysterosalpingography, and intrauterine insemination. Only a fraction of cases of PID result from

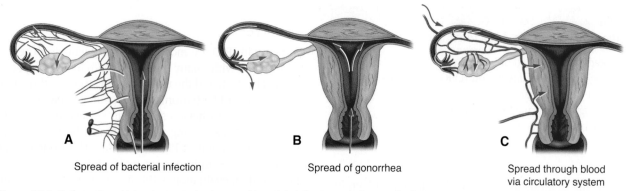

A   Spread of bacterial infection

B   Spread of gonorrhea

C   Spread through blood via circulatory system

Figure 11-1 Pathway by which microorganisms spread in pelvic infections. **A:** Bacterial infection spreads up the vagina into the uterus and through the lymphatics. **B:** Gonorrhea spreads up the vagina into the uterus and then to the tubes and ovaries. **C:** Bacterial infection can reach the reproductive organs through the bloodstream (hematogenous spread).

hematogenous or lymphatic spread or from a transperitoneal source, such as a perforated appendix or intra-abdominal abscess.[9]

PROGRESSION

PID is a progressive disease and its stages are determined by the upward migration of surface-invading bacteria from the cervix to the endometrium to the oviducts to the pelvic peritoneum. The initial spread of infection past the cervical barrier results in endometritis, an intermediate stage of PID.[10] The endometrial cavity is a conduit by which microorganisms reach the fallopian tubes. Varying degrees of salpingitis and ovarian and peritoneal involvement resulting from the spread of infection characterize later PID (Fig. 11-1).[10]

The next stage of PID is characterized by acute salpingitis in which the tube becomes inflamed and edematous. Extension of the inflammatory exudate from the salpinges may involve the broad ligaments (parametritis) and the ovaries (oophoritis). Ovaries affected by past or current PID may be adherent to the uterus. They may be enlarged, usually because of acute oophoritis. If the purulent material formed in the tube drains from the fimbriated opening and over the ovary (perioophoritis), an abscess involving the tubes, the ovary, and adjacent bowel may form. This is referred to as a tuboovarian abscess.[10]

CLINICAL FINDINGS

The patient with pelvic infection is often a young, sexually active woman with a wide range of nonspecific complaints. The clinical presentation ranges from minor complaints to acute, life-threatening illness. The most frequent symptoms are lower abdominal and pelvic pain. Adnexal tenderness, usually diffuse and bilateral, and constant dull pain, usually described as accentuated by movement or sexual activity, are also reported. Onset of symptoms may be rapid (associated more often with *N. gonorrhoeae*) or insidious

(associated more often with *C. trachomatis*). Physical examination may reveal cervical motion tenderness, uterine tenderness, adnexal tenderness, abdominal tenderness with or without guarding, and adnexal masses (Fig. 11-2).[10]

The vague nature of presenting symptoms in patients with PID contributes to a high rate of misdiagnosis. Given the severity and chronicity of the long-term sequelae of the disease, recent recommendations for the initiation of treatment based on relaxed clinical criteria have been introduced. Diagnosis of PID is now recommended for a woman who presents with pelvic or lower abdominal pain and has findings of cervical motion tenderness, uterine tenderness, or adnexal tenderness, whereas previous diagnostic criteria required all three physical findings.[5]

Other findings that support but are not required for the diagnosis include oral temperature over 101°F (38.33°C), mucopurulent cervical discharge, increased white blood cells (WBCs) seen on microscopic evaluation of vaginal discharge, elevated erythrocyte sedimentation rate, elevated C-reactive protein, and *N. gonorrhea* or *C. trachomatis* cervicitis.[5] However, most

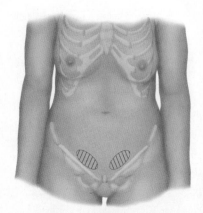

Figure 11-2 The tenderness of acute salpingitis (inflammation of the fallopian tubes) is usually maximal just above the inguinal ligaments. Rebound tenderness and rigidity may be present. On pelvic examination, motion of the uterus causes pain.

PATHOLOGY BOX 11-1

Laboratory Findings Associated with PID

Elevated WBC in blood or vaginal secretions
High erythrocyte sedimentation (ESR)
Elevated C-reactive protein
Positive gonorrhea and/or chlamydia
Positive bacterial vaginosis

specific for diagnosing PID are the findings of endometritis on endometrial biopsy, ultrasound, computed tomography (CT), or magnetic resonance imaging (MRI): thickened, edematous fallopian tubes or TOA and laparoscopic examination consistent with PID.[5] While the invasive techniques of endometrial biopsy and laparoscopic surgery are less often utilized for diagnostic confirmation of the disease, noninvasive imaging modalities and particularly ultrasound are more often employed in this clinical setting. Aside from laparoscopy, ultrasound has been described as the gold standard for the diagnosis of PID and TOA, with a 93% sensitivity and 98% specificity in the diagnosis of TOA.[11]

Some patients may present with pelvic and right-sided upper quadrant pain. Fitz-Hugh-Curtis syndrome is a constellation of clinical findings that includes right-sided pleuritic pain and right-sided upper quadrant pain and tenderness on palpation. Fitz-Hugh-Curtis syndrome is experienced by 5% to 10% of patients with PID and is caused by perihepatic inflammation from peritonitis, as the infected fluid tracks into the subhepatic space from the lower pelvic peritoneal compartments (Fig. 11-3).[12] Often, ultrasound of these patients shows no definitive abnormality, whereas CT scan may exhibit thickening of the liver capsule.[12]

IMAGING FINDINGS

Sonography

Women with PID are most often young women of reproductive age with many years of reproductive capacity ahead. This fact, and the understanding that the three major sequelae of PID (chronic pelvic pain, ectopic pregnancy, and infertility) have a significant impact in the health and lives of these young women, make the timely diagnosis and treatment of PID a necessity. Ultrasonographic evaluation plays an important role in this process. Use of ultrasound for evaluation of PID has improved greatly with the advent of endovaginal imaging with Doppler capability, which has enhanced the ability to image the fallopian tubes and to detect subtle changes in pelvic anatomy that are characteristic of the disease.[13,14] In addition, patients with acute pain may be unable to tolerate the full bladder that is required for optimal transabdominal scanning, making the endovaginal approach preferable.[13]

The sonographic presentation of PID varies with the extent of the infection. Findings may be unremarkable or extremely subtle (as in the case of early, mild disease) or dramatic (as is seen in advanced disease).[43] Findings are also likely to be dynamic, changing rapidly over a short time in response to both progression of disease or treatment.[13] This discussion considers the sonographic appearance of the various stages of infection and their sequelae.

Acute Pelvic Inflammatory Disease: Early and Intermediate Findings

Early sonographic findings are often nonspecific and may not provide a definitive diagnosis of PID. However, a constellation of sonographic findings, in conjunction with the aforementioned signs and symptoms of the disease, support the diagnosis. Early acute infection is concentrated within the endometrium with characteristic uterine findings. The uterus is mildly enlarged and exhibits indistinct margins (Fig. 11-4).[13] The myometrial

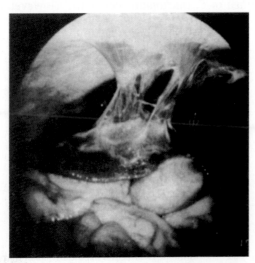

Figure 11-3 Laparoscopic view of perihepatitis, showing scarring and stringlike perihepatic adhesions associated with both gonococcal and chlamydial salpingitis seen with Fitz-Hugh-Curtis syndrome.

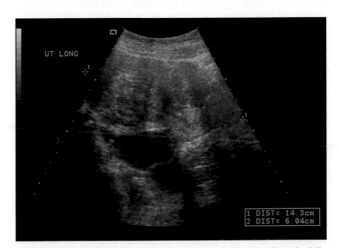

Figure 11-4 Sagital view of the uterus in a patient with early PID. The uterus is enlarged in the longitudinal plane. The borders of the uterus and surrounding tissues are indistinct. The myometrial endometrial junction is poorly defined.

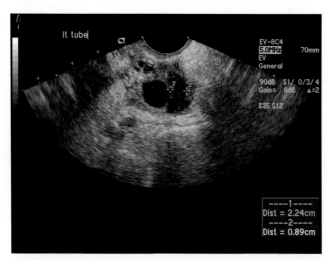

Figure 11-5 Left adnexa seen in a patient with acute salpingitis. The ovoid structure with thickened walls adjacent to the ovary represents a dilated fallopian tube.

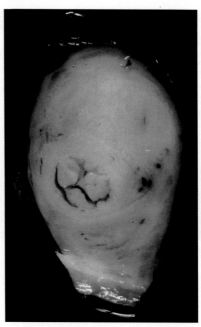

Figure 11-6 Cross-section of a "pus tube" shows thickening of the wall and a lumen swollen with pus seen in this case of gonorrhea of the fallopian tube.

endometrial junction also appears blurred and the endometrium may be thickened and heterogeneous and contain fluid within the cavity.[15-17] Other early findings are indistinct borders of the pelvic structures and posterior cul-de-sac fluid. While some patients will not exhibit free fluid, careful attention should be paid to the presence of any complex fluid or fluid with dependent low-level echogenicity, indicative of purulent accumulation.[13,17]

The normal fallopian tube is not visualized using endovaginal ultrasound unless surrounded by an abnormally large amount of free fluid in the pelvis, as is seen with ascites. However, in the setting of the acute salpingitis of PID, the anatomy of the tube is significantly altered, allowing for distinct sonographic visualization. The acute inflammatory process causes the tubal wall to grow thickened and edematous and therefore enhances visualization on ultrasound (Figs. 11-5 and 11-6).[13] The thickened endosalpingeal folds of the tubal mucosa narrow the tubal lumen and create a purulent exudate that fills and often occludes the tube.[14] Tubal occlusion resulting from purulent material and adhesion formation results in distension of the tube and formation of the pyosalpinx, a thick-walled (≥5 mm) and elongated ovoid structure. Distortion of the fallopian tube leads to the appearance of thickened but incomplete "septa," which project from the tubal wall into the lumen but do not reach to the contralateral side of the dilated structure (Fig. 11-7). The affected tube exhibits the "cogwheel" sign when imaged in cross-section secondary to the thickened endosalpingeal folds that are characteristic of the disease.[13] Fluid within the pyosalpinx may be anechoic or hypoechoic, or they may exhibit a layered appearance.[17] Doppler flow to the thickened tubal walls and incomplete septa is enhanced with a hyperemic appearance.[13] The affected tube is more likely to be found within the posterior aspect of the pelvis in contrast to enlarged ovarian structures that are often

found anterior to the normal uterus.[13] Affected ovaries may appear enlarged and are found adjacent to the uterus in their usual anatomic position.[11]

Acute Pelvic Inflammatory Disease: Advanced Findings of Tubo-ovarian Complex and Tubo-ovarian Abscess

Tubo-ovarian complex results from the escape of purulent exudate beyond the tube. The ovary itself may become involved secondary to bacterial infiltration through the ruptured corpus luteum.[11] In the setting of tubo-ovarian complex, ovarian enlargement and adherence to adnexal structures make the pelvic tissue planes ill defined. However, in contrast to TOA, tubo-ovarian complex refers to the affected ovary and tube that are

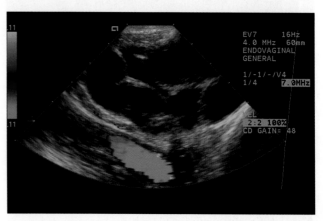

Figure 11-7 Edematous adnexal structure consistent with a pyosalpinx. The fallopian tube has thickened walls and internal debris. The appearance of incomplete septations results from distortion of the dilated tube.

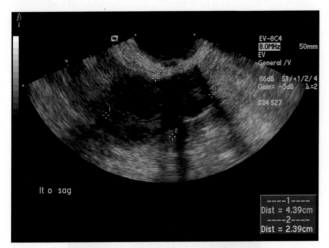

Figure 11-8 Adnexal mass in a patient with a history of PID. The ovary and the adjacent abnormal tubal structure are adherent to one another; however, their individual architecture remains visible on ultrasound, consistent with tubo-ovarian complex.

adherent to one another, but their individual architecture is still identifiable on ultrasound (Fig. 11-8).[11,13,14,17] A true TOA occurs once the ovarian parenchyma is affected and the ovarian and tubal structures cannot be seen separately on ultrasound evaluation. TOA is often a bilateral process of varying size and echogenicity; however, TOA may also be unilateral. Bilateral TOAs may completely fill the pelvis, obscuring the uterine borders. TOA should be suspected when cystic adnexal masses with indistinct, thick walls, internal septations, or complex internal echoes are imaged (Fig. 11-9). The sonographic characteristics of these masses vary according to the stage of abscess formation. TOA may appear as an indistinct, complex mass, whereas a resorbing mass results in a more cystic appearance. As

treatment leads to healing, pelvic structures begin to regain their normal appearances. Color and power Doppler show increased flow in the thickened walled and incomplete septa of the affected tubal complex. TOAs are usually well perfused owing to increased vascularization, and they demonstrate low resistive and pulsatility indices.[13]

Chronic Pelvic Inflammatory Disease

Chronic PID refers to both the sequelae of acute infection and the subacute recurrence of previous inflammation. In the case of the latter, chronic PID may develop from an incompletely treated prior infection. Clinically, patients with chronic PID present with findings of hydrosalpinx on ultrasound, and these findings may develop even when initial imaging at the time of acute disease was normal.[13] Hydrosalpinx develops when fluid accumulates within a scarred, obstructed fallopian tube. It appears as a sausage-shaped or ovoid anechoic adnexal structure with the incomplete septa seen in acute PID.[13] However, unlike acute disease, the hydrosalpinx seen in chronic PID has distinct borders and thin walls (<5 mm), owing to long-standing enlargement and pressure of the edema on the walls of the damaged tube (Fig. 11-10).[13] When seen in cross-section, the hydrosalpinx may exhibit the "beads on a string" sign in which 2-to-3–millimeter (mm) echogenic nodules line the wall of the tube. These nodules are the ultrasonographic representation of the remnants of the thickened endosalpingeal folds seen as the "cogwheel" sign of acute disease. Hydrosalpinx may be difficult to differentiate from an ovarian cyst or small cystadenoma; however, unlike the septations typically seen in ovarian neoplasms, the septa seen within the hydrosalpinx do not extend the diameter of the edematous tube (Fig. 11-11). Like ovarian cysts, hydrosalpinges occasionally undergo torsion.

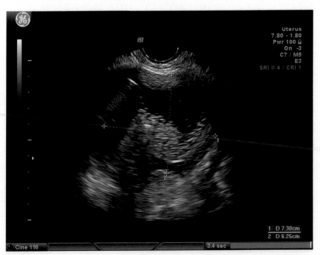

A

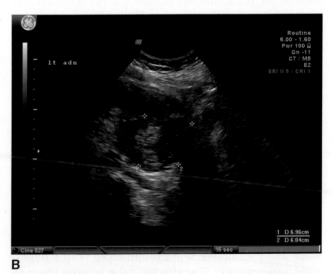

B

Figure 11-9 Bilateral, complex adnexal masses in a patient with prior bilateral TOAs 1 year prior to presentation treated conservatively with intravenous (IV) antibiotics. The masses exhibit indistinct borders and internal echogenicity. Ovarian tissue is not distinctly visualized, a typical appearance of TOA.

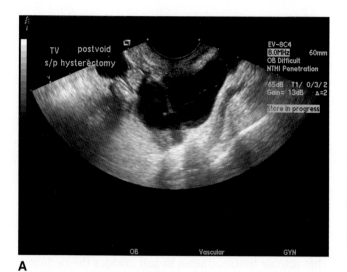 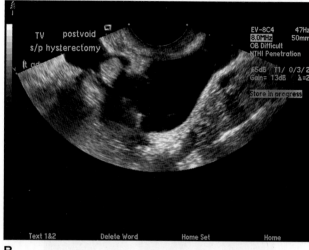

A **B**

Figure 11-10 Sausage-shaped adnexal structures consistent with hydrosalpinges. Both masses are anechoic and thin walled, and they exhibit sharp borders with surrounding pelvic structures. Thin, incomplete septa are seen.

After treatment, serial ultrasonographic examinations demonstrate resolution of pelvic infection by documenting changes in the size and appearance of pelvic structures. If the disease does not respond to conservative therapy, the ultrasound examination provides valuable information on the size and location of abscesses for surgical drainage with or without sonographic guidance. With appropriate treatment, the end result may be a return to a completely normal pelvis or one that is scarred and functionally impaired. Sonographic changes can appear rapidly following treatment, with the resolution of complex fluid and inflammation in surrounding tissues often seen within a few days of therapy.[13]

CT and MRI

Although ultrasound is the standard diagnostic imaging technique in the evaluation of PID, other noninvasive

imaging modalities such as CT and MRI may play a role in making the diagnosis. CT is often employed in the diagnostic evaluation of female patients with diffuse pelvic pain. Early inflammatory changes seen in PID may be better visualized on CT than ultrasound. These early findings include changes in pelvic fat, blurring of fascial planes within the pelvis, thickened uterosacral ligaments, fluid within the enhanced endometrial cavity, enhanced and thickened fallopian tubes, and enhanced and enlarged ovaries.[17] Later in

Figure 11-11 Thin incomplete septa seen in an adnexal mass consistent with hydrosalpinx. In contrast to septations seen within an ovarian mass, the thin, linear septa does not span the entire diameter of the mass. This appearance assists in distinguishing the mass as a hydrosalpinx.

PATHOLOGY BOX 11-2

Ultrasound Findings of Pelvic Inflammatory Disease (PID)

Stage 1: Endometritis
 Nonspecific findings, variable appearance
 Enlarged uterus with indistinct margins
 Thickened, heterogeneous endometrium ± fluid within the cavity
 Cul-de-sac fluid, anechoic or complex
Stage 2: Acute Salpingitis
 Thick-walled, edematous tubal structure (pyosalpinx)
 Hypoechoic or complex, incomplete septa, "cogwheel" sign
 Enhanced Doppler flow to tubal structure
Stage 3: A. Acute Tubo-ovarian Complex
 Ovarian enlargement, adherence to other adnexal structures
 Ill-defined tissue planes, ovary distinctly visualized
B. Acute Tubo-ovarian Abscess
 Indistinct, complex adnexal mass, thick walled, internal septations
 Increased Doppler flow to adnexal mass
C. Chronic disease
 Thin-walled, edematous tubal structure (hydrosalpinx)
 Anechoic, incomplete septa, "beads on a string" sign

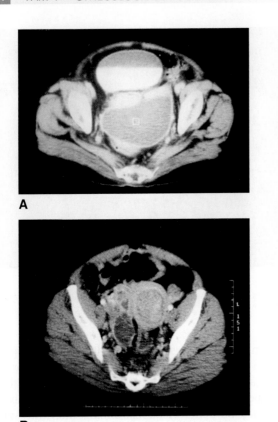

Figure 11-12 A: Axial CT image through the pelvis demonstrating a TOA. **B:** MRI of TOA.

disease progression on CT scan, TOA appears as a low-attenuation multiloculated adnexal mass.[17] MRI may be superior to ultrasound for imaging of TOA, pyosalpinx, and enlarged ovaries as seen in PID. Despite the benefits of CT and MRI, sonography remains the primary diagnostic imaging modality, because it is inexpensive, readily available, does not expose patients to ionizing radiation, and lends itself to serial scanning to follow treatment efficacy (Fig. 11-12).

TREATMENT

In the setting of pelvic or abdominal pain in a sexually active woman with cervical motion tenderness, uterine tenderness, or adnexal tenderness, empiric antimicrobial therapy for PID is indicated in the absence of another discernable etiology for the patient's symptoms. Appropriate empiric therapy involves broad-spectrum antibiotics that treat *C. trachomatis*, *N. gonorrhoeae*, and anaerobes. Hospitalization is recommended for patients who are pregnant, those who cannot tolerate or have not improved clinically on oral antibiotic therapy, those who have high fever, or those in whom surgical emergencies such as appendicitis cannot be definitely ruled out.[5] First-line outpatient therapy includes a combination of a third-generation, and doxycycline with or without metronidazole. Recommended parenteral therapy combines cefotetan or cefoxitin and doxycycline, or

clindamycin and gentamicin. These regimens represent a change in recommended therapy for *N. gonorrhoeae* in response to increasing fluoroquinolone resistance in various regions throughout the United States.[5] For patients who do not respond to parenteral antibiotic therapy, ultrasound-guided percutaneous drainage or surgical intervention for treatment of tubo-ovarian abscess or removal of the affected tubes or ovaries may be indicated.

ENDOMETRIOSIS

Endometriosis is defined as heterotopic growth of the glands and stroma of the endometrium, the lining of the uterus that is shed monthly in menstruating women. This ectopic tissue adheres to and invades the peritoneal surface[18] as it continues to respond to the hormonal influence of the ovulatory cycle.[19] Although the disease is usually regarded as a benign process, cellular activity and progression often lead to adhesion formation and interruption of normal reproduction. Chronic progression can produce a wide range of clinical consequences, including severe cyclic pelvic pain and infertility. Endometriosis is a prevalent disease and is recognized as the third most common reason for gynecologic hospital admission in the United States.[19]

ETIOLOGY

The etiology of endometriosis is uncertain, but several theories have been advanced. The dissemination of endometrial tissue fragments throughout the pelvis because of retrograde menstruation is a common theory. Retrograde menstruation refers to the reflux of sloughed endometrial cells through the fallopian tubes onto the serosal surfaces within the pelvis. Other theories postulate coelomic metaplasia or hematologic or lymphatic spread. Genetic factors are likely to play a role, considering the concordance of endometriosis in monozygotic twins.[19] Further complicating the understanding of the etiology of the disease are the findings that retrograde menstruation occurs in 90% of women and that most women with recognized ectopic endometriotic implants are asymptomatic.[19] The etiology of endometriosis is a well-studied but unsettled area of ongoing research.

Endometriosis and its symptoms are directly related to the cyclic hormonal stimulation and therefore is seen only in reproductive age women. Women who have undergone bilateral oophorectomy experience prompt and complete regression of the ectopically located endometrial tissue followed by relief of symptoms. Natural menopause also gradually brings relief of symptoms. Without the cyclic hormonal stimulation secreted from the ovarian tissue, intrapelvic bleeding of ectopic endometrial implants ceases and leads to a decrease in adhesion formation.

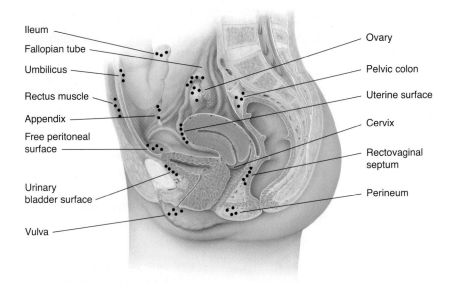

Ileum

Fallopian tube

Umbilicus

Rectus muscle

Appendix

Free peritoneal
surface

Urinary
bladder surface

Vulva

Ovary

Pelvic colon

Uterine surface

Cervix

Rectovaginal
septum

Perineum

Figure 11-13 Common sites of endometriosis.

Endometriosis can be diffuse or focal. The majority of implants are located in the pelvis, and the most common locations are the ovary and the posterior cul-de-sac.[20] Focal implants that have developed into a cystic collection are referred to as endometriomas and are found in 17% to 44% of women with endometriosis.[1] While the definite etiology of endometrioma formation is unknown, it has been suggested that lesions form secondary to progressive invagination of the ovarian cortex in response to cycle bleeding of endometriotic implants on the ovarian surface.[20,21] Endometrioma is the most common type of ovarian cyst found at surgery.[21] The term "chocolate cyst" is used to describe the characteristic appearance of endometriomas, which are filled with old blood from repeated episodes of hormonally stimulated endometrial sloughing within the implant. Endometriomas commonly measure between 5 to 10 centimeters (cm), with cysts greater than 15 to 20 cm being extremely rare.[9,22] Between 30% and 50% of lesions are bilateral,[22,23] with larger lesions more likely to be bilateral.[25] Other pelvic locations where endometrial implants are found include the anterior and posterior cul-de-sac, the broad ligaments, the pelvic lymph nodes, the cervix, vagina, vulva, and the rectrosigmoid colon (Fig. 11-13).[9]

Rarely, implantation occurs in areas of previous surgical incision of the abdominal wall, the umbilicus, bladder, ureter, kidney, extremities, and lung. Pleural endometriosis has been documented.[9] Malignant transformation of endometriosis is highly unusual, occurring most commonly in the ovary at a rate of 0.7% of all cases of endometriosis, with clear cell and endometrioid carcinoma being the most common histologic types.[20,21]

The color, shape, size, degree of inflammation, and associated fibrosis of endometrial implants vary. The differences are associated with cyclic hormonal changes

and length of time the implant has been active. The typically described blue or black lesion represents the bleeding endometriotic implant that has been discolored by hematologic pigment (Fig. 11-14). The inflammatory response to this lesion leads to the destruction and devascularization of the implants, resulting in fibrosis of the lesion and a whitish appearance. Red lesions are the most active lesions and are seen most commonly on the broad and uterosacral ligaments. More subtle lesions may appear white with opacification of the peritoneal surface or thickened, raised lesions. Additionally, endometriosis may be present microscopically without gross findings on direct visualization.[18]

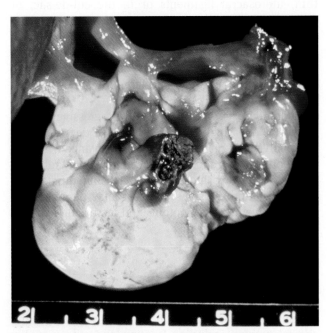

Figure 11-14 Endometriosis. Implants of endometriosis on the ovary appear as red-blue nodules.

CLINICAL FINDINGS

The American Society of Reproductive Medicine categorizes endometriosis according to extent of disease found at laparoscopy as minimal (stage I), mild (stage II), moderate (stage III), and severe (stage IV). However, this scoring system is based only on disease seen on direct visualization and correlates poorly with the severity of patient symptoms.[24] A minimal amount of tissue implantation may result in excruciating pain if it causes peritoneal stretching, whereas extensive endometrial implants in less sensitive locations may create no symptoms. As many as 22% of women in some populations may have no symptoms despite evidence of endometriosis.[24]

Endometriosis presents with a variety of symptoms, including asymptomatic involuntary infertility, dysmenorrhea, dyspareunia, dysuria, pain on defecation, and chronic pelvic pain with and without infertility.[24] From 20% to 50% of infertile women and 40% to 50% of infertile women with chronic pelvic pain exhibit endometriosis.[24]

Dysmenorrhea, or pelvic pain with menses, usually begins 24 to 48 hours before menstruation and lasts for several days, or pain may be chronic, worsening during menses. Descriptions of the pain range from a dull ache to severe unilateral or bilateral pain that may radiate to the lower back, legs, or groin. Patients also report "pelvic heaviness," describing a feeling of swelling or congestion in the pelvic region. Dysmenorrhea associated with endometriosis is less responsive to nonsteroidal anti-inflammatory drugs (NSAIDs) than cyclic pelvic pain in the absence of the disease.[24] Women may complain of dyspareunia because of direct pressure of implantation on the rectovaginal septum, uterosacral ligaments or in the cul-de-sac, or as a result of the immobilization of adherent structures.[24] Dysuria and pain on urination and defecation are seen when the bladder and rectosigmoid colon are involved, respectively.[24] In rare cases, more extensive involvement of the small and large intestines may result in obstruction.[24]

Endometriosis is a chronic and progressive disease of the childbearing years. Although the degree of pelvic involvement may not necessarily advance with age, the depth of infiltration, size of implants, and adhesion formation may progress with increasing duration of illness. This progression of disease may be associated with a worsening of symptoms and increasing need for therapeutic intervention.

IMAGING FINDINGS

Sonography

The goal of ultrasound in the management of endometriosis is to add as much detail as possible to the clinical picture, including location and extent of disease. Ultrasound findings are most useful in the clinical

---

PATHOLOGY BOX 11-3

Common Locations of Deep Endometriotic Implants and Associated Symptoms[7,10,19,27]

Anterior	
Bladder Vesicouterine pouch	Urinary symptoms
Posterior	
Upper vagina	Painful defecation
Rectovaginal septum	Gastrointestinal symptoms
Rectosigmoid colon	
Uterosacral ligaments	Deep dyspareunia
Ureters	
Upper abdomen	
Appendix	Noncyclic pain
Terminal ileum	Gastrointestinal symptoms
Upper sigmoid colon	

---

management of advanced disease and in the determination and planning of appropriate surgical intervention.[25]

As in all scanning protocols for gynecologic sonography, the ideal examination should include examination of the uterus and cervix, ovaries, pelvic vasculature, and bladder, all in at least two planes. The careful delineation of structures as well as viewing images in real time are particularly important when attempting to diagnose diffuse processes, which may produce subtle sonographic changes. Both transabdominal and endovaginal ultrasound techniques are employed.[25] Particularly for the diagnosis of endometriosis, some authors recommend imaging in the late secretory phase of the cycle when lesions may be most prominent.[25] Others suggest the use of bowel preparation prior to ultrasound, which may allow for improved visualization of lesions within the rectosigmoid colon.[25]

The sonographic findings in endometriosis are variable.[23] The uterus usually appears normal in size and echogenicity. Endometriotic lesions are located both on the peritoneal surface (endometriotic implants) and within the ovary (endometrioma). Lesions of the ovary are discussed in further detail below. Endometriotic implants vary in size, echogenicity, and location. Lesions may be a few millimeters to several centimeters in diameter. They vary from hypoechoic to hyperechoic in appearance and may be either cystic in the case of recent hemorrhage or nodular secondary to fibrosis.[23] Peritoneal implants may be superficial (<5 mm of invasion) or deep (>5 mm of invasion) and may be located throughout the pelvis.[26] Small nodules measuring only a few millimeters are most commonly found in the rectovaginal septum and appear hypoechoic. In contrast, larger nodules measuring 1.5 to 2 cm are located most commonly in the bladder wall. Laminar or thin plaquelike lesions are seen within the recto-vaginal septum, the broad ligaments, and the rectal wall as a hypoechoic thickening of the effected pelvic structure.[23]

Focal ovarian endometriosis appears on ultrasound examination as cystic structures termed endometriomas. These structures result from invagination of the ovarian cortex in response to surface endometriotic implants and the resulting adhesion formation (Fig. 11-15). Repeated hemorrhage within the lesions results is the usual "chocolate cyst" appearance described at the time of surgical evacuation. On ultrasound, endometriomas typically appear as discrete, thick-walled, spherical adnexal masses (Fig. 11-16). Most commonly (95% of the time), they exhibit uniform dispersion of low-level internal echoes or a homogeneous "ground glass" appearance, although endometriomas may also appear anechoic or solid.[22,27,28] They are commonly unilocular; however, they may appear multilocular with thin or thick septations and may contain fluid

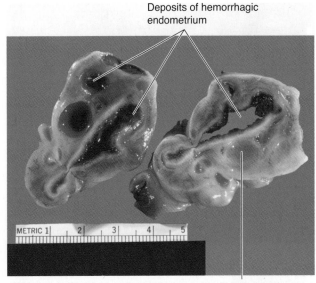

Figure 11-15 Hemorrhagic, cystic deposits of endometrium are visible in this ovary. Note the small follicle.

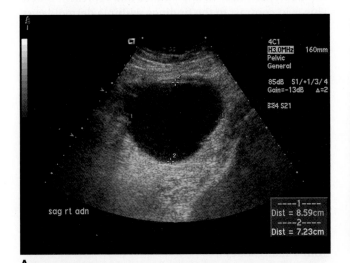

A

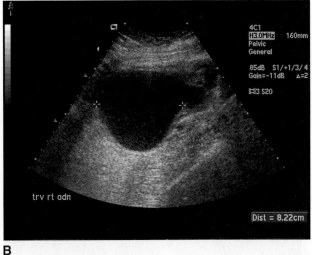

B

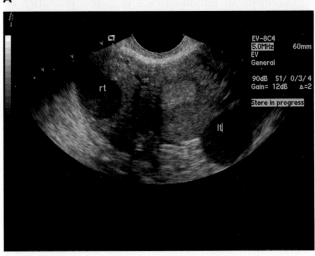

C

Figure 11-16 **A,B:** Sagittal and transverse images of a large adnexal mass consistent with endometrioma. The mass is thick walled and has a unilocular, homogeneous or "ground glass" appearance typically seen in ovarian endometrioma. **C:** Transverse image of the pelvis demonstrating bilateral endometriomas.

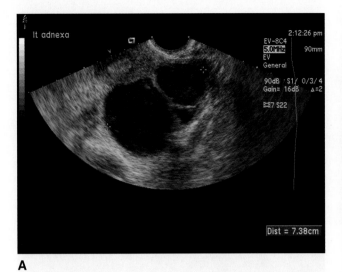

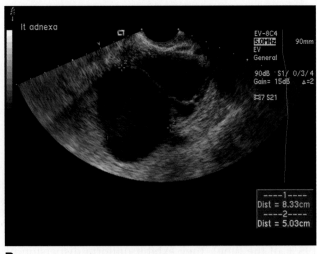

A   **B**

Figure 11-17 Sagittal and transverse images of an ovarian endometrioma. Unlike the more commonly seen unilocular appearance, this mass is multilocular with multiple thin septations. The structure demonstrates the typical appearance seen with endometriomas.

or debris (Fig. 11-17).[22] Some authors have reported small cystic structures with hyperechoic margins located in the peripheral aspect of the endometrioma, as well as small echogenic foci within the wall of the cystic structure.[22,27,28]

In the case of the endometrioma, sonographic findings may be nonspecific. The echo pattern of the endometrioma may mimic that of the hemorrhagic cyst[28] and, less often, benign cystic teratoma or dermoid, both of which may appear as complex structures with variable degrees of solid components (Fig. 11-18). Endometriomas may contain central calcifications frequently seen in dermoid lesions and these calcifications may be indicative of older lesions.[27] Presence of a fluid-fluid level within the cyst will assist in the differentiation between

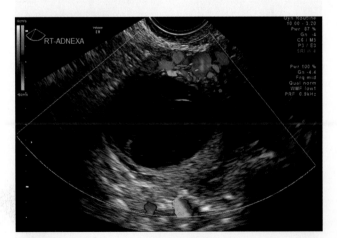

Figure 11-18 Ovarian endometrioma with an atypical appearance. Instead, the adnexal mass may be mistaken for a hemorrhagic cyst with heterogeneous internal debris or a benign cystic teratoma with linear echogenicity. Persistence of the mass over multiple cycles favors the diagnosis of endometrioma or benign cystic teratoma over a hemorrhagic process.

endometrioma and dermoid. When a fluid-fluid level is present within the endometrioma, the dependent layer will be hyperechoic in appearance and represent blood. This is in contrast to the findings within a dermoid cyst, in which the supernatant layer appears echogenic and represents the fatty component of the lesion.[27]

Color Doppler typically demonstrates evidence of pericystic flow around and not within these masses, similar to that noted with a simple cyst (Fig. 11-19).[22] The presence of Doppler flow within the mass should raise suspicion for the uncommon malignant transformation of an endometriotic lesion. In the case of complex cystic structures with solid components and internal Doppler flow, surgical excision and histologic evaluation may be necessary to rule out malignancy.[23] Decidualization of an endometrioma may occur in pregnancy, giving the appearance of internal vascularity and solid elements that are difficult to differentiate from a malignancy.[29]

Diagnosis of endometriosis is based primarily on clinical findings with imaging studies providing supporting or confirmatory information that assist in treatment planning. Endovaginal ultrasound for the diagnosis and exclusion of peritoneal or ovarian endometriosis is both sensitive and specific and should be considered first-line imaging in patients in whom endometriosis is suspected.[30] Endovaginal imaging is more cost-effective, more acceptable to patients, and more feasible than transrectal imaging, given that the latter may require general anesthesia and provides imaging of posterior lesions only.[25]

CT and MRI

Endovaginal ultrasound is also more cost-effective and provides improved resolution of pelvic structures when compared to CT. When ultrasound findings are

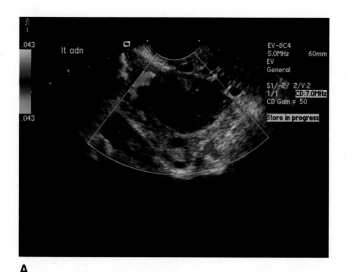

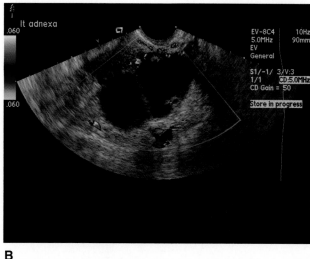

A   **B**

Figure 11-19 When applied to ovarian endometrioma, color Doppler exhibits a pericyclic flow pattern. This is seen in both unilocular lesions and those with septations.

equivocal, MRI may be employed for further evaluation (Fig. 11-20).[23]

TREATMENT

Treatment of the chronic symptoms of endometriosis may take several forms, including surgical excision of endometriotic implants and medical alteration in the hormones that stimulate implant growth. More conservatively, the patient may be observed and her symptoms controlled with analgesics. Endometriosis is a chronic condition, and the main goal of therapeutic intervention is to decrease pain and infertility symptoms and eliminate disease recurrence.

PATHOLOGY BOX 11-4

Ultrasound Findings of Endometriosis

Variable findings
Uterus normal in size and echogenicity

Peritoneal lesions

Vary in size: millimeters to centimeters
Vary in echogenicity: hypoechoic to hyperechoic
Vary in location: bladder, rectovaginal septum, uterosacral ligaments

Ovarian lesions: Endometriomas

Discrete adnexal mass with peripheral Doppler flow
Thick walled
Homogeneous, low level echogenicity
Majority unilocular, occasionally have septations
Less common findings:
Fluid level with dependent hyperechoic level
Central calcifications
Echogenic foci within thick wall
Small peripheral cystic structures with hyperechoic margins

NSAIDs are commonly used for the pain of endometriosis, either in a continuous or cyclic fashion, although evidence of their efficacy in treating the pain of endometriosis is inconclusive.[31] Despite this lack of evidence for their efficacy, NSAIDs are often employed, most likely because they are not habit forming and have few dangerous side effects when taken properly. Narcotic analgesic options are used less frequently given the chronicity of the endometriosis disease process. When NSAIDs are used cyclically, around-the-clock administration should be initiated 24 to 48 hours before the onset of menses for maximum improvement in symptoms.

A number of hormonal medications have been employed in the treatment of endometriosis with varying levels of success. Medications are often started empirically without definitive diagnosis by diagnostic laparoscopy. Oral contraceptive pills are used commonly to inhibit ovulation and treat the symptoms of endometriosis, despite limited evidence for their efficacy in relieving endometriosis symptoms.[32] Gonadotropin-releasing hormone agonists and androgens are also used commonly in clinical practice; however, their use is limited by significant side effects. Gonadotropin-releasing hormone agonists such as leuprolide acetate and nafarelin acetate produce a medical menopause, while androgens such as danazol cause weight gain, increased muscle mass, acne, deepening of voice, and altered libido.[33] Continuous progestins, as well as antiprogestins, have shown promise in treating endometriosis symptoms and are more effective than cyclic progestins used in the luteal phase of the cycle.[34] The progestin-releasing intrauterine device has been suggested as an alternative therapy for the treatment of endometriosis given the success of other continuous progestins; however, its efficacy has not been proven and requires further investigation.[35]

Alternative medications such as aromatase inhibitors, selective progesterone receptors modulators, and tumor

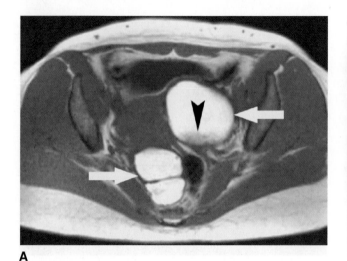

A

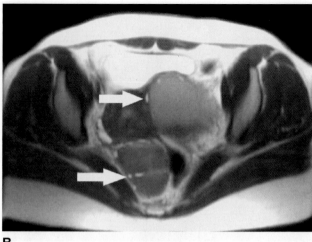

B

Figure 11-20 Bilateral endometriomas. **A:** T1-weighted image through pelvis demonstrates high signal intensity adnexal fluid collections (*arrows*). Signal of collections did not suppress with fat-suppression techniques (not shown). Note debris in left adnexal lesion (*arrowhead*). **B:** Despite their cystic nature, both lesions demonstrate mild signal loss on T2-weighted image (*shading*). Note high signal follicles (*arrows*) draped around both lesions, confirming their ovarian origin. Bilateral ovarian endometriomas found at surgery.

necrosis factor-alpha (TNFα) inhibitors have shown promise in treating endometriosis in animal models, as have medications that influence inflammation, angiogenesis, and matrix metalloproteinase activity. Further studies in humans are needed to confirm their effectiveness in treating the symptoms of endometriosis.[36]

Laparoscopic surgery is the gold standard for the diagnosis of endometriosis and plays an important role in disease treatment as well. Surgical intervention that involves laparoscopic excision of endometriotic implants in symptomatic patients with mild to moderate disease is likely to be more effective in relieving pain than diagnostic laparoscopy alone.[37] In patients with endometrioma, removal of the cystic structure including the cyst wall is associated with a decrease in dysmenorrhea, dyspareunia, pelvic pain, cyst recurrence, and need for future related surgery when compared to ablation of the mass alone.[38] For patients with severe symptoms in whom conservative surgical management and medical therapies have been exhausted, oophorectomy with or without uterine conservation may be considered for relief of symptoms. This results in surgical menopause and subsequent regression of endometriosis and relief of symptoms. However, this intervention should be reserved only for refractory cases given the negative effects of oophorectomy on bone health, vaginal dryness, and vasomotor symptoms. Hormone replacement therapy for women who have undergone oophorectomy as treatment for endometriosis is controversial as it may result in disease recurrence.[39]

Treatment modalities that employ a combination of hormonal regulation and surgical intervention are commonplace in the management of endometriosis. Both preoperative and postoperative medical management has been used in attempts to improve surgical outcomes and delay or eliminate disease recurrence following surgical

intervention. While the postoperative addition of medical therapies that inhibit ovulation may not improve pain symptoms or pregnancy rates in comparison with surgery alone, hormonal regulation following surgery has been shown to decrease the risk of disease recurrence.[40]

ADENOMYOSIS

DEFINITION

Adenomyosis is a uterine condition in which endometrial glands and stroma are located within the uterine myometrium proximal to the basalis layer of the endometrium.[16,29,37] Endometrial glands and stroma are surrounded by hypertrophic myometrial smooth muscle. The uterus is often asymmetrically affected with the posterior wall more commonly involved.[4,29] Adenomyosis is generally considered a variant of endometriosis in that ectopic endometrial tissue grows within the myometrium. Possible etiologies include a defect in the basement membrane separating the myometrial and endometrial layers of the uterus and endometrial migration via vascular or lymphatic spread (Fig. 11-21).[4]

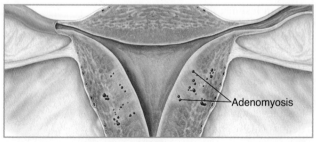

Figure 11-21 Adenomyosis occurs when endometrial cells grow within the wall of the uterus. This may cause heavy and painful menstrual cycles.

CLINICAL FINDINGS

Frequently found in parous women in their 30s and 40s, the common symptoms of Adenomyosis include abnormal bleeding, secondary dysmenorrhea, and an enlarged, tender uterus.[41,42] Because these symptoms are nonspecific, it is not surprising that this benign process is often misdiagnosed clinically; however, up to two-thirds of hysterectomies show adenomyosis.[43] The cause of adenomyosis is not clear, but it is usually associated with multiparity, chronic endometriosis, and often endometriosis. This disease process has two forms, diffuse and nodular (or focal) and is most frequently a diffuse process involving the entire uterine musculature. This results in relatively uniform uterine enlargement. Up to 80% of adenomyotic uteri are associated with such conditions as leiomyomata, endometrial hyperplasia, peritoneal endometriosis, and uterine cancer.[43] The focal form of adenomyosis produces the adenomyoma, occurring as discrete nodules within the myometrium[45-47] or cervix.

IMAGING FINDINGS

Multiple imaging modalities help in the diagnosis of adenomyosis. This includes not only sonography but the radiographic hysterosalpingogram and MRI. The sonographic examination, performed with a high-frequency endovaginal transducer, has a sensitivity of 53% to 89% and a specificity of 68% to 86%, resulting in an accuracy between 78 and 88%.[43,46] The MRI has similar rates; however, sonography is often the first exam performed due to cost-effectiveness and patient comfort.

Sonography

Prior to the availability of endovaginal sonography, ultrasound was not a sensitive tool for use in the diagnosis of adenomyosis, and definitive diagnosis required surgical removal of the uterus and histologic confirmation. However, endovaginal ultrasound has improved both the sensitivity and specificity of ultrasound evaluation

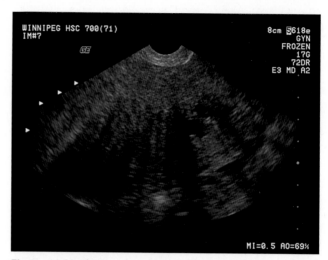

Figure 11-22 This is a sagittal endovaginal image of the uterus. Notice the irregular appearance of the endometrium and the posterior portion of the uterus. (Image courtesy of GE Medical, Wauwatosa, WI.)

for adenomyosis and now plays an important role in the diagnosis of this disease.[41]

Sonographic findings for adenomyosis are nonspecific, including an enlarged uterus with normal contours and an intact endometrial lining.[43] Adenomyosis may result in an asymmetrically enlarged uterus with an abnormal appearance of the myometrium (Fig. 11-22).[41,47] The abnormal echogenicity of the myometrium consists of a heterogeneous echotexture, areas of increased and decreased echogenicity, and anechoic regions or myometrial cysts.[41,48,49] The hypoechoic areas correspond histologically to smooth muscle hyperplasia, whereas the heterogeneous appearance results from heterotopic endometrial tissue and surrounding hypoechoic smooth muscle.[41,48,49] Myometrial cysts represent dilated endometrial glands or areas of hemorrhage and commonly measure less than 5 mm (Fig. 11-23).[49]

Another hallmark of adenomyosis on ultrasound is poor visualization of the junction between the endometrium and the myometrium. The interface appears

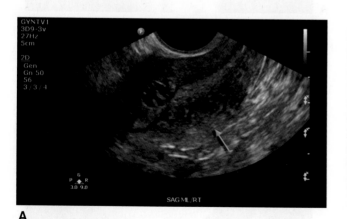

A

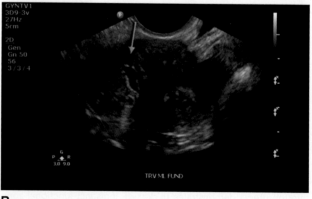

B

Figure 11-23 A: This is a sagittal endovaginal image of the uterus. Notice the heterogenous appearance of the myometrium and the posterior portion of the uterus (arrow). **B:** The same uterus on a transverse plane demonstrates anechoic areas (arrow) within the first two-thirds of the uterine wall. (Images courtesy of Philips Medical Systems, Bothell, WA.)

blurred and results in a pseudowidening of the endometrial measurement.[41,49]

In contrast to the ultrasound appearance of uterine leiomyomata, the sonographic appearance of adenomyosis is marked by lack of a discrete mass seen within the myometrium. Endovaginal color and power Doppler have also proven helpful in differentiating between these two conditions. In the case of adenomyosis, Doppler flow is seen diffusely throughout the myometrium whereas flow is seen in the periphery surrounding discrete leiomyomata.[41,48]

MRI

MRI imaging is also highly sensitive and specific for the diagnosis of adenomyosis.[49,50] Findings of adenomyosis are most notable on T2-weighed images in which the junctional zone representing the interface between the endometrium and myometrium is seen as a poorly defined and enlarged area of low signal intensity.[51] This area corresponds to the smooth muscle hyperplasia seen in adenomyosis. Within this abnormal region of low signal intensity, bright foci are seen in approximately 50% of patients and represent ectopic endometrial tissue with cystic glandular dilation and areas of hemorrhage.[49,50] MRI and ultrasound may be used in concert in confirming the diagnosis of adenomyosis, and MRI may be particularly important for cases in which endovaginal ultrasound is equivocal (Fig. 11-24).[49]

Radiography

Hysterosalpingogram (HSG) images spiculations and myometrial defects in the patient with adenomyosis. This method of imaging has a low accuracy rate because adneomyosis is difficult to differentiate from

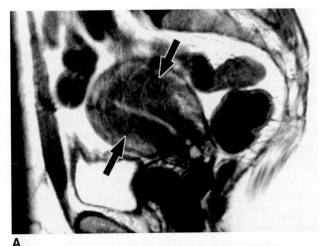

A

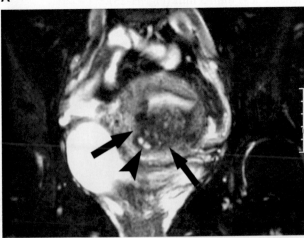

B

Figure 11-24 A: Diffuse adenomyosis. Sagittal T2-weighted image through uterus demonstrates thickened, indistinct junctional zone *(arrows)*. **B:** Focal adenomyosis. Coronal fat-suppressed T2-weighted image through uterus shows focal thickening of junctional zone *(arrows)* containing small high signal foci *(arrowhead)*. Note minimal distortion of endometrial stripe and serosal surface of uterus.

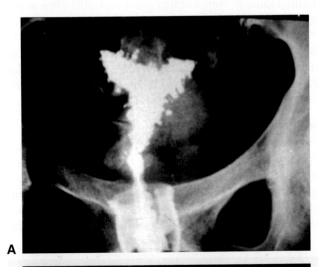

A

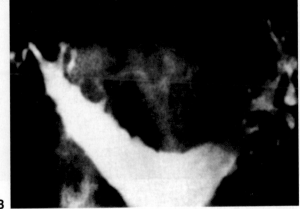

B

Figure 11-25 A,B: Hysterograms show direct signs of adenomyosis. The contrast medium has injected numerous diverticula.

other processes such as vascular or lymphatic extravasation.[52] Definitive diagnosis with this radiographic modality comes with the imaging of a connection between the endometrial cavity and the ectopic endometrial glands (Fig. 11-25).[52] Due to the low sensitivity and specificity, coupled with patient discomfort, HSG is seldom used for diagnosis of adenomyosis.

TREATMENT

Adenomyosis is generally treated surgically, and hysterectomy with or without removal of the ovaries remains the mainstay of definitive therapy. Surgical intervention such as endometrial ablation and uterine artery embolization and medical management with hormonal therapy (GnRH agonists, androgens, and oral contraceptives) are less effective and often fail to adequately relieve patient symptoms.[43]

SUMMARY

- PID is usually the result of sexually transmitted polymicrobal infections.
- A rare complication of PID is the development of perihepatic inflammation resulting in what is called the Fitz-Hugh-Curtis syndrome.

- PID staging correlates with the involvement of the female reproductive organs.
- Acute or early to intermediate PID localizes to the endometrium, resulting in loss of boundary detail on the sonographic image.
- Advanced PID results in salpingitis, tubo-ovarian complex or TOA.
- With a TOA, ovarian and tubal structures cannot be separated on the sonographic image.
- Tubo-ovarian complex demonstrates enlarged ovaries, adhesions, and ill-defined planes; however, structures can still be identified.
- Thin-walled hydrosalpinges are seen with chronic PID.
- Sonographic findings of endometriosis vary and are often nonspecific.
- Endometriomas—large, blood-filled cysts on the ovaries—image as smooth-walled structures with low-level internal echoes.
- Adenomyosis is the invasion of endometrial glands and stroma into the myometrium while endometriosis is the abnormal seeding of endometrial tissue outside of the uterus.

Critical Thinking Questions

1. A patient presents to the imaging department for a sonographic examination of her pelvis. She complains of generalized cyclic pelvic pain with a focal area on the right side. Her last menstrual period was 3 weeks ago and she is G2P1. Though she wishes to become pregnant, she has been unsuccessful for the last year. During the exam a mass imaged on the right side (Fig. 11-26). Color Doppler demonstrated pericytic flow. List differentials for this finding based on the patient symptoms. What other possible benign differentials might apply? Hint: Refer to Chapter 8.

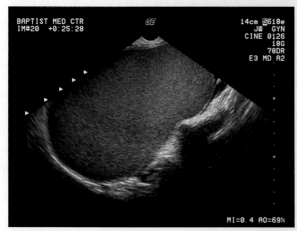

Figure 11-26

ANSWER: This is most likely an endometrioma of the right ovary; however, other differentials include a hemorrhagic cyst, ovarian torsion, teratoma, mucinous or serous cystadenoma, or a fibroma. (Sonographic image courtesy of GE Healthcare, Wauwatosa, WI.)

2. The patient is a 41-year-old female G0 who presents to the emergency room with 4 days of lower abdominal pain, nausea, vomiting, and diarrhea. She denies vaginal discharge, vaginal bleeding, fever, and chills. She has not been sexually active for 4 years and denies a history of sexually transmitted disease. Laboratory evaluation reveals leukocytosis with WBC 14.2. Hemoglobin, hematocrit, platelets, and electrolytes are within normal limits. Gonorrhea and chlamydia cultures are negative.

Transvaginal pelvic ultrasound is performed and reveals bilateral adnexal masses corresponding to the physical exam findings. Internal septations and Doppler flow are not seen within the masses bilaterally. Normal ovarian tissue is not seen distinct from the adnexal masses as described (Fig. 11-27).

(A) Given the clinical presentation and ultrasound findings, list differentials for these findings. (B) Examine image A and B. Explain the reason for the differing sector size and image brightness.

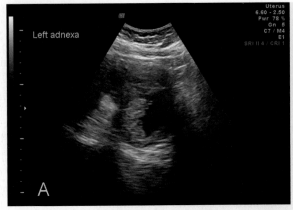
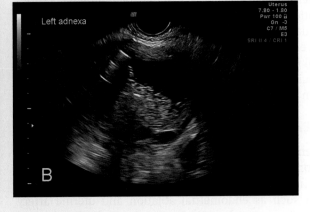

Figure 11-27

ANSWER:

(A) The differential diagnosis includes ovarian neoplasm, such as hemorrhagic cyst, benign cystic teratoma, or serous cystadenoma versus bilateral TOA. The pathology report reveals bilateral ovary and fallopian tubes with acute and chronic inflammation and bilateral fallopian tubes with muscular wall hypertrophy.

(B) In image A the decrease in sector size results in increased line density, thus increasing image detail. This image was obtained transabdominally, while B is an endovaginal image. The overall gain has a higher setting on image A, which can be seen by the setting indicator located in the upper right of the image. The abdominal image uses a gain (GN) setting of 5, while the endovaginal image has a -3 gain setting.

REFERENCES

1. Rein DB, Kassler WJ, Irwin KL, et al. Direct medical cost of pelvic inflammatory disease and its sequelae: decreasing, but still substantial. *Obstet Gynecol.* 2000;95(3):397–402.

2. Simms J, Stephenson JM. Pelvic inflammatory disease epidemiology: what do we know and what do we need to know? *Sex Transm Infect.* 2000;76(2):80–87.

3. Kelly AM, Ireland M, Aughey D. Pelvic inflammatory disease in adolescents: high incidence and recurrence rates in an urban teen clinic. *J Pediatr Adolesc Gynecol.* 2004;17(6):383–388.

4. Barrett S, Taylor C. A review on pelvic inflammatory disease. *Int J STD AIDS.* 2005;16(11):715–721.

5. Center for Disease Control and Prevention. Sexually Transmitted Disease Treatment Guidelines 2006. Available at: http://www.cdc.gov/std/treatment/2006/pid/htm. Updated January 28, 2011. Accessed September 21, 2011.

6. Ness RB, Soper DE, Holley RL, et al. Hormonal and barrier contraception and risk of upper genital tract disease in the PID Evaluation of Clinical Health (PEACH) study. *Am J Obstet Gynecol.* 2001;185(1):121–127.

7. Gareen IF, Greenland S, Morgenstern H. Intrauterine devices and pelvic inflammatory disease: meta-analyses of published studies, 1974–1990. *Epidemiology.* 2000;11(5):589–597.

8. Meirik O. Intrauterine devices—upper and lower genital tract infections. *Contraception.* 2007;75(6 Suppl):S41–S47.

9. Katz VL. *Comprehensive Gynecology.* 5th ed. St. Louis, MO: Consult; 2007.

10. Berek JS. *Berek and Novak's Gynecology.* 14th ed. Philadelphia: Lippincott Williams and Wilkins; 2007.

11. Lambert MJ, Villa M. Gynecologic ultrasound in emergency medicine. *Emerg Med Clin North Am.* 2004;22(3):683–696.

12. Wang C, Guo X, Yuan Z, et al. Radiologic diagnosis of Fitz-Hugh-Curtis syndrome. *Chin Med J.* 2009;122(6):741–744.

13. Horrow MM. Ultrasound of pelvic inflammatory disease. *Ultrasound Q.* 2004;20(4):171–179.

14. Timor-Trisch IE, Lerner JP, Monteagudo A, et al. Transvaginal sonographic markers of tubal inflammatory disease. *Ultrasound Obstet Gynecol.* 1998;12(1):56–66.

15. Ignacio EA, Hill MC. Ultrasound of the acute female pelvis. *Ultrasound Q.* 2003;19(2):86–98.

16. Kamaya A, Shin L, Chen B, et al. Emergency gynecologic imaging. *Semin Ultrasound CT MRI.* 2008;29(5):353–368.

17. Vandermeer FQ, Wong-you-cheong JJ. Imaging of acute pelvic pain. *Clin Obstet Gynecol.* 2009;52(1):2–20.

18. Donnez J, Van Langendonckt A. Typical and subtle atypical presentations of endometriosis. *Curr Opin Obstet Gynecol.* 2004;16(5):431–437.

19. Winkel CA. Evaluation and management of women with endometriosis. *Obstet Gynecol.* 2003;102(2):397–408.

20. Busacca M, Vignali M. Ovarian endometriosis: from pathogenesis to surgical treatment. *Curr Opin Obstet Gynecol.* 2003;15(4):321–326.

21. Alborzi S, Zarel A, Alborzi S, et al. Management of ovarian endometrioma. *Clin Obstet Gynecol.* 2006;49(3):480–491.

22. Bhatt S, Kocakoc E, Dogra VS. Endometriosis: sonographic spectrum. *Ultrasound Q.* 2006;22(4):273–280.

23. Carbognin G, Guarise A, Minelli L, et al. Pelvic endometriosis: US and MRI features. *Abdom Imaging.* 2004;29(5):609–618.

24. Schorge JO, Schaffer JI, Halvorson LM, et al. *Williams Gynecology.* New York: McGraw-Hill; 2008.

25. Goncalves MO, Dias JO, Podgaec S, et al. Transvaginal ultrasound for diagnosis of deeply infiltrating endometriosis. *Int J Gynecol Obstet.* 2009;104(2):156–160.

26. Kinkel K, Frei KA, Balleyguier C, et al. Diagnosis of endometriosis with imaging: a review. *Eur Radiol.* 2006; 16(2):285–298.

27. Asch E, Levine D. Variations in appearance of endometriomas. *J Ultrasound Med.* 2007;26(8):993–1002.

28. Patel MD, Feldstein VA, Chen DC, et al. Endometriomas: diagnostic performance of US. *Radiology.* 1999;210(3): 739–745.

29. Poder L, Coakley FV, Rabban JT, et al. Decidualized endometrioma during pregnancy: recognizing an imaging mimic of ovarian malignancy. *J Comput Assist Tomogr.* 2008;32(4):555–558.

30. Moore J, Copley S, Morris J, et al. A systematic review of the accuracy of ultrasound in the diagnosis of endometriosis. *Ultrasound Obstet Gynecol.* 2002;20(6): 630–634.

31. Allen C, Hopewell S, Prentice A, et al. Non-steroidal anti-inflammatory drugs for pain in women with endometriosis. *Cochrane Database Syst Rev.* 2009;(2):CD004753.

32. Davis LJ, Kennedy SS, Moore J, et al. Oral contraceptives for pain associated with endometriosis. *Cochrane Database Syst Rev.* 2007;(3):CD001019. doi: 10.1002/14761858.

33. Selak V, Farquhar C, Prentice A, et al. Danazol for pelvic pain associated with endometriosis. *Cochrane Database Syst Rev.* 2007;(4):CD000068.

34. Prentice A, Deary A, Bland ES. Progestagens and anti-progestagens for pain associated with endometriosis. *Cochrane Database Syst Rev.* 2000;(2):CD002122.

35. Vercellini P, Vigano P, Somigliana E. The role of levonorgestrel-releasing intrauterine device in the management of symptomatic endometriosis. *Curr Opin Obstet Gynecol.* 2005;17(4):359–365.

36. Ferrero S, Abbamonte LH, Anserini P, et al. Future perspectives on the medical treatment of endometriosis. *Obstet Gynecol Surv.* 2005;60(12):817–826.

37. Jacobson TZ, Duffy JMN, Barlow D, et al. Laparoscopic surgery for pelvic pain associated with endometriosis. *Cochrane Database Syst Rev.* 2009(4):CD001300.

38. Harr RJ, Hickey M, Maouris P, et al. Excisional surgery versus ablative surgery for ovarian endometriomata. *Cochrane Database Syst Rev.* 2008;(2):CD004992.

39. Al Kadri H, Hassan H, Al-Fosan HM, et al. Hormone therapy for endometriosis and surgical menopause. *Cochrane Database Syst Rev.* 2009;(1):CD005997.

40. Yap C, Furness S, Farquhar C, et al. Pre and post operative medical therapy for endometriosis surgery. *Cochrane Database Syst Rev.* 2004;(3):CD003678.

41. Andreotti RF, Fleischer AC. The sonographic diagnosis of adenomyosis. *Ultrasound Q.* 2005;21(3):167–170.

42. Matalliotakis IM, Katsikis IK, Panidis DK. Adenomyosis: what is the impact of fertility? *Curr Opin Obstet Gynecol.* 2005;17(3):261–264.

43. Poder L. Ultrasound evaluation of the uterus. In: *Ultrasonography in Obstetrics and Gynecology.* 5th ed. Philadelphia: Elsevier; 2008.

44. Koskas M, Nizard J, Salmon LJ, et al. Abdominal and pelvic ultrasound findings within 24 hours following uneventful Cesarean section. *Ultrasound Obstet Gynecol.* 2008;32(4):520–526.

45. Krakow D. Medical and surgical complications of pregnancy. In: *Danforth's Obstetrics and Gynecology.* 10th ed. Philadelphia: Lippincott Williams and Wilkins; 2003.

46. Chang YT, Lin JY. Intraperitoneal rupture of mature cystic ovarian teratoma secondary to sit-ups. *J Formos Med Assoc.* 2009;108(2):173–175.

47. Williams PL, Laifer-Narin SL, Ragavendra N. US of abnormal uterine bleeding. *Radiographics.* 2003;23(3):703–718.

48. Dueholm M, Lundorf E. Transvaginal ultrasound or MRI diagnosis of adenomyosis. *Curr Opin Obstet Gynecol.* 2007;19(6):505–512.

49. Reinhold C, Tafazoli F, Mehio A, et al. Uterine adenomyosis: endovaginal US and MR imaging features with histopathologic correlation. *Radiographics.* 1999;19:S147–S160.

50. Tamai K, Togashi K, Ito T, et al. MR Imaging findings of adenomyosis: correlation with histopathologic features and diagnostic pitfalls. *Radiographics.* 2005;25(1):21–40.

51. Wang PH, Su WH, Sheu BC, et al. Adenomyosis and its variance: adenomyoma and female fertility. *Taiwan J Obstet Gynecol.* 2009;48(3):232–238.

52. Cherng-Jye J, Huang S, Shen J, et al. Laparoscopy-guided myometrial biopsy in the definite diagnosis of diffuse adenomyosis. *Human Reprod.* 2007;22(7):2016–2019.

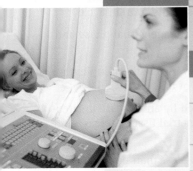

12 Assisted Reproductive Technologies (ART), Contraception, and Elective Abortion

Catheeja Ismail and Molina Dayal

OBJECTIVES

Summarize the role of sonography in the diagnosis and treatment of infertility

Describe the process of conception as it occurs both naturally and with assisted reproductive technologies (ART)

Explain the role of sonography in the many and varied routes to assisted reproduction

Discuss the role of sonography in the three areas of reversible contraception, irreversible contraception, and elective abortion

KEY TERMS

assisted reproductive technologies | infertility | in vitro fertilization | intrauterine insemination | conception | contraception | saline-infusion sonohysterography | hysterosalpingiography | male factor infertility | ovarian hyperstimulation | multifetal reduction | embryo transfer

GLOSSARY

Assisted reproductive technologies (ART) Clinical treatments and laboratory procedures used to establish a pregnancy

Blastocyst transfer Transfer of embryo 5 to 6 days after fertilization.

Cleavage-stage transfer Transfer of embryo 2 to 3 days after fertilization.

Clomiphene citrate Most commonly prescribed fertility medication used for ovulation induction of a single follicle or superovulation of multiple follicles

Controlled ovarian hyperstimulation (COH) Process that stimulates multiple follicle development using clomiphene citrate or gonadotropins

Cryopreservation Process, usually using liquid nitrogen, to freeze embryos or gametes

Embryo transfer (ET) In vitro fertilized embryo transfer into the uterine cavity at the cleavage (2 to 3 days after fertilization) or blastocyst (5 to 6 days after fertilization) stage

Estradiol Primary sex hormone produced by ovarian follicles in women of childbearing age

Fertile window Period during which the viability and survivability of both oocytes and sperm are maximum;

refers to the 4- to 5-day interval ending on the day after ovulation

Fertility Capacity to produce offspring

Follicular phase First half of the ovarian cycle characterized by high levels of circulating follicle-stimulating hormone (FSH), which result in ovarian follicle maturation

Gamete intrafallopian transfer (GIFT) Placement of the sperm and ova (i.e., gametes) directly in the ampullary portion of the fallopian tube, for in vivo fertilization

Human chorionic gonadotropin (hCG) Hormone produced by the trophoblastic cells of the normal developing placenta or by abnormal germ cell tumors, molar pregnancies, and choriocarcinoma

Intrauterine contraceptive device (IUD or IUCD) Products inserted into the uterine cavity as a birth control mechanism to prevent pregnancy

In vitro fertilization (IVF) Formation of a zygote from extracted ova and sperm in a laboratory setting

In vivo fertilization Process whereby ova and sperm come into contact within the body and fuse to form a zygote

Infertility Failure to achieve a successful pregnancy after 12 months or more of regular unprotected intercourse

Intracytoplasmic sperm injection (ICSI) Injection of a single sperm into an ovum

Intrauterine insemination (IUI, aka artificial insemination) Placement of seminal fluid free sperm through the cervix directly into the uterine cavity

Luteal phase Second half of the ovarian cycle, when the corpus luteum secretes high levels of progesterone, which acts on the endometrium

Menstrual phase First 5 days of the menstrual cycle, characterized by endometrial shedding

Microinsert Coil introduction into the fallopian tube, resulting in tissue growth and obliteration of the fallopian tube lumen

Ovarian hyperstimulation syndrome (OHSS) Excessive response to ovulation induction therapy

Ovulation induction Development of a single follicle with administration of fertility medications that, upon reaching optimal size, requires administration of hCG for ovulation

Ovarian reserve Estimation of the quantity and quality of a woman's remaining follicles

Periovulatory period Portion of the cycle spanning the follicular and the luteal phases of the ovarian cycle

Proliferative phase Overlaps the menstrual phase and extends through midcycle

Theca lutein cysts Enlarged ovaries with multiple cysts due to abnormally high levels of hCG

Secretory phase Characterized by an increase in circulating progesterone and endometrial tissue increase and thickening

Subfertility Condition of being less than normally fertile though still capable of achieving fertilization

Sonography plays a key role in interventions designed to assist infertile couples in successfully achieving pregnancy and a somewhat small role in interventions designed to assist women in controlling pregnancy. This chapter will cover the role of sonography in these two areas. Part I comprises the bulk of this chapter, and will cover the role of sonography in assisted reproductive technologies (ART) that aid couples in achieving pregnancy. Part II is shorter and will cover the role of sonography in contraception and elective abortion. In closing, two case studies will help readers assess their application of the material presented in this chapter.

PART I. CONCEPTION: THE ROLE OF SONOGRAPHY IN ASSISTED REPRODUCTIVE TECHNOLOGIES (ART)

This section will first provide an overview of the diagnosis and treatment of infertility. Second, it will describe the anatomy, physiology, pathology, and sonographic assessment of the reproductive system as it pertains to infertility. Third, it will explain the many and varied routes to assisted reproduction, with an emphasis on those treatment options that utilize sonography.

OVERVIEW OF THE DIAGNOSIS AND TREATMENT OF INFERTILITY

The diagnosis of infertility occurs when a couple fails to conceive naturally despite 1 year of unprotected intercourse. The incidence of infertility has remained unchanged over the past three decades.[1] One in five couples in the United States consults with a physician about difficulty conceiving, and half of these couples require specialist care.[2] Etiologies of infertility are divided into 40% due to the female partner, 40% due to the male, 5% to 10% related to both partners, and 5% to 10% idiopathic.[3] In couples, the etiologies of infertility are tubal and pelvic pathology (35%), male problems (35%), ovulatory dysfunction (15%), unexplained infertility (10%), and unusual problems (5%).[1,3,4] Sexually transmitted disease and the delay of childbearing, among other factors, contribute to infertility. Individuals with a variety of etiologies of infertility may in fact achieve pregnancy if their particular etiology can be overcome through treatment options available with the use of ART. Some have referred to these couples as subfertile,[5,6] as they are indeed able to conceive with assistance. In keeping with the more prevalently used language, however, the current authors use the term "infertile" in this chapter.

Sonography is helpful in the diagnosis of infertility. In women, sonography helps diagnose structural anomalies and pathologies of the uterus, tubes, and ovaries that contribute to the female factors of infertility (Fig. 12-1)(Table 12-1). In men, sonography may be of

PATHOLOGY BOX 12-1	
Causes of Infertility in Couples	
Tubal and pelvic pathology	35%
Male problems	35%
Ovulatory dysfunction	15%
Unexplained infertility	10%
Unusual problems	5%

(Modified from Speroff, Leon and Fritz, Marc A., *Clinical Gynecologic Endocrinology and Infertility*, 7 ed. Philadelphia: Lippincott Williams & Wilkins; 2005.)

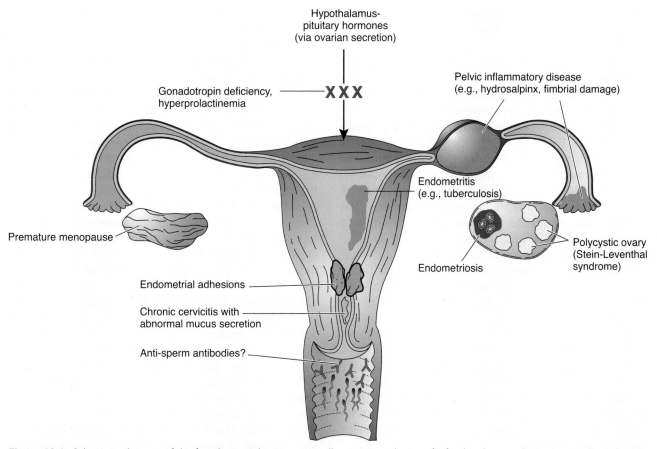

Figure 12-1. Schematic diagram of the female reproductive system illustrating etiologies of infertility that may be overcome through ARTs. The female factors of infertility include hormonal deficiencies that affect the hypothalamus-pituitary-ovary route; tubal diseases that interfere with passage of gametes or conceptus; ovarian diseases that impact on the number or quality of viable ova or their release at mid-cycle; structural abnormalities that interfere with the passage of sperm, ova, or conceptus; endometrial or myometrial abnormalities that interfere with implantation or fetal development; and abnormalities of the chemical environment that adversely affect sperm viability.

TABLE	12-1		
Anatomic Causes of Female Infertility			
Location	**Pathology**	**Etiology**	**Sonographic Findings**
Uterus			
	Subserosal, intramural, submucosal myoma	Unknown	Varies: hyperechoic/hypoechoic with shadowing
	Septate uterus	Congenital anomaly	Septum visualized with 3D sonography
	Endometrial polyp	Unknown	Hyperechoic lesion indenting into endometrial cavity
	Asherman's disease, uterine scarring	Unknown; almost always follows pregnancy loss	Absence or discontinuation of endometrial stripe
Tubes			
	Hydrosalpinx. Blocked or scarred tubes	Infection, prior surgery	Varies: tube-shaped adnexal structure that is sonolucent or has mixed echogenicity
	Adhesions. Scarring around tubes/ovaries	Infection, prior surgery	Varies: fixed, echogenic fluid areas surrounding ovary, tubes
Ovary			
	Endometriosis: ectopic endometrial tissue	Unknown	Low-level internal echoes
	PCOS: Ovarian hyperandrogenism	Unknown	Cysts arranged like a string of pearls

help in diagnosing scrotal pathology that contributes to male factors of infertility. This section describes these sonographic assessments.

Sonography plays a variety of roles valuable in the treatment of infertility. The most central role is the monitoring of follicular growth for women undergoing controlled ovarian hyperstimulation (COH). In this treatment protocol, administration of fertility medication (either FSH injection or clomiphene citrate) is coupled with a schedule of endovaginal sonograms and serum hormone levels to monitor ovarian response. Medication dosages change according to the findings of the sonograms and hormone levels. In this way, the clinician can control the stimulation of the ovaries to achieve optimal size and timing of follicular growth. Following COH, many routes to reproduction are available to infertile couples. COH is coupled with timed intercourse, intrauterine insemination (IUI), or in vitro fertilization (IVF). Sonography also plays a role in the guidance of a needle to retrieve oocytes from mature follicles. In many centers, sonography provides guidance for transferring the embryos into the woman's uterus. Furthermore, sonography plays a continuing role in the assessment of treatment complications (e.g., ovarian hyperstimulation syndrome [OHSS] or multiple gestations), in assessing the early gestation for its viability, and the ongoing gestation for its development until full-term delivery.

In summary, sonography is valuable in the diagnosis and treatment of infertility. Sonography helps in the diagnosis of anatomic abnormalities or disease in the female or the male partner that hinder fertilization or implantation. Sonography aids in monitoring fertility treatment, retrieving oocytes from the ovaries, transferring embryos into the uterus, and in documenting the location, viability, and subsequent development of the pregnancy. Part I of this chapter covers the diagnosis and treatment of infertility through a varied array of ART, emphasizing those procedures and protocols in which sonography plays a role.

DIAGNOSIS OF INFERTILITY

This section will introduce sonographers to the anatomy, physiology, pathology, and scan techniques pertinent to the sonographic diagnosis of infertility. It will first cover conception as it occurs naturally; second, it will give an overview of the ovarian and menstrual cycles; third, it will discuss the sonographic assessment of the ovary; fourth, it will discuss the sonographic assessment of the uterus; and fifth, it will make a brief comment on the role of sonography in diagnosing male infertility.

Conception as It Occurs Naturally

The process of conception is so intricate it is a wonder of nature that a woman does successfully conceive in any given menstrual cycle. Only 20% of couples

engaging in sexual intercourse will conceive in any month when not using contraception.[7] In an ideal world conception occurs naturally as a result of multiple coordinated events (Fig. 12-2). For this to happen, adequate, viable, motile sperm must be deposited into the vagina at the appropriate moment in the mid-cycle fertile window when the cervical mucus is slippery and clear, permitting sperm passage through the cervix and into the uterus. The sperm must then travel the entire length of the uterine cavity, enter the fallopian tube, and continue far into the mid (ampullary) portion of the fallopian tube. Meanwhile, the ovum (egg) must be released out of a follicle in the ovary and swept from the surface of the ovary into the fimbriated end of the fallopian tube and it then must travel to its ampullary portion. Fertilization of one ovum by one sperm must occur in the ampullary portion of the fallopian tube. The resulting zygote must then divide into one blastocyst which must travel down the entire length of the fallopian tube and arrive in the uterine cavity 4 to 5 days after fertilization. In addition, the endometrium must be ready to support and nurture an implanting blastocyst. The implantation must trigger the endometrium to undergo trophoblastic changes that will initiate the development of one chorionic sac and one amniotic sac. One single fetus must develop within the amniotic sac. The fetus must develop a beating heart and continue to develop into a viable fetus, to result in a healthy singleton full-term neonate. If all these events occur, a woman will have conceived and reproduced in a natural and ideal way. Counseling is the first step when couples present to an infertility specialist seeking help, to ensure that all these processes do occur. With such counseling, they may still achieve pregnancy naturally.[8]

If one or more of these processes fail, the couple may be unable to conceive children through an entirely natural process. However, in light of medical advances, this does not preclude the possibility of this couple having children. There are many ART treatment options available. To understand the role of these advances in the diagnosis and treatment of infertility, it is helpful to review some basic concepts in anatomy, physiology, and pathology as they pertain to infertility and assisted reproduction.

Ovarian/Menstrual Cycles

The ovarian cycle and the menstrual cycle are presented together (Fig. 12-3) in this section because they help explain the diagnosis and treatment of infertility and they are best understood as two interrelated cycles working together. The prototypical ovarian/menstrual cycles last 28 days, beginning on the first day of a woman's menses and extending to the first day of her next menses. During a normal cycle, the ovary and endometrium undergo changes in response to a milieu of hormones secreted by the hypothalamus, anterior pituitary, and ovary.

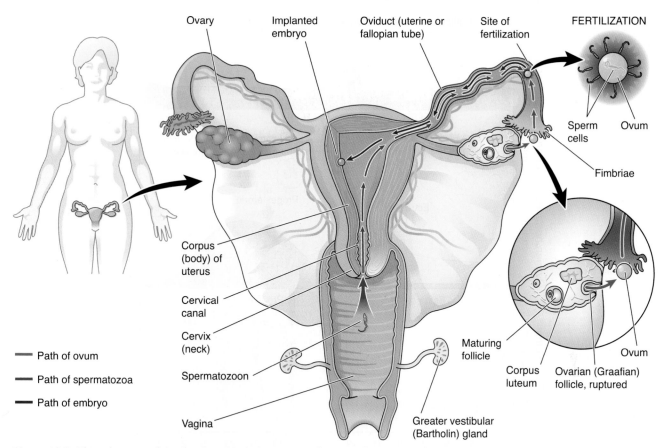

Figure 12-2. This schematic of the female reproductive system illustrates the wonder of nature in the process of conception. Conception occurs as a result of multiple coordinated events illustrated here. Arrows show the pathway of the sperm and ovum, fertilization of the ovum, and implantation of the blastocyst.

Gonadotropin-releasing hormone (GnRH) from the hypothalamus initiates the cycles. GnRH acts on the anterior pituitary gland, causing it to release follicle-stimulating hormone (FSH) into circulating blood. This hormone, which is a gonadotropin, acts on the ovary. Responding to increasing levels of FSH, a cohort of primary follicles in the ovary begins to grow and mature. The follicles that begin to grow during one cycle continue their growth for several months.[9] A fluid-filled cavity called the antrum forms within each of a select few primary follicles, and after about 6 months of growth they become sonographically visible as antral follicles during the first half of the ovarian cycle, the follicular phase. As antral follicles mature, the developing ovum within each follicle is pushed to one side, into a complex called the cumulus oophorus. In a natural cycle, one of these antral follicles matures into a dominant, or Graafian, follicle. Granulosa cells of the growing ovarian follicles (Fig. 12-4) produce the hormone estradiol. The first half of the ovarian cycle is the follicular phase, and the second half is the luteal phase. Just before midcycle, there is a sharp increase in the levels of the gonadotropins luteinizing hormone (LH) and FSH in the blood. Within 12 to 36 hours[10] of the surge in LH, the dominant follicle ruptures and the ovum bursts out of the ovary. This is ovulation. Ovulation occurs approximately 14 days before the onset of

the next menstrual cycle (i.e., day 14 of a 28-day cycle). This begins the second half of the ovarian cycle, the luteal phase. The remnants of the ruptured follicle now become the corpus luteum, which secretes the hormone progesterone into circulating blood. If fertilization does occur during this cycle, the corpus luteum remains active as the corpus luteum of pregnancy. If fertilization does not occur during this cycle, the corpus luteum begins to degenerate about 8 to 10 days after ovulation.

Paralleling the ovarian cycle is the menstrual cycle occurring in the endometrial lining of the uterus (Figs. 12-3 and 12-5). The cycle begins with the shedding of the old endometrium from the previous cycle. This is the menstrual phase of the menstrual cycle. Sonographically, the endometrium is thinnest during the menstrual phase (Fig. 12-5d). As the old endometrium sheds, estradiol produced by the growing ovarian follicles and secreted into the bloodstream causes the proliferation of a new endometrium. This is the proliferative phase of the endometrial cycle. During this phase, the endometrium has a triple layer, or trilaminar, sonographic appearance (Fig. 12-5c). During the periovulatory period, the endometrium exhibits a variety of sonographic appearances spanning across those of the proliferative and the secretory phases. After ovulation, progesterone (secreted by the corpus luteum

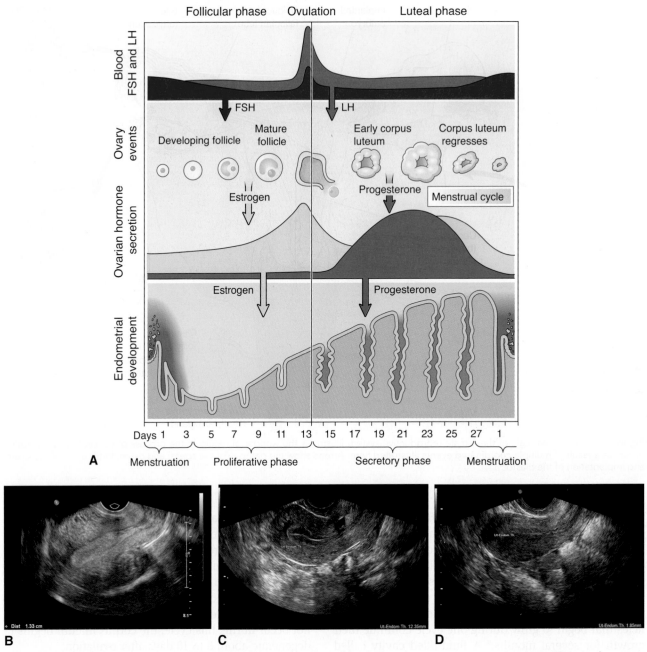

Figure 12-3. A: The anterior pituitary releases FSH and LH into circulating blood. These hormones act on ovarian tissue. FSH stimulates ovarian follicles to grow. A sharp spike in LH precipitates ovulation. During the follicular phase of the ovarian cycle, the developing follicles of the ovary release estrogen (estradiol). During the luteal phase of the ovarian cycle, the corpus luteum of the ovary releases progesterone into the blood. Estrogen and progesterone act on the endometrial tissue lining the uterus. The endometrium has distinctive appearances depending on the time within the cycle. The thin menstrual endometrium **(D)** appears echogenic, while the proliferative endometrium **(C)** has a trilaminar appearance. A thick, hyperechoic endometrium **(B)** indicates the secretory phase of the menstrual cycle.

into circulating blood) rises. Rising progesterone levels cause the endometrial cycle to enter its secretory phase (Fig. 12-5b), during which spiral arteries enlarge, glandular cells store an increasing amount of glycogen, and the endometrium grows to its greatest thickness in preparation for the possible implantation of a blastocyst. Sonographically, the endometrium is thick, homogeneous, and a double hyperechoic layer in this phase. In the sonogram, a thin line reflecting the uterine cavity separates the two layers. If fertilization does not occur, estradiol and progesterone levels drop and

the endometrial tissue degenerates and is shed from the body as the menstrual flow. Although the menstrual flow is the end of this process, the first day of menses designates the first day of the menstrual cycle.

In summary, in the first few days of the ovarian/menstrual cycles, follicles that began to develop during a previous cycle continue to mature into antral follicles, and endometrial tissue that grew during the previous cycle sheds from the uterus. Following this, a single Graafian follicle emerges as the dominant follicle in the ovary and secretes estradiol. Under the

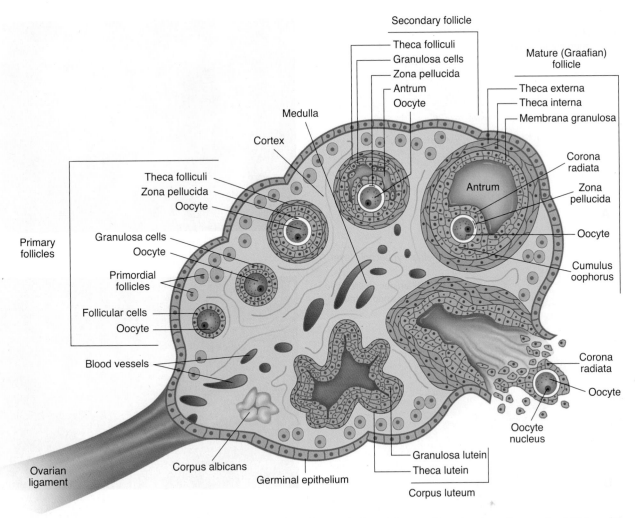

Figure 12-4. Schematic diagram of an ovary showing the sequence of events in the origin, growth, and rupture of an ovarian follicle and the formation and retrogression of a corpus luteum. The atretic follicles are those that show signs of degeneration and death.

influence of estradiol levels, the endometrium proliferates. At midcycle, a sharp rise in the level of LH triggers ovulation. In the second half of the cycle, high levels of progesterone secreted by the ovarian corpus luteum cause the endometrium to enter its secretory phase in anticipation of pregnancy. If no fertilization occurs, this endometrial lining sheds as a new cycle begins. Sonographically, the endometrium is thin in the menstrual phase, triple-layered and thickened during the proliferative phase, and double-layered, homogeneous, hyperechoic, and thickest during the secretory phase.

Sonographic Assessment of the Ovary

Ovaries are well visualized by routine endovaginal sonography (Figs. 12-6 and 12-7). In the evaluation of a patient for infertility, scanning helps assess the appearance and volume of the ovaries.

To perform an endovaginal scan of the ovaries, the sonographer first locates the uterus for reference and then sweeps out sagittally to the left and then the right adnexa, moving out laterally toward the hypogastric vessels to locate each ovary. In a screening sonogram, carefully assess each ovary and the adjacent regions sagittally and coronally. Document the sagittal, anterio-posterior (AP), and coronal measurements of each ovary, noting any cystic or solid lesions.

Varieties of tools help predict ovulation. In routine clinical practice, two-dimensional (2D) sonography aids in serial measurement of follicular size and growth to predict the timing of ovulation. In research-related practice, however, spectral and color Doppler increase the understanding of perifollicular and stromal flow[11] and their impact on ovulation.[5] Along with sonography, indirect tests including measurements of basal body temperature and blood hormone levels (serum LH and progesterone levels) help assess changes occurring in related structures around ovulation. Performance of an endometrial biopsy allows indirect assessment of ovulation.

Ovarian follicles destined to ovulate derive from a cohort of growing follicles, themselves derived from the pool of primordial follicles present since birth. Three types of follicles at different stages of development are

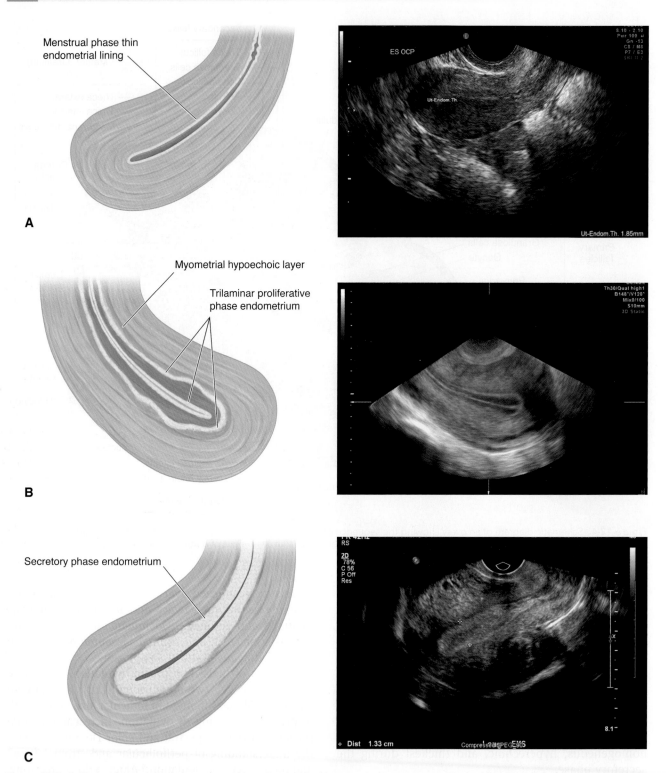

Figure 12-5. A: During the menstrual phase, the endometrium is at its thinnest as it degenerates and is shed from the body. **B:** Proliferative phase trilaminar endometrium (note retroverted uterus in this particular patient). During the proliferative phase, the endometrium has a triple layer, or trilaminar, appearance. As it transitions from the pre- to the postovulatory period, the endometrium may exhibit a variety of appearances. **C:** Secretory phase hyperechoic endometrium. After ovulation the endometrial tissue enters into its secretory phase, during which time the endometrium grows to its greatest thickness in preparation for the possible implantation of a pregnancy. (Images courtesy Washington Radiology Associates.)

primordial, early-growing, and antral follicles.[9] Within 5 days of a natural unstimulated cycle, as the liquor folliculi increases, small antral follicles are sonographically visible as anechoic structures within the ovarian cortex. Antral follicles differ from the rest of the cohort in terms of their greater size and rate of growth. In the natural cycle, follicles that go on to become atretic rarely grow larger than 10 millimeters (mm), and so visualization of a large follicle (Fig. 12-7) suggests that it is likely to be the dominant follicle that will ovulate.

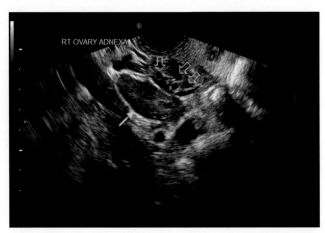

Figure 12-6. Normal ovary *(straight arrow)* with no sonographically visible follicles. Medial to the ovary is the uterus with prominent vasculature *(open arrows)*. (Image courtesy Washington Radiology Associates, Washington, DC.)

Only in 5% of cases will there be two or more dominant follicles in the natural cycle.[6] In the 4 to 5 days preceding ovulation, the dominant follicle grows approximately 1 to 2 mm daily. The growth in diameter of this single dominant follicle is directly proportionate to the rise in serum estradiol. At the time of ovulation, the mean diameter of the dominant follicle in a natural cycle is approximately 15 to 25 mm.[12]

As a woman advances through her reproductive years, her ovaries reduce in baseline antral follicle count (BAFC) and ovarian volume.[12] When performing a diagnostic workup of infertility in a woman, it is helpful to be able to estimate her ovarian reserve, which is defined as the quantity and quality of her remaining follicles. Ovarian reserve decreases with age. The number of small antral follicles observed at the beginning of the ovarian/menstrual cycles reflects the size of a woman's resting follicular pool.[13] Women in their forties may demonstrate a BAFC of as few as two to ten follicles. Women with fewer than five antral follicles

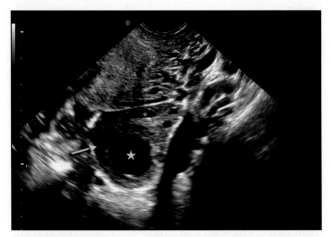

Figure 12-7. Normal ovary *(straight arrow)* with single Graafian follicle *(star)*. (Image courtesy of Washington Radiology Associates, Washington, DC.)

have a greater chance of poor ovarian response.[6] The observation of a BAFC of 10 or fewer follicles is associated with an increased risk of cycle cancellation.[14]

Ovarian reserve predicts the responsiveness of ovaries to fertility drugs and the likelihood of success with fertility treatment. In theory, an accurate measure of quantitative ovarian reserve would entail counting the number of follicles present in the ovaries from an ovarian specimen, only possible after surgical removal of the ovaries.[15] Usually, measurement of ovarian reserve is not through such drastic procedures. Rather, ovarian reserve assessment is made through measurement of serum FSH and estradiol levels in the early follicular (day 3 of the ovarian cycle) period. In addition, sonography may also help predict ovarian reserve (Fig. 12-8) by providing an ovarian volume and estimated BAFC.

Broekmans et al.[9] proposed a scanning protocol by which to determine BAFC. The sonographer counts all identifiable antral follicles of 2 to 10 mm (Fig. 12-9) in both the left and the right ovary, using a high frequency (minimum 7 megahertz [MHz]) endovaginal transducer to systematically sweep through each ovary and locate the largest plane for measuring each follicle. The sonographer then adds the two obtained counts. In addition, the sonographer counts any anechoic structures measuring 10 mm or more and subtracts this value from the total count. This yields the BAFC. For consistency, Broekmans suggests that BAFC should be measured between days 2 and 4 of onset of spontaneous menses.[2,9]

Technological innovations with three-dimensional (3D) volume acquisitions can provide automated counting and measurement of follicles in those labs that have the newer machines. The sonographer acquires a 3D volume dataset, and software automatically counts all follicles in each ovary. The automated 3D acquisition improves the speed, but not the accuracy of the follicle count.[16]

Sonography helps detect ovulatory dysfunction. In some cycles, there is asynchrony between the estradiol peak, the LH surge, and the growth and rupture of ovarian follicles. In such cases, the follicle is usually less than 14 mm in diameter and either ruptures prematurely or ceases to grow, becoming atretic, a process that can be detected with sonographic monitoring.

One common etiology of anovulation is polycystic ovary syndrome (PCOS). This syndrome is associated with irregularly timed menstrual cycles, elevated androgen levels often manifested by increased hair growth, hair loss, or acne, and polycystic-appearing ovaries. Ovaries associated with PCOS (Figs. 12-10, 8-38A, and 8-39A) have an increased surface area (often 2.8 times normal size) and an increased number of growing and atretic follicles as compared to ovaries that are normal. Often, polycystic ovaries have multiple follicles less than 10 mm in size, referred to as a "string of pearls" located in the periphery of the ovary.[17]

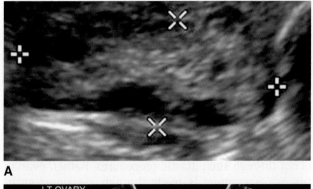

A

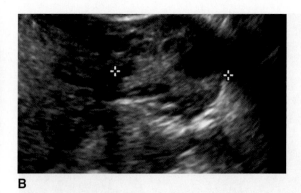

B

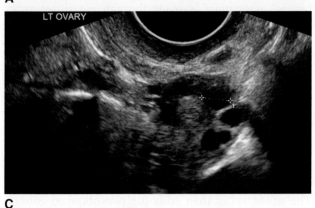

C

Figure 12-8. Ovarian reserve estimation by ovarian volume. The length and height measurements are taken on a sagittal scan (**A**) and the width is taken on a transverse scan (**B**). Ovarian volume is obtained by multiplying L × H × W × 0.52. **C:** The number of follicles measuring between 2 mm and 10 mm are noted for the BAFC.

Sonography visualizes ovarian cystic and solid pathology. This includes endometriosis (Fig. 12-11), an ovarian condition common in infertile women. The presence of an ovarian endometrioma reflects severe endometriosis, which can impact fertility. A rare type of ovulatory dysfunction is ovum entrapment in an unruptured follicle.[6,18] The phenomenon has been termed luteinized unruptured follicle (LUF) syndrome. Although briefly mentioned, neither these entities nor pathologies

such as dermoids, hemorrhagic cysts, or other complex cysts (Figs. 12-12, 12-13, and 12-14) commonly seen in the ovary will be further elaborated on here, as they are covered in detail in other chapters.

Sonographic Assessment of the Uterus

The screening of a patient's uterus during a workup to diagnose and treat infertility involves assessment for structural anomalies as well as pathology of the entire uterus, with attention to the cervix, endometrium, myometrium, and fallopian tubes. This section discusses the sonographic assessment of these entities.

Cervix

The cervix and endocervical canal visualize during endovaginal sonography (Fig. 12-15). First, align the transducer with the endometrial stripe in the longitudinal plane, follow the stripe from the fundus to the cervix, and then angle or withdraw the transducer inferiorly to optimize the view of the cervix.

Routine cervical findings include cervical mucus, which may be physiologic at midcycle, extending from the external os to the uterine cavity[19] produced in response to the elevated periovulatory level of estradiol. Surgical trauma, diethylstilbestrol-related abnormalities, ovulatory dysfunction, or medications can be responsible for the absence of cervical mucus. Although a rare cause of infertility, cervical factor infertility can prevent sperm from ascending into the uterus.

Figure 12-9. Endovaginal scan showing multiple small antral follicles (*stars*) in the periphery of this ovary. Cursors measure the sagittal (1 D) and AP dimensions (2 D) of the ovary. The central echogenic region (*arrow*) of the ovary demonstrates its connective tissue. (Image courtesy of Washington Radiology Associates, Washington, DC.)

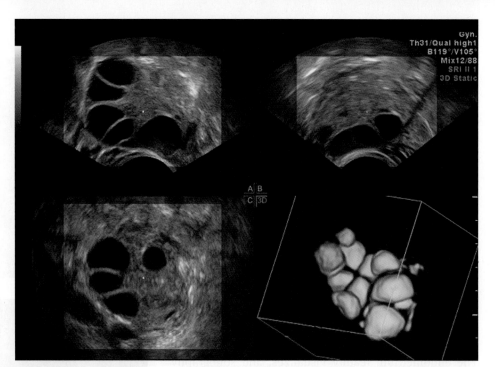

Figure 12-10. Sonograms depicting the "string of pearls" appearance of the cysts in this woman with polycystic ovaries. (Sonographic image courtesy of GE Healthcare, Wauwatosa, WI.)

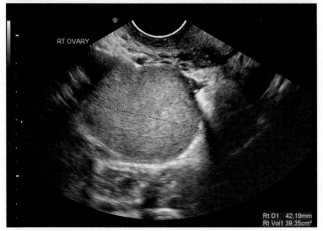

Figure 12-11. Endometriosis on the ovary. This cyst with low-level internal echoes and posterior acoustic enhancement is an endometrioma. (Image courtesy of GE Healthcare, Wauwatosa, WI.)

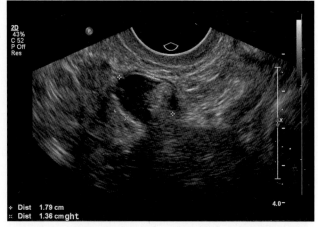

Figure 12-12. Dermoid. (Image courtesy of The George Washington University Hospital.)

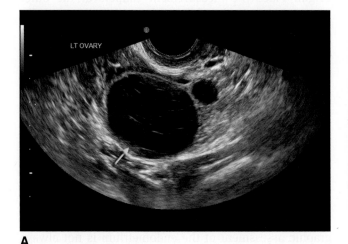

A

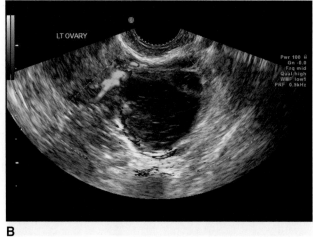

B

Figure 12-13. **A:** 2D grayscale image of a hemorrhagic ovarian cyst *(arrow)*. **B:** Power Doppler image demonstrating peripheral flow. (Image courtesy of Washington Radiology Associates.)

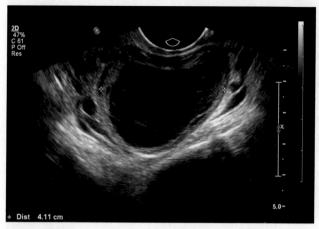

Figure 12-14. Complex ovarian cyst. (Image courtesy of The George Washington University Hospital.)

Endometrium

The endometrium readily visualizes, and sonography aids in extensive research studies of the uterine lining. Although sonography is useful in diagnosing endometrial pathology, many questions remain unanswered.

Because it is critically important that the endometrium be receptive for the blastocyst to successfully implant,[20] much attention has been paid to sonography of the endometrium. Some failures of hormone-induced infertility treatments have been attributed to lack of receptivity of the endometrium.[21] There is, however, some question as to the clinical applications of sonographic findings.[12,21-23] Sonographic findings of the endometrium of interest to sonographers working in the field of infertility are discussed here. These findings are thickness, blood flow, texture, peristaltic movements, presence of intracavitary lesions, and presence of intracavitary fluid.

Measure the thickness of the endometrium across the uterine cavity (Fig. 12-16). Scanning in the longitudinal plane, thickness is measured as an AP measurement, with care being taken to exclude the hypoechoic

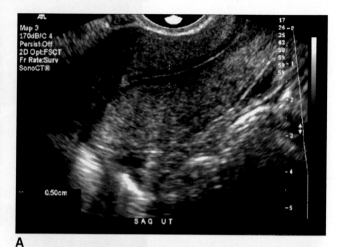

A

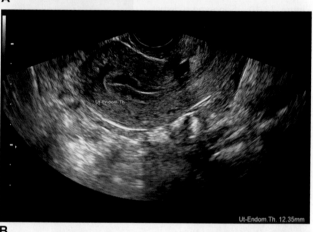

B

Figure 12-16. A and B: Measuring the trilaminar proliferative endometrium. Two images illustrate the different yet similar appearances of the proliferative endometrium. Scanning in the longitudinal plane, thickness is measured as an AP measurement, with care being taken to exclude the hypoechoic halo, which is myometrial rather than endometrial in origin. The measurement calipers should be placed at the outer hyperechoic margins of the endometrium. (Image **A** and **B** courtesy of Washington Radiology Associates, Washington, DC.)

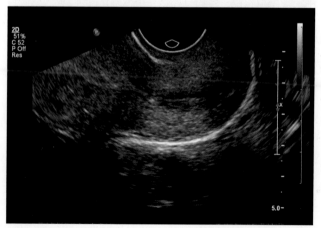

Figure 12-15. Sagittal endovaginal sonogram of the cervix. (Image courtesy of The George Washington University Hospital.)

halo, which is myometrial rather than endometrial in origin. Place the measurement calipers at the outer hyperechoic margins of the endometrium, one anterior and the other posterior to the uterine cavity. In other words, the measurement includes both spans (anterior and posterior) of the endometrium across the (empty) uterine cavity, which the endometrium encompasses. The endometrium, which undergoes cyclic change during the menstrual cycle, varies in thickness and sonographic appearance during the cycle. The endometrium itself consists of two layers, a basal and a functional layer. Hormonal fluctuations occurring during the menstrual cycle result in the changes seen in the functional layer. During the reproductive years, normal endometrial thickness can vary from 3 to 14 mm within the menstrual cycle. Researchers have found that sonographic assessment of the endometrium is not always helpful in predicting the receptivity of the uterus for successful implantation[21] but research does show that endometrial thickness of less than 6 mm is useful in predicting poor implantation rates.[12] Advances in 3D sonographic instrumentation have improved the assessment of the thickness and volume of the endometrium.[23]

Characteristic changes in blood flow dynamics occur during the menstrual cycle. Doppler sonography helps assess blood flow and note physiologic changes involving the uterine artery. Research has shown that spectral Doppler findings of the uterine artery are helpful in predicting severely decreased uterine perfusion as a cause of infertility. Using a pulsatility index cutoff level of 3 to 3.5 for the uterine artery, prediction of a nonreceptive endometrium was 100% specificity and 100% positive predictive value.[21] As such, spectral Doppler is useful in predicting poor receptivity to implantation. It has, however, not been found as useful in predicting good receptivity.

The texture of the endometrium has characteristic sonographic appearances during each of the three phases of the menstrual cycle (Figs. 12-5 and 12-17). The thin endometrium seen during the menstrual phase is due to shedding of the uterine lining. It forms a thin, echogenic interface with the myometrium. Endovaginal sonography may demonstrate physiologic blood (menses) of mixed echogenicity within the uterine cavity. During the proliferative phase, the endometrium thickens and typically becomes triple layered. The triple layer is thought to reflect the growth of endometrial glands with their secretions.[12] Although this triple-line appearance of the endometrium is characteristic of the preovulatory period, it is not a finding exclusive to this period. Research has shown all three endometrial patterns in the periovulatory period.[21] Echogenicity and thickness increase during the secretory phase of the cycle and the endometrium changes from the triple-layer appearance of the proliferative phase to a homogeneous, hyperechoic, thick, double layer during the secretory phase.

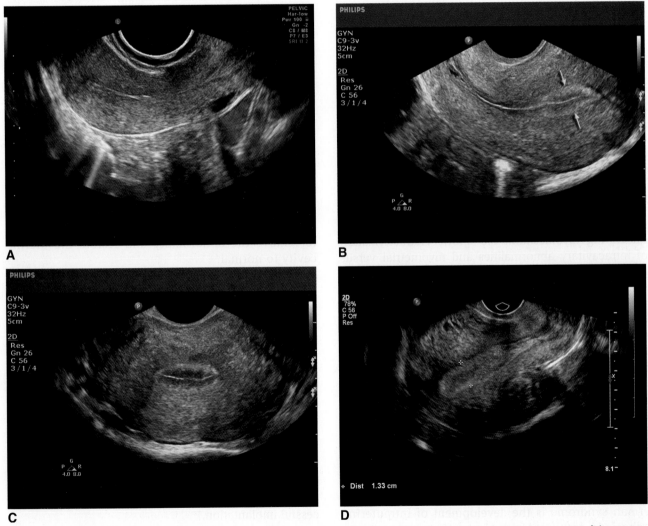

Figure 12-17. A: Menstrual phase endometrium. **B:** Triple-layer endometrium in proliferative phase. Endovaginal sonogram of the preovulatory uterus and endometrium. Measurement of the endometrium includes two thicknesses, from one myometrial interface to the opposite interface *(between arrows)*; texture grading suggests a triple-stripe preovulatory pattern. **C:** Axial or transverse view of the triple layer endometrium. **D:** Secretory phase endometrium. Endovaginal sonogram of the uterus and endometrium. The endometrium is thickened and hyperechoic with respect to the myometrium, characteristic of the secretory luteal-phase endometrium. (Images **A** and **D** courtesy Washington Radiology Associates, Washington, DC. Images **B** and **C** courtesy of Philips Medical, Bothell, WA.)

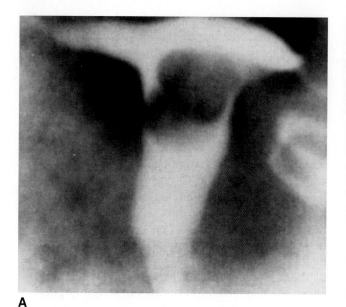

A

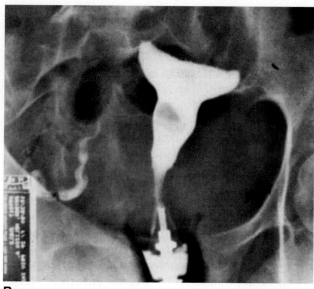

B

Figure 12-18. **A:** HSG demonstrates an endometrial polyp. **B:** Saline infusion sonohysterography of the same submucosal fibroid.

Peristaltic movement of the endometrium has been visualized with sonography.[6,19] Endovaginal sonography has found that increased peristaltic endometrial and myometrial movements appear to occur in women around midcycle. These movements probably enhance sperm propulsion toward the tubal ostia.[24]

Intracavitary lesions (Figs. 12-18, 12-19, and 8-16) may be assessed by routine endovaginal sonography as well as magnetic resonance imaging (MRI), hysterosalpingography, saline-infusion sonohysterography (SIS), and 3D or four-dimensional (4D) sonography.

Lesions may arise from either the endometrium or the underlying myometrium. SIS allows characterization of intracavitary abnormalities and myometrial versus endometrial lesions. These include polyps, myomas, synechiae, retained products of conception, endometrial hyperplasia, and carcinoma. The presence of any clinically significant intracavitary abnormality can decrease the likelihood of pregnancy, with or without fertility treatment, and may increase the likelihood of miscarriage. For these reasons, assessment of the uterine cavity is critical in the evaluation of a couple with infertility. Pelvic sonography also helps in detection of endometrial polyps as well as intracavitary and submucosal myomas.

Often, the endometrium appears heterogeneous, and hyperechoic irregularities may be noted. SIS helps to characterize abnormalities. 3D[23] and 4D sonography can help in diagnoses such as these. Asherman syndrome is the development of intrauterine adhesions resulting from postpartum or postabortal surgical curettage, pelvic inflammatory disease (PID), uterine surgery (cesarean section or myomectomy), or tuberculosis, possibly with concomitant symptoms of hypomenorrhea or amenorrhea. SIS is the preferred method of identifying Asherman syndrome, in which synechiae are demonstrated within the endometrial cavity. Without the infusion of saline, intrauterine adhesions appear as sonolucent defects within the bright, thickened endometrium during the secretory phase, or as an obliteration of the normal endometrium on pelvic sonogram. Many times, however, the endometrium appears normal despite the presence of intrauterine adhesions. Hysterosalpingography (HSG) also helps to assess for intrauterine adhesions (Fig. 12-19). If an intracavitary lesion is present, surgical intervention is undertaken to remove the abnormality and restore the uterine cavity to normal.

Physiologic intracavitary fluid in the form of mucus or blood visualizes with endovaginal sonography. The physiologic presence of intracavitary mucus may accompany midcycle endometrial changes. Intracavitary blood images during the first week of the cycle. Other than the above situations, the presence of endometrial fluid is considered pathologic. The presence of intracavitary fluid at the time of embryo transfer is associated with implantation failure, and it is common clinical practice to postpone the embryo transfer in the presence of fluid. In this situation, embryos are frozen for future use. However, despite the markedly diminished chance of implantation, it has been reported that removal of the fluid with a catheter (Fig. 12-20) and immediately transferring the embryo has yielded successful implantation.[12]

Myometrium

The myometrial layer visualizes well by transabdominal sonography of the uterus and is even better visualized during endovaginal scanning, but these modalities may

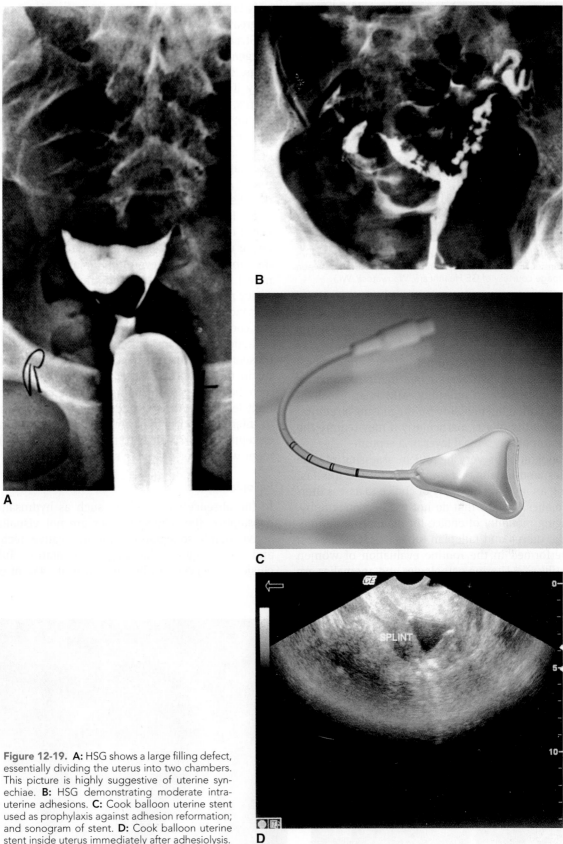

Figure 12-19. A: HSG shows a large filling defect, essentially dividing the uterus into two chambers. This picture is highly suggestive of uterine synechiae. **B:** HSG demonstrating moderate intrauterine adhesions. **C:** Cook balloon uterine stent used as prophylaxis against adhesion reformation; and sonogram of stent. **D:** Cook balloon uterine stent inside uterus immediately after adhesiolysis.

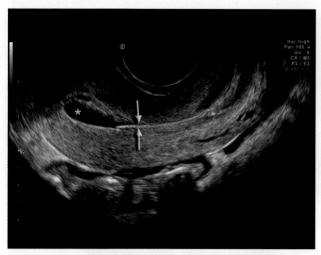

Figure 12-20. Intracavitary fluid *(star)* should be removed before embryo transfer. Hyperechoic line represents the catheter (between arrows). (Image courtesy of GE Healthcare, Wauwatosa, WI.)

only play an ancillary role in the diagnosis of structural uterine etiologies of infertility. Adding saline SIS to the repertoire of studies available to the sonologist makes it possible to distinguish myometrial from endometrial pathology, and to help asses some uterine anomalies that may contribute to infertility. MRI is an excellent noninvasive imaging modality for diagnosing structural anomalies of the uterus, particularly if they require the visualization of the serosal layer or a septum.

3D sonography is very helpful in assessing uterine anomalies, and in labs that utilize this feature it is fast becoming an imaging modality of choice to assess uterine anomalies. In labs that do not use 3D sonography, the imaging modality of choice for diagnosing anomalies of the uterus and fallopian tubes is HSG. This is a study performed in the routine evaluation of women for infertility.[25,26] Uterine pathologies and anomalies are

only briefly reviewed in this chapter, as they are treated in greater detail elsewhere in this book.

Structural uterine abnormalities, which include congenital anomalies, fibroids, and adenomyosis (Figs. 12-21 and 12-22), can have an impact on infertility if they interfere with implantation.[27,28] A septate uterus, which increases a woman's risk of miscarriage, cannot be visualized by conventional sonography but can be diagnosed through SIS. 3D sonography may help diagnose septate uterus if digital reconstruction of the coronal plane of the uterine cavity demonstrates a septum.[12] A septum can be surgically removed to increase the likelihood of a woman carrying a pregnancy to full term. Fibroids can contribute to infertility in several ways: distorting the shape of the uterine cavity, interfering with uterine/endometrial blood flow, occluding the tubal ostia, or preventing implantation. Surgical removal of submucosal fibroids improves clinical pregnancy rates.[26,28] Adenomyosis (Fig. 12-22), which is the presence of endometrial tissue within the myometrium, can coexist with other pathology, including leiomyoma, endometriosis, and endometrial hyperplasia. It can present in a diffuse or focal form. MRI has proven useful in the diagnosis. Varied patterns to adenomyoma have been imaged, including multiple cysts within distinct lesions.[29] Although adenomyosis may contribute to infertility and/or miscarriage, its medical (oral contraceptives) or surgical (often, a hysterectomy) treatment will render a woman subfertile or sterile.

Fallopian Tubes

In the absence of pathology such as hydrosalpinx or pyosalpinx, the fallopian tubes are not visualized by conventional sonography, but innovative techniques and technology are changing this limitation. Tubal occlusion is believed to be the cause of 14% of couples

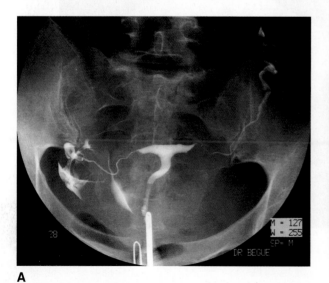

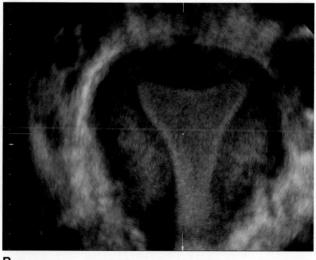

A   **B**

Figure 12-21. A: HSG showing a T-shaped uterus in a diethylstilbestrol-exposed woman. **B:** 3D reconstruction of a coronal view of a normal endometrium reflecting the shape of the normal endometrial cavity, for comparison. (Image courtesy of GE Healthcare, Wauwatosa, WI.)

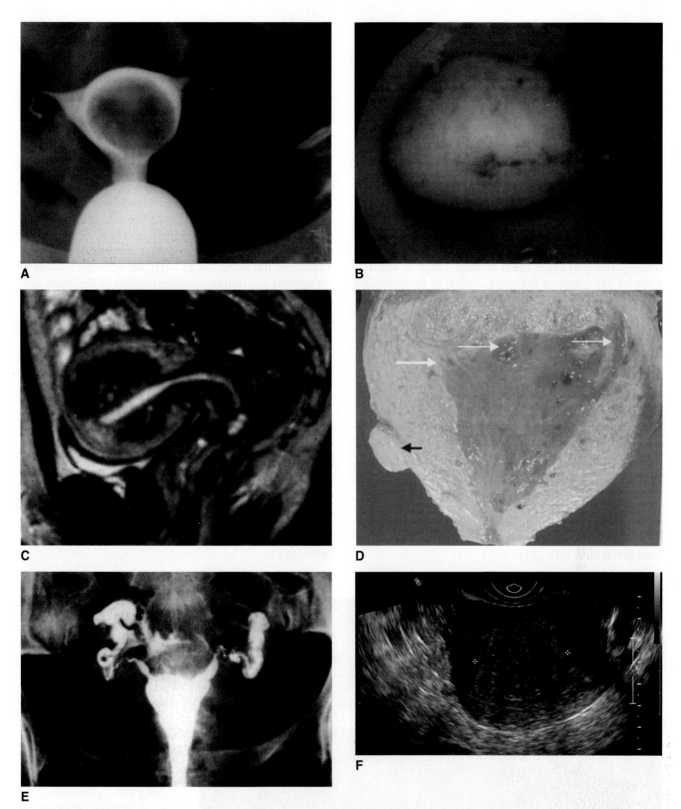

Figure 12-22. A: HSG using a water-soluble contrast medium demonstrates a large, smooth filling defect within the endometrial cavity resulting from an intracavitary fibroid. The mass effect on the study is nonspecific, and only direct visualization can confirm that it is caused by a fibroid. **B:** The hysteroscopic view of this intracavitary leiomyoma. **C:** Sagittal T2-weighted image demonstrates oval areas of thickened junctional zone containing a few hyperintense foci that are characteristic of adenomyosis. **D:** This gross photograph of a bisected supracervical hysterectomy specimen exhibits irregular thickening of the myometrium, characteristic of adenomyosis. Multiple deep myometrial foci of dark blue discoloration mark the sites of adenomyosis *(long white arrows)*. The short black arrow indicates a small leiomyoma. **E:** A direct sign of adenomyosis are the finding of numerous diverticula as seen in Figure 11-26. An indirect sign of adenomyosis is calle "tuba erecta" as seen on this hysterogram. **F:** Endovaginal sonogram of adenomyosis. (Image courtesy of The George Washington University Hospital.)

requiring infertility treatment,[28] and disease or damage of the tube is reported to account for 25% to 35% of infertility.[30]

Laparoscopy is the gold standard[30] and HSG is the imaging procedure of choice to evaluate tubal patency. In some labs SIS plays an increasing role in assessing the patency of fallopian tubes.[6,31] Using this technique, the sonographer evaluates tubal patency by noting the presence of fluid in the cul-de-sac following the infusion of saline into the uterus. In the absence of obstruction, saline that is infused into the uterus flows out of the fimbrial end of the fallopian tube. Diagnosis of at least one tube's patency is through visualization of free fluid in the cul-de-sac. Unfortunately, this technique does not provide information regarding bilateral tubal patency or other tubal disease. Color or spectral Doppler can improve the visualization of fluid flowing out of the fallopian tube into the adnexa.[32,33] Doppler assessments (Fig. 12-23) are further improved in those parts of the world where contrast media is approved for use to enhance the study.[33]

Male Factor Infertility

Semen parameters (i.e., sperm density, motility, morphology/shape) must be adequate for conception to occur. Routine workup of infertile couples includes assessment of sperm quality with a semen analysis. Etiologies for poor semen quality are varied and include testicular failure, vasoepididymal obstruction of congenital or infectious origin, varicocele, systemic disease, and idiopathic causes.[3] Of these, varicoceles are the most common abnormality associated with male factor infertility and are present in a high percentage of men presenting with infertility.[34]

Diagnosis of clinically significant varicocele can be made based on a physical examination alone. Although smaller, subclinical varicoceles visualize by sonography, it is only the larger palpable varicoceles that are typically associated with infertility. Scrotal sonography is only indicated when the physical exam is inconclusive.[34] The scan is performed with a high-frequency linear transducer (7 to 12 MHz) superior to the testicles, where the veins of the pampiniform plexus are visualized as anechoic tubular structures. A classic "bag of worms" appearance of multiple tubular veins superior to the testes (Fig. 12-24) is characteristic of varicoceles. Measure the vessel diameters on the sonogram. The patient is asked to hold his breath and bear down on his belly (i.e., apply the Valsalva maneuver) in an attempt to distend the veins. As an alternate, scan the patient in an upright position to promote pooling of the blood due to the force of gravity, if the veins are indeed varicose. Measurement of three or more veins 3 mm or greater is diagnostic of varicocele, whether visualized with or without the Valsalva maneuver.

Left-sided varicoceles are more common because of the insertion of the left spermatic vein into the left renal vein. The right spermatic vein enters the inferior vena cava directly. Varicoceles are present in a significantly higher percentage of men with secondary infertility (81%) compared to primary (35%) infertility.[35] Semen parameters are often abnormal in the presence of varicocele, with decreases in sperm density and motility and changes in morphology. Perhaps the effects of scrotal temperature, hormonal abnormalities, and biochemical and immunologic factors combine to increase the likelihood of male factor infertility.[36]

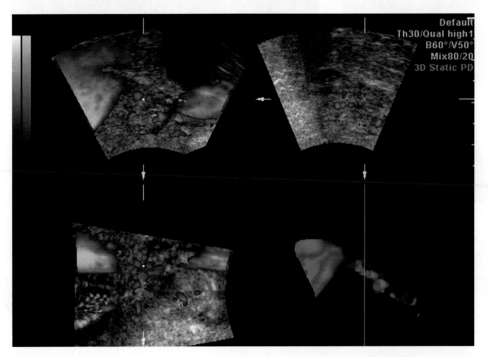

Figure 12-23. Fallopian tube color Doppler saline infusion sonohysterosalpingography to assess tubal patency. 3D power Doppler scan of uterine cavity after injection of isotonic saline. 3D power Doppler rendering allows simultaneous assessment of triangular shape of uterine cavity and proximal part of tube (lower right). Reprinted from Kupesic S, Plavsic, BM. 2D and 3D hysterosalpingo-contrast-sonography in the assessment of uterine cavity and tubal patency. *European Journal of Obstetrics & Gynecology and Reproductive Biology 133*(1) p. 67 (2007). With permission from Elsevier.

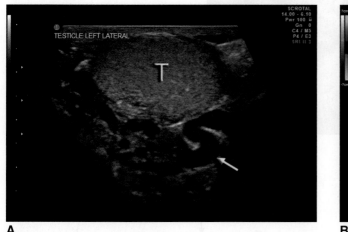

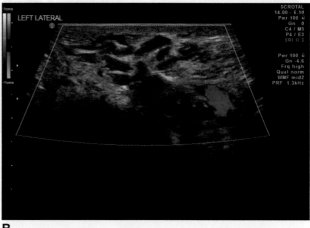

A   B

Figure 12-24. A: 2D "bag of worms" appearance to varicoceles *(arrow)* performed with a trapezoid imaging function, which allows for imaging of peripheral structures. *T*, testicle. **B:** Color Doppler imaging demonstrating flow within the varicosed vein. Varicoceles occur more often on the left side due to the venous termination into the left renal vein. (Images courtesy of Washington Radiology Associates, Washington, DC.)

THE MANY AND VARIED ROUTES TO ASSISTED REPRODUCTION

The scope of infertility treatment has changed dramatically over the last few decades. The birth of Louis Brown in 1978 after in vitro fertilization (IVF) was the first major technological breakthrough for clinically successful birth of a child to an infertile couple.[37] Since then, IVF has become popular worldwide. Approximately 1 in 50 births in Sweden, 1 in 60 in Australia, and 1 in 80 to 100 in the United States are through IVF procedures.[38] Depending on the couple's etiology of infertility, there are many routes available for assisted reproduction. This section gives an overview of the treatments involved in the services of ART.

Fertility treatment[12,28,39] may simply involve the stimulation of follicles in a woman's ovaries followed by timed intercourse or an IUI. Or it may involve controlled stimulation of multiple follicles and aspiration of ova from these follicles followed by any one of additional reproductive technologies.

An IUI is performed after ovarian follicle stimulation if the underlying cause of a couple's infertility is either unexplained or a mild male factor. Typical mild male factors are borderline sperm concentration, motility, or shape. An IUI entails the placement of prewashed sperm directly into the woman's uterus during a routine pelvic exam at the time of ovulation. Many couples undergo IVF if prior IUIs have failed to result in a pregnancy or if either the sperm are poor on semen analysis or the fallopian tubes are diseased (i.e., occluded or have hydrosalpinges).

IVF (Fig. 12-25) is preceded by the stimulation of multiple follicles and retrieval of ova. Ova retrieval occurs with the assistance of endovaginal sonography. An aspiration needle, attached to the biopsy guide of the endovaginal transducer, visualizes on the sonography screen, allowing for real-time guidance of the follicle aspiration. Because ova themselves do not directly visualize by sonography, aspiration of the fluid within each follicle into a small container allows for microscopic assessment for the presence of ova within the adjoining embryology laboratory.

Once ova are aspirated from a woman's follicles, a host of possibilities opens up for assisted reproduction. The ova may be cryopreserved for use in the future or they may be used immediately. Ova may be inserted along with sperm into a woman's fallopian tube (Fig. 12-26) in a procedure known as gamete intrafallopian transfer (GIFT), from which point everything can continue on naturally, with fertilization occurring in vivo. If this treatment technique does not address the couple's etiology of infertility, the fertilization may be conducted in vitro by placing ova and sperm together in a culture dish, where fertilization takes place outside the body. The resulting conceptus, known as a zygote, can then be introduced into the woman's fallopian tube in a technique (very rarely done today) referred to as zygote intrafallopian transfer (ZIFT). Following the transfer, all else occurs naturally, with the conceptus propelled by the fallopian tube into the uterine cavity where it implants in the lining of the uterus, allowing the pregnancy to continue naturally from this point onward. More commonly, following IVF the embryo is allowed to develop for several days and then is transferred (ET) transcervically into the uterus (Fig. 12-27), where implantation can follow naturally. In general, IVF with ET is standard clinical practice, whereas GIFT and ZIFT are uncommonly used.

If a couple's etiology of infertility is due to a male factor (i.e., low sperm count or decreased motility or abnormally shaped sperm on semen analysis), the ability of sperm to fertilize an egg diminishes, despite

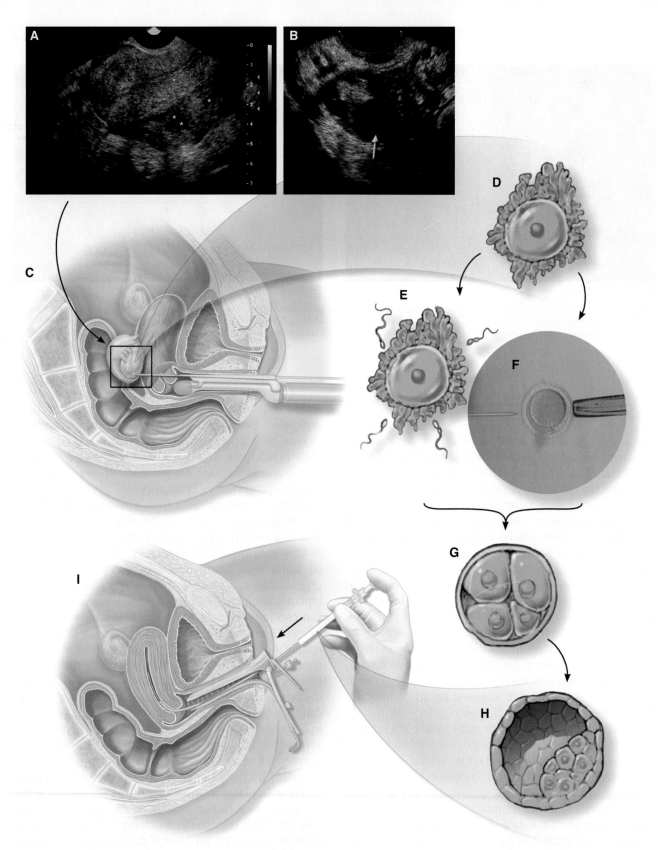

Figure 12-25. Sonographic imaging occurs at many steps of the IVF-ET process. Ovary stimulation is through daily injections of gonadotropins to optimize follicular development. Endovaginal ultrasound helps with monitoring of follicular growth. Sonogram of an unstimulated ovary, located in the posterior cul-de-sac, demonstrates small follicles **(A, star)**. This image demonstrates an ovary with a dominant follicle **(B, arrow)**. Sonographically guided endovaginal egg retrieval follicular fluid aspiration **(C)**. The recovered mature human egg **(D)** is fertilized through egg culturing and introduction of multiple motile sperm **(E)**. Multiple sperm attach to the egg's zona pellucida *(arrows)*. Intracytoplasmic sperm injection fertilization is a technique whereby the injection of a single sperm occurs through use of a thin glass pipette **(F)**. Though developed to solve male-factor infertility, this process is now used in a majority of IVF cycles. Culturing of multiple embryos to the eight-cell embryo takes approximately 3 days **(G)**. Blastocyst embryos take up to 5 days **(H)** before the inner cell mass forms *(arrow)*. The selected embryos are then transferred to the uterus **(I)**. Cryopreserving allows for saving of any remaining good quality embryos for use in future pregnancy attempts.

**Oocyte (egg) retrieval and
GIFT (gamete intrafallopian transfer) or
ZIFT (zygote intrafallopian transfer)**

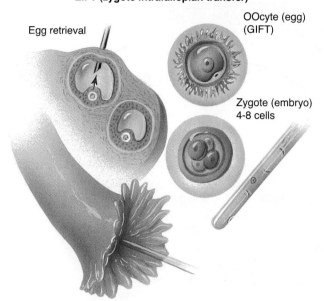

Egg retrieval

OOcyte (egg)
(GIFT)

Zygote (embryo)
4-8 cells

Oocyte and sperm introduced
into tubal ampulla

Figure 12-26. GIFT and ZIFT. Gamete intrafallopian transfer (ova and sperm inserted into fallopian tube) or zygote intrafallopian transfer (ova and sperm fertilized in vitro, and the zygote inserted into the fallopian tube). Both these procedures are rarely performed today. More commonly, embryos are transferred directly into the uterine cavity.

combining both sperm and egg in a dish for IVF. Fortunately for these couples, intracytoplasmic sperm injection (ICSI) is available. ICSI involves the injection of one sperm into the cytoplasm of one egg, thereby increasing the likelihood of egg fertilization and subsequent embryo development.[38,40]

If a couple's etiology of infertility is uterine anomaly or pathology that precludes the woman carrying a pregnancy, the couple may still have a biological child using their own sperm and ovum, using a gestational carrier. Furthermore, donor sperm and/or ova also address a couple's infertility problems through the use of IVF or in vivo fertilization.[41] In rare situations, cryopreserved zygotes and/or embryos are obtained from a donor couple. Indeed, couples who were considered infertile in years gone by may not be infertile at all, but simply subfertile. Clinical procedures overcome these problems, helping them to conceive and have a child.

Depending on the particular infertility center or office, there may be a variety of individuals involved in the services of assisted reproduction (Fig. 12-28). This includes patients (female and male), reproductive endocrinologists, embryologists, andrologists, sonographers, sonologists, geneticists, nurses and medical assistants, egg or sperm donors, psychologists, and obstetricians, to name some of the players who may be involved in interdisciplinary work helping couples overcome infertility. The patients may be infertile heterosexual couples, same-sex couples, or single women seeking parenthood. Volunteers may donate their sperm or eggs. If helping as a gestational carrier, a woman offers to conceive and carry a pregnancy to term in her uterus to help an infertile couple. The role of the sonographer may vary in different settings. Although sonographers typically perform the diagnostic workup and follicular monitoring, sonologists perform the more invasive procedures. Obstetricians or radiologists may perform procedures such as SIS, whereas a reproductive endocrinologist performs endovaginal follicle aspiration for oocyte retrieval and embryo transfers. Sonographers or sonography physician-extenders

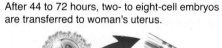

After 44 to 72 hours, two- to eight-cell embryos
are transferred to woman's uterus.

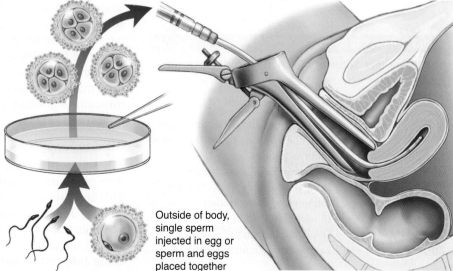

Figure 12-27. Embryo transfer. Ova are fertilized by sperm in a laboratory dish and are then transferred with a catheter directly into a woman's uterus. This (as compared to GIFT or ZIFT) is the more commonly performed procedure.

Outside of body,
single sperm
injected in egg or
sperm and eggs
placed together

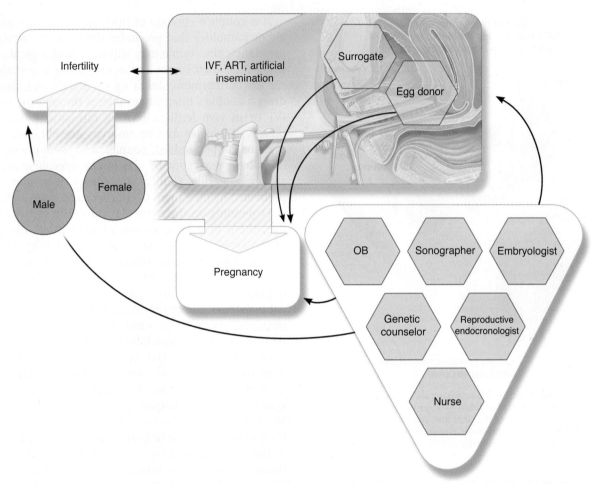

Figure 12-28. This diagram demonstrates the many people involved in the successful pregnancy resulting from infertility treatments.

may perform the sonographic guidance in real-time for the transfer of embryos into a woman's uterus. An embryologist handles the retrieved eggs, the introduction of sperm for fertilization, and the subsequent monitoring and care of embryos; these individuals bring embryos into the procedure room for transfer into the uterus. A nurse assists in the coordination of ovarian stimulation, in the pre- and post-procedure care of patients, and in the counseling of the couple. Working together, interdisciplinary teams[39] help serve the many-faceted needs of couples seeking assisted reproduction.

Treatment of Infertility

Treatment protocols for infertility can include one or more of the following: a baseline sonogram, sonographic monitoring during the follicular phase, sonographic assessment during the periovulatory period, evaluation for complications of OHSS, sonographic guidance for follicle aspiration, sonographic guidance for embryo transfer, documentation of early gestation, multifetal reduction, and sonography of the fetus through its gestation. This section elaborates on these topics.

Baseline Sonogram

A baseline sonogram is performed within the first few days of menstrual flow, before the initiation of therapy. This scan should make note of any existing uterine or adnexal abnormalities, for the record.

When assessing the ovaries, the sonographer should make note of any cystic lesions. This may include polycystic ovaries (PCOs), which often appear

---

PATHOLOGY BOX 12-2

The "Alphabet Soup" of Modern Reproductive Technologies

Acronym	Procedure Described
ART	Assisted reproductive technologies
COH	Controlled ovarian hyperstimulation
ET	Embryo transfer
GIFT	Gamete intrafallopian transfer
ICSI	Intracytoplasmic sperm injection
IUI	Intrauterine insemination
IVF	In vitro fertilization
OI	Ovulation induction
ZIFT	Zygote intrafallopian transfer

as multiple, small cysts (measuring less than 10 mm) along the periphery of the ovary that is enlarged or at the upper limits of normal (Fig. 12-10). Note resolution of all prior follicular development or minimal follicles in this phase of the ovarian cycle. Document cysts such as these for pretreatment precautions to reduce the risk of complications such as ovarian hyperstimulation syndrome (OHSS). This syndrome occurs with either the clomiphene or the gonadotropin regimen, although it is less likely in the former. Any pre-existing cysts may be aspirated in the early follicular phase before the initiation of an IVF cycle has been advocated to facilitate better follicular development and improve clinical pregnancy rates.[28] The effects of cyst aspiration are transient, as these cysts tend to recur. Although easily performed, ovarian cyst aspiration should be contemplated carefully before being carried out. The potential risk of malignancy in cystic ovarian lesions and the consequences of performing vaginal aspiration in such instances are unclear. Endometriomas may be aspirated under sonographic guidance but tend to re-accumulate their contents within the cyst.

Sonographic Monitoring during Follicular Phase

Controlled ovarian hyperstimulation plays a central role in ART available to couples. For most causes of infertility, the first step in treatment is the hyperstimulation of the woman's ovaries to yield single or multiple "dominant" follicles. This opens up a host of treatment options (Table 12-2), some involving sonography. Endovaginal sonography is an important tool for directly visualizing follicular growth and maturation. In fertility treatment, serial scans of the ovarian follicles help monitor follicle growth.

If the infertility evaluation establishes PCOS as the etiology of ovulatory dysfunction, the first line of treatment is ovulation induction using clomiphene citrate. For individuals who do not ovulate on their own, the goal of treatment is to have a single follicle develop and ovulate. Hormonal studies and multiple sonograms assessing follicular growth help determine response or ovulation with clomiphene citrate. This close monitoring of patients provides evidence of nonresponse, adequate response, or overresponse.

If clomiphene does not work, the treatment can be changed to exogenous gonadotropins such as FSH to stimulate follicular growth, coupled with an ovulation "trigger" such as hCG to induce ovulation. Self-administered FSH injections occur on a daily basis. Because women with anovulation are more sensitive and therefore more apt to develop many follicles under the influence of gonadotropins, they require close monitoring of dosage and follicular development. The goals of therapy for women with anovulation with either clomiphene citrate or gonadotropin treatment regimens are to induce satisfactory maturation of a single follicle yet avoid excessive follicular development, OHSS, and multiple-gestation pregnancies.[8]

For couples with unexplained infertility, COH provides a means for superovulation (i.e., the development of multiple follicles). For those women undertaking treatment with an IUI, the goal is to develop three to four dominant follicles at one time. This provides multiple "targets" for sperm to fertilize. Although this approach increases the likelihood of pregnancy, it also increases the risk of a multiple pregnancy. In these patients, for the purpose of ovarian stimulation, use either clomiphene citrate or injectable gonadotropins.

If there is a need for five or more follicles, usually for IVF, clinicians use controlled ovarian hyperstimulation facilitated through the use of injectable gonadotropins. As previously discussed, egg retrieval is achieved with sonographic guidance. The eggs are then fertilized outside the body, and the resultant embryos are returned to the woman's uterus for possible implantation. Severe OHSS is a rare (1% to 2% incidence) complication of IVF, whereas multiple pregnancy is not (25% to 30% of all embryo transfers).[42]

Although the risk of severe OHSS is low[43] with clomiphene citrate therapy, most fertility clinics perform sonograms during the follicular phase to ensure proper response. On occasion, a single endovaginal sonogram is performed 5 days after the last dose of clomiphene to provide documentation of growth of the follicle and help plan the timing of ovulation induction.[12] The rate of follicular growth is approximately 1 to 2 mm increase in mean follicular diameter daily. The mean follicular size at which ovulation occurs is 20 mm in clomiphene citrate–stimulated ovulation induction cycles.

In treatment regimens involving exogenous gonadotropins for follicular hyperstimulation, it is generally accepted that sonographic monitoring is necessary.[6,43,44] Sonography helps evaluate follicular growth and modify dosage of medication accordingly. Protocols of scheduled tests vary, however, between different assisted

TABLE 12-2			
Sequencing of Select Fertility Treatments			
Treatment	Medication	Follicles	Fertilization
Ovulation Induction	Clomiphene	One	Intercourse
COH	Clomiphene	Multiple (2–4)	IUI
COH	Gonadotropin	Multiple (2–4)	IUI
COH	Gonadotropin	Multiple; aspirated	IVF-ET

OI, Ovulation induction; *COH*, Controlled ovarian hyperstimulation; IUI, intrauterine insemination; *IVF*, in-vitro fertilization; *ET*, embryo transfer

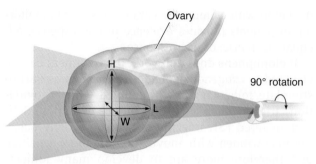

Figure 12-29. Diagram of measurement planes for follicles, illustrating one method in which follicular measurements are made: length plus height plus width (L + H + W/3) = mean follicular diameter. Some laboratories obtain the length measurement on a sagittal and then the AP and transverse on the coronal image. Other labs perform the longitudinal and AP measurement on the sagittal image and the transverse on the coronal ovary measurement. Either method obtains the requisite measurements; however, the sonographer must be sure to obtain three measurements and adhere to the departmental measurement protocol. To improve efficiency in scanning time, many labs today utilize only two dimensions of the follicle off a scan imaged in its largest plane.

PATHOLOGY BOX 12-3

Mean Diameters of Mature Follicles at Ovulation

Type of Cycle	Mean Diameter at Ovulation
Gonadotropin-stimulated cycles	16 to 18 mm
Clomiphene-stimulated cycles	20 mm
Natural cycle	15 mm to 25 mm

reproduction treatment centers. The American Society of Reproductive Medicine recommendation is that one sonogram be performed after 4 to 5 days of treatment and that additional scans be performed at 1- to 3-day intervals, according to response.[45] To help patients manage treatment costs, others have published minimal recommendations for performance of endovaginal scans to evaluate follicular growth at day 7 and day 10 of treatment. If follicles lag in growth, then a third and a fourth additional scan can be added on a case-by-case basis.[44]

Measurement of follicles is through either two or three of the following of each follicle: length (L), height (AP), and width (W) (Fig. 12-29). Calculate a mean follicular diameter by adding the measurements and

dividing the sum by the number of dimensions. Sonography machines used in ART centers may also have software programs that generate a report of the mean diameters of all the measured follicles (Fig. 12-30). Some labs may use three dimensions, whereas most labs will simply average two dimensions measured off an image of the follicle in its largest plane. To obtain such a plane, sweep through each follicle in real time to locate and freeze the optimum view from which to measure that particular follicle before moving on to the next and finding its optimum plane for measurement.

Many follicles are at different stages of development because patients often harbor antral follicles at various stages of growth in FSH-stimulated cycles (Fig. 12-31). Simply count and report the number of follicles measuring less than 10 mm, but individually measure and report mean diameters of each follicle greater than 10 mm in each ovary. Assessment of follicular mean diameter aids in timing ovulation trigger administration, usually when the lead follicles have a mean diameter of 17 mm[44] and most follicles are at least 15 mm[12] in mean diameter. The mean diameter at which follicles are mature (Table 12-2) in gonadotropin-stimulated cycles

Parameter	D1	D2	D3	Mean
B Mode Measurements				
General Gynecology				
Follicle				
Rt Follicle 02	2.19 cm	2.12 cm		2.15 cm
Lt Follicle 01	2.96 cm	1.51 cm		2.23 cm
Lt Follicle 02	1.44 cm	0.86 cm		1.15 cm
Lt Follicle 03	1.30 cm	0.94 cm		1.12 cm
Lt Follicle 04	1.41 cm	0.71 cm		1.06 cm
Lt Follicle 05	2.55 cm	1.37 cm		1.96 cm
Endo	1.34 cm	1.34		

Figure 12-30. Measuring follicles. Machine-generated report. (Image courtesy of Shady Grove Fertility Center, Rockville, MD.)

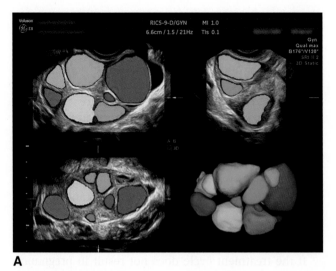
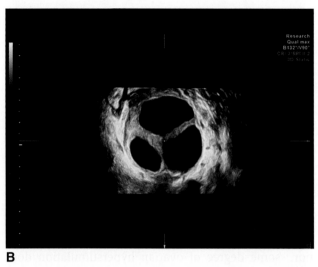

Figure 12-31. A: 3D volume imaging of stimulated ovary, showing multiple follicles, coded in color. **B:** Follicles of varying size are seen. (Sonographic image courtesy of GE Healthcare, Wauwatosa, WI.)

is 16 to 18 mm; in clomiphene-stimulated cycles, the mean diameter at maturity is 20 mm. As a comparison in the natural cycle, ovulation occurs in follicles with mean diameters of 15 to 25 mm.[12]

Recent technological innovations with 3D volume acquisitions can also provide automated counting and measurement of follicles.[16] The sonographer acquires a 3D volume dataset and uses the software to automatically measure and generate a complete report of mean diameters of all follicles in each ovary (Fig. 12-32). The automated 3D acquisition improves the speed of the exam. It also reduces the risk of occupational injury in the sonographer, who may otherwise experience musculoskeletal injury due to uncomfortable ergonomics during intense and prolonged endovaginal scanning.

Sonography during the Periovulatory Period

During this period, scan both the follicles and the endometrium to help evaluate the patient, predict the timing of ovulation, and assess the receptivity of the endometrium for implantation. When sufficient follicles reach average diameters that are considered to be mature, an ovulation trigger in the form of hCG is administered to induce ovulation. Sonography of the endometrium is of little use in predicting favorable implantation outcomes,[21] but research does show that endometrial thickness of less than 6 mm is useful in predicting poor implantation rates.[12]

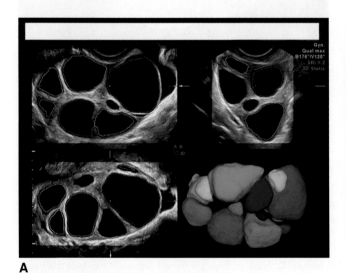

Name	SonoAVC3, 3D				Perf. Phys.			
Pat. ID	034		DOB		Ref. Phys.			
Indication			Sex	Female	Sonogr.			
LMP		Day of Cycle			Gravida		AB	
Day of stim.	11	Expected Ovul.			Para		Ectopic	

Ovary: Total#:	Left 17					Ovary: Total#:	Right 18				
Nr.	d(V) mm	dx mm	dy mm	dz mm	mn. d mm	V cm³	Nr.	d(V) mm	dx mm	dy mm	dz mm	mn. d mm	V cm³
1	29.7	36.1	30.4	26.1	30.9	13.71	1	29.4	35.8	30.0	25.8	30.5	13.27
2	26.4	31.0	29.1	21.7	27.3	9.61	2	25.9	30.4	28.5	21.3	26.7	9.07
3	19.9	24.3	20.1	17.5	20.6	4.14	3	19.6	23.9	19.8	17.2	20.3	3.93
4	19.9	23.9	20.9	17.3	20.7	4.10	4	19.3	23.5	20.2	16.8	20.2	3.76
5	15.6	19.7	17.1	11.6	16.1	1.98	5	15.2	22.8	13.1	13.1	16.3	1.82
6	15.5	23.2	13.4	13.4	16.7	1.95	6	15.1	18.1	16.3	13.8	16.1	1.81
7	15.5	18.6	16.7	13.9	16.4	1.94	7	14.9	19.2	16.3	11.0	15.5	1.73
8	11.9	15.9	14.3	8.5	12.9	0.87	8	11.7	15.7	14.1	8.3	12.7	0.83
9	11.3	20.3	9.6	8.6	12.9	0.76	9	11.2	21.5	9.4	8.2	13.0	0.74
10	8.9	14.8	13.2	3.8	10.6	0.36	10	8.3	12.0	9.4	6.0	9.1	0.30
11	8.8	12.5	9.9	6.4	9.6	0.35	11	8.3	14.2	12.4	3.5	10.0	0.29
	8.6	12.1	9.8	5.6	9.2	0.33	12	8.1	11.7	9.3	5.2	8.7	0.28
13	7.6	10.1	9.1	5.5	8.2	0.23		7.0	9.4	8.5	5.0	7.6	0.18

Figure 12-32. A: New software in sonography machines with 3D volume acquisitions enables automatic counting and measuring of follicles, shown here color-coded. **B:** An automatically generated report provides planar dimensions as well as an average diameter and volume of each follicle. (Sonographic image courtesy of GE Healthcare, Wauwatosa, WI.)

Complications of Controlled Ovarian Hyperstimulation

OHSS and multifetal gestations are serious complications of ovarian hyperstimulation techniques used in assisted reproduction. OHSS can occur in either the clomiphene or the gonadotropin regimens used to hyperstimulate a woman's ovaries as part of her infertility treatment. In general, the risk of severe OHSS is low in patients using clomiphene citrate for ovarian hyperstimulation, whereas gonadotropins slightly increase this complication. Sonography plays an important role in monitoring follicular growth with both regimens, because of the increased incidence of complications such as OHSS and multifetal gestations.

Due to the very nature of the COH treatment option, some degree of ovarian hyperstimulation does occur in patients undergoing follicle stimulation with gonadotropins as part of their assisted reproduction treatment.[45,46] The treatment regimen is not discontinued if the degree of hyperstimulation is clinically insignificant. The symptoms of hyperstimulation range from mild abdominal discomfort to, in its most severe form, circulatory compromise and electrolyte imbalance. In severe OHSS, the ovaries are markedly enlarged (greater than 10 centimeters [cm]) and edematous. Ascites and pleural effusions are present, with concomitant hemoconcentration and oliguria. There is increased risk of ovarian cyst rupture or torsion. Severe OHSS occurs in cycles with enlarged ovaries, high estradiol levels, and many small or intermediate, rather than large, follicles.[47] This situation can be limited by withholding hCG and thus not triggering ovulation. Were OHSS to be diagnosed with these characteristics, the treatment cycles would be canceled (i.e., all available embryos frozen with no embryos being transferred) and any further treatment put off for another menstrual cycle.

If the treatment cycle does not result in pregnancy, the syndrome spontaneously resolves within a few days. The syndrome, however, is most commonly seen with pregnancy (Fig. 12-33), in which case resolution occurs more slowly, over 6 to 8 weeks. Hospitalization and abdominal paracentesis under sonographic guidance are often required.

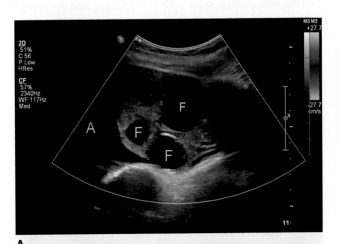

A

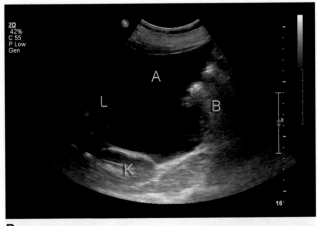

B

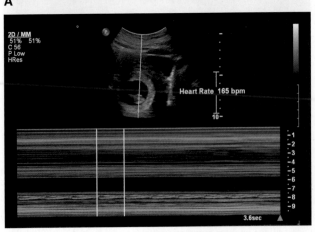

C

Figure 12-33. This scan demonstrates OHSS and pregnancy. **A:** There are multiple large, anechoic follicles and ascites in the left adnexa. *A,* ascites; *F,* follicle. **B:** Large amount of ascites imaged in the right upper quadrant. A paracentesis procedure was used to drain the fluid. Note right kidney posterior to the fluid. *L,* liver; *K,* kidney; *B,* bowel; *A,* ascites. **C:** A live embryo confirmed with an M-mode of the heartbeat. (Image courtesy of The George Washington University Hospital, Washington, DC.)

Aspiration of Follicles Following Controlled Hyperstimulation of Ovaries

Follicle aspiration procedures occur in a surgical suite. Sonography plays an important role in the real-time guidance for retrieval of oocytes by aspiration of hyperstimulated ovarian follicles. Aspiration of the oocyte occurs when a sufficient number of follicles reach an optimum size in the hyperstimulated ovaries with real-time sonographic guidance of the biopsy needle. Most endovaginal transducers have sterilizable biopsy guides, which fix to the transducer. A double dotted line representing the path of the biopsy guide reflects onto the monitor by the software program of the machine. Needles of an appropriate gauge pass through the guide along or between the superimposed dotted guidelines on the monitor. Centimeter lines indicate depth and allow for an estimate of needle depth penetration along the biopsy guideline. Aspirating needles have sonographically marked tips to help with visualization. The needle connects directly to a pump device by intravenous fluid tubing for oocyte retrieval or to a syringe for fluid collection and flushing. Place the needle through the guide, which fastens directly to the transducer. The position of the entire length of the needle remains within the scanning plane, under direct visualization.

Movement of the needle is through manual manipulation or by an automated needle puncture system. In the first method, the needle is placed within the guide and manually advanced into the area of interest along the monitor's superimposed biopsy lines. The target is kept centralized as much as possible between the biopsy needle guides. An automated spring-loaded needle puncture device fixed to the shaft of the vaginal transducer may be used. Precise depth of penetration can be programmed using the same linear biopsy monitor guide. The advantage with this technique is that because of the force with which the needle is directed into the target, a thinner needle can be used, minimizing tissue trauma and pain. Separate vaginal punctures for each target are a main disadvantage of this procedure. The manual technique allows for a single vaginal entry, with change in angulations in the transducer and needle about that point, facilitating targeting and aspiration of multiple areas, as is essential for oocyte retrieval. Occasionally, transuterine puncture is necessary to access an ovary. The patient may experience some discomfort with the aspiration of oocytes,

Sonographically Guided Embryo Transfer

Embryo transfer is performed in an outpatient setting in a lab situated adjacent to an embryology laboratory. Transabdominal sonography can be used routinely for real-time guidance of transcervical embryo transfer (Fig. 12-27).[6,12,48] However, there is controversy as to the usefulness of sonographic guidance for embryo transfer, and some turn to sonography selectively, only in difficult cases.[6]

Embryos can be transferred either as cleavage stage embryos 2 or 3 days after fertilization, or as blastocysts 5 or 6 days after fertilization.[49,50] Whereas in early years of ART, multiple embryos were routinely transferred into a woman's uterus to increase the chances of achieving even one singleton gestation, current recommendations have changed this practice. As clinical experience with assisted reproduction has matured over the past few decades, practitioners around the world have come to reassess the impact of multifetal gestations on maternal health, fetal outcome, and associated costs, and to revise guidelines of the number of embryos transferred during ART procedures. A generally desired outcome of ART is that of a healthy singleton gestation.[49] Italy passed laws strictly limiting the practice to single embryo transfers.[51] The American Society of Reproductive Medicine published guidelines for the number of embryos to transfer, taking into consideration a variety of factors, including a woman's age, her etiology of infertility, and her history of previous failed IVF cycles. The recommendations range from one single embryo (for women under 35 years of age who have favorable prognosis) to five cleavage-stage embryos (for women older than 40 years of age).[49] In collaboration with the reproductive endocrinologist and the embryologist, along with consideration of the published guidelines, the woman receiving IVF treatment signs an informed consent statement as to the number and stage of embryos for transfer.[49,50] Embryos can be transferred into the woman's uterus during the same cycle in which follicles were aspirated, or they can be cryopreserved and transferred at a later date.[52] After obtaining informed consent from the couple, an embryologist draws the embryos into a transfer catheter. With or without sonographic guidance, the reproductive endocrinologist then transfers the embryo(s) into the uterine cavity.

If providing sonographic guidance, the sonographer aligns the view of the cervical canal and the uterus on the monitor, scanning transabdominally with the patient's full bladder as a window, and using a 3 MHz or 4 MHz transducer. The transfer catheter containing the embryos visualizes as echogenic lines in the cervical canal, and the sonographer continues to maintain the catheter tip in clear view to help guide the physician to advance the catheter tip toward the fundus of the uterus and expel the embryos into the cavity. If baseline sonography or prior sonohysterogram have identified this patient as potentially difficult, then a trial run (i.e., a mock procedure) without embryos prior to the scheduled IVF-ET procedure helps determine the best path for the transfer catheter.[6]

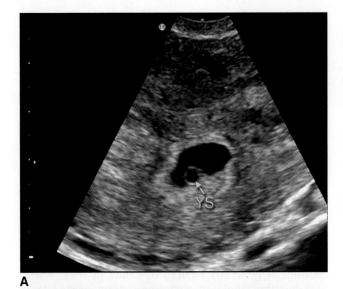

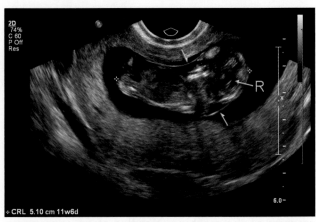

Figure 12-35. Crown rump length (CRL) measurement of an 11-week singleton gestation. Note the thin amnion (arrows) surrounding the embryo. R, rhombencephalon. Image courtesy of The George Washington University Hospital, Washington, DC.

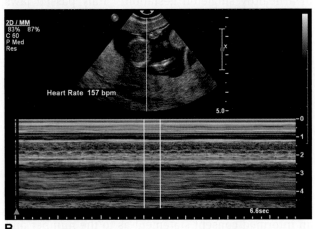

Figure 12-34. A: Early gestation shows a gestational sac, and a yolk sac but no fetal pole. YS, yolk sac. **B:** A fetal pole with heartbeat is demonstrated in this gestation 4 weeks postembryo transfer. (Images courtesy of The George Washington University Hospital, Washington, DC.)

Endovaginal Sonogram to Detect Viable Gestation

Endovaginal sonography routinely aids in detection of the early gestation. A gestational sac is visualized by 5 weeks after a woman's last menstrual period (i.e., it can be visualized as early as 3 weeks after egg retrieval/fertilization). If the gestation is viable, a yolk sac (Fig. 12-34a) can be seen within the gestational sac by 5.5 weeks, and a fetus with heartbeat (Fig. 12-34b) can be seen by 6.5 weeks since the last menstrual period.

Multifetal Reduction

The goal of ART is to help couples have children. Yet a complication of ART procedures is that treatment can result in gestations of too many fetuses, compromising the viability of the entire pregnancy. To preserve the pregnancy, couples with three or more fetuses may elect for selective or multifetal reduction. Sonography guides the reductive procedure. With sonographic guidance, a physician injects saline into one or more of the gestational sacs, selectively aborting particular sacs while preserving the rest of the gestation. The embryo targeted for reduction depends on the ease of access and asymmetry of growth.

Sonography for Continued Assessment of the Ongoing Gestation to Term

Obstetric sonography is routinely performed for ongoing (Fig. 12-35) imaging and evaluation of the gestation. Although briefly mentioned here, it is not elaborated on since it is covered in several other chapters.

PART II: CONTRACEPTION AND ELECTIVE ABORTION

This section describes the role of sonography in interventions designed to control pregnancy. This part of the chapter covers these topic.

THE ROLE OF SONOGRAPHY IN CONTRACEPTION

The concept of IUCDs for use in preventing pregnancy in animals dates back as far as 3,000 years. IUCD use in women began more recently, in the early 20th century.[53]

Popularity of IUCDs increased in the 1960s and 1970s, abated for a while, and has shown signs of an increase in recent years.

Reversible Contraception

Two types of IUCDs currently marketed in the United States allow reversible contraception. These are the ParaGard© (Copper) IUCD and the Mirena© levonorgestrel-releasing IUCD. However, it is important that sonographers be familiar with additional devices, as

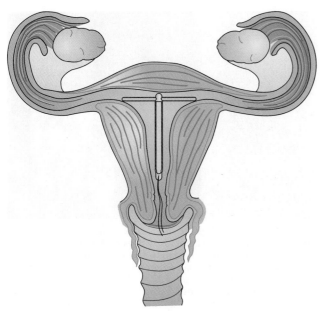

Figure 12-36. Schematic diagram of female reproductive organs with intrauterine device in place in uterus.

patients may present to a sonography lab for evaluation of complications.

The ParaGard and the Mirena devices are both T-shaped (Fig. 12-36). The ParaGard is made of plastic coated in copper, which has a contraceptive action that—while not fully understood—is thought to affect the contractile action of the myometrium[54] and thus prevent pregnancy. The copper may also act as an irritant to the endometrium and possibly has an ovicidal action.[53] The ParaGard IUCD lasts up to 10 years. It is well visualized by sonography as highly reflective intracavitary linear echoes (Fig. 12-37), with a reverberation artifact that draws attention to the IUCD.

The Mirena IUCD, on the other hand, releases the synthetic hormone levonorgestrel and lasts for 5 years.

In addition to its use in contraception, the hormone-releasing Mirena is also prescribed for menorrhagia.[53] The steady release of microdoses of levonorgestrel within the uterus creates an endometrium that is hostile to implantation and cervical mucus that is too thick to permit sperm entry into the uterus. The 32-mm vertical and horizontal stems of the more recent versions of the Mirena IUCD are visible sonographically, though in earlier versions sonographers had difficulty seeing much more than the tips on sonograms.

IUCDs that were in use in the latter half of the 20th century in the United States included both inert and copper-containing devices. They are well visualized by plain film radiography when trying to find an IUCD that has migrated from the uterus or by sonography if there is a suspicion that it is malpositioned but within the uterus. A spiral-shaped device known as the Lippes Loop, a coil-shaped one named the Saf-T coil, and a ring-shaped one named the Dalkon Shield were inert devices that mechanically interfered with implantation of the conceptus (Figs. 12-38 and 12-39). Copper-releasing IUCDs shaped like the number 7 or the letter T were devices that had both a mechanical as well as a chemical contraceptive action. Though no longer marketed in the United States, one of these may be seen in a patient who had it inserted in the past. It should also be noted that there is a ring-shaped (Fig. 12-40) IUCD not marketed in the United States but widely used to date in China.

The string, attached to the tailpiece, extends through the cervix and can be used to locate the normally functioning IUCD. However, the string may retract into the uterus or break at the time of an attempted removal. Sonography has replaced the standard radiograph in assessing such cases, permitting easy identification of the IUCD's location as long as it is within the uterus. Sonography also assesses evidence of perforation,

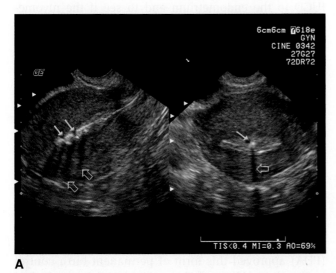

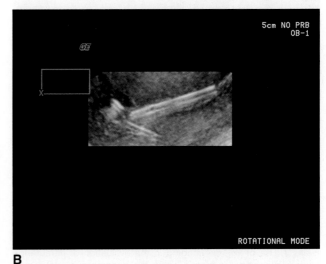

A　　　　　　　　　　　　　　　　　　　　　**B**

Figure 12-37. A: A dual image of an IUCD *(arrows)* with the sagittal (left image) and transverse (right image). Characteristic shadowing *(open arrows)* images posterior to the IUCD. **B:** 3D rendering of a T-shaped IUCD. (Sonographic image courtesy of GE Healthcare, Wauwatosa, WI.)

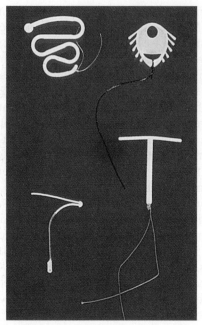

Figure 12-38. Different shapes of intrauterine contraceptive devices marketed in the United States over the years. Clockwise from top: Lippes loop, Dalkon Shield, Copper T, and Copper 7.

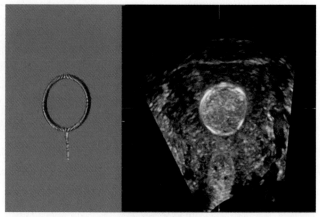

Figure 12-40. Coronal plane (from 3D volume set) of the uterus showing the Chinese ring intrauterine device. (Wilson M, and Whyte-Evans J. Use of volume imaging in the evaluation of intrauterine contraceptive devices placed within the endometrium. *Journal of Diagnostic Medical Sonography*, 2009; 25: p. 39. Reprinted by permission of SAGE Publications.)

malpositioning within the uterine cavity, embedding in the myometrium, or incomplete removal. Difficult removals due to shifts in IUCD positioning in the uterus or its embedding can be anticipated, and removal can be guided with sonography.

Expulsion or partial expulsion of the IUCD from the uterine cavity with resultant embedding of a portion of the IUCD device, especially the stem, can occur without the user being aware. Absence of the string or strong cramping pelvic pain indicates a need for sonographic evaluation. Identification of uterine perforation, though usually occurring at the time of insertion, is rarely identified until later. Endovaginal sonography can tell that

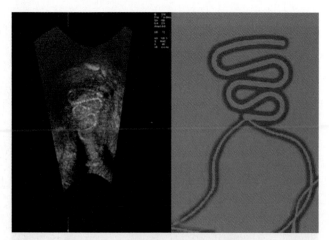

Figure 12-39. 3D reconstruction image. Coronal plane of the uterus showing the Lippes Loop intrauterine device. (Wilson M, and Whyte-Evans J. Use of volume imaging in the evaluation of intrauterine contraceptive devices placed within the endometrium. *Journal of Diagnostic Medical Sonography*, 2009; 25: p. 39. Reprinted by permission of SAGE Publications.)

the device is no longer within the uterus. It had been considered that sonography was rarely of use in localizing an IUCD that had migrated from the uterus, but case reports do show that endovaginal sonography can visualize the IUCD outside the uterus. Correlative imaging with MRI or CT and plain film radiographs helps in these cases, however. Penetration of the IUCD through the uterus and migration to the colon,[55] to an ovarian carcinoma,[56] and to other[57] locations in the abdominopelvic cavity have been reported. Immediate removal is necessary to prevent further complications.

3D and 4D sonography are well suited to assessing the proper placement of the IUCD within the endometrial cavity.[58] Real-time 3D (i.e., 4D) imaging lends itself to a more speedy examination than it would take to perform offline reconstruction of 3D data. The coronal view is readily accessed in real time (i.e., 4D sonography), making it easier to assess the relationship of the IUCD to the endometrium and to see if the myometrium is penetrated. 3D volume imaging also enables the sonographer to visualize the location of the string (Fig. 12-41).

Irreversible Contraception: The Essure© Device

To achieve irreversible birth control, women now have access to an intervention that prevents pregnancy by permanent bilateral occlusion of their fallopian tubes. This occurs when placing Essure microinsert coils into the cornual portion of the fallopian tubes, stimulating tissue growth over them. Over the period of 3 to 6 months, tissue growth around these coils effectively occludes the fallopian tube, resulting in irreversible contraception. In 2002, the Food and Drug Association (FDA) approved this form of permanent birth control in the United States.[59] Current protocol in the United States advocates the use of hysterosalpingography

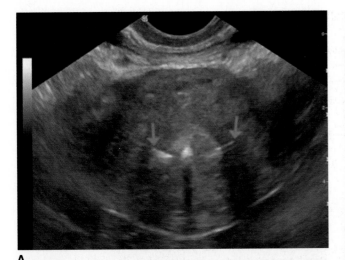

A

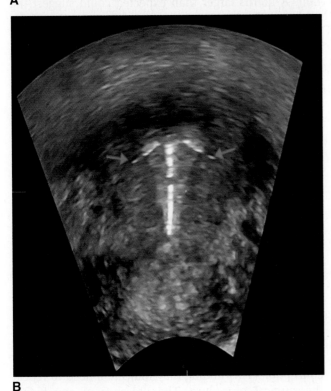

B

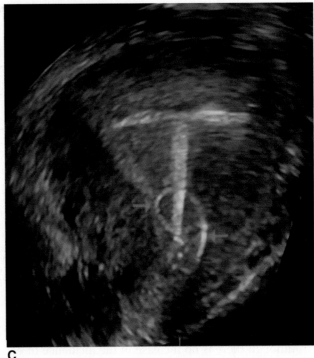

C

Figure 12-41. A: Transverse plane of the uterus in which the cross bars of the IUCD are extending into the myometrium *(red arrow)*. **B:** Note that in this patient, the cross bars are within the endometrium. **C:** In this patient, the string is visualized within the cervix. (Wilson M, and Whyte-Evans J. Use of volume imaging in the evaluation of intrauterine contraceptive devices placed within the endometrium. *Journal of Diagnostic Medical Sonography,* 2009; 25: p. 41. Reprinted by permission of SAGE Publications.)

rather than sonography for the routine 3-month follow-up on the procedure. Literature reports on the value of using 3D and 4D endovaginal sonographic screening after 1 month, or at the patient's first office visit to her health care practitioner.[60] This early screening can verify proper positioning of the coils. Authors report that most patients require no additional evaluation unless the coils are malpositioned. One of the pathways of coil migration is to the fallopian tubes. The authors contend that, if done by experienced sonographers, the use of real-time 3D sonography provides access to the coronal view and to any additional plane that helps instantaneously visualize the microinsert within the cornu, and the proximity of the coil to the endometrium (Fig. 12-42). The use of real-time 3D (i.e., 4D) imaging

makes the exam fast and effective, as it reduces the need for the postprocessing that can be time consuming with 3D reconstruction. The authors performed sonographic screening soon after the procedure for early detection of malposition (See figure 12-43).[60]

Pregnancy and Intrauterine Devices

Pregnancy in the presence of an IUCD poses many serious problems. Removal is recommended if it can be accomplished without significant uterine manipulation. Complications of allowing the IUCD to remain in the uterus include spontaneous abortion, sepsis, premature delivery, and maternal death. Removal early in pregnancy decreases the miscarriage rate. Sonography is essential in locating the device in relation to the ongoing gestation.

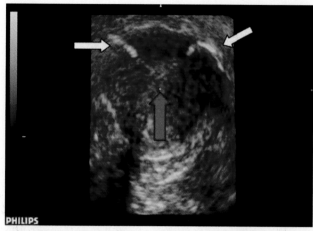

Figure 12-42. Multiplanar reconstruction view of a 3D endovaginal sonogram demonstrating both Essure microinserts *(white arrows)* in relationship to the endometrium *(red arrow)*. (Oliveira M, Johnson D, Switalksi P., et al. Optimal Use of 3D and 4D transvaginal sonography in localizing the Essure contraceptive device. *Journal of Diagnostic Medical Sonography* 2009;25:3 p.165. Reprinted by permission of SAGE Publications.)

Although there is no increase in the incidence of ectopic pregnancy with IUCD use, a high percentage of pregnancies that occur in patients with an IUCD are ectopic. Vaginal bleeding with an IUCD and a suspected pregnancy must be aggressively evaluated by sonography and pregnancy testing.

Questions with regard to associated pelvic infection with the IUCD have been the major deterrent to its more widespread use. Although many believe that the risk and incidence of PID are increased with IUCD use, evidence is confounded by the general increase in the incidence of PID and differences in occurrence rates with different devices and within different relationships

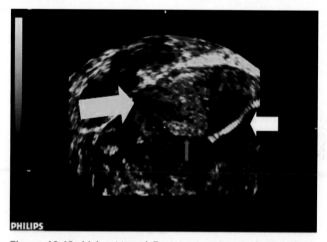

Figure 12-43. Malpositioned Essure microinsert coil. 3D volume rendered view of an endovaginal sonogram demonstrates one Essure microinsert coil *(white arrow)* properly aligned within the left cornu. The thicker yellow arrow demonstrates the absence of any microinsert coil in the right cornu. The thin red arrow points to the endometrium. (Oliveira M, Johnson D, Switalksi P., et al. Optimal Use of 3D and 4D transvaginal sonography in localizing the Essure contraceptive device. *Journal of Diagnostic Medical Sonography* 2009;25:3 p.166. Reprinted by permission of SAGE Publications.)

(e.g., monogamous as opposed to multiple partners). Endovaginal as well as transabdominal sonography may be of use in the diagnosis. Suspicion of pelvic infection *[indicates* or *should lead to]* immediate removal of the IUCD.

ELECTIVE ABORTION

When a patient has made a decision to undergo an elective abortion, sonography can be useful in clinical management before, during, and after the procedure.

Preoperative Evaluation: Use of sonography establishes gestational age before an abortion procedure when there is any discrepancy between menstrual dates (from last menstrual period) and physical examination. A uterus larger than expected could suggest the presence of a leiomyoma, congenital anomalies of the uterus, adnexal cysts, multiple gestations, hydatidiform mole, a date discrepancy, or possibly no pregnancy at all. To help define the true clinical situation, simultaneous quantitative beta-hCG pregnancy testing and sonography become necessary.

Intraoperative Sonographic Guidance: Indications for sonographic guidance of an elective abortion include congenital anomaly of the uterus and cervical abnormalities. Placement of the suction cannula with sonographic direction permits the operator to be certain of reaching the chorionic sac while avoiding injury or perforation. Guidance should be applied when there is any concern on the part of the operator that the procedure was not complete (e.g., absence of villi in the curettings suggestive of an incomplete procedure, congenital anomaly of the uterus, or ectopic pregnancy).

Postoperative Sonography: When, after dilatation and evacuation, a patient complains of immediate or delayed severe pain or bleeding, sonography can be particularly useful in identifying retained products of conception. This finding may indicate a need to repeat the surgical procedure. The presence of any highly echogenic mass within the endometrial cavity with the history of a recent miscarriage or therapeutic abortion should raise this concern.

ACKNOWLEDGMENTS

The authors wish to acknowledge the work of Frances R. Batzer, MD, who wrote this chapter in the previous edition of this volume. His material was used as a base upon which to develop the current rendition of the chapter.

SUMMARY

- Ovarian follicles 10 mm or less usually become atretic
- The mean diameter of a dominant follicle is between 15 and 25 mm

Critical Thinking Question

A patient who presents to the diagnostic imaging department complains of pelvic pain. She has been undergoing infertility treatment for infertility with gonadotropins for COH. List additional views you would obtain in addition to the routine pelvic sonographic examination. Explain the sonographic findings seen in these images (Figure 12-44A-E).

ANSWER: OHSS has the possibility of developing ovarian torsion, ascites, and pleural effusion. Doppler, both color and spectral, helps identify or rule out the torsed ovary. Images of the pleural bases determine the presence or absence of pleural effusion.

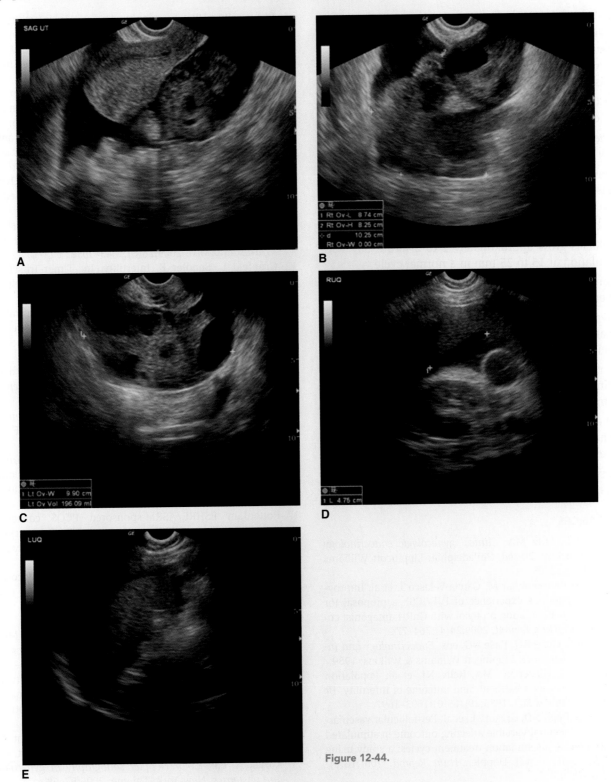

Figure 12-44.

(continued)

In this patient the uterus has a normal appearance. There are two large complex masses posterior to the uterus thought to be enlarged, hyperstimulated ovaries. The anterior and posterior cul-de-sac contains extensive fluid. Ascites extends into the right and left upper quadrants, around the right lobe of the liver and the spleen. Pseudo-Meigs syndrome describes the triad of abdominal ascites, pleural effusion, and ovarian masses. (Sonograms courtesy of Shady Grove Fertility, in Rockville, Maryland.)

- BAFC relates to both ovarian volume and ovarian response
- Asynchronous ovarian and uterine cycles are due to estradiol peak, LH surge, and ovarian follicle growth mismatches
- PCOS, endometriosis, LUF, dermoids, and hemorrhagic or complex ovarian cysts are causes of infertility
- The normal endometrial thickness for a woman in her reproductive years is between 3 and 14 mm
- Spectral Doppler PI of the uterine artery of 3 to 3.5 has 100% specificity and positive predictive value for endometrium receptiveness for pregnancy
- 35% of male primary infertility is due to varicoceles
- Follicles grow approximately 1 to 2 mm a day with ovulation at 15 to 25 mm in a normal cycle
- Sonographic follicular monitoring begins on treatment day 4 or 5
- Ovarian follicles may be measured on two or three planes to calculate a mean follicular diameter as long as interobserver methods remain consistent
- A mature follicle is 16 to 18 mm in a gonadotropin-stimulated cycle and 20 mm in a clomiphene citrate–stimulated ovulation induction cycle
- The modern ParaGard IUCD is made of copper, whereas the Mirena releases synthetic hormones to prevent pregnancy
- Essure is a permanent microcoil form of contraception placed in the fallopian tubes

REFERENCES

1. Speroff L, Fritz MA. *Clinical gynecologic endocrinology and infertility*. 7th ed. Philadelphia: Lippincott Williams & Wilkins; 2005.
2. Devroey P, Aboulghar M, Garcia-Velasco J, et al. Improving the patient's experience of IVF/ICSI: a proposal for an ovarian stimulation protocol with GnRH antagonist co-treatment. *Hum Reprod*. 2009;24(4):764–774.
3. Speroff L, Glass RH, Kase NG, eds. *Endocrinology and infertility*. Baltimore: Lippincott Williams & Wilkins; 1989.
4. Hull MGR, Glazener CMA, Kelly NJ, et al. Population study of causes, treatment, and outcome of infertility. *Br Med J (Clin Res Ed)*. 1985;291(6510):1693–1697.
5. Bhal PS, Pugh ND, Gregory L, et al. Perifollicular vascularity as a potential variable affecting outcome in stimulated intrauterine insemination treatment cycles: a study using endovaginal power Doppler. *Hum Reprod*. 2001;16(8):1682–1689.
6. Pierson RA. Ultrasonographic imaging in infertility. In: Callen PW, ed. *Ultrasonography in obstetrics and gynecology*. Philadelphia: Saunders Elsevier; 2008:986–1019.
7. Mosher WD. The demography of infertility in the United States. *Annu Prog Reprod Med*. 1993:37–43.
8. American Society of Reproductive Medicine, Society for Reproductive Endocrinology and Infertility. Optimizing natural fertility. *Fertil Steril*. 2008;90(Suppl 3):S1–S6.
9. Broekmans FJ, de Ziegler D, Howles CM, et al. The antral follicle count: practical recommendations for better standardization. *Fertil Sterility*. 2009;94(3):1044–1051.
10. American Society of Reproductive Medicine. Ovulation detection. Available at www.asrm.org. Accessed on December 16, 2009 (2006).
11. Hope JM, Long K, Kudla M, et al. Three-dimensional power Doppler angiography of cyclic ovarian blood flow. *J Ultrasound Med*. 2009;28(8):1043–1052.
12. Grunfeld L, Sandler B. Infertility. In: Timor-Tritsch IE, Goldstein SR, ed. *Ultrasound in gynecology*. Philadelphia: Churchill Livingstone; 2007.
13. Scheffer GJ, Broekmans FJM, Dorland M, et al. Antral follicle counts by endovaginal ultrasonography are related to age in women with proven natural fertility. *Fertil Steril*. 1999;72(5):845–851.
14. Nikolaou D, Templeton A. Early ovarian ageing: a hypothesis. Detection and clinical relevance. *Hum Reprod*. 2003;18(6):1137–1139.
15. Broekmans FJ, Kwee J, Hendriks DJ, et al. A systematic review of tests predicting ovarian reserve and IVF outcome. *Hum Reprod Update*. 2006;12(6):685–718.
16. Moawad NS, Gibbons H, Liu J, et al. Comparison of 3- and 2-dimensional sonographic techniques for counting ovarian follicles. *J Ultrasound Med*. 2009;28(10):1281–1288.
17. Rotterdam ESHRE/ASRM-sponsored PCOS consensus workgroup. Revised 2003 consensus on diagnostic criteria and long-term health risks related to polycystic ovary syndrome (PCOS). *Hum Reprod*. 2004;19(1):41–47.
18. Kupesic S, Kurjak A, Zodan T. Abnormalities of corpus luteum function. In: Schmidt WO, Kurjak A, eds. *Color Doppler sonography in gynecology and obstetrics*. New York: Thieme; 2005:77–82.
19. Parsons JH, Steer CV. Infertility. In: Dewbury KC, Meire HB, Cosgrove DO, et al., eds. *Ultrasound in obstetrics and gynecology*. London: Churchill Livingstone; 2001:99–122.
20. Salamonsen LA, Nie G, Hannan NJ, et al. Society for reproductive biology founders' lecture 2009. Preparing fertile soil: The importance of endometrial receptivity. *Reprod Fertil Dev*. 2009;21(7):923–934.
21. Grab D, Sterzik K. Color Doppler sonography for the optimization of assisted reproduction. In: Schmidt WO, Kurjak A, eds. *Color Doppler sonography in gynecology and obstetrics*. New York: Thieme; 2005:57–68.

22. Kovacs P, Matyas S, Boda K, et al. The effect of endometrial thickness on IVF/ICSI outcome. *Hum Reprod.* 2003;18(11):2337–2341.

23. Maymon R, Herman A, Ariely S, et al. Three-dimensional vaginal sonography in obstetrics and gynecology. *Hum Reprod Update.* 2000;6(5):475–484.

24. Abramowicz JS, Archer DF. Uterine endometrial peristalsis: a transvaginal ultrasound study. *Fertil Steril.* 1990;54(3):451–454.

25. Balasch J. Investigation of the infertile couple: investigation of the infertile couple in the era of assisted reproductive technology: a time for reappraisal. *Hum Reprod.* 2000;15(11):2251–2257.

26. American Society of Reproductive Medicine, Society of Reproductive Surgeons. Myomas and reproductive function. *Fertil Steril.* 2008;90(Suppl 3):S125–S130.

27. Clark RL, Keefe B. Infertility: imaging of the female. *Urol Radiol.* 1989;11(4):233–237.

28. Devroey P, Fauser BCJM, Diedrich K. Approaches to improve the diagnosis and management of infertility. *Hum Reprod Update.* 2009;15(4):391–408.

29. Batzer FR, Hansen L. Bizarre sonographic appearance of an adenomyoma and its presentation. *J Ultrasound Med.* 1996;15(8):599–602.

30. American Society of Reproductive Medicine. The role of tubal reconstructive surgery in the era of assisted reproductive technologies. *Fertil Steril.* 2008;90(Suppl 3):S250–S253.

31. McHugo JM. Fallopian tube patency. In: Dewbury KC, Meire HB, Cosgrove DO, et al., Eds. *Ultrasound in obstetrics and gynecology.* London: Churchill Livingstone; 2001:123–130.

32. Huneke B, Kleinkauf-Houcken A, Lindner C, et al. Pulsed Doppler and color duplex sonography in the assessment of tubal patency. In: Schmidt WO, Kurjak A, eds. *Color Doppler sonography in gynecology and obstetrics.* New York: Thieme; 2005:69–76.

33. Chudleigh T, Thilaganathan B. *Obstetric ultrasound: how, why and when.* 3rd ed. London: Elsevier Limited; 2004.

34. American Society of Reproductive Medicine. Report on varicocele and infertility. *Fertil Steril.* 2008;90(Suppl 3):S247–S249.

35. Gorelick JI, Goldstein M. Loss of fertility in men with varicocele. *Fertil Steril.* 1993;59(3):613–616.

36. Chehval MJ, Purcell MH. Deterioration of semen parameters over time in men with untreated varicocele: evidence of progressive testicular damage. *Fertil Steril.* 1992;57(1):174–177.

37. Cohen J, Trounson A, Dawson K, et al. The early days of IVF outside the UK. *Hum Reprod Update.* 2005;11(5):439–460.

38. Van Voorhis BJ. Clinical pratice: in vitro fertilization. *N Engl J Med.* 2007;356(4):379–386.

39. Society for Assisted Reproductive Technology, American Society of Reproductive Medicine. Revised minimum standards for practices offering assisted reproductive technologies. Available at asrm.org. Accessed on December 16, 2009.

40. American Society of Reproductive Medicine. Intracytoplasmic sperm injection (ICSI). Available at asrm.org. Accessed on December 16, 2009.

41. American Society of Reproductive Medicine, Society for Assisted Reproductive Technology. 2008 Guidelines for gamete and embryo donation: a practice committee report. *Fertil Steril.* 2008;90(Suppl 3):S30–S44.

42. Van Voorhis B. Outcomes from assisted reproductive technology. *Obstet Gynecol.* 2006;107(1):183–200.

43. Grunfeld L, Walker B, Bergh PA, et al. High-resolution endovaginal ultrasonography of the endometrium: a noninvasive test for endometrial adequacy. *Obstet Gynecol.* 1991;78(2):200–204.

44. Strawn EY, Roesler M, Rinke M, et al. Minimal precycle testing and ongoing cycle monitoring for in vitro fertilization and fresh pre-embryo transfer do not compromise fertilization, implantation, or ongoing pregnancy rates. *Am J Obstet Gynecol.* 2000;182(6):1623–1628.

45. American Society of Reproductive Medicine. Use of exogenous gonadotropins in anovulatory women: a technical bulletin. *Fertil Steril.* 2008;90(Suppl 3):S7–S12.

46. American Society of Reproductive Medicine. Ovarian hyperstimulation syndrome. *Fertil Steril.* 2008;90(Suppl 3):S188–S193.

47. Blankstein J, Shalev J, Saadon T, et al. Ovarian hyperstimulation syndrome: prediction by number and size of preovulatory ovarian follicles. *Fertil Steril.* 1987;47(4):597–602.

48. Kupesic S, Kurjak A, Ertran AK. Interventional ultrasound in reproductive medicine. In: Schmidt WO, Kurjak A, eds. *Color Doppler sonography in gynecology and obstetrics.* New York: Thieme; 2005:83–93.

49. Society for Assisted Reproductive Technology, American Society of Reproductive Medicine. Guidelines on number of embryos transferred. *Fertil Steril.* 2008;90(Suppl 3):S163–S164.

50. American Society of Reproductive Medicine. Definitions of infertility and recurrent pregnancy loss. Available at asrm.org. Accessed on December 16, 2009.

51. La Sala GB, Nicoli A, Capodanno F, et al. The effect of the 2004 Italian legislation on perinatal outcomes following assisted reproduction technology. *J Perinat Med.* 2009;37(1):43–47.

52. Yeung WSB, Li RHW, Cheung TM, et al. Frozen-thawed embryo transfer cycles. *Hong Kong Med J.* 2009;15(6):420–426.

53. Peri N, Graham D, Levine D. Imaging of intrauterine contraceptive devices. *J Ultrasound Med.* 2007;26(10):1389–1401.

54. Salamanca A, Carrillo MP, Beltran E, et al. Transvaginal sonographic evaluation of subendometrial-myometrial contractility in women using a copper-releasing intrauterine device. *Contraception.* 2008;77(6):444–446.

55. Arslan A, Kanat-Pektas M, Yesilyurt H, et al. Colon penetration by a copper intrauterine device: a case report with literature review. *Arch Gynecol Obstet.* 2009;279(3):395–397.

56. Koo HR, Oh YT, Kim YT, et al. Intrauterine device found in an ovarian carcinoma. *J Comput Assist Tomogr.* 2008;32(1):69–71.

57. Deshmukh S, Ghanouni P, Jeffrey RB. Early sonographic diagnosis of intrauterine device migration to the adnexa. *J Clin Ultrasound.* 2009;37(7):414–416.

58. Wilson M, Whyte-Evans J. Use of volume imaging in the evaluation of intrauterine contraceptive devices. *J Diagn Med Sonography.* 2009;25(1):38–43.

59. Food and Drug Administration. 2002 device approvals. Available at http://www.accessdata.fda.gov/cdrh_docs/pdf2/p020014a.pdf. Accessed on September 5, 2010.

60. Oliveira M, Johnson D, Switalski P, et al. Optimal use of 3D and 4D endovaginal sonography in localizing the Essure® contraceptive device. *J Diagn Med Sonography.* 2009;25(3):163–167.

13 The Use of Ultrasound in the First Trimester

Paula Woletz

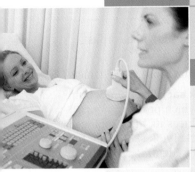

OBJECTIVES

Discuss gamete formation, fertilization, placenta development, and early development of the zygote

Recognize normal sonographic findings in first-trimester pregnancies

Describe sonographic methods of determining gestational age in the first trimester

Explain the safe use of ultrasound during early pregnancy

KEY TERMS

amnion | chorion | crown-rump length | estimated date of delivery (EDD) | gestational age | mean sac diameter (MSD) | nuchal translucency (NT) | umbilical vesicle | yolk sac

GLOSSARY

Acrosome Area located in the head of the sperm containing enzymes to aid in penetration of the oocyte

Amnion Membrane enclosing the amniotic cavity and embryo or fetus

Aneuploidy Abnormal number of chromosomes

Blastocyst Early gestation consisting of a thin outer layer of cells (trophoblast), a fluid-filled cavity, and an inner cell mass (embryoblast)

Chorion Membrane around the chorionic cavity, made up of trophoblast cells and extraembryonic mesoderm

Chorionic villi Budlike outward growths from the trophoblast, some of which give rise to the fetal portion of the placenta

Conceptual age Duration of pregnancy, counted from fertilization (conception), expressed in hours or days. Also called embryonic age or postovulatory age

Conceptus Product of fertilization, including all stages from zygote to fetus

Corpus luteum Progesterone-secreting structure formed by a follicle after releasing its oocyte

Crown-rump length (CRL) Measurement of the longest axis of an embryo to determine gestational age

Estimated date of delivery (EDD) Due date, calculated by adding 280 days to the first day of the

last menstrual period; also called estimated date of confinement (EDC)

Decidualization Changes in the endometrium to allow implantation of a blastocyst.

Estrogen Group of hormones, primarily produced in the ovaries, which affect secondary sex characteristics and the menstrual cycle

Fertilization Penetration of an oocyte by a sperm to form a diploid zygote

Follicle-stimulating hormone (FSH) Hormone produced in the anterior pituitary, which stimulates the maturation of ovarian follicles

Gamete Haploid cell that, when merged with a gamete from the opposite sex, creates a diploid zygote

Gestational age (GA, a.k.a. menstrual age) Duration of pregnancy, counted from the first day of the last menstrual period, expressed in weeks and days or fractions of weeks. A pregnancy typically lasts about 280 days, or 40 weeks, counted from the first day of the last menstrual period, and is commonly divided into three trimesters:

> **First trimester:** 0 days (first day of last menstrual period) to the end of the 13th week
>
> **Second trimester:** 14 weeks to the end of the 27th week
>
> **Third trimester:** 28 weeks to delivery

Gestational sac First sonographic evidence of an intrauterine pregnancy, the fluid-filled blastocyst

Gravidity Number of times a woman has been pregnant

Human chorionic gonadotropin (hCG) Hormone produced by trophoblast cells of the blastocyst, which extends the life of the corpus luteum in the ovary; most pregnancy tests are based on detection of hCG

Last menstrual period (LMP) First day of last menstrual period

Luteinizing hormone (LH) Hormone produced in the anterior pituitary, which triggers ovulation in females

Mean sac diameter (MSD) Average diameter of the gestational sac, used to determine gestational age

Morula Solid cluster of undifferentiated cells formed by repeated cleavage of the single cell that resulted from the fusion of two gametes

Nuchal translucency (NT) Subcutaneous fluid in the posterior region of the neck of embryos and fetuses up to 14 weeks' gestational age; abnormally large NTs have been associated with a higher risk of chromosomal and structural abnormalities

Oocyte Female gamete; also called ovum or egg

Parity Summary of a woman's pregnancy outcomes. The most common description of parity is expressed in four numbers: the first is the number of term deliveries, the second is the number of preterm deliveries (usually after 24 weeks' gestational age), the third is the number of other pregnancies and includes both spontaneous and therapeutic abortions, and the fourth number is the woman's living children.

Pregnancy-associated plasma protein A (PAPP-A) Protein produced by the trophoblasts; abnormal levels of PAPP-A may be associated with an increased risk of chromosomal abnormalities

Progesterone Hormone produced by the corpus luteum and the placenta

Spermatozoon (plural: spermatozoa) Male gamete

Umbilical vesicle (a.k.a. yolk sac) Structure within the cavity of the blastocyst, which provides nourishment to the embryo and produces its first blood cells; the secondary umbilical vesicle (yolk sac) is the first structure to be sonographically identified within the gestational sac

Yolk sac (a.k.a. umbilical vesicle) Structure within the cavity of the blastocyst, which provides nourishment to the embryo and produces its first blood cells. The secondary umbilical vesicle (yolk sac) is the first structure to be sonographically identified within the gestational sac

Zygote Single cell resulting from the fusion of two gametes

The birth of a healthy, normal baby is the result of processes that began long before conception. Since the time fertilization occurs is rarely known, a clinically diagnosed pregnancy is generally dated from the first day of the woman's last normal menstrual period, approximately 2 weeks before she was truly pregnant. Pregnancy typically lasts about 280 days, or 40 weeks, from the first day of the last menstrual period (LMP) and is divided into three trimesters.

During the first trimester of pregnancy, a single cell with genetic components derived from its mother and father develops into a complex organism. When these dramatic changes are occurring, the embryo or young fetus is particularly susceptible to physical and chemical insults that can disrupt its development. Most spontaneous losses occur during the first 12 weeks of pregnancy.

The most pressing concern in the sonographic evaluation of the early pregnancy remains the determination of where implantation has occurred, the gestational age and estimated date of delivery (EDD), and whether the pregnancy is likely to continue to term. Increasingly, sonographers help determine whether the pregnancy is normal in appearance or if the embryo is at risk for structural or chromosomal abnormalities. To that end, the practitioner must have an understanding of the processes that occur from gamete formation and ovulation through the beginning of fetal development.

GAMETE FORMATION

Most human cells are called *diploid*, because they contain two sets of chromosomes, 23 of which originally came from the individual's mother, and 23 from the father. New cells form through a process of duplication and division called *mitosis*, which results in two cells with the same number of chromosomes as the cell from which they originate.

A different process, *meiosis*, reduces the number of chromosomes, resulting in haploid cells containing a single set of 23 chromosomes. These haploid cells are gametes. Male gametes are called *spermatozoa* (singular: spermatozoon) or *sperm*, and female gametes are called *ova* (singular: ovum) or *oocytes*.

The male begins to produce mature sperm around the onset of puberty, and sperm production continues throughout adult life. Sperm development occurs in the seminiferous tubules of the testes. The haploid sperm are stored in the epididymis, where they complete their maturation. Each mature sperm cell has a head and a tail. The head contains the cell nucleus and is topped with a hatlike acrosome with enzymes capable of penetrating the outer layer of an ovum. The tail contains mitochondria to power the whiplike motion that creates sperm motility.

When ejaculation occurs during sexual intercourse, spermatozoa and fluid produced in the seminal vesicles, prostate, and bulbourethral glands are pumped through the urethra of the penis and deposited in the vagina at the external os of the cervix. Hundreds of millions of sperm are released in a single ejaculation, but only a small percentage of them successfully reach the portion of the fallopian tube where fertilization most commonly occurs.[1]

In females, the ovaries and all their rudimentary follicles form long before birth. Within each follicle, there is an immature oocyte surrounded by a layer of follicular cells. At puberty, under the influence of follicle-stimulating hormone (FSH) produced in the pituitary gland, the follicles mature and begin to fill with fluid. The oocyte is not in direct contact with the fluid; it remains surrounded by follicular cells, which produce estrogen. The rising level of estrogen eventually causes the pituitary to release luteinizing hormone (LH), which triggers ovulation—the release of the ovum. In general, only a single follicle matures and releases an ovum at a time. The haploid oocyte has undergone the first stage and part of the second stage of meiosis and is surrounded by a membrane containing glycoproteins (the *zona pellucida*) and a cloudlike cluster of follicular cells (*corona radiata*). The second stage of meiosis is not complete at the time of ovulation.[1]

The moving, fimbriated ends of the fallopian tube help direct the ovum into the tube, and cilia and contractions of the walls of the tube help propel it toward the uterus. Meanwhile, the ruptured follicle fills with a variable amount of blood, and its walls involute, thicken, and begin to secrete progesterone. The ruptured follicle is now called a *corpus luteum*.

FERTILIZATION AND IMPLANTATION

Fertilization usually occurs in the ampullary portion of the fallopian tube, 24 to 36 hours after ovulation, when the zona pellucida is penetrated by a single sperm. Penetration by the sperm causes a change in the chemical composition of the zona pellucida, so no other sperm can enter the ovum. Penetration by the sperm also activates the completion of the second meiotic division of the ovum, forming a mature oocyte. Once inside the ovum, the sperm loses its tail and its nucleus enlarges. The genetic contents of the sperm merge with those of the ovum to form a single diploid cell—the *conceptus* or *zygote* (Fig. 13-1).[1]

Cleavage, the rapid division of cells, begins 24 to 30 hours after fertilization. With each division, the number of cells increases while the size of the cells becomes smaller and smaller. The developing zygote continues to move through the fallopian tube.

Still surrounded and protected by the zona pellucida, the cells continue to divide, forming a solid cluster of cells. This ball of cells, the *morula*, continues its passage through the fallopian tube and reaches the uterine cavity

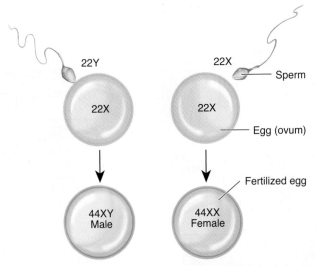

Figure 13-1 Inheritance of gender and the normal diploid chromosome count. Each ovum contains 22 autosomes and an X chromosome. Each spermatozoon (sperm) contains 22 autosomes and either an X chromosome or a Y chromosome; upon fusion of the genetic material, the normal diploid chromosome count results. The sex of the zygote is determined at the time of fertilization by the combination of the sex chromosomes of the sperm (either X or Y) and the ovum (X).

about 4 days after fertilization. Once in the uterus, it is nourished by secretions from the endometrial glands. These secretions cross the zona pellucida and enter the morula, forming a fluid-filled cavity. The structure is now called a *blastocyst* and has three distinct parts:

- The trophoblast, the thin outer layer of cells, part of which will give rise to the embryonic portion of the placenta
- The fluid-filled blastocystic cavity or blastocele
- An inner cell mass or embryoblast, which will develop into the embryo

Implantation has not yet occurred (Fig. 13-2).

The zona pellucida disintegrates, making implantation possible. No longer confined to the limited space within the zona pellucida, the blastocyst begins to grow. However, normal implantation cannot occur unless the blastocyst meets a receptive endometrium.[1,2]

The human endometrium constantly undergoes cyclical changes throughout a woman's reproductive years. The endometrium has two layers: a thin basal layer adjacent to the myometrium and a functional layer of connective tissue (stroma), glands, and capillaries, which are covered by a thin layer of epithelial cells. Initial growth of the endometrium is controlled by rising levels of estrogen. After ovulation, the corpus luteum produces progesterone, which causes differentiation (decidualization) of the endometrial cells, allowing implantation to occur.[3] The period during which the endometrium is able to receive the blastocyst is called the *implantation window*, and it begins 6 to 8 days after ovulation and lasts approximately 4 days. If estrogen and progesterone levels drop, the functional layer of endometrium is shed (menstruation), but the basal layer remains intact,

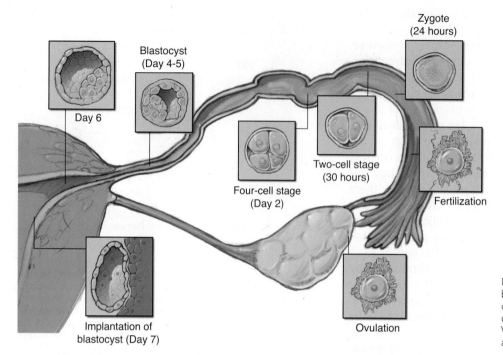

Figure 13-2 After an ovum has been fertilized, it takes about 6 days to reach the lining of the uterus where it becomes implanted. Various stages of cellular division are taking place during this time.

allowing regeneration of the functional layer in the next menstrual cycle. If pregnancy occurs, the endometrium remains decidualized and is now called *decidua*.[2,4-6]

Successful implantation commonly occurs about 6 days after fertilization, when the blastocyst mass attaches to the endometrium. The trophoblast cells over the inner cell mass differentiate into two layers: an inner cytotrophoblast and an outer mass called the *syncytiotrophoblast*. The syncytiotrophoblast produces the hormone human chorionic gonadotropin (hCG), which

extends the life of the corpus luteum. The corpus luteum continues to secrete progesterone for several more weeks, preventing the uterus from shedding its endometrial lining and the rapidly developing products of conception.

The syncytiotrophoblast proliferates, excreting enzymes that erode the endometrial surface and allow the blastocyst to bury itself within the endometrium. The opening it created seals with a blood clot (fibrin coagulum) (Fig. 13-3).[1]

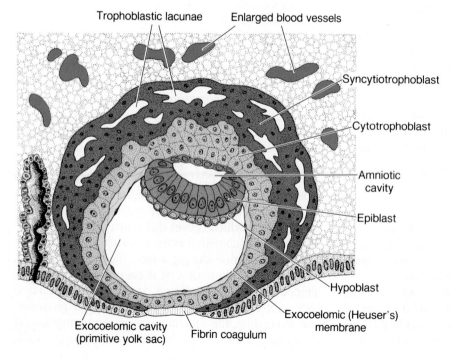

Figure 13-3 A 9-day human blastocyst. The syncytiotrophoblast shows a large number of lacunae. Flat cells form the exocoelomic membrane. The bilaminar germ disc consists of a layer of columnar epiblast cells and a layer of cuboidal hypoblast cells. The original surface defect is closed by a fibrin coagulum.

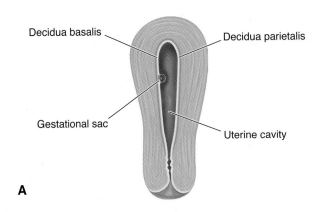

A

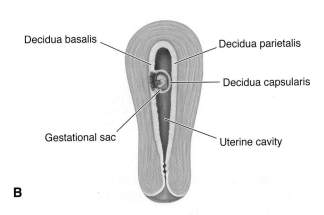

B

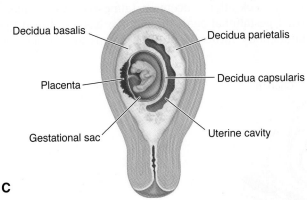

C

Figure 13-4 Implantation of an early embryo. **A:** The blastocyst attaches to and begins to embed itself into the decidua. The blastocyst is too small to be sonographically identified at this time. **B:** The blastocyst is now embedded in a layer of decidua. The point of deepest attachment, where the trophoblasts proliferate, is the decidua basalis. Decidua capsularis surrounds the rest of the blastocyst. Decidua parietalis is on the opposite side of the uterine cavity. A small gestational sac, actually the chorionic cavity, may now be visualized. **C:** As the gestational sac grows, the contour of the decidua capsularis distorts the uterine cavity. The decidua capsularis and the decidua parietalis create the double decidual sac sign.

Decidualized endometrium has three distinct layers defined by their relationship to the blastocyst. At the point of attachment by the blastocyst, the decidua basalis contributes the maternal portion of the placenta. The decidua capsularis closes over and surrounds the burrowing blastocyst. The decidua parietalis, or decidua vera, lines the remainder of the endometrial cavity (Fig. 13-4).

EARLY DEVELOPMENT OF THE CONCEPTUS

The blastocyst's inner cell mass differentiates into two layers: a thick epiblast adjacent to the trophoblast and a thin hypoblast facing the blastocele.

Fluid from the maternal decidua begins to collect within the epiblast, creating the amniotic cavity. Specialized cells from the epiblast form the *amnion*, a membrane around the fluid. The cells of the amnion begin to produce amniotic fluid.

Cells of the hypoblast and adjoining cells lining the exocoelomic cavity form the primary umbilical vesicle, commonly known as the *primary yolk sac*. Cells from the vesicle wall form a layer of extraembryonic mesoderm between the vesicle and the cytotrophoblast.[7]

The primary umbilical vesicle gets smaller and is lined by extraembryonic endoderm cells formed by the hypoblast. It is now called the *secondary umbilical vesicle* or *yolk sac* (Fig. 13-5). The secondary yolk sac is the first structure that can be sonographically visualized within the gestational sac.[8] A slender connection, the *vitelline duct*, eventually connects the umbilical vesicle to the embryonic midgut.

The umbilical vesicle provides nourishment to the conceptus and produces the embryo's first blood cells. These blood cells are carried to and from the embryo via the umbilical vesicle's vitelline veins and arteries. An extension of the umbilical vesicle, the *allantois*, protrudes into the connecting stalk, forming the urachus. The blood vessels of the allantois become the umbilical arteries.[7,9]

Eventually, the yolk sac becomes part of the embryonic gut. Its cells contribute to the development of digestive, respiratory, and urogenital systems of the fetus.

Within the growing extraembryonic mesoderm, fluid spaces form and coalesce to create the chorionic cavity. The chorion, which surrounds the chorionic cavity, is made up of fused mesoderm and trophoblast cells. The umbilical vesicle and the amnion are within the chorionic cavity, connected to the chorion by a stalk. The chorionic sac, also known as the gestational sac, is the first sonographic evidence of an intrauterine pregnancy.

Within the epiblast of the inner cell mass, a line of cells thickens to form a primitive streak. Some cells of the primitive streak become the embryonic mesoderm. Cells from both the primitive streak and the epiblast

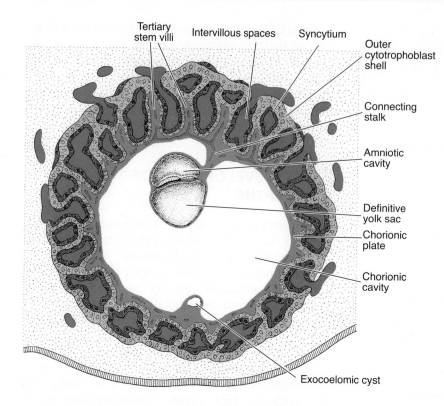

Figure 13-5 Presomite embryo and the trophoblast at the end of the third week. Tertiary and secondary stem villi give the trophoblast a characteristic radial appearance. Intervillous spaces, which are found throughout the throphoblast, are lined with syncytium. Cytotrophoblastic cells surround the trophoblast and are in direct contact with the endometrium. The connecting stalk suspends the embryo in the chorionic cavity.

form embryonic endoderm, and the remainder of the epiblast becomes embryonic ectoderm. The embryonic disc now contains the three germ cell layers from which all future organs and tissues are derived.[7,10]

During the embryonic period, the once-flat embryonic disc folds and further differentiates, and the amniotic cavity expands at the expense of the chorionic cavity (Fig. 13-6). Eventually the amniotic cavity completely fills the chorionic cavity, and the amnion and chorion fuse. The amnion covers the umbilical cord, which develops within the cavity.

The embryonic endoderm, mesoderm, and ectoderm continue to differentiate, and by the end of the eighth week after conception (almost 11 weeks' menstrual/gestational age), the embryo has developed the rudimentary forms of all of its organs and structures.

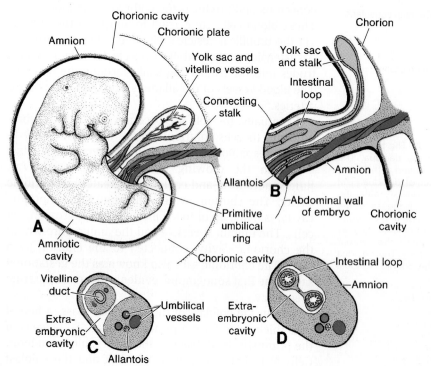

Figure 13-6 A: A 5-week embryo showing structures passing through the primitive umbilical ring. **B:** The primitive umbilical cord of a 10-week embryo. **C:** Transverse section through the structures at the level of the umbilical ring. **D:** Transverse section through the primitive umbilical cord showing intestinal loops protruding in the cord.

The embryonic period is now complete, and the fetal stage, with its rapid growth and maturation of organ systems, commences.[10]

DEVELOPMENT OF THE PLACENTA

Chorionic villi (singular: villus) project outward from the walls of the blastocyst into the decidua. As the gestational sac grows, the chorionic villi associated with the decidua capsularis disappear, leaving smooth chorion laeve. At the point of implantation, however, villi continue to grow and proliferate, forming the chorion frondosum or villous chorion. The chorion frondosum becomes the conceptus's contribution to the formation of the placenta. The erosion from the syncytiotrophoblast causes areas of decidual bleeding, into which the growing villi project.[11] Eventually, the fetal portion of the placenta occupies almost all of the decidua basalis, leaving only the basal layer intact.[12]

Fresh maternal blood is continually supplied to the spaces between the villi by the endometrial spiral arteries and drained by endometrial veins. Over time, fetal capillaries from branches of the umbilical vein and arteries extend into the villi. The membrane covering the villi is thin enough to allow oxygen and nutrients from the maternal blood to reach the fetal capillaries and fetal waste products to enter maternal circulation.

In addition to producing hCG, the placenta also begins to secrete estrogen and progesterone, replacing the hormones that had been synthesized by the no longer functioning corpus luteum.[11]

PREGNANCY TESTS

The glycoprotein hCG, which consists of α and β subunits, enters the maternal circulation and can be detected in a pregnant woman's blood and urine. Because the α subunit is nearly identical to components of other hormones, pregnancy tests rely on identifying the β subunit, commonly called β-hCG.[13] The β subunit is usually part of the intact hCG molecule, but it can also be detected by itself. When the β subunit is found unattached to the α subunit, it is called "free β-hCG."[14]

Urine tests are qualitative; that is, they are negative if β-hCG levels are less than what is seen in men and nonpregnant women and positive if the level meets or exceeds that threshold. Although quantitative and semiquantitative urine β-hCG tests are under investigation, they are not available in the United States at this time.[15-17]

Currently available quantitative pregnancy tests measure the level of β-hCG in maternal serum. In a normal, singleton intrauterine pregnancy, the levels rise quickly. On average, at a gestational age ranging from 22 days to almost 5 weeks, the hCG level more than doubles every day and a half. Between 5 and 6 weeks' gestational age, the hCG level doubles every two and a half days on average. After 6 weeks' gestational age, the hCG level continues to rise, but at a slower rate.[18-20] The hCG level reaches its peak 8 to 12 weeks after the LMP and then plateaus.[21,22]

SONOGRAPHIC FINDINGS IN EARLY PREGNANCY

Because of its microscopic size, the preimplantation development of the conceptus is impossible to detect sonographically. However, as early as 11 days after conception (3 weeks + 4 days' gestational age), when the blastocyst is completely embedded in decidua, one may follow the central linear interface created by the collapsed endometrial cavity between the anterior and posterior layers of endometrium (now decidua) and detect a round fluid collection eccentrically located within an echogenic area adjacent to—not within—the endometrial cavity (Fig. 13-7). This is the intradecidual sign first described by Yeh et al. in 1986.[23] The sonolucent structure is the

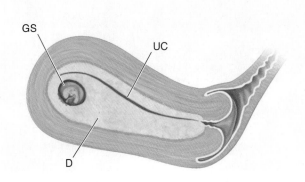

A

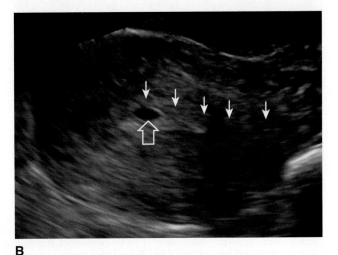

B

Figure 13-7 A: The intradecidual sign. The early gestational sac *(GS)* is eccentrically located adjacent to the interface created by the collapsed endometrial cavity *(UC)* between the anterior and posterior layers of decidua *(D)*. It is not seen within the endometrial cavity. **B:** The *open arrow* points to the early gestational sac, which is adjacent to the linear echo of the endometrial cavity *(solid arrows)*.

chorionic cavity of the blastocyst, and the sonographic term for the sonolucent chorionic cavity seen at this time is the gestational sac. The clinical utility of the intradecidual sign has been confirmed by multiple studies.[23-25]

At approximately 7 weeks' gestational age, as the gestational sac grows and distorts the uterine cavity, two layers of decidua (decidua capsularis and decidua parietalis) may be seen surrounding much of the gestational sac. This is called the *double sac sign* (Fig. 13-8). It should be noted that the interface created by the collapsed uterine cavity is not found between the developing placenta and the decidua basalis.[24,26,27]

In normal pregnancies, only part of the full depth of the decidua basalis is invaded by trophoblasts to become the maternal portion of the placenta. Wong et al. have described the sonographic appearance of the remaining decidua basalis throughout the first trimester (Fig. 13-9).[12]

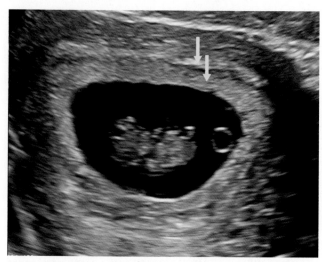

Figure 13-8 The double decidual sac sign. Two layers of decidua can be seen surrounding the gestational sac (arrows).

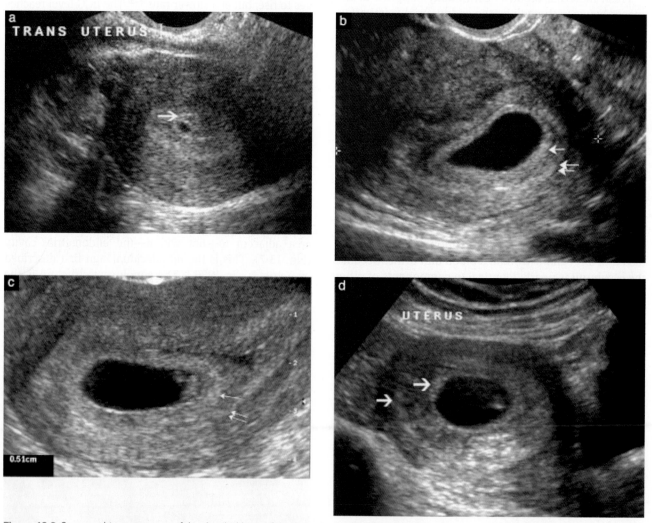

Figure 13-9 Sonographic appearance of the decidual layer of the uterus in the first trimester. **A:** Transverse section at 4 weeks' gestation. The gestational sac is completely embedded in the endometrium. The gestational sac lining appears thicker on the side further away from the uterine cavity (arrow), indicating the possible location of the future placenta. **B:** Longitudinal section at 5 weeks. A uniform echogenic decidual layer (double arrow) can be seen around the gestational sac. The placenta (single arrow) can be distinguished from the rest of the gestational sac lining by its thickness. The placenta, the decidual layer and the myometrium appear as concentric layers. **C:** Sagittal section at 6 weeks. A distinct uniform echogenic layer of decidua basalis (double arrow) can still be seen between the placenta (arrow) and the myometrium. **D:** Transverse section at 7 weeks. The decidual layer (between the two arrows) appears more heterogeneous in echogenicity. However, its thickness remains uniform around the gestational sac. (continued)

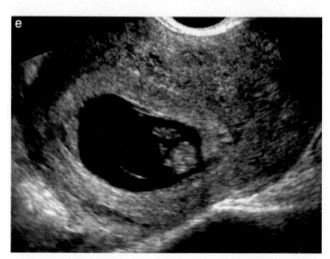

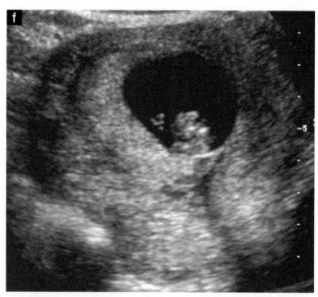

Figure 13-9 *(continued)* **E,F:** Longitudinal sections at 9 weeks. **E:** On transvaginal ultrasound, a distinct decidual layer could not be identified. The placenta appeared to lie next to the myometrium and an interface could be seen. **F:** In another case, on transabdominal ultrasound, a definite decidual layer could not be identified. There was an area between the placenta and the myometrium that appeared partly hypoechoic and partly isoechoic compared with the placenta. Reprinted from Wong HS, Cheung YK, Taits J. Sonographic study of the decidua basalis in the first trimester of pregnancy. *Ultrasound in Obstetrics and Gynecology,* 2009; 33:634-637, with permission.

As noted earlier, the first structure to be seen within the chorionic cavity (the gestational sac) is the secondary umbilical vesicle (secondary yolk sac) (Figs. 13-5, 13-10).[28] This appears as a round, anechoic structure surrounded by a highly reflective echogenic ring. It is seen endovaginally about 5 weeks after the LMP and transabdominally by 6 to 7 weeks post-LMP. At 5 weeks, the internal yolk sac measurement is approximately 2.3 mm in diameter. It gradually grows to about 5.6 mm by 11 weeks and generally disappears by 12 weeks' gestational age.[6,8,28] When its attachment to the vitelline duct is visualized, the appearance is sometimes described as a balloon on a string (Fig. 13-11).

By the end of the fifth week or the beginning of the sixth week gestational, the early embryo may be identified endovaginally, measuring 2 to 4 mm in length. It is first seen as a somewhat straight cluster of echoes adjacent to the yolk sac (Fig. 13-12). The amniotic cavity is seen between 7 and 8 weeks' gestational age.[7,28] The appearance of the small, sonolucent amniotic sac, the yolk sac, and the developing embryo between them have been described as the "double bleb" (Fig. 13-13).[29]

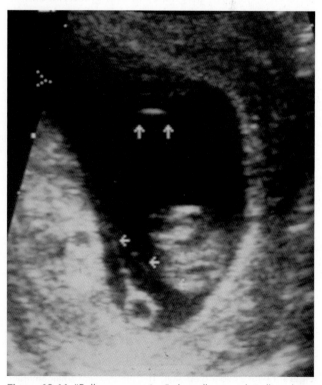

Figure 13-10 The yolk sac within an early gestational sac. This is actually the secondary yolk sac (secondary umbilical vesicle).

Figure 13-11 "Balloon on a string": the yolk sac and vitelline duct.

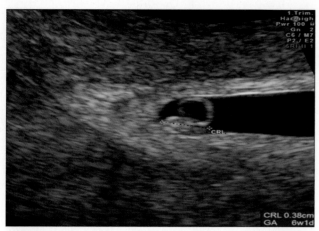

Figure 13-12 An early embryo adjacent to the yolk sac.

The embryo grows at a rate of about 1 to 2 mm per day. By the end of the sixth week, it is shaped like a kidney bean.[8] In the seventh week, the head occupies nearly half of the entire body (Fig. 13-14). The amniotic cavity also grows, occupying a greater proportion of the chorionic cavity (Fig. 13-15). At this stage, it is obvious that the yolk sac is in the chorionic cavity, while the embryo is in the amniotic cavity.[27,28,30]

SONOEMBRYOLOGY

From the use of high-frequency endovaginal transducers to three-dimensional (3D) and four-dimensional (4D) ultrasound, technical advances in the field have enabled us to view the early pregnancy in ever greater detail.[30,31] The identification and evaluation of embryonic anatomy is called *sonoembryology*, a term apparently coined by Dr. Timor-Trisch and colleagues in 1990.[32]

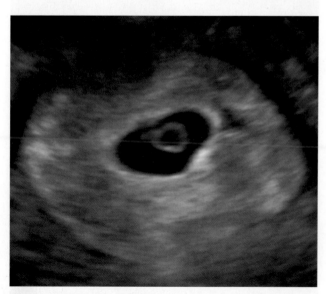

Figure 13-13 Double bleb sign. The embryo and small amniotic cavity are seen adjacent to the yolk sac.

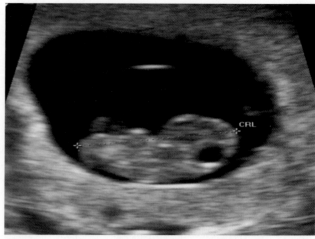

Figure 13-14 The head, with its sonolucent rhombencephalon, can be distinguished from the rest of the body. Note that at this time, the head takes up approximately half of the whole body.

A summary of early sonographic milestones is found in Table 13-1. The following is a discussion of some of the organ systems that can be evaluated in the first trimester.

HEART

As an organism grows in size and complexity, many of its cells are no longer in direct contact with an environment that provides oxygen and nutrients and allows discharge of carbon dioxide and wastes. A means of transportation becomes necessary. This is the role of the cardiovascular system and, not surprisingly, the heart is the first organ to function in the embryo. The primitive heart begins to beat about 23 days after conception (5+ weeks' gestational age). The mean rate of

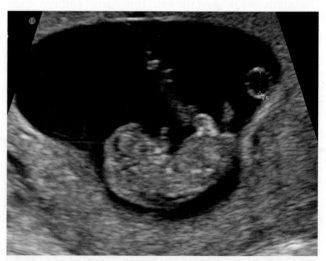

Figure 13-15 The amnion separates the amniotic cavity from the chorionic cavity. The yolk sac is seen within the chorionic cavity, which is filled with fine echoes. The embryo and umbilical cord are seen within the amniotic cavity.

TABLE 13-1

Sonographic Milestones in the Early First Trimester

Gestational Age (Weeks+ days)	Carnegie Stage[58]	Sonographic Findings
4+3 to 5+0	10–11	A small gestation sac (2–5 mm) is seen within the endometrium, adjacent to the uterine cavity interface
5+1 to 5+5	12	Umbilical vesicle (yolk sac) can be seen within the chorionic cavity
5+6 to 6+0	14–17	An embryonic pole measuring 2–4 mm may be identified adjacent to the yolk sac
6+1 to 6+6	18–19	The yolk sac is clearly separate from the embryo. Cardiac activity is visualized by the time the embryonic pole measures 5 mm. It may be possible to distinguish the head from the body
7+0 to 7+6	20–22	The yolk sac images in the chorionic cavity, while the amniotic membrane clearly encloses the embryo in the amniotic cavity. The sonolucent rhombencephalon visualizes in the embryonic head
8+0 to 8+6	23	The CRL is 17–23 mm. The embryonic forebrain, midbrain and hindbrain can be identified and limbs become evident. The physiologic herniation of the midgut may also be visible
9+0 to 10+0	Stages end at 8 weeks' gestation or 10 weeks LMP	Cerebral hemispheres become more distinct, and echogenic choroid plexus can be seen within the lateral ventricles. Hands and feet can be visualized

Adapted from Sawyer E, Jurkovic D. Ultrasonography in the diagnosis and management of abnormal early pregnancy. *Clin Obstet Gynecol.* 2007;1:31–54 and Kurjak A, Pooh RK, Merce LT, et al. Structural and functional early human development assessed by three-dimensional and four-dimensional sonography. *Fertil Steril.* 2005;84:1285–1299.

pulsations increases from 110 beats per minute (bpm) at 5 weeks to 175 bpm by 9 weeks, after which it gradually decreases to 160 to 170 bpm.[6] By the third trimester, the normal resting heart rate is between 110 and 160 bpm.[33]

Cardiac pulsations should be sonographically visualized in all normal embryos measuring 5 mm or larger, and can be documented using M-mode (Fig. 13-16). Failure to detect cardiac activity in embryos measuring less than 5 mm may be a normal finding and warrants a follow-up examination to establish viability.[6]

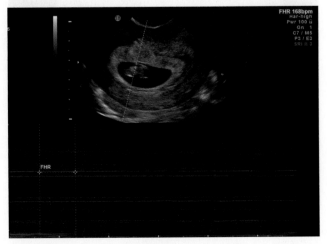

Figure 13-16 An M-mode tracing showing an embryonic heart rate of 168 bpm.

CENTRAL NERVOUS SYSTEM

A section of embryonic ectoderm forms a neural plate, which folds to form the neural tube and the neural crest. The cranial section of the neural tube forms the brain, and the rest of the neural tube forms the spinal cord. [7]

The embryonic brain develops three vesicles: the prosencephalon, or embryonic forebrain, gives rise to the telencephalon and the diencephalon; the mesencephalon is the embryonic midbrain, which remains undivided; and the rhombencephalon, the embryonic hindbrain. The prosencephalon and the rhombencephalon each divide, creating a total of five brain vesicles, which become the lateral ventricles, third ventricle, and the upper and lower parts of the fourth ventricle, and the connections between them.[34,35]

3D ultrasound has improved our ability to assess the embryonic brain, but many structures can be seen on two-dimensional (2D) images. The rhombencephalon may be sonographically identified as early as 7 weeks' gestational age and in a sagittal plane appears as a prominent, diamond-shaped sonolucent structure high in the posterior part of the brain; the diencephalon and mesencephalon appear as an anterior sonolucent crescent (Fig. 13-17). Between 8 and 9 weeks, on an axial view of the head, the hemispheres are seen as crescent-shaped structures occupied by the sonolucent lateral ventricles. Choroid plexus in the roof of the future fourth ventricle first appears as echogenic folds in the rhombencephalon. At 9 to 10 weeks' gestational age,

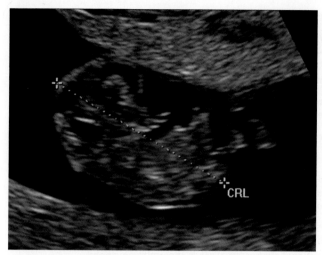

Figure 13-17 The crescent-shaped sonolucency in the anterior aspect of the brain is created by the diencephalon and mesencephalon. Physiologic herniation of the midgut is also seen in this 9-week embryo.

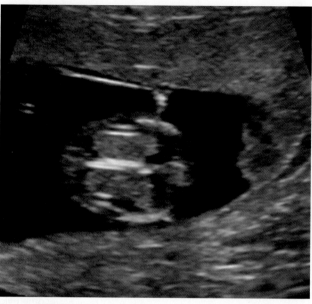

Figure 13-18 The lateral ventricles, largely filled with choroid plexus, appear to occupy most of the hemispheres of the developing brain.

echogenic choroid plexus can be seen within the lateral ventricles, which largely fill the hemispheres (Fig. 13-18). From 10 to 11 weeks, there is notable thickening of the brain cortex, and the cerebellar hemispheres appear to join at the midline after 11 weeks' gestational age.[34–36]

Limited views of the developing spine can be seen by ultrasound as early as 7 to 8 weeks, but the vertebrae are insufficiently ossified to cause acoustic shadowing.[28,30,34]

EXTREMITIES

In the eighth week, limb buds begin to appear (Fig. 13-19), and hands and feet can be identified by 10 weeks' gestational age (Fig. 13-20).[28,37]

GASTROINTESTINAL TRACT/ ABDOMINAL WALL

Around 8 weeks post-LMP, the embryonic gut herniates out of the abdominal cavity into the base of the cord (Fig. 13-21). It then goes through a process of rotation and eventually recedes back into the abdominal cavity by 12 weeks' gestational age.[38,39] This physiologic herniation is a normal process, and as long as the mass measures no greater than 7 mm, this should not be mistaken for an omphalocele.[40]

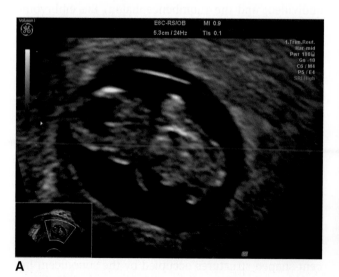

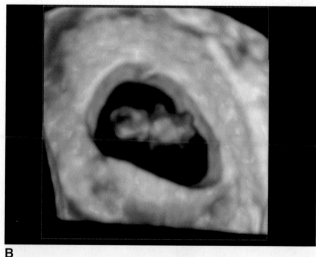

A **B**

Figure 13-19 A: A 2D image demonstrating limb buds. Note the amnion/chorion separation. **B:** A 3D surface reconstruction demonstrating limb buds in an 8-week embryo.

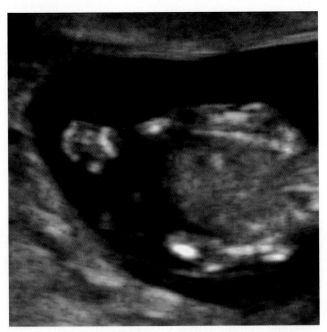

Figure 13-20 The thumb is seen separate from the other digits, but separations have not yet developed between the rest of the fingers.

DETERMINING GESTATIONAL AGE IN THE VERY EARLY PREGNANCY

Before detecting a measurable embryonic pole, the pregnancy can be dated by measuring the gestational sac (Fig. 13-22). To obtain a mean sac diameter (MSD), the height, width, and depth of the fluid portion of the sac taken at the fluid–chorionic tissue interface is measured by scanning in two planes at right angles to one another and calculating an average of the three measurements. Other authors have used the maximal sac diameter, which requires only a single measurement. Gestational sacs as small as 2 to 3 mm, corresponding to a menstrual age of 5 weeks, have been identified. The MSD grows about 1 mm per week.[41]

By endovaginal ultrasound, the embryonic pole frequently visualizes in the sixth week. A crown-rump length (CRL) can be obtained by measuring the embryo along its longest axis, preferably in a sagittal view. The image must be sufficiently enlarged to be certain the yolk sac is not included in the measurement. Appropriate measurement is critical not only for

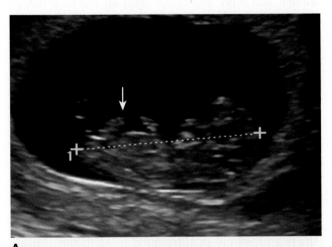

A

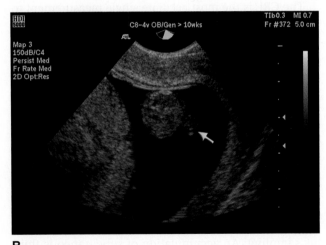

B

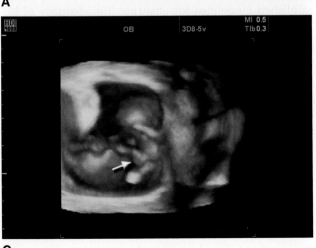

C

Figure 13-21 A: The *arrow* points to the normal physiologic herniation of embryonic midgut into the base of the umbilical cord on this sagittal image. **B:** A transverse image of the abdomen demonstrating the midgut herniation on an 11-week embryo. **C:** A 3D surface rendering of a 10-week gestation with a physiologic herniation (*arrow*) into the base of the umbilical cord.

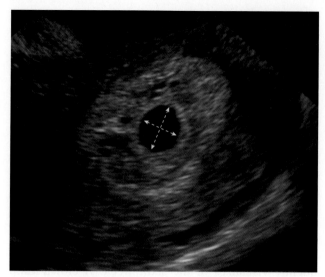

Figure 13-22 Measurement of the MSD.

assigning an EDD, but also because even slight errors can affect the estimation of risk for aneuploidy (see the succeeding discussion of nuchal translucency).[42] Examples of CRL measurements are shown throughout this chapter (Figs. 13-12, 13-14, 13-17, 13-21A).

The CRL is the most accurate single measurement to establish an EDD, although a combination of multiple parameters early in the second trimester approaches the accuracy of the CRL.

Nomograms are available to establish gestational age based on these measurements. Formulas for these measurements are found in Table 13-2. See Chapter 16 for a complete discussion of second- and third-trimester pregnancy dating techniques.

NUCHAL TRANSLUCENCY

In 1990, a letter appeared in the *Lancet* describing an unusual finding that was discovered by scanning the embryos of patients who had undergone chorionic villus sampling. An accumulation of subcutaneous fluid in the nuchal region was seen in seven of seven embryos with trisomy 21. Only 1 of 105 chromosomally normal embryos was found to have a similar appearance.[43] Concurrently, an article in *Prenatal Diagnosis* described the significance of a nonseptated "cystic hygroma" in the first trimester, noting that embryos with this finding had a 50% chance of having chromosomal abnormalities, including trisomy 21.[44] This fluid collection is now known as the *nuchal translucency* (NT).

Around the same time, investigators were looking at biochemical markers in the blood of pregnant women that were associated with an elevated risk of chromosomal defects. In 1999, a meta-analysis of these studies showed that although abnormal levels of two chemicals produced by the trophoblasts—pregnancy-associated plasma protein A (PAPP-A) and the free β subunit of the hCG molecule—detected 65% of fetuses with trisomy 21 with a 5% false-positive rate, "when NT measurement is combined with testing for PAPP-A and free β-hCG, the detection rate increases to 86%" with the same 5% false-positive rate.[45]

The NT images as a sonolucent area enclosed by a membrane that extends from the posterior aspect of the embryo's head to a variable point along the spine (Fig. 13-23). Because an error of less than a millimeter may falsely impact a patient's NT risk assessment, the American Institute of Ultrasound in Medicine (AIUM) published guidelines for ensuring the adequacy of NT measurements (Table 13-3, Fig. 13-24).[46] The NT is performed between about 11 and 14 weeks' gestational age (as determined by the laboratory performing the corresponding maternal blood work).

In light of these developments, the American College of Obstetricians and Gynecologists has revised its Practice Bulletin on screening for chromosomal abnormalities as follows:

- "First-trimester screening using both nuchal translucency measurement and biochemical markers is an effective screening test for Down syndrome in the general population. At the same false-positive rates, this screening strategy results in a higher Down syndrome detection rate than does the second-trimester maternal serum triple screen and is comparable to the quadruple screen."

TABLE   13-2

Formulas for Calculation of First-Trimester Gestational Age[41,59–61]

Anatomy	Formula
MSD in mm	MSD = (length × width × height)/3
Gestational age in days	Menstrual age in days = MSD + 30
Gestational age in weeks	Menstrual age in weeks = Menstrual age in days/7
CRL gestational age	CRL in cm + 6
EDD Naegele's rule	EDD = LMP − 3 months + 7 days

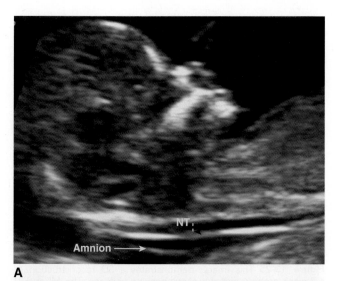

A

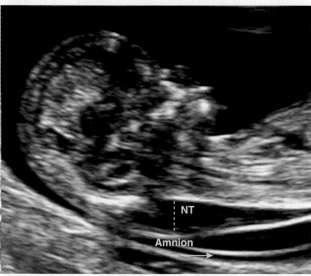

B

Figure 13-23 Correct measurement of the NT. These images display the correct plane and appropriate magnification for measuring the NT, which can be clearly distinguished from the amnion. **A:** Normal NT. **B:** An enlarged NT.

- "Measurement of nuchal translucency alone is less effective for first-trimester screening than is the combined test (nuchal translucency measurement and biochemical markers)."
- "Women found to have increased risk of aneuploidy with first-trimester screening should be offered genetic counseling and the option of chorionic villus sampling or second-trimester amniocentesis."
- "Specific training, standardization, use of appropriate ultrasound equipment, and ongoing quality assessment are important to achieve optimal nuchal translucency measurement for Down syndrome risk assessment, and this procedure should be limited to centers and individuals meeting these criteria."[47]

TABLE	13-3

Guidelines for NT Measurement

1. The margins of the NT edges must be clear enough for proper placement of the calipers.
2. The fetus must be in the midsagittal plane.
3. The image must be magnified so that it is filled by the fetal head, neck, and upper thorax.
4. The fetal neck must be in a neutral position, not flexed and not hyperextended.
5. The amnion must be seen as separate from the NT line.
6. The (+) calipers on the ultrasound must be used to perform the NT measurement.
7. Electronic calipers must be placed on the inner borders of the nuchal space with none of the horizontal crossbar itself protruding into the space.
8. The calipers must be placed perpendicular to the long axis of the fetus.
9. The measurement must be obtained at the widest space of the NT.

From the American Institute of Ultrasound in Medicine. *AIUM Practice Guideline for the Performance of Obstetric Ultrasound Examinations.* Laurel, MD: AIUM, 2007. www.aium.org/publications/guidelines/obstetric.pdf), with permission.

COMPONENTS OF A FIRST-TRIMESTER SONOGRAM

The AIUM *Practice Guideline for the Performance of Obstetric Ultrasound Examinations*, which was developed in collaboration with the American College of Obstetricians and Gynecologists and the American College of Radiologists (ACR), recommends that first-trimester sonograms include images of the uterus and adnexa to identify the presence and location of a gestational sac and the presence or absence of abnormal adnexal masses or fluid in the cul-de-sac. When an intrauterine gestational sac is detected, the images and report should document whether a yolk sac and/or embryo can be seen. If the pregnancy is too early to visualize an embryo, an MSD should be obtained to estimate the gestational age, but once an embryo is evident, measurement of the CRL is preferred. The presence or absence of cardiac activity in the embryo should be mentioned in the report.[46]

Correct placement

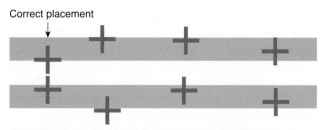

Figure 13-24 Only the first pair of calipers in this diagram shows correct placement when measuring the NT. Source: http://www.aium.org/publications/guidelines/obstetric.pdf. Reproduced with permission from the American Institute of Ultrasound in Medicine.

PRIMUM NON NOCERE: APPLYING THE ALARA PRINCIPLE IN THE FIRST TRIMESTER

Medical students and other students in health care professions are taught, *"Primum non nocere,"* or "First, do no harm." Sonographers and sonologists should be applying the ALARA principle (for *as low as reasonably achievable*) during every sonogram they perform. This is especially true during the first trimester of pregnancy, when development of the embryo or early fetus is at its highest risk of being disrupted. Nevertheless, recent studies show that the majority of sonographers and sonologists do not understand how to implement the ALARA principle during obstetric sonograms.[48,49]

The potential for unwanted bioeffects during a diagnostic ultrasound examination is affected by the duration and level of exposure. Ultrasound is a form of mechanical energy and therefore has the potential to cause damage to cells containing pockets of gas. In addition, as (ultra)sound waves pass through a medium, some of the energy converts to heat, which can also be harmful to cells.

The U.S. Food and Drug Administration's Center for Devices and Radiological Health requires ultrasound machines with the capability of producing excessive acoustic output to display indices showing whether the ultrasound exposure during a given exam is within acceptable limits. These displays are the mechanical index (MI) and the thermal index (TI).[50] Because it is unlikely that the embryo or fetus contains gas bodies, the index of greatest interest during obstetric scanning is the TI.

There are three thermal indices, two of which have applications in obstetric scanning. These are the thermal index for soft tissue (TIS), and the thermal index for structures near bone (TIB). The thermal index for cranial bone (TIC) is used when the transducer is right up against bone and therefore is not used during fetal scanning. The operator must select the appropriate TI and modify it as needed. In the early first trimester, before mineralization of bone occurs, the TIS should be selected. Because bone absorbs heat, sensitive adjacent tissue including brain and spinal cord may also be subject to heating. Therefore, the TIB should be selected from 10 weeks' gestational age onward.[51–53]

The MI and TI can change over the course of an exam. They are affected by factors including output levels, transducer frequency, pulse repetition rates, and scan modes. At otherwise identical settings, the lowest exposures occur during B-mode and M-mode scanning. Exposure increases with the use of color Doppler and is even higher when spectral Doppler is applied. Therefore, Doppler should not be used in the first trimester unless there is a clinical indication to do so.[52–54]

3D ultrasound imaging is derived from a data set comprised of a series of 2D images produced by either a matrix or mechanical transducer. 4D ultrasound correlates the images with the time each was acquired,

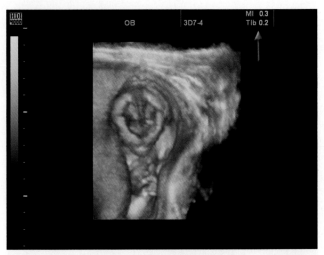

Figure 13-25 This image demonstrates a 3D reconstruction of a 7-week embryo and the accompanying yolk sac. The MI and TI display *(arrow)* indicates exposure of the fetus to ultrasound energy. The British Medical Ultrasound Society safety guidelines indicate display indices should be at 0.5 for the TI and 0.3 for the MI during obstetric imaging to reduce any bioeffects.[56,57]

demonstrating motion. The data sets may be used to obtain traditional 2D images in optimal planes, 3 dimensional surface renderings (Figs. 13.19B, 13.21C, 13-25), and other display modalities. The MI and TI are the same as they would be for traditional 2D scanning.[55] Because the sound beam does not dwell on any one area, the actual exposure may in fact be decreased when 3D data sets are processed to obtain the required components of an exam. One caveat: a sonographer may actually increase the overall exposure time in an effort to produce the ideal 3D keepsake image for the patient (an otherwise acceptable practice when obtained during the course of a medically indicated sonogram). For more information on 3D imaging, refer to Chapter 32.

Critical Thinking Question

View the following first-trimester study.

(Fig. 13-26A–J)

Using the AIUM or ACR protocol standards, critique this study for improvement.

> ANSWER: This study has important images missing, which include;
> - Inadequate bladder filling for the transabdominal images
> - A single measurement of the CRL and gestational sac
> - No documentation of the embryonic heart rate
> - Yolk sac measurement missing
> - Single images, without measurements of the uterus and ovaries
> - Use of incorrect CRL or sac measurement package

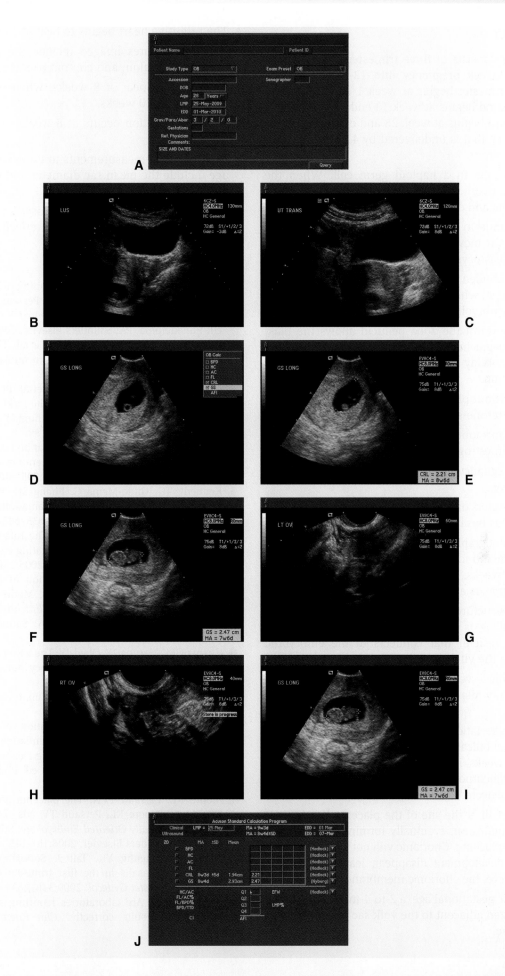

SUMMARY

- Pregnancy consists of three trimesters, dividing the normal 40-week pregnancy into 12-week sections. The first trimester begins at week 1 ending at week 12, the second begins at week 13 ending in week 27, and the third begins at week 28 and ends at delivery. A pregnancy that is undelivered by 42 weeks is considered postterm.

- Meiosis results in a haploid germ cell. When the sperm and ovum unite, a single diploid cell, the zygote, results and divides via mitosis.

- Cells continue to divide creating the morula, a ball of cells, as it moves through the fallopian tube [it's already a blastocyst by the time it reaches the uterus].

- Once a fluid-filled cavity forms, the structure becomes the blastocyst, which contains the trophoblast, blastocele, and embryoblast.

- Disintegration of the zona pellucid allows the blastocyst to begin implantation into the endometrium-during the 4-day implantation window 6 to 8 days postovulation.

- The syncytiotrophoblast produces hCG, extending the progesterone-secreting corpus luteum.

- Placental hormone production includes chorionic gonadotropin, estrogen, and progesterone.

- A urine pregnancy test is qualitative; the blood test is quantitative.

- The three layers of the decidualized endometrium are the deciduas basalis, capsularis, and parientalis.

- The first sonographic evidence of an intrauterine pregnancy is the intradecidual sign, which may be seen as early as 3 weeks, 4 days gestational age. The double sac sign appears at about 7 weeks' gestational age.

- The first structure sonographically seen within the gestational sac is the secondary yolk sac (secondary umbilical vesicle) that connects to the embryonic midgut via the vitelline duct.

- The umbilical vesicle produces the embryo's first blood cells, while the allantois become the umbilical arteries.

- At 5 weeks gestational age, the internal diameter of the yolk sac/umbilical vesicle is approximately 2.3 mm, and by 11 weeks, it measures 5.6 mm. The yolk sac is eventually incorporated into the embryonic gut, and is no longer detected by 12 weeks.

- Chorionic villi at the site of the placenta become the chorion frondosum, eventually forming the fetal portion of the placenta. Chorionic villi not associated with placental development disappear, leaving a smooth chorion laeve, the chorionic membrane.

- By 6 weeks gestational age, a 2-to-4-mm embryo may be visualized adjacent to the yolk sac within the gestational sac.

- The primitive heart begins to beat at 23 days.

- Neural structures imaged include the neural tube, rhombencephalon, and choroid plexus.

- Limb buds appear at 8 weeks, whereas hands and feet image at 10 weeks.

- Midgut herniation occurs at 8 weeks and recede by 12 weeks.

- First-trimester measurements to establish gestational age include the mean sac diameter and the more accurate CRL.

- The nuchal translucency, when used in conjunction with biochemical markers, is an effective screening tool for Down syndrome.

REFERENCES

1. Moore KL, Persaud TVN. The beginning of human development: first week. In: Moore KL, Persaud TV, eds. *The Developing Human: Clinically Oriented Embryology*. 8th ed. Philadelphia, PA: Saunders Elsevier; 2008:14–41.

2. Diedrich K, Fauser BC, Devroey P, et al. The role of the endometrium and embryo in human implantation. *Hum Reprod Update*. 2007;13(4):365–377.

3. Labied S, Kajihara T, Madureira P, et al. Progestins regulate the expression and activity of the forkhead transcription factor FOXO1 in differentiating human endometrium. *Mol Endocrinol*. 2006;20(1):35–44.

4. Maruyama T, Yoshimura Y. Molecular and cellular mechanisms for differentiation and regeneration of the uterine endometrium. *Endocr J*. 2008;55(5):795–810.

5. Kennedy TG, Gillio-Meina C, Phang SH. Prostaglandins and the initiation of blastocyst implantation and decidualization. *Reproduction*. 2007;134(5):635–643.

6. Jauniaux E, Johns J, Burton GJ. The role of ultrasound imaging in diagnosing and investigating early pregnancy failure. *Ultrasound Obstet Gynecol*. 2005;25(6):613–624.

7. Moore KL, Persaud TVN. Formation of the bilaminar embryonic disc: second week. In: Moore KL, Persaud TV, eds. *The Developing Human: Clinically Oriented Embryology*. 8th ed. Philadelphia, PA: Saunders Elsevier; 2008:42–53.

8. Chama CM, Marupa JY, Obed JY. The value of the secondary yolk sac in predicting pregnancy outcome. *J Obstet Gynecol*. 2005;25(3):245–247.

9. Takashina T. Haemopoiesis in the human yolk sac. *J Anat*. 1987;151:125–135.

10. Moore KL, Persaud TVN. Formation of germ layers and early tissue and organ differentiation: third week. In: Moore KL, Persaud TV, eds. *The Developing Human: Clinically Oriented Embryology*. 8th ed. Philadelphia, PA: Saunders Elsevier; 2008:54–71.

11. Moore KL, Persaud TVN. The placenta and fetal membranes. In: Moore KL, Persaud TV, eds. *The Developing Human: Clinically Oriented Embryology*. 8th ed. Philadelphia, PA: Saunders Elsevier; 2008:110–145.

12. Wong HS, Cheung YK, Tait J. Sonographic study of the decidua basalis in the first trimester of pregnancy. *Ultrasound Obstet Gynecol*. 2009;33(6):634–637.

13. Cao Z, Rej R. Are laboratories reporting serum quantitative hCG results correctly? *Clin Chem*. 2008;54(4):761–764.

14. Azzazy HE, Romero LF, Hall L, et al. Two-center clinical evaluation of a new automated flourometric immunoassay for the quantitative analysis of total beta-human chorionic gonadotropin. *Clin Biochem.* 2003;36(7):523–528.

15. Ajubi NE, Nijholt N, Wolthuis A. Quantitative automated human chorionic gonadotropin measurement in urine using the Modular Analytics E170 module (Roche). *Clin Chem Lab Med.* 2005;43(1):68–70.

16. Cole LA, Khanlian SA. The need for a quantitative urine hCG assay. *Clin Biochem.* 2009;42(7–8):676–683.

17. Grossman D, Berdichevsky K, Larrea F, et al. Accuracy of a semi-quantitative urine pregnancy test compared to serum beta-hCG measurement: a possible screening tool for ongoing pregnancy after medication abortion. *Contraception.* 2007;76(2):101–104.

18. Check JH, Weiss RM, Lurie D. Analysis of serum human chorionic gonadotropin levels in normal singleton, multiple and abnormal pregnancies. *Hum Reprod.* 1992; 7(8):1176–1180.

19. Shamonki MI, Fratterelli JL, Bergh PA, et al. Logarithmic curves depicting initial level and rise of serum beta human chorionic gonadotropin and live delivery outcomes with in vitro fertilization: an analysis of 6021 pregnancies. *Fertil Steril.* 2009;91(5):1760–1764.

20. Barnart KT, Sammel MD, Rinaudo PF, et al. Symptomatic patients with an early viable intrauterine pregnancy: hCG curves redefined. *Obstet Gynecol.* 2004;104(1):50–55.

21. Feldkamp CS, Pfeffer WH. The measurement of human chorionic gonadotropin for pregnancy testing. *Henry Ford Hosp Med J.* 1982;30(4):207–213.

22. Braunstein GD, Rasor J, Danzer H, et al. Serum human gonadotropin levels throughour normal pregnancy. *Am J Obstet Gynecol.* 1976;126(6):678–681.

23. Yeh HC, Goodman JD, Carr L, et al. Intradecidual sign: a US criterion of early intrauterine pregnancy. *Radiology.* 1986;161(2):463–467.

24. Yeh HC. Efficacy of the intradecidual sign and fallacy of the double decidual sac sign in the diagnosis of early intrauterine pregnancy. *Radiology.* 1999;210(2):579–582.

25. Chiang G, Levine D, Swire M, et al. The intradecidual sign: is it reliable for diagnosis of early intrauterine pregnancy? *Am J Roentgenol.* 2004;183(3):725–731.

26. Yeh HC. Some misconceptions and pitfalls in ultrasonography. *Ultrasound Q.* 2001;17(3):129–155.

27. Bradley WG, Fiske CE, Filly RA. The double sac sign of early intrauterine pregnancy: use in exclusion of ectopic pregnancy. *Radiology.* 1982;143(1):223–226.

28. Sawyer E, Jurkovic D. Ultrasonography in the diagnosis and management of abnormal early pregnancy. *Clin Obstet Gynecol.* 2007;50(1):31–54.

29. Yeh HC, Rabinowitz JG. Amniotic sac development: ultrasound features of early pregnancy—the double bleb sign. *Radiology.* 1988;166(1 pt 1):97–103.

30. Kurjak A, Pooh RK, Merce LT, et al. Structural and functional early human development assessed by three-dimensional and four-dimensional sonography. *Fertil Steril.* 2005;84(5): 1285–1299.

31. Benoit B, Hafner T, Kurhak A, et al. Three-dimensional sonoembryology. *J Perinat Med.* 2007;30(1):63–73.

32. Timor-Tritsch IE, Peisner DB, Raju S. Sonoembryology: an organ-oriented approach using a high-frequency vaginal transducer. *J Clin Ultrasound.* 1990;18(4):286–298.

33. American College of Obstetricians and Gynecologists. ACOG practice bulletin no. 106: intrapartum fetal heart rate monitoring: nomenclature, interpretation, and general management principles. *Obstet Gynecol.* 2009;114(1): 192–202.

34. Jurkovic D, Gruboeck K, Campbell S. Ultrasound features of normal pregnancy development. *Curr Opin Obstet Gynecol.* 1995;7(6):493–504.

35. Blaas HG, Eik-Nes SH. Sonoembryology and early prenatal diagnosis of neural anomalies. *Prenat Diagn.* 2009; 29(4):312–325.

36. Kim MS, Jeanty P, Turner C, et al. Three-dimensional sonographic evaluations of embryonic brain development. *J Ultrasound Med.* 2008;27(1):119–124.

37. Hata T, Manabe A, Aoki S, et al. Three dimensional sonography in the early first-trimester of human pregnancy: preliminary study. *Hum Reprod.* 1998;13(3):740–743.

38. Blaas HG, Eik-Ness SH, Kiserud T, et al. Early development of the abdominal wall, stomach, and heart from 7 to 12 weeks of gestation: a longitudinal study. *Ultrasound Obstet Gynecol.* 1995;6(4):240–249.

39. Achiron R, Soriano S, Lipitz S, et al. Fetal midgut herniation into the umbilical cord: improved definition of ventral abdominal anomaly with the use of endovaginal sonography. *Ultrasound Obstet Gynecol.* 1995;6(4):256–260.

40. Van Zalen-Sprock RM, Van Vugt JMG, Van Geijn HP. First-trimester sonography of physiological midgut herniation and early diagnosis of omphalocele. *Prenat Diagn.* 1997;17(6):511–518.

41. Filly RA, Hadlock FP. Sonographic determination of menstrual age. In: Callen PW, ed. *Ultrasonography in Obstetrics and Gynecology.* 4th ed. Philadelphia, PA: WB Saunders; 2000:146–170.

42. Salomon LJ, Bernard M, Amarsy R, et al. The impact of crown-rump length measurement error on combined Down syndrome screening: a simulation study. *Ultrasound Obstet Gynecol.* 2009;33(5):506–511.

43. Szabo J, Gellen J. Nuchal fluid collection in trisomy-21 detected by vaginosonography. *Lancet.* 1990;336(8723):1133.

44. Cullen MT, Gabrielli S, Green JJ, et al. Diagnosis and significance of cystic hygroma in the first trimester. *Prenat Diagn.* 1990;10(10):643–651.

45. Cuckle HS, van Lith JMM. Appropriate biochemical parameters in first-trimester screening for Down syndrome. *Prenat Diagn.* 1999;19(6):505–512.

46. American Institute of Ultrasound in Medicine. *AIUM Practice Guideline for the Performance of Obstetric Ultrasound Examinations.* Laurel, MD: AIUM; 2007.

47. American College of Obstetricians and Gynecologists. ACOG practice bulletin no. 77: screening for fetal chromosomal abnormalities. *Obstet Gynecol.* 2007;109(1):217–227.

48. Sheiner E, Shoham-Vardi I, Abramowicz JS. What do clinical users know regarding safety of ultrasound during pregnancy? *J Ultrasound Med.* 2007;26(3):319–325.

49. Sheiner E, Abramovicz JS. Clinical end users worldwide show poor knowledge regarding safety issues of ultrasound during pregnancy. *J Ultrasound Med.* 2008;27(4):499–501.

50. U.S. Department of Health and Human Services Food and Drug Administration Center for Devices and Radiological Health. Information for Manufacturers Seeking Marketing Clearance of Diagnostic Ultrasound Systems and Transducers. Rockville, MD: USDHHS-FDA; 2008.

51. Abramovicz JS, Barnett SB, Duck FA, et al. Fetal thermal effects of diagnostic ultrasound. *J Ultrasound Med.* 2008;27(4):541–559.

52. Nelson TR, Fowlkes JB, Abramovicz JS, et al. Ultrasound biosafety considerations for the practicing sonographer and sonologist. *J Ultrasound Med.* 2009;28(2):139–150.

53. Sheiner S, Freeman J, Abramovicz JS. Acoustic output as measured by mechanical and thermal indices during routine obstetric ultrasound examinations. *J Ultrasound Med.* 2005;24(12):1664–1670.

54. Sheiner E, Shoham-Vardi I, Pombar S, et al. An increased thermal index can be achieved when performing Doppler studies in obstetric sonography. *J Ultrasound Med.* 2007;26(1):71–76.

55. Miller DL. Safety assurance in obstetrical ultrasound. *Semin Ultrasound CT MR.* 2008;29(2):156–264.

56. British Medical Ultrasound Society. Statement on the safe use, and potiential hazards of diagnostic ultrasound. London, October 2007.

57. British Medical Ultrasound Society. Guidelines for the safe use of diagnostic ultrasound equipment. London, UK: British Institute of Radiology; 2000.

58. Swiss Virtual Campus. Module 8 Embryonic phase. University of Fribourg, Lausanne, and Bern (Swizerland). http://www.embryology.ch/anglais/iperiodembry/carnegie01.html. Accessed 2009.

59. SDMS National certification examination review. Abdomen/Obstetrics and Gynecology. 2001, Dallas.

60. Hagan-Ansert S. *Textbook of Diagnostic Ultrasonography.* 6th ed. St. Louis, MO: Mosby; 2006.

61. Shirlina D, Shirish S. Uterine Volume: An aid to determine the rought and technique of hysterectomy. *J Obstet Gynecol.* 2004;54(1):68–72.

14 Sonographic Evaluation of First-Trimester Complications

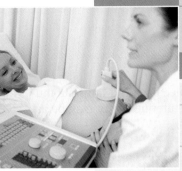

Paula Woletz

OBJECTIVES

Describe the indications for diagnostic ultrasound in the first trimester

Distinguish the sonographic findings of normal early pregnancy from those of early pregnancy failure, spontaneous abortion, and molar pregnancy

Discuss the use of ultrasound to screen for chromosomal abnormalities

Identify structural abnormalities in the first trimester

KEY TERMS

aneuploidy | threatened abortion | anembryonic pregnancy | retained products of conception (RPOC) | subchorionic hemorrhage | hydatidiform mole

GLOSSARY

Abortion Spontaneous or induced termination of an early pregnancy and expulsion of fetal and placental tissues

Amniocentesis Invasive procedure in which a quantity of amniotic fluid is removed from the amniotic sac for analysis of the fetal cells or for the presence of certain chemicals in the fluid itself; may also be performed as a palliative measure in patients with severe polyhydramnios

Anembryonic pregnancy Pregnancy that has failed prior to the development of an identifiable embryo or in which embryonic tissue has been resorbed after early embryo demise

Anemia Deficiency of red blood cells

Blighted ovum Empty gestational sac seen in an anembryonic pregnancy

Bradycardia Abnormally slow heart rate

Chorionic villus sampling Invasive procedure in which the chorionic villi of an early pregnancy are removed for analysis

Complete hydatidiform mole Abnormal fertilization of an oocyte that contains no maternal chromosomes, resulting in the proliferation of swollen chorionic villi and the absence of identifiable embryonic structures

Gestational trophoblastic disease Spectrum of disorders that begin at fertilization and involve abnormal proliferation of the trophoblasts that in a normal pregnancy form the placenta; may become invasive, malignant, and metastasize

Gestational trophoblastic neoplasia Invasive or metastatic form of gestational trophoblastic disease

Hydatidiform mole Form of gestational trophoblastic disease resulting from abnormal fertilization in which there is proliferation of swollen chorionic villi; also called a molar pregnancy

Hyperemesis Excessive vomiting during pregnancy sometimes called hyperemesis gravidarum

Hyperthyroidism Excessive activity of the thyroid

Incomplete abortion Spontaneous abortion in which some products of conception remain in the uterus

Inevitable abortion Failed early pregnancy that is in the process of being expelled from the uterus

Miscarriage Spontaneous failure and expulsion of an early pregnancy

Missed abortion Early failed pregnancy that remains in the uterus

Molar pregnancy Hydatidiform mole

Partial hydatidiform mole Abnormal fertilization resulting in one maternal and two paternal sets of chromosomes (triploidy), leading to the development of an abnormal fetus and placenta

Respiratory insufficiency Inadequate absorption of oxygen and/or inadequate expulsion of carbon dioxide

Subchorionic hemorrhage (a.k.a. subchorionic hematoma) Crescent-shaped sonolucent collection of blood between the gestational sac and the uterine wall

Tachycardia Abnormally rapid heart rate

Theca-lutein cysts Large, often bilateral ovarian cysts, the formation of which is usually stimulated by excessive levels of circulating human chorionic gonadotropin (hCG)

Threatened abortion, threatened miscarriage Vaginal bleeding in a pregnancy of less than 20 weeks; may be accompanied by pain or cramping

Toxemia of pregnancy Pregnancy-induced hypertension, proteinuria, edema, and headache (preeclampsia), which may progress to the development of seizures (eclampsia)

Triploid, triploidy Having three copies of each chromosome.

When a patient reports a problem during the first trimester of pregnancy, or when the clinician perceives an unusual or discrepant finding, ultrasound is often the method of choice to confirm or rule out the clinician's suspicions. The following discussion focuses first on the most commonly presenting clinical symptoms in the first trimester. This is followed by the expanded criteria to predict pregnancy viability, findings that raise the suspicion of chromosomal abnormalities, and the early detection of structural anomalies.

SIZE-DATES DISCREPANCY

If a patient is unsure of her last menstrual period (LMP), or if a clinical examination of the uterus does not agree with the patient's reported LMP, her clinician may request a sonogram to date the pregnancy. The presence of uterine fibroids, maternal obesity, surgical scars, or multiple gestation may make it difficult for the obstetrician to estimate the size of the uterus, from which the gestational age is estimated. Because other aspects of pregnancy management (e.g., establishing the estimated date of delivery, methods of termination, interpretation of maternal serum levels, timing of chorionic villus sampling or amniocentesis) hinge on the correct assessment of the duration of pregnancy, the patient may be sent for ultrasound evaluation in the first trimester.

Ultrasound helps date, establish early pregnancy failure, or an ectopic pregnancy in the finding of a smaller than expected uterus. Once an intrauterine pregnancy (IUP) is identified, careful measurements are taken to establish the gestational age. If the development of the gestational sac and its contents is less advanced than the patient's dates indicate, correlation with human chorionic gonadotropin (hCG) levels may be indicated and serial sonograms performed to establish a normal rate of growth. Early-onset intrauterine growth restriction (defined as a crown-rump length at least two standard deviations below the mean for the expected gestational age) in a woman with a reliable menstrual history is an increased risk for miscarriage (spontaneous abortion).[1]

A uterus that is large for gestational age may be due to incorrect dates, multiple gestation, molar pregnancy, or uterine fibroids (Fig. 14-1). Contrary to earlier reports, most fibroids do not grow during pregnancy. However, fibroids are associated with preterm labor, premature rupture of membranes, and fetal malposition. In the first trimester, retroplacental fibroids may be associated with vaginal bleeding, and large submucosal fibroids that distort the uterine cavity may be associated with pregnancy loss.[2]

EARLY PREGNANCY FAILURE

Most pregnancies are clinically confirmed after a woman has missed a menstrual period and has had a positive urine or serum pregnancy test. An unknown number of pregnancies are spontaneously aborted before a woman has missed her menstrual period, without her or her obstetrician ever being aware of the pregnancy and its loss. As many as 10% to 20% of clinically recognized pregnancies result in spontaneous abortion before 20 weeks' gestational age, with the majority of those occurring before 12 weeks.[3-5] Although pregnancy failure has many causes, 50% to 70% are caused by genetic abnormalities.[6]

When an asymptomatic woman has an early sonogram (i.e., one performed between 6 weeks + 2 days, and 11 weeks + 6 days, gestational age) that demonstrates a singleton pregnancy with a normal heart rate, the subsequent risk of miscarriage drops to 1.6%.[7]

In women with vaginal bleeding or pain, the risk of pregnancy loss increases. Approximately half of patients who experience vaginal bleeding miscarry, with the greatest risk seen in patients with heavy bleeding and pain.[6,8-10] Of those patients whose pregnancies continue, 17% may experience complications later in pregnancy.[9] Other causes of vaginal bleeding in early

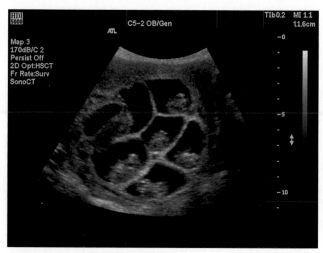

Figure 14-1 First-trimester septuplet pregnancy. (Image courtesy of Philips Medical Systems, Bothell, WA.)

pregnancy include gestational trophoblastic disease, which is covered later in this chapter, and ectopic pregnancy, which is reviewed in Chapter 15.

Vaginal bleeding in a pregnancy of less than 20 weeks is called a *threatened abortion* or *threatened miscarriage*. It is a common complication of pregnancy, and as many as 15% to 27% of pregnancies are complicated by one or more episodes of vaginal bleeding in the first 20 weeks.[8,10–12] Bleeding may be characterized as spotting (frequently occurring at the time of implantation), light, or heavy, and can originate in the uterus, the cervix, or the vagina.

Although factors unrelated to the pregnancy may be the source of the bleeding, first consideration goes to establishing the viability of the pregnancy. The value of ultrasound in threatened abortion lies not in any endeavor to alter the outcome of the pregnancy, but in the ability to predict which pregnancies will continue successfully to term.

The sonographic findings of early pregnancy failure depend on the stage of embryologic development at which they occur, and whether the uterus has begun to expel the products of conception.[3]

In an anembryonic pregnancy (sometimes called a blighted ovum), the pregnancy either ended before a sonographically identifiable embryo formed or the early embryo was resorbed once the pregnancy failed. An empty gestational sac (i.e., a gestational sac devoid of embryo or yolk sac) with a mean sac diameter greater than 20 mm by endovaginal ultrasound is likely to indicate pregnancy failure.[13] A smaller than expected empty gestational sac in a patient with reliable dates may also predict a poor outcome.[14] Because there is some overlap between the measurements of viable and nonviable pregnancies, it may be prudent to do a follow-up examination in a desired pregnancy with a borderline sac measurement (Fig. 14-2).[3,13–15]

As noted in Chapter 13, the first structure to be sonographically identified in a normally developing gestational sac is the secondary yolk sac (secondary umbilical vesicle). Yolk sacs that are too large (greater than two standard deviations above the mean yolk sac diameter for a given gestational age) or too small (more than two standard deviations below the mean yolk sac diameter for gestational age), or those that do not show the characteristic round appearance, are strong predictors of a poor outcome (Fig. 14-3).[16–18]

In normal pregnancies, visualization of the amnion surrounding the early embryo occurs after sonographic identification of the yolk sac. In 2010, Yegul and Filly reported that visualization of an amnion without sonographic evidence of an embryo (the "empty amnion sign") is definitive evidence of pregnancy failure.[19]

Cardiac activity in an embryo measuring 5 mm or greater is generally thought to be a reassuring sign, and the risk of spontaneous abortion is low. However, bradycardia (heart rate <90 beats per minute [bpm] at 6.2 weeks or <110 bpm at 6.3 to 7 weeks) detected between 6 and 7 weeks' gestational age has been associated with an increased risk of pregnancy loss.[20] Tachycardia (≥155 bpm at 6.3 to 7 weeks), on the other hand, has a high likelihood of a normal outcome.[21]

Embryo demise is diagnosed when there is no cardiac activity in an embryo measuring 5 mm or more.[3] Absence of cardiac activity in an embryo that is less than 5 mm and seen within an enlarged amniotic sac may also be a sign of demise. Yegul and Filly call this evidence of early demise the "expanded amnion sign."[22] (Fig. 14-4) Another indication of demise in an embryo that is less than 5 mm and is without a detectable heart beat is when, instead of the "double bleb" sign described in Chapter 13, there is an obvious yolk stalk between the yolk sac and the embryo and amniotic sac (Fig. 14-5).[23]

A patient with an anembryonic pregnancy or embryo demise that has not yet been expelled from the uterus

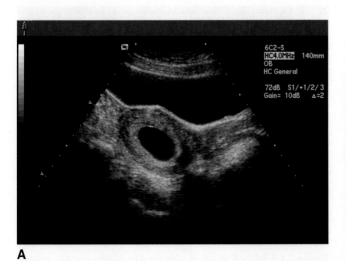

A

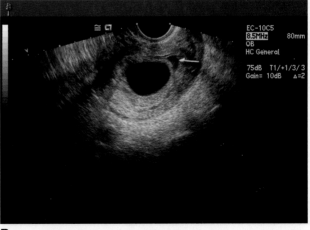

B

Figure 14-2 A: Transabdominal image of a blighted ovum. **B:** Endovaginal image of the same empty sack. Note the beginning of sac separation from the uterine wall *(arrow)*.

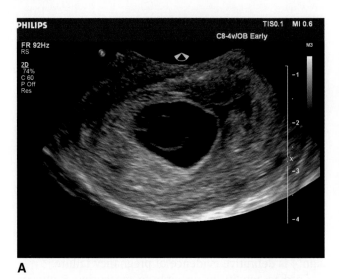

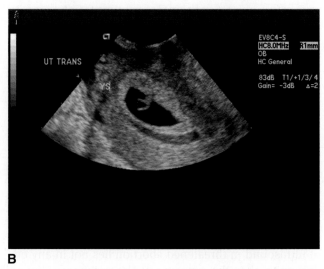

A   **B**

Figure 14-3 Abnormal yolk sacs. **A:** Enlarged yolk sac. **B:** Collapsed, irregular yolk sac. (Image **A** courtesy of Philips Medical Systems, Bothell, WA.)

is said to have a missed or delayed abortion. (Fig. 14-5) An incomplete abortion occurs when some placental or fetal tissue has been expelled but some products of conception remain in the uterus. Sonographically, an incomplete abortion is seen as thickened endometrium or hyperechoic tissue within the uterus.[24] There is little consensus over an endometrial thickness measurement that could be considered diagnostic for retained products of conception (RPOC).[25] The use of color Doppler is helpful in these cases because increased flow within the myometrium may be associated with RPOC (Fig. 14-6).[26]

When a patient is noted to have profuse bleeding and the cervical os has begun to dilate, abortion is said to be inevitable and impending. Sonographically, a gestational sac may be seen in the cervix or vagina as it is expelled (Fig. 14-7).[3]

SUBCHORIONIC HEMORRHAGE

A crescent-shaped sonolucent fluid collection between the gestational sac and the uterine wall is evidence of a subchorionic hemorrhage (or subchorionic hematoma). Its presence increases the risk of spontaneous miscarriage, preeclampsia, placental abnormalities, or preterm delivery. There is no consensus on whether the size of the hemorrhage predicts the likelihood of spontaneous abortion (Fig. 14-8).[27,28] Table 14-1 summarizes the sonographic appearance of the abnormal pregnancy.

GESTATIONAL TROPHOBLASTIC DISEASE

As its name implies, gestational trophoblastic disease encompasses disorders that begin at fertilization and

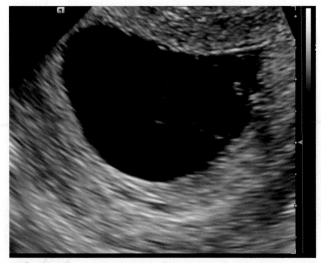

Figure 14-4 Expanded amnion sign. No cardiac activity is detected in the embryonic pole seen within an enlarged amniotic cavity. (Image courtesy of Jiri Sonek, MD.)

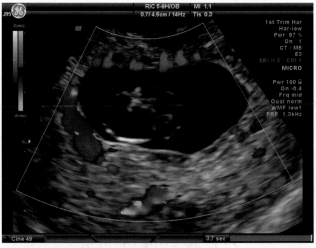

Figure 14-5 Missed abortion with no identifiable cardiac activity. Embryonic membranes and tissue remain in the uterus. (Image courtesy of Jiri Sonek, MD.)

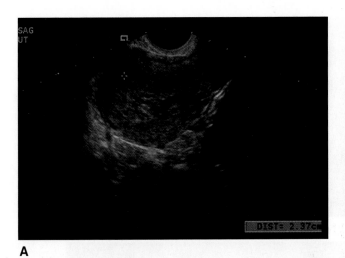

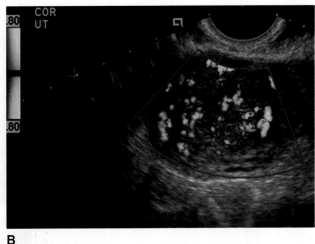

Figure 14-6 RPOCs after a spontaneous abortion. Note the hypervascularity of the myometrium as seen on color Doppler. (Images courtesy of William Lindley Diacon, MD.)

involve abnormal proliferation of the trophoblasts that in a normal pregnancy would have gone on to form the placenta. The most common forms are known as molar pregnancies and include complete hydatidiform mole and partial hydatidiform mole.[29]

Partial hydatidiform mole occurs when an apparently normal oocyte is fertilized by sperm that duplicates itself or, rarely, by two spermatozoa. The result is a triploid pregnancy with 69 chromosomes. An identifiable embryo or fetus may develop, along with a thick, hydropic placenta with focal areas of vesicular swelling.[30-34] (Tripoidy that results from the fertilization of an abnormal, diploid oocyte by a single sperm does not include abnormal proliferation of the trophoblasts and is not classified as a form of gestational trophoblastic disease.[32]) Patients with partial hydatidiform mole may present with a vaginal bleeding and a small-for-date or normal-sized uterus.[31]

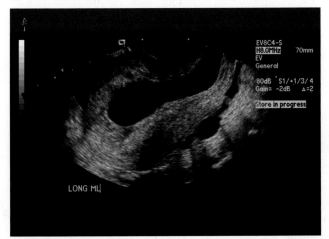

Figure 14-7 Impending abortion. The low position of the gestational sac and the open cervix indicate imminent expulsion of the uterine contents.

The abnormal proliferation of trophoblasts in both complete and, to a lesser extent, partial moles results in the production of excessive levels of hCG, which can be detected by a quantitative serum hCG test.

In early pregnancy, both forms of molar pregnancies may present with vaginal bleeding, although as many as 41% of cases are asymptomatic in the first trimester. In general, the increase in hCG levels and the clinical signs and symptoms associated with complete molar pregnancies are more severe than in partial moles. As pregnancy progresses, patients may experience heavy vaginal bleeding, a large-for-date uterus, hyperemesis, and passage of molar vesicles.[32,34] As many as 46% of patients with complete molar pregnancies develop enlarged ovaries with multiple theca lutein cysts, probably a result of hyperstimulation from the elevated levels of hCG. Theca lutein cysts are usually bilateral and measure between 6 and 12 cm, although some may be as large as 20 cm in diameter.[33]

The diagnosis of molar pregnancy is critical. The trophoblastic vesicles are usually removed by suction and/ or sharp curettage of the uterine cavity. The patient will have weekly blood tests until her hCG levels are normal for three consecutive weeks.[33] Clinical concern is warranted because between 2% and 4% of patients with partial moles and up to 28% of patients with complete molar pregnancies develop either locally invasive or metastatic gestational trophoblastic neoplasia (GTN, also known as choriocarcinoma).[31,33] Early diagnosis and evacuation of molar pregnancies has resulted in earlier normalization of hCG levels, which may be attributed to the growing use of ultrasound in the first trimester.[35]

The sonographic appearance of complete molar pregnancy in the first trimester is variable. In the earliest cases, before discrete villi are discernable, the appearance may mimic that of an early, empty gestational sac or RPOCs associated with a missed or incomplete

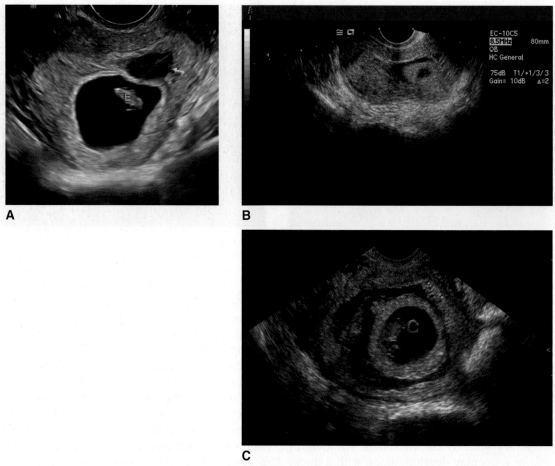

Figure 14-8. A: Complex subchorionic hemorrhage *(arrow)* with embryo *(E)*. **B:** Endovaginal image of a retroverted uterus with an early IUP and subchorionic hemorrhage. **C:** 7-week pregnancy with subchorionic hemorrhage. (Image **A** courtesy of Leeber Cohen, MD.)

abortion.[36,37] However, a case with an intrauterine mass measuring more than 3.45 cm in greatest diameter, thin endometrium (no more than 1.2 cm at its thickest point), and/or low-resistance arterial flow on color or pulsed Doppler is more likely to be a form of gestational trophoblastic disease than a failed pregnancy.[37,38] If available, an elevated level of hCG supports the diagnosis of molar pregnancy.

Most cases are seen as a complex echogenic intrauterine mass with multiple small cystic spaces. This vesicular pattern is typically seen in the second trimester as well. Occasional large cystic spaces and/ or an intrauterine fluid collection may be seen as well, and theca lutein cysts may be seen in one or both ovaries.[36,31] No embryo or fetus is seen in a complete hydatidiform mole (Fig. 14-9).

An early partial mole also has a similarly variable appearance, but if it is far enough along, there will be an identifiable embryo or fetus, and the placenta appears abnormally thick, with focal vesicular changes[36,31] (Fig. 14-10). Table 14-2 summarizes the sonographic appearance of gestational trophoblastic disease.

TABLE 14-1	
Sonographic Appearance of the Abnormal Pregnancy	
Pregnancy Type	**Sonographic Appearance**
Anembryonic pregnancy (blighted ovum)	Empty gestational sac greater than 20 mm, smaller than expected sac size
Embryonic demise	Lack of heart motion, expanded amnion sign, lack of double bleb sign
Incomplete abortion	Thickened endometrium, increased flow in myometrium
Inevitable abortion	Empty low-lying gestational sac, open cervix
Subchorionic hemorrhage	Crescent-shaped sonolucent or complex fluid collection between the gestational sac and uterus

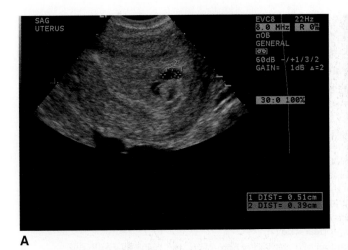

A

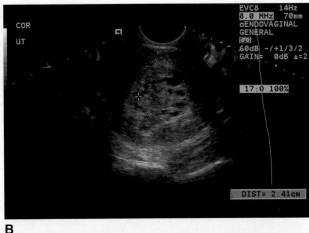

B

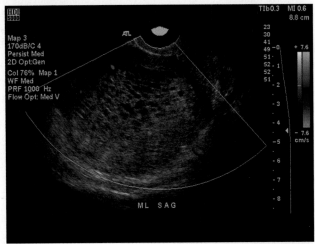

C

Figure 14-9 Complete molar pregnancy. **A:** Initial presentation of a patient with uncertain dates. **B:** Same patient at follow-up, 9 days later. **C:** Another early complete hydatidiform mole. (Images **A** and **B** courtesy of William Lindley Diacon, MD. Image C courtesy of Leeber Cohen, MD.)

FETAL ANEUPLOIDY

As mentioned in Chapter 13, it is now recommended that all pregnant women be offered screening tests to assess their risk of carrying a chromosomally abnormal fetus. In the first trimester, this is done by measuring

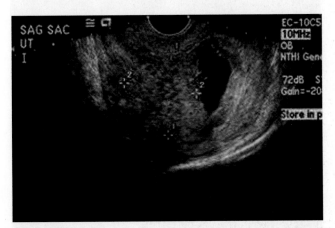

Figure 14-10 Partial mole. The calipers are measuring the abnormal placenta with swollen villi. Note the yolk sac within the gestational sac. (Image courtesy of William Lindley Diacon, MD.)

the crown-rump length, nuchal translucency, and maternal serum biochemistry levels (Fig. 14-11). A number of authors also recommend measuring the nasal bone and obtaining Doppler velocimetry of the ductus venosus. There is no consensus on whether to include maternal age in the risk calculation or whether all the ultrasound markers should be routinely included in the assessment or whether measurements of the nasal bone and ductus venosus should only be performed if the nuchal translucency measurement is abnormal or borderline (Fig. 14-12).[39-43]

STRUCTURAL ABNORMALITIES AND SYNDROMES

Growing familiarity with the normal sonographic appearance of embryonic and fetal structures during the first trimester has led to early identification of a number of structural abnormalities and syndromes.

Central nervous system abnormalities detected in the first trimester include acrania/anencephaly, holoprosencephaly, Dandy-Walker malformation, encephalocele, and spina bifida.[44-49] Cardiac anomalies include ectopia cordis, hypoplastic left heart syndrome,

TABLE 14-2

Sonographic Appearance of Gestational Trophoblastic Disease

Trophoblastic Process	Sonographic Appearance
Hydatidiform mole (first trimester)	May have appearance of a blighted ovum, threatened abortion, or variable echogenicity filling the entire uterus without the characteristic vesicular appearance
Hydatidiform mole (after first trimester)	Large soft tissue mass of low- to moderate-amplitude echoes filling the uterine cavity and containing fluid-filled spaces
Incomplete or partial mole	May present as a gestational sac that is relatively large and intact, surrounded by a thick rim of placentalike echoes with well-defined sonolucent spaces within. It may be empty or may contain a disproportionately small viable or nonviable fetus. Echogenic fetal parts may be visualized with or without normal placenta.
Coexisting mole and fetus	Concurrent presence of normal-appearing placenta and fetus and a separate area of cystic vesicular appearance
Invasive mole	Enlarged uterus with foci of increased echogenicity and cystic spaces in the myometrium
Choriocarcinoma	Cystic to solid areas of necrosis, coagulated blood, or tumor tissue invading and extending as a mass outside the uterine wall with metastatic lesions located in the liver

atrioventricular septal defect, conduction disorders, and heart failure.[47,50–54] Other anomalies include body stalk anomaly, cystic hygroma, multicystic dysplastic kidney, megacystis, omphalocele and gastroschisis, micrognathia, umbilical cord cysts, pleural effusion, polydactyly, hydrops, and clubfoot.[45,47,48,50,55–62] Conjoined twins and twin reversed arterial perfusion (TRAP) sequence have been diagnosed in first-trimester multiple gestations.[45,47,63,64] Walker-Warburg syndrome, Meckel-Gruber syndrome, pentalogy of Cantrell, and Cornelia de Lange syndrome are among the growing number of syndromes that have been diagnosed by first-trimester

sonograms.[47,65–68] Examples of anomalies in the first trimester are seen in Figures 14-13 to 14-25.

Although the first-trimester detection of abnormalities is improving, it is important to note that in a study of over 2,800 pregnant women who underwent detailed scanning between 11 and 14 weeks and again in the second and/or third trimester, abnormalities identified before 14 weeks represented only about 22% of all sonographically detected abnormalities in the study population.[69] Therefore, detailed sonographic evaluation in the first trimester in no way replaces the need for a careful anatomic survey in the second trimester.

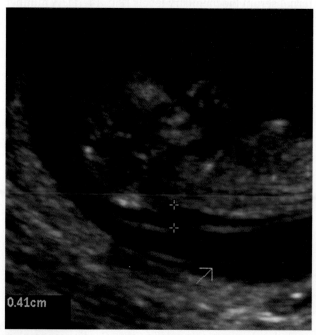

Figure 14-11 Large nuchal translucency. (Image courtesy of Leeber Cohen, MD.)

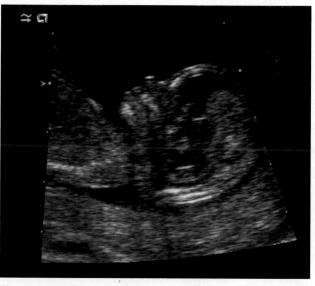

Figure 14-12 Absent nasal bone. (Image courtesy of William Lindley Diacon, MD.)

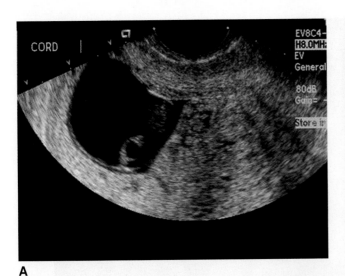

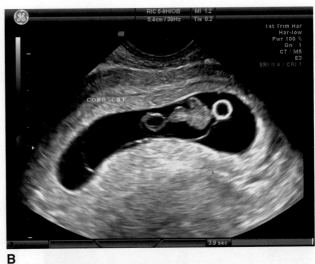

Figure 14-13 Two examples of umbilical cord cysts. **A:** Cyst associated with an early demise. **B:** Cyst eventually resolved. (Image **A** courtesy of William Lindley Diacon, MD. Image **B** courtesy of Leeber Cohen, MD.)

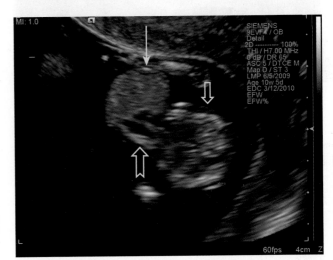

Figure 14-14 A transverse view of the upper abdomen and lower thorax of a fetus with pentalogy of Cantrell at 13 weeks' gestation. The *open arrow* points to the fetal abdomen, the *solid arrow* points to an omphalocele, and the *notched arrow* points to the ectopia cordis. (Image courtesy of Jiri Sonek, MD.)

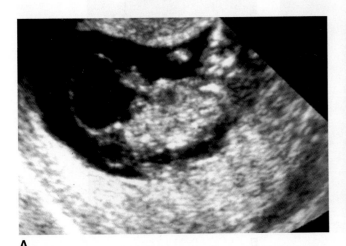

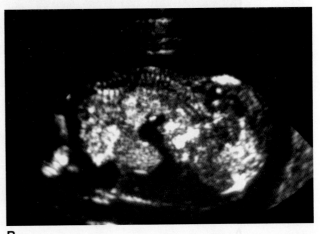

Figure 14-15 A,B: Examples of anomalies associated with amniotic band syndrome. (Images courtesy of Beryl Benacerraf, MD.)

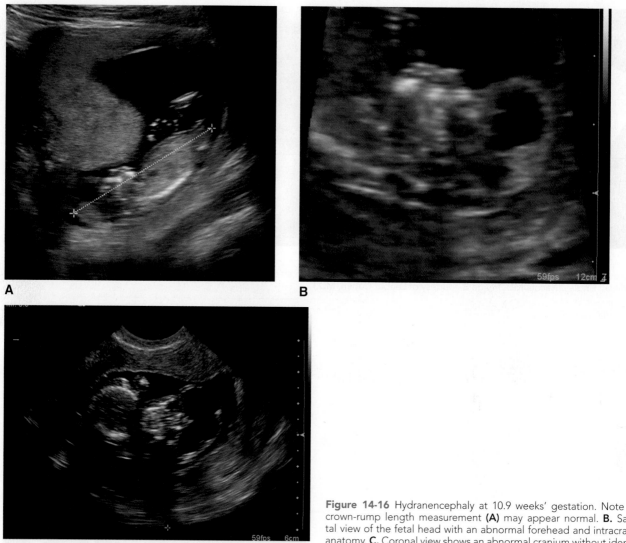

A

B

C

Figure 14-16 Hydranencephaly at 10.9 weeks' gestation. Note the crown-rump length measurement **(A)** may appear normal. **B.** Sagittal view of the fetal head with an abnormal forehead and intracranial anatomy. **C.** Coronal view shows an abnormal cranium without identifiable brain structures. (Images courtesy of Jiri Sonek, MD.)

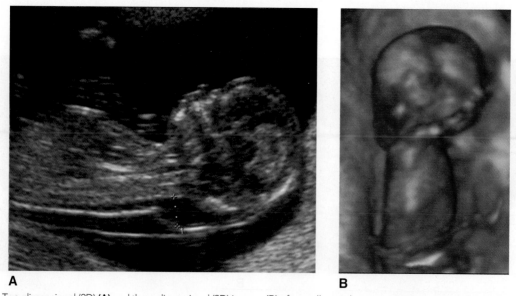

A

B

Figure 14-17 Two-dimensional (2D) **(A)** and three-dimensional (3D) images **(B)** of a small cystic hygroma. (Images courtesy of Beryl Benacerraf, MD.)

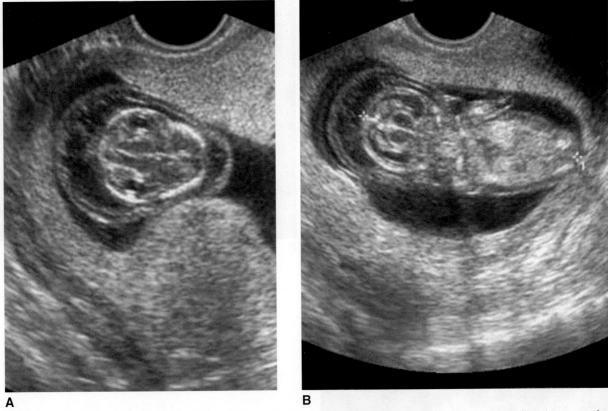

A   B

Figure 14-18 Cystic hygroma and hydrops, possibly due to jugular lymphatic obstructive sequence. (Images courtesy of Beryl Benacerraf, MD.)

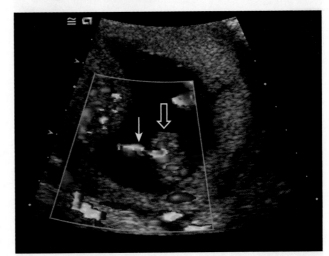

Figure 14-19 A transverse view of a fetal abdomen with a gastroschisis at 11 weeks' gestation (*solid arrow*, cord insertion; *open arrow*, gastroschisis). (Image courtesy of Jiri Sonek, MD.)

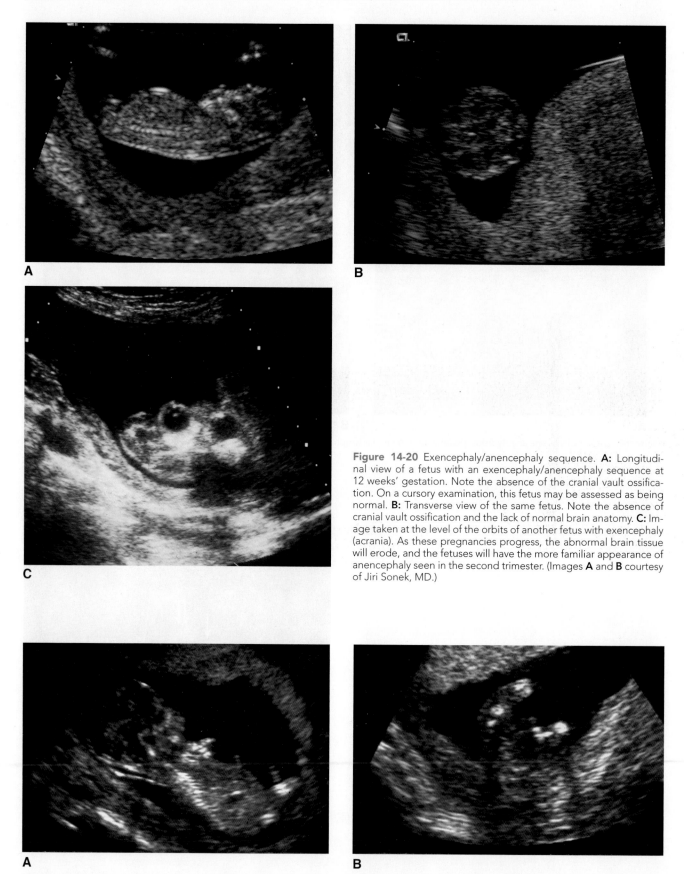

A

B

C

Figure 14-20 Exencephaly/anencephaly sequence. **A:** Longitudinal view of a fetus with an exencephaly/anencephaly sequence at 12 weeks' gestation. Note the absence of the cranial vault ossification. On a cursory examination, this fetus may be assessed as being normal. **B:** Transverse view of the same fetus. Note the absence of cranial vault ossification and the lack of normal brain anatomy. **C:** Image taken at the level of the orbits of another fetus with exencephaly (acrania). As these pregnancies progress, the abnormal brain tissue will erode, and the fetuses will have the more familiar appearance of anencephaly seen in the second trimester. (Images **A** and **B** courtesy of Jiri Sonek, MD.)

A

B

Figure 14-21 Sagittal **(A)** and transverse **(B)** images of a first-trimester fetus with osteogenesis imperfecta. (Images courtesy of Beryl Benacerraf, MD.)

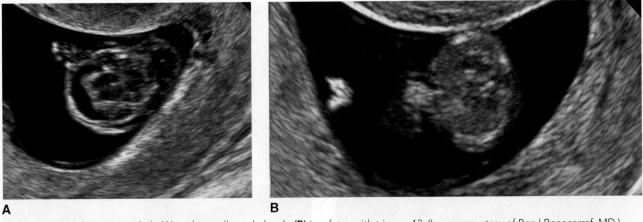

Figure 14-22 Holoprosencephaly **(A)** and a small omphalocele **(B)** in a fetus with trisomy 13. (Images courtesy of Beryl Benacerraf, MD.)

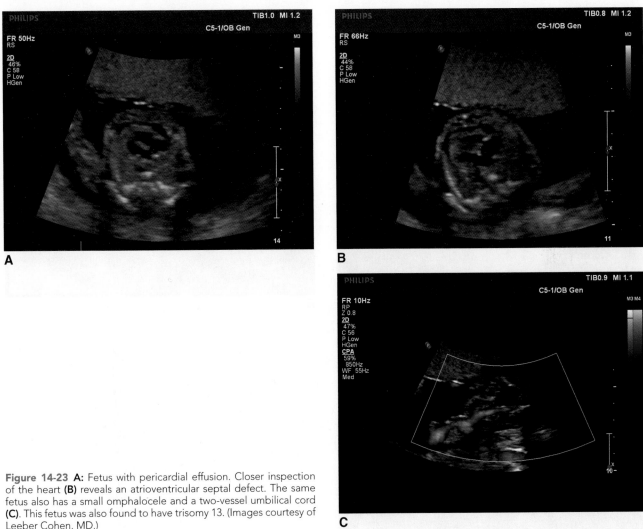

Figure 14-23 A: Fetus with pericardial effusion. Closer inspection of the heart **(B)** reveals an atrioventricular septal defect. The same fetus also has a small omphalocele and a two-vessel umbilical cord **(C)**. This fetus was also found to have trisomy 13. (Images courtesy of Leeber Cohen, MD.)

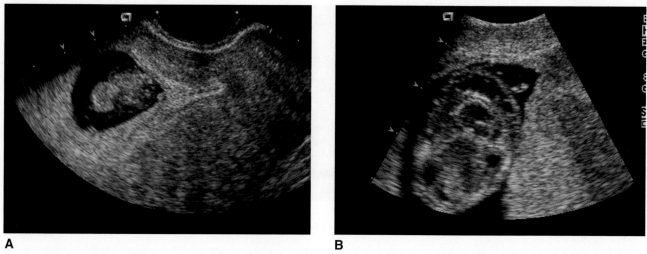

Figure 14-24 A transverse view of the fetal abdomen **(A)** reveals an omphalocele, and a small cystic hygroma **(B)** is also seen in a fetus with trisomy 18. (Images courtesy of William Lindley Diacon, MD.)

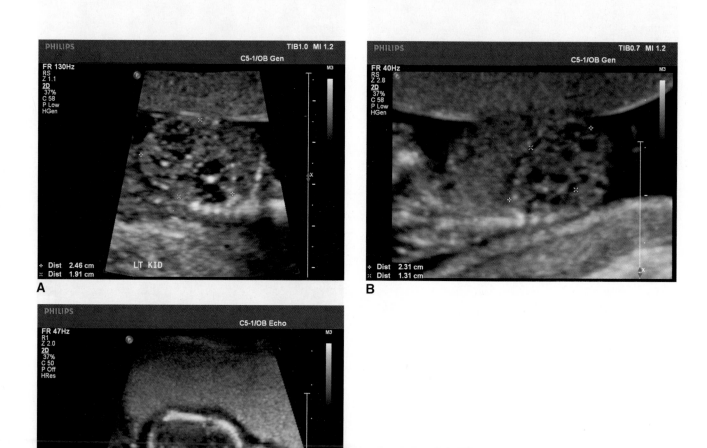

Figure 14-25 A,B: Bilateral enlarged multicystic kidneys. **C:** Occipital encephalocele in a first-trimester fetus with Meckel-Gruber syndrome. (Images courtesy of Leeber Cohen, MD.)

Critical Thinking Questions

1. In the first trimester the liver and portions of the bowel project out of the abdomen into the base of the umbilical cord. This physiologic hernia appears similar to an omphalocele on the sonographic image. How can the sonographer differentiate between the normal physiologic hernia and omphalocele in the first trimester?

   ANSWER: Physiologic herniation is first seen at about 8 weeks gestational age, and and resolves by 12 weeks. During this interval, a mass (measuring no more than 7 mm in greatest diameter) seen at the abdominal cord insertion site and is likely to be caused by this normal process. Resolution of the mass after 12 weeks confirms that the diagnosis of normal physiologic herniation.An omphalocele is usually larger, and will persist beyond 12 weeks gestational age. Omphaloceles may be isolated findings, but they are frequently associated with aneuploidies and other genetic syndromes. The maternal alpha fetoprotein (AFP) level may be elevated, and if the omphalocele is a manifestation of a chromosomal defect, the fetus may have an enlarged nuchal translucency.

2. A patient presents for a first-trimester examination because of a fundal height smaller than expected and vaginal spotting for the last week. Her home and clinician's urine pregnancy test returned positive. During the sonographic examination, there was identification of an empty gestational sac with a mean measurement of 25 mm. A complex mass imaged adjacent to the empty sac and a 2-cm cyst imaged on the left ovary. How can an early pregnancy failure be differentiated from a partial molar pregnancy?

   ANSWER: The patient's symptoms correlate to failure of an early pregnancy with a subchorionic bleed. In the presence of a mole, the patient presents with a small or normal uterus, vaginal bleeding, hyperemesis, and a very high quantitative hCG. A partial hydatidiform mole can demonstrate an empty sac; however, the placenta images differently. The trophoblastic vesicles image as multiple small cystic masses creating a complex mass with low resistance arterial flow. Patients with molar pregnancies can demonstrate multiple, bilateral, theca luteal cysts because of the high levels of hCG. Compare Figures 14-2, 14-9, and 14-10.

SUMMARY

- Any vaginal bleeding in a patient less than 20 weeks is called a threatened abortion or miscarriage.

- A blighted ovum is the failure of an early pregnancy.

- An empty gestational sac measuring greater than 20 mm indicates a pregnancy failure.

- The abnormally shaped yolk sac is an indicator of a poor pregnancy outcome.

- Diagnosis of demise is made through the lack of fetal heart motion in an embryo measuring 5 mm or larger.

- The presence of a subchorionic hemorrhage increases the risk of an adverse outcome.

- Hydatidiform moles are the result of abnormal fertilization.

REFERENCES

1. Mukri F, Bourne T, Bottemley C, et al. Evidence of early first-trimester growth restriction in pregnancies that subsequently end in miscarriage. *BJOG.* 2008;115(10): 1273–1278.
2. Ouyang DW, Economy KE, Norwitz ER. Obstetric complications of fibroids. *Obstet Gynecol Clin North Am.* 2006;33(1):153–169.
3. Chen BA, Creinin MD. Contemporary management of early pregnancy failure. *Clin Obstet Gynecol.* 2007;50(1):67–88.
4. Farquharson RG, Jauniaux E, Exalto N. Updated and revised nomenclature for description of early pregnancy events. *Hum Repro.* 2005;20(11):3008–3011.
5. Eyvazzadeh AD, Levine D. Imaging of pelvic pain in the first trimester of pregnancy. *Radiol Clin North Am.* 2006;44(6):863–877.
6. Dighe M, Cuevas C, Moshiri M, et al. Sonography in first trimester bleeding. *J Clin Ultrasound.* 2008;36(6): 352–366.
7. Tong S, Kaur A, Walker SP, et al. Miscarriage risk for asymptomatic women after a normal first-trimester prenatal visit. *Obstet Gynecol.* 2008;111(3):710–714.
8. Sotiriadis A, Papatheodorou S, Makrydimas G. Threatened miscarriage: evaluation and management. *BMJ.* 2004;329(7458):152–155.
9. Paspulati RM, Bhatt S, Nour S. Sonographic evaluation of first-trimester bleeding. *Radiol Clin North Am.* 2004;42(2):297–314.
10. Hasan R, Baird DD, Herring AH, et al. Association between first-trimester vaginal bleeding and miscarriage. *Obstet Gynecol.* 2009;114(4):860–867.
11. Schauberger CW, Mathiason MA, Rooney BL. Ultrasound assessment of first-trimester bleeding. *Obstet Gynecol.* 2005;105(2):333–338.
12. Snell BJ. Assessment and management of bleeding in the first trimester of pregnancy. *J Midwifery Womens Health.* 2009;54(6):483–491.
13. Sawyer E, Jurkovic D. Ultrasonography in the diagnosis and management of abnormal early pregnancy. *Clin Obstet Gynecol.* 2007;50(1):31–54.
14. Falco P, Zagonari S, Gabrielli S, et al. Sonography of pregnancies with first-trimester bleeding and a small intrauterine gestational sac without a demonstrable embryo. *Ultrasound Obstet Gynecol.* 2003;21(1):62–65.
15. Elson J, Salim R, Tailor A, et al. Prediction of early pregnancy viability in the absence of an ultrasonically detectable embryo. *Ultrasound Obstet Gynecol.* 2003;21(1):57–61.
16. Chama CM, Marupa JY, Obed JY. The value of the secondary yolk sac in predicting pregnancy outcome. *J Obstet Gynaecol.* 2005;25(3):245–247.

17. Varelas FK, Prapas NM, Liang RI, et al. Yolk sac size and embryonic heart rate as prognostic factors of first trimester pregnancy outcome. *Eur J Obstet Gynecol Reprod Biol.* 2008;138(1):10–13.

18. Berdahl DM, Blaine J, Van Voorhis B, et al. Detection of enlarged yolk sac on early ultrasound is associated with adverse pregnancy outcomes. *Fertil Steril.* 2010;94(4):1535–1537.

19. Yegul NT, Filly RA. Further observations on the empty "amnion sign." *J Clin Ultrasound.* 2010;38(3):113–117.

20. Doubilet PM, Benson CB. Outcome of first-trimester pregnancies with slow embryonic heart rate at 6–7 weeks gestation and normal heart rate by 8 weeks at US. *Radiology.* 2005;236(2):643–646.

21. Doubilet PM, Benson CB, Chow JS. Outcome of pregnancies with rapid embryonic heart rates in the early first trimester. *AJR Am J Roentgenol.* 2000;175(1):67–69.

22. Yegul NT, Filly RA. The expanded amnion sign: evidence of early embryonic death. *J Ultrasound Medicine.* 2009;28(10):1331–1335.

23. Filly MR, Callen PW, Yegul NT, et al. The yolk stalk sign: evidence of death in small embryos without heartbeats. *J Ultrasound Medicine.* 2010;29(2):237–241.

24. Abbasi S, Jamal A, Eslamian L, et al. Role of clinical and ultrasound findings in the diagnosis of retained products of conception. *Ultrasound Obstet Gynecol.* 2008;32(5):704–707.

25. Sawyer E, Ofuasia E, Ofili-Yebovi D, et al. The value of measuring endometrial thickness and volume on endovaginal ultrasound scan for the diagnosis of incomplete miscarriage. *Ultrasound Obstet Gynecol.* 2007;29(2):205–209.

26. Mungen E, Dundar O, Babacan A. Postabortion Doppler of the uterus: incidence and causes of myometrial hypervascularity. *J Ultrasound Med.* 2009;28(8):1053–1060.

27. Leite J, Ross P, Rossi AC, et al. Prognosis of very large first trimester hematomas. *J Ultrasound Med.* 2006;25(11):1441–1445.

28. Nagy S, Bush M, Stone J, et al. Clinical significance of subchorionic and retroplacental hematomas detected in the first trimester of pregnancy. *Obstet Gynecol.* 2003;102(1):94–100.

29. Kirk E, Papageorghiou AT, Condous G, et al. The accuracy of first trimester ultrasound in the diagnosis of hydatidiform mole. *Ultrasound Obstet Gynecol.* 2007;29(1):70–75.

30. Altieri A, Franceschi S, Ferlay J, et al. Epidemiology and aetiology of gestational trophoblastic diseases. *Lancet Oncol.* 2003;4(11):670–678.

31. Berkowitz, RS, Goldstein DP. Clinical practice. Molar pregnancy. *N Eng J Med.* 2009;360(16):1639–1645.

32. Barken SS, Skibsted L, Jensen LN, et al. Diagnosis and prediction of parental origin of triploidies by fetal nuchal translucency and maternal serum free b-hCG and PAPP-A at 11–14 weeks of gestation. *Acta Obstetricia et Gynecologica.* 2008;87(9):975–978.

33. Garner EIO, Goldstein DP, Feltmate CM, et al. Gestational trophoblastic disease. *Clin Obstet Gynecol.* 2007;50(1):112–122.

34. Soper JT, Mutch DG, Schink JC. Diagnosis and treatment of gestational trophoblastic disease: ACOG Practice Bulletin No. 53. *Gynecol Oncol.* 2004;93(3):575–585.

35. Kerkmeijer LGW, Massuger LFAG, Ten Kate-Booij MJ, et al. Earlier diagnosis and serum human chorionic gonadotropin regression in complete hydatidiform moles. *Obstet Gynecol.* 2009;113(2 pt 1):326–331.

36. Benson CB, Genest DR, Bernstein MR, et al. Sonographic appearance of first trimester complete hydatidiform moles. *Ultrasound Obstet Gynecol.* 2000;16(2):188–191.

37. Betel C, Atri M, Arenson AM, et al. Sonographic diagnosis of gestational trophoblastic disease and comparison with retained products of conception. *J Ultrasound Med.* 2006;25(8):985–993.

38. Zhou Q, Lei XY, Cardoza JD. Sonographic and Doppler inaging in the diagnosis and treatment of gestational trophoblastic disease: a 12-year experience. *J Ultrasound Med.* 2005;24(1):15–24.

39. Gebb J, Dar P. Should the first-trimester aneuploidy screen be maternal age adjusted? Screening by absolute risk versus adjusted to maternal age. *Prenat Diagn.* 2009;29(3):245–247.

40. Rosen T, D'Alton ME, Platt LD, et al. First-trimester ultrasound assessment of the nasal bone to screen for aneuploidy. *Obstet Gynecol.* 2007;110(2 pt 2):399–404.

41. Nyberg DA, Hyett J, Johnson J, et al. First trimester screening. *Radiol Clin North Am.* 2006;44(6):837–861.

42. Maiz N, Valencia C, Kagan KO, et al. Ductus venosus Doppler in screening for trisomies 21, 18, and 13 and Turner syndrome at 11–13 weeks of gestation. *Ultrasound Obstet Gynecol.* 2009;33(5):512–517.

43. Sahota DS, Leung TY, Chan LW, et al. Comparison of first-trimester contingent screening strategies for Down syndrome. *Ultrasound Obstet Gynecol.* 2010;35(3):286–291.

44. Blass HG, Eik-Nes SH. Sonoembryology and early prenatal diagnosis of neural anomalies. *Prenat Diagn.* 2009;29(4):312–325.

45. Castro-Aragon I, Levine D. Ultrasound detection of first trimester malformations: a pictorial essay. *Radiol Clin North Am.* 2003;41(4):681–693.

46. Chaoui R, Benoit B, Mitkowska-Wozniak H, et al. Assessment of intracranial translucency (IT) in the detection of spina bifida at the 11–13 week scan. *Ultrasound Obstet Gynecol.* 2009;34(3):249–252.

47. Fong KW, Toi A, Salem S, et al. Detection of fetal structural abnormalities with ultrasound during early pregnancy. *Radiographics.* 2004;24(1):157–174.

48. Oztekin O, Oztekin D, Tinar S, et al. Ultrasonographic diagnosis of fetal structural abnormalities in prenatal screening at 11–14 weeks. *Diagn Interv Radiol.* 2009;15(3):221–225.

49. Sepulveda W. Monosomy 18p presenting with holoprosencephaly and increased nuchal translucency in the first trimester. *J Ultrasound Medicine.* 2009;28(8):1077–1080.

50. Bronshtein M, Zimmer EZ, Blazer S. The utility of detailed first trimester ultrasound examination in abnormal fetal nuchal translucency. *Prenat Diagn.* 2008;28(11):1037–1041.

51. Martinez Crespo JM, Del Rio M, Gomez O, et al. Prenatal diagnosis of hypoplastic left heart syndrome and trisomy 18 in a fetus with normal nuchal translucency and abnormal ductus venosus blood flow at 13 weeks of gestation. *Ultrasound Obstet Gynecol.* 2003;21(5):490–493.

52. Sciarrone A, Masturzo B, Botta G, et al. First-trimester fetal heart block and increased nuchal translucency: an indication for early fetal echocardiography. *Prenat Diagn.* 2005;25(12):1129–1132.

53. Barbee K, Wax JR, Pinette MG, et al. First-trimester prenatal sonographic diagnosis of ectopia cordis in a twin gestation. *J Clin Ultrasound.* 2009;37(9):539–540.

54. Tonni G, Azzoni D, Ventura A, et al. Early detection (9+6 weeks) of cardiac failure in a fetus diagnosed as Turner syndrome by 2D endovaginal ultrasound-guided coelocentesis. *J Clin Ultrasound.* 2009;37(5):302–304.

55. Smrcek JM, Germer U, Krokowski M, et al. Prenatal ultrasound diagnosis and management of body stalk anomaly: analysis of nine singleton and two multiple pregnancies. *Ultrasound Obstet Gynecol.* 2003;21(4):322–328.

56. Graesslin O, Derniaux E, Alanio E, et al. Characteristics and outcome of fetal cystic hygroma diagnosed in the first trimester. *Acta Obstet Gynecol Scand.* 2007;86(12):1442–1446.

57. Hashimoto K, Shimizu T, Fukuda M, et al. Pregnancy outcome of embryonic/fetal pleural effusion in the first trimester. *J Ultrasound Med.* 2003;22(5):501–505.

58. Nakamura-Pereira M, Carneiro do Cima L, Llerena JC, et al. Sonographic findings in a case of tetrasomy 9p associated with increased nuchal translucency and Dandy-Walker malformation. *J Clin Ultrasound.* 2009;37(8):471–474.

59. Yonemoto H, Itoh S, Nakamura Y, et al. Umbilical cord cyst detected in the first trimester by two- and three-dimensional sonography. *J Clin Ultrasound.* 2006;34(3):150–152.

60. Jouannic JM, Hyett JA, Pandya PP, et al. Perinatal outcome in fetuses with megacystis in the first half of pregnancy. *Prenat Diagn.* 2003;23(4):340–344.

61. Teoh M, Meagher S. First-trimester diagnosis of micrognathia as a presentation of Pierre Robin syndrome. *Ultrasound Obstet Gynecol.* 2003;21(6):616–618.

62. Van Zalen-Sprock RM, Van Vugt JMG, Van Geijn HP. First-trimester sonography of physiological midgut herniation and early diagnosis of omphalocele. *Prenat Diagn.* 1997;17(6):511–518.

63. Bornstein E, Monteagudo A, Dong R, et al. Detection of twin reversed arterial perfusion sequence at the time of first-trimester screening. *J Ultrasound Med.* 2008;27(7):1105–1109.

64. Vural F, Vural B. First trimester diagnosis of dicephalic parapagus conjoined twins via endovaginal ultrasonography. *J Clin Ultrasound.* 2005;33(7):364–366.

65. Blin G, Rabbe A, Ansquer Y, et al. First trimester diagnosis in a recurrent case of Walker-Warburg syndrome. *Ultrasound Obstet Gynecol.* 2005;26(3):297–299.

66. Ickowicz V, Eurin D, Maugey-Laulom B, et al. Meckel-Gruber syndrome: sonography and pathology. *Ultrasound Obstet Gynecol.* 2006;27(3):296–300.

67. Peixoto-Filho FM, Carneiro do Cima L, Nakamura-Pereira M. Prenatal diagnosis of pentalogy of Cantrell in the first trimester: is 3-dimensional sonography needed? *J Clin Ultrasound.* 2007;37(2):112–114.

68. Chong K, Keating S, Hurst S, et al. Cornelia de Lange syndrome (CdLS): prenatal and autopsy findings. *Prenat Diagn.* 2009;29(5):489–494.

69. Carvalho MHB, Brizot ML, Lopes LM, et al. Detection of fetal structural abnormalities at the 11–14 week ultrasound scan. *Prenat Diagn.* 2002;22(1):1–4.

15 Sonographic Assessment of the Ectopic Pregnancy

Amanda Auckland

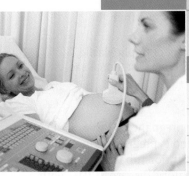

KEY TERMS

interstitial pregnancy | cornual pregnancy | cervical pregnancy | intramural pregnancy | ovarian pregnancy | abdominal pregnancy | heterotopic pregnancy | pelvic inflammatory disease (PID) | assisted reproductive techniques (ART) | beta human chorionic gonadotropin (β-hCG)

GLOSSARY

Abdominal pregnancy Gestation located within the intraperitoneal cavity, apart from tubal, ovarian, or intraligamentous sites

Assisted reproductive techniques (ART) A number of techniques used to aid fertilization, including in vitro fertilization (IVF), intracytoplasmic sperm insertion (ICSI), follicle aspiration, sperm injection, and assisted follicular rupture (FASIAR)

Beta human chorionic gonadotropin (β-hCG) Glycoprotein hormone produced in pregnancy that is made by the developing embryo soon after conception and later by the placenta

Cervical pregnancy Gestation located within the endocervical canal

Cornual pregnancy Gestation located within a rudimentary uterine horn or one horn of a bicornuate or septated uterus

Discriminatory cutoff Level of β-hCG at which a normal intrauterine pregnancy can be seen with sonography

Double decidual sac sign Two concentric hyperechoic rings (representing the echogenic base of the endometrium and the decidua capsularis/chorion laeve) surrounding the anechoic gestational sac in a normal intrauterine pregnancy

Ectopic pregnancy Implantation of a fertilized ovum in any area outside of the endometrial cavity

Heterotopic pregnancy Concomitant intrauterine pregnancy and ectopic pregnancy

Hypovolemic shock Shock due to a decrease in blood volume

Interstitial pregnancy Gestation located in the intra-myometrial segment of the fallopian tube

Intramural pregnancy Gestation located within the myometrium of the uterus

Intrauterine contraceptive device (IUD) Form of birth control; small, plastic or copper, usually T-shaped device with a string attached to the end that is inserted into the uterus

In vitro fertilization (IVF) Laboratory procedure in which sperm are placed with an unfertilized egg in a petri dish to achieve fertilization; the embryo is then transferred into the uterus to begin a pregnancy or cryopreserved for future use

Morison's pouch Hepatorenal recess; deep recess of the peritoneal cavity on the right side extending upward between the liver and the kidney; gravity-dependent portion of the peritoneal cavity when in the supine position

Ovarian pregnancy Gestation located within the ovary

Pelvic inflammatory disease (PID) Infection of the female reproductive tract that results from microorganisms transmitted especially during sexual intercourse or by other means such as during surgery, abortion, or parturition

Pregnancy of unknown location (PUL) Pregnancy in which no signs of an intrauterine pregnancy or ectopic pregnancy are seen by sonography

Sliding sac sign When gentle pressure from the transducer moves the gestational sac

Tubal ring sign Hyperechoic ring of trophoblastic tissue that surrounds an extrauterine gestational sac

An *ectopic pregnancy* is defined as implantation of a fertilized ovum in any area outside the endometrial cavity.[1] It accounts for about 2% of all pregnancies in the United States.[2] The prevalence of ectopic pregnancy has increased from 0.37% of pregnancies in 1948 to about 2% of pregnancies in 1992, and a sixfold increase was seen in the United States between 1970 and 1992.[3] In spite of the rising incidence of ectopic pregnancy in the United States in the last 30 years, maternal mortality and morbidity have declined considerably by almost 90% from 1979 to 1992.[3] Yet, ectopic pregnancy is still the leading cause of maternal death in the first trimester of pregnancy, having a mortality rate of 9% to 14%.[3] The decline in maternal mortality and morbidity can be attributed to routine endovaginal sonography, which is readily available in almost all clinical settings and is an essential tool in the early diagnosis of ectopic pregnancy.[4]

The clinical diagnosis of ectopic pregnancy is made by physical examination in conjunction with diagnostic sonography and human chorionic gonadotropin (hCG) radioimmunoassay. The anatomical information provided by the sonographic images is important in making the diagnosis of ectopic pregnancy. A thorough understanding of sonographic features, implantation sites, scanning technique, and differential diagnoses is necessary for the practitioner to perform a proper sonographic evaluation of a patient at risk for ectopic pregnancy. Knowledge of the physiology of conception and gestation, along with an awareness of the meaning of pertinent laboratory values, clinical symptoms, and clinical histories that predispose one to ectopic pregnancy, supplement the information provided by the sonographic images.

ETIOLOGY

Each fallopian tube is derived from the müllerian duct system. It is the only connection between the peritoneal cavity and the endometrial cavity. As the ovum is expelled from the dominant follicle and is swept up by the fimbriae into the oviduct, certain conditions may impede its normal course and cause it to implant in the fallopian tube or other abnormal locations.[5]

Conditions that prevent or hinder migration of the fertilized ovum to the uterine cavity are major risk factors for ectopic pregnancy; therefore, anything that could cause damage to the fallopian tube increases the subsequent risk of ectopic pregnancy (Table 15-1).[6] The key risk factors for ectopic pregnancy include a history of ectopic pregnancy, prior tubal surgical procedures, and pelvic inflammatory disease (PID), with previous ectopic pregnancy being the strongest associated risk factor.[6,7] The possibility of a repeat ectopic pregnancy increases significantly with the number of prior ectopic pregnancies; women with an ectopic gestation are three times more likely to have had one prior ectopic gestation when compared to women with an intrauterine pregnancy (IUP).[6] Damage to the fallopian tube also occurs from any gynecologic surgery, endometriosis, history of multiple sexual partners, congenital uterine or tubal anomalies, history of placenta previa, history of smoking (affects tubal motility), infertility, use of intrauterine contraceptive device (IUD) (Fig. 15-1), increasing maternal age, and use of assisted reproductive techniques (ARTs).[6–8] However, more than half of ectopic pregnancies are diagnosed in women without known risk factors.[9]

The increased rate of ectopic gestations in the last few decades may be a result of a rise in the incidence of sexually transmitted infections and PID, which result in tubal impairment or blockage.[2] A history of PID is particularly significant, as it raises the threat of an ectopic gestation sevenfold.[4] ARTs have also contributed

TABLE 15-1
Risk Factors Associated with Increased Incidence of Ectopic Pregnancy
History of:
previous ectopic pregnancy
pelvic inflammatory disease
tubal surgical procedure
gynecologic surgery
multiple sexual partners
placenta previa
smoking
Endometriosis
Congenital uterine or tubal anomalies
Infertility
Assisted reproductive techniques
IUD use
Increased maternal age

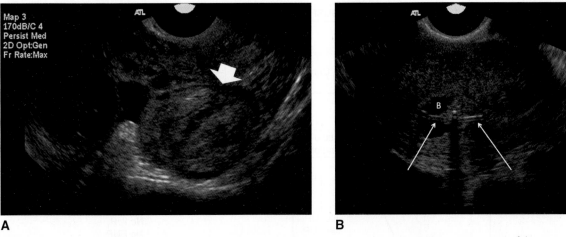

A   **B**

Figure 15-1 A: Ruptured tubal ectopic pregnancy *(white arrowhead)* seen in a patient with an IUD. **B:** Transverse image of the uterus showing the IUD *(white arrows)* located within the endometrial canal surrounded by blood. *B,* blood.

considerably to the increase in ectopic pregnancies, with an ectopic rate of 2.2% to 8.6%, compared to the general population's rate of about 2%.[10] Both in vitro fertilization (IVF) and ovulation induction techniques, particularly with clomiphene citrate, increase the risk of an ectopic gestation because of theoretical variances involving conception via ART and natural conception.[10,11] The risk of ectopic pregnancy in women using ART varies with the type of procedure, the reproductive health of the woman, and the embryo implantation potential.[10] Theories exist that certain embryo factors in abnormal gestations may cause an ectopic pregnancy, though it has been proven that the rate of chromosomal abnormalities are comparable to that expected for women with the same maternal and gestational age.[12,13]

CLINICAL PRESENTATION

The triad of clinical presentation of ectopic pregnancy includes vaginal bleeding, pelvic pain, and a palpable adnexal mass; however, these classic symptoms only arise in less than 45% of women with ectopics.[1] Most patients present with a history of amenorrhea, pelvic pain, and irregular vaginal bleeding, but symptoms may range from completely asymptomatic (up to 50% of patients) to as severe as hypovolemic shock.[1,7,14,15] The amount of pelvic or abdominal pain the patient experiences does not always correlate with the size or location of the ectopic gestation.[15] Findings on physical exam vary with the hemodynamic condition of the patient; hypotension, tachycardia, shoulder pain from diaphragmatic irritation, significant abdominal pain, rebound tenderness and guarding, hypovolemic shock, or even diminished pain may all be signs of tubal rupture and/ or hemoperitoneum[1,9,15,16](Figs. 15-1 and 15-2).

Ectopic pregnancies are typically diagnosed at 6 to 10 weeks of gestation during the first trimester.[9] Pregnancy is determined by the level of either a urine or serum concentration of β-hCG.[9] The β-hCG concentration rises rapidly and reaches a plateau around 9 to 11 weeks.[9,14] In a normal IUP, the β-hCG level should approximately double every 48 hours.[17] A rise of at least 53% should be seen in a normal IUP, if not, ectopic gestation should be considered.[18] Women presenting with ectopic pregnancies tend to have lower than normal β-hCG levels that rise at a much slower rate; however, up to 21% of women with an ectopic gestation have normal doubling times.[2,19,20] Ectopic pregnancies can have normally rising, falling, or a plateau of β-hCG levels; thus, serial measurements of β-hCG are especially valuable.[9]

The "discriminatory cutoff" is the level of β-hCG at which a normal IUP can be seen with ultrasonography.[21] A β-hCG concentration above 1,500 to 2,500 mIU/mL is the discriminatory cutoff using endovaginal sonography; therefore, if a normal IUP is not visualized at this level, it is most likely an abnormal gestation.[22-24] When the β-hCG level is below the discriminatory cutoff and an IUP is not visualized, this could indicate an early normal IUP, a spontaneous abortion, or an ectopic pregnancy.[25] Patients in stable condition with no evidence of a gestational sac by ultrasound should be monitored with serial β-hCG levels and endovaginal sonography using an algorithm (Fig. 15-1 and 15-2) for the evaluation of an ectopic pregnancy.[26,27]

SITES OF ECTOPIC PREGNANCY

A normal intrauterine gestation implants within the uterine cavity above the level of the internal os, medial to the interstitial portion of the fallopian tubes, and frequently, eccentrically within the uterine cavity.[28] Those that do not implant within the uterine cavity are ectopic in location. Ectopic pregnancies implant most often in the fallopian tubes (95%), though interstitial, cornual, cervical, intramural, ovarian, and abdominal ectopics also occur (Fig. 15-3).[7,29] A tubal ectopic gestation usually occurs in the ampullary portion of the tube (70%), or less commonly in the isthmus (12%) or fimbria (11.1%).[29]

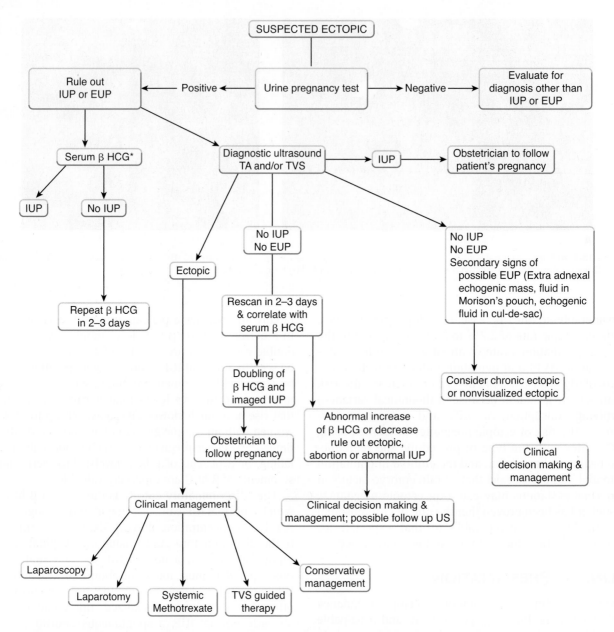

* Intrauterine gestational sac should be seen on TVS with β HCG ≥ 1000 mIU/mL (2nd IS): on TA with β HCG ≥ 2600 mIU/mL (2nd IS). Values of 1000 mIU/mL and 3600 mIU/mL represent the upper limits of the discriminatory zones.

EUP   = Extra Uterine Pregnancy
IUP   = Intrauterine Pregnancy
TA   = Transabdominal Ultrasound
TVS   = Transvaginal Ultrasound
2nd IS = Second International Standard
US   = Ultrasound

Figure 15-2 Management of stable patients with suspected ectopic pregnancy.

Interstitial pregnancy occurs in the intramyometrial segment of the fallopian tube (Fig. 15-4) and accounts for 2% to 4% of all ectopic gestations.[30,31] The intramural segment of the tube in which the interstitial pregnancy implants is completely surrounded by myometrium, allowing for a greater degree of distensibility than other portions of the fallopian tube.[32] This distensibility allows the pregnancy to progress further without symptoms (as late as 16 weeks), leading to rupture at a later gestational age and possible life-threatening hemorrhage.[32]

Because of the proximity of the uterine arteries to the interstitial portion of the tube, hemorrhage can be 2.5 to 5 times greater than in rupture of other types of ectopic pregnancy.[32,33] The maternal morbidity and mortality rate associated with interstitial pregnancy rupture is elevated because of this, as high as 2% to 2.5%.[32] Prior ipsilateral salpingectomy and IVF can increase a woman's risk for interstitial pregnancy, whereas an IUD may actually protect against implantation in the interstitial portion of the tube.[29,31]

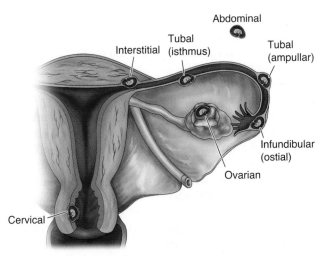

Figure 15-3 Sites of implantation of the fertilized ovum in an ectopic pregnancy.

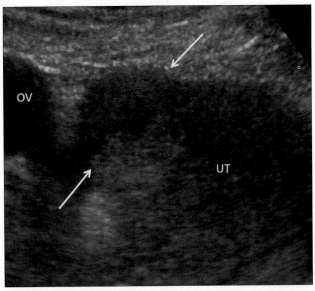

Figure 15-4 Transabdominal sonographic image of an interstitial pregnancy. *OV,* right ovary; *UT,* uterus; *white arrows,* interstitial pregnancy.

The terms *cornual pregnancy* and *interstitial pregnancy* have been used interchangeably in literature, though they are not synonymous.[33] A cornual pregnancy occurs within a rudimentary uterine horn or one horn of a bicornuate or septate uterus (Fig. 15-5).[27,34] Even though it is implanted within the uterine cavity, a cornual pregnancy is classified as an ectopic pregnancy because of its propensity to rupture in the second trimester.[35,36] Cornual pregnancy accounts for less than 1% of ectopic pregnancies.[7] Maternal morbidity and mortality are increased with cornual pregnancy for similar reasons as interstitial pregnancy: It may rupture at a later gestational age and critical hemorrhage could ensue.[7]

Cervical pregnancy occurs when the gestation implants within the endocervical canal (Fig. 15-6).[37] It is rare, accounting for less than 1% of all ectopic pregnancies, and may be linked to risk factors such as previous curettage, anatomic anomalies, endometriosis, IUD use (may accelerate the course of the ovum through the uterus), and IVF.[37–39] Cervical pregnancies can produce significant hemorrhage and be associated with high morbidity and adverse consequences for future fertility.[38,39]

Intramural pregnancy occurs by implantation of the gestation within the myometrium of the uterus.[40] It is extremely rare and accounts for less than 1% of ectopic pregnancies.[40] Intramural pregnancies can be seen following procedures that cause an injury to the myometrium, including curettage, hysteroscopy, myomectomy, metroplasty, and cesarean section, possibly due to tract formation through the myometrium.[41,42] Implantation within the scar from a previous cesarean section may be a result of the endometrial and myometrial disruption and scarring.[41] Cesarean scar pregnancy is

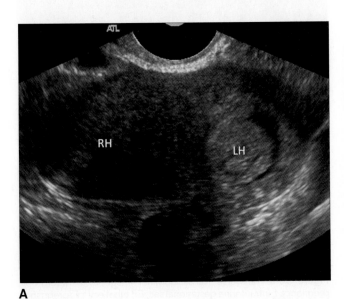

A

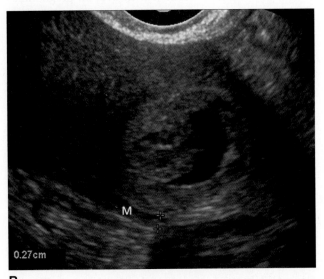

B

Figure 15-5 A: Transverse image of a bicornuate uterus containing a gestational sac in the left horn. *RH,* right horn; *LH,* left horn. **B:** Transverse image of the left horn of the same cornual pregnancy showing very thinned myometrium around the gestation. *M,* myometrium.

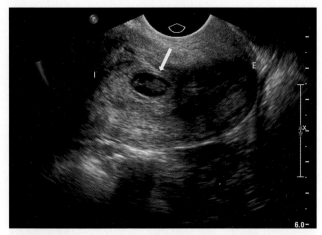

Figure 15-6 Longitudinal endovaginal image of a cervical pregnancy. *I*, internal os; *E*, external os; *white arrow*, cervical pregnancy.

probably the rarest of all ectopic pregnancies, but there has been an increase in the number of cases reported, most likely owing to the great increase in the number of cesarean deliveries in recent years.[43–45] Patients with an intramural pregnancy are at a significant risk for uterine rupture, causing massive hemorrhage and hypovolemic shock.[46,47]

Ovarian pregnancy occurs when the fertilized ovum implants in the ovary (Fig. 15-7), though there is debate on whether it is a result of secondary implantation of the embryo on the ovary or a failure of follicular extrusion.[48–50] It accounts for 1% to 3% of all ectopic gestations and the incidence has been increasing over the last two decades.[48,51] This increase is possibly due to the rise of the rates of sexually transmitted diseases, PID, and use of IUDs; other risk factors for ovarian pregnancy include endometriosis and ART.[48–53] IUD use is strongly associated with ovarian pregnancy; the IUD prevents implantation within the uterus and the fallopian tube but cannot protect against implantation within the ovary.[51,54] Women with ovarian pregnancies

usually present with lower abdominal pain and bleeding, and the pregnancy usually ends with rupture and hemoperitoneum because of the increased vascularity of ovarian tissue.[48]

Abdominal pregnancy occurs when the ovum implants within the intraperitoneal cavity, apart from tubal, ovarian, or intraligamentous sites.[7] It is uncommon and accounts for up to 1.4% of ectopic pregnancies.[55] Abdominal pregnancies can be divided into primary and secondary types; primary abdominal pregnancy occurs when the fertilized ovum implants within the intraperitoneal cavity directly, and secondary abdominal pregnancy occurs when a tubal ectopic pregnancy ruptures or aborts and reimplants within the intraperitoneal cavity.[56] Patients with abdominal pregnancy present with general malaise, nausea, vomiting, vaginal bleeding, and painful fetal movements.[56,57] The risk of abdominal pregnancy is increased with PID, endometriosis, tubal damage, multiparity, and ART.[58,59] Abdominal pregnancy has been reported having implanted on the uterine surface, liver, spleen, diaphragm, bowel, omentum, broad ligament, large vessels, and the pelvic cul-de-sacs.[56,58,60–62] Because of their location, abdominal pregnancies can continue to a much more advanced gestational age; this places the mother at risk for disseminated intravascular coagulation (DIC), bowel obstruction, and severe hemorrhage.[57,62] Significant maternal mortality is associated with abdominal pregnancy, reported as high as 30%, and a perinatal mortality rate as high as 95%.[55,63]

Heterotopic pregnancy occurs when two or more fertilized ova implant, usually an IUP and an ectopic pregnancy (Fig. 15-8).[64] It is exceptionally rare and

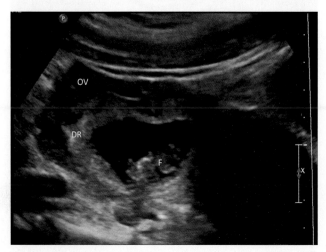

Figure 15-7 Transabdominal image of an ovarian ectopic. *OV*, ovary tissue; *DR*, decidual reaction; *F*, fetus.

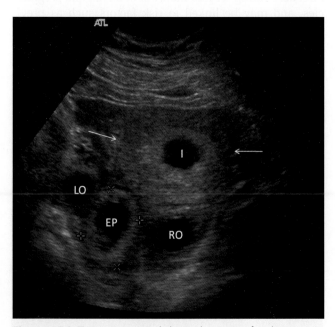

Figure 15-8 Transverse transabdominal image of a heterotopic pregnancy. *I*, intrauterine gestational sac; *EP*, tubal ectopic pregnancy; *LO*, left ovary; *RO*, right ovary; *white arrows*, uterus.

accounts for 1:30,000 natural pregnancies.[65,66] Heterotopic pregnancy increases considerably with ART procedures from ovulation induction and controlled ovarian hyperstimulation, with a rate of 1% to 3% of pregnancies from IVF.[67,68] Abdominal pain is the most frequent symptom seen with heterotopic pregnancy; vaginal bleeding rarely occurs due to the concomitant IUP.[67] A positive outcome of the IUP is seen in about 66% of heterotopic pregnancies.[69]

SONOGRAPHIC PROTOCOL

Optimal visualization of the uterus and adnexa is crucial in the sonographic evaluation of a suspected ectopic pregnancy. The sonographer must be familiar with the patient's medical and surgical history as well as his or her clinical presentation to correlate the sonographic findings and formulate the differential diagnosis. The goal of the sonogram is to establish the presence of an IUP; however, this does not rule out an ectopic gestation.[7,70]

Transabdominal sonography was the principal imaging method used to evaluate for ectopic pregnancy.[1] It is very useful for obtaining more complete views of the adnexa, fundal region, flank areas, and abdomen (Fig. 15-9) and has a diagnostic reliability around 70%.[1] The diagnosis of ectopic pregnancy has been radically improved by the use of endovaginal sonography (Fig. 15-10); it has a sensitivity and specificity of 90.9% and 99.9%, respectively.[4,70] Endovaginal sonography should demonstrate an IUP when β-hCG levels are above the discriminatory zone (1,500 to 2,500 mIU/mL).[22–24] Transabdominal sonography demonstrates an IUP when β-hCG levels are above 6,500 mIU/mL.[15]

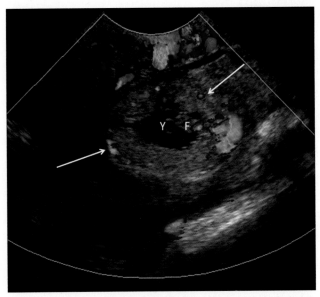

Figure 15-10 Endovaginal image showing the same tubal ectopic pregnancy (*white arrows*) as Figure 15.8. *Y*, yolk sac; *F*, fetus.

Endovaginal sonography allows visualization of the gestational sac with a double decidual sac sign (two concentric hyperechoic rings surrounding the anechoic gestational sac) at 4 1/2 to 5 weeks of gestation in normal IUPs.[71,72] The yolk sac should be visualized by 5 weeks and the fetal pole with possible cardiac motion at 5 1/2 to 6 weeks of gestation.[71]

When the β-hCG is below the discriminatory cutoff and an IUP is not visualized, it could indicate a spontaneous abortion, early IUP, or an ectopic gestation; therefore, follow-up is suggested rather than treatment.[25] When the β-hCG is above the discriminatory cutoff and an IUP is not visualized, the patient may undergo a procedure to evacuate the contents of the uterus to determine whether the pregnancy was an abnormal IUP or an ectopic pregnancy.[2] It is also advised in this situation to monitor the patient with serial β-hCG measurements and sonography examinations before providing treatment.[26,27]

The absence of an IUP with a β-hCG level above the discriminatory cutoff should prompt a thorough investigation with transabdominal and endovaginal sonography to locate the ectopic pregnancy; however, 35% of ectopic gestations do not have a visible adnexal mass or abnormality.[7] If no signs of an IUP or ectopic pregnancy are seen on endovaginal sonography, it is described as a pregnancy of unknown location (PUL).[73] The rate of PULs ranges from 8% to 31% because of the differences in the quality of the sonogram.[73,74] The initial sonographic exam detects up to 90% of ectopic pregnancies; the diagnosis should be found on the visualization of an adnexal mass using endovaginal sonography.[70,75]

The sonographer must systematically evaluate all potential sites of implantation when an ectopic pregnancy is in question. Evaluate the entire uterus in

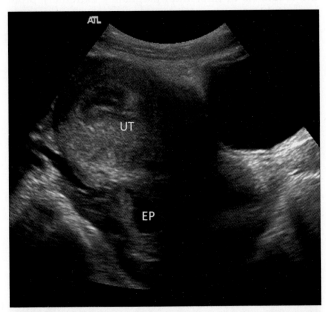

Figure 15-9 Transabdominal image of the uterus in longitudinal showing a tubal ectopic pregnancy in the posterior cul-de-sac. *UT*, uterus; *EP*, tubal ectopic pregnancy.

TABLE	15-2

Scanning Protocol for the Evaluation of an Ectopic Pregnancy

- Be acquainted with the patient's clinical history, pregnancy test results, and last menstrual period
- Use transabdominal sonography to examine the uterus and adnexae in longitudinal and transverse planes
- Evaluate the cul-de-sacs, pericolic gutters, and Morison's pouch for free fluid
- Use endovaginal sonography to evaluate the uterus, adnexae, and cul-de-sacs in coronal and transverse planes
- Describe sonographic findings and establish a preliminary impression

both longitudinal and transverse views and investigate the endometrium to find signs of an IUP or pseudo-sac formation. Inspect both adnexa thoroughly for the identification of any masses; any mass found should be noted, characterized, and treated as a potential ectopic pregnancy until proven otherwise (Table 15-2). An ectopic gestation can be definitively diagnosed when cardiac activity is identified outside of the endometrial cavity (Fig. 15-11).[4] Sonographic evaluation also includes the hepatorenal recess (Morison's pouch) and paracolic gutters to evaluate for the extent of free fluid, such as blood from a ruptured ectopic gestation or peritoneal fluid from a ruptured ovarian cyst (Fig. 15-12).

SONOGRAPHIC CHARACTERISTICS

UTERINE

In the setting of an ectopic pregnancy, the uterus may appear normal. Typically, the endometrium is thickened because of the decidual reaction during pregnancy; an endometrial stripe thickness less than 8 mm can be indicative of an abnormal or ectopic pregnancy.[4] A

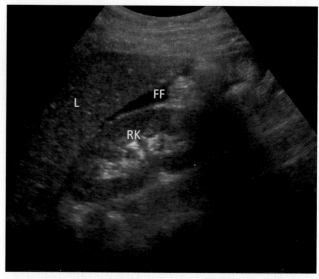

Figure 15-12 Free fluid from a ruptured tubal ectopic pregnancy seen within Morison's pouch. *L,* liver; *RK,* right kidney; *FF,* free fluid.

pseudosac may be seen within the uterus (Fig. 15-13) and must not be confused for a normal gestational sac; a pseudosac is a fluid collection caused by bleeding from the decidualized endometrium.[71] A true gestational sac and a pseudosac can be differentiated by their location within the endometrium; a pseudosac is within the endometrial cavity and a gestational sac abuts the endometrial canal.[71] Also, a pseudosac is surrounded by a single layer of tissue and a gestational sac should have the typical double decidual sac sign.[28]

An interstitial pregnancy demonstrates on sonography as an eccentrically located gestational sac surrounded by a very thin layer of myometrium (less than 5 mm).[7] This layer of myometrium (Fig. 15-14) makes the diagnosis of interstitial pregnancy extremely problematical by sonography; it is the most difficult type of ectopic gestation to diagnose.[28,33] Visualization of the interstitial line, described by Ackerman et al., may be a sensitive sign of an interstitial pregnancy.[76] It is an

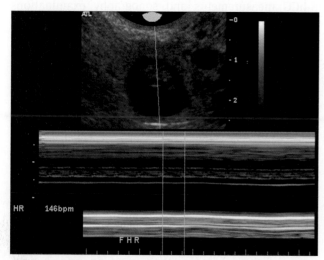

Figure 15-11 Cardiac activity documented with M-mode within the fetus of a tubal ectopic pregnancy.

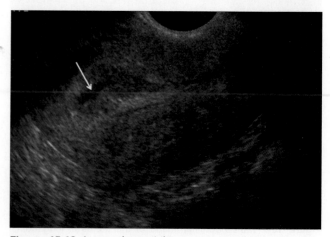

Figure 15-13 A pseudosac *(white arrow)* visualized within the endometrial canal in the presence of an ectopic gestation.

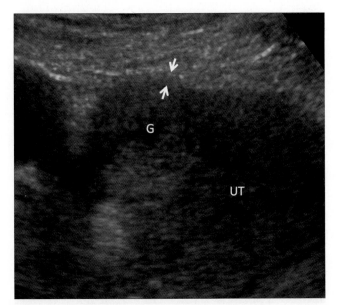

Figure 15-14 Thinned myometrium *(white arrowheads)* surrounding an interstitial pregnancy. *G,* gestational sac; *UT,* uterus.

echogenic line that extends into the midportion of the gestational sac and represents the interstitial portion of the fallopian tube.[76] The diagnosis of interstitial pregnancy can also be aided by the criteria developed by Timor-Tritsch et al.: (1) an empty uterine cavity, (2) a gestational sac greater than 1 cm from the most lateral point of the endometrial cavity, and (3) a gestational sac surrounded by a thin myometrial layer.[77]

A cornual pregnancy can be diagnosed by visualizing a single interstitial portion of the fallopian tube, a gestational sac surrounded by myometrium separate from the uterus, and by demonstrating a vascular peduncle adjoining the gestational sac to the unicornuate uterus.[28] A gestational sac seen in one horn of a bicornuate uterus is also considered a cornual pregnancy.[33]

A cervical pregnancy frequently presents during the sonographic exam as an hourglass-shaped uterus from the gestation expanding the cervical canal.[7] If a gestational sac is seen within the cervix and cardiac activity is visualized below the level of the internal os (Fig. 15-15), a cervical pregnancy is evident.[78] The sliding sac sign is very useful in the diagnosis of cervical pregnancy; if gentle pressure from the transducer can move the gestational sac, it is not implanted in the cervical canal and is most likely an abortion in progress.[79]

An intramural pregnancy demonstrates a gestational sac completely surrounded by myometrium with no communication with the endometrial cavity.[38] A cesarean scar pregnancy can be diagnosed by using the criteria proposed by Vial et al.: (1) the trophoblast is located between the bladder and the anterior uterine wall, (2) fetal parts are not present in the uterine cavity, and (3) in a sagittal view, no myometrium is seen between the gestational sac and the urinary bladder, illustrated by the lack of continuity of the anterior uterine wall.[47]

EXTRAUTERINE

Adnexal masses can be visualized as a tubal ring, a complex or solid adnexal mass, a nonliving embryo or yolk sac, or a live embryo with cardiac motion.[4] The adnexal mass is more explicitly an ectopic pregnancy when a yolk sac or embryo is seen within it.[4] A tubal ectopic pregnancy is usually seen as the tubal ring sign (Fig. 15-16), which is a hyperechoic ring that surrounds an extrauterine gestational sac; this should move independently from the adjacent ovary.[4,80]

An ovarian pregnancy is surrounded by ovarian cortex.[28] Pathologic criteria, described by Spiegelberg, can assist with the diagnosis of ovarian pregnancy: (1) the tube must be entirely normal, (2) the gestational sac has to be anatomically located in the ovary, (3) the ovary and the gestational sac have to be connected to the uterine ovarian ligament, and (4) placental tissue has to be mixed with ovarian cortex.[28] The sonographic image demonstrates a wide echogenic ring (Fig. 15-17), possibly containing a yolk sac or fetus, on the ovary.[51]

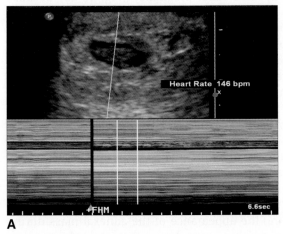

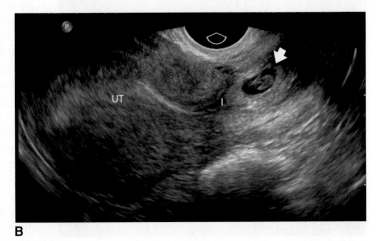

Figure 15-15 A: Positive fetal cardiac activity seen within a cervical pregnancy. **B:** Longitudinal endovaginal image of the same cervical pregnancy *(white arrowhead). UT,* uterus; *I,* internal os.

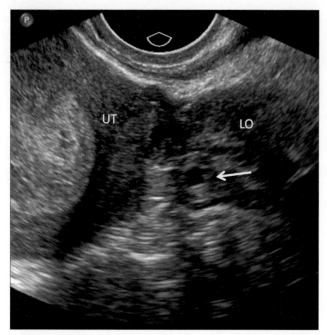

Figure 15-16 Tubal ring sign *(white arrow)* seen in a transverse endovaginal image of an early unruptured tubal ectopic pregnancy. *UT,* uterus; *LO,* left ovary.

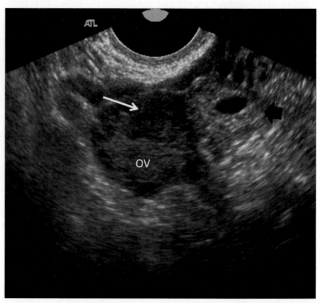

Figure 15-18 Corpus luteum *(white arrow)* appearing hypoechoic on the ovary and tubal ectopic pregnancy *(black arrowhead)* appearing more hyperechoic adjacent to the ovary. *OV,* right ovary.

Ovarian pregnancies are frequently confused with corpus luteum cysts, which are more hypoechoic than the echogenic decidual reaction of the ovarian pregnancy (Fig. 15-18).[49,81]

Abdominal pregnancy can be diagnosed using the criteria described by Allibone et al.: (1) demonstration of a fetus in a gestational sac outside the uterus, (2) failure to visualize the uterine wall between the fetus and urinary bladder, (3) close proximity between the fetus and the anterior abdominal wall, and (4) localization of the placenta outside the confines of the uterine cavity.[82] Extended field of view (EFOV) or panoramic

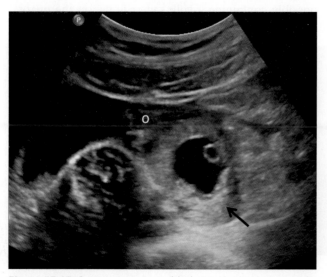

Figure 15-17 Ovarian pregnancy *(black arrow)* seen on a transabdominal image of the right ovary. *O,* ovarian cortex.

sonography is a useful tool for visualizing an abdominal pregnancy.[56]

Heterotopic pregnancy is diagnosed with sonography upon visualization of an IUP and a concomitant extrauterine pregnancy (Fig. 15-19).[7] When an IUP is seen, the ectopic gestation could be easily missed or confused with the corpus luteal cyst.[83] One must continue to search for a possible ectopic gestation, especially in patients undergoing ART; though this may be difficult because of ovarian hyperstimulation and the multiple luteal cysts that result.[67]

Acute rupture of an ectopic pregnancy images as a formation of a complex mass-like area representing hemorrhage (Fig. 15-20); when there is a partial or complete rupture, a variety of sonographic appearances visualize. The adnexal mass is larger in patients with a ruptured tubal pregnancy (Fig. 15-21) versus an unruptured tubal pregnancy (Fig. 15-22) because of the blood and gestational contents comprising the larger adnexal mass.[84] Free fluid (Fig. 15-23) is the most obvious indicator of a ruptured ectopic pregnancy, though it is nonspecific and could be the result of a ruptured ovarian cyst. Hematosalpinx, hemoperitoneum, fluid within Morison's pouch, pelvic cul-de-sacs (Fig. 15-24), or paracolic gutters are all findings that help with the diagnosis of a suspected ectopic pregnancy.[7] Pelvic hemorrhage is a very specific finding for a ruptured ectopic pregnancy, with up to a 93% positive predictive value when there is an abnormal β-hCG level.[7] Yet in one study, up to 21% of patients with tubal rupture had no signs of intraperitoneal fluid, and therefore, the appearance of the adnexal mass during the sonographic exam does not necessarily correlate with tubal rupture.[84]

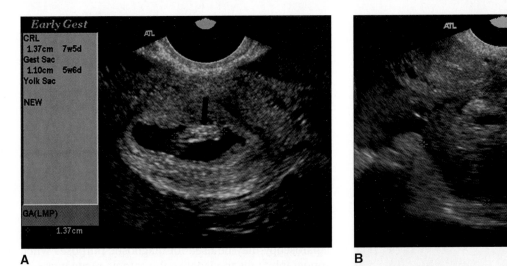

A

B

Figure 15-19 A: Crown-rump length of the fetus *(black arrow)* in an intrauterine pregnancy. **B:** The concomitant ruptured tubal ectopic pregnancy (between calipers) seen medial to the left ovary.

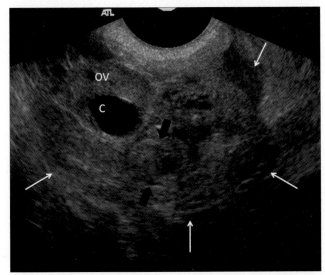

Figure 15-20 Ruptured tubal ectopic pregnancy *(black arrows)* is not easily seen because of the blood and clot material *(white arrows)* within the right adnexa. *OV*, right ovary; *C*, corpus luteal cyst.

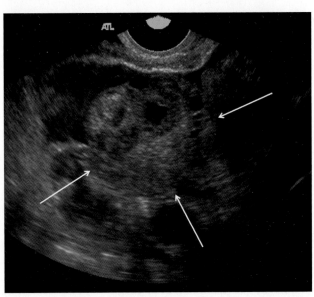

Figure 15-21 Adnexal mass *(white arrows)* seen in a patient with a ruptured tubal ectopic pregnancy.

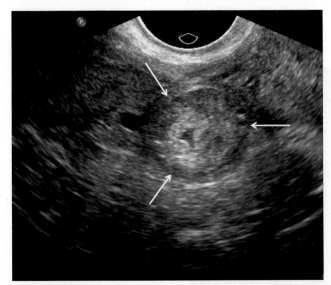

Figure 15-22 Adnexal mass *(white arrows)* seen in a patient with an unruptured tubal ectopic pregnancy.

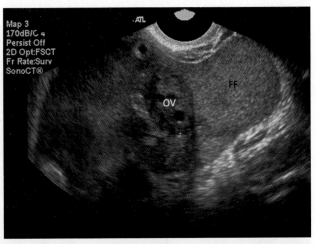

Figure 15-23 Free fluid seen within the right adnexa in the presence of a ruptured ectopic pregnancy. *FF*, free fluid; *OV*, right ovary.

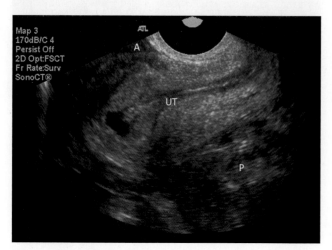

Figure 15-24 Complex free fluid within the anterior and posterior cul-de-sacs. *A,* anterior cul-de-sac; *UT,* uterus; *P,* posterior cul-de-sac.

COLOR DOPPLER

The detection of vascularity with color Doppler around a questionable adnexal mass may be useful in the diagnosis of an ectopic pregnancy.[85] The "ring of fire" sign is frequently described as a finding in an ectopic pregnancy; this represents the increased blood flow surrounding an ectopic gestation.[86] A pulsed spectral Doppler of this flow usually shows a low resistive index, which is a proposed indicator of an ectopic pregnancy.[85] Color Doppler is limited, though, in its diagnostic properties, as the corpus luteum may also have a similar color Doppler pattern and resistive index and could therefore be mistaken for an ectopic pregnancy (Fig. 15-25).[87]

Color Doppler is also useful in determining if a gestation is an abortion in progress versus a cervical pregnancy or cesarean scar pregnancy. An aborting gestational sac is avascular and a viable gestation is well perfused when visualized with color Doppler.[41] This technique could also be helpful in determining the difference between a pseudosac and a viable gestation within the uterus.[7]

ALTERNATE DIAGNOSTIC MODALITIES

Other diagnostic modalities may be employed for the evaluation of ectopic pregnancy when the sonographic findings are equivocal. If it is an undesired pregnancy, a uterine curettage may help with the diagnosis to determine if chorionic villi are present within the uterus or not.[88] Culdocentesis was once widely used to diagnose hemoperitoneum in patients with a suspected ectopic pregnancy, but it has a very limited value with the technology we now utilize.[89] Laparotomy was often used for the diagnosis of ectopic pregnancy in the past; today, laparoscopy may be used for diagnostic purposes when sonography fails to visualize the ectopic pregnancy.[2]

Less invasive diagnostic modalities now exist for the evaluation of ectopic pregnancy. CT and MRI are used when endovaginal sonography is unable to locate an ectopic gestation or differentiate it from a spontaneous abortion. MRI can confirm or better define an ectopic pregnancy with its superior tissue contrast (Fig. 15-26); it also provides information on the maturity of blood that is present within the pelvis and abdomen.[90] It is considered the gold standard for diagnosing abdominal pregnancy because of its accurate localization of sites of abnormal implantation and is therefore also extremely informative in cases of possible intramural/cesarean scar pregnancies.[38,56]

TREATMENT

Therapeutic treatment options for ectopic pregnancy include expectant management, medical therapy, and surgery.[91] Most ectopic pregnancies are detected early in gestation before tubal rupture since the advent of endovaginal sonography and rapid access to quantitative β-hCG testing; this allows for more conservative methods of treatment to be utilized in hemodynamically stable patients.[92]

Expectant management follows the natural history of the ectopic pregnancy, with the thought that the ectopic

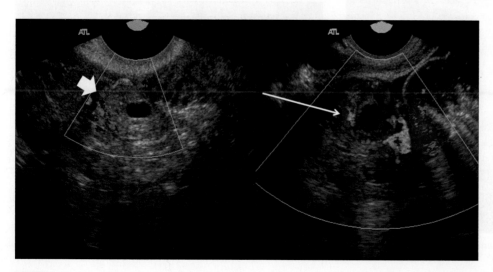

Figure 15-25 "Ring of fire" *(white arrowhead)* seen surrounding a tubal ectopic pregnancy and similar color Doppler *(long white arrow)* flow seen around the corpus luteal cyst.

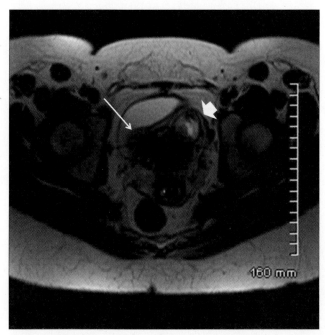

Figure 15-26 MRI image showing the gravid left uterine horn (*white arrowhead*) and empty right uterine horn (*long white arrow*) in a bicornuate uterus.

gestation can resolve spontaneously by regression or tubal abortion.[9,93] A good number of ectopic pregnancies diagnosed with endovaginal sonography would not have been detected in the past, and some of these would have resolved with no treatment.[93] The success rate of expectant management ranges from 7% to 40%; the success is increased with a lower initial β-hCG level, decreasing trend in β-hCG levels, and an absent gestational sac.[93,94]

Medical treatment with the antimetabolite cytotoxic drug methotrexate (MTX) has changed the treatment of ectopic pregnancy and facilitated a more conservative management technique.[95] MTX is a folic acid antagonist that impedes DNA synthesis in dividing cells.[9] It can be administered systemically as a single dose or multiple doses or can be directly injected into the ectopic gestation.[95] When administered properly, MTX has a success rate up to 94%; multiple-dose therapy has a greater success rate than single dose but with the consequence of more side effects.[9] Medical treatment with MTX is indicated when the patient is hemodynamically stable, has a β-hCG level less than 5,000 mIU/mL, is willing to follow up with monitoring after treatment, and when there is no fetal cardiac activity.[9]

Surgical management of ectopic pregnancy is performed on patients who have contraindications to medical treatment, have had medical treatment failure, or are hemodynamically unstable.[9] The most successful treatment for a tubal ectopic pregnancy is laparoscopic surgery—it is more cost-effective; has less operative time, blood loss, and anesthetic need, a faster recovery time; and fewer postoperative complications than laparotomy.[9,91] Salpingostomy or salpingectomy can be performed during the laparoscopy; salpingostomy is preferred for women desiring future fertility, but salpingectomy may be required in women with tubal rupture, recurrent ectopic pregnancy in the same tube, a severely damaged tube, or in cases where the diameter of the gestational sac exceeds 5 cm.[9] Laparotomy is still necessary for some cases of abdominal pregnancy, cornual and interstitial pregnancy, and cervical pregnancy, and also in severely hemodynamically unstable patients.[56,92,96]

SUMMARY

- An ectopic pregnancy is the implantation of a fertilized ovum outside of the endometrial cavity.
- The three biggest risk factors are a history of ectopic pregnancy, prior tubal surgical procedure, and PID.
- b-hCG levels rise slower with an ectopic pregnancy than with an IUP.
- Discriminatory cutoff is the level of b-hCG when an IUP can be visualized with sonography.
- Ectopic pregnancies occur most often in the fallopian tube, but can also be interstitial, cornual, cervical, intramural, ovarian, or abdominal.
- Heterotopic pregnancy occurs when two or more fertilized ova implant, usually an IUP and an ectopic pregnancy.
- The double decidual sac sign can be visualized with endovaginal sonography at 4 1/2 to 5 weeks of gestation.
- The yolk sac should be visualized by five weeks gestation.
- The fetal pole should be visualized by 5 1/2 to 6 weeks of gestation, possibly with cardiac motion.
- An ectopic pregnancy can be diagnosed when cardiac activity is identified outside of the endometrial cavity.
- A pseudosac within the uterus with an endometrial stripe thickness of less than 8 mm is suspicious for an ectopic pregnancy.
- An interstitial pregnancy is visualized as an eccentrically located gestational sac surrounded by myometrium measuring less than 5mm.
- A cornual pregnancy is diagnosed by visualizing a single interstitial portion of the fallopian tube, a gestational sac surrounded by myometrium separate from the uterus, and a vascular peduncle adjoining the gestational sac to the unicornuate uterus or one horn of a bicornuate uterus.
- A cervical pregnancy may present as an hourglass-shaped uterus due to the gestation expanding the cervical canal.
- An intramural pregnancy is visualized as a gestational sac completely surrounded by myometrium with no communication to the endometrial cavity.

Critical Thinking Questions

1. A primigravida patient presents to the department for a routine size and dates examination. Her only complaint was some bleeding and pain early in pregnancy, which has since resolved. The sonographic examination revealed a 20-week gestation with dates appropriate for last menstrual period (LMP). The placenta appears to be implanted over a pelvic mass. The amniotic fluid measures normal; however, there is either no or very thinned uterine walls. Explain the findings.

   ANSWER: This is an ectopic pregnancy that ruptured and reimplanted on the uterine fundus. The absence of the uterine wall was a clue to the type of pregnancy. This was an actual case that was carried to 35 weeks and delivered by caesarian section. A hysterectomy was performed simultaneously.

2. Review the following patient history and sonographic findings.

Patient history

- Infertility due to PID
- LMP 6 weeks ago
- ART with placement of three embryos
- Abdominal pain
- β-hCG twice the expected level

Sonographic findings

- Gestational sac with a yolk sac and live embryo within the uterus
- Crown-rump length measurements appropriate for dates
- Complex masses in the right and left adnexa
- Color flow identified surrounding the right adnexal mass
- Spectral Doppler tracings demonstrate a low Resistive Index (RI) in the right adnexal mass
- Fluid in the right pelvis and paracolic gutters extending into Morison's pouch

a. From this history and findings, identify the type of ectopic pregnancy.

b. What do the other findings tell us?

   ANSWER a: Heterotopic pregnancy

   ANSWER b: The high β-hCG tells us that there is more than one pregnancy. The level of twice the normal value raises suspicion for a twin pregnancy. The complex masses can confuse things, as both an ectopic and corpus luteal cyst have similar appearances. Since only one mass, the right one, demonstrated flow, it is likely the ectopic pregnancy is on this side. The fluid is another clue. An assumption is that the fluid is due to a ruptured ectopic pregnancy on the right side, which has resulted in hemorrhaging.

- Extrauterine ectopic pregnancies may be visualized as a tubal ring, a complex or solid adnexal mass, a nonliving embryo or yolk sac, or alive embryo with cardiac motion.

- Ovarian cortex surrounds an ovarian pregnancy

- Abdominal pregnancies are diagnosed when a fetus is visualized outside of the uterus, if no uterine wall can be seen between the fetus and the urinary bladder, if there is close proximity between the fetus and the anterior abdominal wall, or if a placenta is found outside of the uterine cavity.

- Color Doppler may demonstrate a "ring of fire" around an ectopic pregnancy, but a corpus luteum may also have a similar color Doppler pattern.

- MRI can confirm or better define an ectopic pregnancy; it is the gold standard for diagnosing abdominal pregnancy.

- Treatment options for ectopic pregnancy include expectant management, medical therapy, and surgery.

REFERENCES

1. Lehner R, Kucera E, Jirecek S, et al. Ectopic pregnancy. *Arch Gynecol Obstet*. 2000;263(3):87–92.
2. Seeber BE, Barnhart KT. Suspected ectopic pregnancy. *Obstet Gynecol*. 2006;107(2 pt 1):399–413.
3. Centers for Disease Control and Prevention. Ectopic pregnancy—United States, 1990–1992. *MMWR Morb Mortal Wkly Rep*. 1995;44(3):46–48.
4. Gurel S, Sarikaya B, Gurel K, et al. Role of sonography in the diagnosis of ectopic pregnancy. *J Clin Ultrasound*. 2007;35(9):509–517.
5. Hill GA, Herbert CM. Ectopic pregnancy. In: Copeland LJ, ed. *Textbook of Gynecology*. Philadelphia, PA: WB Saunders; 1993:242.
6. Barnhart KT, Sammel MD, Gracia CR, et al. Risk factors for ectopic pregnancy in women with symptomatic first-trimester pregnancies. *Fertil Steril*. 2006;86(1):36–43.
7. Lin EP, Bhatt S, Dogra VS. Diagnostic clues to ectopic pregnancy. *Radiographics*. 2008;28(6):1661–1671.
8. Ankum WM, Mol BW, van der Veen F, et al. Risk factors for ectopic pregnancy: a meta-analysis. *Fertil Steril*. 1996;65(6):1093–1099.
9. Murray H, Baakdah H, Bardell T, et al. Diagnosis and treatment of ectopic pregnancy. *CMAJ*. 2005;173(8):905–912.
10. Clayton HB, Schieve LA, Peterson HB, et al. Ectopic pregnancy risk with assisted reproductive technology procedures. *Obstet Gynecol*. 2006;107(3):595–604.
11. Fernandez H, Gervaise A. Ectopic pregnancies after infertility treatment: modern diagnosis and therapeutic strategy. *Hum Reprod Update*. 2004;10(6):503–513.
12. Goddijn M, van der Veen F, Schuring-Blom GH, et al. Cytogenic characteristics of ectopic pregnancy. *Epidemiology*. 1993;4:252–258.
13. Coste J, Fernandez H, Joye N, et al. Role of chromosome abnormalities in ectopic pregnancy. *Fertil Steril*. 2000;74(6):1259–1260.
14. Lipscomb GH, Stovall TG, Ling FW. Nonsurgical treatment of ectopic pregnancy. *N Eng J Med*. 2000;343(18):1325–1329.

15. Attar E. Endocrinology of ectopic pregnancy. *Obste Gynecol Clin North Am*. 2004;31(4):779–794.

16. Mol BW, Hajenius PJ, Ankum WM, et al. Screening for ectopic pregnancy in symptom-free women at increased risk. *Obstet Gynecol*. 1997;89(5 pt 1):704–707.

17. Daya S. Human chorionic gonadotropin increase in normal early pregnancy. *Am J Obstet Gynecol*. 1987;156(2):286–290.

18. Seeber BE, Sammel MD, Guo W, et al. Application of redefined human chorionic gonadotropin curves for the diagnosis of women at risk for ectopic pregnancy. *Fertil Steril*. 2006;86(2):454–459.

19. Kaplan BC, Dart RG, Moskos M, et al. Ectopic pregnancy: prospective study with improved diagnostic accuracy. *Ann Emerg Med*. 1996;28(1):10–17.

20. Kohn MA, Kerr K, Malkevich D, et al. Beta-human chorionic gonadotropin levels and the likelihood of ectopic pregnancy in emergency department patients with abdominal pain or vaginal bleeding. *Acad Emerg Med*. 2003;10(2):119–126.

21. Barnhart K, Mennuti MT, Benjamin I, et al. Prompt diagnosis of ectopic pregnancy in an emergency department setting. *Obstet Gynecol*. 1994;84(6):1010–1015.

22. Barnhart K, Esposito M, Coutifaris C. An update on the medical treatment of ectopic pregnancy. *Obstet Gynecol Clin North Am*. 2000;27(3):653–667.

23. Fylstra DL. Tubal pregnancy: a review of current diagnosis and treatment. *Obstet Gynecol Surv*. 1998;53(5):320–328.

24. Pisarska MD, Carson SA, Buster JE. Ectopic pregnancy. *Lancet*. 1998;351(9109):1115–1120.

25. Mehta TS, Levine D, Beckwith B. Treatment of ectopic pregnancy: is a human chorionic gonadotropin level of 2,000 mIU/mL a reasonable threshold? *Radiology*. 1997;205(2):569–573.

26. Sauer MV, Gorrill MJ, Rodi IA, et al. Nonsurgical management of unruptured ectopic pregnancy: an extended clinical trial. *Fertil Steril*. 1987;48(5):752–755.

27. Dialani V, Levine D. Ectopic pregnancy: a review. *Ultrasound Q*. 2004;20(3):105–117.

28. Jurkovic D, Mavrelos D. Catch me if you scan: ultrasound diagnosis of ectopic pregnancy. *Ultrasound Obstet Gynecol*. 2007;30(1):1–7.

29. Bouyer J, Costa J, Fernandez H, et al. Sites of ectopic pregnancy: a 10 year population-based study of 1800 cases. *Hum Reprod*. 2002;17(12):3224–3230.

30. Webb EM, Green GE, Scoutt LM. Adnexal mass with pelvic pain. *Radiol Clin North Am*. 2004;42(2):329–348.

31. De Boer CN, van Dongen PW, Willemsen WN, et al. Ultrasound diagnosis of interstitial pregnancy. *Eur J Obstet Gynecol Reprod Biol*. 1992;47(2):164–166.

32. Malinowski A, Bates SK. Semantics and pitfalls in the diagnosis of cornual/interstitial pregnancy. *Fertil Steril*. 2006;86(6):1764.e11–e14.

33. Kun W, Tung WK. On the look out for rarity—interstitial/cornual pregnancy. *Eur J Emerg Med*. 2001;8(2):147–150.

34. Lau S, Tulandi T. Conservative medical and surgical management of interstitial ectopic pregnancy. *Fertil Steril*. 1999;72(2):207–215.

35. DeNicola RR, Peterson MR. Pregnancy in rudimentary horn of uterus. *Am J Surg*. 1947;73:382–386.

36. Nahum GG. Rudimentary uterine horn pregnancy. The 20th-century worldwide experience of 588 cases. *J Reprod Med*. 2002;47(2):151–163.

37. Hofmann HM, Urdi W, Hofler H, et al. Cervical pregnancy: case reports and current concepts in diagnosis and treatment. *Arch Gynecol Obstet*. 1987;241(1):63–69.

38. Molinaro TA, Barnhart KT. Ectopic pregnancies in unusual locations. *Semin Reprod Med*. 2007;25(2):123–130.

39. Kraemer B, Abele H, Hahn M, et al. Cervical ectopic pregnancy on the portio: conservative case management and clinical review. *Fertil Steril*. 2008;90(5):2011.e1–e4.

40. Bernstein HB, Thrall M, Clark W. Expectant management of intramural ectopic pregnancy. *Obstet Gynecol*. 2001;97(5 pt 2):826–827.

41. Rotas MA, Haberman S, Levgur M. Cesarean scar ectopic pregnancies. *Obstet Gynecol*. 2006;107(6):1373–1381.

42. Karakok M, Balat O, Sari I, et al. Early diagnosed intramural ectopic pregnancy associated with adenomyosis; report of an unusual case. *Clin Exp Obstet Gynecol*. 2002;29(3):217–218.

43. Lee CL, Wang C, Chao A, et al. Laparoscopic management of an ectopic pregnancy in a cesarean section scar. *Hum Reprod*. 1999;14(5):1234–1236.

44. Valley MT, Pierce JG, Daniel TB, et al. Cesarean scar pregnancy: imaging and treatment with conservative surgery. *Obstet Gynecol*. 1998;91(5 pt 2):838–840.

45. Leitch CR, Walker JJ. The rise in cesarean section rate: the same indications but a lower threshold. *Br J Obstet Gynaecol Surv*. 1998;105(6):621–626.

46. Graesslin O, Dedecker F, Quereux C, et al. Conservative treatment of ectopic pregnancy in a cesarean scar. *Obstet Gynecol*. 2005;105(4):869–871.

47. Vial Y, Petignat P, Hohlfeld P. Pregnancy in a cesarean scar. *Ultrasound Obstet Gynecol*. 2000;16(6):592–593.

48. Hiroshi I, Ishihara A, Koita H, et al. Ovarian pregnancy: report of four cases and review of the literature. *Pathology International*. 2003;53(11):806–809.

49. Bontis J, Grimbizis G, Tarlatzis BC, et al. Intrafollicular ovarian pregnancy after ovulation induction/intrauterine insemination: pathophysiological aspects and diagnostic problems. *Hum Reprod*. 1997;12(2):376–378.

50. Marret H, Hamamah S, Alonso AM, et al. Case report and review of the literature: primary twin ovarian pregnancy. *Hum Reprod*. 1997;12(8):1813–1815.

51. Comstock C, Huston K, Lee W. The ultrasonographic appearance of ovarian ectopic pregnancies. *Obstet Gynecol*. 2005;105(1):42–45.

52. Einenkel J, Baier D, Horn LC, et al. Laparoscopic therapy of an intact primary ovarian pregnancy with ovarian hyperstimulation syndrome. *Hum Reprod*. 2000;15(9):2037–2040.

53. Ghi T, Banfi A, Marconi R. Three-dimensional sonographic diagnosis of ovarian pregnancy. *Ultrasound Obstet Gynecol*. 2005;26(1):102–104.

54. Fuse Y. Case study of ovarian pregnancies. *Pract Gynecol Obstet*. 1992;41:501–507.

55. Atrash HK, Friede A, Hogue CJ. Abdominal pregnancy in the United States: frequency and maternal mortality. *Obstet Gynecol*. 1987;69(3 pt 1):333–337.

56. Gaither K. Abdominal pregnancy—an obstetrical enigma. *South Med J*. 2007;100(4):347–348.

57. Rahman MS, Al-Suleiman S, Rahman J, et al. Advanced abdominal pregnancy—observations in 10 cases. *Obstet Gynecol*. 1982;59(3):366–372.

58. Ludwig M, Kaisi M, Bauer O, et al. The forgotten child—a case of heterotopic, intraabdominal and intrauterine pregnancy carried to term. *Hum Reprod*. 1999;14(5):1372–1374.

59. Tsudo T, Harada T, Yoshioka H, et al. Laparoscopic management of early unruptured abdominal pregnancy. *Obstet Gynecol*. 1997;90(4 pt 2):687–688.

60. Dover RW, Powell MC. Management of a primary abdominal pregnancy. *Am J Obstet Gynecol*. 1995;172(5):1603–1604.

61. Varma R, Mascarenhas R, Jame D. Successful outcome of advanced abdominal pregnancy with exclusive omental insertion. *Ultrasound Obstet Gynecol*. 2003;21(2):192–194.

62. Fisch B, Peled Y, Kaplan B, et al. Abdominal pregnancy following in vitro fertilization in a patient with previous bilateral salpingectomy. *Obstet Gynecol*. 1996;88(4 pt 2): 642–643.

63. Ramachandran K, Kirk P. Massive hemorrhage in a previously undiagnosed abdominal pregnancy presenting for elective Cesarean delivery. *Can J Anaesth*. 2004;51(4): 57–61.

64. Louis-Sylvestre C, Morice P, Chapron C, et al. The role of laparoscopy in the diagnosis and management of heterotopic pregnancies. *Hum Reprod*. 1997;12(5):1110–1112.

65. Chin HY, Chen FP, Wang CJ, et al. Heterotopic pregnancy after in-vitro fertilization—embryo transfer. *Int J Gynaecol Obstet*. 2004;86(3):411–416.

66. Reece EA, Petrie RH, Sirmans MF, et al. Combined intrauterine and extrauterine gestations: a review. *Am J Obstet Gynecol*. 1983;146(3): 323–330.

67. Oliveira FG, Abdelmassih V, Costa AL, et al. Rare association of ovarian implantation site for patients with heterotopic and with primary ectopic pregnancies after ICSI and blastocyst transfer. *Hum Reprod*. 2001;16(10):2227–2229.

68. Fernandez H, Gervaise A. Ectopic pregnancy after infertility treatment: modern diagnosis and therapeutic strategy. *Hum Reprod Update*. 2004;10(6):503–513.

69. Pistofidis GA, Mastrominas MJ, Dimitropoulos K. Laparoscopic management of heterotopic pregnancies. *J Am Assoc Gyneco Laparosc*. 1995;2:S42–S43.

70. Condous G, Okaro E, Khalid A, et al. The accuracy of transvaginal ultrasonography for the diagnosis of ectopic pregnancy prior to surgery. *Hum Reprod*. 2005;20(5):1404–1409.

71. Ahmed AA, Tom BD, Calabrese P. Ectopic pregnancy diagnosis and the pseudo-sac. *Fertil Steril*. 2004;81(5): 1125–1128.

72. Morin L, Van den Hof MC. SOGC clinical practice guidelines: ultrasound evaluation of first trimester pregnancy complications. *Int J Gynecol Obstet*. 2006;93(1):77–81.

73. Condous G, Timmerman D, Goldstein S, et al. Pregnancies of unknown location: consensus statement. *Ultrasound Obstet Gynecol*. 2006;28(2):121–122.

74. Condous G, Kirk E, Lu C, et al. Diagnostic accuracy of varying discriminatory zones for the prediction of ectopic pregnancy in women with a pregnancy of unknown location. *Ultrasound Obstet Gynecol*. 2005;26(7): 770–775.

75. Kirk E, Papageorghiou AT, Condous G, et al. The diagnostic effectiveness of an initial transvaginal scan in detecting ectopic pregnancy. *Hum Reprod*. 2007;22(11): 2824–2828.

76. Ackerman TE, Levi CS, Dashefsky SM, et al. Interstitial line: sonographic finding in interstitial (cornual) ectopic pregnancy. *Radiology*. 1993;189(1):83–87.

77. Timor-Tritsch IE, Monteagudo A, Matera C, et al. Sonographic evolution of cornual pregnancies treated without surgery. *Obstet Gynecol*. 1992;79(6):1044–1049.

78. Kung FT, Lin H, Hsu TY, et al. Differential diagnosis of suspected cervical pregnancy and conservative treatment with the combination of laparoscopy-assisted uterine artery ligation and hysteroscopic endocervical resection. *Fertil Steril*. 2004;81(6):1642–1649.

79. Jurkovic D, Hacket E, Campbell S. Diagnosis and treatment of early cervical pregnancy: a review and a report of two cases treated conservatively. *Ultrasound Obstet Gynecol*. 1996;8(6):373–380.

80. Blaivas M, Lyon M. Reliability of adnexal mass mobility in distinguishing possible ectopic pregnancy from corpus luteum cysts. *J Ultrasound Med*. 2005;24(5):599–603.

81. Chang FW, Chen CH, Liu JY. Early diagnosis of ovarian pregnancy by ultrasound. *Int J Gynecol Obstet*. 2004;85(2):186–187.

82. Allibone GW, Fagan CJ, Porter SC. The sonographic features of intra-abdominal pregnancy. *J Clin Ultrasound*. 1981;9(7):383–387.

83. Barrenetxea G, Barinaga-Rementeria L, Lopez de Larruzea A, et al. Heterotopic pregnancy: two cases and comparative review. *Fertil Steril*. 2007;87(2):417.e9–e15.

84. Frates MC, Brown DL, Doubliet PM, et al. Tubal rupture in patients with ectopic pregnancy: diagnosis with transvaginal US. *Radiology*. 1994;191(3):769–772.

85. Fukami T, Emoto M, Tamura R, et al. Sonographic findings of transvaginal color Doppler ultrasound in ectopic pregnancy. *J Med Ultrasonics*. 2006;33:37–42.

86. Blaivas M. Color Doppler in the diagnosis of EP in the emergency department: is there anything beyond a mass and fluid? *J Emerg Med*. 2002;22(4):379–384.

87. Atri A. Ectopic pregnancy versus corpus luteum cyst revisited: best Doppler predictors. *J Ultrasound Med*. 2003;22(11):1181–1184.

88. Nyberg D, Filly R, Laing F, et al. Ectopic pregnancy diagnosis by sonography correlated with quantitative hCG levels. *J Ultrasound Med*. 1987;6(3):145–150.

89. Vermesh M, Graczykowski JW, Sauer MV. Reevaluation of the role of culdocentesis in the management of ectopic pregnancy. *Am J Obstet Gynecol*. 1990;162(2):411–413.

90. Tamai K, Koyama T, Tagashi K. MR features of ectopic pregnancy. *Eur Radiol*. 2007;17(12):3236–3246.

91. Mol F, Mol BW, Ankum WM, et al. Current evidence on surgery, systemic methotrexate and expectant management in the treatment of tubal ectopic pregnancy: a systematic review and meta-analysis. *Hum Reprod Update*. 2008;14(4):309–319.

92. Jermy K, Thomas J, Doo A, et al. The conservative management of interstitial pregnancy. *Int J Obstet Gynecol*. 2004;111(11):1283–1288.

93. Elson J, Tailor A, Banerjee S, et al. Expectant management of tubal ectopic pregnancy: prediction of successful outcome using decision tree analysis. *Ultrasound Obstet Gynecol*. 2004:23(6):552–556.

94. Kirk E, Condous G, Bourne T. The non-surgical management of ectopic pregnancy. *Ultrasound Obstet Gynecol*. 2006;27(1):91–100.

95. Kirk E, Condous G, Haider Z, et al. The conservative management of cervical ectopic pregnancies. *Ultrasound Obstet Gynecol*. 2006;27(4):430–437.

96. Verma U, Goharkhay N. Conservative management of cervical ectopic pregnancy. *Fertil Steril*. 2009;91(3):671–674.

16 Assessment of Fetal Age and Size in the Second and Third Trimester

Susan Johnston

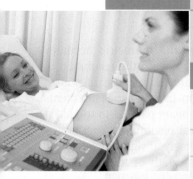

OBJECTIVES

Recognize the correct level for obtaining standard second and third trimester biometric measurements

Explain the use of multiple biometric parameter accuracy in fetal dating

Summarize the use of alternate dating methods such as humerus, forearm, lower leg, cerebellar, and ocular measurements

Discuss the correct method for measuring fetal biometry

Calculate estimated fetal weight

List fetal ratios that help determine normal growth of the fetus

KEY TERMS

biparietal diameter (BPD) | head circumference (HC) | abdominal circumference (AC) | femur length (FL) | cephalic index (CI) | binocular distance (BOD) | humeral length (HL) | HC/AC ratio

GLOSSARY

Axial resolution Minimum distance between two bright echoes along the path of the ultrasound beam, which is half the spatial pulse length

Cephalic index (CI) Ratio of the BPD to the OFD

Lateral resolution Minimum distance between two bright echoes at right angles (perpendicular) to the ultrasound beam path directly related to the beam width and focal zone

Marcrosomia Fetus over 4,000 grams (g) (8 pounds, 13 oz)

Occipito-frontal diameter (OFD) Measurement from the frontal to the occipital obtained at the same level as the BPD

Predictive value Precision rate or the probability of disease

A critical portion of any obstetrical sonographic examination involves measuring various parameters of the pregnancy. These measurements have two objectives: to estimate the fetal age and to determine the size and development of the fetus. These interrelated objectives indicate not only fetal size but dating of the pregnancy, assuming a normal pregnancy. Obstetric patient management requires accurate evaluation and fetal age determination.

Two terms used to indicate the expected birth date are the estimated date of confinement (EDC) or estimated delivery date (EDD). Fetal age calculation based on this date is often called the gestational age, although it is actually counted from the first day of the last menstrual period (LMP) and not from the date of conception. The dates of the pregnancy are important for planning the mode and date of delivery, screening evaluation for aneuploidy, determining dates of possible termination, gauging fetal growth, and suggesting whether or not the pregnancy is progressing normally. An important indicator of fetal health is the estimated size.

Sonographic measurements (biometry) aid in estimation of the fetal size and dates. The parameters discussed were selected because they are relatively accurate and easy to obtain. No single measurement consistently dates all fetuses, resulting in the use of several measurements. Using more than one or two fetal parameters also improves the accuracy in assessing dates and fetal size.[1–4]

GENERAL SCANNING METHODOLOGY AND USE OF FETAL AGE CHARTS

All normal fetuses originate from a single fertilized egg and grow to a birth size that varies from infant to infant. Early measurements of the embryo result in the most accurate dating, as individual differences have yet to become evident.[1] Because of this, once the gestational age has been determined and confirmed by an ultrasound, this date should never change. Growth individuation takes place later in gestation.

Normal human fetuses tend to be uniform in morphology with an ethnic group.[2,5,6] Although there may be some differences in various normal growth parameters due to altitude, genetics, maternal smoking, and other influences, such differences are small in most cases. This is especially true of the average fetus early in gestation. Variations in any single parameter's prediction of age will usually be less than ±10% of the age at any given time in pregnancy (±2 weeks at midpregnancy and ±4 weeks at term). This means that virtually any published chart derived with valid scientific methodology can be used to estimate fetal age. It is important that the user know how the measurements were generated to compose a given chart. If, for example, the chart was created using biparietal diameter (BPD) measurements that were taken from the outer edge to the inner edge of the skull, it will produce valid age estimates only if the BPD for the fetus being examined is measured in the same manner. In other words, if the sonographer does not know how the author of a particular chart took the measurements and did the calculations to produce that chart, then the use of that chart may lead to error.

Some experts recommend measuring a parameter several times and averaging for the measurement of record[7] and others believe that one single "correct" measurement is sufficient.[8] The former is the preferred measurement method. Multiple measurements (three or more) are made of any given parameter and are observed for a "cluster" with a range of <2 or 3 millimeters (mm). Any measurements that fall outside the cluster are discarded and the remaining measurements are averaged for the measurement of record.

There are generally two ways of listing fetal age in charts. One is to list the estimated age in weeks and days; the other is to use weeks and tenths of weeks; either method is valid. Fetal age is usually computed in "menstrual weeks" because of the historical precedent of using the date of the LMP for calculating the dates of the pregnancy. Normally conception takes place about 2 weeks after the LMP. Birth normally occurs 40 weeks from the LMP (a 38-week gestation ±2 to 3 weeks). In this chapter fetal age is given as the number of weeks since the LMP, unless otherwise stated (i.e., *28 weeks LMP* means the pregnancy has completed the 28th but not the 29th week after the LMP). The term *last normal menstrual period* (LNMP) is used only for the first day of the last period as reported by the woman.

ACCURACY OF SONOGRAPHIC MEASUREMENTS

Image resolution determines the biometric accuracy of any sonogram. Two factors govern the resolution of a sonographic beam, axial and lateral (beam width) resolution.[9–11] Axial resolution involves measurements along the axis or path of the beam parallel to the ultrasound beam direction. Lateral resolution governs any dimension measured transversely at right angles to the beam direction, or across the path of the beam. The focal range of a sonographic transducer is the depth at which the sound beam width (lateral resolution) is narrowest or best focused (Fig. 16-1).

Axial resolution is related directly to the frequency of the sound and the pulse length and reproduction rate of those pulses producing the sonographic beam. Short and frequent pulses yield the greatest axial resolution. An ultrasound system cannot distinguish the echoes from two structures separated by less than the length of a single pulse. This explains why transducers that produce higher frequency sound usually produce shorter pulses and therefore have better axial resolution.[14] Accordingly, a sonographer should use the

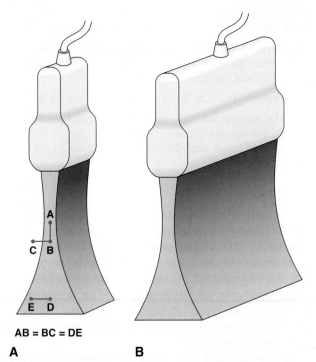

AB = BC = DE

A   **B**

Figure 16-1 Axial and lateral resolution. A stylized drawing of the shape of a linear array transducer beam and the resulting field of view (FOV). The focal range is at the narrowest portion of the beam. In this image, there is equal distance between various points. AB = CB = ED. Lateral resolution images points C & B and E & D; however, the decreased distance between D & E fails to demonstrate separate echoes due to the thickness of the beam width. Axial resolution demonstrates separation of points A & B. (From DuBose TJ. Fetal Sonography, Philadephia, WB Saunders, 1996; p 73.)

highest-frequency transducer that produces adequate penetration and diagnostic-quality images.

Lateral resolution is related to beam width. In general, the wider the beam of sound, the wider a single echo in the image will appear. An ultrasound system cannot separate echoes that are closer together than the width of the beam. A beam width artifact tends to make measurement points a bit fuzzy.[9,12] Cursors should be placed at the edge of the most definite echo observed but should not include the beam width artifact.

It is important for the sonographer to understand how the orientation of a measured fetal structure affects fetal measurement accuracy with regard to axial and lateral resolution. In general, images obtained along the beam axis using the axial resolution have the least measurement error, whereas measurements taken transversely to the beam using lateral resolution have the greatest errors. Usually only the BPD and the diameter of the fetal abdomen that are parallel to the beam can take advantage of the lesser measurement errors obtained using axial resolution. Almost all other parameters are measured using lateral resolution and exhibit some indistinctness at the edges owing to beam width artifact. To obtain measurements of the greatest accuracy, the sonographer must exercise judgment and skill to select the appropriate transducer, obtain images, and place cursors for measurements.

Although any modern real-time transducer can be used effectively for fetal measurements, curvilinear and linear-array transducers, with their larger near field of view, make measurements easier to obtain in advanced pregnancy.[13] All transducers used to obtain measurements should be tested for accuracy. Sonographers can test for proper equipment function using an American Institute of Ultrasound in Medicine (AIUM) Standard Test Object or other acceptable phantoms. If measurements on the test object appear inaccurate, the machine should be recalibrated by an authorized service person. Generally, sonographic measurement errors in the range of 1% to 2% (1 or 2 mm/10 cm) may be expected.[14] These standard errors may be due to beam width, machine calibration, and cursor placement variation.[14-16]

MULTIPLE FETAL PARAMETERS TECHNIQUE

Because all fetuses are proportioned differently, it must be recognized that any single fetal parameter, used alone, may not be as specific an indicator of fetal age as desired. This is especially true later in pregnancy. This can be an important consideration with serial studies for fetal growth and development, because in subsequent examinations fetal position or other changing conditions may preclude exact replication of a set of fetal measurements used in earlier examinations. It has been found that in cases of premature rupture of the membranes, the external uterine pressure on the fetal skull can produce measurement errors in BPD as well as the cephalic index in as many as 45% of the cases.[17-19]

Other problems may occur in progressive diseases such as hydrocephalus or maternal diabetes. If only one or two measurement parameters are used, then in the event of progressive abnormalities or changing fetal or intrauterine conditions one may have difficulty comparing biometric information on follow-up examinations. For this reason, it is recommended that the following measurements be obtained routinely as a minimum: head measurements (BPD and HC), abdominal circumference (AC), and the length of at least one extremity long bone, preferably the femur. As a rule, the more measurements obtained and averaged, the more accurate the fetal age estimate.

In 1983, Hadlock and coworkers[20] found that throughout pregnancy an average gestational age determined from multiple fetal parameters (BPD, HC, AC, and the femoral diaphysis length [FL]) yielded a more accurate estimation of fetal age throughout gestation than any single parameter used alone. They referred to this average age as the multiple fetal parameter (MFP) average age.[20,21] This research was replicated and confirmed in 1986 by Ott.[22] The average of MFP is a more accurate indicator of fetal age for two reasons. Fetal parameters obtained early in gestation are so small that any error in measurement due to the limits of resolution in the sonographic instrument used or to operator error will be relatively larger. In addition, late in gestation there is more molding of the fetal skull, leading at times to relative dolichocephaly and brachycephaly, and other individuation of fetal proportions (i.e., some fetuses are fatter, some thinner, some longer, and some shorter). Using multiple parameters tends to minimize these errors and average out normal individual variations.[1,3] Inherent in the concept of estimating age from an average of MFPs is the idea that no single parameter is a perfect indicator of fetal age.[1,2] This is because all people have slightly different proportions.

Fetal parameter ages can also be estimated using polynomial formulas.[1] Sonographic equipment often uses these complex formulas as built-in software to estimate fetal ages and weights. The operator only needs to take the parameter measurement and the formula calculations are invisible to the sonographer.

MEASUREMENT TECHNIQUES IN THE SECOND AND THIRD TRIMESTER

FETAL HEAD MEASUREMENTS

Biparietal Diameter

The fetal BPD has long been a primary sonographic measurement for determining fetal age. The BPD is usually easy to obtain, has a distinctive appearance, and provides a relatively accurate measurement.

The BPD measurement carries a small interobserver variance or error (usually <2 mm), but molding and normal morphologic variations of the fetal head have a greater effect on the accuracy of BPD in assessing age. These effects and the lesser reliability of the BPD measurements tend to be greatest after the 33rd menstrual week, when extrinsic pressure on the fetal skull is greatest. The resulting fetal skull molding makes the BPD a less accurate parameter for fetal age after that time. The BPD can also be affected by oligohydramnios, which can enhance molding of the skull.[18,19,23]

Most of the published BPD charts were created using leading edge measurements (outer skull table to inner skull table) obtained in a transverse view with a lateral approach (Fig. 16-2). The plane of this transverse view has been widely described. Accurate measurements at this level are obtained through the use of the leading edges of the parietal bones, which reflect very sharp, specular echoes enhanced by the axial resolution of the sound beam. The normally circular shape of the skull in the coronal plane makes the BPD easy to obtain and relatively accurate in normally shaped heads.[17]

Measurement Methods

The BPD can be measured routinely from 12 weeks' gestation and occasionally earlier. The sonographer must first identify the fetal lie. Beginning transversely at the base of the fetal cranium, the sonographer locates the base X formed by the sphenoid bones (bilateral anteriorly) and petrous bones (bilateral posteriorly) (Fig. 16-3). The proper plane for the BPD lies parallel to and above this base X.[24-26] From the base X, move the plane of view higher in the skull until the thalamus and cavum septi pellucidi appear.[2,24-26] For an optimal measurement, the entire calvarium forms a complete oval. A transverse plane that includes the top of the cerebellum is too low in the posterior portion of the image.

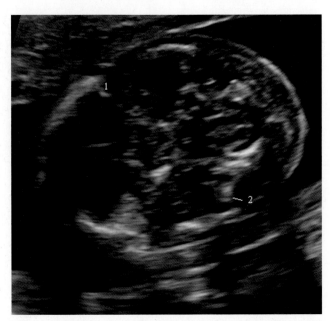

Figure 16-3 Transverse fetal head at the base of the skull demonstrates the base X formed by the bilateral sphenoid bones (1) anterior and the bilateral petrous (2) bones posterior.

The BPD is measured from the fetal parietal bones that form the lateral walls of the skull (Fig. 16-4 and 19-2). Measure the BPD at the widest transverse diameter of the skull, just above the ears. The view for the BPD measurement should be made perpendicular to the interhemispheric fissure (midline) in either the transverse or coronal plane and should include the thalamus.[1,2] Exclude the soft tissue of the scalp when measuring from the leading edge of the parietal bone. Decreasing the system overall gain helps distinguish soft tissue from bone; the bone echoes persist at the lower settings.

If the fetus's face is turned directly toward or away from the maternal spine or if the fetus's head is low in the pelvis, behind the maternal pubic bone, measurement of the BPD may be difficult. When the fetus's head is low in the pelvis, a slight Trendelenburg position (maternal pelvis elevated, head lowered) sometimes helps to bring the head out of the mother's pelvis. The fetus may move to a more convenient position in response to the mother's changing position or if the sonographer proceeds with other parts of the examination and returns later to try the measurement again. As uncooperative as fetuses may be, an experienced sonographer should be able to obtain accurate BPD measurements at least 95% of the time. In the rare event of an extremely uncooperative fetus when no satisfactory BPD can be obtained, other fetal parameters may serve as indicators of fetal age. If the fetal head is very low in the pelvis, an endovaginal transducer may allow BPD measurements.[17]

The accuracy of the predictive value of the BPD (Table 16-1) has been reported by some authors as ±3 weeks

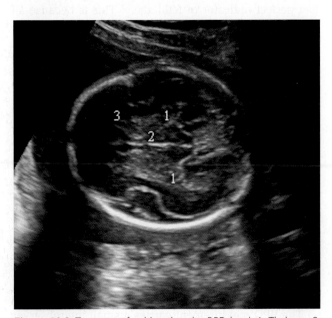

Figure 16-2 Transverse fetal head at the BPD level. 1. Thalmus. 2. Falx. 3. Cavum septum pellucidum.

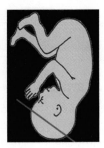

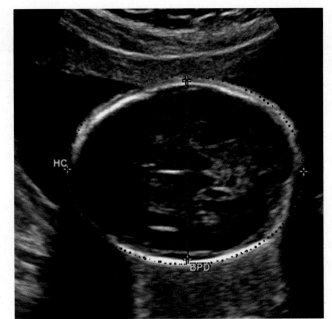

Figure 16-4 Transverse fetal head measuring BPD and HC. These measurements should be performed on the same image. Measurement of the BPD is from the outer margin of the nearest calvarium margin to the inner margin of the furthest calvarium margin. Measure the HC at the outer margin of the calvaria.

TABLE	16-1

BPD Tables - Hadlock 84

BPD (mm)	GA (wks)	+/- 2 SD	BPD (mm)	GA (wks)	+/- 2 SD	BPD (mm)	GA (wks)	+/- 2 SD	BPD (mm)	GA (wks)	+/- 2 SD
<14	na	——	36	17.0	1.2	59	24.1	2.2	82	33.0	3.1
14	11.9	1.2	37	17.3	1.2	60	24.5	2.2	83	33.4	3.1
15	12.1	1.2	38	17.6	1.2	61	24.8	2.2	84	33.8	3.1
16	12.3	1.2	39	17.9	1.2	62	25.2	2.2	85	34.2	3.1
17	12.5	1.2	40	18.1	1.7	63	25.5	2.2	86	34.7	3.1
18	12.8	1.2	41	18.4	1.7	64	25.9	2.2	87	35.1	3.1
19	13.0	1.2	42	18.7	1.7	65	26.3	2.2	88	35.6	3.1
20	13.2	1.2	43	19.0	1.7	66	26.6	2.2	89	36.0	3.2
21	13.4	1.2	44	19.3	1.7	67	27.0	2.2	90	36.5	3.2
22	13.6	1.2	45	19.6	1.7	68	27.4	2.2	91	36.9	3.2
23	13.8	1.2	46	19.9	1.7	69	27.7	2.2	92	37.4	3.2
24	14.1	1.2	47	20.2	1.7	70	28.1	2.2	93	37.8	3.2
25	14.3	1.2	48	20.5	1.7	71	28.5	2.2	94	38.3	3.2
26	14.5	1.2	49	20.8	1.7	72	28.9	2.2	95	38.7	3.2
27	14.8	1.2	50	21.1	1.7	73	29.3	2.2	96	39.2	3.2
28	15.0	1.2	51	21.5	1.7	74	29.7	2.2	97	39.7	3.2
29	15.2	1.2	52	21.8	1.7	75	30.1	3.1	98	40.2	3.2
30	15.5	1.2	53	22.1	1.7	76	30.5	3.1	99	40.6	3.2
31	15.7	1.2	54	22.4	1.7	77	30.9	3.1	100	41.1	3.2
32	16.0	1.2	55	22.8	1.7	78	31.3	3.1	101	41.6	3.2
33	16.3	1.2	56	23.1	1.7	79	31.7	3.1	102	42.1	3.2
34	16.5	1.2	57	23.4	1.7	80	32.1	3.1	103	42.6	3.2
35	16.8	1.2	58	23.8	1.7	81	32.5	3.1	>103	na	——

Hadlock FP, Deter RL, Harrist RB, et al. Estimating fetal age: computer-assisted analysis of multiple fetal growth parameters, *Radiology.* 1984;152(2):497–501.

TABLE 16-1 (continued)											
BPD - Jeanty											

					GA (WKS + DAYS)						
BPD (cm)	**5%**	**50%**	**95%**	**BPD (cm)**	**5%**	**50%**	**95%**	**BPD (cm)**	**5%**	**50%**	**95%**
1.00	6w4d	9w1d	11w6d	4.00	14w4d	17w2d	1 9w6d	6.90	24w0d	26w5d	29w3d
1.10	6w6d	9w4d	12w1d	4.10	14w6d	17w4d	20w1d	7.00	24w3d	27w1d	29w6d
1.30	7w2d	10w0d	12w5d	4.20	15w1d	17w6d	20w4d	7.10	24w6d	27w4d	30w1d
1.40	7w4d	10w2d	12w6d	4.30	15w3d	18w1d	20w6d	7.20	25w1d	27w6d	30w4d
1.50	7w6d	10w4d	13w1d	4.40	15w5d	18w3d	21w1d	7.30	25w4d	28w2d	30w6d
1.60	8w1d	10w6d	13w3d	4.50	16w0d	18w5d	21w3d	7.40	26w0d	28w5d	31w2d
1.70	8w3d	11w1d	13w5d	4.60	16w2d	19w0d	21w5d	7.50	26w3d	29w1d	31w5d
1.80	8w4d	11w2d	14w0d	4.70	16w4d	19w2d	22w0d	7.60	26w6d	29w4d	32w1d
1.90	8w6d	11w4d	14w1d	4.80	16w6d	19w4d	22w2d	7.70	27w1d	29w6d	32w4d
2.00	9w1d	11w6d	14w4d	4.90	17w1d	19w6d	22w4d	7.80	27w4d	30w2d	33w0d
2.10	9w3d	12w1d	14w6d	5.00	17w4d	20w2d	22w6d	7.90	28w0d	30w5d	33w3d
2.20	9w5d	12w3d	15w0d	5.10	17w6d	20w4d	23w1d	8.00	28w4d	31w1d	33w6d
2.30	9w6d	12w4d	15w2d	5.20	18w1d	20w6d	23w4d	8.10	28w6d	31w4d	34w2d
2.40	10w1d	12w6d	15w4d	5.30	18w4d	21w1d	23w6d	8.20	29w2d	32w0d	34w5d
2.50	10w4d	13w1d	15w6d	5.40	18w6d	21w4d	24w1d	8.30	29w6d	32w4d	35w1d
2.60	10w5d	13w3d	16w1d	5.50	19w1d	21w6d	24w4d	8.40	30w1d	32w6d	35w4d
2.70	11w0d	13w5d	16w3d	5.60	19w4d	22w1d	24w6d	8.50	30w5d	33w3d	36w0d
2.80	11w2d	14w0d	16w4d	5.70	19w6d	22w4d	25w1d	8.60	31w1d	33w6d	36w4d
2.90	11w4d	14w1d	16w6d	5.80	20w1d	22w6d	25w4d	8.70	31w4d	34w2d	37w0d
3.00	11w6d	14w4d	17w1d	5.90	20w4d	23w1d	25w6d	8.80	32w1d	34w6d	37w3d
3.10	12w1d	14w6d	17w3d	6.00	20w6d	23w4d	26w1d	8.90	32w4d	35w2d	37w6d
3.20	12w2d	15w1d	17w5d	6.10	21w1d	23w6d	26w4d	9.00	33w0d	35w5d	38w3d
3.30	12w4d	15w2d	18w0d	6.20	21w4d	24w1d	26w6d	9.10	33w4d	36w1d	38w6d
3.40	12w6d	15w4d	18w2d	6.30	21w6d	24w4d	27w1d	9.20	34w0d	36w5d	39w3d
3.50	13w1d	15w6d	18w4d	6.40	22w1d	24w6d	27w4d	9.30	34w4d	37w1d	39w6d
3.60	13w4d	16w1d	18w6d	6.50	22w4d	25w2d	27w6d	9.40	35w0d	37w5d	40w3d
3.70	13w5d	16w3d	19w1d	6.60	22w6d	25w4d	28w2d	9.50	35w4d	38w2d	40w6d
3.80	14w0d	16w5d	19w3d	6.70	23w2d	26w0d	28w4d				
3.90	14w2d	17w0d	19w5d	6.80	23w5d	26w3d	29w0d				

Jeanty P, Romero R. *Obstetrical Ultrasound.* McGraw-Hill Book Company; 1984;57–61.

from 29 weeks LMP to term.[2] However, many consider the BPD reliable to (±2 weeks) only until about 30 weeks' LMP.[2] Consequently, if the BPD is going to be used to estimate fetal age, the measurement should be obtained before 33 weeks LMP.[2]

Transverse Head Circumference

The transverse head circumference (HC) was first suggested as an indicator of fetal age by Levi and Erbsman in 1975.[27] Many authors have suggested that the BPD may be inaccurate owing to normal variations in head shape and molding.[1-3,14,18,23,25-30] The consistency of the fetal head has been referred to as plastic.[28] If pressure against the external lateral wall(s) of the skull shortens the BPD, the long and/or vertical axis is displaced and lengthened. Likewise, if the long and/or vertical axis is compressed, the width (BPD) of the skull is enlarged to compensate. Therefore, two-dimensional (2D) circumferences of the fetal skull are more accurate than one-dimensional (1D)

diameters. Hadlock and colleagues found that using the two diameters in the formula for the circumference resulted in essentially the same measurement as direct outlining methods, if the BPD and occipito-frontal diameter (OFD) are measured outer edge to outer edge.[50] Because hand-tracing outlining methods are tedious and slow, the use of ellipse drawing tools or the two-diameter method to calculate the circumference is generally recommended (Fig. 16-4). Whatever method is employed, a chart that was generated using the same method should be used to evaluate fetal age (Table 16-2). If one wishes to measure the HC using the perimeter tracing method, the measurement should be made around the outer edge of the calvarium. The head circumference should be measured on the same image used for the BPD. This transverse view should include the cavum septi pellucidi, interhemispheric fissure (midline), and thalamus. The greatest source of error in measuring the HC is selection of a calvarial image in an improper or angled plane.

TABLE 16-2

Hadlock 84

HEAD CIRCUMFERENCE (CM)											
HC (mm)	GA (wks)	+/− 2SD	HC (mm)	GA (wks)	+/− 2SD	HC (mm)	GA (wks)	+/− 2SD	HC (mm)	GA (wks)	+/− 2SD
<55	n/a	——	135	17.0	1.2	215	23.6	1.5	290	31.9	3.0
55	12.0	1.2	140	17.3	1.2	219	23.9	1.5	295	32.6	3.0
60	12.3	1.2	145	17.7	1.2	220	24.0	2.1	300	33.3	3.0
65	12.6	1.2	149	18.0	1.2	225	24.5	2.1	305	33.9	3.0
70	12.8	1.2	150	18.1	1.5	230	25.0	2.1	310	34.6	3.0
75	13.1	1.2	155	18.4	1.5	235	25.5	2.1	315	35.3	3.0
80	13.4	1.2	160	18.8	1.5	240	26.1	2.1	319	35.9	3.0
85	13.7	1.2	165	19.2	1.5	245	26.6	2.1	320	36.1	2.7
90	14.0	1.2	170	19.6	1.5	250	27.1	2.1	325	36.8	2.7
95	14.3	1.2	175	20.0	1.5	255	27.7	2.1	330	37.6	2.7
100	14.7	1.2	180	20.4	1.5	260	28.3	2.1	335	38.3	2.7
105	15.0	1.2	185	20.8	1.5	265	28.9	2.1	340	39.1	2.7
110	15.3	1.2	190	21.3	1.5	270	29.4	2.1	345	39.9	2.7
115	15.6	1.2	195	21.7	1.5	274	29.9	2.1	350	40.7	2.7
120	16.0	1.2	200	22.2	1.5	275	30.0	3.0	355	41.6	2.7
125	16.3	1.2	205	22.6	1.5	280	30.7	3.0	360	42.4	2.7
130	16.6	1.2	210	23.1	1.5	285	31.3	3.0	>360	n/a	——

Hadlock FP, Deter RL, Harrist RB, et al. Estimating fetal age: computer-assisted analysis of multiple fetal growth parameters. *Radiology*. 1984;152(2):497–501.

Jeanty

HEAD CIRCUMFERENCE (CM)						
GA (wks)	5%	50%	95%	GA (wks)	5%	50%	95%
10	2.60	5.00	7.40	26	21.80	24.20	26.60
11	3.80	6.30	8.70	27	22.80	25.20	27.70
12	5.10	7.50	10.00	28	23.80	26.20	28.60
13	6.40	8.80	11.20	29	24.70	27.10	29.60
14	7.60	10.10	12.50	30	25.60	28.10	30.50
15	8.90	11.30	13.80	31	26.50	28.90	31.30
16	10.10	12.60	15.00	32	27.30	29.70	32.20
17	11.40	13.80	16.30	33	28.10	30.50	32.90
18	12.60	15.10	17.50	34	28.80	31.20	33.60
19	13.80	16.30	18.70	35	29.40	31.90	34.30
20	15.00	17.50	19.90	36	30.00	32.50	34.90
21	16.20	18.70	21.10	37	30.60	33.00	35.50
22	17.40	19.80	22.30	38	31.10	33.50	35.90
23	18.50	21.00	23.40	39	31.50	33.90	36.40
24	19.60	22.10	24.50	40	31.90	34.30	36.70
25	20.70	23.20	25.60				

Jeanty P, Cousaert E, Hobbins JC, et al. A longitudinal study of fetal head biometry. *Am J Perinatol*. 1984;1(2):118–128.

A shortened HC measurement can result if the proper transverse plane is not used

Measurement Methods

The HC can be measured directly from the frozen image using an ellipse-drawing function to trace the outline of the skull or by measuring two perpendicular diameters and calculating the circumference. The average of two diameters of the fetal skull—the outer-to-outer axial measurement and an outer-to-outer frontal to occipital measurement taken at the same level as the BPD—is used in the following formula for the circumference of a circle: Circumference = $(D1 + D2) \times 1.57$

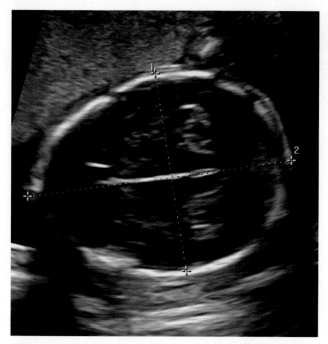

Figure 16-5 Measurements of fetal cranium. BPD *(1)* and OFD *(2)*.

The OFD is measured outer edge to outer edges of the middle of the frontal bone and the occipital bone echoes (Fig. 16-5).[1,2,14]

Cephalic Index

Normal skulls have variable shapes. The cephalic index (CI = BPD/FOD × 100) is used to determine if the shape of the transverse fetal skull can allow a reliable BPD measurement. The CI does not address the variation of the vertical axis of the head.[14] Usually, the normal CI is <80% (±9%) in about 95% of fetuses. These percentages vary somewhat from investigator to investigator, depending on how the head measurements are taken.[2,14]

A fetus with a long and narrow or dolichocephalic head has a relatively short BPD measurement, and the CI is below normal. A fetus whose BPD is relatively wide and whose FOD is short is called brachycephalic; the CI is greater than normal and again suggests an unreliable BPD measurement (CI > 89%). Other fetal head dysmorphisms such as acrocephaly, turricephaly, and oxycephaly in which the calvarium is relatively high (a sort of "cone-headedness") may be missed using the CI, in that all have vertical diameters of the cranium that are greater or less than normal.[2,14] An apparent reverse oxycephaly is called platycephaly. It often occurs late in pregnancy or when crowding of the fetus puts pressure on the vertex of the skull, causing shortening of the vertical dimension of the skull and widening of both diameters of the transverse plane (BPD and OFD), which may not affect the CI (Fig. 16-6).

Transverse Cerebellum Measurement

Another commonly used measurement for gestational age and growth is the transverse cerebellar diameter (Figs. 16-7 and 19-3). The cerebellum maintains a relationship to the gestational age and is independent of the shape of the cranium.[31] Cerebellar size is also relatively unaffected by fetal growth disturbances (Table 16-3).[31,32]

Measurement Method

Beginning transversely at the base of the fetal cranium, the sonographer again locates the base X formed by the sphenoid bones (bilateral anteriorly) and petrous bones (bilateral posteriorly) (Fig. 16-3). The correct plane for the cerebellum lies parallel to and above this base X.

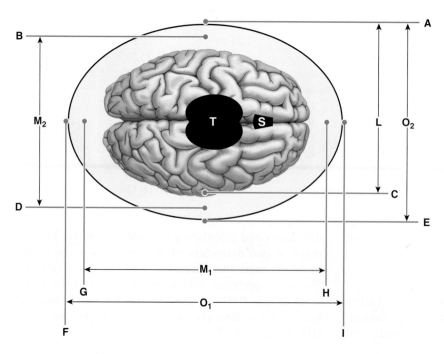

Figure 16-6 Transverse head circumference demonstrating various locations to measure the fetal skull. Here O_1 = outer-to-outer FOD; M_1 = mid-to-mid FOD; O_2 and M_2 = outer-to-outer and mid-to-mid BPDs. L = leading-edge to leading-edge BPD; t = thalamus and S = cavum septum pellucid. Algebraically $O_2/O_1 = M_2/M_1$ and $L = M_2$; therefore $O_2/O_1 = L/M_1$. The most common measurement technique is the leading-edge to leading-edge BPD (L). Beam width artifacts tend to exaggerate the outer-to-outer FOD; however, use of the mid-to-mid FOD (M_1) preserves the normal ratio increasing the accuracy of M_1. The same physics applies to the use of the ellipse tools to trace AHCG or BHDG. (From DuBose TJ. Fetal Sonography, Philadephia, WB Saunders, 1996; p 73.)

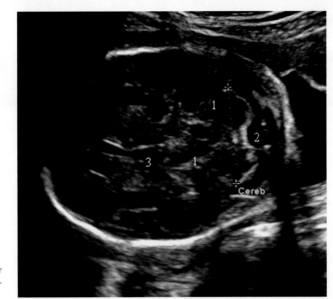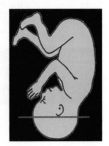

Figure 16-7 Transverse cerebellar diameter (measured). Cerebellar hemispheres *(1)*. Cisterna Magna *(2)*. Falx *(3)*.

TABLE	16-3

Transverse Cerebellar Diameter

CEREBELLUM (CM)							
GA (wks)	10%	50%	90%	GA (wks)	10%	50%	90%
15	1.00	1.40	1.60	28	2.70	3.10	3.40
16	1.40	1.60	1.70	29	2.90	3.40	3.80
17	1.60	1.70	1.80	30	3.10	3.50	4.00
18	1.70	1.80	1.90	31	3.20	3.80	4.30
19	1.80	1.90	2.20	32	3.30	3.80	4.20
20	1.80	2.00	2.20	33	3.20	4.00	4.40
21	1.90	2.20	2.40	34	3.30	4.00	4.40
22	2.10	2.30	2.40	35	3.10	4.05	4.70
23	2.20	2.40	2.60	36	3.60	4.30	5.50
24	2.20	2.50	2.80	37	3.70	4.50	5.50
25	2.30	2.80	2.90	38	4.00	4.85	5.50
26	2.50	2.90	3.20	39	5.20	5.20	5.50
27	2.60	3.00	3.20				

Goldstein I, Reece EA, Pilu G, et al. Cerebellar measurement with ultrasonography in the evaluation of fetal growth and development. *Am J Obstet Gynecol.* 1987;156(5):1065–1069.

CEREBELLUM (CM)					
GA (wks)	Mean	+/− 2SD	GA (wks)	Mean	+/− 2SD
15	1.50	0.30	28	3.30	0.40
16	1.60	0.20	29	3.40	0.40
17	1.70	0.20	30	3.70	0.40
18	1.80	0.20	31	3.90	0.40
19	2.00	0.20	32	4.10	0.50
20	2.00	0.30	33	4.30	0.50
21	2.20	0.30	34	4.60	0.90
22	2.30	0.30	35	4.70	0.70
23	2.40	0.30	36	4.90	0.90
24	2.60	0.40	37	5.10	1.10
25	2.80	0.40	38	5.10	1.21
26	3.00	0.40	39	5.20	1.00
27	3.00	0.40	40	5.20	0.80

Hill LM, Guzick D, Fries J, et al. The transverse cerebellar diameter in estimating gestational age in the large for gestational age fetus. *Obstet Gynecol.* 1990;75(6):981–985.

TABLE 16-4 Fetal Orbital Diameter Binocular Distance (BOD) (mm)							
GA (wks)	5%	50%	95%	GA (wks)	5%	50%	95%
11	5	13	20	26	36	44	51
12	8	15	23	27	38	45	53
13	10	18	25	28	39	47	54
14	13	20	28	29	41	48	56
15	15	22	30	30	42	50	57
16	17	25	32	31	43	51	58
17	19	27	34	32	45	52	60
18	22	29	37	33	46	53	61
19	24	31	39	34	47	54	62
20	26	33	41	35	48	55	63
21	28	35	43	36	49	56	64
22	30	37	44	37	50	57	65
23	31	39	46	38	50	58	65
24	33	41	48	39	51	59	66
25	35	42	50	40	52	59	67

Romero R, Pilu G, Jeanty P, et al. *Prenatal Diagnosis of Congenital Anomalies.* Norwalk, CT, Appleton & Lange, 1988; p 83.

From the base X, the plane of view is moved higher in the skull until the hemispheres of the cerebellum are located (Fig. 16-7).

Binocular Measurement

The distance from the outer edges of the left and right fetal eyes is called the binocular distance (BOD).[14] The BOD is useful when fetal position makes the BPD or other measurements difficult to obtain (Table 16-4). To measure the BOD, both orbits must be imaged at their greatest diameters. The outer orbit-to-outer-orbit (OOD) distance is measured from the edges of the skeletal orbit (Fig. 16-8 and 19-9). It must be pointed out that this measurement may also be difficult to obtain at times owing to fetal position. Late in gestation, fetal nasal bones tend to shadow the detail of the eye farthest from the transducer during lateral scans. These shadowing effects of the nasal bones may cause the observer to measure to the inside of the lateral retina at times or to the inner surface of the zygoma at other times.

The diameters of the individual globes of the eyes and the interocular (between the eyes) distance (IOD) have also been used to estimate fetal growth.[3] Because these measurements are relatively small, any error in cursor placement will cause a relatively large percentage error. For this reason, the larger BOD is favored.

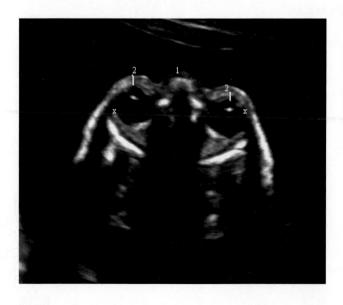

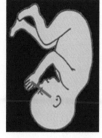

Figure 16-8 Fetal orbits. Nasal bone *(1)*, Lenses of the eyes *(2)*, binocular distance *(x)*.

FETAL BODY MEASUREMENTS

Abdominal Circumference

AC is a valuable indicator of fetal growth because it reflects the development of abdominal organs such as the liver and spleen. Few other fetal parameters are so often mismeasured as the AC. Because most modern formulas for estimating fetal weight rely heavily on this measurement, its importance cannot be overemphasized. Abdominal measurements can also be affected by the degree of spinal flexion, fetal breathing motion, sonographic technique, and accurate visualization of the skin line.

The measurement of the AC is performed at the standard transverse abdominal level where the umbilical and portal veins are confluent. This is usually the largest transverse section of the abdomen and is also reflective of the size of the spleen, and particularly the liver, which are indicators of fetal health and well-being. The liver is proportionately larger in the fetus than in the adult.[33] The AC measurement also reflects the amount of subcutaneous fat, which has a large influence on fetal weight. The AC is considered more important as an indicator of fetal weight and health than as an indicator of fetal age (Table 16-5).[2,14]

Measurement Methods

The standard view for obtaining the AC is at the level of the umbilical vein junction with the portal vein and perpendicular to the spine.[2,14] The AC should be circular. If the plane used to measure the AC is oblique to the spine, one axis will be elongated, resulting in an erroneously large measurement.

A successful measuring technique for obtaining the fetal AC is to first visualize the long axis of the fetal spine. After the lie of the spine is observed, the transducer field of view is turned perpendicular to the midportion of the spine; the fetal stomach and umbilical vein are then located. The favored view will demonstrate the confluence of the umbilical and portal veins in the fetal liver, called the "hockey stick" or "J" view by some. If these veins cannot be visualized owing to fetal position or maternal obesity, then a section demonstrating the fluid-filled fetal stomach is acceptable. It is important, however, when using the stomach as a landmark, not to mistake fluid in the lower gastrointestinal tract for the stomach. Measurements above or below the standard hockey stick view may produce an erroneously small AC.[2,14] Observation of heart motion indicates a plane superior to the proper AC plane. Visualization of both fetal kidneys is an indication that the section is too low for accurate AC

TABLE 16-5											
Hadlock 84											
AC											
AC (mm)	GA (wks)	+/− 2SD	AC (mm)	GA (wks)	+/− 2SD	AC (mm)	GA (wks)	+/− 2SD	AC (mm)	GA (wks)	+/− 2SD
<50	na	——	135	19.0	2.1	225	26.9	2.2	315	35.4	3.0
50	12.0	1.7	140	19.4	2.1	230	27.4	2.2	320	35.9	3.0
55	12.4	1.7	145	19.8	2.1	235	27.8	2.2	321	36.0	3.1
60	12.8	1.7	150	20.2	2.1	240	28.3	2.2	325	36.4	3.1
65	13.2	1.7	155	20.7	2.1	245	28.7	2.2	330	36.9	3.1
70	13.6	1.7	160	21.1	2.1	250	29.2	2.2	335	37.4	3.1
75	14.0	1.7	165	21.5	2.1	255	29.7	2.2	340	37.9	3.1
80	14.4	1.7	170	22.0	2.1	258	30.0	2.2	345	38.4	3.1
85	14.8	1.7	175	22.4	2.1	259	30.1	3.0	350	38.9	3.1
90	15.2	1.7	180	22.9	2.1	260	30.2	3.0	355	39.4	3.1
95	15.6	1.7	185	23.3	2.1	265	30.6	3.0	360	39.9	3.1
100	16.0	1.7	190	23.7	2.1	270	31.1	3.0	365	40.4	3.1
105	16.4	1.7	192	23.9	2.1	275	31.6	3.0	370	40.9	3.1
110	16.9	1.7	193	24.0	2.2	280	32.0	3.0	375	41.4	3.1
115	17.3	1.7	195	24.2	2.2	285	32.5	3.0	380	42.0	3.1
120	17.7	1.7	200	24.6	2.2	290	33.0	3.0	385	42.5	3.1
123	17.8	1.7	205	25.1	2.2	295	33.5	3.0	>385	na	——
124	18.0	2.1	210	25.5	2.2	300	34.0	3.0			
125	18.1	2.1	215	26.0	2.2	305	34.5	3.0			
130	18.5	2.1	220	26.4	2.2	310	34.9	3.0			

Hadlock FP, Deter RL, Harrist RB, et al. Estimating fetal age: computer-assisted analysis of multiple fetal growth parameters. *Radiology*. 1984;152(2):497–501.

TABLE 16-5 (continued)

Jeanty

CM					
AC (cm)	GA (w+d)	AC (cm)	GA (w+d)	AC (cm)	GA (w+d)
5.00	11w2d	14.00	19w6d	23.00	28w3d
5.50	11w5d	14.50	20w2d	23.50	29w0d
6.00	12w1d	15.00	20w6d	24.00	29w3d
6.50	12w5d	15.50	21w2d	24.50	30w0d
7.00	13w1d	16.00	21w5d	25.00	30w4d
7.50	13w4d	16.50	22w2d	25.50	31w1d
8.00	14w1d	17.00	22w5d	26.00	31w5d
8.50	14w4d	17.50	23w1d	26.50	32w2d
9.00	15w0d	18.00	23w5d	27.00	32w6d
9.50	15w4d	18.50	24w1d	27.50	33w3d
10.00	16w0d	19.00	24w4d	28.00	34w1d
10.50	16w3d	19.50	25w1d	28.50	34w6d
11.00	17w0d	20.00	25w4d	29.00	35w4d
11.50	17w3d	20.50	26w0d	29.50	36w2d
12.00	17w6d	21.00	26w4d	30.00	37w0d
12.50	18w3d	21.50	27w0d	30.50	37w6d
13.00	18w6d	22.00	27w3d	31.00	38w6d
13.50	19w2d	22.50	28w0d	31.50	39w6d

Jeanty P, Cousaert E, Cantraine F. Normal growth of the abdominal perimeter. *Am J Perinatol.* 1984;1(2):129–135.

measurement.[14] The lower ribs may normally be observed bilaterally and, if seen, should be symmetric.

After the AC view is obtained and the image frozen, two options for circumference calculation are available: a trace or ellipse calculation of the fetal abdomen for circumference calculation or using perpendicular abdominal diameters (Fig. 16-9). All measurements are from the outer skin lines. Using abdominal diameter measurements, the transverse diameter (TAD) is measured from side to side, and the antero-posterior abdominal diameter (APD) is taken from the skin line above the umbilical cord insertion to the skin line just behind the spine. Care must be taken to measure to the skin line so that the resulting circumference is not underestimated. The formula for two-point calculation is AC = $1.57 \times (d_1 + d_2)$, where d_1 and d_2 are the two diameters of the abdomen.[1,14] The resulting AC will be in the same units as the diameters (i.e., diameters measured in millimeters will yield an AC in millimeters).

Acoustic shadowing from extremities or the spine can also make the skin line difficult to see in some segments of the AC. The ellipse drawing function of modern machines can also be used. It often helps to look at the "full circle" of the abdomen rather than to focus attention on a single area. The abdominal circumference can also be manually traced, but this method is subject to error and very cumbersome. Measurements should be taken several times and observed for a cluster range, eliminating any measurements falling outside of the "best" cluster. The best measurements are averaged for the measurement of record.

Sonographers should be sure that the measurements extend to the outer abdominal wall and not just to the fetal peritoneal lining. This error is most common when a lateral approach to the abdomen is used and when positioning the caliper for the deep abdominal wall. The peritoneal cavity wall and ribs often generate very strong specular echoes. This may lead to errors resulting in underestimation of the AC by excluding the hypoechoic skin, muscle, and baby fat from the measurement.

FETAL EXTREMITIES MEASUREMENTS

Long Bones

The fetal long bones are good indicators of fetal growth. Although the head and abdomen may be subject to changes in shape resulting from molding or position, the long bones are not. A limiting factor in using long bones for measurements is that they are affected by the genetic pool; tall parents tend to have long babies. The accuracy of the humerus, tibia, and ulna measurements in predicting fetal age are considered by some researchers to be approximately ±3 weeks at term. Femur length dating accuracy is better in the first part of pregnancy because phenotypic differences (i.e. tall, short) do not exhibit as much as in the third trimester. At term, the femur length accuracy is about ± 2.2 weeks.[2] Fetal femur length has been shown to correlate both with fetal age and crown-heel length at birth.[34] Visualization and measurement of any fetal long bone or other linear structure with sonography require some mental

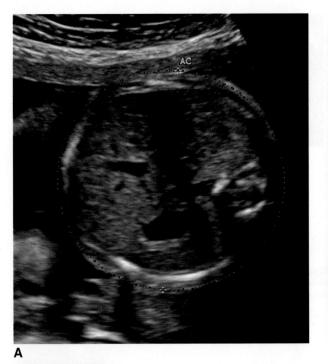

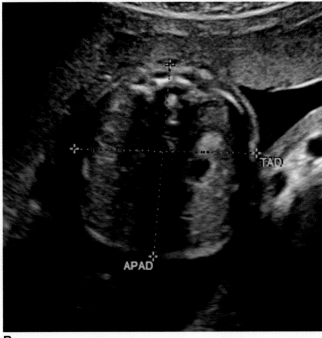

A

B

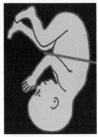

Figure 16-9 A: Transverse fetal abdomen with measurement for abdominal circumference. **B:** Transverse abdomen with APD measurement and transverse diameter measure. The spine is anterior and shadows the umbilical vein landmark.

gymnastics involving eye-hand coordination. The greatest source of error in measuring any long bone occurs when the transducer is positioned slightly oblique to the bone rather than along its axis and, therefore, does not include both ends of the bone. An attempt to exclude the effects of beam width artifacts at the ends of linear structures must be made whenever measurements are taken.

The measurement of the long bones is best accomplished by obtaining several measurements and averaging them for the measurement of record. Usually the average measurement of a single bone is all that is necessary for estimating fetal age. However, all fetal extremities should be visually examined to confirm symmetry and normal morphology.

Femoral Length

The femur is among the most commonly used parameters for estimating fetal age and may be more accurate than the BPD late in pregnancy.[2,14] The femur can be reliably used after 14 weeks' gestation.[3] It is usually called a femur length measurement (FL), but this is a misnomer. The femoral measurement used in obstetric sonography is actually the length of the osseous femoral diaphysis, or shaft, of the bone (Fig. 16-10). This measurement does not include the cartilaginous femoral head or distal femoral condyles (Table 16-6).

To locate the femur, it is first necessary to determine the fetal position (head, spine, and rump). The sonographer can locate the femurs by scanning transversely along the spine until the echogenic, obliquely oriented iliac bones are visible. The transducer is then moved along the iliac bone until the echogenic linear echo produced by the femur is seen. Once the femur's general location is identified, it becomes necessary to angle the transducer until a linear echo with a clean acoustic shadow is generated. The femur may have a slightly curved or bowed appearance when viewed from the posteromedial aspect, but this does not normally affect its length relative to age.[35] The femur nearest the transducer should always be measured.

Humeral Length

The humerus nearest to the transducer is usually easy to find in relationship to the head and spine, but the humerus deep to the transducer is often obscured by the fetal ribs or spine. The humerus has similar measurements to the femur (Table 16-6).[14]

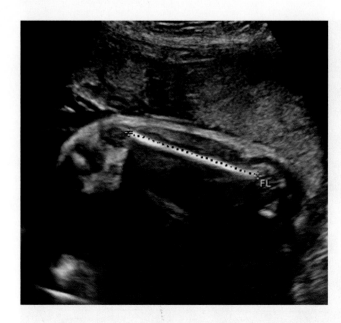

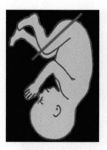

Figure 16-10 This long axis view of the femur demonstrates measurement (calipers) from the proximal end near the femoral neck to the distal epiphyses, including only the ossified portions.

TABLE	16-6								
	Femur (mm)			Tibia (mm)			Fibula (mm)		
GA (wks)	5%	50%	95%	5%	50%	95%	5%	50%	95%
12	3.9	8.1	12.3	3.3	7.2	11.2	1.7	5.7	9.6
13	6.8	11.0	15.2	5.6	9.6	13.6	4.7	8.7	12.7
14	9.7	13.9	18.1	8.1	12.0	16.0	7.7	11.7	15.6
15	12.6	16.8	21.0	10.6	14.6	18.6	10.6	14.6	18.6
16	15.4	19.7	23.9	13.1	17.1	21.2	13.3	17.4	21.4
17	18.3	22.5	26.8	15.6	19.7	23.8	16.1	20.1	24.2
18	21.1	25.4	29.7	18.2	22.3	26.4	18.7	22.8	26.9
19	23.9	28.2	32.6	20.8	24.9	29.0	21.3	25.4	29.5
20	26.7	31.0	35.4	23.3	27.5	31.6	23.8	27.9	32.0
21	29.4	33.8	38.2	25.8	30.0	34.2	26.2	30.3	34.5
22	32.1	36.5	40.9	28.3	32.5	36.7	28.5	32.7	36.9
23	34.7	39.2	43.6	30.7	34.9	39.1	30.8	35.0	39.2
24	37.4	41.8	46.3	33.1	37.3	41.6	33.0	37.2	41.5
25	39.9	44.4	48.9	35.4	39.7	43.9	35.1	39.4	43.6
26	42.4	46.9	51.4	37.6	41.9	46.2	37.2	41.5	45.7
27	44.9	49.4	53.9	39.8	44.1	48.4	39.2	43.5	47.8
28	47.3	51.8	56.4	41.9	46.2	50.5	41.1	45.4	49.7
29	49.6	54.2	58.7	43.9	48.2	52.6	42.9	47.2	51.6
30	51.8	56.4	61.0	45.8	50.1	54.5	44.7	49.0	53.4
31	54.0	58.6	63.2	47.6	52.0	56.4	46.3	50.7	55.1
32	56.1	60.7	65.4	49.4	53.8	58.2	47.9	52.4	56.8
33	58.1	62.7	67.4	51.1	55.5	60.0	49.5	53.9	58.4
34	60.0	64.7	69.4	52.7	57.2	61.6	50.9	55.4	59.9
35	61.8	66.5	71.2	54.2	58.7	63.2	52.3	56.8	61.3
36	63.5	68.3	73.0	55.8	60.3	64.8	53.6	58.2	62.7
37	65.1	69.9	74.7	57.2	61.8	66.3	54.9	59.4	64.0
38	66.6	71.4	76.2	58.7	63.2	67.8	56.0	60.6	65.2
39	68.0	72.8	77.7	60.1	64.7	69.3	57.1	61.7	66.3
40	69.3	74.2	79.0	61.5	66.1	70.7	58.1	62.8	67.4

| TABLE | 16-6 | (continued) | | | | | | | |

Long Bones									
	Humerus (mm)			Radius (mm)			Ulna (mm)		
GA (wks)	5%	50%	95%	5%	50%	95%	5%	50%	95%
12	4.8	8.6	12.3	3.0	6.9	10.8	2.9	6.8	10.7
13	7.6	11.4	15.1	5.6	9.5	13.4	5.8	9.7	13.7
14	10.3	14.1	17.9	8.1	12.0	16.0	8.6	12.6	16.6
15	13.1	16.9	20.7	10.5	14.5	18.5	11.4	15.4	19.4
16	15.89	19.7	23.5	12.9	16.9	20.9	14.1	18.1	22.1
17	18.5	22.4	26.3	15.2	19.3	23.3	16.7	20.8	24.8
18	21.2	25.1	29.0	17.5	21.5	25.6	19.3	23.3	27.4
19	23.8	27.7	31.6	19.7	23.8	27.9	21.8	25.8	29.9
20	26.3	30.3	34.2	21.8	25.9	30.0	24.2	28.3	32.4
21	28.2	32.8	36.7	23.9	28.0	32.2	26.5	30.6	34.8
22	31.2	35.2	39.2	25.9	30.1	34.2	28.7	32.9	37.1
23	33.5	37.5	41.6	27.9	32.0	36.2	30.9	35.1	39.3
24	35.7	39.8	43.8	29.7	34.0	38.2	33.0	37.2	41.5
25	37.9	41.9	46.0	31.6	35.8	40.0	35.1	39.3	43.5
26	39.9	44.0	48.1	33.3	37.6	41.9	37.0	41.3	45.6
27	41.9	46.0	50.1	35.0	39.3	43.6	38.9	43.2	47.5
28	43.7	47.9	52.0	36.7	41.0	45.3	40.7	45.0	49.3
29	45.5	49.7	53.9	38.3	42.6	46.9	42.5	46.8	51.1
30	47.2	51.4	55.6	39.8	44.1	48.5	44.1	48.5	52.8
31	48.9	53.1	57.3	41.2	45.6	50.0	45.7	50.1	54.5
32	50.4	54.7	58.9	42.6	47.0	51.4	47.2	51.6	56.1
33	52.0	56.2	60.5	44.0	48.4	52.8	48.7	53.1	54.5
34	53.4	57.7	62.0	45.2	49.7	54.1	50.0	54.5	59.0
35	54.8	59.2	63.5	46.4	50.9	55.4	51.3	55.8	60.3
36	56.2	60.6	64.9	47.6	52.1	56.6	52.6	57.1	61.6
37	57.6	62.0	66.4	48.7	53.2	57.7	53.7	58.2	62.8
38	59.0	63.4	67.8	49.7	54.2	58.8	54.8	59.3	63.9
39	60.4	64.8	69.3	50.6	55.2	59.8	55.8	60.4	64.9
40	61.9	66.3	70.8	51.5	56.2	60.8	56.7	61.3	65.9

Derived from compilation of data: Jeanty P, Cousaert E, Cantraine F, et al. A longitudinal study of fetal limb growth. *Am J Perinatol.* 1984;1(2):136–144; Merz E, Grubner A, Kern F. Mathematical modeling of fetal limb growth. *J Clin Ultrasound.* 1989;17(3):179–185; and Exacoustos C, Rosati P, Rizzo G, et al. Ultrasound measurements of fetal limb bones. *Ultrasound Obstet Gynecol.* 1991;1(5):325–330. Nyberg DA, McGahan JP, Pretorius DH, et al. *Diagnostic Imaging of Fetal Anomalies.* Philadelphia: Lippincott Williams & Wilkins, 2003.

Measurement Method

The humerus is best located by first imaging the fetal head and spine to assess the fetal lie. The transducer is then moved caudal from the head until the neck region is located. As the transducer is moved in a caudal direction, the shoulder appears. At this point, the transducer should be rotated until a well-defined linear echo is imaged from the shoulder to the elbow (Fig. 16-11). To make sure that this is the single bone of the humerus, cross-plane rocking[61] of the transducer from side to side is used to avoid confusion with the two linear bone echoes of the forearm, representing the radius and ulna.

In some projections the distal end of the humerus appears to have a split or relatively echo-free, central Y-shaped portion. The Y shape is caused by scanning coronally through the humerus, showing the coronoid fossa between the lateral and medial epicondyles. The recommended measurement includes the entire ossified portion of the humerus to the end of the longest epicondyle.

Distal Extremity Bones

The distal long bones of the arms and legs can be difficult to measure because the fetus, particularly if active, may move them frequently and not allow a reliable prediction as to their relationship to the spine or head. Once the bone is located, measuring it is not difficult. If one encounters a fetus with a disparity in the more-often measured parameters, the distal bone measurements can be used to resolve any conflict in age estimates (Table 16-6). Routine measurements of the

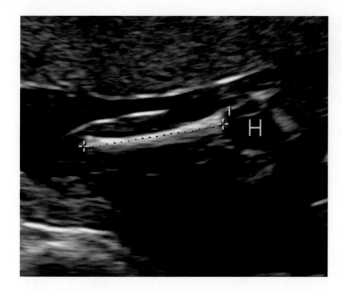

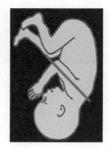

Figure 16-11 As the humerus may resemble the femur, care must be taken to scan from the adjacent bony thorax, through the anechoic humeral head *(H)* and into the arm to properly identify the humerus for measurement (calipers).

distal long bones are not necessary for most sonographic examinations, but the bones should be observed for normal morphology and contralateral symmetry.

Forearm

To measure the bones of the forearm, the sonographer should do a survey scan of the fetus to locate the head, spine, and humerus. The sonographer follows the humerus out to the elbow. There it can be determined whether the elbow is flexed or extended, and the forearm can be followed out to the hand. The sonographer should be aware that there are two bones in the forearm, the ulna and radius, and both bones can be measured. The ulna is the larger of the two and is anatomically medial in location (Fig. 16-12). The increased length of the ulna over the length of the radius is most obvious at the proximal or elbow end of the bones. The radius is imaged lateral to the ulna (Fig. 16-12). If the

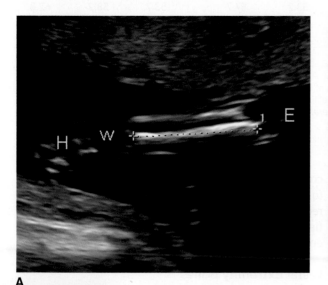

A

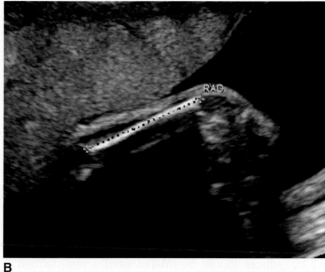

B

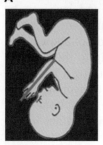

Figure 16-12 Fetal forearm. **A:** While the ulna (measured) extends further into the elbow *(E)* than the radius (lateral), both bones end at approximately the same level at the wrist *(w)*. Lack of wrist bone ossification results in a hypo to anechoic area between the forearm and hand *(H)*. **B:** Fetal radius. Note longer ulna is seen medial.

fetal wrist and hand are rotated, the ulna and radius will be crossed rather than parallel.[14]

Lower Leg

The lower leg also has two bones, the tibia and fibula, and can be difficult to image, depending on fetal position and activity. To locate the lower leg, the sonographer follows the femur from the hip out to the knee and determines whether the knee is flexed or extended. The tibia is the larger of the two bones in the lower leg and is located medially (Fig. 16-13).[14]

FETAL WEIGHT

CALCULATION FROM MEASUREMENT PARAMETERS

Weight is one of the most often sought parameters of fetal growth in obstetrics.[1-3,14] This is because low birth weight, or intrauterine growth restriction (IUGR), has been associated with higher incidences of neonatal morbidity and death. Macrosomia or large birth weight babies, commonly defined as a birth weight 4,000 grams or higher, are also at increased risk of maternal and neonatal morbidity.[36,37] Therefore, an estimate of the relative fetal weight is important to alert the obstetrician to developing problems and to assist in subsequent management of the pregnancy. An indication of the importance of this parameter is the fact that a U.S. National Library of Medicine National Institutes of Health search (pubmed.gov) resulted in over 2,300 titles in multiple languages with articles dating as far back as 1967. Most current ultrasound machines calculate fetal weight from measurements obtained during an examination. Table 16-7 uses the BPD and AC for estimating fetal weight for manual calculations. Results from various weight-prediction methods can result in high error rates in ether singleton or multiple pregnancies with 2D imaging[38-40]; however, the use of three-dimensional (3D) imaging has shown an increase in weight prediction accuracy through measurement of soft tissue such as thigh volumes.[14,41,42]

Recent research has found that the mean fetal weight varies in populations. This research studied birth weights for more than 38,000 singleton, sonographically dated, term pregnancies. Using stepwise multiple regression analysis the researchers found that, "Apart from gestational age and sex, the maternal height, weight at first visit, ethnic group, parity and smoking all have significant and independent effects on birth weight."[43] This means that much of the variation and standard errors in fetal weight estimates can be accounted for by these variables.

Most of the multiple-parameter fetal weight estimation formulas are a variation of a theme that uses parameters of the fetal head or abdomen or other sonographic parameters to estimate the relative fat content, as well as the size of the head and liver and the fetus's length. This works because the brain is the

(text continued on page 390)

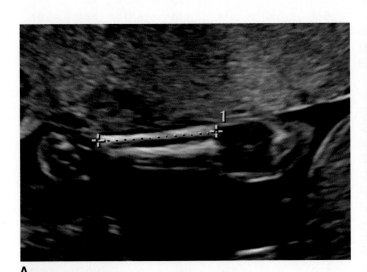

A

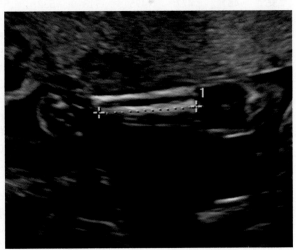

B

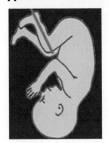

Figure 16-13 Fetal lower leg. Long axis view of the leg demonstrates the ossified portions of the fibula (measured in **A**) and fibula (measured in **B**) Tibia (measured). Fibula is seen lateral to tibia.

TABLE	16-7

Estimation of Fetal Weight (in grams) by Biparietal Diameter (BPD) and Abdominal Circumference (AC)*

BPD (mm)	AC (MM)												
	155	160	165	170	175	180	185	190	195	200	205	210	215
31	224	234	244	255	267	279	291	304	318	332	346	362	378
32	231	241	251	263	274	286	299	312	326	340	355	371	388
33	237	248	259	270	282	294	307	321	335	349	365	381	397
34	244	255	266	278	290	302	316	329	344	359	374	391	408
35	251	262	274	285	298	311	324	338	353	368	384	401	418
36	259	270	281	294	306	319	333	347	362	378	394	411	429
37	266	278	290	302	315	328	342	357	372	388	404	422	440
38	274	286	298	310	324	337	352	366	382	398	415	432	451
39	282	294	306	319	333	347	361	376	392	409	426	444	462
40	290	303	315	328	342	356	371	386	403	419	437	455	474
41	299	311	324	338	352	366	381	397	413	430	448	467	486
42	308	320	333	347	361	376	392	408	424	442	460	479	498
43	317	330	343	357	371	387	402	419	436	453	472	491	511
44	326	339	353	367	382	397	413	430	447	465	484	504	524
45	335	349	363	377	393	408	425	442	459	478	497	517	538
46	345	359	373	386	404	420	436	454	472	490	510	530	551
47	355	369	384	399	415	431	448	466	484	503	524	544	565
48	366	380	395	410	426	443	460	478	497	517	537	558	580
49	376	391	406	422	438	455	473	491	510	530	551	572	594
50	387	402	418	434	451	468	486	505	524	544	565	587	610
51	399	414	430	446	463	481	499	518	538	559	580	602	625
52	410	426	442	459	476	494	513	532	552	573	595	618	641
53	422	438	455	472	489	508	527	547	567	589	611	634	657
54	435	451	468	485	503	522	541	561	582	604	627	650	674
55	447	464	481	499	517	536	556	577	598	620	643	667	691
56	461	477	495	513	532	551	571	592	614	636	660	684	709
57	474	491	509	527	547	566	587	608	630	653	677	701	727
58	488	505	524	542	562	582	603	625	647	670	695	719	745
59	502	520	539	558	578	598	619	642	664	688	713	738	764
60	517	535	554	573	594	615	636	659	682	706	731	757	784
61	532	550	570	590	610	632	654	677	700	725	750	777	804
62	547	566	586	606	627	649	672	695	719	744	770	797	824
63	563	583	603	624	645	667	690	714	738	764	790	817	845
64	580	600	620	641	663	686	709	733	758	784	811	838	867
65	597	617	638	659	682	705	728	753	778	805	832	860	889
66	614	635	656	678	701	724	748	773	799	826	853	882	911
67	632	653	675	697	720	744	769	794	820	848	876	905	935
68	651	672	694	717	740	765	790	816	842	870	898	928	958
69	670	691	714	737	761	786	811	838	865	893	922	952	983
70	689	711	734	758	782	807	833	860	888	916	946	976	1,008
71	709	732	755	779	804	830	856	883	912	941	971	1,002	1,033
72	730	763	777	801	827	853	880	907	936	965	996	1,027	1,060
73	751	775	799	824	850	876	904	932	961	991	1,022	1,054	1,087
74	773	797	822	847	874	901	928	957	987	1,017	1,049	1,081	1,114
75	796	820	845	871	898	925	954	983	1,013	1,044	1,076	1,109	1,143
76	819	844	870	896	923	951	980	1,009	1,040	1,072	1,104	1,137	1,172
77	843	868	894	921	949	977	1,007	1,037	1,068	1,100	1,133	1,167	1,202
78	868	894	920	947	975	1,004	1,034	1,065	1,096	1,129	1,162	1,197	1,232
79	893	919	946	974	1,003	1,032	1,062	1,094	1,126	1,159	1,193	1,228	1,264

TABLE 16-7 (continued)

Estimation of Fetal Weight (in grams) by Biparietal Diameter (BPD) and Abdominal Circumference (AC)*

	AC (MM)												
BPD (mm)	155	160	165	170	175	180	185	190	195	200	205	210	215
80	919	946	973	1,002	1,031	1,061	1,091	1,123	1,156	1,189	1,224	1,259	1,296
81	946	973	1,001	1,030	1,060	1,090	1,121	1,153	1,187	1,221	1,256	1,292	1,329
82	974	1,001	1,030	1,059	1,089	1,120	1,152	1,185	1,218	1,253	1,288	1,325	1,363
83	1,002	1,030	1,059	1,089	1,120	1,151	1,183	1,217	1,251	1,286	1,322	1,359	1,397
84	1,032	1,060	1,090	1,120	1,151	1,183	1,216	1,249	1,284	1,320	1,356	1,394	1,433
85	1,062	1,091	1,121	1,151	1,183	1,216	1,249	1,283	1,318	1,355	1,392	1,430	1,469
86	1,093	1,122	1,153	1,184	1,216	1,249	1,283	1,318	1,354	1,390	1,428	1,467	1,507
87	1,125	1,155	1,186	1,218	1,250	1,284	1,318	1,353	1,390	1,427	1,465	1,505	1,545
88	1,157	1,188	1,220	1,252	1,285	1,319	1,354	1,390	1,427	1,465	1,504	1,543	1,584
89	1,191	1,222	1,254	1,287	1,321	1,356	1,391	1,428	1,465	1,503	1,543	1,583	1,625
90	1,226	1,258	1,290	1,324	1,358	1,393	1,429	1,456	1,504	1,543	1,583	1,624	1,666
91	1,262	1,294	1,327	1,361	1,396	1,432	1,468	1,506	1,544	1,584	1,624	1,666	1,708
92	1,299	1,332	1,365	1,400	1,435	1,471	1,508	1,546	1,586	1,626	1,667	1,709	1,752
93	1,337	1,370	1,404	1,439	1,475	1,512	1,550	1,588	1,628	1,668	1,710	1,753	1,796
94	1,376	1,410	1,444	1,480	1,516	1,554	1,592	1,631	1,671	1,712	1,755	1,798	1,842
95	1,416	1,450	1,486	1,522	1,559	1,597	1,635	1,675	1,716	1,758	1,800	1,844	1,889
96	1,457	1,492	1,528	1,565	1,602	1,641	1,680	1,720	1,762	1,804	1,847	1,892	1,937
97	1,500	1,535	1,572	1,609	1,547	1,686	1,726	1,767	1,809	1,852	1,895	1,940	1,986
98	1,544	1,580	1,617	1,654	1,693	1,733	1,773	1,815	1,857	1,900	1,945	1,990	2,037
99	1,589	1,625	1,663	1,701	1,740	1,781	1,822	1,864	1,907	1,951	1,996	2,042	2,089
100	1,635	1,672	1,710	1,749	1,789	1,830	1,871	1,914	1,958	2,002	2,048	2,094	2,142

BPD (mm)	220	225	230	235	240	245	250	255	260	265	270	275	280
31	395	412	431	450	470	491	513	536	559	584	610	638	666
32	405	423	441	461	481	502	525	548	572	597	624	651	680
33	415	433	452	472	493	514	537	560	585	611	638	666	693
34	425	444	463	483	504	526	549	573	598	624	652	680	710
35	436	455	475	495	517	539	562	587	612	638	666	695	725
36	447	466	486	507	529	552	575	600	626	653	681	710	740
37	458	478	498	519	542	565	589	614	640	667	696	725	756
38	470	490	510	532	554	578	602	628	654	682	711	741	772
39	482	502	523	545	568	592	616	642	669	697	727	757	789
40	494	514	536	558	581	606	631	657	684	713	743	773	806
41	506	527	549	572	595	620	645	672	700	729	759	790	828
42	519	540	562	585	609	634	660	688	716	745	776	807	841
43	532	554	576	600	624	649	676	703	732	762	793	825	859
44	545	567	590	614	639	665	692	719	749	779	810	843	877
45	559	581	605	629	654	680	708	736	765	796	828	861	896
46	573	596	620	644	670	696	724	753	783	814	846	880	915
47	588	611	635	660	686	713	741	770	801	832	865	899	934
48	602	626	650	676	702	730	758	788	819	851	884	919	954
49	617	641	666	692	719	747	776	806	837	870	903	938	975
50	633	657	683	709	736	765	794	824	856	889	923	959	996
51	649	674	699	726	754	783	812	843	876	909	944	980	1,017
52	665	690	717	744	772	801	831	863	895	929	964	1,001	1,039
53	682	708	734	762	790	820	851	883	916	950	986	1,023	1,061
54	699	725	752	780	809	839	870	903	936	971	1,007	1,045	1,084
55	717	743	771	799	828	859	891	924	958	993	1,030	1,068	1,107

TABLE 16-7 *(continued)*

Estimation of Fetal Weight (in grams) by Biparietal Diameter (BPD) and Abdominal Circumference (AC)*

BPD (mm)	220	225	230	235	240	245	250	255	260	265	270	275	280
56	735	762	789	818	848	879	911	945	979	1,015	1,052	1,091	1,131
57	753	780	809	838	869	900	933	966	1,001	1,038	1,075	1,114	1,155
58	772	800	829	858	889	921	954	989	1,024	1,061	1,099	1,139	1,180
59	792	820	849	879	911	943	977	1,011	1,047	1,085	1,123	1,163	1,205
60	811	840	870	900	932	965	999	1,035	1,071	1,109	1,148	1,189	1,231
61	832	861	891	922	955	988	1,023	1,058	1,095	1,134	1,173	1,214	1,257
62	853	882	913	945	977	1,011	1,046	1,083	1,120	1,159	1,199	1,241	1,284
63	874	904	935	967	1,001	1,035	1,071	1,107	1,145	1,185	1,226	1,268	1,311
64	896	927	958	991	1,025	1,059	1,096	1,133	1,171	1,211	1,253	1,295	1,339
65	919	950	982	1,015	1,049	1,084	1,121	1,159	1,198	1,238	1,280	1,323	1,368
66	942	973	1,006	1,039	1,074	1,110	1,147	1,185	1,225	1,266	1,308	1,352	1,397
67	965	997	1,030	1,065	1,100	1,136	1,174	1,213	1,253	1,294	1,337	1,381	1,427
68	990	1,022	1,056	1,090	1,126	1,163	1,201	1,241	1,281	1,323	1,367	1,411	1,458
69	1,015	1,048	1,082	1,117	1,153	1,190	1,229	1,269	1,310	1,353	1,397	1,442	1,489
70	1,040	1,074	1,108	1,144	1,181	1,219	1,258	1,298	1,340	1,383	1,427	1,473	1,521
71	1,066	1,100	1,135	1,171	1,209	1,247	1,287	1,328	1,370	1,414	1,459	1,505	1,553
72	1,093	1,128	1,163	1,200	1,238	1,277	1,317	1,358	1,401	1,445	1,491	1,538	1,586
73	1,121	1,156	1,192	1,229	1,267	1,307	1,348	1,390	1,433	1,478	1,524	1,571	1,620
74	1,149	1,184	1,221	1,259	1,297	1,338	1,379	1,421	1,465	1,511	1,557	1,605	1,655
75	1,178	1,214	1,251	1,289	1,328	1,369	1,411	1,454	1,499	1,544	1,592	1,640	1,690
76	1,207	1,244	1,281	1,320	1,360	1,401	1,444	1,487	1,533	1,579	1,627	1,676	1,727
77	1,238	1,275	1,313	1,352	1,393	1,434	1,477	1,522	1,567	1,614	1,663	1,712	1,764
78	1,269	1,306	1,345	1,385	1,426	1,468	1,512	1,557	1,603	1,650	1,699	1,749	1,801
79	1,301	1,339	1,378	1,418	1,460	1,503	1,547	1,592	1,639	1,687	1,737	1,787	1,840
80	1,333	1,372	1,412	1,453	1,495	1,538	1,583	1,629	1,676	1,725	1,775	1,826	1,879
81	1,367	1,406	1,446	1,488	1,531	1,575	1,620	1,666	1,714	1,763	1,814	1,866	1,919
82	1,401	1,441	1,482	1,524	1,567	1,612	1,657	1,704	1,753	1,803	1,854	1,906	1,960
83	1,436	1,477	1,518	1,561	1,605	1,650	1,696	1,744	1,793	1,843	1,895	1,948	2,002
84	1,473	1,513	1,555	1,599	1,643	1,689	1,735	1,784	1,833	1,884	1,936	1,990	2,045
85	1,510	1,551	1,594	1,637	1,682	1,728	1,776	1,825	1,875	1,926	1,979	2,033	2,089
86	1,548	1,589	1,633	1,677	1,722	1,769	1,817	1,866	1,917	1,969	2,022	2,077	2,134
87	1,586	1,629	1,673	1,717	1,764	1,811	1,859	1,909	1,960	2,013	2,067	2,122	2,179
88	1,626	1,669	1,714	1,759	1,806	1,854	1,903	1,953	2,005	2,058	2,113	2,169	2,226
89	1,667	1,711	1,756	1,802	1,849	1,897	1,947	1,998	2,050	2,104	2,159	2,216	2,274
90	1,709	1,753	1,799	1,845	1,893	1,942	1,992	2,044	2,097	2,151	2,207	2,264	2,322
91	1,752	1,797	1,843	1,890	1,938	1,988	2,039	2,091	2,144	2,199	2,255	2,313	2,372
92	1,796	1,841	1,888	1,936	1,984	2,035	2,086	2,139	2,193	2,248	2,305	2,363	2,423
93	1,841	1,887	1,934	1,982	2,032	2,083	2,135	2,188	2,242	2,298	2,356	2,414	2,475
94	1,887	1,934	1,982	2,030	2,080	2,132	2,184	2,238	2,293	2,350	2,407	2,467	2,527
95	1,935	1,982	2,030	2,080	2,130	2,182	2,235	2,289	2,345	2,402	2,460	2,520	2,582
96	1,984	2,031	2,080	2,130	2,181	2,233	2,287	2,342	2,398	2,456	2,515	2,575	2,637
97	2,033	2,082	2,131	2,181	2,233	2,286	2,340	2,396	2,452	2,510	2,570	2,631	2,693
98	2,085	2,133	2,183	2,234	2,286	2,340	2,395	2,451	2,508	2,567	2,627	2,688	2,751
99	2,137	2,186	2,237	2,288	2,341	2,395	2,450	2,507	2,565	2,624	2,684	2,746	2,810
100	2,191	2,241	2,292	2,344	2,397	2,452	2,507	2,564	2,623	2,682	2,743	2,806	2,870

TABLE	16-7	(continued)

Estimation of Fetal Weight (in grams) by Biparietal Diameter (BPD) and Abdominal Circumference (AC)*

BPD (mm)	AC (MM)												
	285	290	295	300	305	310	315	320	325	330	335	340	345
31	696	726	759	793	828	865	903	943	985	1,029	1,075	1,123	1,173
32	710	742	774	809	844	882	921	961	1,004	1,048	1,094	1,143	1,193
33	725	757	790	825	861	899	938	979	1,022	1,067	1,114	1,163	1,214
34	740	773	806	841	878	916	956	998	1,041	1,087	1,134	1,183	1,235
35	756	789	823	858	896	934	975	1,017	1,061	1,107	1,154	1,204	1,256
36	772	805	840	876	913	953	993	1,036	1,080	1,127	1,175	1,226	1,278
37	788	822	857	893	931	971	1,012	1,056	1,101	1,147	1,196	1,247	1,300
38	805	839	874	911	950	990	1,032	1,076	1,121	1,168	1,218	1,269	1,323
39	822	856	892	930	969	1,009	1,052	1,096	1,142	1,190	1,240	1,292	1,346
40	839	874	911	949	988	1,029	1,072	1,117	1,163	1,212	1,262	1,315	1,369
41	857	892	929	968	1,008	1,049	1,093	1,138	1,185	1,234	1,285	1,338	1,393
42	875	911	948	987	1,028	1,070	1,114	1,159	1,207	1,256	1,308	1,361	1,417
43	893	930	968	1,007	1,048	1,091	1,135	1,181	1,229	1,279	1,331	1,385	1,442
44	912	949	987	1,027	1,069	1,112	1,157	1,204	1,252	1,303	1,355	1,410	1,467
45	932	969	1,008	1,048	1,090	1,134	1,179	1,226	1,275	1,326	1,380	1,435	1,492
46	951	989	1,028	1,069	1,112	1,156	1,202	1,249	1,299	1,351	1,404	1,406	1,518
47	971	1,010	1,049	1,091	1,134	1,178	1,225	1,273	1,323	1,375	1,430	1,486	1,545
48	992	1,031	1,071	1,113	1,156	1,201	1,248	1,297	1,348	1,401	1,455	1,512	1,571
49	1,013	1,052	1,093	1,135	1,179	1,225	1,272	1,322	1,373	1,426	1,482	1,539	1,599
50	1,034	1,074	1,115	1,158	1,203	1,249	1,297	1,347	1,399	1,452	1,508	1,566	1,626
51	1,056	1,096	1,138	1,181	1,226	1,273	1,322	1,372	1,425	1,479	1,535	1,594	1,655
52	1,078	1,119	1,161	1,205	1,251	1,298	1,347	1,398	1,451	1,506	1,563	1,622	1,683
53	1,101	1,142	1,185	1,229	1,276	1,323	1,373	1,425	1,478	1,533	1,591	1,651	1,713
54	1,124	1,166	1,209	1,254	1,301	1,349	1,399	1,452	1,506	1,562	1,620	1,680	1,742
55	1,148	1,190	1,234	1,279	1,327	1,376	1,426	1,497	1,534	1,590	1,649	1,710	1,773
56	1,172	1,215	1,259	1,305	1,353	1,402	1,454	1,507	1,562	1,619	1,678	1,740	1,803
57	1,197	1,240	1,285	1,332	1,380	1,430	1,482	1,535	1,591	1,649	1,709	1,770	1,835
58	1,222	1,266	1,311	1,358	1,407	1,458	1,510	1,564	1,621	1,679	1,739	1,802	1,866
59	1,248	1,292	1,338	1,386	1,435	1,486	1,539	1,594	1,651	1,710	1,770	1,834	1,899
60	1,274	1,319	1,366	1,414	1,464	1,515	1,569	1,624	1,682	1,741	1,802	1,866	1,932
61	1,301	1,346	1,393	1,442	1,493	1,545	1,599	1,655	1,713	1,773	1,835	1,899	1,965
62	1,328	1,374	1,422	1,471	1,522	1,575	1,630	1,686	1,745	1,805	1,868	1,932	1,999
63	1,356	1,403	1,451	1,501	1,552	1,606	1,661	1,718	1,777	1,838	1,901	1,967	2,034
64	1,385	1,432	1,481	1,531	1,583	1,837	1,693	1,751	1,810	1,872	1,935	2,001	2,069
66	1,444	1,492	1,542	1,594	1,647	1,702	1,759	1,817	1,878	1,941	2,006	2,073	2,142
67	1,474	1,523	1,574	1,626	1,679	1,735	1,792	1,852	1,913	1,976	2,042	2,109	2,179
68	1,505	1,555	1,606	1,658	1,713	1,769	1,827	1,887	1,949	2,012	2,078	2,147	2,217
69	1,537	1,587	1,639	1,692	1,747	1,803	1,862	1,922	1,985	2,049	2,116	2,184	2,255
70	1,570	1,620	1,672	1,726	1,781	1,839	1,898	1,959	2,022	2,087	2,154	2,223	2,295
71	1,603	1,654	1,706	1,761	1,817	1,875	1,934	1,996	2,059	2,125	2,193	2,262	2,334
72	1,636	1,688	1,741	1,796	1,853	1,911	1,971	2,044	2,098	2,164	2,232	2,302	2,375
73	1,671	1,723	1,777	1,832	1,890	1,948	2,009	2,072	2,137	2,203	2,272	2,343	2,416
74	1,706	1,759	1,813	1,869	1,927	1,987	2,048	2,111	2,176	2,244	2,313	2,384	2,458
75	1,742	1,795	1,850	1,907	1,965	2,025	2,087	2,151	2,217	2,265	2,354	2,426	2,501
76	1,779	1,833	1,888	1,945	2,004	2,065	2,127	2,192	2,258	2,326	2,397	2,469	2,544
77	1,816	1,871	1,927	1,985	2,044	2,105	2,168	2,233	2,300	2,369	2,440	2,513	2,588
78	1,855	1,910	1,966	2,025	2,085	2,146	2,210	2,275	2,343	2,412	2,484	2,557	2,633
79	1,894	1,949	2,006	2,065	2,126	2,188	2,252	2,318	2,386	2,456	2,528	2,603	2,679

TABLE 16-7 (continued)

Estimation of Fetal Weight (in grams) by Biparietal Diameter (BPD) and Abdominal Circumference (AC)*

BPD (mm)	| AC (MM) 285	290	295	300	305	310	315	320	325	330	335	340	345
80	1,934	1,990	2,048	2,107	2,168	2,231	2,296	2,362	2,431	2,501	2,574	2,649	2,725
81	1,975	2,031	2,089	2,149	2,211	2,275	2,340	2,407	2,476	2,547	2,620	2,695	2,773
82	2,016	2,073	2,132	2,193	2,255	2,319	2,385	2,462	2,522	2,594	2,667	2,743	2,821
83	2,059	2,116	2,176	2,237	2,300	2,364	2,431	2,499	2,569	2,641	2,715	2,791	2,870
84	2,102	2,160	2,220	2,282	2,345	2,410	2,477	2,546	2,617	2,689	2,764	2,841	2,920
85	2,146	2,205	2,266	2,328	2,392	2,457	2,525	2,594	2,665	2,739	2,814	2,891	2,970
86	2,192	2,251	2,312	2,375	2,439	2,505	2,573	2,643	2,715	2,789	2,864	2,942	3,022
87	2,238	2,298	2,359	2,423	2,488	2,554	2,623	2,693	2,765	2,840	2,916	2,994	3,074
88	2,285	2,346	2,408	2,472	2,537	2,604	2,673	2,744	2,817	2,892	2,968	3,047	3,128
89	2,333	2,394	2,457	2,521	2,587	2,655	2,725	2,796	2,869	2,944	3,021	3,101	3,182
90	2,382	2,444	2,507	2,572	2,639	2,707	2,777	2,849	2,923	2,998	3,076	3,155	3,237
91	2,433	2,495	2,559	2,624	2,691	2,760	2,830	2,903	2,977	3,053	3,131	3,211	3,293
92	2,484	2,547	2,611	2,677	2,744	2,814	2,885	2,958	3,032	3,109	3,187	3,268	3,350
93	2,536	2,599	2,664	2,731	2,799	2,869	2,940	3,014	3,089	3,166	3,245	3,326	3,409
94	2,590	2,653	2,719	2,786	2,854	2,925	2,997	3,070	3,146	3,224	3,303	3,384	3,468
95	2,644	2,709	2,774	2,842	2,911	2,982	3,054	3,129	3,205	3,283	3,362	3,444	3,528
96	2,700	2,765	2,831	2,899	2,969	3,040	3,113	3,188	3,264	3,343	3,423	3,505	3,589
97	2,757	2,822	2,889	2,958	3,028	3,099	3,173	3,248	3,325	3,404	3,484	3,567	3,651
98	2,815	2,881	2,948	3,017	3,088	3,160	3,234	3,309	3,387	3,466	3,547	3,630	3,715
99	2,874	2,941	3,009	3,078	3,149	3,222	3,296	3,372	3,450	3,529	3,600	3,694	3,779
100	2,935	3,002	3,070	3,140	3,211	3,285	3,359	3,436	3,514	3,594	3,676	3,759	3,845

BPD (mm)	350	355	360	365	370	375	380	385	390	395	400
31	1,225	1,279	1,336	1,396	1,458	1,523	1,591	1,661	1,735	1,812	1,893
32	1,246	1,301	1,258	1,418	1,481	1,546	1,615	1,686	1,761	1,838	1,920
33	1,267	1,323	1,381	1,441	1,504	1,570	1,639	1,711	1,786	1,865	1,946
34	1,289	1,345	1,403	1,464	1,528	1,595	1,664	1,737	1,812	1,891	1,973
35	1,311	1,367	1,426	1,488	1,552	1,619	1,689	1,762	1,839	1,918	2,001
36	1,333	1,390	1,450	1,512	1,577	1,645	1,715	1,789	1,865	1,945	2,029
37	1,356	1,413	1,474	1,536	1,602	1,670	1,741	1,815	1,893	1,973	2,057
38	1,379	1,437	1,498	1,561	1,627	1,696	1,768	1,842	1,920	2,001	2,086
39	1,402	1,461	1,523	1,586	1,653	1,722	1,794	1,870	1,948	2,030	2,115
40	1,426	1,486	1,548	1,612	1,679	1,749	1,822	1,898	1,977	2,059	2,145
41	1,451	1,511	1,573	1,638	1,706	1,776	1,849	1,926	2,005	2,088	2,174
42	1,475	1,536	1,599	1,664	1,733	1,804	1,878	1,954	2,035	2,118	2,205
43	1,500	1,562	1,625	1,691	1,760	1,832	1,906	1,984	2,064	2,148	2,236
44	1,526	1,588	1,652	1,718	1,788	1,860	1,935	2,013	2,094	2,179	2,267
45	1,552	1,614	1,679	1,746	1,816	1,889	1,964	2,043	2,125	2,210	2,298
46	1,579	1,641	1,706	1,774	1,845	1,918	1,994	2,073	2,156	2,241	2,330
47	1,605	1,669	1,734	1,803	1,874	1,948	2,024	2,104	2,187	2,273	2,363
48	1,633	1,697	1,763	1,832	1,904	1,976	2,055	2,136	2,219	2,306	2,396
49	1,661	1,725	1,792	1,861	1,934	2,009	2,086	2,167	2,251	2,339	2,429
50	1,689	1,754	1,821	1,891	1,964	2,040	2,118	2,200	2,284	2,372	2,463
51	1,718	1,783	1,851	1,922	1,995	2,071	2,150	2,232	2,317	2,406	2,498
52	1,747	1,813	1,882	1,953	2,027	2,103	2,183	2,266	2,351	2,440	2,532
53	1,777	1,843	1,913	1,984	2,059	2,136	2,216	2,299	2,386	2,475	2,568
54	1,807	1,874	1,944	2,016	2,091	2,169	2,250	2,333	2,420	2,510	2,604
55	1,838	1,906	1,976	2,049	2,124	2,203	2,284	2,368	2,456	2,546	2,640

TABLE 16-7 (continued)

Estimation of Fetal Weight (in grams) by Biparietal Diameter (BPD) and Abdominal Circumference (AC)*

BPD (mm)	350	355	360	365	370	375	380	385	390	395	400
56	1,869	1,938	2,008	2,082	2,158	2,237	2,319	2,403	2,491	2,582	2,677
57	1,901	1,970	2,041	2,115	2,192	2,272	2,354	2,439	2,528	2,619	2,714
58	1,934	2,003	2,075	2,150	2,227	2,307	2,390	2,475	2,564	2,657	2,752
59	1,966	2,037	2,109	2,184	2,262	2,342	2,426	2,512	2,602	2,694	2,790
60	2,000	2,071	2,144	2,219	2,298	2,379	2,463	2,550	2,640	2,733	2,829
61	2,034	2,105	2,179	2,255	2,334	2,416	2,500	2,588	2,678	2,772	2,869
62	2,069	2,140	2,215	2,291	2,371	2,453	2,538	2,626	2,717	2,811	2,909
63	2,104	2,176	2,251	2,328	2,408	2,491	2,577	2,665	2,757	2,851	2,949
64	2,140	2,213	2,288	2,366	2,446	2,530	2,616	2,705	2,797	2,892	2,991
65	2,176	2,250	2,326	2,404	2,485	2,569	2,656	2,745	2,838	2,933	3,032
66	2,213	2,287	2,364	2,443	2,524	2,609	2,696	2,786	2,879	2,975	3,075
67	2,251	2,326	2,403	2,482	2,564	2,649	2,737	2,827	2,921	3,018	3,117
68	2,290	2,365	2,442	2,522	2,605	2,690	2,778	2,869	2,964	3,061	3,161
69	2,329	2,404	2,482	2,563	2,646	2,732	2,821	2,912	3,007	3,104	3,205
70	2,368	2,444	2,523	2,604	2,688	2,774	2,863	2,955	3,050	3,149	3,250
71	2,409	2,485	2,564	2,646	2,730	2,817	2,907	2,999	3,095	3,193	3,295
72	2,450	2,527	2,607	2,689	2,773	2,861	2,951	3,044	3,140	3,239	3,341
73	2,491	2,569	2,649	2,732	2,817	2,905	2,996	3,089	3,186	3,285	3,386
74	2,534	2,612	2,693	2,776	2,862	2,950	3,041	3,135	3,232	3,332	3,435
75	2,577	2,656	2,737	2,821	2,907	2,996	3,088	3,182	3,279	3,380	3,483
76	2,621	2,700	2,782	2,866	2,953	3,042	3,134	3,299	3,327	3,428	3,531
77	2,666	2,746	2,828	2,912	3,000	3,090	3,128	3,277	3,376	3,477	3,581
78	2,711	2,792	2,874	2,959	3,047	3,137	3,230	3,326	3,425	3,526	3,631
79	2,757	2,838	2,921	3,007	3,095	3,186	3,279	3,376	3,475	3,576	3,681
80	2,804	2,886	2,969	3,056	3,144	3,235	3,329	3,426	3,525	3,627	3,733
81	2,852	2,934	3,018	3,105	3,194	3,286	3,380	3,477	3,577	3,679	3,785
82	2,901	2,983	3,068	3,155	3,244	3,336	3,431	3,529	3,629	3,732	3,838
83	2,950	3,033	3,118	3,206	3,296	3,388	3,483	3,581	3,682	3,785	3,891
84	3,001	3,084	3,169	3,257	3,348	3,441	3,536	3,634	3,735	3,839	3,945
85	3,052	3,135	3,221	3,310	3,401	3,494	3,590	3,688	3,790	3,894	4,000
86	3,104	3,188	3,274	3,363	3,454	3,548	3,644	3,743	3,845	3,949	4,056
87	3,157	3,241	3,328	3,417	3,509	3,603	3,700	3,799	3,901	4,005	4,113
88	3,210	3,295	3,383	3,472	3,565	3,659	3,756	3,855	3,958	4,063	4,170
89	3,265	3,351	3,438	3,528	3,621	3,716	3,813	3,913	4,015	4,120	4,228
90	3,321	3,407	3,495	3,585	3,678	3,773	3,871	3,971	4,074	4,179	4,287
91	3,377	3,464	3,552	3,643	3,736	3,832	3,930	4,030	4,133	4,239	4,347
92	3,435	3,522	3,611	3,702	3,795	3,891	3,989	4,090	4,193	4,299	4,408
93	3,494	3,581	3,670	3,761	3,855	3,951	4,050	4,151	4,254	4,361	4,469
94	3,553	3,641	3,738	3,822	3,916	4,013	4,111	4,213	4,316	4,423	4,532
95	3,614	3,701	3,791	3,884	3,978	4,075	4,174	4,275	4,379	4,486	4,595
96	3,675	3,763	3,854	3,946	4,041	4,138	4,237	4,339	4,443	4,550	4,659
97	3,738	3,826	3,917	4,010	4,105	4,202	4,302	4,404	4,508	4,615	4,724
98	3,802	3,890	3,981	4,074	4,170	4,267	4,367	4,469	4,573	4,680	4,790
99	3,866	3,956	4,047	4,140	4,236	4,333	4,433	4,536	4,640	4,747	4,857
100	3,932	4,022	4,113	4,207	4,303	4,400	4,501	4,603	4,708	4,815	4,924

* Estimated fetal weights: Log (birth weight) $= -1.7492 + 0.166$ (BPD) $+ 0.046$ (AC) $- 2.646$ (AC + BPD)/1,000.

(From Shepard MJ, Richards VA, Berkowitz RL, et al. An evaluation of two equations for predicting fetal weight by ultrasound. *Am J Obstet Gynecol.* 1982; 147:47–54. Used by permission.)

most uniform organ in humans, whereas the size of the abdomen indicates fat content and liver size, and the femur length is usually proportional to fetal length.[1] The caveat for these methods is that they cannot detect "symmetric IUGR" in a single examination. The sonographer should be particularly careful when taking measurements to be used in weight estimates, particularly those involving abdominal diameter and AC. It is easy to err on the small side and underestimate fetal weight.

FETAL PARAMETER RATIOS

Ratios of various parameters have been historically used to assess fetal proportionality. The ratio or index is a powerful statistical tool for comparing the relative sizes of two parameters. This is because many fetal parameters grow at different rates and it is difficult to compare their sizes directly. However, at any given time in gestation the ratio of their sizes is normally fairly consistent. This means that calculating the ratio of the two measurements provides an idea of their relative sizes, one to the other.

In a ratio, the parameter that is the so-called "standard" is usually the denominator.[68] As the comparative numerator becomes larger, the ratio also increases, and vice versa. This standard is not always followed and either parameter can be used as the numerator as long as the observer understands the relationships in the ratio.[45] It is best if ratios compare like measurements; that is to say, compare linear to linear measurements, circumferences to circumferences, or volumes to volumes. A consideration for the use of ratios to evaluate proportions is in the case where a particular ratio is abnormal. The observer must then determine if the numerator or the denominator of the ratio is the abnormal parameter.

Ratio = numerator/denominator

Percentage = 100(numerator/denominator)

ABDOMEN TO HEAD RATIO

Many ratios have been proposed to evaluate the proportionality of fetal parameters. One of the most common is the transverse head circumference/abdominal circumference ratio (HC/AC)[45,46] With this ratio, as the

TABLE 16-8									
Fetal Biometric Ratios									
	HC/AC			AC/FL			BPD/FL		
GA (wks)	5th	50th	95th	5th	50th	95th	5th	50th	95th
14	1.12	1.23	1.33	4.82	5.40	6.04	1.70	1.87	2.06
15	1.11	1.22	1.32	4.64	5.19	5.81	1.62	1.78	1.95
16	1.10	1.21	1.31	4.49	5.03	5.62	1.55	1.70	1.87
17	1.09	1.20	1.30	4.37	4.89	5.47	1.49	1.64	1.80
18	1.09	1.19	1.29	4.27	4.78	5.34	1.45	1.59	1.74
19	1.08	1.18	1.29	4.19	4.69	5.24	1.41	1.54	1.69
20	1.07	1.17	1.28	4.13	4.62	5.16	1.37	1.51	1.66
21	1.06	1.16	1.27	4.08	4.56	5.10	1.35	1.48	1.62
22	1.05	1.15	1.26	4.05	4.53	5.06	1.33	1.46	1.60
23	1.04	1.14	1.25	4.03	4.50	5.04	1.31	1.44	1.58
24	1.03	1.13	1.24	4.02	4.49	5.02	1.30	1.43	1.57
25	1.02	1.12	1.23	4.02	4.49	5.02	1.29	1.42	1.56
26	1.01	1.11	1.22	4.02	4.50	5.03	1.29	1.41	1.55
27	1.00	1.10	1.21	4.04	4.51	5.05	1.28	1.41	1.54
28	0.99	1.09	1.20	4.05	4.53	5.07	1.28	1.40	1.54
29	0.98	1.08	1.19	4.08	4.56	5.10	1.28	1.40	1.54
30	0.97	1.08	1.18	4.10	4.58	5.13	1.28	1.40	1.54
31	0.96	1.07	1.17	4.12	4.61	5.16	1.27	1.40	1.53
32	0.95	1.06	1.16	4.15	4.64	5.19	1.27	1.39	1.53
33	0.94	1.05	1.15	4.17	4.66	5.22	1.27	1.39	1.53
34	0.93	1.04	1.14	4.19	4.69	5.24	1.26	1.37	1.52
35	0.92	1.03	1.13	4.20	4.70	5.26	1.25	1.36	1.51
36	0.91	1.02	1.12	4.21	4.71	5.27	1.24	1.34	1.49
37	0.90	1.01	1.11	4.21	4.70	5.27	1.22	1.32	1.47
38	0.89	1.00	1.10	4.20	4.68	5.26	1.20	1.30	1.45
39	0.88	0.99	1.09	4.18	4.66	5.23	1.18	1.28	1.42

From Snijders RJ, Nicolaides KH. Fetal biometry at 14–40 weeks' gestation. *Ultrasound Obstet Gynecol.* 1994;4(1):34–48.

Critical Thinking Questions

1. At term the fetal head descends into the maternal pelvis, resulting in either molding or difficulty in imaging the brain structures. Some fetal malformations result in abnormal brain structures and caldarium size. What alternative measurements allow for determining gestational age and fetal growth in these cases?

   ANSWER: Multiple biometric parameters; OOD, IOD, cerebellum measurements, and long bone measurements aid in determining fetal age in the absence of the BPD and HC.

2. A 34-year-old patient presents to the department for a third-trimester follow-up sonographic examination. The routine 24-week exam demonstrated a normal head and abdomen with slightly shorter than expected femur length. Today's exam demonstrates appropriate interval growth of the head and abdomen and continued lagging of the femurs. List additional measurements that would aid in dating.

   ANSWER: In this case, the humerus, tibia/fibula, and radius/ulna would need to be measured. If these limbs also measure short, these findings raise concern for a skeletal dysplasia.

3. A 22-year-old patient presents at 20 weeks' gestation for a general anatomy scan. This patient had a previous exam at 10 weeks confirming her EDC. The current exam shows no abnormalities, but fetal size is more consistent with 18 weeks. Should the EDC be adjusted?

   ANSWER: No. Earlier dating has an accuracy of ±1 week. In the second trimester the accuracy decreases to ±2 weeks. An EDC confirmed by an early exam is the date used for all consecutive exams. The insufficient growth seen since the first exam warrants further examination.

4. A 26-year-old patient, G3P1A1, presents for her first ultrasound exam with uncertain dates and late prenatal care. Fetal head and femur measurements are consistent with 34 weeks' gestation but the abdomen is consistent with 28 weeks. Which due date should be used?

   ANSWER: The fetal abdomen is the first measurement that lags with IUGR. Since fetal head and femur are consistent with 34 weeks, this should be used for dating—keeping in mind that dating in the third trimester is +/− 3 weeks. With the abdomen lagging behind, this fetus should be evaluated for IUGR.

abdomen becomes larger, relative to the head, the ratio becomes smaller, and vice versa. The HC/AC ratio is normally 1:1 (299 mm/299 mm = 1.0) at ~34 LMP weeks. This ratio should normally be over 100% before 34 weeks and less after that time (Table 16-8).

OTHER BODY RATIOS

Other ratios that are useful in the study of fetal proportions are ratios comparing the femur length, the BPD, and the abdominal AC (Table 16-8).

SUMMARY

Factors that the sonographer should be particularly aware of are as follows:

- To use any fetal parameter size-age chart, the user must know how the measurements were taken and must take measurements by the methods used by the author to construct the chart.

- The use of multiple fetal parameter average ages and the range of the ages produce more accurate dates and are more likely to expose abnormal parameters or erroneous measurements than is the use of single fetal parameters.

- Any two fetal parameter ages from the same examination should not have a range in weeks over 20% of the fetal age (range of ages = maximum age − minimum age).

- All parameter ages from an examination should be within ±10% of the average fetal parameter age.[1]

- Age estimates from fetal head parameters normally have about half the error (variance) of body parameter ages.

- Long bone (femur, humerus) sonographic measurements should include only the osseous portions of the bone diaphysis (shaft). The sonographer should be careful not to include beam width artifacts or the DFP or PHP in the measurement.

- If the transverse cephalic index is normal and the coronal skull shape is a circle, then the BPD is a good estimator of dates; otherwise, the HC is recommended as head molding increases. When taking measurements the sonographer should always use the transducer and focal range that give the highest resolution.

- Once EDC has been confirmed with ultrasound, it should not be changed.

REFERENCES

1. Benson CB, Doubilet PM. Fetal measurements – normal and abnormal fetal growth. In: Rumack CM, Wilson SR, Charboneau JW, et al., eds. *Diagnostic ultrasound*. 3rd ed. St. Louis: Elsevier Mosby; 2005.
2. Galan HL, Pandipati S, Filly RA. Ultrasound evaluation of fetal biometry and normal and abnormal fetal growth. In: Callen PW, ed. *Ultrasonography in obstetrics and gynecology*. 5th ed. Philadelphia: Saunders Elsevier; 2008.
3. Nyberg DA, McGahan JP, Pretorius DH, et al. *Diagnostic imaging of fetal anomalies*. Philadelphia: Lippincott Williams & Wilkins; 2003.
4. Kurtz AB, Goldberg BB. Combined fetal head and body measurements. In: Kurtz AB, Goldberg BB, eds. *Obstetrical*

measurements in ultrasound: a reference manual. 2nd ed. Chicago: Mosby; 2006.

5. Firoozabadi RD, Ghasemi N, Firoozabadi MD. Sonographic fetal weight estimation using femoral length: Honarvar equation. *Ann Saudi Med.* 2007;27(3):179–182.

6. Salpou D, Kiserud T, Rasmussen S, et al. Fetal age assessment on 2nd trimester ultrasound in Africa and the effect of ethnicity. *BMC Pregnancy Childbirth.* 2008;8:48.

7. Birnholz JC. Ultrasonic measurements. In: Deter RL, Harrist RB, Birnholz JC, et al. eds. *Quantitative obstetrical ultrasonography.* New York: John Wiley & Sons; 1986:10.

8. Jeanty P. Basic baby II. *J Ultrasound Med.* 1987;6:548.

9. Kremkau FW. *Diagnostic ultrasound: physical principles & exercises.* St. Louis: Saunders Elsevier; 2006:76–81.

10. Martinez DA, Barton JL. Estimation of fetal body and fetal head volumes: description of technique and nomograms for 18 to 41 weeks of gestation. *Am J Obstet Gynecol.* 1980;137(1):78–84.

11. Winter J, Kimme-Smith C, King W III. Measurement accuracy of sonographic sector scanners. *AJR Am J Roentgenol.* 1985;144(3):645–648.

12. Zagzebski JA. Physics and instrumentation. In: Sabbagha RE, ed. *Diagnostic ultrasound, applied to obstetrics and gynecology.* 3rd ed. Philadelphia: JB Lippincott; 1994.

13. Bartrum RJ, Crow HC. *Real-time ultrasound: a manual for physicians and technical personnel.* 2nd ed. Philadelphia: WB Saunders; 1983:147.

14. DeBose TJ, Hagen-Ansert SL. Obstetric measurements and gestational age. In: Hagen-Ansert SL, ed. *Textbook of diagnostic ultrasonography.* 6th ed. St. Louis: Mosby Saunders; 2006.

15. DuBose TJ. A simple test of excessive B scanner transducer ring. *Med Ultrasound.* 1983;7:169–172.

16. Zador IE, Sokol RJ, Chik L. Interobserver variability: a source of error in obstetric ultrasound. *J Ultrasound Med.* 1988;7(5):245–249.

17. DuBose TJ. Fetal cranial biometry. In: *Fetal sonography.* Philadelphia: WB Saunders; 1996:157–199.

18. Kurtz AB, Goldberg BB. Fetal head measurements. In: Kurtz AB, Goldberg BB, eds. *Obstetrical measurements in ultrasound: a reference manual.* Chicago: Year Book Medical Publishers; 1988;22–35.

19. O'Keeffe DF, Garite TJ, Elliott JP, et al. The accuracy of estimated gestational age based on ultrasound measurements of biparietal diameter in preterm premature rupture of the membranes. *Am J Obstet Gynecol.* 1985;151(3):309–312.

20. Hadlock FP, Deter RL, Harrist RB, et al. Computer-assisted analysis of fetal age in the third trimester using multiple growth parameters. *J Clin Ultrasound.* 1983;11(6):313–316.

21. Hadlock FP, Deter RL, Harrist RB, et al. Estimating fetal age: computer-assisted analysis of multiple fetal growth parameters. *Radiology.* 1984;152(2):497–501.

22. Ott WJ. Accurate gestational dating. *Obstet Gynecol.* 1985; 66(3):311–315.

23. Sabbagha RE, Barton FB, Barton BA. Sonar biparietal diameter I. Analysis of percentile growth differences in two normal populations using same methodology. *Am J Obstet Gynecol.* 1976;126(4):479–484.

24. Bowie JD. Real-time ultrasonography in the diagnosis of fetal anomalies. In: Winsburg F, Cooperberg PL, eds. *Clinics in diagnostic ultrasound.* New York: Churchill Livingstone, 1982;228.

25. McLeary RD, Kuhns LR, Barr M. Ultrasonography of the fetal cerebellum. *Radiology.* 1984;151(2):439–442.

26. Fiske CE, Filly RA. Ultrasound evaluation of the normal and abnormal fetal neural axis. In: Callen PW, ed. *Ultrasonography in obstetrics and gynecology.* Philadelphia: WB Saunders; 1983:100.

27. Law RG, MacRae KD. Head circumference as an index of fetal age. *J Ultrasound Med.* 1982;1(7):281–288.

28. Cunningham F, Leveno K, Bloom S, et al. *Williams obstetrics.* 23rd ed. New York: McGraw-Hill Professional; 2009.

29. Hadlock FP, Deter RL, Harrist RB, et al. Fetal head circumference: relation to menstrual age. *Am J Roentgenol.* 1982;138(4):649–653.

30. Hill LM, Breckle R, Gehrking WC. The variable effects of oligohydramnios on the biparietal diameter and the cephalic index. *J Clin Ultrasound.* 1984;3(2):93–95.

31. Pilu G. Ultrasound evaluation of the fetal neural axis. In: Callen PW, ed. *Ultrasonography in obstetrics and gynecology.* 5th ed. Philadelphia: Saunders Elsevier; 2008.

32. Gottlieb A, Galan H. Nontraditional sonographic pearls in estimating gestational age. *Semin Perinatol.* 2008;32(3): 154–160.

33. Filly RA, Feldstein VA. Ultrasound evaluation of normal fetal anatomy. In: Callen PW, ed. *Ultrasonography in obstetrics and gynecology.* 5th ed. Philadelphia: Saunders Elsevier; 2008.

34. Hadlock FP, Deter RL, Roecker E, et al. Relation of fetal femur length to neonatal crown-heel length. *J Ultrasound Med.* 1984;3(1):1–3.

35. DuBose TJ. Fetal extremities. In: *Fetal sonography.* Philadelphia: WB Saunders; 1996:237–244.

36. Pates JA, McIntire DD, Casey BM, et al. Predicting macrosomia. *J Ultrasound in Med.* 2008;27(1):39–43.

37. Melamed N, Yogev Y, Meizner I, et al. Sonographic prediction of fetal macrosomia: the consequences of false diagnosis. *J Ultrasound in Med.* 2010;29(2):225–230.

38. Diaz-Garcia C, Bernard JP, Ville Y, et al. Validity of sonographic prediction of fetal weight and weight discordance in twin pregnancies. *Prenat Diagn.* 2010;30(4):361–367.

39. Pineau JC, Grange G, Kapitaniak B, et al. Estimation of fetal weight: accuracy of regression models versus accuracy of ultrasound data. *Fetal Diagn Ther.* 2008;24(2):140–145.

40. Melamed N, Yogev Y, Meizner I, et al. Sonographic fetal weight estimation: which model should be used? *J Ultrasound Med.* 2009;28(5):617–629.

41. Schild RL, Maringa M, Siemer J, et al. Weight estimation by three-dimensional ultrasound imaging in the small fetus. *Ultrasound Obstet Gynecol.* 2008;32(2):168–175.

42. Yu J, Wang Y, Chen P. Fetal ultrasound image segmentation system and its use in fetal weight estimation. *Med Biol Eng Comput.* 2008;46(12):1227–1237.

43. Rose BI. Abbreviated tables for estimating fetal weight with ultrasound. *J Reprod Med.* 1988;33(3):298–300.

44. Hadlock FP, Deter RL, Roecker E, et al. Relation of fetal femur length to neonatal crown-heel length. *J Ultrasound Med.* 1984;3(1):1–3.

45. Sokal RR, Rohlf FJ. Biometry. *The principles and practice of statistics in biological research.* 3rd ed. New York: WH Freeman; 1994.

46. Campbell S, Thomas A. Ultrasound measurements of the fetal head to abdomen circumference in assessment of growth retardation. *Br J Obstet Gynaecol.* 1977;84(3): 165–174.

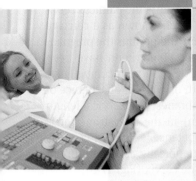

17 The Fetal Environment

Malka Stromer

GLOSSARY

Abruptio placentae Premature separation of the placenta from the uterus

Annular placenta Bandlike placenta encircling the internal uterus

Battledore placenta Placenta with the umbilical cord inserted into the border

Bilobed placenta (succenturiate lobe) Extra placental lobe smaller than the placenta

Braxton-Hicks Uterine contractions that do not lead to labor

Cerclage Stitch placed into the incompetent cervix to prevent opening

Circumvallate placenta Abnormally attached placenta with a peripheral raised ring

Cotyledons Lobule or subdivision of the maternal placenta containing fetal vessels, chorionic villi, and the intervillous space

Cord prolapse Delivery of the cord before the fetus

Intervillous thrombosis Clot in the intervillous spaces of the placenta

Intervillous spaces (sinus) Placental spaces that communicate with maternal vessels

Nuchal cord 360 degree wrapping of the umbilical cord around the fetal neck

Placenta accreta, increta, and percreta Abnormal attachment of the placenta to the uterus with

different terms used to describe the depth of placental invasion

Placenta hydrops Abnormal fluid accumulation coexisting with fetal hydrops

Placenta previa Low uterine implantation of the placenta resulting in total or partial covering of the cervix

Retroplacental Area between the myometrium and placenta

Placental infarction Tissue death resulting from circulatory obstruction

Placenta membranacea Fetal membranes covered by chorionic villi due to failure of chorion differentiation into the chorion laeve and chorion frondosum

Trophoblast Extraembryonic tissue that develops into the placenta

Valsalva Inhalation and suspension of breath coupled with abdominal muscle contraction to increase abdominal pressure

Vasa previa Crossing of the cervix by the umbilical cord coexisting with a velamentous cord insertion or placental succenturiate

Velamentous insertion Cord attachment to the edge of the placenta

Vernix caseosum White, cheeselike coating of fetal skin

Wharton's jelly Mucous tissue surrounding the umbilical cord

During the second and third trimesters, the obstetric sonographic examination is usually performed trans-abdominally. The examination should include a full evaluation of the fetus, including assessment of fetal anatomy, size, position, and state, as well as examination of the uterus, placenta, and amniotic fluid. Although normal ovaries are often not visible in the second and third trimesters because the enlarging uterus obscures them, both adnexal areas should be scanned for residual corpus luteal cysts and/or disease. If the mother has flank pain or other symptoms or signs related to the kidneys, they should be included in the sonographic examination.

UTERUS: CERVIX AND LOWER SEGMENT

The imaging examination of the cervix and lower uterine segment looks for evidence of cervical incompetence or placenta previa. Individuals with a history of premature labor and/or birth, premature rupture of membranes, uterine anomalies, or multiple gestations should undergo cervical evaluation. Assessment of the lower segment and cervix is traditionally performed transabdominally through a partially full maternal bladder, but when the fetal head is low and obscures the cervix, translabial/transperineal or endovaginal scanning may be useful. The overfull bladder may appose the anterior and posterior walls of the lower uterine segment, thereby creating the false appearance of placenta previa or falsely elongating the cervical measurement (Fig. 17-1). Due to this potential of distortion, the endovaginal technique allows for a more accurate measurement of the cervical length (internal os to external os) (Fig. 17-2).[1] Historically, application of fundal pressure or Valsalva techniques have been used to evaluate cervical length. These are no longer deemed necessary.[2]

The cervix normally remains tightly closed until the time of delivery. Dilatation of the cervix before term can lead to second trimester spontaneous abortion or premature delivery. Cervical incompetence is the painless cervical dilatation. Placement of a stitch, known as a cerclage loop, prevents further dilatation and permits the pregnancy to continue.[3] Several sonographic criteria have been proposed for early detection of cervical incompetence. Opening of the internal os with or without observance of protruding or herniating membranes, or a cervical length less than 2.5 centimeters (cm) in the third trimester is suggestive of cervical incompetence.[1,4] Once a cerclage is in place, it is visible sonographically as several bright echoes within the muscle of the cervix (Fig. 17-3).

Marked dilatation of the cervix with bulging of membranes through the external os is a poor prognostic sign. Take special care while imaging the contents of the fluid and membranes protruding into the cervical canal. The presence of any part of the umbilical cord within the cervical canal is a serious threat to the fetus, an obstetric emergency requiring immediate intervention (Fig. 17-4).[5]

THE UTERUS: BODY

The muscular myometrium composes most of the uterine body while an inner layer, the endometrium, lines the uterine cavity. During pregnancy, the smooth muscle of the myometrium stretches and hypertrophies rapidly. Myometrial vessels also proliferate and enlarge greatly.[6]

On sonographic examination, the myometrium appears as a band of tissue surrounding the gestational sac that is less echogenic than the placenta. The uterine vessels are most abundant along the lateral uterine wall and may alter the echogenicity of the myometrium as they enlarge.

Myometrial thickness should be uniform around the gestational sac. Any evidence of thinning inferior to the placenta may indicate an abnormally adherent placenta such as placenta accreta, increta, or percreta (Fig. 17-5).[7]

Throughout the pregnancy, focal areas of smooth muscle in the uterine wall contract, causing a bulging into

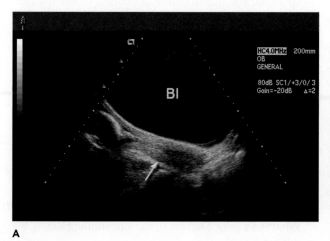

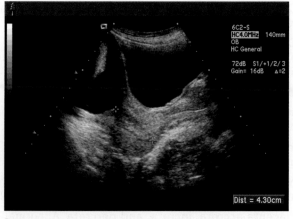

A

B

Figure 17-1 A: The cervix and lower uterine segment *(arrow)* compress with an overfull bladder. *Bl,* bladder **B:** An appropriately filled bladder and cervical length measurement.

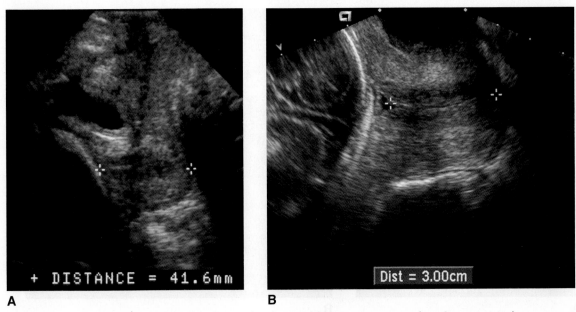

Figure 17-2 The normal cervix in the translabial **(A)** and endovaginal **(B)** image measures at least 3 cm on sagittal measurements.

the amniotic cavity. These Braxton-Hicks contractions should not be confused with fibroids or altered placental patterns such as abruption or infarction. The muscle contractions appear homogeneous in echotexture and should disappear within 30 to 45 minutes (Fig. 17-6).

Uterine leiomyomas, or fibroids, may be located in the wall of the uterus. They tend to be hypoechoic, round, and somewhat heterogeneous. They may distort the outer or inner contour of the uterus, but unlike myometrial contractions they do not change during the course of a sonographic examination. Fibroids sometimes enlarge during pregnancy and may become symptomatic owing to degeneration or increased uterine irritability. Location of fibroids is important, as those in a retroplacental position may increase risk of

placental abruption. Large fibroids positioned in the lower uterine segment may obstruct delivery, forcing a C-section (Fig. 17-7).[8]

Occasionally a subchorionic hematoma may mimic a fibroid or uterine contraction. Within several days, this subchorionic collection becomes cystic as the hematoma breaks down and no longer confuses the diagnosis.[9]

THE PLACENTA AND UMBILICAL CORD

Accurate assessment of the placenta and umbilical cord is of considerable importance in an obstetric sonographic evaluation. Placental pathology and/or abnormal placental development can result in a variety of complications to the pregnancy.[10] The sonographer has the

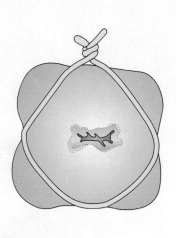

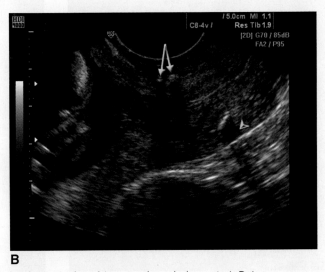

Figure 17-3 A: Cervical cerclage. Inferior view of a cervix that has been cerclaged (as seen through the vagina). **B:** Incompetent cervix with cerclage. Longitudinal endovaginal sonogram demonstrating dilated internal cervical os to the level of the cerclage represented by bright echoes in the distal cervix *(arrows)* and characteristic posterior shadowing *(arrowhead)*. (Image courtesy of Philips Medical Systems, Bothell, WA.)

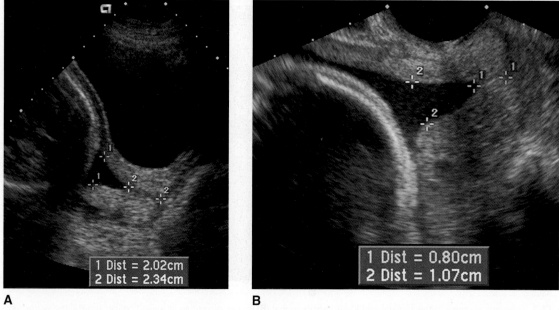

A   **B**

Figure 17-4 Short funneled cervix. **A:** Transabominal view demonstrates a dilated cervix measuring 20.2 mm (+1 calipers) at the internal os. The length of the residual closed cervix is 23.4 mm (+2 calipers). **B:** Endovaginal view of the cervix (in another case) demonstrates a dilated cervix measuring 10.7 mm dilated (+2 calipers) at the internal os. Residual closed cervix measures 8.0 mm (+1 calipers).

tools to perform a detailed evaluation of placental morphology, placental localization, and fetoplacental hemodynamics. Although detection of placental pathology is often nonspecific, findings lead the health care team toward further investigation to minimize risks to fetal outcomes.[11] Structural lesions (e.g., umbilical cord compression, placental tumor, or lesions consequent to maternal diseases such as hypertension or diabetes) can result in vascular resistance changes, severely compromising the fetus. Moreover, the morphology and vascular condition of the placenta and umbilical cord may suggest the presence of coincident fetal anomalies.

The extensive technological advances that have facilitated detailed sonographic study of the placenta include Doppler spectral analysis, color flow Doppler, and endovaginal and transperineal ultrasound. Many sonography departments now consider endovaginal sonography to be a routine part of first-trimester evaluation, and it has become a staple in the evaluation of complications such as placenta previa and vasa previa late in pregnancy.

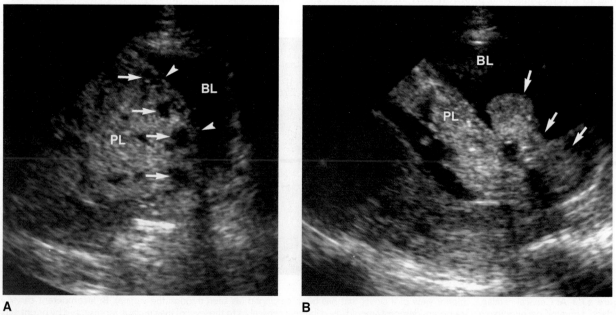

A   **B**

Figure 17-5 Placenta accreta or increta. **A:** Sagittal view of the lower uterus demonstrates markedly thinned myometrium (*arrows*) beneath the placenta (*PL*). **B:** Compare the normal hypoechoic myometrium of a sagittal image of the lower uterine segment (LUS).

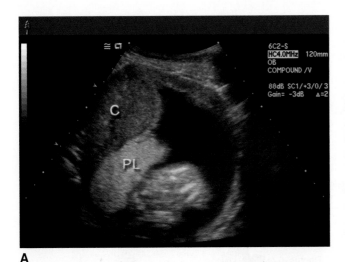

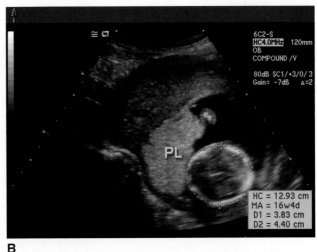

A **B**

Figure 17-6 **A:** Transverse image of a right lateral placenta demonstrates a contraction (C) inferior to the placenta (PL). **B:** The same area later in the exam demonstrates relaxation of the contraction.

Color flow Doppler and conventional Doppler, used judiciously, have revolutionized fetoplacental sonography and greatly increased our understanding of normal and abnormal gestational hemodynamics. A further benefit of these advances has been to render established techniques (such as amniocentesis) quicker, safer, and easier to perform. In addition, a variety of newer ultrasound-guided invasive procedures such as percutaneous umbilical blood sampling, chorionic villus sampling, and placental biopsy have added to the fetal diagnostic repertoire.

PLACENTAL STRUCTURE AND FUNCTION

Development of the Placenta

The placenta is composed of both a maternal (arising from the endometrium) and fetal (arising from a section of the chorionic sac) portion. Decidua is the term used to describe the functional layer of the endometrium in the gravid woman. The decidua is further named according to the specific anatomic relationship to the implanted conceptus: 1) the decidual basalis lies deep to the conceptus and develops into the maternal side of the placenta; 2) the decidua capsularis overlies the conceptus, and; 3) the decidua parietalis/vera encompasses all of the remaining decidua.[12]

Cells known as trophoblasts, which arise from the implanting conceptus, invade the decidua and are therefore involved in early placental development. This is the beginning of the intercommunicating lacunar network that later becomes placental intervillous spaces. Some of the trophoblasts form the chorionic sac, whose surface is covered by tiny projections known as chorionic villi. As the chorionic sac grows, the villi in close proximity to the decidua capsularis eventually becomes compressed, and a smooth, bare, avascular area called the smooth chorion emerges. On the other hand, the villi associated with the decidua basalis (maternal side of placenta) persist and proliferate into the villous chorion or chorion frondosum, the fetal side of the placenta.[12]

Placental Function

The placenta is the link between the mother and the fetus. It is where all nutritional, respiratory, and excretory exchanges that ensure fetal growth and development take place. The placenta also has various metabolic functions, synthesizing sugars, fats, and hormones (human chorionic gonadotropin, estrogen, and progesterone).[12] Fetal well-being depends on an intact and uncompromised uteroplacental vascular supply.[13] Maternal disease or vascular abnormalities can affect the size, vascularization, and function of the placenta, which in turn may compromise fetal well-being.

Size, Shape, and Location

The placenta is a flattened, circular, vascular organ that weighs about 480 to 600 grams (g) at term (one-sixth to one-seventh of fetal weight). Attachment to the uterine

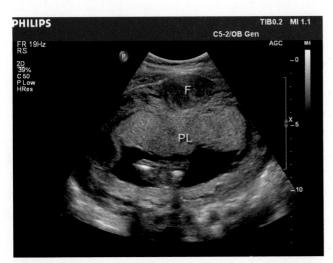

Figure 17-7 A fibroid (F) has a focal hypoechoic mass appearance inferior to the anteriorly located placenta (PL). (Image courtesy of Philips Medical Systems, Bothell, WA.)

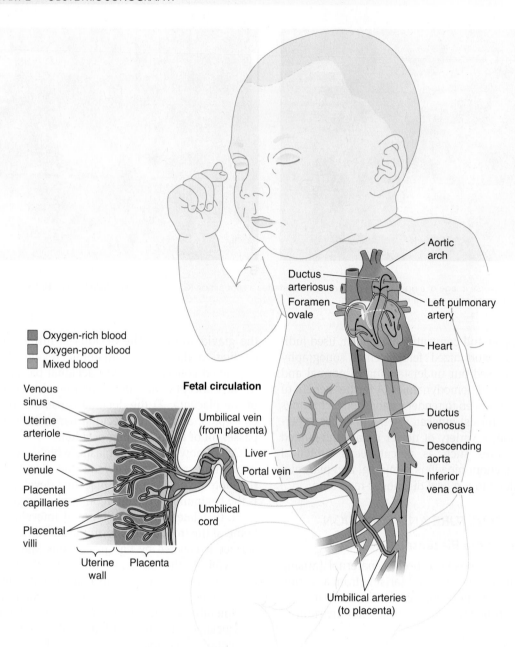

Oxygen-rich blood
Oxygen-poor blood
Mixed blood

Fetal circulation

Venous sinus
Uterine arteriole
Uterine venule
Placental capillaries
Placental villi

Uterine wall   Placenta

Umbilical vein (from placenta)
Liver
Portal vein
Umbilical cord

Aortic arch
Ductus arteriosus
Foramen ovale
Left pulmonary artery
Heart
Ductus venosus
Descending aorta
Inferior vena cava

Umbilical arteries (to placenta)

Figure 17-8 Fetal circulation and section of placenta. Colors show relative oxygen content of blood.

wall can occur anywhere within the uterine cavity. At the fetal side is a fused layer of amnion and chorion (chorionic plate) with underlying fetal vessels. At the maternal side are about 20 functional lobes, or cotyledons, composed of maternal sinusoids and chorionic villous structures (Fig. 17-8).[14] The placenta is a relatively homogeneous organ that may exhibit varying degrees of calcification and anechoic spaces (lacunae) in later pregnancy.

By the end of the fourth month sonography helps identify the final shape of the placenta. It is usually discoid. The normal cord insertion is approximately in the central portion, but it may insert eccentrically near the margins (battledore placenta) or below the edge of the placenta (velamentous insertion) (Fig. 17-9).[10,14] In general, the wider the base of attachment, the thinner the placenta. Evaluation of placental length, volume,

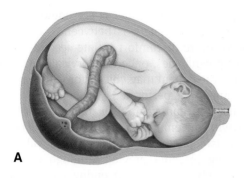

A

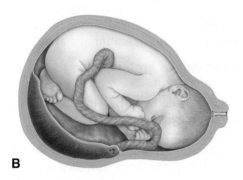

B

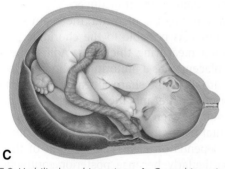

C

Figure 17-9 Umbilical cord insertions. **A:** Central insertion of cord into placenta. **B:** Battledore insertion. Cord is inserted near the margin or edge of the placenta. **C:** Velamentous insertion. Cord is inserted into chorioamniotic membranes, which extend beyond the placental parenchmya and lie along the uterine wall. Location of this type of insertion near the lower uterine segment can lead to complications such as vasa previa.

and thickness allows for pregnancy outcome correlation. In general, a placental thickness of greater than 4 cm prior to 24 weeks' gestation is considered abnormal, and further investigation for causal effect should be considered.[10]

PATHOLOGY BOX 17-1

The Placenta

480–600 grams
20 functional lobes/cotyledons
Discoid shape
Central cord insertion
Normal placenta 2–4 cm thick

Placental Circulation

The maternal and fetal circulations are separate.[14] Oxygenated maternal blood is pumped through spiral arterioles within the decidua basalis and enters the intervillous spaces (sinus) surrounding and bathing the villi. Gases and nutrients exchange across the walls of the villi, allowing nutrition, respiration, and waste removal to take place. Deoxygenated fetal blood, carried to the placenta by the umbilical arteries, circulates through capillaries in the chorionic villi within the placental lobes. The resulting oxygenated blood within the villous capillaries returns to the fetus through the umbilical vein.[14]

During pregnancy, maternal blood volumes increase to satisfy fetal needs. The many vascular channels and sinusoidal structure of the placenta create a low-impedance system, even lower than other fetal vascular beds, at least until late in pregnancy.[14] Doppler investigation of maternal and fetal vessels demonstrates the low-resistance nature of the placenta. Anything that causes increased placental resistance or placental insufficiency can have profound effects on the developing fetus. The term "placental insufficiency" is often used with reference to nonspecific placental deficiencies. These usually relate to increased vascular resistance within the placenta, caused by either maternal or placental alterations. Doppler evaluation in compromised pregnancies provides much needed information, leading to improved management of these patients. Fetoplacental Doppler is discussed in depth in Chapter 24.

SCANNING TECHNIQUES

Transabdominal, Endovaginal, Transperineal, 3D Imaging, and Doppler

Transabdominal scanning with a curvilinear transducer provides excellent delineation of placental structure and location. Endovaginal transducers allow visualization of the placenta and umbilical cord earlier than with transabdominal imaging. In addition, due to transducer placement within the vagina directly adjacent to the uterus, there is no need for a full bladder. The proximity to the os, and an empty bladder, make the endovaginal approach ideal for evaluating questionable previas late in pregnancy.

Transperineal ultrasound is a valuable adjunct to obstetric ultrasound protocols when endovaginal imaging is contraindicated or not available, particularly in evaluating the relationship between the placental edge and the internal os of the cervix.[15] Often in late second or third trimester pregnancies, the endocervical canal is obscured transabdominally, because of obstructive fetal parts and the inability to maintain a full bladder. With transperineal ultrasound, this area can be clearly imaged in most cases. With the transducer placed directly on the maternal perineum, it is possible to obtain an image similar to that obtained endovaginally, with less discomfort to the patient.[16]

In the past few years, valuable information has been obtained from conventional and color flow Doppler studies of the umbilical cord and placenta. For example, evaluation of the systolic-diastolic ratio in the uterine artery and evaluation for the persistence of an early diastolic notch have been demonstrated to be effective predictors of perinatal outcome, because they relate directly to increased placental or umbilical impedance.[10] Use of pulsed-wave Doppler may expose the fetus to higher energy intensities than are consistent with safety. It is suggested that Doppler be used on the fetus only when a study is clinically indicated, and that power output, color sector size, and examination time be kept to a minimum.[10]

Three-dimensional (3D) ultrasound complements two-dimensional (2D) and Doppler ultrasound, especially in the assessment of placental abnormalities. 3D evaluation allows for more accurate detailing of anatomic relationships and internal architecture.[17]

Is a Full Bladder Important?

For most transabdominal applications, the answer is a qualified "yes." A properly full bladder enhances placental visualization in early pregnancy and improves imaging of the lower uterine segment later in gestation. This latter point is particularly relevant when a diagnosis of placenta previa is being considered. An empty bladder may preclude visualization of the cervical os, but an overdistended bladder can cause a false-positive appearance of placenta previa. A very full bladder causes close apposition of the anterior and posterior walls of the lower uterine segment, producing what appears to be the internal cervical os at a falsely superior location. The sonographer can improve patient comfort and reduce the possibility of false-positive images of placenta previa by varying the degree of bladder distention during the examination (i.e., start with full bladder, then have the patient empty 1 cup of urine at a

time).[18] In general, a bladder is considered adequately full when cervical length is between 3 and 5 cm.[18,19] To relieve severe discomfort in late second- and third-trimester pregnancies, once the cervical area has been evaluated, the patient may void before the remainder of the examination is performed.

Because the endovaginal examination is best performed with an empty bladder, it may be better tolerated in late pregnancy and can be a valuable tool in assessing placenta previa. Although there are no confirmed adverse effects of endovaginal imaging, in some laboratories endovaginal scanning is prohibited if vaginal bleeding has occurred during the pregnancy. In such cases, transperineal scanning may suffice.[20]

Transducer, Angle, Frequency, and Gain Settings

A 3- or 3.5-megahertz (MHz) transducer is adequate for most routine imaging of the placenta. A lower-frequency transducer improves the image in several instances, such as in large patients, during third-trimester imaging, or when the fetus lies over a posterior placenta. Real-time units allow the user to control the electronic focal zone of the transducer.

When scanning the placenta, the beam should be as perpendicular as possible to the chorionic plate, especially when measuring thickness. Adjust the gains so that the placenta has a uniform and homogeneous granular texture. Both the sharp, linear acoustic interface of the chorionic plate and the hypoechoic retroplacental zone should be seen clearly (Fig. 17-10). Differentiation of placental tissue from that of a uterine contraction or myoma depends on clear visualization of these structures, particularly because posterior contractions may appear as echogenic as placental tissue. In such cases, other than waiting 20 to 30 minutes for disappearance of a contraction, the only way to prove that a particular tissue mass is placental is to demonstrate areas of placental

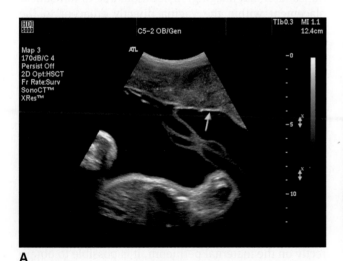

A

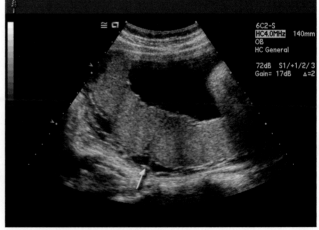

B

Figure 17-10 **A:** Curved linear image of an anterior placenta showing the distinct chorionic plate (*arrow*). **B:** Posterior placenta demonstrating the hypoechoic retroplacental zone (*arrow*). (Image **A** courtesy of Philips Medical Systems, Bothell, WA.)

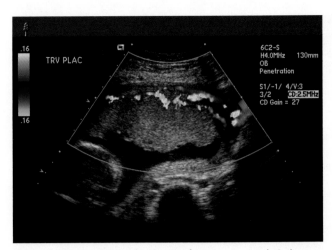

Figure 17-11 Color Doppler image of an anterior grade I placenta demonstrating retroplacental vascularity.

demarcation.[20] The gains may have to be reduced with posterior placentas to offset enhanced acoustic transmission from the overlying amniotic fluid. It is also important not to confuse a retroplacental contraction with the retroplacental complex of maternal veins. Increasing the gain to visualize flowing blood during real-time observation can be useful in distinguishing placental lakes or retroplacental vascular structures from other hypoechoic placental or retroplacental masses. The use of color Doppler aids in this evaluation (Fig. 17-11).

Measurement of Placental Thickness

The sonographer should first identify the placentomyometrial interface in an unobstructed midpoint position. The measurement should exclude the myometrium and retroplacental complex. Ideally, the transducer should be perpendicular to the placenta lest the resultant measurement be falsely high.[22] Evaluation of this measurement should take into consideration the shape of the

placenta. For example, a broad-based placenta may be thinner and a narrow-based placenta thicker, without indicating the presence of any lesion. 3D volumes may become a more important measurement for the evaluation of the placenta (Figure 17-12).

NORMAL SONOGRAPHY OF THE PLACENTA

Scanning Protocol

Placental evaluation should be part of every obstetric scan with documentation of the placental location of the placenta in relation to the internal cervical os. In the case of an accessory (succenturiate) lobe, note the location along with the position of the connecting tissue or membranes. Evaluate the structural texture, morphology, and any abnormalities of the placenta and the insertion site of the cord. Placental thickness should be determined and correlated with clinical data (Table 17-1). If there has been any vaginal bleeding or abdominal pain, examine the retroplacental area for possible areas of elevation.

Morphology

Endovaginal sonography can identify trophoblast development as a distinct echogenic ring, as early as 4 to 5 weeks.[21] The placenta is easily visualized transabdominally by 8 to 10 weeks as focal thickening of the decidua surrounding the gestational sac (Fig. 17-13). By 12 weeks, the placenta clearly visualizes as a discoid structure with a homogeneous echotexture. This stage also allows for identification of the sharp, linear acoustic interface of the chorionic plate on the fetal side of the placenta.[10] Other than the site of cord insertion, the subchorionic area usually appears smooth and uninterrupted throughout most of pregnancy. However, later in pregnancy this chorionic interface becomes less smooth as fetal vessels develop just below the placental surface.[12] Doppler assessment of the umbilical

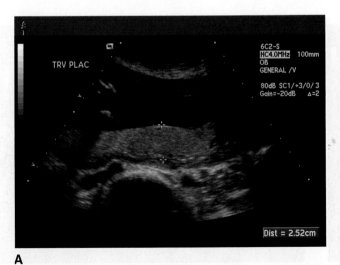

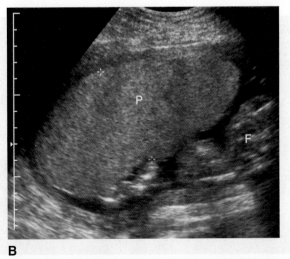

A   **B**

Figure 17-12 A: Curved linear image of a normal posterior placenta showing placement of cursors for measurement of placental thickness with a posterior placenta. The measurement excludes the retroplacental complex. **B:** Placement of the calipers for a lateral or fundal placenta is perpendicular to the placenta, not the beam. This placenta, taken at 25 weeks' gestation, is thickened at 6.3 cm. *P*-placenta; *F*-fetus.

TABLE 17-1			
Disease States in Relation to Placental Appearance[10,21,47]			
Increased Placental Thickness (>4 cm)	**Decreased Placental Thickness (<2 cm)**	**Early Placental Maturation**	**Delayed Placental Maturation**
Diabetes (nonvascular types)	Pre-eclampsia	IUGR	Gestational diabetes
Rh incompatibility (hydropic changes)	IUGR	Hypertension	Rh disease
Cytomegalovirus infection	Juvenile diabetes (vascular forms)		
Abruption*	Placentation abnormality (memraneous placenta)		
Chorioangioma			
Multiple gestation			
Syphilis			
Chromosomal abnormality (triploidy)			

*Apparent thickening due to retroplacental clot, isoechoic with placenta.[16,55]

artery has demonstrated the low-resistance, high diastolic blood flow characteristic of the normal placenta as early as 5 weeks' gestation.[23] Increasing gain settings allows visualization of red blood cell movement. In this manner, subchorionic and intraplacental vascular structures may be differentiated from other, nonvascular, pathologic entities.[24] In addition, 3D power Doppler is now being used to assess the angiographic features of placental masses.[25] Turning the transducer 90 degrees to demonstrate the tubular nature of an unknown structure provides another clue to suggest that it is vascular. Occasionally, an area of the chorionic plate may be seen that appears separated from the placenta. This could represent an area of prior placental (subchorionic) hemorrhage and may be correlated with a previous episode of vaginal bleeding.

Intraplacental Texture

Placental texture changes from an echogenic focal thickening of the wall of the gestational sac early in pregnancy to the fine, granular, homogeneous texture seen from the end of the first trimester. This texture continues throughout most of the pregnancy and usually images in the older placenta. However, in the second and third trimesters, intraplacental and subchorionic vascular spaces may sometimes be seen and should be assessed carefully. Although they usually have no clinical significance (Fig. 17-14), any areas of varied echogenicity (e.g., a multiple cystic or vesicular appearance; irregular, hypoechoic areas; or highly echogenic areas with hypoechoic margins) should be carefully documented. There is an association between increased levels of serum alpha-fetoprotein and the findings of large vascular spaces. A late third-trimester placenta may exhibit cystic areas located centrally within clearly delineated lobes. These nonvascular areas may represent areas of necrosis.[21]

The Retroplacental Complex

No assessment of the placenta is complete without evaluation of the retroplacental complex (RPC). This zone is composed of the decidua basalis and portions of the

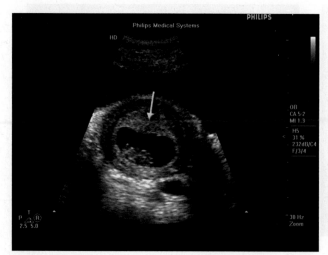

Figure 17-13 This transabdominal image of a 9-week gestation demonstrates focal thickening (*arrow*), representing early placental formation. (Image courtesy of Philips Medical Systems, Bothell, WA.)

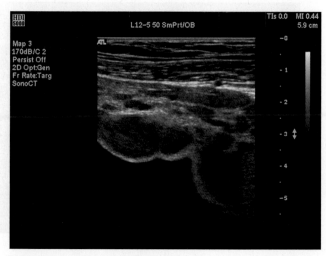

Figure 17-14 Placental lakes appear as hypoechoic areas within the anterior placenta. Blood often images swirling within these structures. (Image courtesy of Philips Medical Systems, Bothell, WA.)

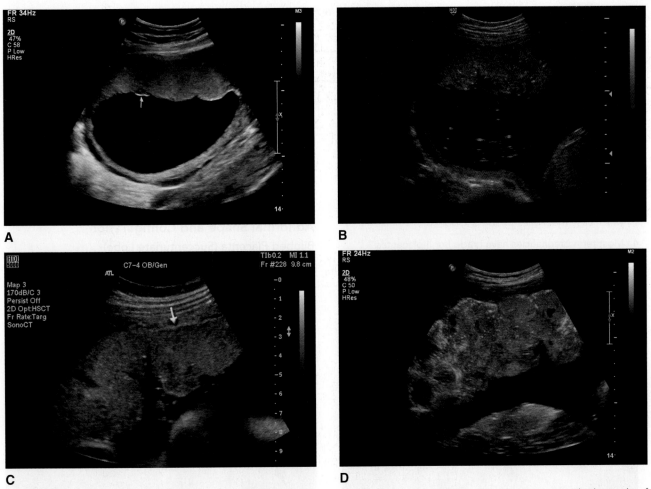

Figure 17-15 A: Anterior grade 0 placenta demonstrating the characteristic smooth, homogeneous texture. The perpendicular angle of incidence allows for imaging of the chorionic plate *(arrow)*. **B:** This grade I placenta contains scattered calcifications with the beginning of lobulations developing on the fetal side. **C:** In the grade II placenta lobulations increase with the basal layer *(arrow)* appearing irregular due to small calcifications. **D:** The grade III placenta demonstrates interlobar and septal calcifications.

myometrium, including maternal veins draining the placenta. Identifiable as early as 14 weeks, this typically hypoechoic area is 10 to 20 millimeters (mm) deep to the placenta.[26] Proper identification of this area is important. A prominent anterior RPC can lead to excessive bleeding during invasive procedures such as amniocentesis or cesarean section. In addition, the RPC can mimic abruptio placentae, degenerating fibroids, or hydatidiform mole. Real-time visualization of blood flow in this area helps distinguish the normal RPC from the aforementioned pathologic conditions.[1,27,28]

Large venous channels may be visualized within the complex, most commonly in posteriorly located placentas, where the effects of gravity-induced pressure can overdistend the veins. The appearance of large venous channels may also occur when the beam strikes tangentially, as with a fundal or lateral placenta.[29]

Normal Placental Calcification

Placental calcium deposition is a normal physiologic process occurring throughout pregnancy. More than 50% of placentas show some degree of macroscopic calcification after 33 weeks.[30] Although the degree of normal calcification is variable, it usually increases throughout pregnancy, becoming more prominent as first the basal area and then the interlobar septa calcify. Calcium may also be found in the villous, perivillous, and subchorionic spaces.[29,31,32] Intraplacental calcifications are imaged sonographically as strong acoustic echoes without significant acoustic shadowing.[30,32]

PLACENTAL GRADING

A grading system based on the degree of placental calcification (Table 17-2) was at one time thought to be an indicator of fetal pulmonary maturity. It is now known that multiple factors, including smoking, low maternal age, parity, and even season of the year can affect the degree of placental calcification,[10] and it is no longer considered a marker for lung maturity.

More to the point, assessment of placental calcification is important in certain serious maternal and fetal conditions. For example, premature placental calcification can occur in maternal hypertensive states and in association

TABLE	17-2

Placental Grading Based on Placental Calcifications[10,33,94]

1. Placental Grading

   Grade 0 No calcifications (to about 31 wk)

      I Scattered calcifications (31–36 wk)

      II Basal calcifications with increase in lobulations (36–38 wk)

      III Basal and interlobar septal calcifications (38 wk to term)

2. The placenta matures considerably after the 40th week.

3. Two parts of the placenta may have different grades, in which case the highest grade is assigned.

4. Most term pregnancies have grade I or II placentas.

5. Only about 10%–15% of term placentas are grade III.

with intrauterine growth retardation/restriction; other conditions such as gestational diabetes or fetal cardiopulmonary disorders may retard the rate of placental calcification. Evaluating placental calcifications in relation to the age of gestation can give additional important input to the entire clinical picture, even though in recent studies placental grading has not been found to be the most reliable predictor of placental function (Fig. 17-15).[33]

ABNORMALITIES OF THE PLACENTA

Table 17-3 lists the common placental abnormalities and their sonographic appearances.

Abnormal Shape and Configuration

Bilobed Placenta (Succenturiate Lobe)

Although it usually consists of one mass, the placenta may be bilobed or have a smaller accessory, succenturiate lobe. This is visualized in up to 6% of cases

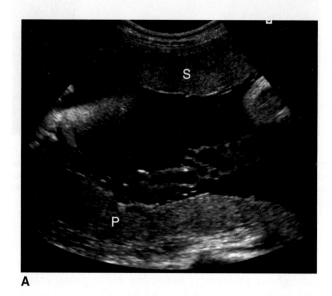

A

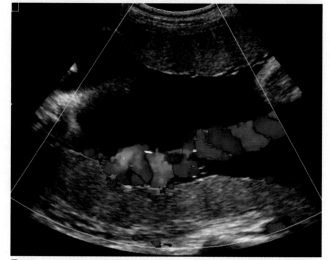

B

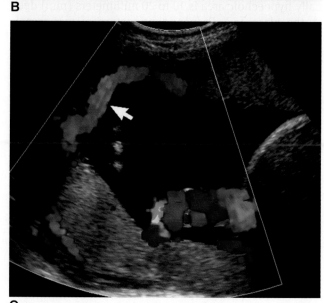

C

Figure 17-16 Succenturiate placentation. **A:** Sonogram demonstrating a succenturiate lobe (S) separate from the anterior placenta (P). **B:** The umbilical cord inserts normally into the posterior lobe. **C:** Anastomotic vessels (arrow) shown with color-flow imaging supply the succenturiate lobe.

TABLE 17-3

Sonographic Characteristics of Placental Abnormalities[16,21,29,30,40,58,60–62,65–67,69,95,96]

Abnormality	Description	Sonographic Characteristics	Differential Diagnosis
Placenta previa	Placental tissue obstructing internal os. Most common cause of bleed in 2nd and 3rd trimester	Placental tissue seen to cover internal os—whether completely, partially, or marginally	Uterine contraction, fibroid, overdistended bladder may falsely suggest previa
Abruption	Premature separation of all or part of the placenta	Elevated portion of placenta or extramembranous retroplacental, subchorionic, or intraplacental, hypoechoic or complex, transonic mass of varying echogenicity. May appear as normal placenta. May appear as thickened placenta	Retroplacental thrombosis, normal placenta, abnormally thick placenta, normal intraplacental complex
Placenta accreta	Decidual formation defect with abnormal placental attachment to uterine wall	Normal retroplacental hypoechoic area not visualized	Myometrial scar
Hypoechoic lesions			
Fibrin depositions	Secondary to vascular thrombosis and cystic degeneration of fibrin	Hypoechoic areas in intervillous spaces beneath chorion. Lack of real-time evidence of blood flow	Venous lakes, hematoma
Hematoma	Area of retroplacental or intraplacental clot	May be hypoechoic or of varied echogenicity depending on age of clot. Lack of real-time evidence of blood flow	Venous lakes, fibrin deposition
Intervillous thrombi	Interplacental areas of hemorrhage and pooling of blood; increase in Rh isoimmunization	Hypoechoic areas of varying size throughout placenta	Hematoma
Breus' mole	Massive subchorionic thrombosis-secondary to extreme venous obstruction; unrelated to fibrin deposition	Extensive hypoechoic hematoma without evidence of venous flow	Placental tumor, fibroid, hematoma
Infarct	Result of obstruction of spiral arteries	No confirmed sonographic appearance, but necrotic infarct may appear hypoechoic or show placental thinning	Retroplacental hematoma, fibrin deposition
Placental lake	Subchorionic blood-filled spaces	Subchorionic, anechoic, tubular spaces. Flow may be demonstrated	Fibrin depositions
Neoplastic lesions			
Chorioangioma	Benign tumor resulting from vascular malformation, most common placental tumor, may be multiple, small, or single large; associated with fetal edema	Usually hypo- or hyperechoic well-circumscribed masses, often with cystic spaces; placenta may show as placental thickening without discrete mass. Large mass may extend from fetal surface of placenta. Associated with hydramnios; may see vascular channels within mass	Fibroid, Breus' mole
Teratoma	Rare, benign to highly malignant germ cell tumor	Complex, heterogeneous mass; may have calcifications	Fibroid

(Fig. 17-16).[29,34] The accessory lobe is connected to the main placental mass either by vessels within a membrane or by a bridge of membranes.[34] The main placental mass tends to be larger than the accessory lobe and is most commonly where the umbilical cord inserts.[29] Identification of an accessory lobe is clinically relevant because of the increased risk of infarction, placenta previa, vasa previa, postpartum, and hemorrhage associated with retained accessory lobes.[29] Perinatal mortality can reach 100% if vasa previa goes undiagnosed, because hemorrhaging may lead to fetal anemia and/or shock.[34] Therefore, sonographic delineation of placental tissue in more than one area of the uterus—and, if possible, the connecting bridge between the two placental masses, especially if it overlies the cervical os—is a valuable contribution to the management of obstetric patients.[29,34] Care should be taken not to confuse a fold in the placenta with an extra lobe.

Circumvallate Placenta

In up to 11% of deliveries, the area of placental implantation extends beyond the limits of the chorionic plate.[35] Therefore, a rim forms around this margin of placenta that does not have associated chorion. The rim consists of fibrinoid tissue with hyaline degeneration of villi. Presence of circumvallate placenta may be associated with maternal bleeding, placental abruption, preterm loss, and oligohydramnios and could potentially be involved in amniotic band syndrome. However, most cases tend to be difficult to visualize later in pregnancy and have no clinical significance.[35,36] Sonographically, circumvallate placenta may be seen as irregular subchorionic or subamniotic marginal cystic structures or infolding of the placental margin into the uterine cavity.[36]

Abnormal Membranes/Amniotic Bands

Before fusion at about 16 weeks' gestation, the amniotic and chorionic membranes are separated by the extraembryonic coelom. A floating membrane seen before this time is thought to represent the not-yet-fused amnion. Floating membranes seen after 16 weeks may represent a separation of the fused membranes or separation of both membranes from the decidua. This may be present without complications or may be associated with vaginal bleeding of varying degrees. Before 16 weeks, the amnion itself may rupture and collapse, leaving the fetus to develop as an "extra-amniotic pregnancy" within the extra-amniotic coelom.[14,37,38]

Sonographically, a collapsed amnion images as multiple wavy linear echoes in the dependent portion of the uterus. Amniotic bands, on the other hand, are linear echoes traversing the amniotic cavity; they may not visualize at all. The consequences of amniotic bands to the fetus vary widely. Although in most cases they do not disturb the fetus, fetal entanglement with these membranes, referred to as the amniotic band syndrome, can result in limb deformities and spine and facial abnormalities of varying degrees of severity, and may even result in amputation of compromised body parts.[39,40] A variant of the amniotic band, the amniotic sheet or shelf, is seen as a thicker and broader floating membrane with only one free edge (Fig. 17-17). This is thought to represent a deep fold of the chorion and may restrict fetal movement.[41,42] Follow-up sonographic evaluations help document any fixation of fetal parts.

Annular Placenta and Placenta Membranacea

Annular placenta refers to a ring-shaped placenta that attaches circumferentially to the myometrium. Placenta membranacea refers to a rare condition in which there is no differentiation of chorion frondosum from chorion laeve, and placental villi cover all or most of the surface of the gestational membranes. The placenta is usually much thinner than normal.[43,44] Both the annular placenta and placenta membranacea have been associated with antepartum and postpartum hemorrhage. A

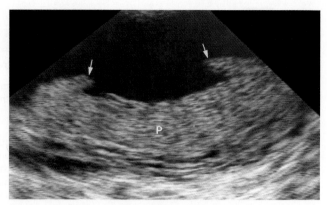

Figure 17-17 Image demonstrates infolding margins *(arrows)* of placenta *(P)* consistent with circumvillate placenta.

placenta membranacea would be diagnosed if placental tissue were seen over most of the uterine cavity.[44]

Abnormal Placental Size

Variation in placental size may be indicative of several important fetal and maternal pathologic conditions (Table 17-1). Much research has been conducted to determine the best sonographic means of assessing placental size in relation to gestational age. Although surface area and volumetric measurements show this relationship best, their determination may be quite time consuming, even with 3D technology. There has been mathematical volumetric work using 2D sonography, which has improved efficiency in determining weight[45]; however, because it is easier to measure, thickness is used more routinely (even though thickness is more variable and less accurate than volume, being a function of gestational age, placental location, and transducer angle).[22,46]

Generally, a normal placenta should be between 2 and 4 cm in thickness.[21] An abnormally thick placenta can be seen in association with maternal gestational diabetes (due to villous edema) or in any case of placental hydrops, which is associated with fetal cardiac overload.[21] A thin placenta (less than 2 cm) may be seen in pregnancies complicated by essential maternal hypertension and pre-eclampsia, and with intrauterine growth retardation and placental infarction.[21,47] Abnormal placental thickness, whether it be thin or thick, can also be associated with intrauterine infection and chromosomal abnormalities.[47]

Placental Hydrops

The abnormal thickness (greater than 5 cm) of a hydropic placenta is due to fluid overload, usually secondary to high-output cardiac failure in the fetus.[47] This can occur in erythroblastosis fetalis, fetomaternal and twin-to-twin transfusion syndromes, chorioangioma (in which fetal blood is shunted through the placental circulation), and vascular obstruction such as umbilical vein thrombosis.[39,47] Sonography of the hydropic placenta shows it to be abnormally thick with a rigid, bulbous

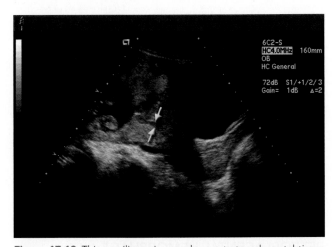

Figure 17-18 This curvilinear image demonstrates placental tissue attaching to the uterine wall completely covering the os. Arrows indicate the slightly echogenic mucosa of the endocervical canal.

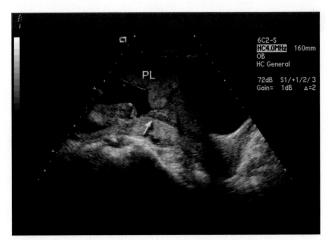

Figure 17-19 Curvilinear image of a marginal previa demonstrates an anterior placenta (PL) with the edge ending next to the hypoechoic cervical os (*arrow*).

appearance. The normal placental architecture is lost and a "spongy" appearance is seen.[47]

ABNORMAL PLACENTAL LOCATION (PLACENTA PREVIA)

Placenta previa is the instance when the placenta partially or completely covers the internal cervical os. Total placenta previa occurs when implantation of the placenta completely crosses the internal os. Sonographically, the body of the placenta covers the os entirely (Fig. 17-18). When just the edge of the placenta is seen to abut or cover the os, it is described as a marginal or partial placenta previa (Fig. 17-19). In these cases, implantation does not cross the os. If the edge of the placenta is near but not abutting the os, it is classified as a low-lying placenta (Fig. 17-20).[21]

Placenta previas tend to be uncommon (less than 0.5% of full-term gestations), yet because of the increase in caesarean sections being performed, there has been an associated increase in previas.[28] Additionally, women with increased maternal age and/or multiple gestations are also at increased risk. Patients tend to present with painless vaginal bleeding requiring sonographic evaluation in the second or third trimester, yet many individuals are asymptomatic.[48] Indeed, placenta previa is said to be one of the most common causes of third-trimester bleeding.[49] It is more common in patients with previous lower uterine incisional scars for cesarean section or myomectomy. Placenta previa seems to be more prevalent in older women and in multiparas. It is thought that myometrial scarring leads to the development of a poorly vascularized, thinner placenta, which occupies a greater uterine surface area, increasing the probability of encroachment on the cervical os.[21]

Although a sonographic diagnosis of placenta previa can be made quite easily, the accuracy of the diagnosis is dependent upon gestational age and whether there is complete or partial previa. The positive predictive value is higher the later the detection via sonography.[50] The

Figure 17-20 Diagram of three types of placentae previa. **A:** In low-lying placenta, the edge of the placenta is visualized near the os. **B:** In marginal or partial previa, placental tissue may cover the os but is not attached to the wall at the other side. **C:** In complete previa, placental tissue completely covers the internal os and is attached to the uterine wall on both sides of the os.

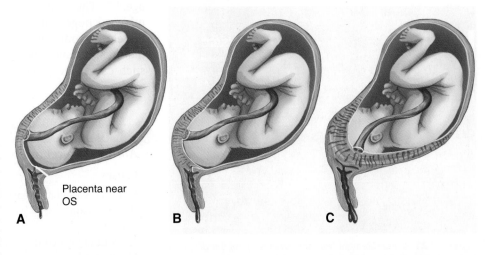

Placenta near OS

A   Marginal

B   Partial

C   Complete

PATHOLOGY BOX 17-2

Risk Factors for Placenta Previa

Advanced maternal age (AMA)
Multiple gestation
History of cesarean section
Previous myomectomy
Multiparity

reason for this is that in most suspected second-trimester placenta previa cases, apparent "placental migration" (caused by late second– and early third–trimester differential growth of the lower uterine segment) results in a normal implantation at term.[51]

The clinical course and outcome of placenta previa relate to the degree of cervical os encroachment. It is important for the sonographer to try to establish the degree of previa that is present. A placenta located less than 2 cm from the internal os usually requires a cesarean section because of the risk of maternal bleeding (Fig. 17-21).[21]

The knowledge of several technical points and ultrasound techniques can help in the diagnosis of placenta previa. A focal, symmetric, lower uterine segment contraction can be mistaken for placenta previa.[28] Repeat scanning after waiting for a half hour should show in the case of a contraction that it has subsided. The sonographer can vary the degree of bladder distention to decrease the rate of false-positive diagnoses. This technique can also help to determine more accurately the type of previa present. In late pregnancy, it may be necessary to scan through a fairly empty bladder, making transabdominal visualization of the cervical area difficult. As a rule of thumb, if a third-trimester placenta is at the uterine fundus, chances of a previa are low, because most placentas are unlikely to extend from the fundus to the cervix.[52] Exceptions to this may occur if the placenta is thin and flat, covering a greater area of the intrauterine surface, or if an accessory lobe is present in association with the lower segment. Endovaginal or transperineal scanning provides additional, more accurate diagnostic information.

When in doubt, it is most important to err on the side of caution and assume the presence of placenta previa. A false-positive diagnosis early in pregnancy, with later reassessment, does not harm the mother or fetus, whereas a missed diagnosis is potentially catastrophic. The usual causes of missed diagnosis are poor technique and poor visualization of a posterior placenta obscured by an overlying fetal head.

RETROPLACENTAL HEMORRHAGE: PLACENTAL ABRUPTION

Placental abruption refers to the premature separation of all or part of the placenta from the underlying myometrium. Abruption has been associated with, among other things, maternal vascular disease, maternal hypertension, trauma, a short umbilical cord, and increased maternal age.[21] Abruption may manifest itself in three ways: as external bleeding without significant intrauterine hematoma, as the development of a retroplacental or marginal hematoma with or without external bleeding, and as formation of a submembranous clot at a distance from the placenta, with or without external bleeding.[21] Clinically, patients may be asymptomatic or may be quite ill with acute hemorrhage and shock, presenting with a rigid abdomen and severe uterine contractions. Perinatal mortality has been found to be up to 60% with abruption, and rarely maternal death may occur.[53] It is important to recognize that the bleeding associated with abruption is usually painful (especially when retroplacental in location). Although it is classically described as one of the leading causes of third-trimester bleeding, it can occur earlier in pregnancy as well.[49,54]

The sonographic appearance of retroplacental hemorrhage is varied, depending on its location, size, and age.[16,40] The hematoma is usually hypoechoic or of mixed echogenicity, and its echogenicity increases as the clot becomes more organized.[16,40] As the hematoma matures, it may appear isoechoic with the placenta. In such cases, the placenta at first glance may appear to

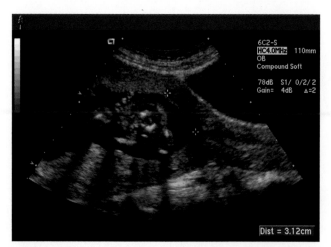

Figure 17-21 A measurement from the lower edge of the placenta to the internal cervical os helps determine the presence or absence of placenta previa. A measurement of 2 cm or greater rules out previa.

PATHOLOGY BOX 17-3

Abruptio Placentae

Causes	Symptoms
Maternal vascular disease	Asymptomatic
Hypertension	External bleeding
Trauma	Pain
Short umbilical cord	Shock
Maternal age	Rigid abdomen

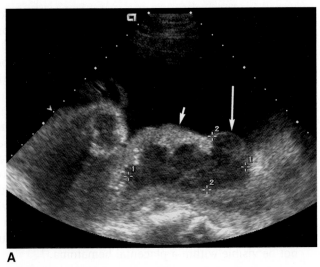
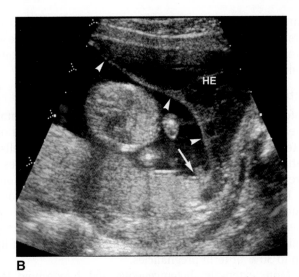

A   **B**

Figure 17-22 Placental abruption. **A:** There is a hypoechoic, retroplacental hematoma *(long arrow and calipers)* lifting the edge of the placenta *(short arrow)*. **B:** The hypoechoic hematoma *(HE)* lifts the edge of the placenta *(arrow)* under the chorionic membrane *(arrowheads)*.

be abnormally thick; however, moving the patient to her side helps in differentiation of the placenta from the underlying clot. This provides a different angle of access to the ultrasound beam and may allow for visualization of the interface between the hematoma and the placenta. If the hematoma is near the lower uterine segment, transperineal ultrasound may provide more diagnostic information (Fig. 17-22).[16,55]

The diagnosis of retroplacental abruption is usually based on clinical symptoms such as painful vaginal bleeding, fetal distress, acute abdominal pain, and tense and tender uterus. Sonography is diagnostic only if a clot or elevation of part of the placenta can be visualized.[56]

An interesting example of a secondary finding that might alert the sonographer to look for evidence of an abruption is a case report of an echogenic mass within the fetal stomach in a patient with retroplacental hemorrhage.[57] Presumably, some intra-amniotic bleeding must have occurred from the abruption, which was then ingested by the fetus. However, many normal fetuses may have intraluminal debris in their stomach from ingested vernix caseosum. It should be emphasized that sonography cannot be relied on to exclude the diagnosis if no hematoma is seen.[16] Many cases of abruption of the placenta may look normal, especially late in pregnancy.[16,58] Assessing the fetal heart rate pattern has been found to reflect the severity of the abruption, with bradycardia and irregularity reflecting the most severe cases.[59]

The clinical outcome depends on the size of the abruption and its location. For example, a paraplacental (marginal) clot has much less clinical importance than a large retroplacental hematoma associated with placental separation, which has a far greater likelihood to lead to premature delivery or miscarriage. The differential diagnosis of a retroplacental hemorrhage includes normal maternal veins in the retroplacental complex, hydatidiform mole, chorioangioma, and leiomyoma.[30,58]

ABNORMAL PLACENTAL ATTACHMENT (PLACENTA ACCRETA, INCRETA, PERCRETA)

Some relatively uncommon conditions are the result of defective decidua formation causing abnormal attachment of the placenta to the uterine wall. In these cases, there is no decidua basalis between the trophoblast and the myometrium.[21] As with placenta previa, the presence of uterine scarring seems to predispose patients to the development of this condition. In fact, up to 70% of cases occur in association with placenta previa and in patients with a history of prior cesarean section. In placenta accreta, the chorionic villi are in direct contact with the myometrium. Placenta increta and percreta are more severe forms. With increta, the villi invade the myometrium as far as the serosa; with percreta the villi penetrate the uterine wall, and their presence can lead to uterine rupture.[21,60,61]

Sonography may reveal obliteration or focal disruption of the normal retroplacental hypoechoic complex; perhaps with a focal mass-like extension of placental tissue into the uterine wall or even the bladder wall (Fig. 17-5).[62] Antenatal detection of this condition is difficult but extremely important. If it is not treated (usually by hysterectomy), it can lead to maternal exsanguination.[63] Power and color flow Doppler have been found to be effective in diagnosis.[63]

ABNORMALITIES OF PLACENTAL ECHOGENICITY—HYPOECHOIC PLACENTAL LESIONS

Subchorionic Lakes

Subchorionic lakes are tubular, anechoic lesions found beneath the chorionic plate that correspond to blood-filled spaces found at delivery. There is some question as to whether these represent normal mature villi or an early stage of intervillous thrombosis or fibrin deposition. It has been suggested that increased flow in these areas is related to decreased fibrin deposition or maternal chronic hypoxia due to high altitudes.[44,64]

Intervillous Thrombosis

Intervillous thrombosis represents an intraplacental area of hemorrhage and clot. It is probably the result of a tear in the villi causing leakage of fetal red blood cells, which in turn stimulate maternal coagulation.[30] These areas of thrombosis appear sonographically as anechoic or hypoechoic lesions of varying sizes that may contain linear echogenicities representing fibrin deposits. They are most commonly found midway between the chorionic and basal plates of the placenta and are present in up to 30% of term pregnancies.[65]

More extensive, heterogeneous and hypoechoic lesions may represent massive subchorionic hematoma or thrombosis (Breus' mole), a rare occurrence secondary to venous obstruction.[66] These lesions often separate the chorionic plate from the underlying villous tissue and may bulge into the amniotic cavity. The blood in these cases is generally of maternal origin and there is an associated large placenta. These are usually found in missed abortions, premature deliveries, and neonatal demise and are associated with maternal diabetes and hypertension.[29,67]

Fibrin Deposition

Fibrin deposition is an apparently insignificant clinical event that is probably the end result of intervillous and subchorionic thrombosis, which results from pooling and stasis of maternal blood in the perivillous and subchorionic spaces.[30,31] Fibrin deposits have been variously reported as sonographically hypoechoic lesions in the subchorionic area or within the placental mass.[30]

Placental Infarction

It is thought that placental infarcts result from obstruction of the spiral arterioles and are usually found at the periphery of the placenta.[31,68] They may be associated with retroplacental hemorrhage and may occur in up to 25% of term placentas.[31] Although they usually have no clinical significance, they appear to be more common in association with intrauterine growth retardation (IUGR) and mothers with pre-eclampsia.[31] Sonographic appearances of placental infarcts are nonspecific but have been seen as anechoic placental lesions that may eventually calcify.[62]

NONTROPHOBLASTIC PLACENTAL TUMORS

Chorioangioma and teratoma represent the two primary nontrophoblastic tumors of the placenta.

Chorioangioma

A chorioangioma is a benign hypervascular malformation found in up to 1% of examined placentas.[21,69] Small chorioangiomas may be nonsymptomatic, whereas large chorioangiomas may result in the development of maternal toxemia, polyhydramnios, premature labor, IUGR, fetal hydrops, or fetal demise.[21] In addition, there may be significant shunting of blood through the tumor, which has been documented with Doppler.[69]

Sonographically, small chorioangiomas image as hypo- or hyperechoic, well-circumscribed placental masses. Often the lesions also contain cystic spaces.[69] The single, large chorioangioma, seen less often, may appear as a well circumscribed, complex mass on the fetal surface of the placenta, adjacent to the cord insertion[70] or protruding into the amniotic cavity (Fig. 18-19).[69] Color Doppler is effective for demonstrating vascular channels within the mass, which would not be visible within a placental hematoma.[69]

Teratoma

Teratomas of the placenta are very rare and are benign. Sonographically, they appear as a complex mass.[71]

Gestational Trophoblastic Disease

Gestational trophoblastic disease (GTD) is a designation given to several disorders arising from either normal or abnormal fertilization of an ovum, resulting in neoplastic changes in the trophoblastic elements of the developing blastocyst. GTD classifications include hydatidiform mole, either complete or partial; nonmetastatic disease or invasive mole; and metastatic disease or choriocarcinoma.[72] GTD is treated extensively in Chapters 9 and 13.

THE UMBILICAL CORD

DEVELOPMENT

The umbilical cord originates from fusion of the yolk sac stalk and the omphalomesenteric duct at approximately 7 weeks' gestation. The urachus, an outpouching from the urinary bladder, forms the allantois and thus the definitive umbilical vessels.

STRUCTURE AND FUNCTION

The umbilical cord normally contains two arteries and one vein surrounded by a mucoid connective tissue (Wharton's jelly), all enclosed in a layer of amnion.[9] The vein brings fresh, oxygenated blood to the fetus and the arteries carry deoxygenated blood from the fetus to the placenta. The umbilical arteries are longer than the vein and wind around it. The vessels are longer than the cord itself, resulting in twisting and bending of the cord and vessels (see Fig. 17-8).[10] The cross-sectional area of the cord has been found to correlate with gestational age, up until it reaches a plateau at 32 weeks.[30] At term, the average length of the cord is about 51.5 to 61 cm, with a mean circumference of 3.8 cm.[29,73]

The Umbilical Cord

2 arteries/1 vein
Covered by Wharton's jelly
Coiled
51.5–61 cm/20.3–24 inches long
3.8 cm/1.5 inches in circumference

SCANNING TECHNIQUE

The umbilical cord visualizes best in the late second and early third trimester, when amniotic fluid volume is at its peak. Because of the extreme length of the cord, it is difficult, on a routine basis, to scan it in its entirety to rule out abnormalities. If a lesion is suspected, every effort must be made to view as much of the cord as possible. Changing the mother's position from side to side may help shift the position of the fetus in relation to the cord. The placental insertion site of the cord, as well as its entry site to the fetus (to rule out, for example, omphalocele) should be imaged and documented routinely. Document the presence of three vessels within the cord. Visualization of the number of cord vessels is difficult when there is oligohydramnios, and it may be troublesome in the third trimester even in a normal fetus because of the relative lack of fluid and the presence of potentially obstructing fetal parts. Any abnormality in cord appearance, size, position, degree of coiling, or attachment sites to placenta or fetus should be noted.[30]

Normal Sonographic Appearance

In early pregnancy, the umbilical cord may appear as a series of short, linear echoes extending from the fetus to the placenta (Fig. 13-15). It tends to be seen as the same length as the fetal pole.[74] As pregnancy progresses, transverse images through the cord reveal the three circles representing the larger vein and two smaller arteries. Longitudinal images at this stage reveal a series of parallel linear echoes within the amniotic fluid that may exhibit the characteristic twisted appearance of the cord (Figs. 18-27 and 18-28). The "stack of coins" appearance refers to visualization of several portions of cord folded on each other (Fig. 17-23).[75] Arterial pulsations may be demonstrated within the umbilical arteries. The insertion of the umbilical cord into the placenta should be easily identifiable sonographically, especially with the use of color Doppler (Fig. 18-28).[76]

ABNORMALITIES OF THE UMBILICAL CORD

Table 17-4 lists the common umbilical cord abnormalities and their sonographic appearances.

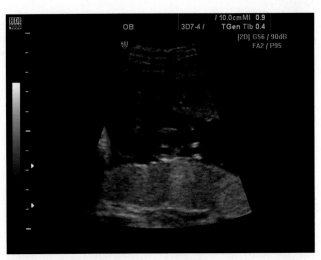

Figure 17-23 When several portions of the cord fold on top of one another, this "stack of coins" appearance is seen. (Image courtesy of Philips Medical Systems, Bothell, WA)

ABSENCE OF UMBILICAL CORD

Complete absence of the umbilical cord (agenesis or acordia) or presence of a very short cord has been associated with the limb-body wall complex, a syndrome of severe fetal structural anomalies.[77] Body stalk anomaly, a fatal condition, has been linked to maternal cocaine abuse.[78] Sonographically, no cord would be seen, but rather an extraembryonic membranous sac in direct apposition to the chorionic plate.[47]

ABNORMALITIES OF CORD INSERTION

The umbilical cord usually inserts in the center of the placenta; however, it may be marginal or velamentous (Fig. 17-9). In the latter case, vessels are found lying on the surface of the chorioamniotic membranes. This condition is associated with various fetal anomalies, a lower birth weight, and more intrapartum complications, often due to umbilical cord malpresentation, such as vasa previa.[79] For this reason, careful examination of the placental insertion site is important (Fig. 17-24).

TRUE AND FALSE KNOTS

The differences in umbilical vein, umbilical artery, and cord stromal length give rise to bending and twisting of the umbilical cord. Sometimes this twisting may appear as a false knot, which has no clinical significance. It can, however, be sonographically confused with a true knot of the cord, which occurs when the fetus actually passes through a loop of cord. This potentially hazardous situation occurs in up to 3% of deliveries.[80] It is difficult to detect sonographically, but has been associated with a "cloverleaf" pattern of the cord.[80] Color Doppler may aid in the diagnosis.

TABLE 17-4

Sonographic Characteristics of Umbilical Abnormalities[77,80,89,90,97–100]

Abnormality	Description	Sonographic Characteristics	Differential Diagnosis
Excessive Wharton's jelly	Diffuse or focal deposits of excess Wharton's jelly; may liquefy and get very large	Variably echogenic, soft tissue mass with three vessels visible within, usually near fetal abdomen, may be cystic if liquefied	Hernia, tumor, hematoma, cysts
Umbilical hernia	Small protrusion of abdominal contents into umbilical cord seen after 17 wk	Small mass adjacent to abdomen. Usually regresses spontaneously	Small omphalocele
Omphalocele	Protrusion of abdominal structures (liver, bowel) into base of cord-covered by peritoneum; high incidence of associated congenital abnormalities	Mass adjacent to anterior abdominal wall, covered by membrane, into apex of which cord appears to insert. Sac may be distended by ascites	Gastroschisis, hematoma
False knot	Folding of vessels that are longer than covering membrane, or simple dilatation of vessels	Irregular protrusion from cord	
True knot	Results from excessive fetal movement, especially with a long cord, or polyhydramnios; may become tightened and occlude umbilical vessels; associated increased incidence of congenital anomalies	Irregular protrusion from cord	May see cloverleaf pattern of cord
Stricture	Localized narrowing of cord, disappearance of Wharton's jelly, torsion of cord or thickening of vessel walls with narrowing of lumen	Narrowing of cord close to fetus with edematous area distal	
Umbilical vein thrombosis	Occlusion of umbilical vein secondary to localized increase of resistance in umbilical circulation; associated with maternal diabetes, arthritis, nonimmune hydrops	Increased echogenicity of umbilical vessels or echoic material within lumen	Artifact
Cystic masses			
Allantoic cyst (developmental urachal cyst)	Fluid-filled remnant of allantoid duct associated with patent urachus and lower tract obstructions	Usually small, mild focal dilatation of cord	Omphalomesenteric cyst
Omphalomesenteric cyst	Vestigal patency and dilatation of duct seen after 16 wk	Cystic dilatation up to 6 centimeters, usually located close to fetus	Hematoma, liquefied Wharton's jelly
Solid masses			
Hemangioma	Benign tumor of vessels or Wharton's jelly—if large can cause vascular obstruction; may be associated with increased amniotic fluid and α-fetoprotein and nonimmune hydrops[99]	Varied appearance; hyperechoic mass with smooth, lobulated contours, up to 15 cm; may have small, ovoid lucencies or numerous, small, highly echoic reflectors. Surrounding cord may appear edematous; usually located near placental margin	Hematoma, teratoma
Complex masses			
Hematoma	Rare; result of extravasation of blood into Wharton's jelly from rupture of umbilical vein; may be due to congenital weakness of vessel wall, or iatrogenic; associated with perinatal loss	May be septated, hyperechoic, or hypoechoic depending on age of clot, may be more irregular than other cystic lesions. May appear as enlargement of cord with constriction of vessels. Has been reported as large, hypoechoic, septated mass adjacent to fetal abdomen	Tumors, cysts
Teratoma	Rare germ cell tumor	Disorganized, heterogeneous mass, up to 9 cm in diameter, may have calcifications, found at any point along the cord	Hemangioma, hematoma

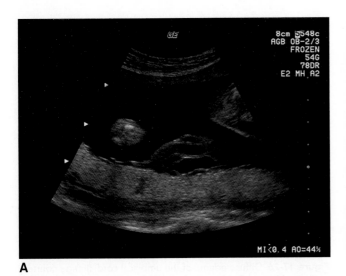

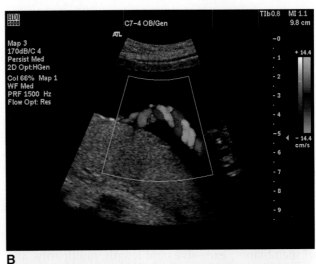

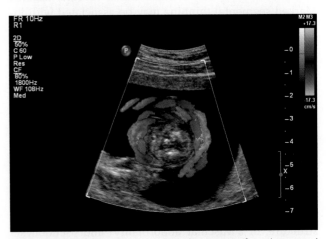

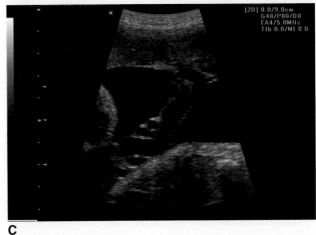

Figure 17-24 Sonographic appearance of cord insertion into placenta. **A:** Curvilinear image of a centrally inserted umbilical cord. **B:** Color Doppler image of a three-vessel cord insertion. **C:** Marginal (battledore) insertion into placenta. (Images **A** and **C** courtesy of Philips Medical Systems, Bothell, WA. Image **B** courtesy of GE Healthcare, Wauwatosa, WI.)

ABNORMAL CORD POSITION

Nuchal Cord

In up to 36% of all deliveries, the umbilical cord is looped around the neck of the fetus one or more times.[81,82] Multiple looping has been associated with increased incidence of complications, such as shoulder dystocia, decreased fetal breathing, movement, and birth weight.[82] These complications are usually the result of cord compression. Meconium-stained amniotic fluid has also been associated with nuchal cord, usually when coincident with oligohydramnios.[81] In most cases, however, the cord is loosely looped around the fetal neck and is clinically insignificant. Routine imaging allows for identification of the presence of a nuchal cord (Fig. 17-25). Color Doppler is more sensitive in detecting nuchal cord than gray-scale imaging.[82] This diagnosis should be considered whenever the umbilical cord is imaged around or near the fetal neck.

Cord Prolapse and Vasa Previa

There are several forms of umbilical cord prolapse. Occult prolapse refers to loops of cord adjacent to the fetal presenting part.[83] Vasa previa refers to a situation in which a segment of umbilical cord is located between the presenting fetal part and the lower pole of intact membranes. Frank or overt prolapse refers to cord protrusion into the cervix, usually through ruptured membranes.[84] Vasa previa, although rare, can be responsible for severe fetal complications during delivery.[63] In some instances, prolapse or vasa previa may be due to velamentous insertion of the cord into membranes that do not overlie

Figure 17-25 Transverse, color Doppler image of cord wrapped around the fetal neck (nuchal cord). (Image courtesy of Philips Medical Systems, Bothell, WA)

placental tissue and that may cross the cervical os before joining the placenta. Prolapse may also be due to abnormal vessels extending from the placental surface.[63]

Sonographic detection of prolapse is clinically important because it may lead to cord compression and fetal vascular compromise, a potentially fatal situation. It can also place these vessels at risk for rupture.[79] Visualization of loops of cord between the presenting part and the cervix or within the cervical canal greatly improves with use of the endovaginal transducer and color flow Doppler.[79] If there is associated velamentous insertion of the umbilical cord or a low-lying placenta, it should be documented.[79] Predisposing factors to the development of umbilical cord prolapse include fetal malpresentation, polyhydramnios, premature rupture of membranes, excessive cord length, multiparity, and cephalopelvic disproportion.[85]

SINGLE UMBILICAL ARTERY

A two-vessel cord representing an umbilical vein and a single umbilical artery (SUA) is seen in 0.2% to 1.1% of all pregnancies and is thought to be due to either primary agenesis of one of the embryonic umbilical arteries or atrophy of a previously normal umbilical artery.[86] A small percentage of fetuses with SUA have associated IUGR, or anomalies of the central nervous, cardiovascular, and genitourinary systems. There have also been associations with trisomy 13 and 18.[86] On sonographic investigation (which is better made closest to the fetal end of the cord, as the arteries can fuse by the placental insertion site),[86] only two vessels are viewed transversely (Fig. 18-28). Often, the SUA measures more than 4 mm in diameter.[86]

UMBILICAL CORD SIZE

Thinning of the Umbilical Cord

Segmental thinning of the cord is an infrequent finding. It is usually caused by absence of a portion of the muscle in the wall of the artery or vein. The placentas in these cases may contain similar vascular lesions. Marked segmental thinning may be associated with increased congenital anomalies and perinatal distress.[31]

Enlargement of the Umbilical Cord

Enlargement of the cord is very rare. It may be a normal variant due to an abnormality of the vitelline duct, or it can be due to focal tumors, cysts, vascular anomalies, or diffuse edema (Fig. 17-26).[77]

UMBILICAL CORD MASSES

Cystic Masses

Cystic masses of the cord are categorized as true cysts (usually related to the vestigial patency of an embryonic structure, or a vascular abnormality) and pseudocysts (localized edema or an area of degenerated Wharton's jelly) (Fig. 17-27).[87]

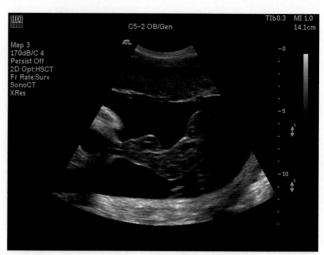

Figure 17-26 Diffuse edema of the umbilical cord. (Image courtesy of Philips Medical Systems, Bothell, WA.)

Cyst discovery begins the use of serial examinations to verify normal fetal growth and to note any change in the size of the cyst, because an expanding cyst (or any mass on the cord) may compress blood vessels. Doppler evaluation may be helpful in such cases.

Umbilical cord hematomas are rare and have been found to be associated with predisposing factors such as cord torsion, short cords, infection, and cysts. There is increased risk of perinatal death.[88] Hematomas appear echogenic when acute but may also appear hypoechoic or even cystic later on. Differentiation from other cystic masses may be difficult, but hematomas are often irregular, septated, and more complex than other cystic lesions. They may also appear as an edematous portion of the cord.

Solid Masses

Solid masses of the umbilical cord include hemangiomas, angiomyxomas, dermoids, and teratomas.[77] Sonographic diagnosis of hemangioma is through the visualization of a hyperechoic mass, usually present at the distal end of the cord near the placenta.[77] When any mass on the cord visualizes, careful examination of the anterior abdominal wall of the fetus helps identify associated abnormalities of abdominal wall formation. The sonographer should also examine the mass for the presence of vessels within. With any mass of the cord, mechanical compression and impairment of circulation is a possible consequence, especially if the mass arises from the vascular tissue itself.[77] The presence of calcifications in a disorganized, heterogeneous mass anywhere along the length of the cord is suggestive of a teratoma.[77]

UMBILICAL VEIN AND ARTERIAL THROMBOSIS

Umbilical vein thrombosis and occlusion is a serious condition found in stillbirths and has been associated with increased perinatal mortality. This condition is

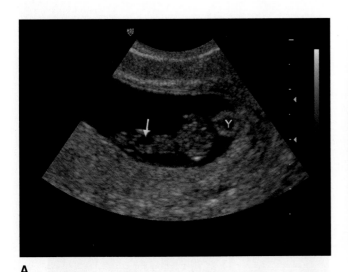

A

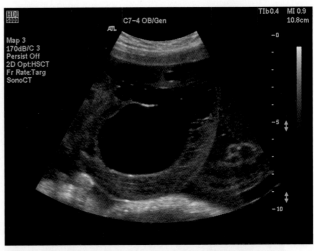

B

Figure 17-27 A: The umbilical cord cyst *(arrow)* images as an anechoic area within the cord of this 9-week gestation. *Y,* yolk sac. **B:** Large cord cyst. (Images courtesy of Philips Medical Systems, Bothell, WA.)

related to maternal diabetes, severe infection, smoking, and coagulation abnormalities, in addition to anatomic abnormalities such as cord torsion and knotting. Although not as common as that in the veins, thrombosis may also occur in the umbilical arteries, with associated aneurysmal dilatation.[89] Fetal mortality is even more likely with umbilical artery thrombosis than with venous thrombosis.[90] Sonographically, the thrombus may present as increased echogenicity and distention of the umbilical vessels.[90]

AMNIOTIC FLUID

Maintenance of a normal amniotic fluid volume is essential to the development of a fetus, as it allows for free fetal movement, protects against injury, maintains

a consistent temperature for the fetus, and is vital for fetal lung development.[47]

Amniotic fluid is normally anechoic (Fig. 17-28) in the first and second trimesters. In the third trimester, it is normal to see floating echogenic particles within the amniotic fluid, representing vernix, which is the result of sloughing of fetal skin.[91] If the vernix becomes highly concentrated, the amniotic fluid may become diffusely echogenic. Pathologic conditions, such as acute bleeding into the amniotic cavity or meconium staining, may also cause the amniotic fluid to appear echogenic. In the third trimester, it is impossible to differentiate these pathologic states sonographically from normally echogenic, vernix-filled amniotic fluid (Fig. 17-29).[91]

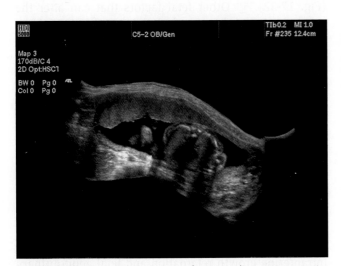

Figure 17-28 Placenta. Sonogram of a second trimester anterior placenta with characteristic homogeneous echopattern. The amniotic fluid in the cavity is anechoic. (Image courtesy of Philips Medical Systems, Bothell, WA)

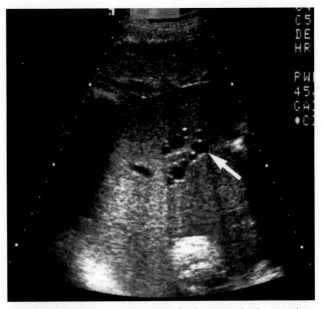

Figure 17-29 Echogenic amniotic fluid surrounds the anechoic umbilical cord.

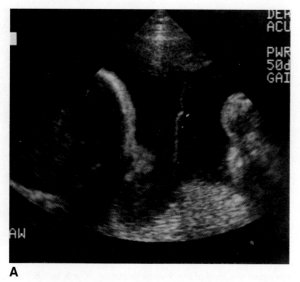
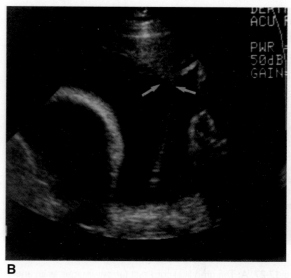

A   **B**

Figure 17-30 Amniotic sheet. **A:** Sonogram demonstrating a membrane crossing a portion of the amniotic cavity. **B:** The edge of the membrane at the uterine wall is broad-based (*arrows*).

Occasionally, a membranous structure images floating in the amniotic cavity or extending across the cavity (Fig. 17-30). Membranes occur either with the amniotic band syndrome or because of a uterine synechia, a fibrous band, or scar in the uterine cavity. In the former, the membranes adhere to the fetus and cause fetal malformations, often severe. In the latter, more common situation, intact amnion and chorion are reflected over a synechia, producing a membrane that traverses part of the amniotic cavity. Sonographic characterization of the uterine synechia is through visualization of a band with a broad-based origin at the uterine wall and focal thickening of the membrane at its free edge, and by the fact that it does not adhere to the fetus.[40]

Altered amounts of amniotic fluid may be an indicator of abnormal fetal or maternal conditions. It is therefore important to include assessment of fluid volume as part of every sonographic examination. Experienced sonographers and sonologists find that subjective determination of the fluid volume is the best and most accurate method. This requires careful sonographic evaluation, comparing the observed amount of fluid with that expected at the current gestational age. The best approach for quantifying amniotic fluid levels is through measurement of fluid pockets. The vertical depth of the best pocket of fluid is measured and correlated with gestational age, or the amniotic fluid index is calculated as the sum of the deepest pocket measurements from the four quadrants of the uterus (Fig. 17-31).[10]

The volume of amniotic fluid increases to its maximum at 36 to 38 weeks, then decreases until delivery. The amniotic fluid volume surrounding the fetus is maintained by a balance of several fetal and maternal factors. The epithelium of the amnion produces amniotic fluid early in pregnancy, and throughout the gestation, the fetal membranes and umbilical cord are involved in fluid and electrolyte exchange.[47] After 16 weeks' gestation, most of the fluid production is through excretion of fetal urine. Fetal swallowing allows absorption of amniotic fluid through the gastrointestinal tract.[14] Abnormalities of either the genitourinary tract or the gastrointestinal tract, or of fetal swallowing can affect the amniotic fluid volume. Obstruction of the esophagus, duodenum, or proximal small bowel, or impairment of swallowing due to a central nervous system lesion or a thoracic mass, lead to polyhydramnios. Diminished or absent urine output, which can result from bilateral renal agenesis, abnormal kidneys (e.g., autosomal recessive polycystic kidney disease), or urinary tract obstruction, leads to oligohydramnios (Fig. 17-32).[92,93] Other fetal factors that can alter the amniotic fluid volume include intrauterine growth retardation, which is associated with oligohydramnios, and fetal hydrops, which is often associated with polyhydramnios.[93]

The single deepest pocket method for assessing amniotic fluid volume can be used to diagnose polyhydramnios when the pocket is greater than 8 cm and oligohydramnios when the pocket is less than 2 cm.[10]

Polyhydramnios is idiopathic in the majority of cases and results from fetal structural anomalies in a much smaller number. Maternal factors account for a small percentage of cases as well, the most common factor being maternal diabetes.

Oligohydramnios is rarely unexplained. The most common cause is premature rupture of membranes. Intrauterine growth retardation and fetal genitourinary anomalies account for most cases of oligohydramnios with intact membranes.[93]

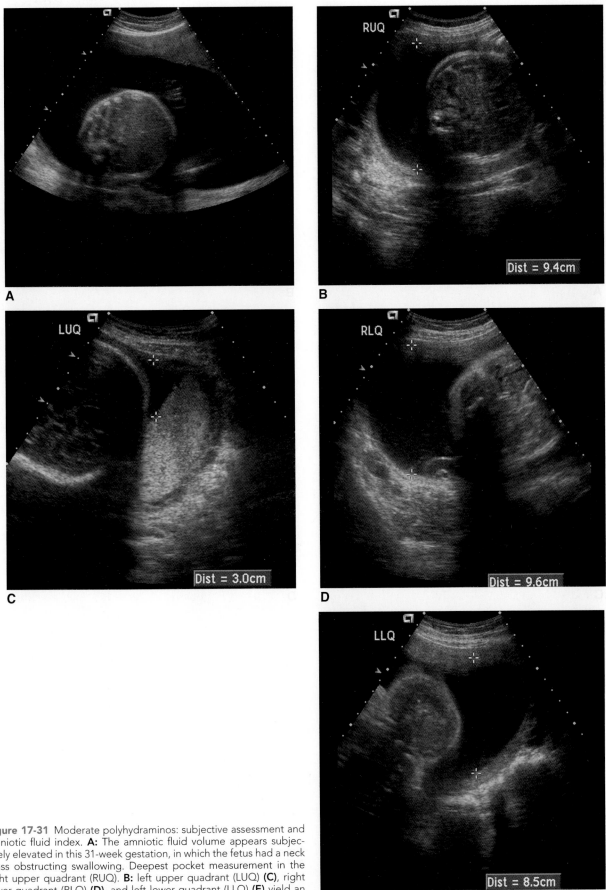

Figure 17-31 Moderate polyhydraminos: subjective assessment and amniotic fluid index. **A:** The amniotic fluid volume appears subjectively elevated in this 31-week gestation, in which the fetus had a neck mass obstructing swallowing. Deepest pocket measurement in the right upper quadrant (RUQ). **B:** left upper quadrant (LUQ) **(C)**, right lower quadrant (RLQ) **(D)**, and left lower quadrant (LLQ) **(E)** yield an amniotic fluid index of 37.5 (9.4 + 10.0 + 9.6 + 8.5).

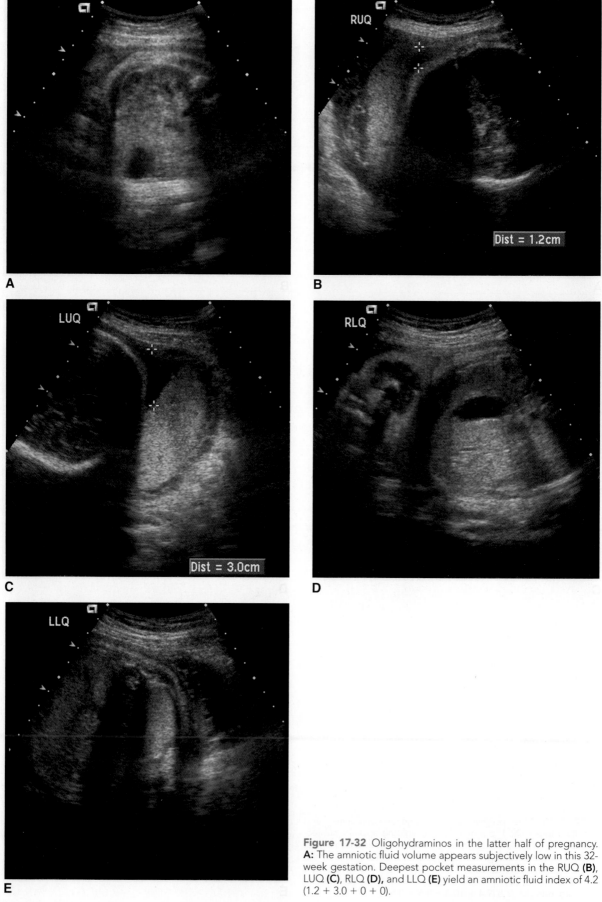

Figure 17-32 Oligohydraminos in the latter half of pregnancy. **A:** The amniotic fluid volume appears subjectively low in this 32-week gestation. Deepest pocket measurements in the RUQ **(B)**, LUQ **(C)**, RLQ **(D)**, and LLQ **(E)** yield an amniotic fluid index of 4.2 (1.2 + 3.0 + 0 + 0).

SUMMARY

- Bladder fullness influences the detection of placenta previa, cervical length, and competence.

- When imaging the placenta, cord, or cervix, use an angle of incidence as close to 90 degrees as possible to ensure optimal image detail and measurements.

- Cervical length in the second semester of greater than 2.5 cm/1 inch rules out cervical incompetence.

- In the case of an incompetent cervix, a cerclage prevents opening of the cervix.

- Nutrient exchange between the fetus and mother occurs within the villi in the placenta.

- The hypoechoic retroplacental complex has a vascular appearance with imaging on 2D and color Doppler ensuring the normal placental/uterine adherence.

Critical Thinking Questions

1. **Examine the placental images and determine placental grade, location, and appropriateness of measurements. Explain your reasoning.**

    ANSWER: (A) This left lateral, grade II placenta has an incorrect measurement technique. Though the best measurements occur with the angle of incidence perpendicular, this is not always possible. In this case, the measurement needs to be perpendicular to the placenta at the thickest point, not perpendicular to the beam. (B) This measurement includes the retroplacental complex and is nonperpendicular to the posterior, grade I placenta. Both of these errors would result in a thicker placental measurement. (C) This correctly measured right lateral, grade I placenta excludes the retroplacental complex and is done perpendicular to the main placental tissue. (D) This anterior grade II placenta images easily in a perpendicular plane. The measurement would also follow this same path; however, this image demonstrates an oblique measurement.

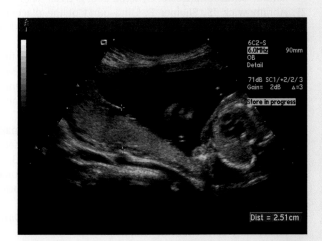

A

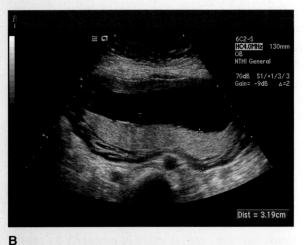

B

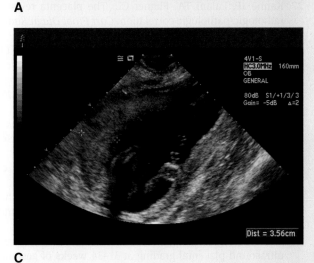

C

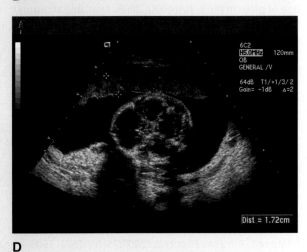

D

- The placenta may locate anywhere within the uterus; however, a low implantation (previa) raises concern for bleeding and delivery before the fetus.
- Thinning of the myometrium inferior to the placenta raises suspicion of placenta accreta, increta, or percreta
- A placenta greater than 2 cm from the internal cervical os rules out previa.
- Familiarity with the sonographic appearance of contractions, fibroids, and subchorionic hematomas prevents confusion with other extraplacental variations or pathology.
- Amniotic bands are fetal in origin, with connections in several locations may trap and amputate fetal anatomy.
- Amniotic sheets, shelf, or synechia are maternal in origin, connecting on only one edge.
- A centrally located cord insertion into the placenta is considered normal.
- Color flow Doppler aids in identifying the cord insertion, vessel number, fetal pelvic insertion, and the presence of a nuchal cord.
- Marginal cord insertions are either a battledore placenta or velamentous insertion.
- Visualization of a two-vessel cord leads the sonographer to search for trisomy 13 and 18 sonographic markers.
- Anechoic amniotic fluid aids in fetal development with abnormal amounts due to fetal or maternal conditions.
- A single pocket depth measurement of greater than 8 cm is diagnostic for polyhydramnios; one less than 2 cm is diagnostic for oligohydramnios.

REFERENCES

1. Kaakaji Y, Nghiem HV, Nodell C, et al. Sonography of obstetric and gynecologic emergencies: Part I, Obstetric Emergencies. *AJR*. 2000;174:641–649.
2. The Royal Australian and New Zealand College of Obstetricians and Gynaecologists. College Statement C-Obs 27: measurement of cervical length in pregnancy for prediction of preterm birth. RANZOG, 2008. Available at: http://www.ranzcog.edu.au/component/content/article/503-c-obs/418--measurement-of-cervical-length-in-pregnancy-for-prediction-of-preterm-birth-c-obs-27.html
3. Chestnut DH. *Obstetric Anesthesia: Principles and Practice*. 3rd ed. Philadelphia: Mosby, Inc; 2004.
4. Ressel GW. ACOG releases bulletin on managing cervical insufficiency. *Am Fam Physician*. 2004;69(2):436–439.
5. Takai N, Nishida M, Urata K, et al. Successful cerclage in two patients with advanced cervical dilatation in the second trimester. *Arch Gynecol Obstet*. 2003;268(2):102–104.
6. Osol G, Mandala M. Maternal uterine vascular remodeling during pregnancy. *Physiology*. 2009;24(1):58–71.
7. Kim KR, Jun SY, Kim JY. Implantation site intermediate trophoblasts in placenta cretas. *Mod Pathol*. 2004;17:1483–1490.
8. Evans P, Brunsell S. Uterine fibroid tumors: diagnosis and treatment. *Am Fam Physician*. 2007;75(10):1503–1508.
9. Kinare A. Fetal environment. *Indian J Radiol Imaging*. 2008;18(4):326–344.
10. Rumack CM, Wilson SR, Charboneau JW, Eds. *Diagnostic Ultrasound*. 3rd ed. St. Louis: Mosby, Inc; 2005.
11. Roberts DJ. Placental pathology, a survival guide. *Arch Pathol Lab Med*. 2008;132(4):641–651.
12. Moore KL, Persaud TVN. *Before We Are Born: Essentials of Embryology and Birth Defects*. 7th ed. Philadelphia: Saunders; 2008.
13. Vause S, Saroya DK. Functions of the placenta. *Anaesthesia & Intensive Care Medicine*. 2005;6(3):77–80.
14. Blackburn ST. *Maternal, Fetal, & Neonatal Physiology: A Clinical Perspective*. St. Louis: Saunders; 2007.
15. AIUM. AIUM practice guideline for the performance of obstetric ultrasound examinations. *J Ultrasound Med*. 2010;29:157–166.
16. Benson CB, Bluth EI, eds. *Ultrasonography in Obstetrics and Gynecology: A Practical Approach to Clinical Problems*. 2nd ed. New York: Thieme Medical Publishers, Inc; 2008.
17. Hata T, Kanenishi K, Inubashiri E, et al. Three-dimensional sonographic features of placental abnormalities. *Gynecol Obstet Invest*. 2004;57:61–65.
18. Malone FD. Placenta accreta percreta. *Contemporary Ob/Gyn*. 2002;4:116–142.
19. Angtuaco TL, Gupta N, Andreotti RF, et al. ACR appropriateness criteria assessment of gravid cervix. *ACR*. 2008;5.
20. Oyelese Y. Placenta previa: the evolving role of ultrasound. *Ultrasound Obstet Gynecol*. 2009;34:123–126.
21. Abramowicz JS, Sheiner E. Ultrasound of the placenta: a systematic approach. Part I: Imaging. *Placenta*. 2008;29(3):225–40.
22. Tongsong T, Boonyanurak P. Placental thickness in the first half of pregnancy. *J Clin Ultrasound*. 2004;32(5):231–234.
23. Abramowicz JS, Sheiner E. Ultrasound of the placenta: a systematic approach. Part II: Functional assessment (Doppler). *Placenta*. 2008;29(11):921–929.
24. Prapas N, Liang RI, Hunter D, et al. Color Doppler imaging of placental masses: differential diagnosis and fetal outcome. *Ultrasound Obstet Gynecol*. 2000;16:559–563.
25. Hata T, Inubashiri E, Kanenishi K, et al. Three-dimensional power Doppler angiographic features of placental chorioangioma. *J Ultrasound Med*. 2004;23(11):1517–1520.
26. Evans MI, Johnson MP, Yaron Y, et al., eds. *Prenatal Diagnosis*. New York: McGraw-Hill; 2006.
27. Kanne JP, Lalani TA, Fligner CL. The placenta revisted: radiologic-pathologic correlation. *Curr Probl Diagn Radiol*. 2005;34(6):238–255.
28. Gibbs RS, Karlan BY, Haney AF, et al., eds. *Danforth's Obstetrics and Gynecology*. 10th ed. Philadelphia: Lippincott Williams & Wilkins; 2008.
29. Benirschke K, Kaufman P. *Pathology of the Human Placenta*. 4th ed. New York: Springer-Verlag; 2000.
30. Kurjak A, Chervenak FA, eds. *Donald School Textbook of Ultrasound in Obstetrics and Gynecology*. 2nd ed. New Delhi: Jaypee Brothers Medical Publishers Ltd; 2008.
31. Fox H, Sebire NJ. *Pathology of the Placenta*. 3rd ed. Philadelphia: Elsevier Limited; 2007.
32. Sebire NJ, Sepulveda W. Correlation of placental pathology with prenatal ultrasound findings. *J Clin Pathol*. 2008;61:1276–1284.
33. Yin TT, Loughna P, Ong SS, et al. No correlation between ultrasound placental grading at 31–34 weeks of gestation and a surrogate estimate of organ function at term obtained by stereological analysis. *Placenta*. 2009;30(8):726–730.

34. Quintero RNA, Kontopoulos EV, Bornick PW, et al. In utero laser treatment of type II vasa previa. *J Matern Fetal Neonatal Med.* 2007;20(12):847–851.

35. Suzuki S. Clinical significance of pregnancies with circumvallate placenta. *J Obstet Gynaecol Res.* 2008;34(1):51–54.

36. Shen O, Golomb E, Lavie O, et al. Placental shelf—a common, typically transient and benign finding on early second-trimester sonography. *Ultrasound Obstet Gynecol.* 2007;29:192–194.

37. Verma A, Mohan S, Kumar S. Late presentation of amniotic band syndrome—case report. *J Clin Diagn Res.* 2007;2:65–68.

38. Hill DS. Extensive nonunion of the amnion: an unusual presentation of amniotic band syndrome? *JDMS.* 2010;26(5):263–265.

39. Benacerraf B. *Ultrasound of Fetal Syndromes.* 2nd ed. Philadelphia: Churchill Livingstone; 2008.

40. Nyberg DA, McGahan JP, Pretorius DH, et al. *Diagnostic Imaging of Fetal Anomalies.* Philadelphia: Lippincott Williams & Wilkins; 2003.

41. Necas M, Worrall JA, DuBose TJ. Recognizing intra-amniotic band-like structures on obstetric ultrasound. 1999. Available at: http://www.obgyn.net/us/cotm/9909/bands.htm. Accessed October 10, 2010.

42. Tan KBL, Tan TYT, Tan JVK, et al. The amniotic sheet: a truly benign condition? *Ultrasound Obstet Gynecol.* 2005;26:639–643.

43. Ahmed A, Gilbert-Barness E. Placenta membranacea: a developmental anomaly with diverse clinical presentation. *Pediatr Dev Pathol.* 2003;6(2):201–203.

44. Faye-Petersen OM, Heller DS, Joshi VV. *Handbook of Placental Pathology.* 2nd ed. Oxon: Taylor & Francis; 2006.

45. Azpurua H, Funai EF, Coraluzzi LM, et al. Determination of placental weight using two-dimensional sonography and volumetric mathematic modeling. *Amer J Perinatol.* 2010;27:151–155.

46. Ohagwu CC, Abu PO, Ezeokeke UO, et al. Relationship between placental thickness and growth parameters in normal Nigerian fetuses. *AJB.* 2009;8(2):133–138.

47. Merz E, Bahlmann F. *Ultrasound in Obstetrics & Gynecology; Volume 1: Obstetrics.* 2nd ed. New York: Thieme; 2005.

48. Goodwin TM, Montoro MN, Muderspach L, et al., eds. *Management of Common Problems in Obstetrics and Gynecology.* 5th ed. Oxford: Blackwell Publishing Ltd; 2010.

49. Beckmann CRB, Ling FW, Barzansky BM, et al., eds. *Obstetrics and Gynecology.* 6th ed. Philadelphia: Lippincott Williams & Wilkins; 2010.

50. Dashe JS, McIntire DD, Ramus RM, et al. Persistence of placenta previa according to gestational age at ultrasound detection. *Obstet Gynecol.* 2002;99(5):692–697.

51. Agrawal V, Kulshresta S. Importance of placental localization in early pregnancy. *N J Obstet Gynaecol.* 2007;2(2):16–19.

52. Datta S, ed. *Anesthetic and obstetric management of high-risk pregnancy.* 3rd ed. New York: Springer-Verlag; 2004.

53. Ananth CV, Wilcox AJ. Placental abruption and perinatal mortality in the United States. *Am J Epidemiol.* 2001;153(4):332–337.

54. Sakornbut E, Leeman L, Fontaine P. Late pregnancy bleeding. *Am Fam Physician.* 2007;75(8):1199–1206.

55. Rani PR, Haritha PH, Gowri R. Comparative study of transperineal and transabdominal sonography in the diagnosis of placenta previa. *J Obstet Gynaecol Res.* 2007;33(2):134–137.

56. Elsasser DA, Ananth CV, Prasad V, et al. Diagnosis of placental abruption: relationship between clinical and histopathological findings. *Obstet Gynecol Surv.* 2010;65(5):297–299.

57. Walker JM, Ferguson DD. The sonographic appearance of blood in the fetal stomach and its association with placental abruption. *J Ultrasound Med.* 1988;7:155–161.

58. Bluth EI, Benson CB, Ralk PW, et al., eds. *Ultrasound: a practical approach to clinical problems.* 2nd ed. New York: Thieme Medical Publishers, Inc; 2008.

59. Usui R, Matsubara S, Ohkuchi A, et al. Fetal heart rate pattern reflecting the severity of placental abruption. *Arch Gynecol Obstet.* 2008;277(3):249–253.

60. Tantbirojn P, Crum CP, Parast MM. Pathophysiology of placenta creta: the role of decidua and extravillous trophoblast. *Placenta.* 2008;29(7):639–645.

61. Kayem G, Grange G, Schmitz T. Clinical aspects and management of morbidly adherent placenta. *Eur Clin Obstet Gynaecol.* 2006;2(3):139–145.

62. Sanders RC, Winter TC III, eds. *Clinical Sonography: A Practical Guide.* 4th ed. Baltimore: Lippincott Williams & Wilkins; 2007.

63. Oyelese Y, Smulian JC. Placenta previa, placenta accreta, and vasa previa. *Obstet Gynecol.* 2006;107(4):927–941.

64. Muramatsu K, Itoh H, Yamasaki T, et al. A case of a huge placental lake; prenatal differential diagnosis and clinical management. *J Obstet Gynaecol Res.* 2010;36(1):165–169.

65. Kurman RJ, ed. *Blaustein's Pathology of the Female Genital Tract.* 5th ed. New York: Springer-Verlag; 2002.

66. Hiroyasu K, Nobuya U, Rika H, et al. A case of massive subchorionic thrombohematoma (Breus' mole) associated with acute maternal hemorrhage and preshock. *Japanese Journal of Obstetrical, Gynecological & Neonatal Hematology.* 2004;13(2):44–47.

67. Chang KTE. Pathological examination of the placenta: *Raison d'être,* clinical relevance of medicolegal utility. *Singapore Med J.* 2009;50(12):1123–1133.

68. Kofinas A, Kofinas K, Sutija V. The role of second trimester ultrasound in the diagnosis of placental hypoechoic lesions leading to poor pregnancy outcome. *J Matern Fetal Neonatal Med.* 2007;20(12):859–866.

69. Kirkpatrick AD, Podberesky DJ, Gray AN, et al. Placental chorioangioma. *Radiographics.* 2007;27:1187–1190.

70. Willard DA, Moeschler JB. Placental chorioangioma: A rare cause of elevated amniotic fluid alphafetoprotein. *J Ultrasound Med.* 1986;5:221–222.

71. Ahmed N, Kale V, Thakkar H, et al. Sonographic diagnosis of placental teratoma. *J Clin Ultrasound.* 2004;32(2):98–101.

72. Sebire NJ, Secki MJ. Gestational trophoblastic disease: current management of hydatidiform mole. *BMJ.* 2008;337:a1193,a1473.

73. Baergen RN, Malicki D, Behling C, et al. Morbidity, mortality, and placental pathology in excessively long umbilical cords: retrospective study. *Pediatr Dev Pathol.* 2001;4:144–153.

74. Sepulveda W. Beware of the umbilical cord 'cyst'. *Ultrasound Obstet Gynecol.* 2003;21:213–214.

75. Fleischer AC, Gordon AN. Sonography of trophoblastic dieases. In: Flesicher AC, Romero R, Manning MD, Jeanty P, James AE, eds. *The Principles and Practices of Ultrasonography in Obstetrics and Gynecology.* 4th ed. Norwalk: Appleton-Century-Crofts; 1991:501–508.

76. Jantarasaengaram S, Suthipintawong C, Kanchanawat S, et al. Ruptured vasa previa in velamentous cord insertion placenta. *J Perinatol.* 2007;27(7):457–459.

77. Stevenson RE, Hall JG, eds. *Human Malformations and Related Anomalies.* 2nd ed. New York: Oxford University Press Inc; 2006.

78. Kähler C, Humbsch K, Schneider U, et al. A case report of body stalk anomaly complicating a twin pregnancy. *Arch Gynecol Obstet.* 2003;268(3):245–247.

79. Shamas AG, Kambhapati L, Abu-Ghazza O, et al. Prenatal diagnosis of velamentous cord insertion and vasa praevia using ultrasound and magnetic resonance imaging—a case report. *Ultrasound.* 2008;16(1):15–17.

80. Srinivasan A, Graves L. Four true umbilical cord knots. *J Obstet Gynaecol Can.* 2006;28(1):32–35.

81. Shrestha NS, Singh N. Nuchal cord and perinatal outcome. *KUMJ.* 2007;5:360–363.

82. Ogueh O, Al-Tarkait A, Vallerand D, et al. Obstetrical factors related to nuchal cord. *Acta Obstet Gynecol Scand.* 2006;85:810–814.

83. Belogolovkin V, Eddleman K. Is it imbilical cord prolapse? *Contemporary OB/GYN.* 2005;50(10):68,70,72.

84. Murray ML, Huelsmann GM. *Labor and Delivery Nursing: Guide to Evidence-Based Practice.* New York: Springer Publishing Company, LLC; 2009.

85. Dilbaz B, Ozturkoglu E, Dilbaz S, et al. Risk factors and perinatal outcomes associated with umbilical cord prolapse. *Arch Gynecol Obstet.* 2006;274:104–107.

86. Weissman A, Drugan A. Sonographic findings of the umbilical cord: implications for the risk of fetal chromosomal anomalies. *Ultrasound Obstet Gynecol.* 2001;17:536–541.

87. Arias MP, Lorenzo FG, Sanchez MM, et al. Enteric duplication cyst resembling umbilical cord cyst. *J Perinatol.* 2006;26(6):368.

88. Sepulveda W, Wong AE, Gonzalez R, et al. Fetal death due to umbilical cord hematoma: a rare complication of umbilical cord cyst. *J Matern Fetal Neonatal Med.* 2005;18(6):387–390.

89. Avagliano L, Marconi AM, Candiani M, et al. Thrombosis of the umbilical vessels revisited. An observational study of 317 consecutive autopsies at a single institution. *Hum Pathol.* 2010;41:971–979.

90. Rubabaza P, Persadie RJ. Two cases of umbilical vein thrombosis, one with associated portal vein thrombosis. *J Obstet Gynaecol Can.* 2008;30(4):338–343.

91. Creasy RK, Resnik R, Iams JD, eds. *Maternal-Fetal Medicine: Principles and Practice.* 5th ed. Philadelphia: Saunders, 2004.

92. O'Brien W, ed. *Top 3 Differentials in Radiology: A Case Review.* New York: Thieme Medical Publishers, Inc; 2010.

93. Fortner KB, Szmanski LM, Fox HE, et al., eds. *The Johns Hopkins Manual of Gynecology and Obstetrics.* 3rd ed. Philadelphia: Lippincott Williams & Wilkins; 2007.

94. Grannum P, Hobbins JC. The placenta. In: Callen PW, ed. *Ultrasonography in Obstetrics and Gynecology.* Philadelphia: WB Saunders; 1983:141–157.

95. Graham D, Guidi S, Sanders RC. Sonography of the placenta. In: Saunders RC, Hill MC, eds. *Ultrasound Annual.* New York: Raven Press; 1984:121–137.

96. Spirt BA, Gordon LP, Kagen EH. Sonography of the placenta. In: Fleisher AC, Manning FA, Jeanty P, et al., eds. *The Principles and Practice of Ultrasonography in Obstetrics and Gynecology.* 5th ed. Stamford: Appleton & Lange; 1996:173–202.

97. Allen M. Diagnostic challenge: I. Excessive amount of Wharton's jelly. *J Diagn Med Sonogr.* 1987;3:27,29,30.

98. Ramanathan K, Epstein S, Yaghoobian J. Localized deposition of Wharton's jelly: Sonographic findings. *J Ultrasound Med.* 1986;5:339–340.

99. Romero R, Pilu G, Jeanty P, et al. The umbilical cord. In: Romero R, Pilu G, Jeanty P, et al., Eds. *Prenatal Diagnosis of Congenital Anomalies.* Norwalk: Appleton & Lange; 1988:385–402.

100. Mishriki YY, Vanyshelbaum Y, Epstein H, et al. Hemangioma of the umbilical cord. *Pediatr Pathol.* 1987;7:49.

18 Abnormalities of the Placenta and Umbilical Cord

Lisa M. Allen

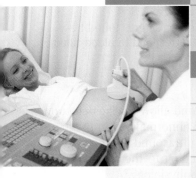

OBJECTIVES

Recognize the sonographic appearance of placental and umbilical cord anomalies

Discuss developmental variations in placental size, shape, and configuration

Identify placenta previa classifications

Explain placental abruption and the associated risk factors

List placenta accreta classifications and known risk factors

Name the various abnormalities of umbilical cord insertion into the placenta

Describe cystic and solid masses of the umbilical cord

KEY TERMS

succenturiate lobe | circummarginate placenta | circumvallate placenta | placenta previa | placental abruption | placenta accreta spectrum | chorioangioma | amniotic band syndrome | uterine synechiae | marginal insertion | battledore placenta | velamentous insertion | true knot | false knot | nuchal cord | cord prolapse | vasa previa | single umbilical artery | cord entanglement | umbilical cord hemangioma | umbilical cord coiling | umbilical coiling index

GLOSSARY

Aneurysm Focal dilatation of an artery

Bilobed placenta Placenta where the lobes are nearly equal in size and the cord inserts into the chorionic bridge of tissue that connects the two lobes

Body stalk anomaly Fatal condition associated with multiple congenital anomalies and absence of the umbilical cord

Breus' mole Very rare condition where there is massive subchorionic thrombosis of the placenta secondary to extreme venous obstruction

Extrachorial placenta Attachment of the placental membranes to the fetal surface of the placenta rather than to the underlying villous placental margin

False knot Bending, twisting, and bulging of the umbilical cord vessels mimicking a knot in the umbilical cord

Gastroschisis Periumbilical abdominal wall defect, typically to the right of normal cord insertion, that allows for free-floating bowel in the amniotic fluid

Limb–body wall complex Condition characterized by multiple complex fetal anomalies and a short umbilical cord

Marginal insertion (a.k.a. battledore placenta) Occurs when the umbilical cord inserts at the placental margin instead of centrally

Mickey Mouse sign Term used to describe the cross-section of the three-vessel umbilical cord or the portal triad (portal vein, hepatic artery, common bile duct)

Omphalocele Central anterior abdominal wall defect of the umbilicus where abdominal organs are contained by a covering membrane consisting of peritoneum, Wharton's jelly, and amnion

Placentomegaly Term that refers to a thickened placenta

Synechia (Asherman's syndrome) Linear, extra amniotic tissue that projects into the amniotic cavity with no restriction of fetal movement

Thrombosis Intraplacental area of hemorrhage and clot

True knot Result of the fetus actually passing through a loop or loops of umbilical cord creating one or more knots in the cord

Umbilical coiling index (UCI) Method of assessing the degree of umbilical cord coiling, defined as the number of complete coils per centimeter length of cord

Umbilical cord Vascular structure connecting the fetus and placenta that normally contains two arteries and one vein surrounded by Wharton's jelly

Umbilical hernia Failure of the normal physiologic gut herniation to regress into the abdomen, resulting in a small amount of bowel protruding into the base of the umbilical cord

Venous lakes Tubular, anechoic structures found beneath the chorionic plate that correspond to blood-filled spaces found at delivery

This chapter is dedicated to the prenatal identification and classification of abnormalities of the placenta and umbilical cord. In the past few decades, there have been significant technological advances in the field of prenatal ultrasound. There is substantial clinical potential to evaluate the fetus and its surroundings in unsurpassed sonographic detail. Historically, the fetus has been the main focus of the obstetrical ultrasound exam, with minimal attention paid to the placenta and umbilical cord. These structures are often overlooked in the routine evaluation of a normal gestation. With the technologies currently available, in addition to the ability to evaluate the anatomic structure of the fetus, we can interrogate and gain valuable information concerning the environment that supports the developing fetus.

Although uncommon, abnormalities of the placenta and umbilical cord are important to recognize prenatally because of the potential for maternal and fetal morbidity and mortality.[1] Imaging techniques such as spectral, color, and power Doppler imaging aid in the analysis of blood flow physiology. Three-dimensional (3D) and four-dimensional (4D) sonography can be utilized to further complement standard two-dimensional (2D) gray-scale imaging, as it permits scanning in several planes with more precise depiction of internal vasculature as well as increased volume assessment accuracy. These applications continue to expand our knowledge and understanding of the structure and function of the placenta and umbilical cord and allow for the detection and evaluation of associated abnormalities in pregnancy. In the future, the use of ultrasound contrast agents may bring further understanding to the placental implantation process and pathophysiology.[2]

ABNORMALITIES OF THE PLACENTA

ABNORMAL PLACENTAL SIZE

The *placenta* is named for its appearance (Greek *plakuos*, meaning "flat cake") and is responsible for the nutritive, respiratory, and excretory functions of the fetus.[1] The normal human placenta typically increases in thickness and volume with advancing gestation (Fig. 18-1). The overall appearance changes with fetal maturity, and visible progressive deposition of calcifications can be observed sonographically (Fig. 18-2). Significant placental calcifications are rarely seen on ultrasound prior to 37 weeks' gestation, and early maturation of the placenta has been reported to increase the risk of adverse fetal outcomes.[2]

Placental size is expressed in terms of thickness in the midportion of the organ and should be approximately between 2 and 4 cm.[1] Placental thinning has been described in maternal hypertension, preeclampsia, placental infarctions, and intrauterine growth restriction (IUGR). In addition, thin placentas are characteristic in annular placentas and placenta

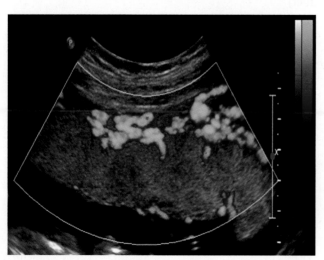

Figure 18-1 Power Doppler angiography of a anterior placenta demonstrating normal placental vascular pattern.

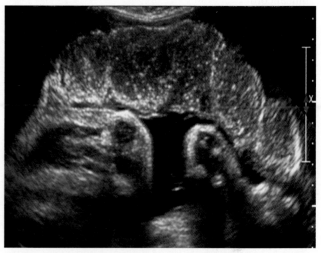

Figure 18-2 Sagittal ultrasound image of a mature anterior placenta with intraparenchymal calcification.

TABLE 18-1

Maternal and Fetal Conditions Associated with Abnormalities of Placental Thickness and Maturation

Increased Placental Thickness (>5 cm)	Decreased Placental Thickness (<1.5 cm)	Early Placental Maturation	Delayed Placental Maturation
1. Maternal diabetes 2. Rh disease 3. Congenital infections 4. Abruption 5. Placental tumors 6. Multiple gestation 7. Chromosomal abnormality/triploidy 8. Gestational trophoblastic disease 9. Mesenchymal dysplasia 10. Placental insufficiency 11. Maternal or fetal anemia 12. Fetal hydrops of any etiology 13. Congenital neoplasms 14. Beckwith-Wiedemann syndrome 15. Confined placental mosaicism	1. Maternal hypertension/preeclampsia 2. Intrauterine growth restriction 3. Juvenile diabetes 4. Placental abnormality (annular placenta and placenta membranacea)	1. Intrauterine Growth Restriction 2. Hypertension	1. Gestational Diabetes 2. Rh disease

membranacea. Thicker placentas of greater than 4 cm may be nonspecific and are usually associated with a normal outcome. However, there are several conditions that are associated with increased placental thickness, decreased placental thickness, and early or delayed placental maturation (Table 18-1). In placental hydrops, the abnormal thickness is due to fluid overload, usually secondary to high-output cardiac failure in the fetus. This can occur in conditions such as fetal hydrops (immune or nonimmune), antepartum infections (particularly syphilis and cytomegalovirus), maternal diabetes, maternal anemia, fetomaternal and twin-to-twin transfusion syndromes, chorioangioma, sacrococcygeal teratomas, and vascular obstruction such as umbilical vein thrombosis. A hydropic placenta assumes a more bulbous appearance and the normal placental architecture is lost to a "ground-glass" appearance. Placentomegaly is also a feature of gestational trophoblastic disease, Beckwith-Wiedemann syndrome, confined placental mosaicism, and mesenchymal dysplasia. Placental thickening can be simulated by myometrial contractions, underlying uterine fibroids, or various forms of abruption (Fig. 18-3).[1]

In some cases of IUGR, the placenta may sonographically appear thickened, with patchy areas of hypoechogenicity and abnormal texture. It may appear to "wobble" in an abnormal fashion, which is termed "jellylike placenta." This may be associated with massive perivillous fibrin deposition and intervillous or subchorionic thrombosis in some cases.[3]

VARIATIONS IN PLACENTAL SHAPE AND CONFIGURATION

Although the placenta usually consists of one placental mass, occasionally, it may be bilobed or have one or more accessory lobes. Abnormalities of placental shape are most often secondary to the disappearance of villi. The placenta normally develops where the chorionic villi interfacing the decidua basalis grow and the remaining villi undergo atrophy. The selective loss of parts of the placenta and growth of other parts is referred to as *trophoblastic trophotropism* and helps explain placental conditions such as velamentous insertion and placental migration. This phenomenon is presumed to occur because the placenta preferentially grows where there is sufficient decidua and vascular supply and atrophies where conditions are less favorable. Ultrasound detection of these placental anomalies affects clinical management and obstetric outcome (Fig. 18-4).[4]

A *succenturiate lobe* is the presence of one or more small accessory lobes that develop in the membranes at a distance from the periphery of the main placenta.[5] This occurs in 0.14% to 3.0% of cases, and the

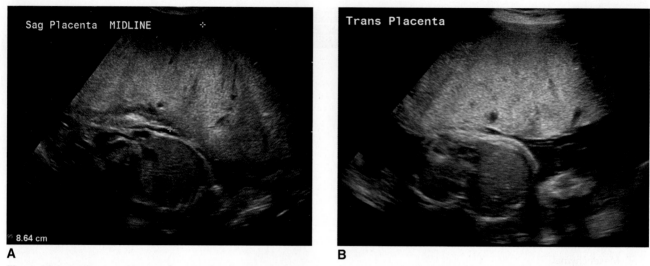

Figure 18-3 A: Ultrasound image of an anterior placenta demonstrating placentomegaly. The electronic calipers denote a maximum thickness exceeding 8 cm. **B:** Ultrasound image of an enlarged, thickened anterior placenta associated with nonimmune fetal hydrops.

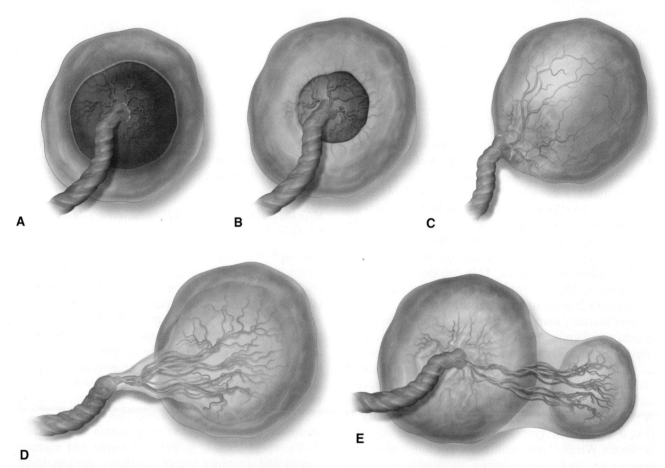

Figure 18-4 Abnormalities of umbilical cord or membrane insertion into the placenta. **A:** Circummarginate placenta. Flat transition of the membranes inserting at some distance in from the placental margin. **B:** Circumvallate placenta. Rolled peripheral edge of the membranes as they insert at some distance in from the placental edge. **C:** Marginal insertion. The umbilical cord inserts at the placental margin, also known as a battledore placenta. **D:** Velamentous cord insertion. The umbilical cord inserts into the membranes at some distance from the placental mass, and the umbilical vessels course through the membranes to the placental disk. **E:** Succenturiate placentation. There is the presence of an accessory lobe of the placenta at a distance from the main placental disk and umbilical vessels course through the membranes connecting the two placental masses.

accessory lobe is connected to the main placental mass by vessels within the membranes. A succenturiate lobe is distinguished from a bilobate placenta, which shows communication of placental tissue between the lobes and central cord insertion into the chorionic bridge of tissue. There is an increased frequency of succenturiate lobes in women of advanced maternal age (35 years and older) and a history of infertility with in vitro fertilization. A succenturiate lobe can be detected sonographically, and the prenatal recognition is clinically important, because retained accessory lobes can be associated with postpartum hemorrhage and infection (Fig. 18-5). There is also a risk of massive intrapartum fetal bleeding secondary to rupture of connecting vessels between the lobes. Most importantly, succenturiate lobes are associated with an increased incidence of velamentous insertion of the umbilical cord and vasa previa, conditions that have significant maternal and fetal complications.[4]

An *annular placenta* refers to a ring-shaped placenta that attaches circumferentially to the myometrium and can be associated with antenatal or postpartum hemorrhage most likely due to poor separation.[4] Placenta membranacea (PM) is an exceedingly rare anomaly with an incidence of 1:20,000 to 1:40,000 pregnancies. In this condition, there is no differentiation of the primitive trophoblastic shell into chorion frondosum and chorion laeve at 8 to 10 weeks. With PM, functioning placental villi are retained beneath the membranes and may cover all (diffuse PM) or part (partial PM) of the gestational sac, and the placenta develops as an abnormally thin membranous structure. Histologically, the amniotic and chorionic membranes are absent, which are then replaced by placental villi. Frequently, however, completely formed villi are not seen, but rather a trophoblastic layer invading the membranes. These pregnancies are complicated by antepartum and postpartum hemorrhage in 50% to 83% of cases and by abnormal placental adherence in approximately 30% of cases. Fetal outcome with PM ranges from preterm birth to stillbirth to neonatal death and usually occurs because of vaginal bleeding. Live births occur in more than 50% of cases.[6,7] Both annular placenta and PM are associated with placenta previa.

Placenta extrachorialis, a term that includes both placenta circummarginate and placenta circumvallate, is defined as the placenta extending beyond the limits of the chorionic plate with attachment of the placental membranes to the fetal surface of the placenta, inward from the edge, rather than to the underlying villous placenta margin (Fig. 18-6). The placenta is termed *circummarginate* if the fetal membrane insertion is flat and may be found in up to 20% of placentas. More often, the transition where the fetal membranes of the chorionic plate terminate has a raised or rolled edge, termed *circumvallate*. Circumvallate placenta, which is characterized by thickened rolled chorioamniotic membranes peripherally, occurs in 1% to 7% of deliveries (Fig. 18-7). In general, circummarginate and partial circumvallate placentas are of no clinical significance.[8,9] However, complete circumvallation of the placenta may be associated with an increased risk of maternal bleeding, placental abruption, premature labor and delivery, IUGR, perinatal death, and fetal anomalies.[10,11] Although difficult to diagnose prenatally, circumvallate placenta may be seen as irregular subchorionic marginal cystic structures or infolding of the placental margin with thick, curled peripheral edge. The classic ultrasound feature of a rolled-up placental edge can appear on some views as a linear structure protruding into the fluid-filled amniotic cavity and thus can be misinterpreted as a uterine synechia (Fig. 18-8).[8] Some authors

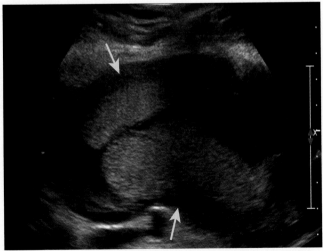
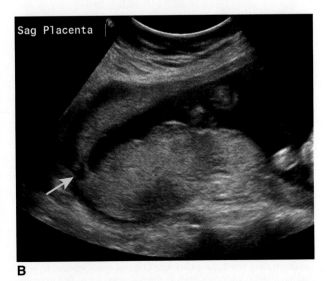

A   **B**

Figure 18-5 Variations in placental shape. **A:** Ultrasound image demonstrating two placental masses (*arrows*) consistent with a succenturiate lobe of the placenta. **B:** Ultrasound image showing two masses of placental tissue connected by a bridge of chorionic tissue (*arrow*) consistent with bilobate placenta.

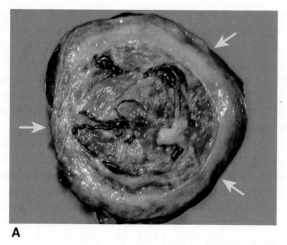
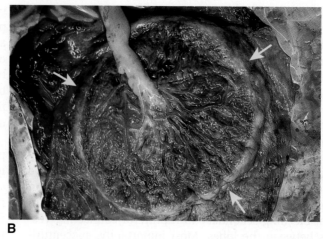

A   **B**

Figure 18-6 A: Gross pathologic specimen of a circummarginate placenta showing the flat transition of the membranes as they insert some distance in from the placental edge *(arrows).* **B:** Gross pathologic specimen of a circumvallate placenta with the characteristic thick rolled edge at the insertion of the membranes on the placental disk *(arrows).*

have referred to this as a *placental shelf*, which is typically a transient and benign finding on early second-trimester sonography. In most cases, the shelf is no longer visible by the late second trimester.[12]

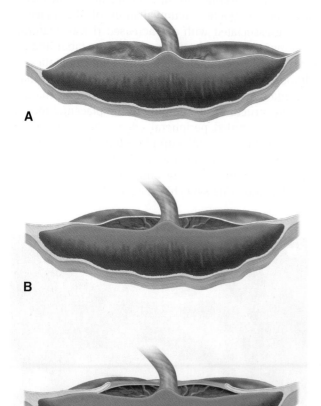

A

B

C

Figure 18-7 Extrachorial placentation. **A:** Normal placentation demonstrating the appropriate transition of membranous to villous chorion inserting appropriately at the placental edge. **B:** Circummarginate placenta with smooth transition from membranous to villous chorion at some distance in from the placental edge. **C:** Circumvallate placenta, similar to circummarginate, except there is a thick rolled edge at the transition.

ABNORMAL PLACENTAL LOCATION

Placenta previa refers to the implantation of the placenta in the lower part of the uterus, thus delivering before the fetus.[13] There are several classifications described in the literature including no previa, low-lying placenta, marginal previa, partial previa, complete previa, and complete central previa (Fig. 18-9).[14] There is some confusion in the literature regarding the correct terminology. A low-lying placenta occurs when the inferior margin of the placenta is within 2 cm of the internal cervical os and is present in around 25% of pregnancies at 20 weeks, but placenta previa at term only affects 1% because of the expansion of the lower uterine segment with advancing gestation.[3] Endovaginal sonography is the method of choice to establish the relationship between the inferior placental margin and the internal cervical os. This is due to several reasons, including the empty maternal bladder does not compress the lower uterine segment, and the close proximity of the transducer to evaluated structures. In addition, the higher frequency endovaginal transducer improves image resolution of the internal cervical os and placental edge, especially in the case of a low fetal head and posterior placenta. (Fig. 18-10). Magnetic resonance imaging (MRI) may be used when clinically indicated to clarify placental position and evaluate for placental invasion (Fig. 18-11). Placenta previa is an important cause of bleeding in the second half of pregnancy, occurring in 1 in 200 to 250 pregnancies.[2] Risk factors for placenta previa include advanced maternal age, previous cesarean section or uterine scar, multiple gestations, previous elective abortions, smoking, cocaine use, and multiparity.[4,13]

ABNORMAL PLACENTAL ATTACHMENT

The placenta accreta spectrum includes placenta accreta, increta, and percreta. This condition involves a defect in the decidua basalis, which allows the chorionic

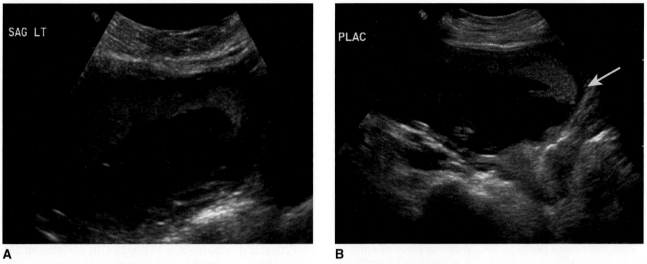

Figure 18-8 Ultrasound images of circumvallate placenta. **A:** Ultrasound image of a circumvallate placenta demonstrating the characteristic rolled-up placental edge. **B:** Ultrasound image of a circumvallate placenta appearing as a linear structure in the amniotic cavity. This can be misinterpreted as a uterine synechia *(arrow)*.

villi to invade into the myometrium and occasionally extend into the tissues beyond (Fig. 18-12).[15] Placenta accreta occurs when the chorionic villi become abnormally adherent to the uterine myometrium rather than the uterine decidua. Placenta increta occurs when there is villous infiltration into the myometrial surface. Placenta percreta occurs when the chorionic villi infiltrate

and penetrate through the entire myometrium, breaching the serosa and potentially invading the surrounding maternal organs.[16-18] The term *placenta accreta* is often used to include all potential forms of placental invasion, as prenatal distinction is not always possible.

The prevalence of placenta accreta has risen tenfold in the United States over the past 50 years, primarily

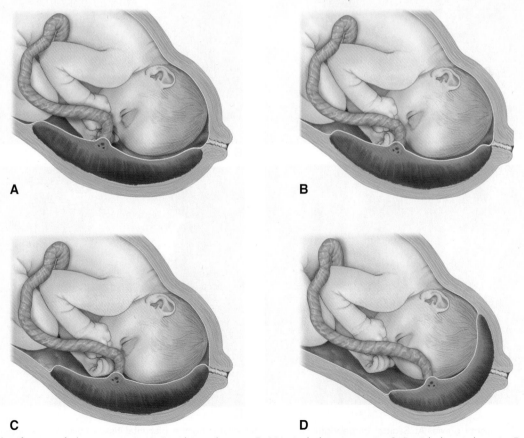

Figure 18-9 Classification of placenta previa: **A:** Low-lying placenta. **B:** Marginal placenta previa. **C:** Partial placental previa. **D:** Complete central placental previa.

PATHOLOGY BOX 18-1

Classifications of Placenta Previa

Subtype	Description
Low-lying placenta	Inferior margin of the placenta is within 2 cm of the internal cervical os
Marginal previa	Placental tissue extends to the edge of the internal cervical os but does not cover it
Partial previa	Placental tissue partially covers the internal os
Complete previa	Placental tissue entirely covers the internal cervical os
Complete central previa	A central placenta mass is implanted directly over the internal cervical os

due to the increasing percentage of pregnant patients undergoing primary and repeat cesarean sections. It has been reported that placenta accreta now occurs in approximately 1 per 1,500 to 2,500 deliveries.[16,19] It is a significant cause of maternal morbidity and mortality and is currently the most common reason for an emergency postpartum hysterectomy. Placenta previa and previous cesarean section delivery are the two most important known risk factors for placenta accreta. In the presence of placenta previa, increasing numbers of prior cesarean deliveries exponentially increase the risk of placenta accreta.[15] Advanced maternal age, uterine anomalies, smoking, myomectomy, previous uterine surgery, and previous dilatation and curettage have also been associated with placenta accreta.[15,17,20]

Prenatal diagnosis is a key factor in optimizing the counseling, treatment, and outcome of patients with placental invasion.[15] Ultrasonography remains the diagnostic standard for the screening and evaluation of this

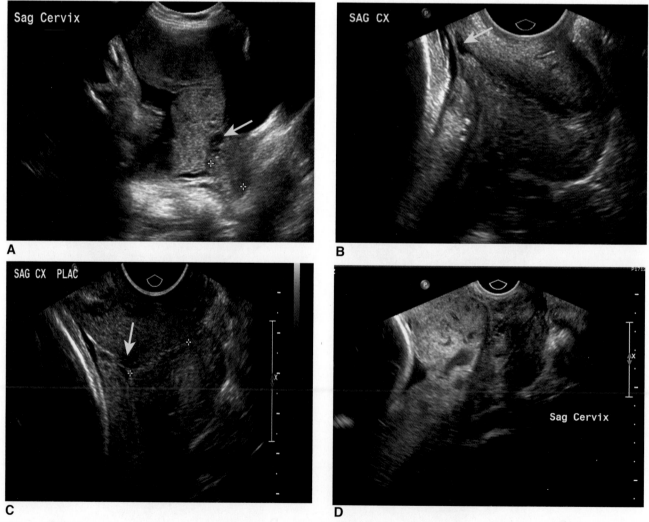

Figure 18-10 Placenta previa. **A:** Sagittal transabdominal image demonstrating the placental tissue covering the internal cervical os. **B:** Endovaginal image with marginal placenta previa. The *arrow* points to the internal cervical os. **C:** Endovaginal image with partial placenta. The *arrow* points to the internal cervical os. **D:** Complete central placenta previa with accreta on an endovaginal image.

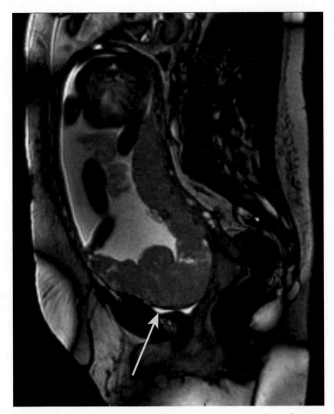

Figure 18-11 T2-weighted MRI demonstrating a complete placenta previa *(arrow)*.

PATHOLOGY BOX 18-2

Classifications of Placental Invasion: The Placenta Accreta Spectrum

Subtype	Description
Placenta accreta	Chorionic villi are attached to but do not invade the myometrium
Placenta increta	Chorionic villi partially invade the myometrium
Placenta percreta	Chorionic villi infiltrate up to or beyond the uterine serosa

sensitivity in the diagnosis of placenta accreta, allowing identification in 78% to 93% of cases after 15 weeks' gestation.[17] Patients may be referred for MRI when there is a high clinical suspicion for placenta accreta or ultrasound findings are equivocal (Fig. 18-14).[18,20] Due to the multiplanar imaging abilities and excellent soft tissue resolution, the use of MRI may be superior to ultrasonography in the assessment of adjacent organ involvement (Fig. 18-15).[14,15,18,20]

The resulting abnormal implantation prevents the normal mechanisms of placental separation and hemostasis. Thus, the clinical consequence of placenta accreta is massive, life-threatening hemorrhage at the time of attempted placental separation. Blood loss averages 3 to 5 L and can lead to disseminated intravascular coagulopathy, adult respiratory distress syndrome, and renal failure. As many as 90% of patients require transfusion and 40% require greater than 10 units of packed red blood cells.[15] Hysterectomy is required in up to 90% of patients with placenta accreta, leading to serious comorbidities such as cystectomy (15.4% of cases), ureteral injury (2.1%), and pulmonary embolus (2.1%), with 26.6% of patients admitted to the intensive care unit.[17] Maternal mortality with placenta accreta has been reported to be as high as 7%.[15]

condition. Sonographic signs suspicious for placenta accreta include a concomitant placenta previa, large numerous placental vascular lacunae (tornado-shaped vessels), absent lower uterine segment myometrium at the placenta/bladder interface, and turbulent flow at the junction between the myometrium and placenta using color flow Doppler (Fig. 18-13). The most common location for placenta accreta is anteriorly at the lower uterine segment. Placental lacunae and abnormal color Doppler imaging patterns are the two most helpful ultrasound markers for this condition. According to the literature, visualization of lacunae has the highest

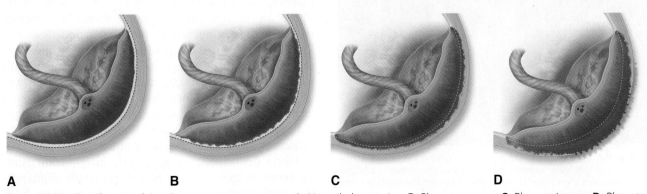

A   **B**   **C**   **D**

Figure 18-12 Classification of the placenta accreta spectrum. **A:** Normal placentation. **B:** Placenta accreta. **C:** Placenta increta. **D:** Placenta percreta.

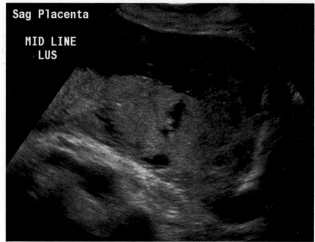

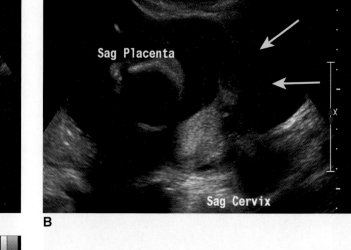

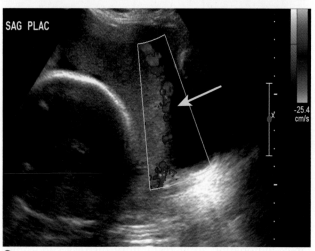

Figure 18-13 Ultrasound criteria for the diagnosis of placental invasion. **A:** Sagittal image of the lower uterine segment demonstrating placenta previa and large numerous placental vascular lacunae. **B:** Irregular interface between the myometrium and the maternal bladder (arrows). **C:** Color Doppler sonography showing turbulent blood flow at the junction between the myometrium of the anterior lower uterine segment and the maternal bladder (arrow).

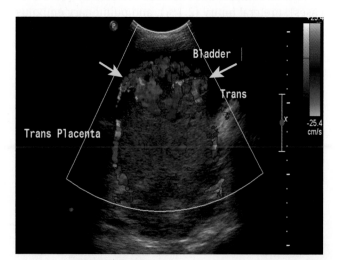

Figure 18-14 Transverse, color Doppler ultrasound image at the junction of the lower uterine, segment, and the maternal bladder with turbulent blood flow at the interface as demonstrated by color Doppler sonography (arrows).

ABNORMALITIES OF PLACENTAL ECHOGENICITY: HYPOECHOIC PLACENTAL LESIONS

Focal cystic and sonolucent lesions of the placenta are frequently encountered by sonography during the dating and anomaly screening examinations. Placental lakes are irregular anechoic structures within the placental parenchyma that are found beneath the chorionic plate. These are thought to correspond to villous vascular spaces with swirling jets of maternal blood flow at a low velocity that can be appreciated with real-time scanning (Fig. 18-16). The lesions are more prevalent with increasing gestational age, and Doppler scanning will fail to demonstrate blood flow. A finding of placental lakes during the second-trimester ultrasound scan does not appear to be associated with uteroplacental complications or an adverse pregnancy outcome.[21]

Fibrin deposition, an apparently insignificant clinical event, is speculated to be the end result of intervillous and subchorionic thrombosis, which results from

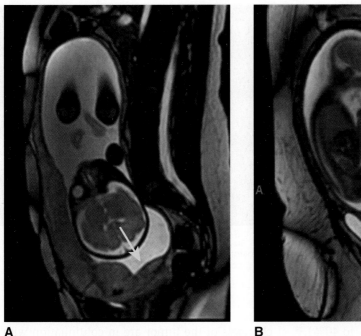
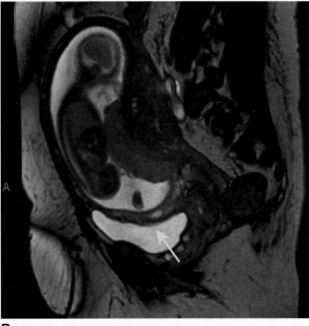

A   **B**

Figure 18-15 MRI of placenta percreta. **A:** T2-weighted MRI image of placenta percreta with obvious placenta previa, appreciable vascular lacunae, and abnormal interface between the lower uterine segment and maternal bladder wall *(arrow)*. **B:** T2-weighted image demonstrating placental invasion *(arrow)*.

pooling and stasis of maternal blood in the perivillous and subchorionic spaces. Fibrin deposits may appear sonographically as hypoechoic lesions in the subchorionic area or within the placental mass, or as linear echogenic streaks within an anechoic lesion.

Intervillous thrombosis represents an intraplacental area of hemorrhage and clot. These areas of thrombosis appear sonographically as hypoechoic placental lesions of varying size that may contain linear echogenicities representing fibrin deposits. They are most commonly found midway between the subchorionic and basal areas of the placenta and are present in up to 50% of term pregnancies. More extensive, heterogeneous, and hypoechoic lesions may represent massive subchorionic hematoma and thrombosis (Breus' mole), a rare occurrence secondary to venous obstruction.

Placental infarction occurs as a result of obstruction of the spiral arteries and is usually found at the periphery of the placenta. Placental infarctions may be associated with retroplacental hemorrhage in up to 25% of term placentas. Although they usually have no clinical significance, they may be associated with IUGR and mothers with preeclampsia. The diagnosis is often pathological and there is no specific sonographic appearance; however, necrotic infarct may appear hypoechoic or show placental thinning.

Subchorionic or septal cysts of the placenta may form at the fetal surface and are thought to be venous in origin. They are usually multiple and near the cord insertion site into the placenta (Fig. 18-17).

PLACENTAL MASSES AND TUMORS

Chorioangiomas and teratomas represent the two primary nontrophoblastic tumors of the placenta. A *chorioangioma* is a benign vascular malformation of the placenta arising from primitive chorionic mesenchyme and is found in about 1% of examined placentas. They can be associated with elevated maternal serum α-fetoprotein or β-human chorionic gonadotropin levels.[22] Small solitary chorioangiomas may be asymptomatic and of little clinical significance, whereas multiple or large chorioangiomas (>5 cm) have been reported to be associated with maternal and fetal complications in 30% to 50% of cases.[23] Chorioangiomas contain arteriovenous shunts that can lead to severe fetal complications such as anemia, heart failure, nonimmune hydrops, thrombocytopenia, polyhydramnios, IUGR, prematurity, and placental abruption. These complications are responsible for the high fetal and neonatal mortality rates

---

PATHOLOGY BOX 18-3

Differential Considerations for Intraplacental Sonolucent Lesions

Placental lakes
Fibrin deposition
Intervillous thrombosis
Placental infarction
Septal cysts

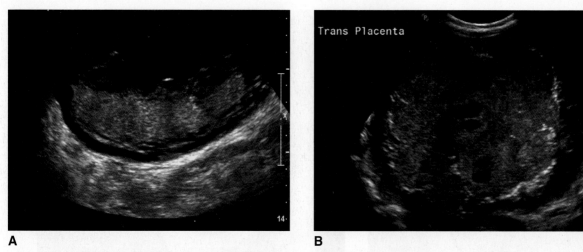

Figure 18-16 Hypoechoic lesions of the placenta. **A:** Ultrasound image of a posterior placenta showing scattered hypoechoic lesions beneath the chorionic plate. Real-time sonography demonstrated swirling blood flow, consistent with venous lakes. **B:** Transverse scan of a fundal placenta with venous lakes.

associated with large chorioangiomas (18% to 40%).[24] The likelihood of a poor outcome is generally correlated with the amount of additional vascularized tissue that the fetal cardiovascular system must perfuse.[22]

Typically, chorioangiomas present sonographically as a well-circumscribed hyperechoic or hypoechoic ovoid mass protruding from the fetal surface of the placenta near the cord insertion.[23] Calcifications and necrosis are occasionally observed (Fig. 18-18). The presence of calcifications in the chorioangioma has been associated with reduced blood flow, improved clinical symptoms, and good outcome.[22] Color Doppler is used to differentiate between other masses such as placental hematoma, degenerating fibroid, placental teratoma, partial hydatidiform mole, infarcts, and intervillous thrombosis. 3D power Doppler can demonstrate that the vascular

channels of the tumor are in continuation with the fetal circulation.[25] The sonographic diagnosis of chorioangioma is based on increased vascularity or a large feeding vessel inside the tumor with the same pulsation rate as the umbilical cord.[26] The vascularization of the chorioangioma, supplied by the fetal circulation through arteriovenous shunts from the umbilical cord, is responsible for fetal anemia and further complications. The Doppler measure of the peak systolic velocity in the middle cerebral artery (MCA) is useful in the diagnosis and management of fetal anemia (Fig. 18-19). Therefore, when ultrasound examination identifies a placental mass consistent with chorioangioma, a close antenatal surveillance should be taken every 7 to 14 days, including MCA peak systolic velocity measurement, as this has been shown to be an excellent tool for

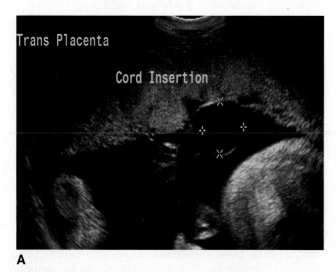

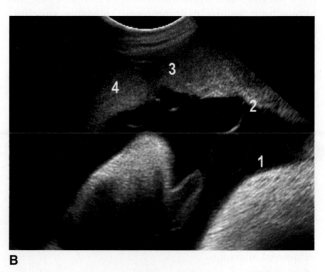

Figure 18-17 Subchorionic or septal cysts of the placenta. **A:** Cyst of the placenta noted at the site of the umbilical cord insertion into the placenta. **B:** Ultrasound image showing multiple cysts at the fetal surface of the placenta. These cysts resolved spontaneously and the fetus was normal at delivery.

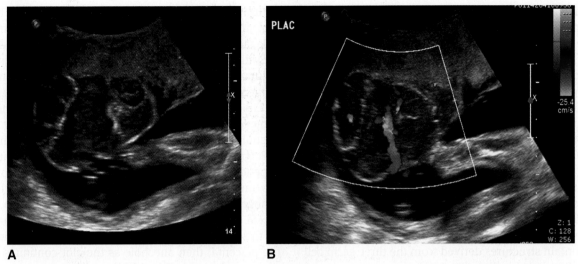

Figure 18-18 Chorioangioma. **A:** Large ovoid mass protruding from fetal surface of the placenta with internal calcifications consistent with a chorioangioma. **B:** As a vascular tumor of the placenta, the chorioangioma demonstrates multiple vascular channels within the mass on color Doppler sonography.

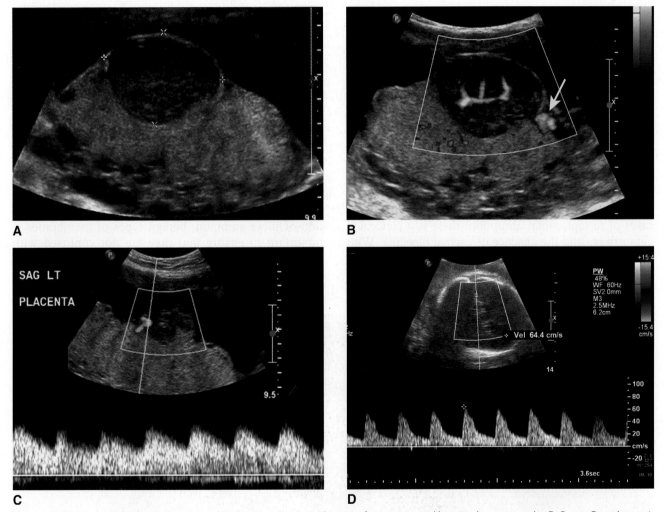

Figure 18-19 Evaluation of a chorioangioma by sonography. **A:** Evaluation of tumor size and location by sonography. **B:** Power Doppler angiography demonstrating vascular channels and an umbilical feeding vessel *(arrow)*. **C:** Color and spectral Doppler interrogation of the feeding vessel to the tumor demonstrates the same pulsation rate as the umbilical cord. **D:** Color and spectral Doppler ultrasound is used to obtain the peak systolic flow of the middle cerebral artery in the evaluation of fetuses at risk for anemia.

early detection of fetal anemia secondary to a large chorioangioma.[24] A placental chorioangioma can increase in size rapidly, leading to progressive heart failure in the fetus. In such cases, Doppler echocardiographic evaluation of the fetal circulation is paramount in assessing the degree of cardiovascular impairment.[22] In situations in which maternal or fetal complications necessitate intervention, there are several possible treatment options; however, most of these cases have a dismal prognosis. Possible interventions include serial fetal blood transfusions, fetoscopic laser coagulation of vessels supplying the tumor, chemosclerosis with absolute alcohol, and endoscopic surgical devascularization.[23]

Teratomas of the placenta are very rare and are usually benign, but they can also be highly malignant. They may contain structures derived from the three germ cell layers. Sonographically, placental teratomas present as a complex mass of the placenta with cystic and solid components; calcifications may be present.

PLACENTAL ABRUPTION

Placental abruption complicates approximately 1% of pregnancies and is defined as a premature separation of all or part of the placenta from the underlying myometrium. Placental abruption has been classified according to the location of separation. The resulting hemorrhage may occur as a retroplacental, intraplacental, marginal, or subchorionic blood clot (Fig. 18-20). Abruption may manifest itself in three ways: as vaginal bleeding without significant intrauterine hematoma, as the development of a retroplacental or marginal hematoma with or without vaginal bleeding, or as formation of a submembranous clot at a distance from the placenta with or without vaginal bleeding. In some cases of retroplacental abruption, there is a concealed hemorrhage and the absence of vaginal bleeding. With placental abruption, the patient may present clinically with acute abdominal and pelvic pain, vaginal bleeding, uterine tenderness, and fetal distress. Numerous risk factors have been associated with this condition, including maternal hypertension, cocaine use, smoking, trauma, uterine anomalies, and premature rupture of membranes.[4]

The diagnosis of abruption is mainly a clinical one, and detection by ultrasound is limited. The sensitivity of ultrasound to detect a placental abruption is approximately 50% because of the variable sonographic appearance, depending on the size and location of the separation and the timing of the evaluation. Acute hemorrhage is highly echogenic. As the hematoma progresses, the blood is of mixed echogenicity as the clot becomes more organized. As the hematoma matures, it may appear isoechoic with the placenta, then anechoic as the clot continues on to resorb and resolve (Fig. 18-21).

Prognosis depends on several factors, including the degree of placental detachment and gestational age. Marginal abruption has much less clinical importance than a large retroplacental hematoma. The gravest prognosis is associated with significant retroplacental hemorrhage involving over 30% to 40% of the placenta and may include fetal growth restriction, oligohydramnios, preterm delivery, and fetal demise.[4]

FETAL MEMBRANE ABNORMALITIES

Various intrauterine membranes, septations, and bands have been demonstrated with sonography in and about the amniotic cavity. The most commonly identified structures or conditions include chorioamniotic separation, elevation due to subchorionic hemorrhage, membranes associated with multiple gestations and blighted ova, and intrauterine synechiae. Recognition of these common, benign types of membranes is important to ensure that they are not confused with amniotic bands.

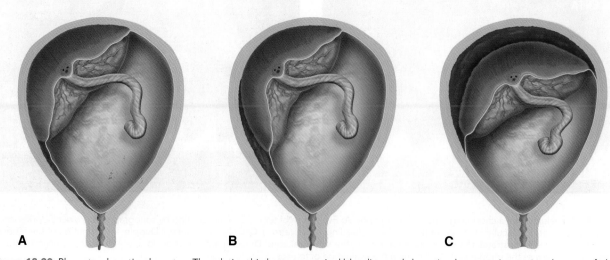

Figure 18-20 Placenta, abruptio placentae. The relationship between vaginal bleeding and abruptio placentae. Increasing degrees of placental separation are shown. **A:** Marginal separation. **B:** Partial separation. **C:** Complete separation.

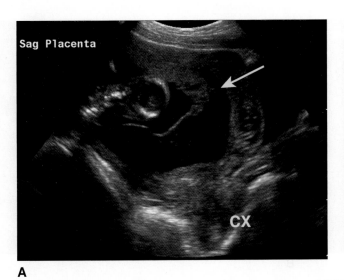

Sag Placenta

CX

A

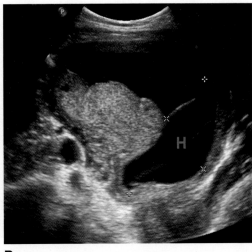

H

B

Figure 18-21 Placental abruption. **A:** Sagittal ultrasound image with partial separation of the placenta from the uterine wall. Note the raised placental edge *(arrow)* with a large accumulation of blood adjacent to the cervix *(CX)*. **B:** Sagittal ultrasound image of a subchorionic hemorrhage with the layering of blood products within the clot formation *(H)*.

The placental (chorion) and fetal (amnion) membranes are separate early in gestation and fuse together at about the 14th week of gestation. In rare instances, chorioamniotic separation can occur later in gestation. This can be focal or extensive and is usually the result of intervention such as amniocentesis, although it may be sporadic. Sporadic cases have been associated with both chromosomal and developmental abnormalities of the fetus. Sonographic diagnosis is possible when the amnion is visible as a discrete, free-floating membrane separate from the chorion surrounding the fetus (Fig. 18-22).[1]

Amniotic sheets or intrauterine synechiae are linear, extra-amniotic tissues that project into the amniotic cavity. These are usually an incidental finding and occur in approximately 1 in 200 pregnancies and in up to 15% to 49% of women who have had uterine curettage performed.[27] Although they appear to be within the amniotic fluid, they are anatomically external to the amniotic sac. On ultrasound, they appear as linear protrusions continuous with and of the same echogenicity as the placenta. Synechiae do not

cause fetal entrapment, or adhere to the fetus, and are not associated with fetal anomalies. Typically, they are no longer visible in the late third trimester secondary to obliteration or compression. Prenatal 3D ultrasound with MRI assessment has been reported to provide exceptional imaging evaluation of this condition (Fig. 18-23).[28] Differential should include a uterine septum, subchorionic hemorrhage, circumvallate placenta, and a multiple gestation with absence of a fetus in one sac.

Amnion rupture sequence or amniotic band syndrome is a sporadic condition that is thought to occur as a result of rupture of the amnion without rupture of the chorion, leading to transient oligohydramnios and passage of the fetus from the amniotic to the chorionic cavity. Early rupture can lead to severe malformations of the cranium, central

---

PATHOLOGY BOX 18-4

Differential Diagnosis for Intrauterine Septations, Bands, and Membranes

Chorioamniotic separation
Amniotic band syndrome
Subchorionic hemorrhage
Multiple gestations
Intrauterine synechia
Uterine septum
Circumvallate placenta

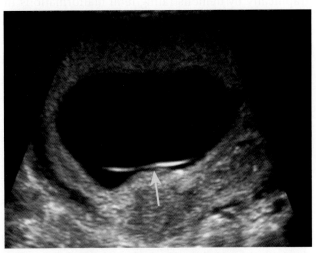

Figure 18-22 Transverse ultrasound image of the uterus denoting posterior chorioamniotic separation.

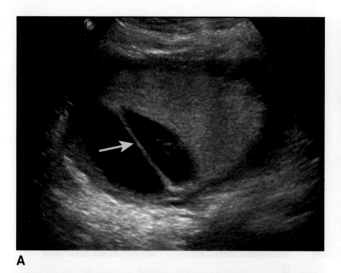

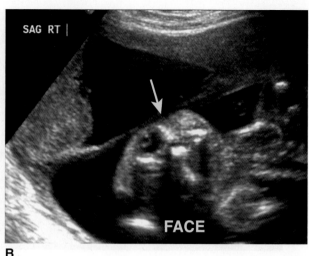

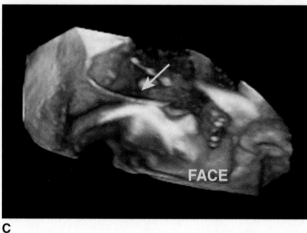

Figure 18-23 Uterine synechia. **A:** Ultrasound image lateral to midline demonstrating a thick linear structure continuous with the placenta in a singleton pregnancy, consistent with an uterine synechia *(arrow)*. This should not be misinterpreted as a circumvallate placenta. **B:** Oblique ultrasound image of a uterine synechia traversing across the fetal face *(arrow)*. **C:** 3D surface rendering in the same patient as **B** showing the synechia superior to the fetal face *(arrow)*. There was no entrapment of fetal parts and the pregnancy outcome was normal.

nervous system, face, and viscera. Amniotic bands may tear or disrupt previously normally developed structures, leading to congenital amputations, constriction rings, and bizarre nonanatomic facial clefts. Amniotic band syndrome may be detected sonographically by demonstrating fetal malformations in a nonembryonic distribution and by direct visualizations of the amniotic bands (Fig. 18-24).[4] For a detailed description, see Amniotic Band Sequence section in Chapter 28.

GESTATIONAL TROPHOBLASTIC DISEASE

Gestational trophoblastic disease (GTD), or gestational trophoblastic neoplasia, is the designation given to several disorders arising from either normal or abnormal fertilization of an ovum, resulting in neoplastic changes in the trophoblastic elements of the developing blastocyst. GTD has been classified into complete or partial hydatidiform mole and metastatic disease or choriocarcinoma. Complete hydatidiform mole, or molar pregnancy, is characterized by chorionic villi that

are markedly hydropic and swollen, and proliferation of the trophoblast cell resulting in excessive production of β-human chorionic gonadotropin levels. Other clinical symptoms include rapid uterine enlargement, excessive uterine size for gestational age, and hyperemesis gravidarum. Sonographically, hydatidiform mole has a very characteristic presentation. There is distention of the uterine cavity by a heterogeneous echogenic mass with a snowstorm appearance.[1] The enlarged uterus is filled with multiple variable-sized small anechoic cysts (Fig. 18-25). In the case of complete mole, there is absence of both amniotic fluid and a fetus. With partial hydatidiform mole, there is the presence of a coexisting fetus along with an enlarged, thickened placenta with multiple cystic spaces. Severe IUGR and fetal anomalies may be present, as triploidy is noted in up to 90% of cases.[4]

Invasive moles represent deep growth of the abnormal tissue into and beyond the myometrium and are considered locally invasive nonmetastasizing neoplasms. Choriocarcinomas are similar to invasive moles; however, they are capable of metastasizing. Approximately 50% of choriocarcinomas arise after

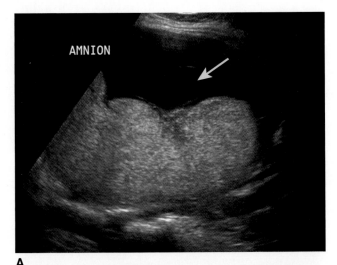

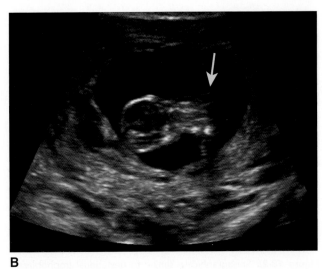

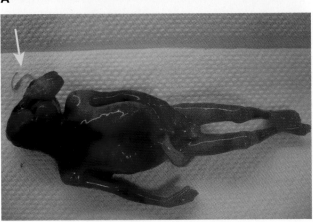

Figure 18-24 Amniotic band syndrome. **A:** Ultrasound image of free-floating amniotic membranes *(arrow)* noted within the uterine cavity in this late second trimester pregnancy. **B:** Ultrasound evaluation of a fetus at 14 weeks of gestation revealed multiple amniotic bands *(arrow)* associated with the fetal head and neck. Limb anomalies, scoliosis, and an anterior abdominal wall defect were also observed. **C:** Postnatal photograph of a different fetus at 15 weeks of gestation with amniotic band syndrome. Note the band of tissue adhered to the significantly deformed fetal head and face with bizarre facial cleft *(arrow)* characteristic of amniotic band syndrome. (Image courtesy of Pathology Associates of Syracuse, Crouse Hospital.)

molar pregnancy, 25% arise after abortion, and 25% arise after normal pregnancy. At sonography, both appear as heterogeneous, echogenic, and hypervascular masses.[1] For a detailed description of gestational trophoblastic neoplasia and choriocarcinoma, see Chapter 9.

Placenta mesenchymal dysplasia (PMD) is a relatively recently recognized, rare placental vascular anomaly characterized by mesenchymal stem villous hyperplasia. This condition presents as an enlarged placenta and may be mistaken for molar pregnancy both clinically and macroscopically because of the presence of "grapelike vesicles." It may be associated with a completely normal fetus, a fetus with gross restriction, or a fetus with features of Beckwith-Wiedemann syndrome.[29–31] The sonographic features of PMD include placentomegaly, dilatation of chorionic vessels, and large areas of cystic villous changes along with areas of normal placenta (Fig. 18-26). 3D reconstruction may reveal a multicystic placental mass clearly separated from, but adjacent to, a normal-appearing placenta. In addition, multiple fluid-filled cysts that do not appear to communicate with each other may be displayed on an inversion mode rendering of the 3D image. The differential diagnosis of PMD includes either partial hydatidiform mole or a complete mole with coexisting fetus, chorioangioma, subchorionic hematoma, placental infarcts, and spontaneous abortion with hydropic changes.[26]

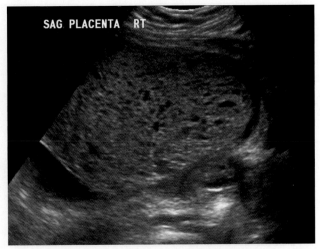

Figure 18-25 Ultrasound image of the intrauterine contents in a case of complete hydatidiform mole. Uterine enlargement is present, with multiple diffuse small cysts dispersed throughout the placental parenchyma. These cysts represent the hydropic chorionic villi associated with this condition. Note the absence of a fetus and amniotic fluid.

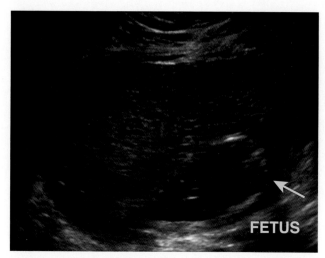

FETUS

Figure 18-26 Sonographically similar to gestational trophoblastic disease, mesenchymal dysplasia also presents with placentomegaly with multiple small cystic areas along with areas of normal placental tissue.

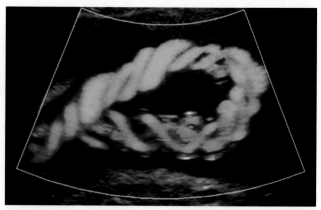

Figure 18-27 Power Doppler angiography ultrasound image demonstrating a three-vessel umbilical cord with normal coiling pattern.

ABNORMALITIES OF THE UMBILICAL CORD

Historically, the evaluation of the fetal umbilical cord during routine obstetric examination has been limited to the documentation of the number of vessels. Recommendations for a systemic evaluation of the umbilical cord at the midtrimester anatomy scan have been suggested. One proposed classification system includes evaluation of the number of blood vessels, measurement of the umbilical cord area, assessment of placental umbilical cord insertion site, and determination of the coiling pattern (Fig. 18-27).[32]

ABNORMAL UMBILICAL VESSEL NUMBER

The umbilical cord normally contains two arteries and one vein surrounded by a mucoid connective tissue called *Wharton's jelly*, all enclosed in a layer of amnion. Evaluation of cord vessel number is performed as part of the routine obstetric exam, and the three vessels are easily distinguishable in 2D imaging ("Mickey Mouse" sign). 2D imaging can demonstrate the presence of a single umbilical artery (SUA) (Fig. 18-28). The increase in the diameter of the umbilical artery relative to the umbilical vein has been reported in cases of SUA.[33] With the use of color Doppler, the application of color within the vessel lumen allows for easy distinction of umbilical cord vessel number (Fig. 18-29). An alternative sonographic method to demonstrate the umbilical cord vessel number is to obtain a transverse image of the fetal pelvis. The application of color Doppler shows

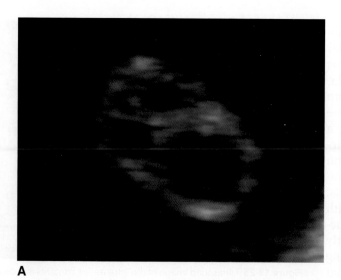

A

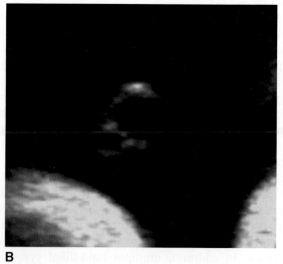

B

Figure 18-28 Transverse view of the umbilical cord. **A:** 2D cross-sectional ultrasound image of a three-vessel umbilical cord, the "Mickey Mouse" sign. **B:** 2D cross-sectional ultrasound image of a two-vessel umbilical cord.

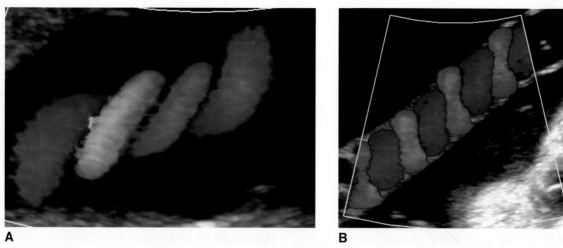

Figure 18-29 Color Doppler of the umbilical cord. **A:** Sagittal ultrasound image showing color Doppler applied to a three-vessel umbilical cord demonstrating two arteries and a single vein with appropriate cord coiling. **B:** Sagittal ultrasound image of a two-vessel umbilical cord with a single umbilical artery.

the presence or absence of umbilical arteries coursing on either side of the fetal urinary bladder (Fig. 18-30). An SUA is one of the most common congenital anomalies, with a reported incidence of about 1% of all singleton pregnancies and 4.6% of twin gestations.[33] Possible mechanisms for SUA include primary agenesis of one artery, atrophy or atresia of a previously present artery, or persistence of the original allantoic artery in the body stalk of the embryo. The left umbilical artery is more commonly absent, and this developmental abnormality has no known recurrence risk.[4,33] In 96% of all umbilical cords, there is an anastomosis; in 3%, there is even fusion of the two umbilical arteries within 1.5 cm of the placental insertion site.[34] Despite the diagnostic methods available for the detection of an SUA and its relatively common occurrence, the antenatal detection

rate is reported to be poor with only one-third of the cases identified.[33]

Fetuses with SUA have a high rate of structural anomalies, ranging from 18% to 68%. According to reports by several investigators, a variety of congenital anomalies have been associated with SUA, including cardiovascular malformations, central nervous system defects, gastrointestinal or genitourinary defects, and musculoskeletal malformations.[33,35] Chromosomal abnormalities are reported in 8% to 11% of fetuses with SUA, particularly trisomies 13 and 18, whereas trisomy 21 does not have a clear association with this anomaly. In a recent study, all chromosomally abnormal fetuses with SUA were found to have associated malformations detected by ultrasound. The presence of isolated SUA is associated with clinically significant fetal

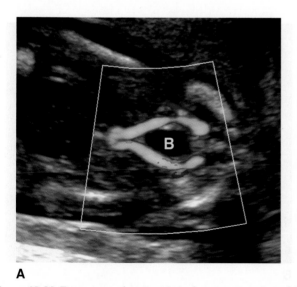

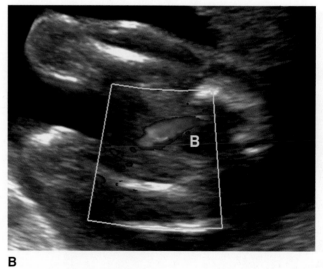

Figure 18-30 Transverse pelvis view. **A:** In the transverse view of the fetal pelvis, two umbilical arteries can be seen coursing around the fetal urinary bladder using power Doppler angiography confirming the presence of a three-vessel umbilical cord. **B:** In the same view, only one umbilical artery is identified adjacent to the fetal bladder consistent with a two-vessel umbilical cord. *B,* bladder.

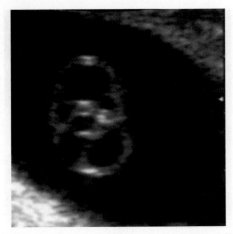

Figure 18-31 Supernumerary vessels. A cross-sectional ultrasound image of an umbilical cord demonstrating multiple vessels in a case of conjoined twinning.

growth restriction, prematurity, and increased perinatal mortality rate.[33,35,36]

Supernumerary vessels are the presence of more than three blood vessels in the umbilical cord. This exceedingly rare condition is almost exclusively associated with various forms of conjoined twinning and is considered an important sonographic landmark for the prenatal diagnosis of conjoined twins (Fig. 18-31). This may represent an abnormal splitting of the umbilical vessels between the third and fifth week of development. On rare occasions, a four-vessel cord has been found in normal neonates but also in association with multiple anomalies.

Persistent right umbilical vein (PRUV), a relatively common vascular variant, is a condition where the right umbilical (portal) vein, rather than the left-sided umbilical vein, remains open. This occurs with an incidence of 0.2%, and the diagnosis is not difficult but often overlooked. On sonographic evaluation, the umbilical vein curves toward the left-sided stomach rather than toward the liver (Fig. 18-32). In addition, the gallbladder will be located medial to the vein rather than its normal lateral position. It is usually an isolated finding but may have a risk of associated anomalies including cardiac malformations.[9]

An umbilical vein varix may be present and is described as a focal dilatation of the umbilical vein. Varix of the umbilical vein is usually seen in the intra-abdominal, extrahepatic portion of the umbilical vein (Fig. 18-33). Color Doppler imaging permits the diagnosis of umbilical vein varix (Fig. 18-34). Diagnostic criteria include an abdominal vein diameter of greater than 9 mm or an enlargement of the varix of at least 50% larger than the diameter of the intrahepatic umbilical vein. Although most cases have a normal outcome, some studies have shown an association with other anomalies, aneuploidy, perinatal death, and hydrops.[9]

ABNORMALITIES OF STRUCTURE

Body stalk anomaly (complete absence of the umbilical cord) and limb body wall complex (a very short cord) are rare occurrences that are associated with severe structural anomalies. Body stalk anomaly is a fatal condition that has been linked to maternal cocaine abuse. Sonographically, no cord would be identified, but rather an extraembryonic sac in direct apposition to the chorionic plate. Again, severe fetal malformations would be obvious on sonographic evaluation, the most common being scoliosis, abdominal wall defects, and neural tube defects (Fig. 18-35).

The average length of the umbilical cord is 55 cm in a normal term newborn. The length of the umbilical

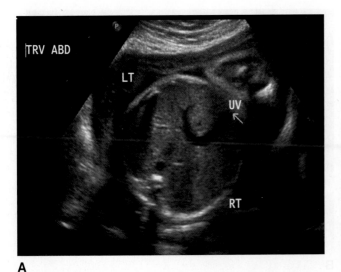

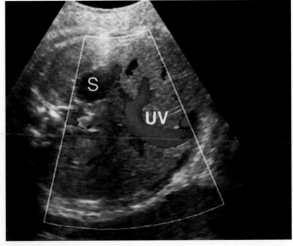

A

B

Figure 18-32 Persistent right umbilical vein. **A:** Transverse view of the fetal abdomen, labeled right and left, showing the umbilical vein coursing to the fetal left. **B:** Color Doppler image of the fetal abdomen demonstrates the umbilical vein curving toward the fetal stomach rather than the fetal liver. *UV,* umbilical vein; *S,* stomach.

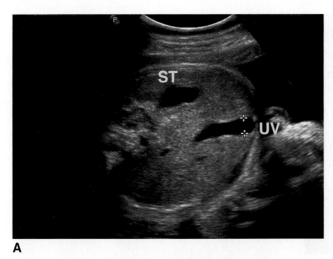
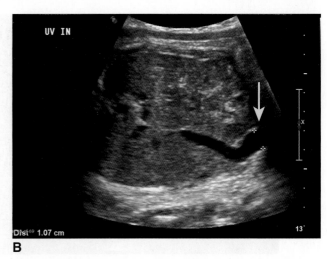

A   **B**

Figure 18-33 Umbilical vein varix. **A:** Transverse section of the fetal abdomen showing focal dilatation of the fetal umbilical vein as it enters the fetal abdomen. **B:** Similar case of umbilical vein varix where the intra-abdominal portion of the umbilical vein measures 11 mm *(arrow)*. *UV,* umbilical vein; *ST,* stomach.

cord is considered an index of fetal activity and is dependent on the tension created by the freely mobile fetus primarily during the first and second trimesters. Currently, measurements of umbilical cord length are not widely applied in obstetrics. A short cord has been defined as 35 cm or less and has been associated with fetal anomalies (often lethal) in which fetal movement is limited or absent, such as body stalk anomaly, limb–body wall complex, restrictive dermopathy, ichthyosis, Neu Laxova syndrome, and fetal akinesia/hypokinesia (Pena-Shokeir syndrome) sequence. It is also considered a significant marker for developmental abnormalities, including trisomy 21. In addition, normal fetuses with short umbilical cords are reported to manifest an increased risk of adverse antenatal and intrapartum complications, including umbilical cord rupture, failure to descend, umbilical vessel hematomas, thrombosis,

thrombocytopenia, cord compression, variable heart decelerations, instrumental and operative deliveries, and fetal demise.[37] An abnormally long umbilical cord may predispose to vascular occlusions by thrombi and true knots, stricture, nuchal cord, cord entanglement, and cord prolapse during labor.[38]

ABNORMALITIES OF CORD INSERTION

Typically, the umbilical cord inserts at or near the center of the placental disc in over 90% of cases (Fig. 18-36).[4] The placental umbilical cord insertion site can be readily determined by sonography at the time of the 11- to 14-week scan (Fig. 18-37). Sonographic evaluation at this early gestational age provides the opportunity for screening for abnormal cord insertion into the placenta in the first trimester, allowing for close surveillance of

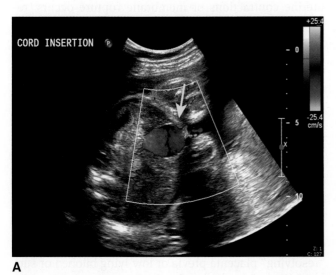
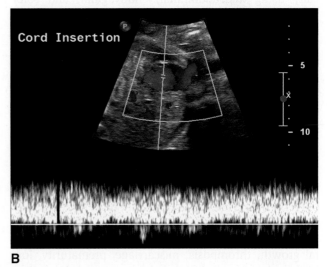

A   **B**

Figure 18-34 Umbilical vein varix. **A:** Color Doppler imaging showing turbulent flow in the cystic dilatation of the umbilical vein as it enters into the fetal abdomen *(arrow)*. **B:** Spectral Doppler demonstrates venous flow within this structure confirming the diagnosis of an umbilical vein varix.

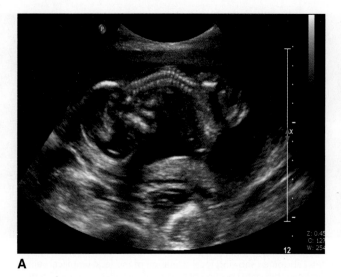

A

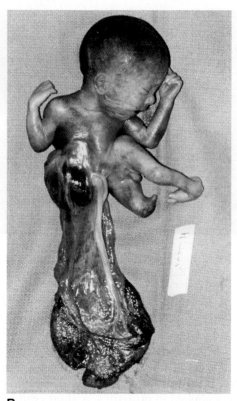

B

Figure 18-35 Limb–body wall complex. **A:** Ultrasound image of a fetus with multiple anomalies including scoliosis, anterior abdominal wall defect, and neural tube defect. Postnatal diagnosis was consistent with limb–body wall complex. **B:** Postnatal photograph of a fetus with limb–body wall complex. Note the multiple malformations, short umbilical cord, and fusion of the placenta to the anterior abdominal wall defect.

the pregnancy for potential complications associated with this condition.[39] Developmental abnormalities of the placenta and umbilical cord have been noted to occur frequently in cases where the cord insertion site into the developing placenta is in the lower third of the uterus in the first trimester of pregnancy. It has been suggested that screening for the cord insertion at 9 to 11 weeks of gestation may be useful for predicting those cases that will have abnormalities of the cord and placenta at delivery.[40] Abnormalities of the umbilical cord insertion into the placenta can be detected sonographically using transabdominal, endovaginal, and color Doppler techniques, with screening for the cord insertion site can improve perinatal outcomes (Fig. 18-38).[41] Marginal insertion of the umbilical cord into the placenta, also known as battledore placenta, occurs when the cord inserts within a centimeter of the placental margin rather than centrally and occurs in 5% to 7% of term pregnancies (Fig. 18-39).[4]

Velamentous insertion occurs in 1% to 2% of term singleton pregnancies and is more frequent in multiple gestations. In this situation, the umbilical vessels separate and course between the amnion and chorion at a distance from the placental margin surrounded only by a fold of amnion devoid of Wharton's jelly (Fig. 18-40).[4,42] Clinically, velamentous cord insertion has been associated with cord compression, poor fetal growth, thrombosis, miscarriage, prematurity, low birth weight, fetal malformation, perinatal death, low Apgar scores, placenta previa, vasa previa, and retained placenta.[4,39] It has been demonstrated that atypical variable deceleration in the first stage of labor is a characteristic fetal heart-rate pattern for velamentous cord insertion and hypercoiled cords.[43]

In vasa previa, some of the velamentous fetal vessels run in the lower uterine segment unprotected by Wharton's jelly. These umbilical vessels traverse within the fetal membranes on or near the region of the internal cervical os (Fig. 18-41). Because these unsupported fetal vessels lie inferior to the presenting fetal part, they are easily compressed or ruptured when uterine contractions or membrane rupture occurs, resulting in fetal hypoxia or exsanguination.[39,44-47] Since bleeding from vasa previa is of fetal origin, the associated fetal morbidity and mortality are extremely high, ranging from 50% to 60% with intact membranes, and 70% to 100% with ruptured membranes. The incidence of vasa previa is estimated to be about 1 in 1,200 to 5,000 pregnancies.[44,48] Risk factors for vasa previa include the ultrasound diagnosis velamentous insertion, bilobed or succenturiate placenta, multiple gestation, suspicion of aberrant vessels, low-lying placenta or placenta previa at earlier gestation, cord insertion into the lower uterine segment, and in vitro fertilization.[44,49]

It has been suggested that a combination of endovaginal sonography in the late first or early second trimester with targeted sonography in patients with "resolving" placenta previa or low-lying bilobed or succenturiate placenta may be the best way to screen for vasa previa. Sonographic identification of the umbilical

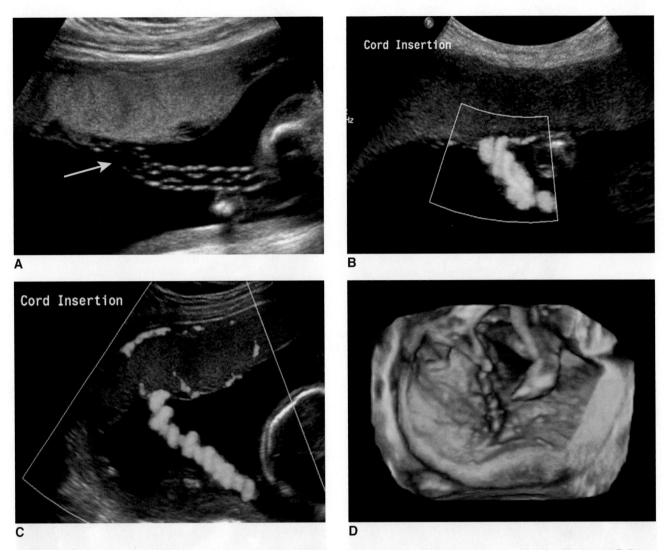

Figure 18-36 Normal cord insertion into the placenta. **A:** 2D image denoting central cord insertion into an anterior placenta *(arrow)*. **B:** Power Doppler angiography applied to the same image showing the helical arrangement of the blood vessels of the cord as it inserts centrally. **C:** Power Doppler angiography demonstrating a paracentric or eccentric umbilical cord insertion into the placenta. **D:** 3D surface rendering of a placenta with a central cord insertion.

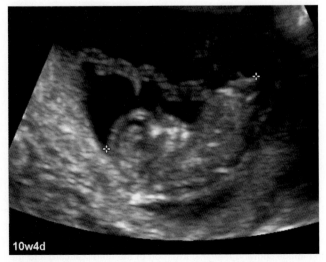

Figure 18-37 Ultrasound image showing normal first trimester sonogram showing cord insertion into the placenta.

cord insertion site in the first trimester could have important implications for pregnancy management.[41] Although it can be missed, the most useful tool for the prenatal diagnosis of vasa previa is a combination of endovaginal sonography and color Doppler examination (Fig. 18-42).[47,50,51] Prenatal diagnosis and evaluation of vasa previa with 3D sonography and power angiography have been reported.

3D ultrasonography in the multiplanar mode allows the evaluation of the spatial relationship between the aberrant vessel and the uterine cervix. 3D in power Doppler or power angiography mode allows mapping of the vessels, which may have value in the surgical section of the uterus.[45,52–54] In cases of prenatally diagnosed vasa previa, it has been suggested that the key to a good outcome is close follow-up with possible hospitalization from 32 gestational weeks onward. Prompt surgery should be carried out in cases of vaginal bleeding,

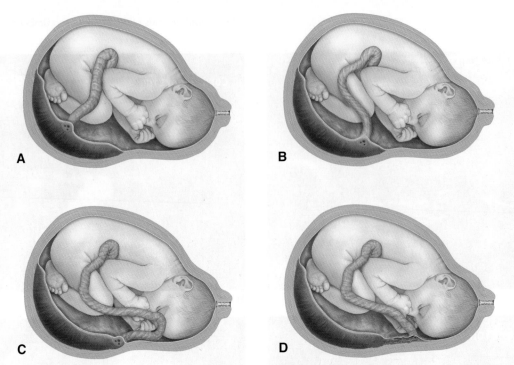

Figure 18-38 Cord insertion into the placenta. **A:** Central cord insertion. **B:** Eccentric cord insertion. **C:** Marginal cord insertion (battledore placenta). **D:** Velamentous cord insertion.

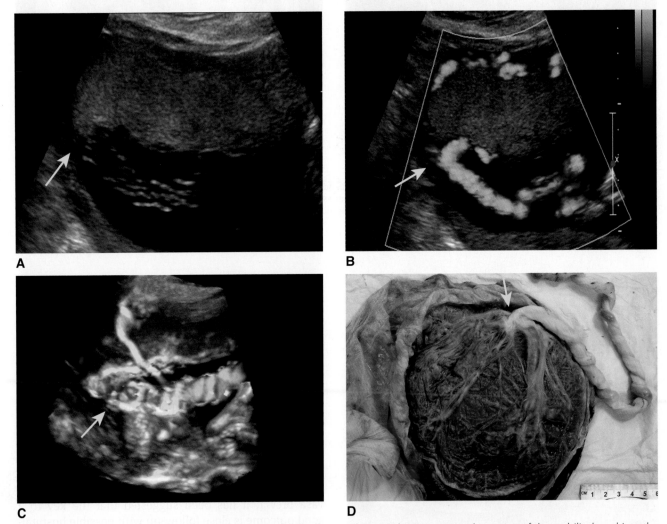

Figure 18-39 Marginal insertion or battledore placenta. **A:** 2D ultrasound image showing marginal insertion of the umbilical cord into the placental disk *(arrow)*. **B:** Power Doppler angiography of the same case demonstrating the marginal insertion site *(arrow)*. **C:** 3D color Doppler of marginal cord insertion *(arrow)*. **D:** Gross pathology specimen with marginal cord insertion into the placenta *(arrow)*. (Image courtesy of Pathology Associates of Syracuse, Crouse Hospital.)

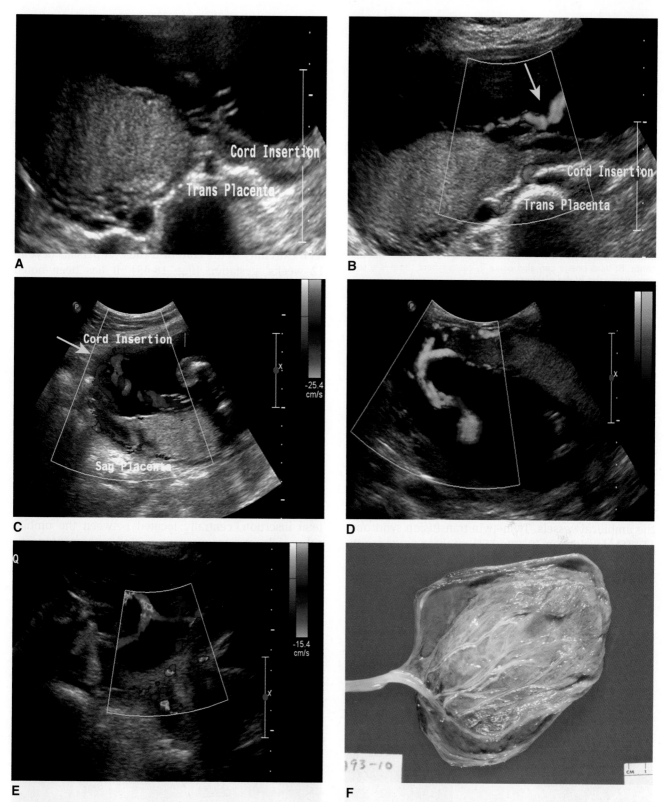

Figure 18-40 Velamentous insertion. **A:** 2D ultrasound image showing a placenta with a velamentous cord insertion (*arrow*). **B:** Image of the same placenta with power Doppler application to show the vessels entering the membranes prior to reaching the placental mass. **C:** Another example of velamentous cord insertion (*arrow*) with color Doppler applied to demonstrate the vessels inserting into the membranes. **D:** Power Doppler of the umbilical cord with velamentous insertion. **E:** Sagittal image of the lower uterine segment with the umbilical vessels insertion into the membranes and branching prior to reaching the placenta. This case also was confirmed to have a vasa previa. **F:** Gross pathology specimen of a placenta with velamentous insertion.

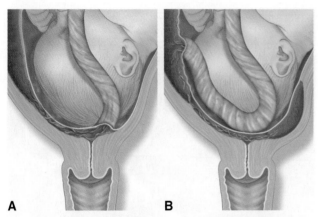

A   **B**

Figure 18-41 Vasa previa is a condition where umbilical vessels run within the membranes near or across the internal cervical os. **A:** Vasa previa in association with velamentous cord insertion into the placenta. **B:** Vasa previa can also occur in cases where there is a succenturiate lobe of the placenta.

ruptured membranes, or onset of labor. Elective cesarean section should be considered when fetal lung maturity has been documented.[45,47,54]

With furcate insertion of the umbilical cord, the umbilical cord blood vessels lose their protective cover of Wharton's jelly before entering the chorionic plate. Owing to the splaying of vessels and their wide distribution, the vessels are exposed to external trauma. During labor and delivery, they may rupture, twist, and consequently compromise the placental circulation, resulting in stillbirth.[55]

Monochorionic twin pregnancies can share the same placenta and often have anastomoses between the umbilical vessels. Twin–twin transfusion syndrome (TTTS) develops in 10% to 15% of these pregnancies. This condition is characterized by discordant fetal size, with polyhydramnios around the larger twin and severe oligohydramnios associated with the smaller "stuck" twin. By color Doppler sonography, anastomosis may be visualized between the cords on the placental surface.[13]

CYSTIC CORD MASSES

In the first trimester, *umbilical cord cysts* are defined as an echolucent area within the umbilical cord with the yolk sac defined as a separate structure. The presence of umbilical cord cysts between 7 and 13 weeks' gestation has been reported at 3%, with more than 20% of the cases having an association with chromosomal or structural defects. The fetus may be more likely to be abnormal if a cyst is located near the placental or fetal extremity of the cord or if the cyst persists beyond 12 weeks' gestation (Fig. 18-43). It has been noted that the appearance of umbilical cord cysts coincides with the onset of coiling of the umbilical cord and the formation of physiologic hernia; therefore, it has been proposed that these cystlike structures result from transient fluid accumulation because of the coiling process or herniation of the bowel interfering with fluid exchange within the cord.[56]

Umbilical cord cysts are defined as true cysts or pseudocysts. True cysts, derived from embryonic remnants of the allantois and the omphalomesenteric duct, have no increased risk of chromosomal anomalies. These cysts represent vestigial patency of an embryonic structure and are typically located near the cord insertion into the fetal abdomen.[56] These cysts are easily detectable on ultrasound, with allantoic cysts close to the fetal insertion, centrally located between the umbilical vessels, and are often associated with spontaneous resolution (Fig. 18-44).[3] Pseudocysts have no epithelial lining and represent localized edema of Wharton's jelly

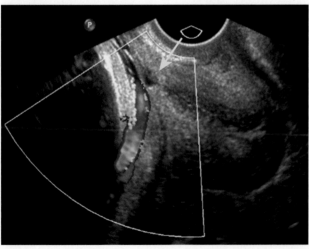

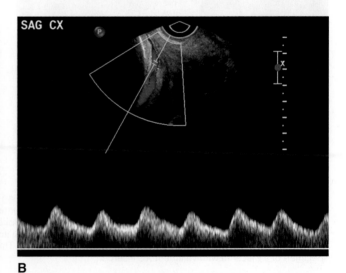

A   **B**

Figure 18-42 Vasa previa. **A:** Endovaginal image of the maternal cervix using color Doppler to document the presence of fetal vessels coursing adjacent to the internal cervical os *(arrow)* in a case with a succenturiate lobe of the placenta. **B:** The addition of a spectral Doppler tracing of the blood vessels demonstrates fetal origin, consistent with vasa previa.

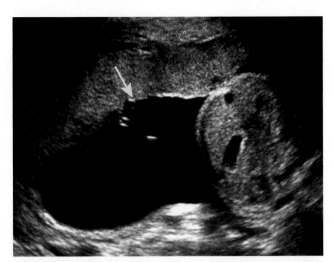

Figure 18-43 Umbilical cord cyst. Ultrasound image of an anechoic cystic structure located adjacent to the umbilical cord insertion site into the placenta consistent with an umbilical cord cyst *(arrow)*. The pregnancy outcome was normal.

or aneurysm of an umbilical artery or vein. Excessive deposits of Wharton's jelly, which appears as a soft tissue mass, may liquefy and present sonographically as a large, cystic mass (Fig. 18-45). Pseudocysts show a positive association to structural and chromosomal defects, particularly trisomy 18 and 13. Prenatal management should include serial ultrasound examinations to assess the size and growth of the cyst. Doppler evaluation may be helpful to assess blood flow patterns since large umbilical cord cysts may compress blood vessels and impair umbilical circulation causing intrauterine demise of the fetus.[57]

Prenatally detected mass lesions in the cord appear as hyperechogenic, solid, and cystic lesions, usually representing hematomas, varices, aneurysms, thrombosis, and rarely tumors such as hemangiomas and teratomas.[3,58] With any cord mass, mechanical compression and impairment of fetal circulation is a potential consequence, especially if the mass arises from the vascular tissue.

Umbilical cord hemangiomas are an extremely rare benign tumor, with less than 50 cases reported in the literature. Also referred to as angiomyxoma, myxangioma, hemangiofibromyxoma, and myxsarcoma, umbilical cord hemangiomas have been associated with congenital anomalies such as capillary vascular malformations of the skin and an SUA. There is also an association with increased maternal serum α-fetoprotein levels, polyhydramnios, preterm labor, and increased perinatal mortality, particularly intrauterine deaths.[58,59] Sonographically, hemangiomas are typically seen as fusiform swellings in the cord with the presence of an angiomatous nodule and are usually located near the placental insertion of the cord. They range in size from 0.2 to 18 cm in diameter and are often surrounded by localized cystic degeneration and edema of the Wharton's jelly distinct from the tumor.[58] In a suspected case of umbilical cord hemangioma, serial ultrasound examinations have been recommended involving amniotic fluid volume assessment, tumor size measurement, and Doppler flow studies of each umbilical vessel separately, with special attention to the segment of cord within the tumor. Since a sudden vascular accident cannot be ruled out, delivery should be considered if fetal lung maturity has been established or assumed. Differential diagnosis includes hematomas and teratomas of the umbilical cord, and abdominal wall defects.[59]

Umbilical cord teratomas, which are usually benign lesions, are very rare and may contain tissues derived from all three germ cell layers. Sonographically, they have a disorganized polymorphic appearance.

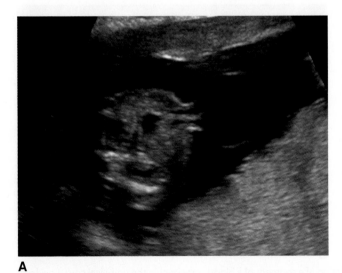

A

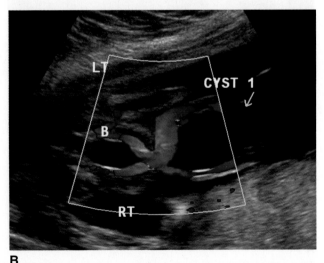

B

Figure 18-44 Allantoic cyst. **A:** 2D ultrasound image of a cyst within the umbilical cord at the site of insertion into the fetal abdomen. **B:** Color Doppler sonography demonstrates the umbilical vessels coursing around the cyst, consistent with an allantoic cyst. The cyst resolved prior to delivery and the fetus was normal.

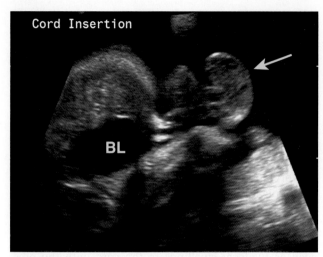

Figure 18-45 Edematous Wharton's jelly. Transverse sonogram of the fetal abdomen at the site of cord insertion into the fetal abdomen. A soft tissue mass of the cord was noted with areas of cystic degeneration consistent with edematous Wharton's jelly *(arrow)*. This fetus had trisomy 18 and the pregnancy outcome resulted in an intrauterine fetal demise at 37 weeks of gestation.

Generally, a complex umbilical cord mass containing cystic areas, solid components, and internal calcifications is suggestive of a teratoma. Because of its heterogeneous appearance, a hemangioma with associated cystic degeneration of Wharton's jelly can appear similar to a teratoma, and distinction between the two presents a challenge.[58]

Most umbilical cord hematomas are the result of either inadvertent laceration at the time of amniocentesis or intentional mechanical penetration of the umbilical vein during cordocentesis.[60] Spontaneous hematomas of the umbilical cord are rare but have a high mortality rate. On sonographic examination, hematomas can have a similar appearance to that of hemangiomas, although hematomas have no preferred location within the cord, nor are they associated with cystic structures. Umbilical cord hematomas have been described as a fusiform hyperechoic structure noted within the umbilical cord. Color flow imaging may be helpful in distinguishing the thrombus within a hematoma from solid vascular lesions such as teratomas and hemangiomas.[58]

Umbilical cord artery and vein thrombosis with occlusion is extremely rare and has been associated with a high perinatal mortality. Sonographically, this condition presents as echogenic material within the lumen of the blood vessel. In the case of a thrombosis of the umbilical artery, sonographic findings associated with this diagnosis may consist of a single-artery umbilical cord with an additional collapsed echogenic third vessel that had previously been described as a three-vessel cord on prior exam.[60] This condition has been associated with nonimmune hydrops and maternal diabetes. Thrombosis may also form secondary to mechanical cord impairment such as torsion, knotting, compression, hypercoiling, or hematoma (Fig. 18-46).

Normally, the physiologic herniation of the midgut into the proximal segment of the umbilical cord resolves by the 14th week. Occasionally, this finding may persist into the second trimester and is consistent with an umbilical hernia. Sonographically, this presents as a small, irregular echogenic soft tissue mass identified in the base of the umbilical cord (Fig. 18-47). This finding has been associated with chromosome abnormalities. An umbilical hernia should not be confused with a gastroschisis or omphalocele, which are congenital anterior abdominal wall defects (Fig. 18-48). The differential diagnosis for a small soft tissue mass located at the base of the umbilical cord would include hematoma, hemangioma, and small omphalocele.

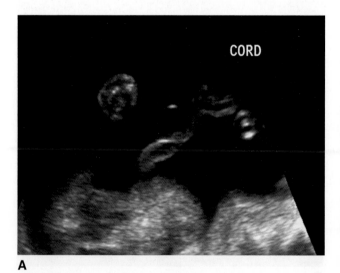

A

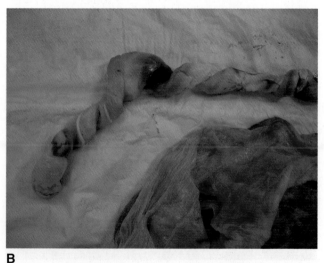

B

Figure 18-46 Cord thrombosis. **A:** Ultrasound image showing focal dilation of a segment of a blood vessel within the umbilical cord. Low-level echoes are noted within the area of thrombosis. There was also hypercoiling of this two-vessel umbilical cord. **B:** Gross pathology specimen of this umbilical cord confirms hypercoiling and umbilical artery thrombosis. (Image courtesy of Pathology Associates of Syracuse, Crouse Hospital.)

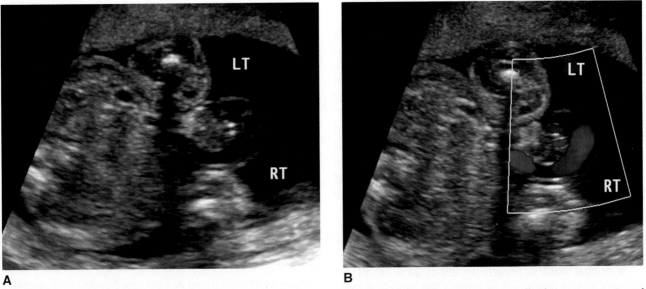

Figure 18-47 Umbilical hernia. **A:** Transverse ultrasound image at the level of the umbilicus demonstrating a small echogenic protrusion of fetal bowel into the base of the umbilical cord. **B:** Color Doppler sonography was used to show the relationship of the fetal umbilical vessels to the umbilical hernia.

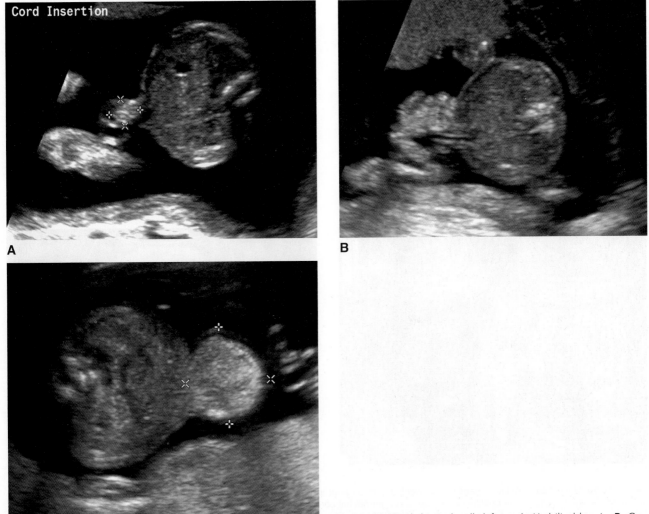

Figure 18-48 Abdominal wall defects. **A:** Umbilical hernia. **B:** Gastroschisis. **C:** Omphalocele.

ABNORMAL CORD POSITION

Fetal compromise of umbilical cord circulation is suspected in at least 20% of stillbirths at autopsy. Any type of force that compresses umbilical cords may lead to diminished blood flow in the umbilical vessels and subsequent fetal hypoxia or circulatory compromise. Mechanical cord compression or "cord" accident can be caused by nuchal/body cords, cord prolapse, or cord entanglements. This can also occur from an abnormal configuration of the cord, such as true knots, hypercoiling/twisting, abnormally long cords, abnormal cord insertions, or strictures.[61] Many intrapartum complications and adverse perinatal outcomes have been associated with such cord abnormalities and likely depend on the duration and degree of occlusion.

A nuchal cord is present in about 24% of all deliveries and is described as having the umbilical cord loop around the neck of the fetus one or more times (Fig. 18-49). In most cases, the cord is loosely looped and is considered clinically insignificant. Only rarely is a nuchal cord associated with significant perinatal complications. Nuchal cords come and go during pregnancy and the rate of nuchal cords increases with increasing gestational age. The presence of a nuchal cord may be demonstrated during routine sonography, and color Doppler is helpful in differentiating it from other neck masses and may also have a particular advantage in cases of low amniotic fluid (Fig. 18-50). A nuchal cord is usually suspected by ultrasound, with the presence of the cord in the transverse and sagittal planes of the neck and lying around at least three of the four sides of the neck.[44] Given the common occurrence of nuchal cord and its association with a favorable

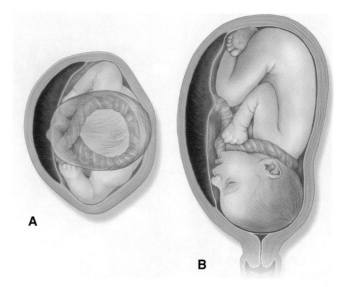

Figure 18-49 Nuchal cord. **A:** Transverse drawing of a fetus with the umbilical cord noted around the fetal neck. **B:** Longitudinal drawing of the fetus with the umbilical cord noted around the fetal neck.

outcome, scanning for and reporting this condition remains controversial.

Funic or cord presentation is a situation where the umbilical cord is the presenting part, usually noted when the fetus is in the transverse of breech positions. This finding is not of clinical significance throughout the progressing pregnancy but may lead to prolapse of the cord during active labor.[56]

Cord prolapse is defined as presentation of the umbilical cord in advance of the fetal presenting part during labor and delivery (Fig. 18-51).[55] This is usually detected by digital exam in cases of fetal distress after rupture of membranes. Sonographic detection of cord

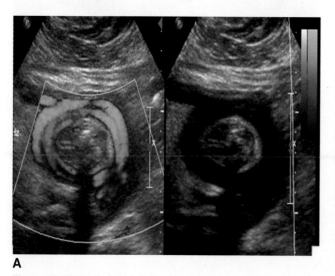

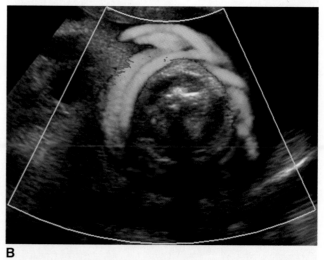

Figure 18-50 Nuchal cord. **A:** Dual image with power Doppler angiography application in a case of nuchal cord. In addition, oligohydramnios and multiple genitourinary abnormalities were noted. A tight nuchal cord times two was documented and noted at the time of delivery. The fetus did not survive secondary to congenital anomalies. **B:** Another case of nuchal cord with power Doppler application to demonstrate the umbilical vessels coursing circumferentially around the fetal neck. Pregnancy outcome was normal.

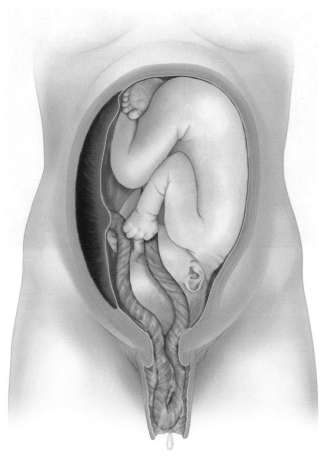

Figure 18-51 Cord prolapse. This diagram demonstrates the presence of segment of umbilical cord extending into the dilated cervical canal prior to the fetal presenting part during labor and delivery.

prolapse is clinically important because it may lead to cord compression and fetal vascular compromise, which can lead to an obstetric emergency with potentially fatal results. Color Doppler sonography is used to demonstrate the blood flow within the umbilical cord within the dilated endocervical canal and vagina.

Differences in the umbilical vein, umbilical arteries, and cord stromal length give rise to bending and twisting of the umbilical cord. Sometimes this bending, twisting, and bulging may appear as a false knot, which has no clinical significance. A focal bulge or vascular protuberance along the cord may be observed sonographically. A true knot of the umbilical cord occurs when the fetus actually passes through a loop or loops of cord. The incidence of true knots of the umbilical cord is approximately 1% to 2% of all deliveries, and fetuses with true knots are at a fourfold risk of stillbirth.[62] In most cases, the knot is either loose in utero or forms during birth, having only marginal impact on the perinatal outcome. However, during active labor, there is the possibility that the knot may tighten during fetal movements or descent, in which time it can potentially lead to decreased umbilical blood flow, fetal asphyxia, and perinatal death.[63] This anomaly has

been associated with advanced maternal age, multiparity, previous miscarriages, obesity, prolonged gravidity, meconium-stained fluid, male fetus, low Apgar scores, long cords, and maternal anemia.[62] The prenatal diagnosis of a true knot of the umbilical cord is challenging because of the difficulty in assessing the whole length of the cord in utero, the distinctive spatial configuration of the umbilical cord in the amniotic cavity, and the lack of characteristic antenatal 2D and color Doppler sonographic features. Sonographically, this condition is often missed or overdiagnosed. The suspicion of a true knot arises where a "cloverleaf" pattern of the cord is observed (Fig. 18-52). Prenatal visualization of a segment of cord closely surrounded by a loop, known as the "hanging noose" sign, has been recently reported as a highly specific sonographic feature in this condition. Both 3D power Doppler and 4D sonography are useful in the evaluation of this condition, where a volumetric view of the knot may sharpen the diagnosis.[62,63]

The umbilical cord exhibits a helical course, which is well established by 9 weeks of gestation. Observational data suggest that fetal movements play a role not only in the development of the cord length (with absent or decreased movements associated with short cords) but also in helical formation.[64] With the assumption that the average umbilical cord is 50 to 60 centimeters long, an average of 0.2 coils per centimeter would predict 10 to 12 vascular coils in a given cord. The generally accepted method of assessing the degree of the umbilical cord coiling is by calculation of the *umbilical cord index* (UCI), defined as the number of complete coils per centimeter length of cord. Using this criterion, the normal UCI is around 0.2 in the postpartum setting following examination of the delivered placenta and umbilical cord (pUCI), and 0.4 when determined antenatally by sonography. This apparent discrepancy, with increased cord coiling observed in utero, is suggested to be a reflection of the fact that the umbilical vessels are distended with blood that may result in a tighter apparent coiling of helical vessels.[64,65]

The cord coiling makes the umbilical cord a structure that is both flexible and strong, and provides resistance to external forces (i.e., tension, compression, entanglement) that could compromise blood flow (Fig. 18-53).[34] Fetuses whose umbilical coiling index values fall outside the normal limits have been shown to have higher rates of suboptimal outcomes (Fig. 18-54). It has been recommended that the cord coil index become part of the routine placental pathology examination, while antenatal evaluation of cord coiling requires further study. An abnormal UCI may be predictive of adverse fetal outcomes and, in the future, prenatal evaluation of the umbilical cord and the UCI may become an integral part of the fetal assessment in high-risk pregnancies.[34] This addition to clinical practice could reduce fetal death rates significantly if guidelines were established for elective delivery at appropriate gestational age in

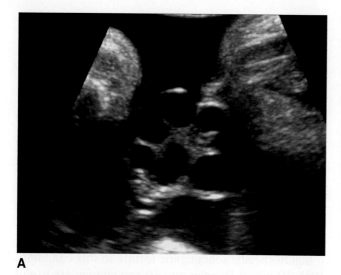

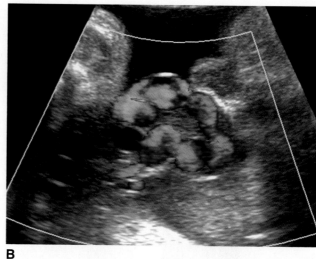

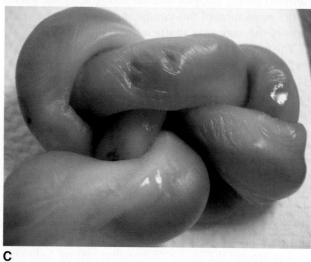

Figure 18-52 True knot. **A:** 2D ultrasound image of a suspected true knot of the umbilical cord. **B:** Power Doppler angiography is applied to the complex structure within the umbilical cord. **C:** Postnatal gross pathology specimen of the umbilical cord demonstrating a true knot. (Image courtesy of Pathology Associates of Syracuse, Crouse Hospital.)

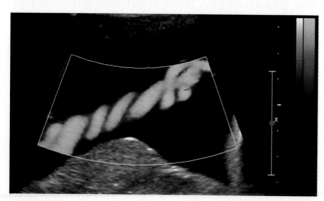

Figure 18-53 Power Doppler angiography image showing normal coiling pattern in this three-vessel umbilical cord.

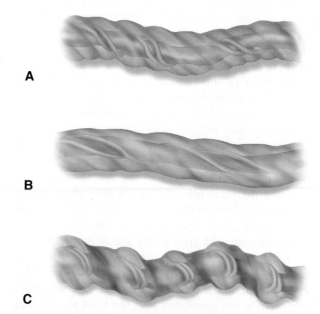

Figure 18-54 Umbilical cord coiling. **A:** Normal umbilical cord coiling pattern (UCI between 0.1 and 0.3 coils per cm). **B:** Hypocoiled umbilical cord (UCI less than 0.1 coil per cm). **C:** Hypercoiled cord (UCI greater than 0.3 coils per cm).

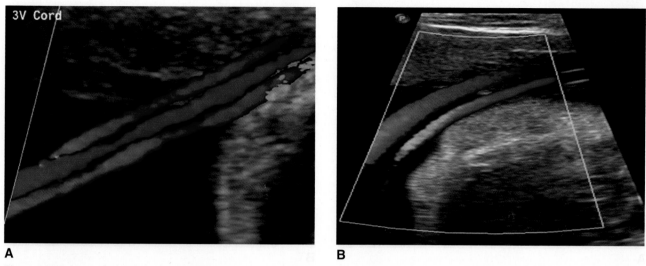

A

B

Figure 18-55 Noncoiled umbilical cords. **A:** Sagittal color Doppler image of a noncoiled three-vessel umbilical cord. **B:** Sagittal color Doppler image of noncoiled two-vessel umbilical cord.

the presence of cord coil abnormality and evidence of vascular compromise.[66]

Roughly 5% of all fetuses have complete absence of umbilical vascular coiling (Fig. 18-55). A variety of perinatal risks have been attributed to fetuses with noncoiled or straight umbilical vessels, including increased rate of fetal anomalies, aneuploidy, fetal heart rate (FHR) decelerations, meconium passage, preterm delivery, IUGR, oligohydramnios, and fetal demise.[4,64] It appears that hypocoiled or undercoiled cords (UCI ≤ 0.1 coils per centimeter) are predominantly associated with an increased frequency of intrauterine death, FHR decelerations, operative delivery for fetal distress, preterm delivery, low Apgar score, the presence of fetal congenital anomalies, aneuploidy, oligohydramnios, meconium staining, and other abnormalities of placental development such as velamentous insertion and the presence of an SUA.[64,65] Hypercoiled or overcoiled cords (UCI ≥ 0.3 coils per centimeter) are associated with aneuploidy, fetal demise, fetal intolerance to labor, operative delivery for fetal distress, IUGR, meconium staining, and chorioamnionitis. Overcoiled cords are also strongly associated with vascular thrombosis of the chorionic plate, umbilical venous thrombosis, and in many cases of cord stenosis and stricture. (Fig. 18-56).[64,66]

Entanglement of the umbilical cords is a potential complication in monoamniotic twins. Occurring in up to 70% of cases of monoamniotic twins, this phenomenon appears sonographically as a "mass" of the umbilical cord, toward which each separate cord can be traced (Fig. 18-57). Using color Doppler, it is important to trace both cords into the entangled mass as a prerequisite for real-time diagnosis of cord entanglement. With compression of the blood vessels, flow may be impaired or greatly reduced, resulting in placental congestion and an additional increase in intraplacental resistance. It has been suggested that in cases of cord

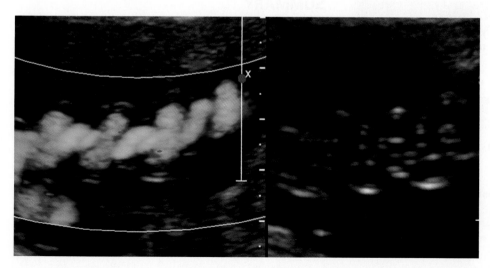

Figure 18-56 Dual-screen ultrasound image showing power Doppler and 2D imaging of a hypercoiled umbilical cord.

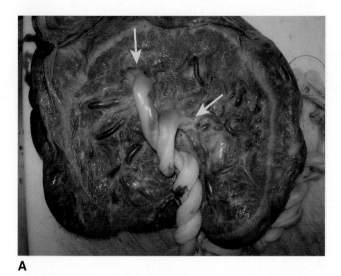

A

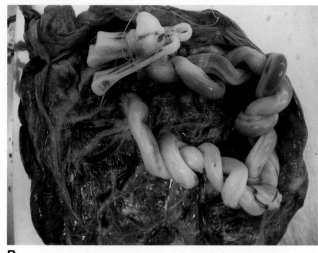

B

Figure 18-57 Cord entanglement. **A:** Gross pathology photograph of a monoanmiotic twin placenta showing entanglement of the umbilical cords. Note the origin of each umbilical cord at the placental surface *(arrows)*. **B:** Significant entanglement of the twin umbilical cords is appreciated in this monoamniotic placenta. (Images courtesy of Pathology Associates of Syracuse, Crouse Hospital.)

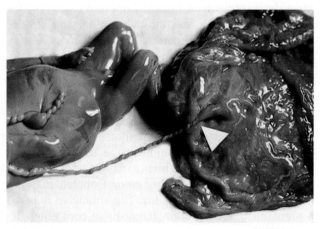

Figure 18-58 Cord stricture. Postnatal photograph of a fetus with umbilical cord stricture. Note the long, narrow umbilical cord.

PATHOLOGY BOX 18-5

Conditions Associated with Mechanical Vascular Obstruction or Compression of the Umbilical Cord Vessels

Long umbilical cord
Narrow umbilical cord with diminished Wharton's jelly
Stricture
Nuchal/body cords
True knots of the umbilical cord
Umbilical cord prolapse
Hypercoiled umbilical cord
Abnormal umbilical cord insertion into the placenta
• Velamentous cord insertion
• Vasa previa
• Succenturiate lobe

---

entanglement, a notch in the umbilical artery flow velocity waveform may identify pregnancies at immediate risk for cord accidents and may be a useful clinical application in the antepartum management of this unique situation. 3D ultrasound can be used to acquire volume data comprising information on umbilical color Doppler flow, providing a very graphic depiction of the cord entanglement.[60,67]

Stricture of the umbilical cord occurs when there is localized narrowing of the cord with disappearance of Wharton's jelly (Fig. 18-58). There will be associated torsion of the cord or thickening of the vessel walls with narrowing of the lumen. This often occurs with long umbilical cords and hypercoiled cords, and in highly active fetuses. Sonographically, it may present as narrowing of the cord close to the fetus with edematous area distal to the site.

SUMMARY

- The placenta increases in both volume and thickness as the gestation progresses.

- The normal placental thickness is between 2 and 4 cm.

- A bilobed placenta has connected areas of placental tissue.

- A succenturiate lobe has a location distant from the main placenta.

- Placental extension beyond the chorionic plate includes placenta circummarginate and circumvallate.

- Implantation of the placenta within 2 centimeters of the internal cervical os is considered a low-lying placenta.

- Placenta accreta results with invasion of the chorionic villi into the myometrium.

- A history of uterine surgery increases the risk of placenta accreta development.
- Anechoic structures inferior to the chorionic plate with real-time imaging of swirling jets are normal placental lakes.
- Hypoechoic fibrin deposits are a normal finding in the placenta.
- Small hypoechoic hemorrhagic areas within the placenta occur in half the pregnancies at midterm.
- Massive subchorionic hematoma and thrombosis of the placenta is a rare occurrence called a *Breus' mole.*
- IUGR has an association with placental infarction.
- Large chorioangiomas, vascular malformations of the placenta, have an association with multiple fetal complications.
- Placental and cord teratomas have a similar cellular makeup seen with this tumor in other areas of the body.

- Placental abruption has a limited diagnosis with ultrasound.
- Amniotic band syndrome is the rupture of fetal membranes with entrapment of fetal parts.
- Uterine synechiae are extra tissue outside the amniotic sac without fetal entrapment.
- Placenta mesenchymal dysplasia mimics a molar pregnancy.
- The average umbilical cord length is 55 cm (21.7 in).
- The normal umbilical cord insertion is at the placental disk and at the fetal midabdomen.
- Wharton's jelly covers the outside of the umbilical cord.
- An umbilical cord with an SUA is associated with an increased incidence of chromosomal anomalies.
- The presence of more than three umbilical cord vessels has a relationship to conjoined twins and singleton pregnancies with multiple anomalies.

Critical Thinking Questions

1. **A thick placenta images during a routine obstetric examination. Explain the significance of this finding. Describe the placental, maternal, and fetal conditions that coexist with a thick placenta.**

   ANSWER: A thick placenta measures greater than 4 cm at the midportion and may be a nonspecific finding. Usually, a thick placenta is of no concern; however, placental or fetal hydrops, fetal growth restriction, maternal infection, diabetes or anemia, transfusion syndromes, placental or fetal masses, and placental vascular obstruction may result in this finding.

2. **A 36-year-old G4P2A1 patient presents to the department with complaints of bright spotting. This non-smoking patient had a lower segment emergency**

cesarean section with her second pregnancy and dilation and curettage with her miscarriage. What is the most likely differential for the finding on this longitudinal low image? What further steps would confirm the diagnosis?

ANSWER: This image demonstrates a placenta previa on the anterior lower segment of the uterus. This patient has had a lower segment cesarean section resulting in a scar at the same level as the placenta. Combined with her history of a dilation and curettage, anteriorly located placenta, and advanced maternal age, the most likely diagnosis would be placenta accreta. The next step would be to provide color or power Doppler images of the placenta to evaluate for turbulent flow at the myometrial/placental boundary.

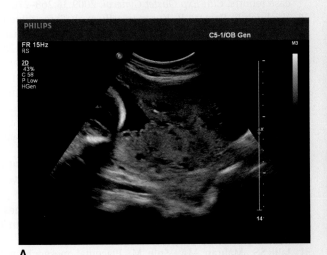

A

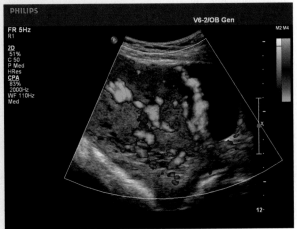

B

- Umbilical vein curvature to the left side indicates a possible persistent right umbilical vein.
- The umbilical cord varix is a focal dilatation within the umbilical vein that is greater than 9 mm.
- The complete absence of the umbilical cord results in limb–body wall complex.
- Abnormal cord insertions into the placenta include marginal insertion, velamentous insertion, vasa previa, and furcated insertion.
- Abnormal cord insertions into the fetal abdomen are either due to an omphalocele or gastroschesis.
- Cysts of the umbilical cord can be either true cysts or pseudocysts.
- Color Doppler helps identify a nuchal cord.
- Cord prolapse occurs at birth if the cord presents before the fetus.
- UCI calculations help identify fetuses at risk for an adverse outcome.
- Monochorionic/monoamniotic twins have an increased incidence of umbilical cord entanglement.
- Torsion or vessel wall thickening of the umbilical cord is the result of cord strictures.

REFERENCES

1. Elsayes KM, Trout AT, Friedkin AM, et al. Imaging of the placenta: a multimodality pictorial review. *Radiographics*. 2009;29:1371–1391.
2. Abramowicz JS, Sheiner E. In utero imaging of the placenta: importance for diseases of pregnancy. *Placenta Suppl*. 2007;21:S14–S22.
3. Sabire NJ, Sepulveda W. Correlation of placental pathology with prenatal ultrasound findings. *J Clin Pathol*. 2008;61:1276–1284.
4. Marino T. Ultrasound abnormalities of the amniotic fluid, membranes, umbilical cord, and placenta. *Obstet Gynecol Clin N Am*. 2004;31:177–200.
5. Suzuki S, Igarashi M. Clinical significance of pregnancies with succenturiate lobes of the placenta. *Arch Gynecol Obstet*. 2008;277:299–301.
6. Ahmed A, Gilbert-Barness E. Placenta membranacea: a developmental anomaly with diverse clinical presentation. *Pediatr Dev Pathol*. 2003;201–203.
7. Greenberg JA, Sorem KA, Shifren JL, et al. Placenta membranacea with placenta accreta: a case report and literature review. *Obstet Gynecol*. 1991;78:512–514.
8. Feldstein VA, Harris RD, Machin, GA. Ultrasound evaluation of the placenta and umbilical cord. In: Callen PW, ed. *Ultrasonography in Obstetrics and Gynecology*. 5th ed. Philadelphia, PA: Saunders Elsevier; 2008;721–757.
9. Sepulveda W, Sohaey R, Nyberg DA. The placenta, umbilical cord, and membranes. In: Nyberg DA, McGahan JP, Pretorius DH, et al., eds. *Diagnostic Imaging of Fetal Anomalies*. Philadelphia, PA: Lippincott Williams & Wilkins. 2003;85–132.
10. Harris RD, Wells, WA, Black WC, et al. Accuracy of prenatal sonography for detecting circumvallate placenta. *AJR*. 1996:1603–1608.
11. Suzuki S. Clinical significance of pregnancies with circumvallate placenta. *J Obstet Gynecol Res*. 2008;34:51–54.
12. Shen O, Golomb E, Lavie O, et al. Placental shelf—a common, typically transient and benign finding on early second-trimester sonography. *Ultrasound Obstet Gynecol*. 2007;29:192–194.
13. Gugmundsson S, Dubiel M, Sladkevicius P. Placental morphologic and functional imaging in high-risk pregnancies. *Semin Perinatol*. 2009;33:270–280.
14. Oyelese Y, Smulian JC. Placenta previa, placenta accreta, and vasa previa. *Obstet Gynecol*. 2006;107:927–941.
15. Warshak CR, Ramos GA, Eskander R, et al. Effect of predelivery diagnosis in 99 consecutive cases of placenta accreta. *Obstet Gynecol*. 2010;115:65–69.
16. Bauer ST, Bonanno C. Abnormal placentation. *Semin Perinatol*. 2009;33:88–96.
17. Baughman WC, Corteville JE, Shah RR. Placenta accreta: spectrum of US and MR imaging findings. *Radiographics*. 2008;28:1905–1916.
18. Ophir E, Singer-Jordan J, Odeh M, et al. Abnormal placental invasion-a novel approach to treatment. *Obstet Gynecol Surv*. 2009;64:811–822.
19. Woodring TC, Klauser CK, Bofill JA, et al. *J Matern Fetal Neonatal Med*. 2010 (in press).
20. Teo TH, Law YM, Tay KH, et al. Use of magnetic resonance imaging in evaluation of placental invasion. *Clin Radiol*. 2009;64:511–516.
21. Thompson MO, Vines SK, Aquilina J, et al. Are placental lakes of any clinical significance? *Placenta*. 2002;23(8–9):685–690.
22. Taori K, Patil P, Attarde V, et al. Chorioamngioma of placenta: sonographic features. *J Clin Ultrasound*. 2008;36:113–115.
23. Kirkpatrick AD, Podberesky DJ, Gray AE, et al. Placental chorioangioma. *Radiographics*. 2007;27:1187–1190.
24. Escribano D, Galindo A, Arbués J, et al. Prenatal management of placental chorioangioma: value of the middle cerebral artery peak systolic velocity. *Fetal Diagn Ther*. 2005;21:489–493.
25. Kondi-Pafiti A, Bakalianou K, Salakos N, et al. Placental chorioangioma and chorioangiosis. Clinicopathological study of six unusual vascular lesions of the placenta—case reports. *Clin Exp Obstet Gynecol*. 2009;36:268–270.
26. Vaisbuch E, Romero R, Kusanovic JP, et al. Three-dimensional sonography of placental mesenchymal dysplasia and its differential diagnosis. *J Ultrasound Med*. 2009;28:359–368.
27. Salzani A, Yela DA, Gabiatti JR, et al. Prevalence of uterine synechia after abortion evacuation curettage. *Sao Paulo Med J*. 2007;125:261–264.
28. Bäumler M, Faure J-M, Couture A, et al. Prenatal 3D ultrasound and MRI assessment of horizontal uterine synechia. *Prenat Diagn*. 2008;28:874–875.
29. Parveen Z, Tongson-Ignacio J, Fraser CR, et al. Placental mesenchymal dysplasia. *Arch Pathol Lab Med*. 2007;131:131–137.
30. Ang DC, Rodríguez Urrego PA, Prasad V. Placental mesenchymal dysplasia: a potential misdiagnosed entity. *Arch Gnyecol Obstet*. 2009;279:937–939.
31. Jalil SS, Mahran MA, Sule M. Placental mesenchymal dysplasia—can it be predicted prenatally? A case report. *Prenat Diagn*. 2009;29:713–714.

32. Sepulveda W, Wong AE, Gomex L, et al. Improving sonographic evaluation of the umbilical cord at the second-trimester anatomy scan. *J Ultrasound Med.* 2009;28:831–835.

33. Dane B, Dane C, Kiray M, et al. Fetuses with single umbilical artery: analysis of 45 cases. *Clin Exp Obstet Gynecol.* 2009;36:116–119.

34. de Laat MW, Franx A, van Alderen ED, et al. The umbilical coiling index, a review of the literature. *J Matern Fetal Neonatal Med.* 2005;17:93–100.

35. Mu SC, Lin CH, Chen YL, et al. The perinatal outcomes of asymptomatic isolated single umbilical artery in full-term neonates. *Pediatr Neonatol.* 2008;49:230–233.

36. Deshpande SA, Jog S, Watson H., et al. Do babies with isolated single umbilical artery need routine postnatal renal sonography. *Arch Dis Child Fetal Neonatal Ed.* 2009;94:F265–F267.

37. Sherer DM, Dalloul M, Ajayi O, et al. Prenatal sonographic diagnosis of short umbilical cord in a dichorionic twin with normal fetal anatomy. *J Clin Ultrasound.* 2010;38:91–93.

38. Graham DG, Fleischer AC, Sacks GA. Sonography of the umbilical cord and intrauterine membranes. In: Fleischer AC, Romero R, Manning FA, et al., eds. *The Principles and Practice of Ultrasonography in Obstetrics and Gynecology.* 4th ed. Norwalk, CT: Appleton & Lange, 1991;159–170.

39. Sepulveda W. Velamentous insertion of the umbilical cord—a first trimester sonographic screening study. *J Ultrasound Med.* 2006;25:963–968.

40. Hasegawa J, Matsuoka R, Ichizuka K, et al. Cord insertion into the lower third of the uterus in the first trimester is associated with placental and umbilical cord abnormalities. *Ultrasound Obstet Gynecol.* 2006;28:183–186.

41. Hasegawa J, Matsuoka R, Ichizuka K, et al. Umbilical cord insertion into the lower uterine segment is a risk factor for vasa previa. *Fetal Diagn Ther.* 2007;22:358–360.

42. Hasegawa J, Matsuoka R, Ichizuka K, et al. Velamentous cord insertion: significance of prenatal detection to predict Perinatal complications. *Taiwan J Obstet Gynecol.* 2006;45:21–25.

43. Hasegawa J, Matsuoka R, Ichizuka K, et al. Atypical variable deceleration in the first stage of labor is a characteristic fetal heart-rate pattern for velamentous cord insertion and hypocoiled cords. *J Obstet Gynecol Res.* 2009;35:35–39.

44. Hasegawa J, Matsuoka R, Ichizuka K, et al. Ultrasound diagnosis and management of umbilical cord abnormalities. *Taiwan J Obstet Gynecol.* 2009;48:23–27.

45. Canterino JC, Mondestin-Sorrentino M, Muench MV, et al. Vasa previa: prenatal diagnosis and evaluation with 3-dimensional sonography and power angiography. *J Ultrasound Med.* 2005;24:721–724.

46. Catanzarite V, Maida C, Thomas W, et al. Prenatal sonographic diagnosis of vasa previa: ultrasound findings and obstetric outcomes in ten cases. *Ultrasound Obstet Gynecol.* 2001;18:109–115.

47. Smorgick N, Tovbin Y, Ushakov F, et al. Is neonatal risk from vasa previa preventable? The 20-year experience form a single medical center. *J Clin Ultrasound.* 2010;38:118–122.

48. Stafford IP, Neumann DE, Jarrell H. Abnormal placental structure and vasa previa: confirmation of the relationship. *J Ultrasound Med.* 2004;23:1521–1522.

49. Gandhi M, Cleary-Goldman J, Ferrara L, et al. The association between vasa previa, multiple gestations, and assisted reproductive technology. *Am J Perinatol.* 2008;25:587–590.

50. Lijoi AF, Brady J. Vasa previa diagnosis and management. *J Am Board Fam Pract.* 2003;16:543–548.

51. Gagnon R, Morin L, Bly S, et al. Guidelines for the management of vasa previa. *J Obstet Gynaecol Can.* 2009;31:748–760.

52. Araujo E Jr, Filho HA, Pires CR, et al. Prenatal diagnosis of vasa previa through color Doppler and three-dimensional power Doppler ultrasonography. A case report. *Clin Exp Obstet Gynecol.* 2006;33:122–124.

53. Lee W, Kirk JS, Comstock CH, et al. Vasa previa: prenatal detection by three-dimensional ultrasonography. *Ultrasound Obstet Gynecol.* 2000;16:384–387.

54. Oyelese Y, Catanzarite V, Prefumo F, et al. Vasa previa: the impact of prenatal diagnosis on outcomes. *Obstet Gynecol.* 2004;103:937–942.

55. Reddy UM, Goldenberg R, Silver R, et al. Stillbirth classification—developing an international consensus for research. *Obstet Gynecol.* 209;114:901–914.

56. Sherer DM, Anyaegbunam A. Prenatal ultrasonographic morphologic assessment of the umbilical cord: a review. Part I. *Obstet Gynecol Surv.* 1997;52:506–514.

57. Weichert J, Chiriac A, Kaiser M, et al. Prenatal management of an allantoic cyst with patent urachus. *Arch Gynecol Obstet.* 2009;280:321–323.

58. Iyoob SD, Tsai A, Ruchelli ED, et al. Large umbilical cord hemangioma: sonographic features with surgical pathologic correlation. *J Ultrasound Med.* 2006;25:1495–1498.

59. Papadopoulos VG, Kourea HP, Adonakis GL, et al. A case of umbilical cord hemangioma: Doppler studies and review of the literature. *Eur J Obstet Gynecol Reprod Biol.* 2009;144:8–14.

60. Sherer DM, Anyaegbunam, A. Prenatal ultrasonographic morphologic assessment of the umbilical cord: a review: part II. *Obstet Gynecol Surv.* 1997;52:515–523.

61. Tantbirojn P, Saleemuddin A, Sirois K, et al. Gross abnormalities of the umbilical cord: related histology and clinical significance. *Placenta.* 2009;30:1083–1088.

62. Ramón y Cajal CL, Martinez RO. Four-dimensional ultrasonography of a true knot of the umbilical cord. *Am J Obstet Gynecol.* 2006;195:896–898.

63. Hasbun J, Alcalde JL, Sepulveda W. Three-dimensional power Doppler sonography in the prenatal diagnosis of a true knot of the umbilical cord. *J Ultrasound Med.* 2007;26:1215–1220.

64. Strong TH, Jarles DL, Vega JS, et al. The umbilical coiling index. *Am J Obstet Gynecol.* 1994;170:29–32.

65. Sebire NJ. Pathophysiological significance of abnormal umbilical cord coiling index. *Ultrasound Obstet Gynecol.* 2007;30:804–806.

66. Machin GA, Ackerman J, Gilbert-Barness E. Abnormal cord coiling is associated with adverse perinatal outcomes. *Pediatr Dev Pathol.* 2000;3:462–471.

67. Henrich W, Tutschek B. Cord entanglement in monoamniotic twins: 2D and 3D colour Doppler studies. *Ultraschall in Med.* 2008;29:271–272.

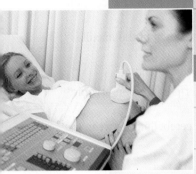

19 Sonographic Assessment of the Fetal Neural Tube Structures

Susan Raatz Stephenson and Roa M. Qato

KEY TERMS

microcephaly | microcephaly | hypotelorism | hypertelorism | microphthalmia | macroglossia | micrognathia | cleft lip | cleft palate | meroanencephaly | hydranencephaly | holoprosencephaly | agenesis of the corpus callosum | Dandy-Walker malformation | schizencephaly | lissencephaly | cephalocele | iniencephaly | Arnold-Chiari malformation | ventriculomegaly | hydrocephalus | cystic hygroma | choroid plexus cysts | porencephaly | intracranial hemorrhage | aneurysm of the vein of Galen, spina bifida | scoliosis | kyphosis | caudal regression syndrome | sacrococcygeal teratoma

GLOSSARY

Anophthalmia Congenital absence of one or both eyes

Brachycephaly Short broad head due to premature suture fusion

Cebocephaly Congenital anomalies of the head due to teratogens or development disruptions of the nervous system

Clinodactyly Abnormal position of the fingers or toes

Colpocephaly Congenital brain anomaly resulting from a migrational defect of the occipital horns of the lateral ventricles leading to ventricular enlargement

Conus medullaris Terminal portion of the spine caudal to lumbar vertebrae 1 and 2

Cryptorchidism Failure of one or both testis to descend from the abdomen into the scrotal sac

Dysgenesis Abnormally formed organs

Dysmorphic Malformation of an organ or structure

Dolichocephaly Long narrow head

Ectasia Dilatation or distention of a hollow structure

Gastroschisis Herniation of abdominal contents without a covering into the amniotic fluid

Lipoma Tumor composed of fat

Lymphangiectasia Combination of nonimmune fetal hydrops and a cystic hygroma

Nares Nostrils

Neuropore Either the rostral or caudal end of the neural tube

Nomogram Graph

Meningocele Spinal defect where the meninges protrude

Myelomeningoceles (aka myelomeningocele) Protrusion of a sac from a spinal defect which contains spinal cord and meninges

Myeloschisis Incomplete fusion of the neural tube resulting in a cleft spinal cord

Omphalocele Herniation of the abdominal contents with a membranous cover

Pathognomonic Disease characteristic

Pluripotent Ability of embryonic cells to differentiate into any type of cell

Rachischisis Complete exposure of the spinal cord due to lack of spinal fusion

Retrognathia Posterior displacement of the maxilla and mandible

Rostral Toward the cephalic or head end

Teratogen Substance that interferes with embryonic development

Vermis Central portion of the cerebellum between the hemispheres

Some of the most common congenital abnormalities involve the central nervous system. These occur in approximately one to two cases per 1,000 births.[1] Some studies have revealed an incidence as high as one in 100 births.[2] Because of the frequency of neural tube defects, a comprehensive and systematic approach to sonographic examination of the complex region of the head, neck, and spine becomes important. Early detection of fatal and nonfatal fetal anomalies allows patients to make early decisions regarding the pregnancy.

Each section in this chapter begins with an explanation of the normal embryogenesis of the brain, face, or neural tube. A basic protocol for examining the neural axis, pausing at various points to provide a detailed description of observed anatomy, provides the examination foundation for neural tube structures. In the second part of this review, a discussion of various abnormalities of the fetal head, neck, and spine allow for recognition of congenital anomalies.

EMBRYOLOGY OF THE BRAIN

Neural plate development completes at approximately days 18 to 23.[1,2] During the endovaginal exam, a hypoechoic region within the echogenic decidua identifies the coelomic cavity of the gestational sac. At approximately 6 menstrual weeks the neural tube differentiates into the primitive brain and spinal cord. Three segments make up the brain: the prosencephalon (forebrain), the mesencephalon (midbrain), and the rhombencephalon (hindbrain) (Fig. 19-1). Identification of these primary vesicles occurs at approximately 7 to 8 weeks, with the rhombencephalon imaging as an anechoic structure in the fetal head (Fig. 13-17).[5]

The forebrain becomes the telencephalon and diencephalon, resulting in the development of the thalami, third ventricle, cerebral hemispheres, and the lateral ventricles. Invagination of the choroid plexus into the ventricles results in almost complete filling of the anechoic ventricles with the hyperechoic plexus (Fig. 13-18).[1,3] As the brain develops, the choroid plexus takes its position in the posterior area of the lateral ventricles.

The metencephalon and myelencephalon arise from the anechoic rhombencephalon. The upper portion of the fourth ventricle, pons, and cerebellum originate from the metencephalon, whereas the medulla and rest of the fourth ventricle originate from the myelencephalon.

Anatomy such as the corpus callosum, cerebellar vermis, sulci, gyri, migration of the germila matrix, and myelination, develop after 15 weeks' gestation.[5] Even later, at about 18 to 20 weeks, development of the corpus callosum completes.[5] This includes the boxlike cavum septum pellucidum (CSP). Brain sulci and gyri image by 28 weeks; however, some of the larger sulci may image earlier.[5]

Many structures develop between week 3 and 16, resulting in this time frame being identified as the critical period of brain development.[2] The rapid growth of the brain throughout gestation and the first 2 years of life allows for teratogens or nutritional deficits to influence the brain.[2] The causes of congenital anomalies are not well understood, though an association with several environmental factors has been found. These include lack of folic acid (shown to correlate with an increase in central nervous system anomalies)[4] and exposure to *Toxoplasma gondii* and high levels of radiation (Table 19-1).[2]

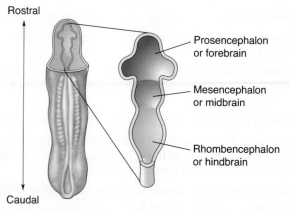

Figure 19-1 The three primary brain vesicles. The rostral end of the neural tube differentiates to form the three vesicles that give rise to the entire brain. This view is from above, and the vesicles have been cut horizontally so that we can see the inside of the neural tube.

TABLE 19-1					
Embryonic Development Chart for the Brain, Spine, and Face.[1–3,76,77]					
Days Post-ovulation/ Carnegie Stage	**Undifferentiated Neural Development**	**Brain**	**Spine**	**Face**	**Embryo Size**
First Trimester					
16 days/7	Neural crest cells organize in the neural tube				0.04 cm
18 days/8	Ectoderm has become the neural plate, which develops the neural groove				0.1–0.15 cm
22 days/10		Brain folding beginning in stage 9 continues	Neural folds begin to fuse forming the neural tube	Cells which become eyes and ears appear lateral to the neural folds	0.15–0.3 cm
24 days/11		Forebrain completely closed	Vasculature to the spine develops	Stomodeum develops	0.25–0.3 cm
26 days/12 Brain and spine combined form the largest portion of the embryo		Forebrain continues growing	Neural tube completely closed	Facial arches appear; eye and ear begin forming	0.3–0.5 cm
32 days/14 Gestational sac seen with ultrasound		Ridges develop separating the midbrain, forebrain, and hindbrain		Mandibular arches and nasal plate develop	0.5–0.7 mm
36 days/15		Brain increased in size by 1/3 from stage 14, fourth ventricle forms	Rostral (cephalic) neuropore closes	Mandibular prominence fuses, external ears and nasal pits begin to appear	0.7–0.9 mm
38 days/16		Cerebral hemispheres and hindbrain begin to develop	Caudal neuropore closes	Mandible demarcates, nasal pits rotate ventrally, median palatine process appears	0.9–1.1 cm
43 days/17 Embryo with heart beat images with ultrasound				Teeth buds form, palatine processes in a horizontal position	1.0–1.3 cm
52 days/21				Eyes developed but still on lateral head, ears low set, tongue development completes	1.7–2.2 cm
57 days/23 Imaging of neural tube possible with ultrasound				Palate and nasal septum begin fusion, ear formed	2.3–2.6 cm

(continued)

Days Post-ovulation/ Carnegie Stage	Undifferentiated Neural Development	Brain	Spine	Face	Embryo Size
Second trimester					
10 weeks		Formation complete, brain size increases to 6.1 cm		Eyelids fused, intermaxillary segment continues fusion	3.1–4.2 cm
12th week		Head about half CRL		Palate fusion completes	6.1 cm
14th week			Development and ossification of dorsal spinal components	Philtrum of lip forms	
16 weeks				Eyes and ears move to final location	
28 weeks		Gyrus and sulci begin forming			

ANATOMIC LANDMARKS AND BIOMETRY

AXIAL VIEWS OF THE HEAD

Biparietal Diameter Level

The fetal biparietal diameter (BPD) was the first sonographic measurement used to determine gestational age.[6] Initially defined as the widest distance between the parietal eminences, the BPD measurement levels are consistent between medical facilities. Basically, any plane of section through a 360-degree arc that passes through the thalami and third ventricle is acceptable for measuring the BPD (Fig. 19-2B).[1] Thus, the anatomic landmarks that delineate the longest BPD show the thalamic bodies (which appear somewhat oval) or the cavum septum pellucidum (which is outlined by two short anterior lines parallel to the midline) or both.[6] Other structures commonly observed in the same plane and near the midline are, from posterior to anterior; the great cerebral vein, or vein of Galen, and its ambient cistern sitting above the cerebellum,[3] the midbrain, the third ventricle between the thalami, and the frontal horns of the lateral ventricles. Laterally placed in the same plane are the spiral hippocampal gyri[4] posteriorly and the bright paired echoes of the insulae with pulsating middle cerebral arteries.

To obtain a properly measured BPD, orient the transducer in two planes: perpendicular to the parietal bones and positioned at the correct cephalocaudal position to intersect the third ventricle and thalami. Callen[1] describes three sonographic rules for obtaining the BPD. The first two criteria define the precise plane of section, while the third describes the proper end points of measurement. First, the correct plane of section is through the third ventricle and thalami. Second, the calvaria are smooth and symmetric bilaterally. Third, position the cursors in one of the three following ways: outer edge of near calvarial wall to inner edge of far calvarial wall, inner edge of near calvarial wall to outer edge of far calvarial wall, or the middle of the near calvarial wall to the middle of the far calvarial wall.[1,5]

The BPD maintains its closest correlation with gestational age in the first and early second trimester. However, this accuracy is lost in the third trimester because of variations in the shape of the fetal skull. As the pregnancy progresses and the head conforms to the pelvis, the result is either a doliochocephalic or brachycephalic head shape.[1] The head circumference (HC) or head perimeter is shape independent and can be used as an alternative measurement (Fig. 19-2A,C).

Microcephaly/Microencephaly

The literal meaning of microcephaly is "small head." Its diagnosis, therefore, is based on biometry rather than on morphology. Consequently, diagnosis requires accurate dating. Although different biometric standards have been described to define microcephaly, a reliable indicator is a head perimeter two to three standard deviations or more *below* the mean for gestational age.[1,5]

Identifying fetal microcephaly can be challenging. Since head measurements alone may be hampered by incorrect dating or intrauterine growth restriction, alternative measurements have been described to aid in the diagnosis. A nomogram of head circumference as a function of gestational age has been shown to be of great predictive value in the diagnosis of microcephaly.[1]

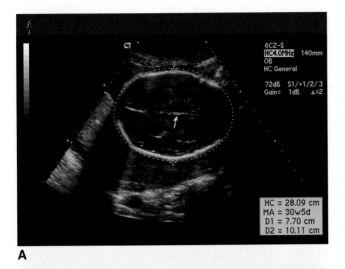

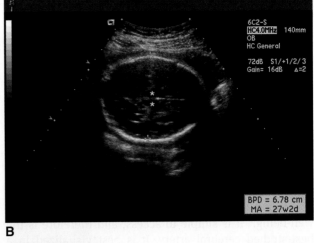

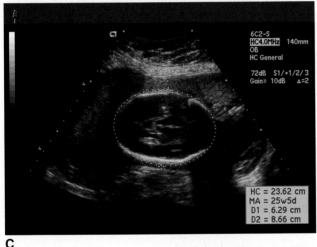

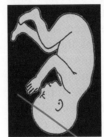

Figure 19-2 A: The brachycephalic fetal head has a shortened occipital-frontal distance and a larger BPD. The slitlike third ventricle *(arrow)* images between the anterior portion of the two thalami. **B:** The normal-shaped head demonstrating the hypoechoic thalamus *(stars)*. This is the main indicator for the BPD and HC measurement level. **C:** The long narrow head, dolichocephaly, would result in a smaller than gestational age BPD measurement and a lengthened occipital-frontal distance.

Further aids to diagnosis include nomograms of ratios of head circumference to abdominal circumference and of femur length to head circumference. Multiple fetal measurements should be used for greater accuracy.[5] Nonetheless, both high false positive and false negative diagnoses occur frequently. Since the predictive value of ultrasound biometry has significant limitations, a qualitative evaluation of the intracranial structures is a necessary supplement to making the diagnosis.[3]

Microcephaly is featured sonographically by a typical disproportion in size between the skull and the face. The forehead slopes and the brain is small, with the cerebral hemispheres affected to a greater extent than the diencephalic and rhomboencephalic structures. Abnormal convolutional patterns, including macrogyria, microgyria, and agyria are frequently found, and the ventricles may be enlarged. Microcephaly is frequently found in cases of porencephaly, lissencephaly, and holoprosencephaly.[1]

Microcephaly is not considered a single clinical entity, but rather it is a symptom of many etiologic disturbances. It may be associated with environmental factors such as prenatal infections (e.g., rubella, cytomegalovirus) or prenatal exposure to drugs or chemicals (e.g., alcohol, hydantoin). It also may be associated with genetic factors such as chromosomal abnormalities (e.g., aneuploidy) or single-gene defects (e.g., Bloom syndrome).

The prognosis for microcephaly varies, but most affected infants have a significantly increased risk of neurologic compromise, and there is a correlation with the size of the head. In general, the smaller the head, the worse the prognosis. As with other malformations, the association with other anomalies increases the likelihood of a poor outcome. Risk of recurrence depends on underlying causes.

Macrocephaly

Macrocephaly or "large head" is defined as a head circumference two to three standard deviations *above* the mean for gestational age and sex.[3] Most often, an enlarged ventricular system (hydrocephalus) or other intracranial anomalies result in macrocephaly. In such cases, the person is usually severely retarded.[1]

Internal Carotid Artery Level

Another important area for evaluation located at a plane parallel but inferior to the BPD is the level of the internal carotid artery. From the BPD, the transducer is moved in a parallel plane toward the base of the skull until the cerebral peduncles, the most rostral portions of the midbrain, appear. An oblique cross-section of the internal carotid artery is obtained at the division of the middle and anterior cerebral arteries, which lie anterior to the cerebral peduncles.

The middle cerebral artery (MCA), a major branch of the circle of Willis in the fetal brain, is a critical structure to visualize, as it carries more than 80% of cerebral blood flow and thus can be used to assess fetal well-being.[8] It is simple to access, and therefore is the best-studied cerebral artery. It is best visualized in a transverse plane at the base of the skull (Fig. 27-7).

Doppler evaluation of the MCA has been shown to be a useful adjunct in the evaluation of the growth-restricted fetus, particularly when the pulsatility index of the MCA is compared to that of the umbilical artery. High-resistance umbilical artery blood flow appears to precede a compensatory, or brain-sparing, cerebral vasodilatation seen in intrauterine growth restriction caused by placental insufficiency. The presence of a normal pulsatility index in the carotid artery with a high-resistance umbilical artery waveform suggests maintenance of normal cerebral circulation. As fetal hypoxia worsens, the internal carotid artery pulsatility index decreases.[8] Recently, Mari et al.[9] have noted that the peak MCA velocity was a better predictor of perinatal death than an elevated pulsatility index in the same vessel.

To obtain the MCA peak velocity, image the fetal head in a transverse plane. To prevent a false elevation peak due to fetal heart accelerations, interrogate the MCA during a period of fetal apnea and absent fetal movement. Color or power Doppler aids in identification of the MCA overlying the anterior wing of the sphenoid bone near the base of the skull. Use an angle of insonation less than 15 degrees; typically, moving the transducer on the maternal abdomen helps obtain an angle of incidence closer to zero degrees. Sonographers usually use the fetal MCA closest to the anterior uterine wall; however, acceptable sampling occurs in the contralateral MCA. To obtain the sample, place a 2-millimeter (mm) pulsed Doppler gate over the vessel just as it bifurcates from the carotid siphon. Peripheral placement of the gate results in a falsely low peak value. Take at least three measurements, using the highest as the final value. During the measurement, adjust the Doppler baseline on the display close to zero; change the pulse repetition frequency (PRF) to change the approximate peak velocity and thus the displayed scale. These adjustments optimize the appearance of the waveform, making the true peak velocity discernible. Use the electronic calipers to measure the peak systolic; automated measurement software that traces the waveform typically underestimates the true peak velocity (Fig. 27-9).[10]

Cerebellar Level

The cerebellum may also visualize in a plane parallel and inferior to the BPD level. Once they are located, the cerebellar structures are obtained through rotation of the transducer inferior to the BPD plane. Imaging of the cerebellum, with its brightly echogenic, centrally placed vermis and two relatively nonechogenic hemispheres resembling a peanut, indicate the correct measurement level. The midbrain may be seen in front of the vermis. Measurement of the cisterna magna is obtained through placement of calipers anteroposteriorly in the midline, between the vermis and the inner table of the occipital bone.[3] Anything less than 10 mm is considered a normal measurement (Fig. 19-3).

Biometry

Between 16 and 24 weeks of gestation, the transverse cerebellar diameter measured in millimeters correlates 1:1 with the gestational age. Even in cases of suspected intrauterine growth retardation (IUGR), the relationship of this transverse diameter to gestational age holds steady and can be relied on for dating due to brain sparing.[1] This diameter becomes useful with the fetus occiput anterior. This is due to the closeness of the posterior fossa to the transducer and in cases of abnormal fetal head shape. Imaging the cerebellar hemispheres on the axial view provides the easiest identification for the lateral placement of measurement calipers.[11]

Lateral Ventricle Level

In an endovaginal approach, the lateral ventricles can be clearly seen by 12 to 13 weeks as ovoid structures largely filled with choroid plexus. Using the transabdominal approach, the lateral ventricles readily image by 16 weeks' gestation as paired anechoic areas within

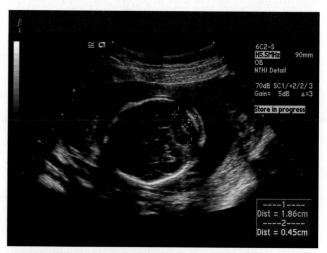

Figure 19-3 The cerebellum (Dist 1) and cisterna magna (Dist 2) lie on the same plane, allowing for simultaneous measurements.

the brain substance. The ventricle farthest from the transducer has better definition because of the lack of reverberation artifacts, which often obscure the anatomy of the closer hemisphere. The lateral wall of the ventricle visualizes consistently as the first echogenic line on the distal edge of the echo-spared ventricle. The medial wall of the ventricle is visualized less consistently. A prominent echogenic area is often seen within the lateral ventricle, which represents the choroid plexus, a highly vascular epithelial proliferation arising within the ependyma of the ventricle that produces and reabsorbs cerebrospinal fluid.

In early fetal life, the ventricular system fills a large portion of the developing brain and has the form of two smooth, curved tubes joined above the third ventricle. As gestation progresses, the shape of the ventricular system increasingly resembles the normal adult brain, occupying a decreasing proportion of the brain's volume. This evolution has been documented sonographically by several authors who have generated nomograms comparing the width of the lateral ventricle to the width of the cerebral hemisphere at various gestational ages.[1,3,5]

Biometry

In 1988, Cardoza and colleagues introduced the measurement of the lateral ventricle's width at its atrium located at an axial plane angled just superiorly to the BPD.[12] Because atrial width does not change during pregnancy, this technique obviates the need for accurate menstrual dating. It also is the earliest site of ventricular dilatation in developing hydrocephalus. The atrium can be readily seen at the level of the BPD; however, the widest measurement is usually obtained in a view that demonstrates the continuity of the atrium of the lateral ventricle with the occipital horn. Measure the widest diameter of the atrium through the choroid

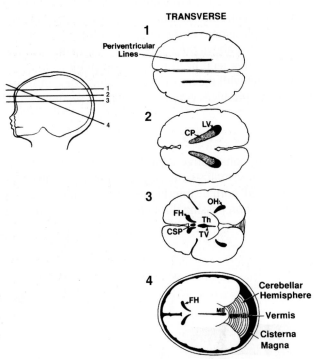

NORMAL VENTRICLES

Figure 19-5 Schematic drawing of normal ventricles and intracranial anatomy on the transverse view. 1: At this level the periventricular lines image within the cerebrum. 2: The choroid plexus images within the ventricles. 3: The BPD and HC measurement level. 4: Level for measurement of the cerebellum, cistern magna, and nuchal fold. 2–4: Recommended as part of a routine obstetric examination in the second and third trimester. *ACP*, choroid plexus; *CSP*, cavum septum pellucidum; *FH*, frontal horn; *LV*, lateral ventricle; *MB*, midbrain; *OH*, occipital horns; *Th*, thalamus; *TV*, third ventricle. (Reproduced with permission from Nyberg DA, Pretorius PH. Cerebral malformations. In: Nyberg DA, Mahony BS, Pretorius DH, eds. *Diagnostic Ultrasound of Fetal Anomalies; Text and Atlas*. Chicago: Year Book; 1990:83–145.)

plexus (Fig. 19-4). A normal measurement should not exceed 10 mm, which is said to be two to three standard deviations from the norm (Fig. 19-5).[13]

Base of the Skull Level

The base of the skull level may be identified by an echogenic "X" formed by the lesser wings of the sphenoid bone and the petrous pyramid. These bony ridges demarcate the anterior, middle, and posterior fossa.

CORONAL AND SAGITTAL VIEWS OF THE HEAD

Transabdominal imaging allows for imaging of fetal intracranial anatomy on the coronal and sagittal planes; however, previously described fetal or maternal factors may limit visualization of structures. In recent years, proponents of endovaginal sonography have been able to obtain intracranial images in coronal and sagittal planes similar to those used in the evaluation of the neonatal brain. In a technique described by Monteagudo

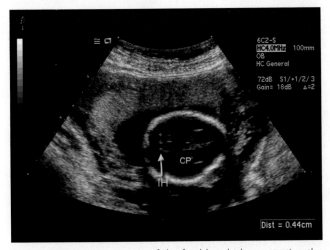

Figure 19-4 Transverse scan of the fetal head, demonstrating the lateral ventricle's atrium in continuity with the occipital horn. This is usually the view in which the widest diameter of the atrium can be measured (*calipers*) through the choroid plexus (*CP*). *IH*, interhemispheric fissure.

and colleagues, a 5.0- to 6.5-megahertz (MHz), slowly advanced endovaginal transducer allows imaging of the fetal brain. Once the transducer aligns with the anterior fontanel, placement of the examiner's free hand on the abdomen just above the symphysis pubis helps manipulate the vertex fetal head to bring the anterior fontanel into contact with the transducer. Rotating the transducer 90 degrees produces coronal and sagittal sections.[14]

CORONAL SECTIONS

A series of consecutive coronal sections from anterior to posterior visualizes the corpus callosum, ventricular system, and normal interhemispheric relationships. A coronal section passing through the level of the anterior

horns of the lateral ventricles demonstrates the interhemispheric fissure, the corpus callosum crossing the midline, the cavum septi pellucidi, and the third ventricle straddled by the thalami (Fig. 19-6). Early in the second trimester, the fissure appears relatively straight. As new sulci and gyri develop with advancing gestation, the interhemispheric fissure becomes irregular. The hypoechoic area between the skull and the cerebral cortex represents the subarachnoid space. This space diminishes in size throughout gestation as the cerebral cortical matter expands to fill the cranial vault. A posterior coronal plane images the occipital horns of the lateral ventricles. In this last view, the cerebellum visualizes inferior to the fourth ventricle and superior to the cisterna magna (Fig. 19-7).

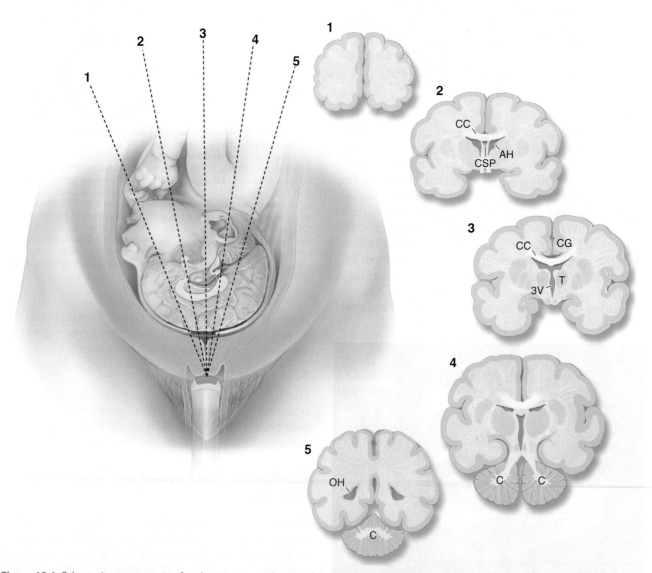

Figure 19-6 Schematic representation for obtaining coronal scans of the second- and third-trimester fetal head through the acoustic window of the anterior fontanel. Plane 1: anterior to the corpus callosum; plane 2: at the level of the anterior horns of the lateral ventricle; plane 3: at the level of the third ventricle; plane 4: posterior plane through the peduncles; plane 5: the posterior coronal plane through the occipital horns. *CC,* corpus callosum; *AH,* anterior horns of the lateral ventricle; *CSP,* cavum septi pellucidi; *3V,* third ventricle; *C,* cerebellum; *OH,* occipital horn of the lateral ventricle; *CG,* cingulate gyrus. (Reprinted with permission from Monteagado A, Timor-Tritsch IE, Reuss ML, et al. Transvaginal sonography of the second- and third-trimester fetal brain. In: Timor-Tritsch IE, Rottem S, Eds. *Transvaginal Sonography.* 2nd ed. New York: Elsevier; 1991:393–426.)

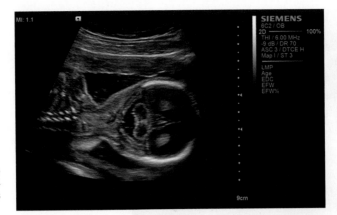
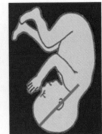

Figure 19-7 A coronal image through the posterior fetal brain correlating with plane 4 in Figure 19-6. (Image courtesy of Siemens Medical, Mountain View, CA.)

SAGITTAL AND PARASAGITTAL SECTIONS

By 18 to 20 weeks' gestation, the corpus callosum is nearly fully developed. In a midsagittal section, it appears as a prominent, semilunar structure composed of three parts, from front to back: the genu, the body, and the splenium (Fig. 19-8). Above and below the corpus callosum are the cingulate gyrus and the sonolucent cavum septi pellucidi, respectively. The posterior fossa contains the cerebellum, the fourth ventricle, and the cisterna magna. The midsagittal view also helps in evaluation of the cerebral hemispheres, surface contour. During the second trimester, the surface is smooth. Echodense lines on the cerebral cortex, seen in the third trimester, represent new gyri and sulci.

Parasagittal sections taken to the right or left of midline allow study of the anterior horns and bodies of the lateral ventricles. Normally, all the various segments of the lateral ventricle—the body and the anterior, posterior, and temporal horns—cannot be seen in a single plane. If all segments image in a single plane, this suggests ventricular dilatation. The bright echogenic arc separating the caudate nucleus from the thalamus images on the parasagittal view. This is known as the caudothalamic groove, which lies posterior to the germinal matrix. The germinal matrix, a highly vascular tissue in the ependyma of the lateral ventricle, only images when abnormal. Most intracranial hemorrhages originate in this area in the preterm neonate.

THE FACE

ORBITS AND EYES

A transverse axial scan slightly caudal to the one commonly used for determination of the biparietal diameter easily reveals orbits and eyes. Measurement of the

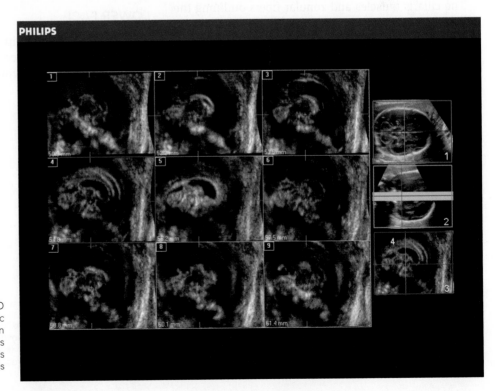

Figure 19-8 The acquisition of a 3D data set allows for a tomographic sequential display of fetal brain structures on the sagittal plane. This sequence demonstrates the corpus callosum. (Image courtesy of Philips Medical Systems, Bothell, WA.)

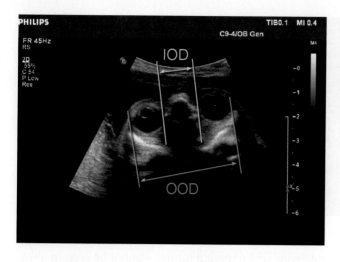

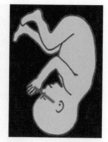

Figure 19-9 Axial image demonstrating the technique for measuring outer orbital and inner orbital diameters. Note the circular lens seen in each eye. (Image courtesy of Philips Medical Systems, Bothell, WA.)

distance between the bony orbits may be useful for determining gestational age and searching for abnormally spaced orbits. Hypotelorism or closely spaced orbits, and hypertelorism, wide spaced orbits image on this plane.[16] Depending on the position of the fetal head, gestational age determination through the use of the inner and outer orbital distances allows for an alternative dating measurement in the absence of malformed cranial structures. Figure 19-9 illustrates the technique for obtaining these measurements. The outer orbital distance is the more valuable measurement because it is the larger of the two measurements and thus has a greater range of normal variation across gestational age compared to the inner orbital distance. This increases confidence concerning the normality of a given measurement.

The ciliaris muscles and zonular fibers outlining the lens of the fetal eye image as a circular area on the front of the globe (Fig. 19-10). On occasion, the vitreous humor, extraocular muscles, and the ophthalmic artery and nerve may be recognized.[17] The hyaloid artery is a branch of the ophthalmic artery and may image within the fetal globe (Fig. 9-11).

EARS

Sonography easily images the pinna of the ear and the development of its cartilages.[17] Visualization of the ears increases with the use of a three-dimensional (3D) surface rendering.[1,3] The pinna is initially smooth but becomes increasingly ridged as gestation progresses (Fig. 19-12). Occasionally, even the basal turn of the cochlea or superior semicircular canal found within the petrous portion of the temporal bone may be imaged.[17] Studies have found that ear length follows a linear growth pattern, resulting in the use of length as an alternative biometric measurement.[3]

LOWER FACE

The nares and upper lip visualize in a coronal scan (Fig. 19-13), and the face can be searched for cleft lip or palate. Fetal swallowing and tongue motion image

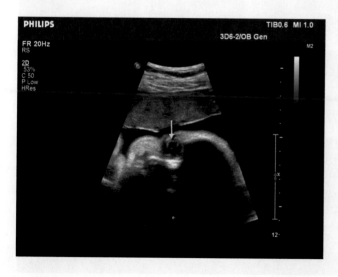

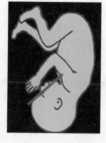

Figure 19-10 Coronal view of the fetal face demonstrating the lens (arrow) within the orbit. (Image courtesy of Philips Medical Systems, Bothell, WA.)

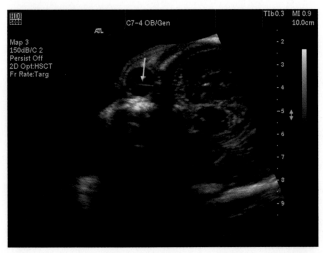

Figure 19-11 The hyaloid artery (*arrow*) extends from the ophthalmic artery located within the optic nerve to the posterior lens. This vessel usually regresses before birth when the need for blood supply to the developing lens is no longer needed. (Image courtesy of Philips Medical Systems, Bothell, WA.)

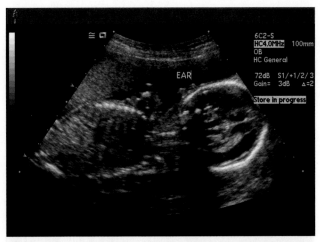

Figure 19-12 Smooth pinna of the fetal ear at 18 weeks' gestation.

easily during the routine sonographic examination. The fetal profile (i.e., a midline sagittal view) verifies the shape and position of the nose and chin, as well as the contour of the face (Fig. 19-14). Isaacson and Birnhoz described a method to document normal fetal breathing by demonstrating color flow due to amniotic fluid motion through the fetal nares (Fig. 19-15).[18]

THE NECK

During the neck examination, careful study of the surface contours helps rule out a variety of lesions that may extend from this area. As early as the 18th week of gestation, the cervical structure size allows for the detailed investigation of cervical structures. Coronal images are considered best for evaluating structures of the fetal neck.[15] The centrally located trachea and the more peripherally located carotid bifurcation images within the substance of the neck (Fig. 19-16). Visualization of

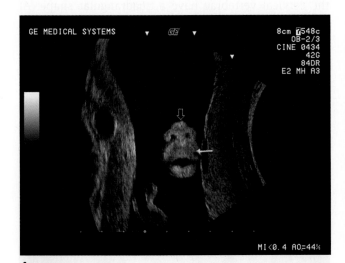

A

B

Figure 19-13 A: Coronal scan of the fetal face demonstrating the nares (*open arrow*) and the upper lip (*arrow*). **B:** 3D surface rendering of the face allows for scrutiny of the upper lip to rule out clefting. (Sonographic images courtesy of GE Healthcare, Wauwatosa, WI.)

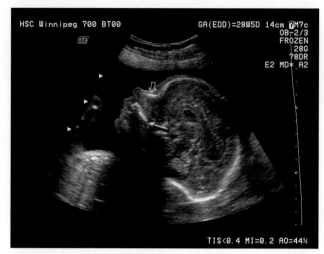

Figure 19-14 The midline profile of this fetus allows for visualization of the normal profile, maxilla (arrow), and nasal bone (open arrow). (Sonographic image courtesy of GE Healthcare, Wauwatosa, WI.)

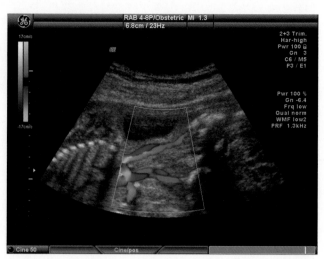

Figure 19-16 A coronal view demonstrating both carotid arteries (red) and jugular veins (blue). (Sonographic image courtesy of GE Healthcare, Wauwatosa, WI.)

the carotid artery and other structures may be difficult because of flexion of the head and an unfavorable position of the fetus.

THE SPINE

SONOGRAPHY OF THE FETAL SPINE

An appreciation of the variability in the shapes of the vertebral bodies and the changing sonographic appearance of the spine during gestation is necessary to differentiate small defects of the spine from normal anatomic variations.[1,2] The fetal spine images as individual vertebrae, with three brightly echogenic ossification centers in the transverse plane by the 16th week of gestation. Two of these ossification centers lie posterior to the spinal canal within the laminae, and one is anterior within the vertebral body (Fig. 19-17).

The systematic examination of the spine begins with a transverse sweep of the transducer along the entire length of the spine. Three types of scanning planes help with the evaluation of spinal integrity: transverse, coronal, and sagittal.

The spinal anatomic configuration changes depending on the level. This becomes evident while obtaining vertebral images on the transverse planes. Three ossification centers surround the neural canal. Beginning at the cervical level, the posterior ossification centers of the cervical vertebrae have a quadrangular shape. At the triangular thoracic and lumbar level, these image in an inverted triangle with the base toward the dorsum of the fetus. Finally, at the level of the sacrum, the posterior ossification centers have a wider placement than the upper vertebrae (Fig. 19-18). The vertebral body, pedicles, transverse processes, posterior laminae,

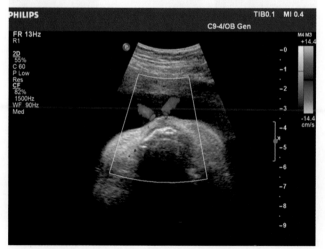

Figure 19-15 Axial view of the fetal face demonstrating fetal breathing through the use of color Doppler. (Image courtesy of Philips Medical Systems, Bothell, WA.)

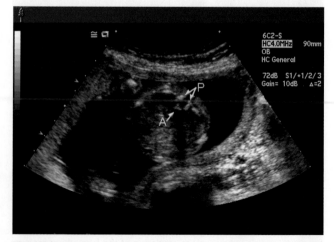

Figure 19-17 Transverse scan of the thoracic fetal spine at 18 weeks' gestation demonstrating the two posterior (P) and one anterior (A) ossification centers.

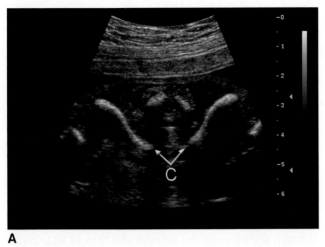

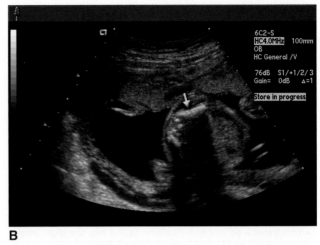

Figure 19-18 A: The transverse cervical spine taken at the level of the clavicles (*C*). **B:** The normal posterior sacral ossification centers have a slightly wider spacing than the thoracic and lumbar spine. The iliac bone (*arrow*) helps identify the correct image level.

and spinous process all image as echogenic structures, which improves as gestation progresses. In addition, the spinal canal and intervertebral foramina may be seen as anechoic areas.

The sagittal plane provides the classic spinal image demonstrating the spine, often in its entirety, as a parallel structure ending in the pointed sacrum (Fig. 19-19). These parallel lines represent the two ossification centers, the vertebral body and posterior arch. The fetus in the prone or supine position allows imaging on a true sagittal image when directing the sonographic beam through the unossified spinous processes. This plane images the neural tube in the first trimester and the spinal cord during the remaining trimesters. In the second and third trimester, the conus medullaris images at the second and third lumbar spine level.[1]

In the coronal plane, the two echogenic posterior ossification centers can be followed progressively from the cervical region to the base of the spine (Fig. 19-20). The posterior ossification centers are normally parallel to each other or converge as they are followed from the lumbar to the sacral regions. Divergence of the posterior elements suggests abnormality, probably a meningocele or meningomyelocele.

Determination of spinal normalcy is through identification of an intact neural canal, normal location and shape of spinal ossification centers, and an intact dorsal skin contour. Imaging the conus medullaris on the sagittal plane increases confidence of normal spinal development. An anatomic survey of the fetus includes, at a minimum, transverse (axial) and longitudinal views of the spine (Table 19-2).[1]

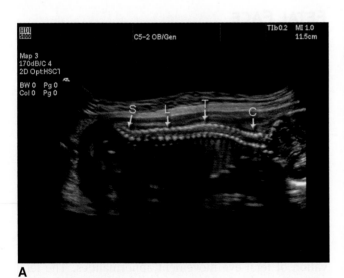

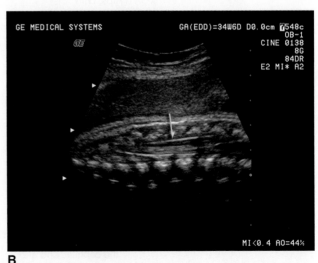

Figure 19-19 A: Panoramic image of the fetal spine. *C*, cervical; *T*, thoracic; *L*, lumbar; *S*, sacrum. **B:** Terminal spine demonstrating nerve roots. (Image **A** courtesy of Philips Medical Systems, Bothell, WA; Image **B** courtesy of GE Healthcare, Wauwatosa, WI.)

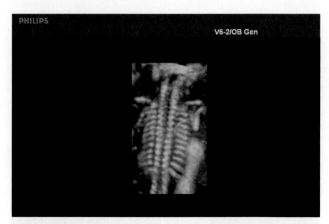

Figure 19-20 A 3D reconstruction of the cervical and thoracic spine demonstrates a normal spinal column flaring into the skull. (Image courtesy of Philips Medical Systems, Bothell, WA.)

ANOMALIES OF THE FETAL HEAD, NECK, AND SPINE

There are myriad schemes for grouping and reviewing abnormalities of the fetal head, neck, and spine. This chapter uses characterization of visualized structures to form the basis for developing a diagnosis. The following four categories differentiate the types of anomalies in this section: (1) absence of a structure normally present; (2) herniation through a structural defect; (3) dilatation behind an obstruction; and (4) presence of an additional structure.

CLINICAL ASSOCIATIONS

Screening for neural tube defects includes not only sonography but also biochemical testing. Alpha-fetoprotein (AFP) is a glycoprotein secreted by the yolk sac and then by the fetal liver. AFP found in amniotic fluid occurs initially through diffusion across immature skin, and later through secretion by the kidneys and thus in fetal urination. The fetus swallows the amniotic fluid AFP, resulting in recirculation, with eventual degradation by the fetal liver. Maternal Serum AFP (MSAFP) levels occur through diffusion across the placenta and amnion.

Structural defects such as anencephaly or spina bifida result in higher levels of AFP entering the amniotic fluid, leading to higher levels in the maternal serum. Levels of AFP are elevated in amniotic fluid and maternal serum only when such defects are open—that is, when the neural tissue is exposed or covered by only a thin membrane. Skin-covered or closed neural tube defects (NTDs) prevent AFP from escaping fetal circulation, resulting in a normal amniotic AFP level. The MSAFP varies with gestation and therefore needs to be expressed as multiples of the median (MoM). Typically, 2.5 MoM is used as the level for a positive screen.[3,19]

It is important to note that AFP is elevated in conditions other than NTD. Such disorders include other open fetal defects, such as omphalocele and gastroschisis, as well as skin disorders that increase diffusion of AFP through fetal skin.[2] Of note, fetuses with Down syndrome have been shown to have a lower mean MSAFP.[2,20]

FETAL FACE

Facial images of the developing fetus are often one of the highlights for parents during the sonographic examination. Though often cute, these images provide valuable information into congenital anomalies of not only the face but related anatomy. Utilization of basic face embryology allows for understanding of the origin of not only congenital facial anomalies but often coexisting cardiac malformations, holoprosencephaly, or syndromes.[3,15]

Improved ultrasound technology allows for the study of smaller parts of the fetus, such as the orbit and lens. It is now possible to evaluate the orbit and lens early in the second trimester of pregnancy to help rule out various genetic diseases or malformations through observation of fetal eye movement abnormalities. The fetal orbit images as an echogenic circle of the lens within an echolucent globe.[2]

TABLE 19-2		
Minimum Brain, Face, and Spine Views Obtained During the Sonographic Examination		
	Plane	**Anatomy Imaged**
Brain	Axial - BPD	Thalami, third ventricle, cavum septum pellucidum
	Axial - Cerebellum	Cerebellum, cisterna magna, vermis
	Axial - Ventricles	Ventricles, choroid plexus
Face	Coronal - Face	Soft tissues of the nose, lips, chin
	Sagittal - Profile	Confirm correct symmetry of forehead, nose, lips, chin
Spine	Axial	Document correct location, ossificiation, and placement of the vertebral body, spinous and transverse processes at the cervical, thoracic, lumbar, and sacral spine
	Sagittal	Obtain views of the spine from the cervical to sacral portions, confirming slight widening at the cephalic end and tapering at the caudal end of the fetus

Lens and orbit diameters, circumferences, and surfaces have been shown to be significantly correlated with gestational age, and thus may be used to detect orbital anomalies.[22]

EMBRYOLOGY OF THE EYE

The eyes develop as lateral projections from the telencephalon called optic vesicles at approximately day 28. By the end of the first month, these become optic cups positioned at the end of an optic stalk. This structure progresses to the lens placode (the developing eye), lens pit, pigmented eye, and then finally the eye at approximately 48 days. Early in gestation the primitive eye structures lie on the lateral portion and dorsal to what becomes the fetal face. As the facial structures migrate to midline the eyes follow suit, locating in the normal location by the end of the first trimester (Fig. 19-21).[2]

Hypotelorism is a decreased interorbital distance and is almost always found in association with other severe anomalies, most commonly with holoprosencephaly.[3] Prognosis for these fetuses and neonates is poor due to the associated anomalies.[15]

Hypertelorism is an increased orbital distance, occurring in either isolation, with malformations, or as part of a syndrome. Extreme cases of hypertelorism increase the chances of mental retardation, often accompanying other facial malformations such as orbital teratomas, anterior encephaloceles, median cleft face syndrome, cleft lip, and agenesis of the corpus callosum.[15,23] Syndromes associated with increased orbital distance include Apert, Crouzon, Noonan, Pena-Shokeir, and Pfeiffer syndromes.[15,23]

Microphthalmia demonstrates decreased orbit size, while absence of the eye is called anophthalmia. The latter is a pathologic diagnosis, as anophthalmia includes not only the orbit but the optic nerves, chiasma, and tracts.[15] Either a unilateral or bilateral process, microphthalmia is usually part of a syndrome.[15,23] Microphthalmia can be an isolated anomaly due to chromosomal abnormalities or intrauterine infections.[15] Prenatal diagnosis of microphthalmia can be detected by ultrasound measurement of the orbit.[3] It is defined as an orbital diameter smaller than the 5th percentile for gestational age.[22]

Macroglossia in a fetus images as the tongue extending beyond the teeth or alveolar ridge.[15] This protrusion may be due to either large size or hypotonia.[3] The profile view of fetuses with trisomy 21 and Beckwith-Weidmann syndrome image with macroglossia during the sonographic examination.[3,15,23] It has also been seen in patients with hypothyroidism, storage diseases, neurofibromatosis, genetic syndromes, and sublingual masses (Fig. 19-22).[15,23]

Micrognathia is defined as a severely hypoplastic mandible. In 40%[15] of cases, micrognathia is an isolated finding, but it is also frequently seen as part of syndromes such as Pierre Robin sequence and hemifacial microsomia (e.g., Treacher-Collins syndrome). Other associated malformations include skeletal dysplasias, aneuploidies such as trisomy 18 and 13 and other chromosomal anomalies (e.g., gene deletions or translocations), and teratogen exposure (e.g., alcohol).[24]

Fetuses with such mandible anomalies are at risk of acute neonatal respiratory distress, since the tongue may obstruct the upper airways and lead to suffocation at delivery. Antenatal recognition is critical. Various ultrasound descriptions have been described but are mostly subjective, such as prominent upper lip and small chin; subjective impression of a small jaw or posterior displacement of the mandible; or an unusually small mandible resulting in a receding chin. Some authors have attempted to describe more objective measures of retrognathia and micrognathia. Rotten et al.[24]

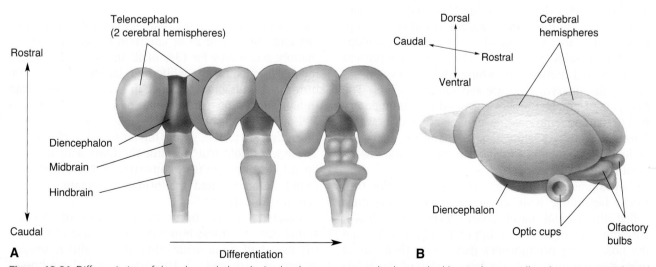

Figure 19-21 Differentiation of the telencephalon. **A:** As development proceeds, the cerebral hemispheres swell and grow posteriorly and laterally to envelop the diencephalon. **B:** The olfactory bulbs sprout off the ventral surfaces of each telencephalic vesicle.

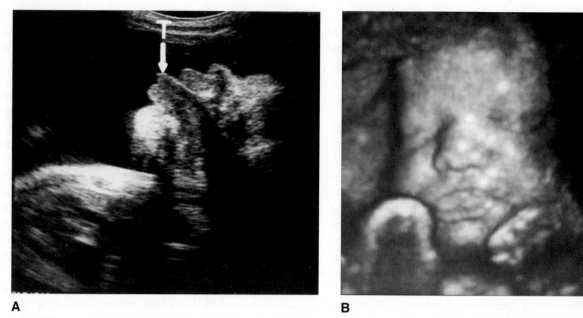

A   **B**

Figure 19-22 Macroglossia. **A:** Sagittal view in the third trimester shows macroglossia with protruding tongue (*T*) in a fetus who proved to have Beckwith-Wiedmann syndrome. **B:** 3D surface rendering of a fetus demonstrating an enlarged tongue protruding beyond the teeth. (Image **A** courtesy of L. Hill, MD, Pittsburgh, PA.)

describe the use of inferior facial angle and mandible width/maxilla width ratio to characterize fetal retrognathic and micrognathic mandibles. Another proposed objective measure is described by Palladini et al. using the jaw index, which is computed as the ratio between the anteroposterior mandibular diameter and the biparietal diameter.[25]

FACIAL CLEFTS

Embryology of the Lower Face

Facial development begins with neural crest cells migrating into the head and neck area, forming the brachial arches. There are a total of six sets of arches; four (also called pharyngeal arches) develop in the fourth and fifth week of embryonic life. The first set, sometimes called the mandibular arches, result in development of the face. The second, or hyoid arch, develops into the muscles of the face. These arches represent mesenchymal tissue outpouchings, which develop lateral to the pharynx and are separated by clefts. The first pair of brachial arches surround the rudimentary mouth (stomodeum) at the end of the fourth week. This arch gives rise to the maxilla, mandible, incus and malleus of the middle ear, maxillary artery, and the trigeminal nerve.[2,3]

Development of the face occurs during the fifth week, beginning with the appearance of swellings called the frontal nasal prominences (Fig. 19-23). Forming what becomes the upper mouth, maxilla, and the nose, these prominences move from their lateral origins to the midline of the face. Fusion of this intermaxillary segment results in a normal facial structure.

The paired mandibular processes (also originating from the first arch) merge, resulting in the formation of the lower face.

The maxillary and one of the five prominences forming the nose develop into the upper lip, incisors, and primary palate. Lack of fusion or persistence of the embryologic grooves in either the maxillary or intermaxillary segment (medial nasal prominence) leads to either a unilateral or bilateral cleft palate or lip.[1,2,3] One type of split occurs between the lateral incisors and the canine teeth in the paramesial position of the upper lip. Incomplete merging of the intermaxillary segments results in a midline cleft.[3]

CLEFT LIP AND PALATE

Facial clefts are the most frequent craniofacial anomalies and the second most common congenital malformation, accounting for 13% of all anomalies. Published incidence rates for the white population are 1 in 1,000 births, with a higher incidence in males.[3,15,23] American Indian populations show a rate of 1:300,[3] with Asians at 1:600.[3] Persons of African descent have an incidence of clefting at 1:2,500, with a higher female incidence.[3,23] These rates hold true only for the fetus with the cleft lip (CL)/cleft palate (CP) combination. Clefting defects found as an isolated malformation remain constant across ethnic groups.[3]

Isolated CL may occur independently of chromosomal abnormalities; however, in the case of CL and CP, over half occur with other abnormalities, usually as part of a trisomy.[15,23] Approximately 350 syndromes have been linked with facial clefting, some of which

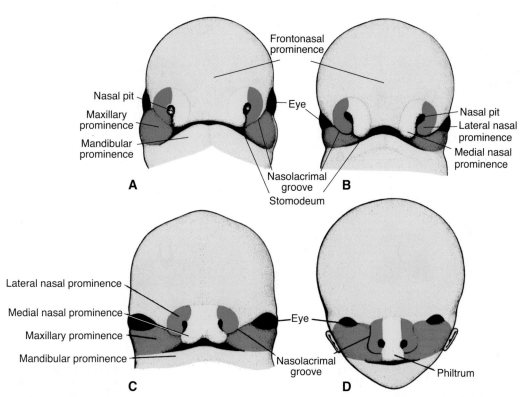

Figure 19-23 The face comes together when the five swellings rotate together. The lower jaw solidifies early, but the upper jaw, lip, and nose merge over a period of weeks. The middle of the upper lip is formed by continuation of the frontonasal prominence **(A, B)**. The maxillary and mandibular swellings merge enough to reduce the breadth of the mouth **(C)**. The pharyngeal arch and mesenchymal swellings rotate in concert with expansion of the brain and rotation of the orbits toward stereoscopy **(D)**. (From Sadler TW. *Langman's Medical Embryology*. 10th ed. Baltimore: Lippincott Williams & Wilkins; 2006. Figure 16.22A,B, p. 263; Figure 16.23A,B, p. 264.)

are lethal or include severe morbidity.[26] Even with this strong correlation to syndromes,[15] CL and CP is a multifactorial process, possibly resulting from teratogenic factors.[2] Club foot is the most frequent anomaly with the finding of an isolated CL or CP.[15] With the combination of CL and CP, polydactyly is the most common finding. Regardless of the clefting malformation, congenital heart disease is likely.[15]

CP is a different process than the combination of palate and lip clefting. Approximately half are a combination of CL and CP, with a third as isolated CP, and the rest CL alone.[15,23] Females have a greater likelihood of an isolated CP, whereas males demonstrate the combination of CL/CP.[3] Cases of isolated CP and CL/CP are specific malformations differing in type. A posterior defect of the posterior portion with an intact upper lip and anterior palate is considered a CP.

Classification of clefting defects depends on the severity of the malformation. Though this malformation occurs in any part of the face, most often the nostril and central posterior palate connect via the defect.[3] In severe cases, CL/CP extends through the hard palate and alveolar ridge, involving the nasal cavity, and possibly the orbit (Fig. 19-24).[15]

Obtaining an image on an anterior coronal or axial plane demonstrates CL by ultrasound. The coronal or tangential plane allows imaging of the linear defect as it extends from the nose to the oral rim, demonstrating any distortion of the upper lip and nose (Fig. 19-25). For an axial or transverse view to demonstrate the defect, place the lower portion of the face closest to the transducer (anterior). An axial image of the maxilla helps in demonstration of the defect into the palate (CL-CP) (Fig. 19-26). To evaluate the defect extension into the face, angle the transducer to image the entire palate. Useful adjunctive findings in the fetus with a CL include undulating tongue movements,[27] hypertrophied tissue at the edge of the cleft,[28] and hypertelorism.[28] Color Doppler imaging may help in diagnosis of the clefts due to the distortion of the normal nasal architecture (Fig. 19-27).

Facial bone shadowing increases the difficulty in diagnosing the isolated CP. 3D ultrasound (3DUS) has been shown to be superior to two-dimensional ultrasound (2DUS) for the prenatal diagnosis of CL and CP. Potential advantages of 3DUS over 2DUS include

---

PATHOLOGY BOX 19-1

Sonographic Features of Cleft Lip/Palate

Axial	Linear defect through the maxilla/lip
Coronal	Linear defect from nose to oral rim

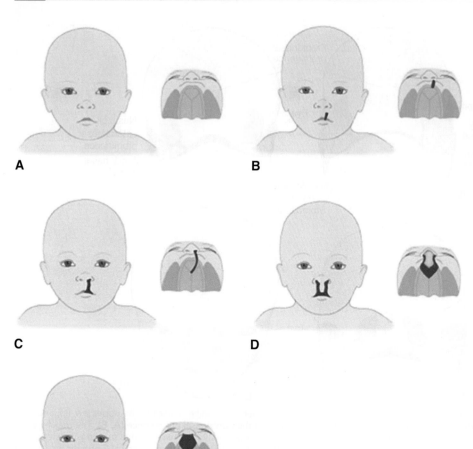

Figure 19-24 Classification of common types of clefts. **A:** Normal. **B:** Unilateral cleft lip (type 1). **C:** Unilateral cleft lip and palate (type 2). **D:** Bilateral cleft lip and palate (type 3). **E:** Median cleft lip and palate (type 4). Not shown are slash-type defects (type 5). (Adapted from Nyberg DA, Sickler GK, Hegge FN, Kramer DJ, Kropp RJ. Fetal cleft lip with and without cleft palate: US classification and correlation with outcome. *Radiology.* 1995;195:677–683.)

(1) the display of a true coronal view of the lips, even with a different acquisition plane; (2) ease in demonstration of the teeth in the alveolar ridge of the maxilla; and (3) accurate localization of the maxillary tooth-bearing alveolar ridge decreasing the chance of

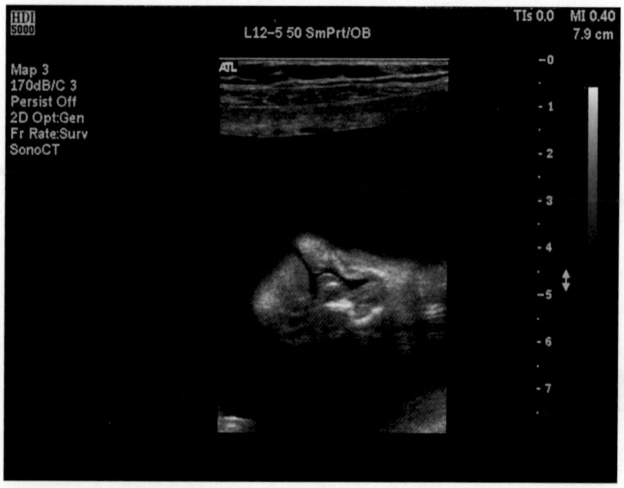

Figure 19-25 The hypoechoic linear defect extends from the nostril to the lip. (Image courtesy of Philips Medical Systems, Bothell, WA.)

confusion with the mandibular ridge (Fig. 19-28).[15] Because of the subtlety of facial changes in clefting malformations, varying 3D techniques describe diagnosis of cleft palate. Campbell et al. have described a technique called the 3D reverse face view. This technique consists of rotating the volume data set 180 degrees around the vertical axis to examine the secondary palate.[29]

FETAL HEAD AND BRAIN

ABSENCE OF A STRUCTURE NORMALLY PRESENT

Meroanencephaly/Anencephaly/Acrania

Meroanencephaly designates the partial development of the brain, which describes the neural tube defect commonly described as anencephaly. Since the latter term describes a fetus without a brain, and in actuality the fetus has some functioning brain tissue and a rudimentary brain stem, meroanencephaly correctly describes the malformation.[2]

Meroanencephaly represents the most common neural tube defect, which is always lethal. Its incidence

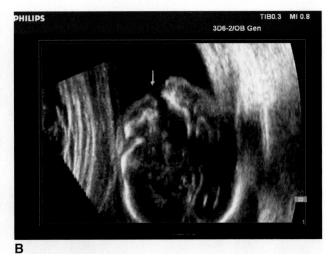

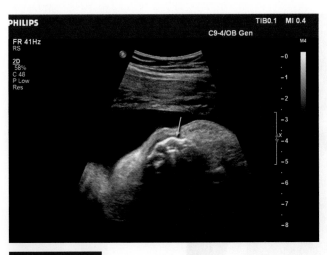

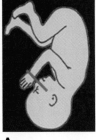

Figure 19-26 A: Normal palate *(arrow)*. **B:** Unilateral CL-CP *(arrow)*. (Image courtesy of Philips Medical Systems, Bothell, WA.)

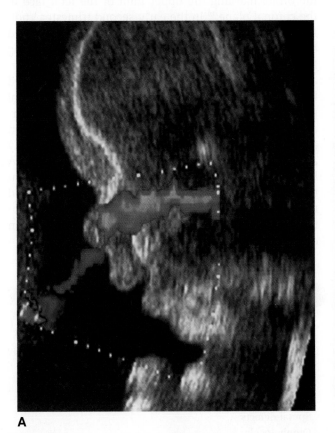

A

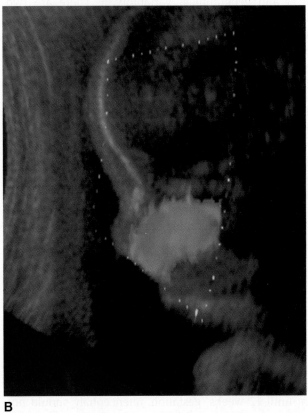

B

Figure 19-27 Normal and cleft palate. **A:** Color-flow imaging of normal fetus with respiratory activity shows amniotic fluid in the nasopharynx, separated from the oral pharynx inferiorly by the intact palate. **C:** Similar view in a fetus with cleft palate shows the nasopharynx and oral pharynx communicating in a single cavity. (Image courtesy of Gianluigi Pilu, MD, Bologna, Italy.)

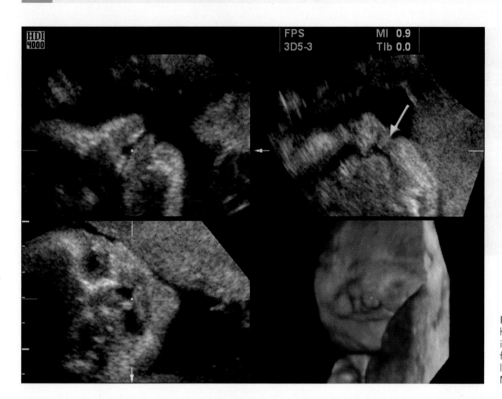

Figure 19-28 The B MPR view helps to confirm the intact palate in this fetus *(arrow)*, while the surface rendering demonstrates the lip cleft. (Image courtesy of Philips Medical Systems, Bothell, WA.)

is approximately 1:1,000, with female predominance (4:1) and geographical variability.[3,23] There are two theories explaining the origin of how this defect occurs with basically the same outcome. One form of meroanencephaly is considered to arise from acrania as a consequence of disruption of abnormal brain tissue unprotected by the calvarium.[30] Acrania refers to the absence of the entire skull, including the skull base, thus only a thin layer, if any, covers the brain. Due to the abnormal structure and vascularization of the ex-encephalic brain, degeneration occurs.[2] Another form results from the failure of the rostral (cephalic) neuropore to close.[2] Though the mechanism of this malformation differs from a meroanencephalic fetus resulting from acrania, the differentiation may be merely academic as the sonographic appearance is quite similar as is the prognosis.

On ultrasound evaluation, acrania usually shows an abnormally shaped cephalic pole. Another feature that has been described in the late embryonic period before 10 weeks' gestation is the altered appearance of the brain cavities, which have a decreased fluid content and thus seem "empty."[30] Sonographic diagnosis of anencephaly is usually possible in the early second trimester (10 to 14 weeks gestational age).[1] However, since ossification of the skull vault is not always apparent until 12 weeks' gestation, anencephaly should not be diagnosed before this time.[19] In the first trimester, ultrasound findings include an absent cranial vault, reduced crown-rump length, exposed neural tissue with a lobulated appearance (exencephaly) or absent neural tissue, and a loss of the normal head contour with

the orbits marking the upper limit of the fetal face in the coronal plane.[19] In the early second trimester, rudimentary brain tissue (area cerebrovasculosa) covered by a membrane but not bone may be seen protruding from the base of the skull, and this gradually degenerates to the characteristic appearance of the flattened head behind the facial structures. Facial views reveal prominent bulging eyeballs, giving a froglike appearance (Fig. 19-29). In the late second to third trimester, associated polyhydramnios[3] usually develops, likely as a result of absent or ineffective fetal swallowing. A high degree of fetal activity is often observed.[23] Conventional 2DUS is accurate in diagnosing anencephaly, and the sensitivity is virtually 100% after 14 weeks' gestation.[3,31] 3DUS has been shown to be equally effective in detecting anencephaly.[32]

> **PATHOLOGY BOX 19-2**
>
> ### Sonographic Features of Meroanencephaly (Anencephaly)
>
> Abnormally shaped cephalic pole
>
> Absent neural tissue
>
> Loss of normal head contour
>
> Froglike eye appearance
>
> Spinal defects
>
> Omphalocele
>
> Club foot
>
> Cleft lip/palate
>
> Polyhydramnios

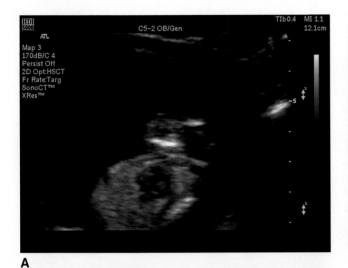

A

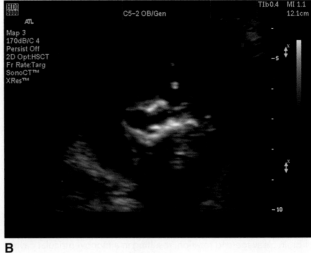

B

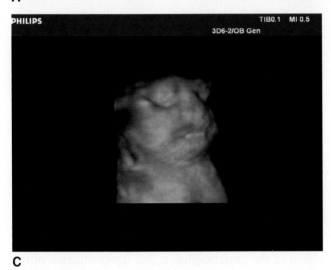

C

Figure 19-29 A: Profile of an anencephalic fetus demonstrating the lack of neural tissue above the orbits. **B:** Axial view of the orbits with bulging eyes creating the froglike appearance typical of the anencephalic face. **C:** 3D surface rendering of an anencephalic fetus. (Images courtesy of Philips Medical Systems, Bothell, WA.)

As with many lethal anomalies, the risk of recurrence in subsequent pregnancies, as with most polygenic or multifactorial anomalies, increases with the number of previously affected fetuses.[3] Associated malformations are common and include spina bifida, cleft lip/palate, club foot, and omphalocele. As with other neural tube defects, a folic acid supplement greatly reduces the occurrence.[3]

Hydranencephaly

Complete or near complete absence of the cerebral cortex characterizes hydranencephaly.[33] This rare congenital cerebral abnormality occurs in less than 1 in 10,000 births. The thalami, lower brain centers, and cerebellum are usually intact. The etiology of hydranencephaly is unclear, but the lesion is thought to represent destruction of a previously normal brain that is subsequently replaced by fluid. Causes of the third trimester brain destruction include maternal toxoplasmosis,[1,5] cytomegalovirus,[1,5] herpes simplex,[3] and carbon monoxide[3] exposure. Other reported causes include intrauterine occlusion of the middle cerebral[3] and internal carotid

arteries.[1,5] The head may be small, of normal size, or extremely enlarged.

Prenatal diagnosis of hydranencephaly is suspected when there is a large fluid collection in the head with no recognizable cerebral cortex. It can be differentiated sonographically from holoprosencephaly by identifying the presence of dural attachments and distinctly separate thalami. In severe hydrocephalus, a rim of cerebral cortex around the cystic cavity and enlargement of the third ventricle may be visualized.[33] Color Doppler imaging of the base of the brain demonstrates lack of flow in the anterior and middle cerebral arteries with normal posterior cerebral artery flow.[3]

Holoprosencephaly

Holoprosencephaly describes a variety of abnormalities of the brain and face due to incomplete cleavage and rotation of the embryonic forebrain,[2,19] resulting in a single, centrally located ventricle and a missing falx (Fig. 19-30).[37] The relatively uncommon defect has multiple causes, such as poorly controlled maternal diabetes and teratogens (such as alcohol), which disrupt

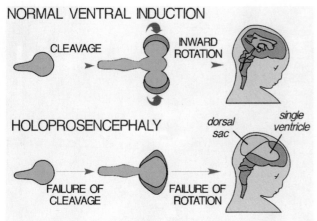

NORMAL VENTRAL INDUCTION

CLEAVAGE — INWARD ROTATION

HOLOPROSENCEPHALY

dorsal sac — single ventricle

FAILURE OF CLEAVAGE — FAILURE OF ROTATION

Figure 19-30 The process of ventral induction in normal fetuses and in holoprosencephaly. In alobar holoprosencephaly, there is failure of brain cleavage and rotation, resulting in a monoventricular cavity.

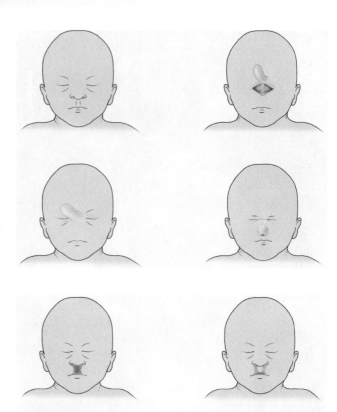

development in the third week.[2] In most cases, it is isolated and sporadic, whereas in other cases, chromosomal abnormalities have been found (trisomy 13 and 18 and polyploidy). Anatomic anomalies such as hypotelorism and other facial malformations accompany holoprosencephaly.[2]

Holoprosencephaly is divided into alobar, semilobar, and lobar varieties, defined by the degree of separation of the cerebral hemispheres (Fig. 19-31).[37] The alobar form is the worst, showing no evidence of division of cerebral cortex into separate hemispheres. Thus, the falx cerebri and interhemispheric fissures are absent and there is a single common ventricle and fused thalami.[37] Alobar holoprosencephaly has been further categorized into the pancake, cup, and ball types (Fig. 19-32). The semilobar and lobar varieties represent greater degrees of brain development. The semilobar type demonstrates partially separated brain, whereas the lobar type shows almost complete separation of the hemispheres, although the frontal horns of the lateral ventricles are fused, as are the thalami.[37]

Figure 19-32 The many faces of holoprosencephaly. From top, left to right, cyclopia, ethmocephaly, cebocephaly, median cleft lip and palate, and bilateral cleft lip and palate.

The prechordal mesoderm, an embryonic connective mass between the oral cavity and the undersurface of the neural tube, is thought to be responsible for both the division of the prosencephalon and the production of the nasofrontal process. Failure of the sagittal division of the prosencephalon is thought to result in holoprosencephaly (Fig. 19-33).[38] The nasofrontal process gives rise to the ethmoid, nasal, and premaxillary bones and to the vomer

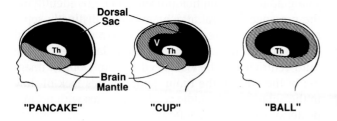

Dorsal Sac

Th

Brain Mantle

"PANCAKE"   "CUP"   "BALL"

V   Th   Th

Figure 19-31 Diagram of three morphologic types of alobar holoprosencephaly (and semilobar holoprosencephaly) in sagittal view. Pancake type: The flattened residual brain mantle at the base of the brain with a correspondingly large dorsal sac. Cup type: This type has more brain mantle but it does not cover the monoventricle. The dorsal sac communicates widely with the monoventricle. Ball type: Brain mantle completely covers the monoventricle, and a dorsal sac may or may not be present. *Th,* thalami; *V,* ventricle. (Modified from McGahn JP, Ellis W, Lindfors KK, et al. Congenital cerebrospinal fluid-containing intracranial abnormalities: sonographic classification. *J Clin Ultrasound.* 1988;16:531–544.)

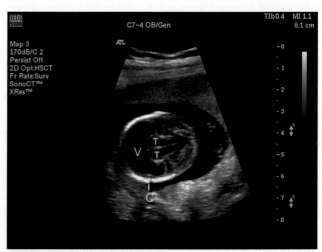

Figure 19-33 Alobar holoprosenceplaphaly demonstrating a single common ventricle (*V*), compressed cerebral cortex (*C*), and prominent thalamus (*T*). (Image courtesy of Philips Medical Systems, Bothell, WA.)

PATHOLOGY BOX 19-3

Sonographic Features of Holoprosencephaly

Alobar	Semilobar	Lobar
Single ventricle	Posterior partial separation of hemispheres and ventricles	Absence of septum pellucidum
Prominent fused thalami	Incomplete fusion of the thalami	Fusion of the frontal horns
Crescent-shaped frontal cortex	Rudimentary occipital horns	Variable fusion of the cingulated gyrus
Absent falx, corpus callosum, interhemispheric fissures	Microcephaly	DWC
Cyclopia		Enlarged posterior fossa
Median cleft lip		High tentorium
Hypotelorism		Upward displacement of the lateral sinuses
Ethmocephaly		Torcular heophili
Cebocephaly		Vermian aplasia or hypoplasia
Microcephaly		Cystic dilatation of the fourth ventricle
		Dandy-Walker variant
		Vermian hypoplasia
		Cystic dilation of the fourth ventricle
		Normal posterior fossa
		Mega cisterna magna
		Enlarged cisterna magna
		Normal cerebellar vermis and fourth ventricle
		Arachnoid cyst
		Anterior displacement of the fourth ventricle and cerebellum
		Signs of Arnold-Chiari malformation
		Cisterna magna absent
		Banana-shaped deformation of the cerebellum
		Lateral ventricular dilatation

---

and the nasal septum. Failure of these structures to develop normally can result in varying degrees of hypotelorism, CL and CP, and nasal malformation. Therefore, individuals with holoprosencephaly often have associated midline facial anomalies. Certain facial anomalies are characteristic of the alobar and semilobar types of holoprosencephaly and are rarely encountered in the lobar form. Cyclopia, the presence of a single median bony orbit with a fleshy proboscis above it, is the most severe malformation. In cebocephaly, hypotelorism is associated with a normally placed nose but with a single nostril. The diagnosis is also suggested by the presence of median cleft lip and microcephaly. The abnormally small head is usually present owing to decreased cortical mass, but macrocephaly may be seen if hydrocephalus develops.[36]

The prognosis of the holoprosencephalies depends largely on the form. The alobar forms of holoprosencephaly carry a poor prognosis. Recurrence rates increase with associated chromosomal abnormalities or autosomal recessive and, rarely, autosomal dominant genetic syndromes. The severe forms are usually associated with neonatal death. Some of the mildest forms (single front incisor) may have mild to moderate mental retardation and are at risk for pituitary dysfunction. Prognosis is also related to associated anomalies. Termination can be offered for the severe cases (semilobar, alobar). Cases diagnosed in utero with lobar holoprosencephaly have also had extremely poor neurologic development (Fig. 19-34).[36]

Agenesis of the Corpus Callosum

The corpus callosum is a large neural commissure connecting the two cerebral hemispheres. This structure begins development at about 12 weeks, originating from the lamina terminalis at the anterior portion of the third ventricle. This bundle of fibers connects the two hemispheres, developing from anterior to posterior. The two septi pellucidi and cavum septi pellucidi associate with the corpus callosum as development progresses.[5]

Agenesis of the corpus callosum (ACC) is a rare congenital disorder in which there is a complete or partial absence of the corpus callosum.[1,2] Development of this structure completes at about 20 weeks, making earlier diagnosis difficult.[5] It can occur as an isolated anomaly, but 80% of cases are associated with other anomalies such as trisomy 13 and 18, hydrocephalus,

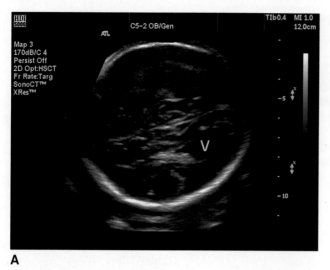

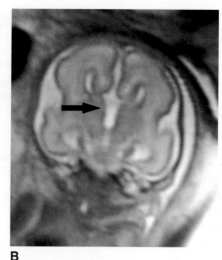

A   **B**

Figure 19-34 A: Axial view of the fetal brain demonstrating the characteristic teardrop shape of the ventricle *(V)* seen with agenesis of the corpus callosum. **B:** Coronal T2-weighted image through the brain at 19 weeks' gestation demonstrates agenesis of the corpus callosum and high-riding third ventricle. (Image **A** courtesy of Philips Medical Systems, Bothell, WA.)

Dandy-Walker complex, Arnold-Chiari malformation, and holoprosencephaly.[5] Aicardi syndrome is specific to females with ACC and results in mental retardation, seizures, spinal malformations, and retinal lesions. Multiple studies confirm the association with ACC and genetics, teratogens, schizophrenia, prematurity, and maternal age.[5,40-42]

Ultrasound diagnosis of ACC requires several planes of study. At the BPD level, the cavum septi pellucidi are absent and the third ventricle, now occupying the usual space of the cavum septi pellucidi, appears widened.

Because of the absence of the corpus callosum, the third ventricle rides high and may be visualized at the lateral ventricle level. There is disproportionate enlargement of the occipital horns, resulting in a characteristic teardrop appearance of the lateral ventricles (termed colpocephaly), which also display laterally displaced medial walls and widened atria (Fig. 19-35).[3] Endovaginal sonography has proved a useful adjunct to improve the diagnosis of complete or partial agenesis of the corpus callosum. The pathognomonic lesion is the "sunburst" lesion seen on midsagittal section, representing radial orientation of the

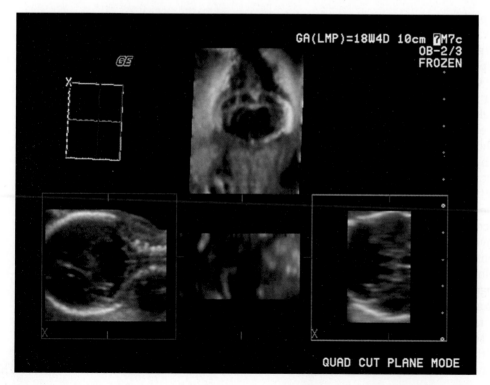

Figure 19-35 MPR images of the large posterior fossa seen with the Dandy-Walker malformation. (Image courtesy of GE Healthcare, Wauwatosa, WI.)

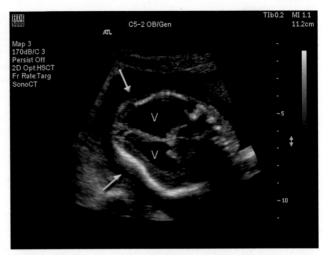

Figure 19-36 Frontal deformities (*arrows*) often referred to as the "lemon sign." *V,* ventricles. (Image courtesy of Philips Medical Systems, Bothell, WA.)

gyri and sulci to the third ventricle rather than paralleling the absent corpus callosum.[5] Certain ultrasound features may not be seen until late in gestation, therefore diagnosis cannot always be made at the usual time of anatomy scan (16 to 22 weeks of gestation).[3] Color Doppler imaging aids in confirming the abnormal course of the cingulated and pericallosal arteries.[3,5]

ACC is frequently a part of syndromes or multiple malformations, thus prognosis depends on associated anomalies. The isolated ACC child has a normal to borderline intellectual development[2,5] and may suffer from seizures as the only symptom.[2,3] Studies indicate a progressive decrease in intelligence and difficulties in school as the child matures.[3,39]

Dandy-Walker Malformation

The term Dandy-Walker complex (DWC) refers to a continuum of abnormalities of the posterior fossa that are distinct entities themselves—Dandy-Walker malformation, Dandy-Walker variant, and mega cisterna magna.[43] Differentiation between the malformations may not be possible with imaging studies. It is believed that the three categories of this malformation are a progression of developmental anomalies that are grouped under the term Dandy-Walker complex.[45] Dandy-Walker malformation, the most severe form, is a rare anomaly of the posterior fossa that consists of marked cystic dilatation of the fourth ventricle, which may fill much of the posterior fossa, complete or partial agenesis of cerebellar vermis, and elevated tentorium. Dandy-Walker variant is a less severe form referring to a partial agenesis of the vermis without a large dilated cystic fourth ventricle. Mega cisterna magna demonstrates a normal cerebellar vermis, and fourth ventricle.[43]

DWC abnormalities are a group of sporadic brain malformations that results from dysgenetic development of the roof of the rhombencephalon and not from a failure of formation of the outlets of the fourth ventricle, as was previously thought.[44] They can occur as an isolated finding or in association with a wide range of different malformations and genetic syndromes. There is a 1:3 male to female ratio. The prognosis depends on

the specific abnormality. As an isolated finding, mega cisterna magna carries a good prognosis with a high chance of normal neurodevelopmental outcome.[5,43] On the other hand, the majority of pregnancies with a Dandy-Walker malformation or Dandy-Walker variant end in termination. This is because fetuses with these abnormalities have poor outcomes, even as isolated findings.[43,44]

During the sonographic exam, obtaining images on the median plane begins the diagnostic process. Sagittal and coronal planes demonstrate the superior displacement of the cystic fourth ventricle, displacement of the frequently hypoplastic cerebellar vermis, and elevation of the tentorium above its normal position. The compressed cisterna becomes a potential space between the dilated fourth ventricle and the dura mater. The hypoplastic, anterolaterally displaced cerebellum images anterior to the large posterior fossa cyst. Hydrocephalus, although frequently seen in cases of Dandy-Walker malformation, is not necessary for the diagnosis (Fig. 19-36). There may also be spina bifida,[5] CL/CP,[3] and absence of the corpus

Normal Values (Mean ± SD) of the Cerebellar Vermis

Gestational Age	Anteroposterior Diameter (mm)	Superoinferior Diameter (mm)	Circumference (mm)	Area (cm²)
21–22	10.6 ± 1.4	11.1 ± 1.1	43.8 ± 3.3	0.9 ± 0.2
23–24	12.9 ± 1.1	12.3 ± 1.4	47.5 ± 5.5	1.2 ± 0.2
25–26	13.5 ± 2.1	13.6 ± 0.3	50.9 ± 4.4	1.4 ± 0.2
27–28	16.3 ± 2.7	13.0 ± 1.6	58.9 ± 6.8	2.0 ± 0.5
29–30	17.5 ± 2.2	17.7 ± 2.1	64.7 ± 6.5	2.3 ± 0.4
31–32	19.0 ± 1.9	19.2 ± 1.1	70.7 ± 6.9	2.8 ± 0.4
33–34	19.2 ± 1.9	21.2 ± 2.3	72.7 ± 8.3	3.0 ± 0.8
35–36	21.4 ± 1.5	19.8 ± 1.0	77.6 ± 5.1	3.4 ± 0.3
37–38	22.1 ± 3.8	23.0 ± 4.6	80.7 ± 9.9	3.9 ± 1.4
39–40	25.7 ± 2.3	25.0 ± 2.6	86.7 ± 7.0	4.9 ± 0.7

Adapted from Malinger G, Ginath S, Lerman-Sagie T, Watemberg N, Lev D, et al. The fetal cerebellar vermis: normal development as shown by transvaginal ultrasound. *Prenat Diagn.* 2001;21:687–692.

callosum,[46] to name a few of the congenital malformations accompanying the DWC.

Due to incomplete development of the posterior fossa, the diagnosis of a Dandy-Walker malformation occurs after 18 weeks' gestation.[3] Measurement of the posterior fossa from the posterior cerebellum to the anterior, internal portion of the skull is less than 10 mm in the normal fetal brain.[3,47] The cisterna magna size changes with gestational age, as indicated in Table 19-3. In a case of mega cisterna, the cerebellum measurement is greater than 10 mm; however, the ventricles measure within normal limits.[5]

Schizencephaly

Schizencephaly is a cerebral developmental disorder that involves disordered neuronal migration.[5] This results in unilateral and bilateral clefts in the cerebral hemisphere.[48] It is manifested on ultrasound by fluid-filled clefts that are lined by gray matter within the cerebral cortex. There is a strong association between absent cavum septum pellucidum and absence of corpus callosum with schizencephaly.[5,48]

Lissencephaly

Lissencephaly is a rare cortical dysplasia that results from impaired neuronal migration during the 12th and 16th weeks of gestation.[52] Failure of neuronal migration into the cerebral cortex results in a broad spectrum of anomalies. Depending on the point in gestation at which the disruption takes place, the fetal cortex can completely lack sulci and gyri (lissencephaly),[5] can have very few gyri (pachygyria),[5,34] or have very small gyri (microgyria).[35] The migrational process may be arrested by environmental factors (ischemia, teratogens), but a genetic predisposition is clearly present at least for some anomalies.[1]

An absence or paucity of gyri results in the characteristic smooth cerebral surface seen with lissencephaly. Other cranial and noncranial abnormalities may also occur in association with lissencephaly. The prognosis is often poor and is manifested by mental retardation, seizures, and often death in infancy or early childhood.[49] Other cranial and extracranial abnormalities also may occur in association with lissencephaly such as minimal or no hydrocephalus, a wide cortical mantle, and characteristic dysmorphic features.[50]

Sulci remain smooth until about 20 weeks' gestation, making sonographic diagnosis difficult in the first half of pregnancy.[50,52] Because of the lack of opercularization of the insulate, diagnosticians assumed that abnormalities of sulcal development could not be diagnosed until the seventh month.[1,5] The earliest gestational ages at which specific sulci could be seen in all fetuses ranged from 18.5 to 27.9 weeks' gestation.[1,51]

The inability to identify sulcations beyond 28 weeks raises concern.[1,5,51] In the third trimester, the occurrence of polyhydramnios associated with IUGR is an expected finding. Facial dysmorphism is characterized by prominent foreheard, short nose, broad and flat nasal bridge, and protuberant upper lip. It is associated with duodenal atresia, urinary tract abnormalities, congenital heart defects, cryptorchidism, inguinal hernia, clinodactyly, and ear anomalies.[5,50]

The prognosis is poor and usually involves severe mental retardation, failure to thrive, infantile spasms, and seizures; death occurs usually within the first 2 to 6 years of life.[5] Since the ultrasound diagnosis is not usually made until the third trimester, termination is not an option. Standard prenatal care is not altered.[50]

HERNIATION THROUGH A STRUCTURAL DEFECT

Cephalocele/Encephalocele

Cephaloceles are protrusions of the meninges and frequently of brain substance through a defect in the cranium.[1] The term encephalocele describes a lesion containing brain tissue. A cranial meningocele is the protrusion of the meninges only through the defect. Occipital lesions make up 80% of cephaloceles in Caucasians of European descent.[1,3] The frontoethmoidal region is the common location for cephaloceles in southeastern Asia populations.[1] The least common form, parietal cephaloceles, occur with significant underlying brain abnormalities.[1]

Although cephaloceles usually result from a defect in neural tube closure, and thus are isolated abnormalities, they may also occur as part of a genetic or nongenetic syndrome. They may be seen in the amniotic band syndrome or in association with various malformation syndromes (i.e., amniotic band, cerebellar dysgenesis, cryptophthalmos, syndrome, Meckel syndrome, etc.).[3]

Sonographically, a cephalocele appears as a paracranial mass not covered with bone.[1] Imaging a skull defect is the only method to definitively diagnose a cephalocele. However, visualization of a small defect may be difficult. In the presence of a defect, determination of the position is achieved through the use of the bony structures of the face and spine, and through identification of brain anatomy. Microcephaly results when a large portion of the brain extrudes through a defect.[3] Hydrocephalus develops because of impaired cerebrospinal fluid circulation.[23] When brain tissue herniates, the result is a saclike complex mass due to the contained solid brain tissue. Ultrasound has not been particularly reliable in differentiating between meningoceles and encephaloceles when there is only a small amount of contained brain tissue.

Routine sonography, occasionally aided by endovaginal technique, must attempt to differentiate cephaloceles from such simulators as cystic hygroma, hemangiomas, teratomas, and branchial cleft cysts.[3] Indirect clues can assist the diagnosis. Cranial cephaloceles are very often associated with ventriculomegaly. Furthermore, cystic hygromas arise from the region of the neck, have multiple internal septations and a thick wall, and are often associated with generalized soft tissue edema and hydrops.[5] Encephaloceles, in general, carry a poor prognosis. Pure meningoceles may have a more favorable prognosis.

Iniencephaly

Iniencephaly is a rare anomaly in which there is a defect in the occiput of the cranium involving the foramen magnum with marked retroflexion of the fetal head and frequently a shortened spine. This malformation occurs at approximately the third week of gestation, the same time as the anencephalic and included rachischisis of the cervical and thoracic spine.[3] Diagnosis is based on visualization of the markedly retroflexed neck, such that the cranium may still be viewed during transverse scanning of the fetal thorax, and on an inability to visualize the entire spine.[3] Other associated anomalies include hydrocephalus, encephalocele, diaphragmatic hernia, and omphalocele.[3]

Arnold-Chiari Malformations

The Arnold-Chiari malformations are a group of anomalies of the hindbrain prolapsing below the level of the foramen magnum. The incidence is about 1 in 1,000 births and often has accompanying spina bifida with meningomyelocele or myeloschisis, and hydrocepehaly.[2]

There are four types of Arnold-Chiari malformations. Usually an incidental computed tomography finding, type I is a mild form where the cerebellar tonsils displace more than 4 mm into the foramen magna and the posterior fossa contains the fourth ventricle.[52] Type II is a congenital deformity characterized by displacement of cerebellar tonsils, parts of the cerebellum, fourth ventricle, pons, and medulla oblongata through the foramen magnum into the spinal canal.[52] Hydrocephalus and myelomeningoceles accompany the type II malformation in over 90% of cases.[52,53] Type III is the most severe form and is associated with large herniation of the posterior fossa contents with myelomeningocele and hydrocephalus.[57] The most important of these is the Chiari type II malformation, which is rarely found without the accompanying spina bifida.[52,57] Type IV accompanies the hypoplastic cerebellum with further herniation of the brain into the spinal canal.[78]

On ultrasound, Chiari type II has a variable displacement of a tongue of tissue derived from the inferior cerebellar vermis into the upper cervical spinal canal. Displacement of the cerebellum inferiorly changes its shape and effaces the cisterna magna, thereby producing the characteristic sonographic finding, the "banana sign."[52] This refers to the flattened, centrally curved, bananalike appearance of the cerebellar hemispheres. There is a similar caudal displacement of the medulla and fourth ventricle. In extreme cases, the cerebellar hemispheres may be absent from view during fetal head scanning.

The cranial findings associated with the Chiari II malformation are found exclusively in fetuses with myelomeningocele.[3] Therefore, identification of features of the Chiari II malformation virtually ensures the presence of a myelomeningocele. Although the dominant features of the Chiari II malformation relate to the hindbrain, many supratentorial abnormalities have also been described. Included in these are callosal dysgenesis, a small third ventricle, enlarged interthalamic adhesions, a "beaked" tectum, polymicrogyria, heterotopias, skull deformities (the "lemon" sign),[3] colpocephaly, and other causes of ventriculomegaly (Fig. 19-37).[56] Important among these is ventriculomegaly, because visualization of the lateral ventricle is required on all routine sonograms. However, ventriculomegaly is considerably less common before 24 weeks than after 24 weeks in fetuses affected with myelomeningocele.[56] Therefore, supratentorial abnormalities are also important in the prenatal recognition that myelomeningocele is present. A major sign that has been discussed is the "lemon sign." During the second trimester, a scalloping of the frontal bones can be seen in axial section of the head, giving a lemonlike configuration to the skull of an affected fetus.[53] The caudal displacement of the cranial

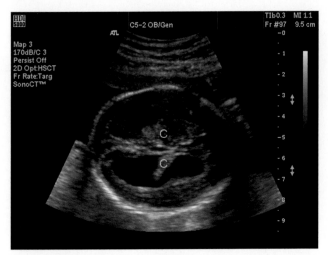

Figure 19-37 Enlarged ventricles allow the choroid to move toward the dependent portion of the brain, resulting in a "dangling choroid." *C,* choroid. (Image courtesy of Philips Medical Systems, Bothell, WA.)

contents within the pliable fetal skull is thought to produce this scalloping effect. However, the lemon sign is frequently not present in later pregnancies and can be seen in healthy fetuses and in other conditions.[3,53,56] Callen et al. have also described an abnormality in the shape of the occipital horn in fetuses with myelomeningocele as having a pointed contour instead of the normal rounded contour.[56]

Dilatation Behind an Obstruction

Ventriculomegaly and Hydrocephalus

Ventriculomegaly, an abnormal increase in the volume of the cerebral ventricles, has many different causes and is a nonspecific finding.[1] Ventriculomegaly may be caused by intraventricular or extraventricular obstruction, a relative decrease in the amount of brain substance, or, rarely, an increase in cerebrospinal fluid production. The term hydrocephalus describes ventriculomegaly, with increased intracranial pressure and head size.[5] Hydrocephalus is frequently associated with spina bifida.[3]

Although an abnormally increased head circumference or BPD may suggest the diagnosis of ventriculomegaly, examination of the intracranial contents is necessary for accurate diagnosis. Enlargement of the ventricles and cerebrospinal fluid displacement of the choroid plexus results in a process termed the "dangling choroid plexus." This choroid plexus displacement within the enlarged lateral ventricle precedes cranial enlargement and is encountered with many different cerebral anomalies.[3] To determine normalcy of the ventricle, sonographers obtain measurements of the internal width of the atrium of the lateral ventricle at the level of the choroid plexus glomus.[3,5] Normally, the measurement is less than 10 mm; a value between 10 to 15 is considered mild ventriculomegaly. Severe ventriculomegaly measures greater than 15 mm and is often associated with intracranial malformations.[5,58] An alternate delineation has classified mild as 10 to 12 mm and moderate as 12.1 to 15 mm. This is due to the poor outcome for ventricles measuring greater than 12 mm.[1,3,59]

Aqueductal stenosis, a congenital obstruction to flow of cerebrospinal fluid through the aqueduct of Sylvius connecting the third and fourth ventricles, accounts for 43% of cases, communicating hydrocephalus accounts for 38%, and Dandy-Walker malformations accounts for 13%.[5] Other causes include agenesis of the corpus callosum, arachnoid cysts, and arteriovenous malformations such as a vein of Galen aneurysm.[1] Ventriculomegaly is also known to be associated with chromosome disorders and intrauterine infections.[58]

Cystic Hygroma

Fetal lymphatic vessels normally drain into two large sacs lateral to the jugular veins. If these jugular lymph sacs fail to communicate with the venous system, they may enlarge as they fill with lymph and form cystic hygromas.[2,15] This failure in lymphatic drainage may accompany hydrops fetalis, resulting in a process called lymphangiectasia.[63]

PATHOLOGY BOX 19-6

Sonographic Features of Arnold-Chiari Malformations

Type I	Type II	Type III	Type IV
Displacement of cerebellar tonsils more than 4 mm into the foramen magna	Inferior displacement of the cerebellar tonsils, fourth ventricle, pons and medulla oblongata through the foramen magnum into the spinal canal. Displacement of the cerebellum results in the banana sign. Lemon sign Myelomeningocele	Large herniation of posterior fossa contents into the foramen magnum, myelomeningocele, hydrocephalus	Cerebellar hypoplasia with further herniation into the spinal canal

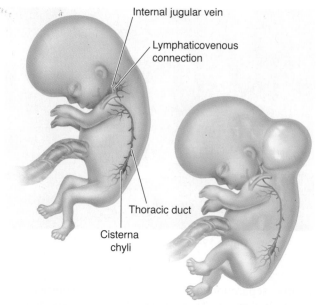

Internal jugular vein

Lymphaticovenous connection

Thoracic duct

Cisterna chyli

Figure 19-38 Schematic representation of the lymphatic drainage system in the normal fetus *(left)* and the failed lymphaticovenous connection in cystic hygroma *(right)*. (Chervenak FA, Isaacson G, Blakemore KJ, et al. Fetal cystic hygroma: cause and natural history. *N Engl J Med.* 1983;309:822.)

Cystic hygromas appear as either single or multiloculated fluid-filled cavities. The most common location is in the lateral neck region, but they can be seen in the chest, axilla, and other areas (Fig. 19-38).[15]

There is an association between cystic hygromas and many chromosomal anomalies and anatomic defects. Autosomal trisomies and trisomy 21 demonstrate an increased incidence of hygromas in the first trimester.[15,62] By midpregnancy, Turner syndrome is the predominant finding.[15,60,63] The large veins linked to the development of cystic hygromas are due to the increased volume of blood flow resulting from the lack of lymphatic drainage. This results in a high incidence of flow-related cardiac defects[3] related to lymphatic distension of the aorta in the ascending portion.[61] Associated nonimmune hydrops manifests sonographically as ascites, pleural effusion, pericardial effusion, and skin edema.[63]

Several sonographic features aid in the diagnosis of fetal cystic hygromas. Hygromas are usually located on the posterolateral neck and have a cystic appearance, and they frequently demonstrate random septa.[15] A midline septum represents the nuchal ligament, which forms between the paired jugular lymph sacs (Fig. 19-39).[15]

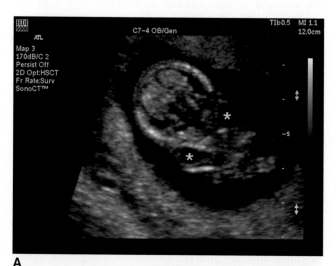

A

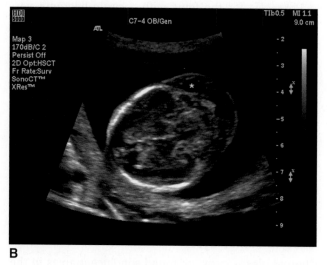

B

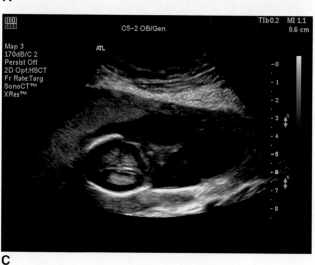

C

Figure 19-39 Cystic hygromas. **A:** Cystic hygromas *(star)* imaged on the lateral neck in a late first trimester exam. **B:** Small unilateral hygroma *(star)* within the nuchal fold in a second trimester fetus. **C:** Large cystic hygroma demonstrating a midline septum. (Images courtesy of Philips Medical Systems, Bothell, WA.)

TABLE 19-4	
Sonographic Comparison of a Cystic Hygroma and a Cephalocele	
Cephalocele	**Cystic hygroma**
Complex paracranial mass	Cystic mass with septa
No bone coverage	Located posterolateral neck region
May demonstrate microcephaly	Nuchal ligament forms midline segment
Hydrocephalus	

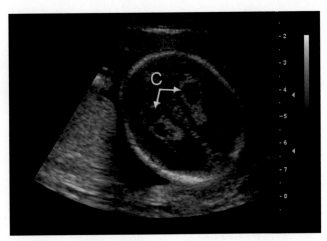

Figure 19-40 Choroid plexus cysts (C).

Within the cystic structure, thinner septa probably represent fibrous structures of the neck and deposits of fibrin, resulting in the typical honeycomb appearance. Most cases seen in the second trimester have decreased amounts of amniotic fluid (oligohydramnios), and a few have either normal fluid or polyhydramnios.[15] Hygroma sizes vary greatly from small collections of fluid to enormous cysts larger than the fetus. Other craniocervical masses that must be differentiated from cystic hygromas include cystic teratomas, cephalocele, hemangioma, branchial cleft cyst, and nuchal edema (Table 19-4).[15]

Prognosis for the fetus with a cystic hygroma varies depending on gestational age, association with hydrops, and coexisting anomalies. The fatal combination of a hygroma with nonimmune hydrops has a strong association with abnormal karyotypes, resulting in a midgestation mortality rate close to 100%.[23,60] In the case of an isolated hygroma, the fetus may have a good outcome. The redevelopment or drainage of the lymphatic channels into the venous system results in reabsorbtion of the fluid collections, with the redundant skin becoming the webbed neck seen in many genetic and nongenetic conditions such as Turner syndrome.[3]

PRESENCE OF AN ADDITIONAL STRUCTURE

Choroid Plexus Cysts

Choroid plexus cysts are round sonolucent areas in the substance of the choroid plexus of the lateral ventricles (Fig. 19-40). They are noted in 1% to 6% of all fetuses and are usually transient and without clinical significance, resolving before the end of the second trimester without sequelae.[5] These cysts have an association with trisomy 18 and other karyotypic abnormalities.[3,5] Many of these fetuses may have other structural anomalies.

Choroid plexus cysts develop in one or both choroids and may be multiple. Typically, the cysts develop within the atria of the lateral ventricles in the normal fetal brain. To classify the rounded, anechoic area as a choroid plexus cyst the area must measure greater than 2 mm.[1,5] It can be difficult to differentiate a large choroid plexus cyst slightly distending the cavity of a ventricle from primary ventriculomegaly. When this

occurs, separation of the cyst from the ventricle becomes important. These choroid plexus cysts demonstrate internal septations and echogenic thick walls.[1]

Porencephaly/Porencephalic Cysts

Porencephaly is a destructive lesion of the brain that appears as one or several hypoechoic, cystic areas in the cerebral cortex, usually communicating with the ventricle, believed to be related to an in utero ischemic event.[1] Though uncommon, multiple pregnancy fetuses have a greater chance of developing porencephaly.[3] It is thought that areas of prior intracranial hemorrhage or tissue necrosis resorb, leaving behind porencephalic cysts. This bilateral, symmetric process usually occurs only in the third trimester and is frequently associated with microcephaly.[1] Studies indicate that congenital infections, intrauterine narrowing, and internal carotid artery and middle cerebral artery occlusion are causative factors in the development of porencephaly.[1,3]

Intracranial Hemorrhage

Intracranial hemorrhage (ICH) refers to bleeding anywhere in the fetal cranium and may be described as a germinal matrix, interventricular or intraparenchymal hemorrhage, or a subdural hematoma.[3] An interventricular hemorrhage is the most common type seen in the fetus. Most frequently seen in the preterm and term neonate 48 to 72 hours after birth, it may occur antenatally as a consequence of coagulopathy, amniocentesis, drug use, trauma, or other unexplained factors.[1,3]

Hemorrhage into the ventricles usually originates in the germinal matrix because of the thin-walled vessels within the matrix. Classification of the bleed uses four grades to describe the location and severity of the hemorrhage (Fig. 19-41). Use of this nomenclature defines a hemorrhage in either the fetus or neonate.

To ensure accurate imaging of the fetal head, begin with a symmetric, nonangled view of the head on an axial plane. The normal choroid plexus imaged on an asymmetric plane may result in simulation of a

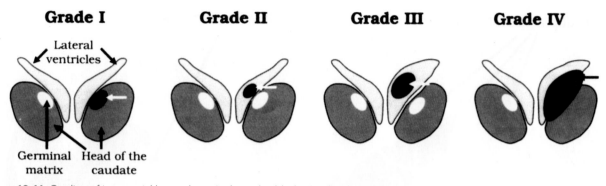

Figure 19-41 Grading of intracranial hemorrhage (indicated in black). Grade I, hemorrhage remains confined to the germinal matrix *(arrow)*; grade II is an intraventricular hemorrhage *(arrow)*; grade III is an intraventricular hemorrhage *(arrow)* and ventricular dilatation; and grade IV represents extension of the hemorrhage into the brain parenchyma *(arrow)*. (Modified from Malinger G, Katz R, Amsel S, Gewurtz G, Zakut H. Brain hemorrhage, germinal matrix. *The Fetus.* 1992;1:1–4.)

germinal matrix hemorrhage. Sonographic diagnosis of ICH varies, depending on the location, severity, and clot age. The acute hemorrhage has a similar echogenicity to the choroid plexus, making separation of the structures difficult.[3] As the clot begins to resolve, the sonographic appearance changes to a retracted hypoechoic mass with an anechoic core. This grade III hemorrhage has an increased incidence of ventricular dilatation.[1,3] In the grade IV hemorrhage, infarcts and white matter destruction complicates diagnosis.[1] This process may develop into a porencephalic cyst or hydranencephaly.[3] Doppler sampling of the middle cerebral artery with a grade IV hemorrhage demonstrates reverse diastolic flow. A typical antenatal hemorrhage is usually seen as a hyperechogenic mass in the region of the germinal matrix or within the lateral ventricles (Fig. 19-42).

Aneurysm of the Vein of Galen

The vein of Galen aneurysm describes three types of cerebral arteriovenous malformations (AVMs). The initial finding is the isolated AVM, a secondary

finding includes the AVM with vein of Galen Ectasia, with the third as a varix of the vein.[1] Imaging an elongated cystic structure at the level of the cistern of the vein of Galen in the third trimester represents the dilated, end-to-end arteries and veins without intervening capillaries (Fig. 19-43).[1,3] Doppler studies demonstrate the characteristic turbulent venous and arterial blood flow through the structure.[1,3] Increased intracranial blood flow due to the artriovenous malformation results in enlargement of the dural sinus and neck vessels. (Fig. 19-44).[1,3,5] This may lead to cardiac overload; therefore cardiomegaly, hepatosplenomegaly, soft tissue edema, polyhydramnios, and nonimmune hydrops may be present in the affected fetus.[1,5,65]

Prognosis is poor for these fetuses, resulting in a high neonatal mortality rate due to heart failure.[1,5] The outcome depends on associated anomalies and the extent of the AVM.

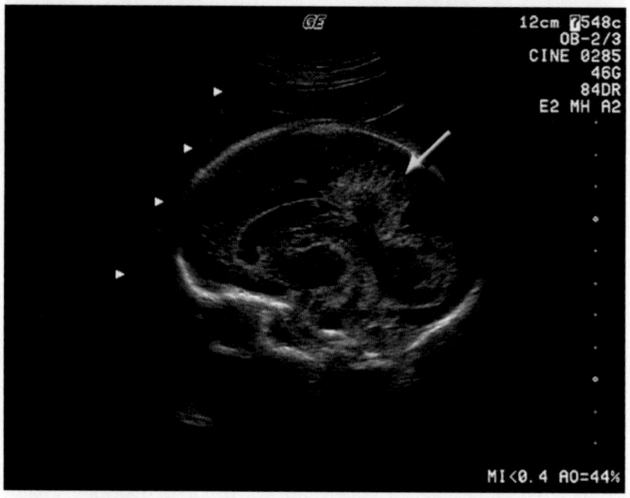

FETAL SPINE

EMBRYOLOGY OF THE SPINE

The central nervous system begins as the neural tube in the embryo. Infolding of the slipper-shaped ectoderm of the neural plate during the third week of embryonic life forms the neural tube (Fig. 19-45).[2] The neural groove fuses to form the neural tube beginning at midembryo and completing at the cranial and caudal neuropore. Any disruption of this 2-day process[2] by infections, drugs, or genetic factors results in closure failure at either end of the neural tube, demonstrating the connection between spinal bifida and caudal defects.[3] If the neural tube fails to fuse, spina bifida with myeloschisis develops.[1,2,3]

Approximately a month after a missed period, the spine begins mineralization.[3] The centrum (vertebral body) and dorsum centers/neural processes form laterally. The transverse, spinous, and articular processes develop from the neural processes, creating the posterior bony structures of the spine.[2] This process, which

Figure 19-42 Sagittal image of 34-week fetus with an intracranial hemorrhage *(arrow)*. (Image courtesy of GE Healthcare, Wauwatosa, WI.)

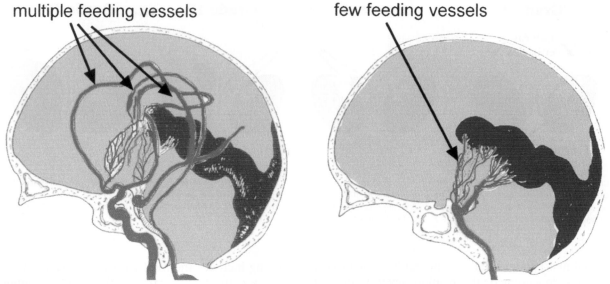

A   **B**

Figure 19-43 Vein of Galen malformation. The vein of Galen malformation comprises in reality a spectrum of vascular anomalies sharing a common dilatation of the vein of Galen. **A:** In the most severe and complicated form, a complex AVM with multiple anomalous arterial vessels arises from the circle of Willis. This condition results in significant vascular compromise, with a steal of blood from the cortex, infarction, hemorrhage, and high-output cardiac failure manifested during fetal life. **B:** Dilatation of the vein of Galen with few arterial vessels occurs in the simplest form. This condition is unlikely to cause vascular compromise and may become symptomatic (excessive head growth, headache) only postnatally. (Adapted from Mori. *Neuroradiology and Neurosurgery.* New York. New York: Theime-Stratton, 1985.)

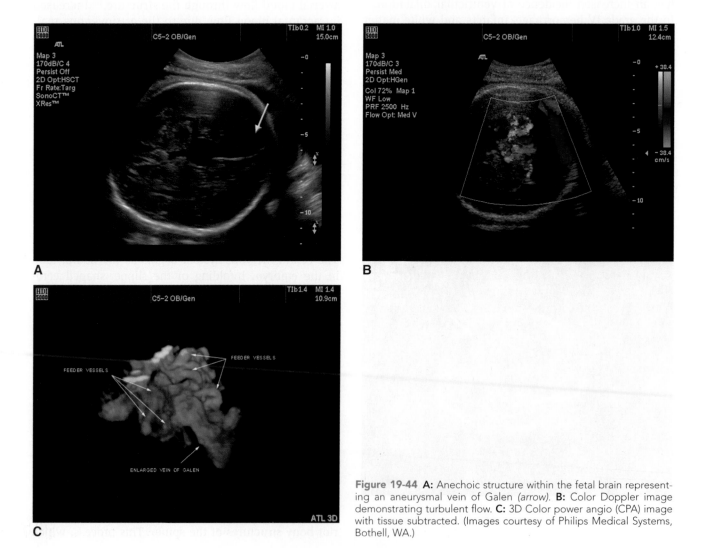

Figure 19-44 A: Anechoic structure within the fetal brain representing an aneurysmal vein of Galen *(arrow).* **B:** Color Doppler image demonstrating turbulent flow. **C:** 3D Color power angio (CPA) image with tissue subtracted. (Images courtesy of Philips Medical Systems, Bothell, WA.)

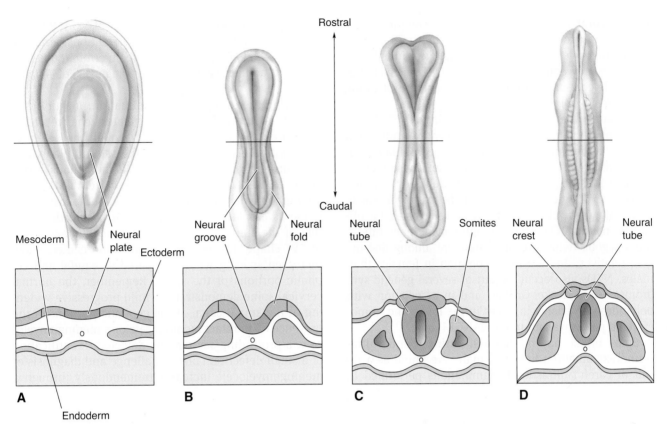

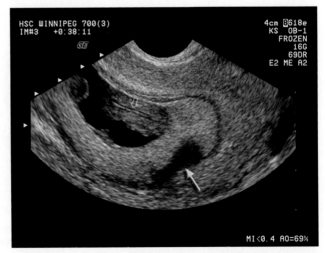

Figure 19-45 Formation of the neural tube and neural crest. These schematic illustrations follow the early development of the nervous system in the embryo. The drawings above are dorsal views of the embryo; those below are cross-sections. **A:** The primitive embryonic central nervous system (CNS) begins as a thin sheet of ectoderm. **B:** The first important step in the development of the nervous system is the formation of the neural groove. **C:** The walls of the groove, called neural folds, come together and fuse, forming the neural tube. **D:** The bits of neural ectoderm that are pinched off when the tube rolls up are called the neural crest, from which the PNS will develop. The somites are mesoderm that will give rise to much of the skeletal system and the muscles.

begins at 13 weeks and completes in the third trimester, explains the development mechanism that fails resulting in spina bifida.[3]

THE ABNORMAL SPINE

Spina Bifida

Spina bifida is a neural tube defect resulting from incomplete closure of the bony elements of the spine (lamina and spinous processes) posteriorly. Two types of lesions, ventral and dorsal, occur. The ventral defect involves vertebral body splitting and development of a neurogenic origin cystic structure.[3] These lesions occur higher in the spine at the lower cervical and upper thoracic spine and are quite uncommon.[3]

The dorsal types of spina bifida have subdivisions of open (defect not covered by skin) and closed (defect covered by skin) forms. Closed spina bifida, or spina bifida occulta, has the split vertebrae covered by skin.[1,3] Spina bifida occulta is the simplest form, in which there is a failure of the dorsal portions of the vertebrae to fuse with one another.[2] The expected location of this abnormality is at the sacrolumbar level. It has a skin covering and is not noticeable on the surface, except for the presence of a small tuft of hair

or other dermal lesion over the affected area.[2,3] It is usually an incidental radiologic finding that is without consequence (Fig. 19-46).[66]

Open spina bifida, or spina bifida aperta, is a full-thickness defect of the skin, underlying soft tissues,

Figure 19-46 The neural tube at 8 weeks (*open arrow*). Formation of the neural structures is complete at approximately 32 days (Carnegie stage 13). Note the subchorionic hemorrhage (*arrow*). (Sonographic image courtesy of GE Healthcare, Wauwatosa, WI.)

and vertebral arches—thus exposing the neural canal.[3] This lesion occurs in 85%[3] of all spina bifida cases. The menigocele lesion has a thin menigeal membrane that does not contain neural tissue.[3] The myelomeningocele contains neural tissue inside the protruding sac. (Fig. 19-47)[2,3]

Although the causative mechanism of NTDs remains poorly understood, genetic factors, nutritional factors, environmental factors, or a combination of these are known to play a definite role. These include diabetes mellitus, obesity, and folate deficiency, among others.[67,68] The genetic factors in the pathogenesis of NTDs are not well defined but are suggested by observations that NTDs have a high concordance rate in monozygotic twins, are more frequent among first-degree relatives, and are more common in females than males. NTDs also occur as part of several genetic syndromes (e.g., Meckel-Gruber) and in association with polymorphic variants in genes in the folate and homocysteine pathways and in the VANGL1 gene.[67,68]

Spina bifida may be detected during routine ultrasound examination; however, many are found as a result of careful ultrasound examinations performed in

pregnancies found to have elevations of MSAFP levels. Because MSAFP elevates in other conditions, amniotic fluid AFP and acetylcholinesterase determinations may have an adjunctive role in the diagnosis of smaller lesions.[70]

During the sonographic examination, location and severity of the defect has the greatest chance of detection on the sagittal views.[1] Although the defect of spina bifida visualizes well on the sagittal plane, ruling out smaller defects requires a meticulous transverse examination of the entire vertebral column. Sonographically, spina bifida images on the transverse plane as a splaying of the posterior ossification centers of the spine, giving the vertebral segment a "U" or "V" shape. The posterior ossification centers show increased spacing when compared to caudal and cephalic portions of the spine. Remember, the normal cervical spine demonstrates a mild progressive widening of the spinal canal at the cephalic portion. In the presence of an intact meningocele or a meningomyelocele, a protruding sac may be detected. Identification of a small defect remains a challenge and diagnosis of meningomyelocele increases tremendously through a

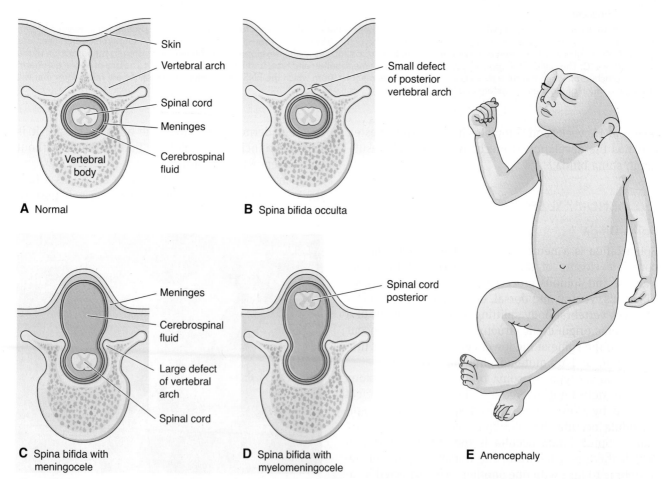

Figure 19-47 Neural tube defects. Cross-section studies of spine. **A:** Normal vertebra and spinal cord. **B:** In occult (minimal) spina bifida (spina bifida occulta) the posterior vertebral arch fails to form. It is usually asymptomatic. **C:** In spina bifida with meningocele, the meninges protrude through the defect. **D:** In spina bifida with myelomeningocele, the meninges and spinal cord protrude through the defect. **E:** In anencephaly, almost all of the brain and spinal cord fail to form.

nearly 100% association with the Arnold-Chiari malformation. Viewing of the actual meningomyelocele, however, is the only definitive way to make a diagnosis (Fig. 19-48).[3]

Examination of the fetal head aids in diagnosis of open spina bifida because of the associated cranial abnormalities. Displacement of cranial structures (cerebellar cermis, fourth ventricle, medulla oblongata) into the foramen magnum and the superior cervical canal is due to cerebrospinal fluid leakage (see section on Chiari type II).[1,3] Sonographically, this results in the characteristic findings of myelomeningocele—the "banana sign" and front "lemon sign."[1,3] The observation of a normal appearance of the cerebellum and cisterna magna virtually excludes a myelomeningocele.[3] Second-trimester

hydrocephalus occurs in 70% of cases[1,2] and in all neonates with spina bifida aperta.[1] Quite often these fetuses also demonstrate bilateral club feet, rocker bottom feet, and hip deformities.[3]

Normal brain anatomy and AFP result in low prenatal diagnosis of a closed spina bifida.[1,3] With the finding of a meningocele or lipoma, the presence of spina bifida occulta becomes suspect.[1,3] The differentiation between open and closed forms is best shown by the sonographic demonstration of abnormal or normal cranial anatomy.[3]

The prognosis for spina bifida depends on the level of the lesion. There is a high association with stillbirths, and a fifth of live-born infants die in the first year.[3] Within another 4 years, 35% die. If the child lives beyond the age of 5, there is a chance of mental

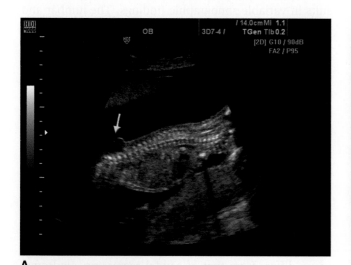

A

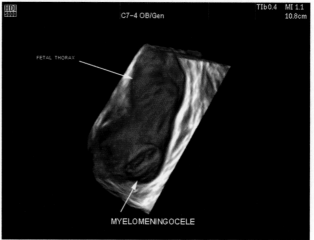

B

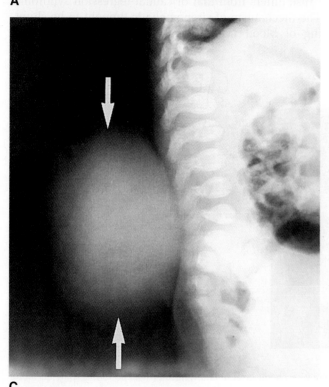

C

Figure 19-48 A: Sagittal image demonstrating a meningomyelocele *(arrow)* in the sacral region. **B:** 3D surface rendering of a sacral defect. **C:** Spina bifida vera with myelomeningocele. Lateral lumbar spine. Note the large myelomeningocele posterior to the lower lumbar spine and upper sacral area *(arrows).* (Images **A** and **B** courtesy of Philips Medical Systems, Bothell, WA.)

retardation, paralyzed limbs, lower limb dysfunction. bowel and bladder dysfunction, inability to walk, and complications due to associated hydrocephalus.[3]

Scoliosis and Kyphosis

Congenital scoliosis is an abnormal lateral curvature of the spine[5] due to anomalous development of the vertebrae, either failure of formation or segmentation. Congenital scoliosis can be associated with various cardiac, genitourinary, and skeletal abnormalities.[71] An abnormal anterior angulation of the spine is called kyphosis.[3,5] Kyphoscoliosis is the combination of the abnormal lateral and anterior curvature. Identification of scoliosis and kyphosis becomes plane dependent because of the spinal curvature. Longitudinal images demonstrate the spine well with scoliosis imaging from the lateral plane and kyphosis from the posterior plane.[5]

Scoliosis, which may also be seen with hemivertebrae,[53,71] meningomyelocele,[3] and multiple other syndromes and malformations, may occur as an isolated defect of the spine. Hemivertebrae, caused by aplasia or dysgenesis of one of the two chondrification centers forming the vertebral bodies, identify sonographically by lateral displacement of the anterior ossification centers or improperly aligned vertebral bodies (Fig. 19-49).[53] These may occur as an isolated entity but are more often seen in association with neural tube defects. In the absence of other anomalies, bends in the vertebral column should reach the extreme of 90 degrees and should be unchanging in serial scans.

Caudal Regression Syndrome

Caudal regression syndrome is a broad term that refers to a heterogeneous group of congenital anomalies affecting the caudal spine and spinal cord, the hindgut, the urogenital system, and the lower limbs. It can range from agenesis of the coccyx to absence of sacral, lumbar, and lower thoracic vertebrae. In the general population, the incidence is less than 1 in 10,000 births; however, a diabetic mother increases the risk by 250 times.[37,52] Other abdominal wall, genitourinary, and cardiac anomalies may also be found.

Disruption of the embryonic process of canalization in the third week of gestation results in the varying degrees of caudal regression. In the normal embryo the conus, filum terminale, sacral nerve roots, and lower genitourinary structures originate from the caudal mesoderm. The disruption of this normal development occurs with a genetic component, or in insulin-dependent mothers.[55]

The severity and extent of the caudal regression results in variable sonographic findings. The lumbar and sacral spine may have isolated anomalies or coexist with clubbed feet and knee and hip contractures. Typically, the sagittal and transverse views of the spine uncover vertebral absence, fused iliac wings, decreased femoral head distance, short femurs, and club feet.[52,53] Because of the lack of spine, and thus, the nerves, lower extremity movement decreases. Associated anomalies include renal and gastrointestinal anomalies.[53] During the first trimester, a short crown-rump length and an abnormal yolk sac has been found to indicate the presence of this syndrome.[52]

Sirenomelia, the main differential for caudal regression syndrome, was once considered a severe form.[55] Increased understanding of this malformation has led sirenomelia to receive a unique classification, as the cause differs from that of caudal regression syndrome. The mechanism of sirenomelia is thought to be shunting of blood from the aorta through the umbilical

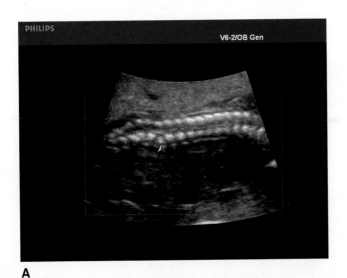

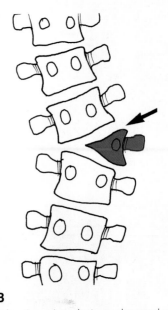

A   B

Figure 19-49 Sagittal image taken from a 3D data set of the spine. The unfused hemivertebra *(arrow)* results in an abnormal spine curvature called scoliosis. (Image courtesy of Philips Medical Systems, Bothell, WA.)

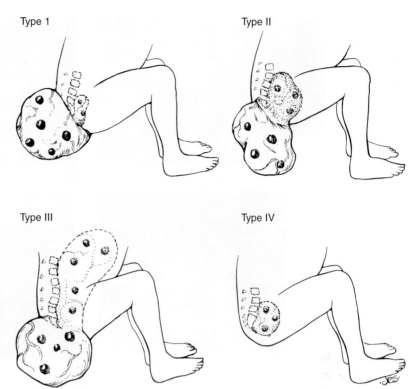

Type 1   Type II

Type III   Type IV

Figure 19-50 Types of sacrococcygeal teratomas. Sacrococcygeal teratomas may be almost entirely external or combined internal and external, or, as in type III, mainly internal. Those that are mainly external are less commonly malignant, whereas type IV tumors, which are mainly internal, usually have a delayed diagnosis and often are malignant. (Reproduced with permission from Altman RP, et al. *Sacrococcygeal teratomas.* American Academy of Pediatrics Surgical Section Survey, 1973.)

artery, resulting in a vascular steal.[55] The main finding for sirenomelia, or mermaid syndrome, is the fusion of the legs.[52]

Sacrococcygeal Teratoma

In the fetus, teratomas develop in the gonads,[53] umbilical cord,[3] placenta,[72] or anywhere on the neural tube, with the caudal end (sacrococcygeal) the most common location.[53] Arising from the presacral area of the spine, this rare germ cell tumor has an occurrence rate of 1 in 40,000; however, it is the most common neoplasm in the newborn.[53] Seventy-five percent of affected infants are female,[3,53] with male fetuses having an increased incidence of developing the malignant form.[3] The American Academy of Pediatric Surgery classification separates the masses on the contents, and the internal or external location of the tumor (Fig. 19-50). Most sacrococcygeal teratomas are Type I or II.

The origin of a sacrococcygeal tumor is unclear but the neoplasm is thought to be a remnant of the primitive streak leading to the inclusion of various embryonic tissue types within the tumor.[2] The germ layers—ectoderm, mesoderm, and endoderm—result in neural, gastrointestinal, and respiratory tissue within the neoplasm.[2,5] The location of teratomas depends on the cells from which they originate.[74] In the case of the sacrococcygeal tumor, the pluripotent tissue derived from the area around Hensen's node migrates rostrally to lie in the coccyx.[3,74] Other authors have suggested the teratoma is the result of failed twinning.[3,74]

On ultrasound, the tumor mass images as a protrusion between the anus and the coccyx, although some tumors develop in the presacral space of the pelvis. The sagittal plane images the masses extending from the spine. Tumors may be solid or complex with cystic components.[53] The choroid plexus tissue secretes the cerebrospinal fluid contained within the tumor mass, resulting in a cystic component (Fig. 19-51). Prenatally, these fetuses are at risk of developing congestive heart failure and hydrops which is thought to be due to vascular arterial-venous shunting within the mass.[53,73] Color and power Doppler demonstrate this vascularity within the solid teratoma.[3]

3DUS has also been used in the prenatal assessment of sacrococcygeal tumors. As an adjunct to 2D sonography, 3D imaging increases visualization of the skeleton and pelvic bones and allows for delineation of the tumor into the pelvis. 3D color sonography also assists in Doppler mapping the mass's blood supply, even in small tumors where 2D sonography fails to identify the mass.[74]

Perinatal mortality and morbidity are most strongly related to high-output cardiac failure because of arteriovenous shunting within the tumor, subsequent fetal hydrops, polyhydramnios, and preterm delivery.[3] Therefore, intrauterine surgery has been described as a treatment option for prenatally diagnosed sacrococcygeal teratomas to interrupt the tremendous vascular shunting through the tumor. This may involve in utero debulking, complete resection, or percutaneous coagulation of the main blood supply with radiofrequency ablation. However, fetal intervention is invasive and may cause significant morbidity to the mother and fetus.[75]

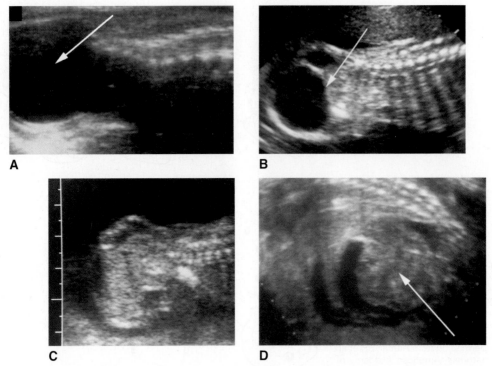

Figure 19-51 The spectrum of sacrococcygeal teratomas. **A:** Type I with predominately cystic teratoma *(arrow)*. **B:** Type II teratomas with cystic and solid elements *(arrow)*. **C:** Type II solid teratoma. **D:** Type IV teratomas presenting as nonimmune fetal hydrops with a large intra-abdomanal mass *(arrow)*.

SUMMARY

- The neural tube segements that become the brain are the prosencephalon, mesencephalon, and rhomben-cephalon.

- Most of the brain, spine, and facial structures develop in the first few weeks of embryogenesis; however, structures continue to form throughout gestation.

- The BPD level anatomy includes axial images of the thalami and third ventricle, a smooth calvarial wall, and brain/calvarium symmetry.

- Microcephaly is a small head in proportion to the fetal face.

- The large fetal head is macroceophaly.

- The MCA carries 80% of flow to the brain structures

- Axial measurements of the cerebellum correlate to gestational age on a one-to-one ratio.

- A measurement of greater than 10 mm of the ventricles obtained at the level of the atrium would be considered abnormal.

- Obtaining sagittal and coronal images of brain anatomy establishes normalcy or detects deviations from the norm.

- Inner ocular distance (IOD) and outer ocular distance (OOD) help date a gestation with either missing or abnormal head structure.

- The normal fetal spine has three ossification centers: the centrum, right, and left neural processes.

- Sagittal images of the spine include the vertebral body, lateral ossification centers, caudal end tapering, skin integrity, and examination of the spinal curvature.

- Transverse (axial) views of the spine are the best plane to identify spinal defects.

- Elevated MSAFP of 2.4 MoM raises suspicion for an open neural tube or abdominal wall defect.

- Hypertelorism exists with holoprosencephaly, cephaloceles, craniosynostosis, median cleft syndrome, and trisomy 18.

- A tongue extending beyond the maxilla (macroglossia) has been found with trisomy 21 and Beckwith-Wiedemann syndrome.

- Micrognathia, the hypoplastic mandible, is associated with Pierre Robin syndrome, trisomy 13, trisomy 18, and musculoskeletal syndromes.

- Clefts are the most common facial abnormality.

- These malformations may be unilateral or bilateral.

- The two major groupings of CP and CL are a cleft involving the upper lip and anterior maxilla with or without involvement of soft and/or hard palate; and a cleft involving hard and soft without CL.

- Meroencephaly or anencephaly is the absence of the skull and cerebral hemispheres.

- Meroencephaly demonstrates bulging fetal orbits with a froglike appearance on the sonographic image.
- Polyhydramnios, facial bones, and increased fetal activity is seen with the meroanencephalic fetus.
- Acrania is the absence of the skull and may or may not have coexisting brain tissue.
- Hydranencephaly is a destructive lesion of the brain resuting in a large anechoic area within the cranial vault surrounded by midbrain and basal ganglia.
- Holoprosensephaly, seen with trisomy 13, is an abnormal development of the fetal brain.
- Agenesis of the corpus callosum is failure of all or part of the corpus callosum.
- DWC demonstrates a large cisterna magna, with an enlarged fourth ventricle and flattened cerebellar hemispheres.
- Abnormal clefting of the brain is termed schizencephaly.
- A smooth brain is said to demonstrate lissencephaly.
- Caudal regression syndrome results in lack of sacral development.

- The herniation of intracranial contents through a cranial defect is a cephalocele.
- Arnold-Chiari malformations are the displacement of posterior fossa brain structures through the foramen magna into the cervical canal.
- Large ventricles, ventriculomegaly, is due to multiple causes and often called hydrocephalus.
- Cystic hygromas are the result of lymph vessel obstruction, usually occurring in the head or neck region.
- Isolated choroid plexus cysts have no significance and usually resolve by the third trimester.
- Intracranial hemorrhage is an uncommon intrauterine occurrence and has the same grading system as seen in a neonatal patient.
- Spina bifida is an open spinal defect that has varying degrees of severity.
- Scoliosis and kyphosis are abnormal curvatures of the spine and may be due to skeletal dysplasias or a hemivertebrae.
- Sacrococcygeal teratomas are germ cell tumors found in the sacral area.

Critical Thinking Questions

1. A 35-year-old G4P3A0 patient presents to your department with a diagnosis of large for gestational age. Her first trimester sonographic dating exam at six weeks dates her at 26 weeks. The exam finds a fetus without brain structures, a froglike face, and polyhydramnios. At what stage of pregnancy does this abnormality develop? What is the cause of the excess fluid? List other malformations that may accompany this finding. How would the sonographer date the pregnancy in the absence of a BPD?

   ANSWER: Meroanencephaly is the result of the rostral neuropore failing to close. Though this occurs at about 36 days (approximately 5 weeks), the embryo is too small to differentiate normal from abnormal development. As the pregnancy progresses, the portion of the brain that helps the fetus swallow fluid lacks development, thus the fetus fails to swallow the amniotic fluid, resulting in polyhydramnios. To date a pregnancy without a head, use the ocular distance, femur length, and abdominal circumference. A search for accompanying malformations may find spinal defects of varying degrees.

2. During alcohol rehabilitation, your next patient discovered she was pregnant. With a history of poorly controlled gestational diabetes, she has a high level of anxiety pertaining to birth defects with this pregnancy. The sonographic examination demonstrated a single common ventricle with a fused thalami without discernable brain mantle. The BPD measurement is two standard deviations below the norm and the facial views demonstrated a hypoechoic linear lucency in the midline of the lip. What malformation do these findings suggest? Explain the process that results in the brain malformation.

   ANSWER: Alobar holoprosencephaly of the pancake form. A small head measurement suggests microcephaly while the facial finding is probably a median CL. Holoprosencephaly results from incomplete separation and rotation of the forebrain.

3. A patient is sent for an examination from a small tertiary hospital with a diagnosis of agenesis of the corpus callosum. What sonographic views would confirm this diagnosis? List image findings seen in the brain with agenesis of the corpus callosum.

   ANSWER: In the axial or transverse plane, the BPD and ventricular level demonstrate the absent cavum septi pellucidi with the third ventricle occupying the space. The ventricle demonstrates a teardrop shape with widened atria and displaced medial walls. In the sagittal plane, lateral to midline, the gyri and sulci form a characteristic sunburst lesion due to radial orientation. Coronal views of the brain also image the ventricular changes. Endovaginal imaging helps with the fetal head in the pelvis; however, views are often restricted to the coronal and sagittal planes.

REFERENCES

1. Pilu G. Ultrasound evaluation of the fetal neural axis. In: Callen PW, ed. *Ultrasonography in Obstetrics and Gynecology*. 5th ed. Philadelphia: Saunders Elsevier; 2008.
2. Moore KL, Persaud TVN. *The Developing Human*. 7th ed. Philadelphia: Saunders Elsevier, 2003.
3. Nyberg DA, McGahan JP, Pretorius DH, et al. *Diagnostic Imaging of Fetal Abnormalities*. Philadelphia: Lippincott Williams & Wilkins, 2003.
4. Blencowe H, Cousens S, Modell B, et al. Folic acid to reduce neonatal mortality from neural tube disorders. *Int J Epidemiol*. 2010;39(Suppl 1):i110–i121.
5. Toi A. The fetal head and brain. In: Rumack CM, Wilson SR, Charboneau JW, et al., eds. *Diagnostic Ultrasound*. 3rd ed. St. Louis: Elsevier Mosby; 2005.
6. Degani S. Fetal biometry: clinical, pathological, and technical considerations. *Obstet and Gynecol Survey*. 2001;3:56.
7. McGahan JP, Phillips HE, Ellis WG. The fetal hippocampus. *Radiology*. 1983;147:201.
8. Abuhamad AZ. The role of Doppler ultrasound in obstetrics. In: Callen PW, ed. *Ultrasonography in Obstetrics and Gynecology*. 5th ed. Philadelphia: Saunders Elsevier; 2008.
9. Mari G, Hanif F, Kruger M, et al. Middle cerebral artery peak systolic velocity: a new Doppler parameter in the assessment of growth-restricted fetuses. *Ultrasound Obstet Gynecol*. 2007;29:310–316.
10. Moise KJ Jr. The usefulness of middle cerebral artery Doppler assessment in the treatment of the fetus at risk for anemia. *Am J Obstet Gynecol*. 2008;198:161.e1–e4.
11. Gottlieb A, Galan H. Nontraditional sonographic pearls in estimating gestational age. *Semin Perinatal*. 2008;32:154–160.
12. Cardoza JD, Goldstein RB, Filly RA. Exclusion of fetal ventriculomegaly with a single measurement: the width of the lateral ventricular atrium. *Radiology*. 1988;169:711–717.
13. Almog B, Gamzu R, Achiron R, et al. Fetal lateral ventricular width: what should be its upper limit? A prospective cohort. *J Ultrasound Med*. 2003;22:39–43.
14. Monteagudo A, Timor-Tritsch IE, Reuss ML, et al. Endovaginal sonography of the second- and third-trimester fetal brain. In: Timor-Tritsch IE, Rottem S, eds. *Endovaginal Sonography*. 2nd ed. New York: Elsevier; 1991:393–426.
15. Pilu G, Segata M, Perolo A. Ultrasound evaluation of the fetal face and neck. In: Callen PW, ed. *Ultrasonography in Obstetrics and Gynecology*. 5th ed. Philadelphia: Saunders Elsevier; 2008.
16. Rotten D, Levaillant JM. Two and three-dimensional sonographic assessment of the fetal face. *Ultrasound Obstet Gynecol*. 2004;23:224.
17. Filly RA, Feldstein VA. Ultrasound evaluation of normal fetal anatomy. In: Callen PW, ed. *Ultrasonography in Obstetrics and Gynecology*. 5th ed. Philadelphia: Saunders Elsevier; 2008.
18. Isaacson G, Birnhoz J. Human fetal upper respiratory tract function as revealed by ultrasonography. *Ann Otol Rhinol Laryngol*. 1991;100(9 pt 1):743–747.
19. Cameron M, Moran P. Prenatal screening and diagnosis of neural tube defects. *Prenat Diagn*. 2009;29:402–411.
20. Norton ME. Genetics and prenatal diagnosis. In: Callen PW, ed. *Ultrasonography in Obstetrics and Gynecology*. 5th ed. Philadelphia: Saunders Elsevier; 2008.
21. Dilmen G, Köktener A, Turhan NO, et al. Growth of the fetal lens and orbit. *Int J Gynaecol Obstet*. 2002;76(3):267–271.
22. Sukonpan K, Phupong V. A biometric study of the fetal orbit and lens in normal pregnancies. *J Clin Ultrasound*. 2009;37(2):69–74.
23. Monhide P, Mernagh J. The fetal face and neck. In: Rumack CM, Wilson SR, Charboneau JW, et al., eds. *Diagnostic Ultrasound*. 3rd ed. St. Louis: Elsevier Mosby; 2005.
24. Rotten D, Levaillant JM, Martinez H, et al. The fetal mandible: a 2D and 3D sonographic approach to the diagnosis of retrognathia and micrognathia. *Ultrasound Obstet Gynecol*. 2002;19(2):122–130.
25. Paladini D. Objective diagnosis of micrognathia in the fetus: jaw index. *Obstet Gynecol*. 1999;93:382.
26. Offerdal K, Jebens N, Syvertsen T, et al. Prenatal ultrasound detection of facial clefts: a prospective study of 49,314 deliveries in a non-selected population in Norway. *Ultrasound Obstet Gynecol*. 2008;31(6):639–646.
27. Christ JE, Meininger MG. Ultrasound diagnosis of cleft lip and cleft palate before birth. *Plast Reconstr Surg*. 1981;6:854.
28. Chervenak FA, Tortora M, Mayden K, et al. Antenatal diagnosis of median cleft face syndrome: sonographic demonstration of cleft lip and hypertelorism. *Am J Obstet Gynecol*. 1984;149:94.
29. Campbell S, Lees C, Moscoso G, Hall P. Ultrasound antenatal diagnosis of cleft palate by a new technique: the 3D "reverse face" view. *Ultrasound Obstet Gynecol*. 2005;25:12.
30. Blaas HG, Eik-Nes SH. Sonoembryology and early prenatal diagnosis of neural anomalies. *Prenat Diagn*. 2009;29:312–325.
31. Lyons EA, Levi CS. The first trimester. In: Rumack CM, Wilson SR, Charboneau JW, et al., eds. *Diagnostic Ultrasound*. 3rd ed. St. Louis: Elsevier Mosby; 2005.
32. Yanagihara T, Hata T, Three-dimensional sonographic visualization of fetal skeleton in the second trimester of pregnancy. *Gynecol Obstet Invest*. 2000;49(1):12–16.
33. Lam YH, Tang MH. Serial sonographic feature of a fetus with hydranencephaly from 11 weeks to term. *Ultrasound Obstet Gynecol*. 2000;16:77–79.
34. Jissendi-Tchofo P, Kara S, Barkovich AJ. Midbrain-hindbrain involvement in lissencephalies. *Neurology*. 2009;3;72(5):410–418.
35. Dorland's Medical Dictionary. 31st ed. Philadelphia: Saunders; 2007.
36. Blaas HG, Eriksson AG, Salvesen KA, et al. Brains and faces in holoprosencephaly: pre and postnatal description of 30 cases. *Ultrasound Obstet Gynecol*. 2002;19:24.
37. Peregrine E, Pandya P. Structural anomalies in the first trimester. In: Rumack CM, Wilson SR, Charboneau JW, et al., eds. *Diagnostic Ultrasound*. 3rd ed. St. Louis: Elsevier Mosby; 2005.
38. Rumack CM, Drose JA. Neonatal and infant brain imaging. In: Rumack CM, Wilson SR, Charboneau JW, et al., eds. *Diagnostic Ultrasound*. 3rd ed. St. Louis: Elsevier Mosby; 2005.
39. Moutard ML. Agenesis of corpus callosum: prenatal diagnosis and prognosis. *Childs Nerv Syst*. 2003;19:471.
40. McGrath JJ, Richards LJ. Why schizophrenia epidemiology needs neurobiology—and vice versa. *Schizophr Bull*. 2009;35(3):577–581.

41. Tang PH, Bartha AI, Norton ME, et al. Agenesis and dysgenesis of the corpus callosum: clinical, genetic and neuroimaging findings in a series of 41 patients. *AJNR*. 2009;30(2):257–263.

42. Glass HC, Shaw GM, Ma C, et al. Agenesis of the corpus callosum in California 1983–2003: a population-based study. *Am J Med Genet A*. 2008;1;146A(19):2495–2500.

43. Long A, Moran P, Robson S. Outcome of fetal cerebral posterior fossa anomalies. *Prenat Diagn*. 2006;26:707–710.

44. Forzano F, Mansour S, Ierullo A, et al. Posterior fossa malformation in fetuses: a report of 56 further cases and a review of the literature. *Prenat Diagn*. 2007;27:495–501.

45. Sasaki-Adams D, Elbabaa SK, Jewells V, et al. The Dandy-Walker variant: a case series of 24 pediatric patients and evaluation of associated anomalies, incidence of hydrocephalus, and developmental outcomes. *J Neurosurg Pediatrics*. 2008;2(3):194–199.

46. Cakmak A, Zeyrek D, Cekin A, et al. Dandy-Walker syndrome together with occipital encephalocele. *Minerva Pediatr*. 2008;60(4):465–468.

47. Phillips JJ, Mahony BS, Siebert JR, et al. Dandy-Walker malformation complex: correlation between ultrasonographic diagnosis and postmortem neuropathology. *Obstet Gynecol*. 2006;107(3):685–693.

48. Lee W, Comstock C, Kazmierczak C, et al. Prenatal diagnostic challenges and pitfalls for schizencephaly. *J Ultrasound Med*. 2009;28(10):1379–1384.

49. Aslan H, Gungorduk K, Yildirim D, et al. Prenatal diagnosis of lissencephaly: a case report. *Clin Ultrasound*. 2009;37(4):245–248.

50. Ghai S, Fong KW, Toi A. Prenatal US and MR Imaging findings of lissencephaly: review of fetal cerebral sulcal development. *Radiographics*. 2006;26(2):389–405.

51. Toi A. How early are fetal cerebral sulci visible at prenatal ultrasound and what is the normal pattern of early fetal sulcal development? *Ultrasound Obstet Gynecol*. 2004;24:706.

52. Leite JM, Granese R, Jeanty P. Fetal syndromes. In: Callen PW, ed. *Ultrasonography in Obstetrics and Gynecology*. 5th ed. Philadelphia: Saunders Elsevier; 2008.

53. Sauerbrei EE. The fetal spine. In: Callen PW, ed. *Ultrasonography in Obstetrics and Gynecology*. 5th ed. Philadelphia: Saunders Elsevier; 2008.

54. Caudal Regression. Medcyclopaedia™ Standard Edition. Available at: http://www.medcyclopaedia.com/library/topics/volume_vii/c/caudal_regression_syndrome.aspx .Accessed June 2010.

55. Smith AS, Grable I, Levine D. Case 66: Caudal regression syndrome in the fetus of a diabetic mother. *Radiology*. 2004;230:229–233.

56. Callen AL, Filly RA. Supratentorial abnormalities in the Chiari II malformation, I: the ventricular "point." *J Ultrasound Med*. 2008;27(1):33–38.

57. Sicuranza GB, Steinberg P, Figueroa R. Arnold-Chiari malformation in a pregnant woman. *Obstetrics & Gynecology*. 2003;102:1191–1194.

58. Manganaro L, Savelli S, Francioso A, et al. Role of fetal MRI in the diagnosis of cerebral ventriculomegaly assessed by ultrasonography. *Radiol Med*. 2009;114:1013–1023.

59. Gaglioti P, Danelon D, Bontempo S, et al. Fetal cerebral ventriculomegaly: outcome in 176 cases. *Ultrasound Obstet Gynecol*. 2005;25:372.

60. Malone FD, Ball RH, Nyberg DA, et al. First-trimester septated cystic hygroma: prevalence, natural history, and pediatric outcome. *Obstet Gynecol*. 2005;106(2):288–294.

61. Gedikbasi A, Gul A, Sargin A, et al. Cystic hygroma and lymphangioma: associated findings, perinatal outcome and prognostic factors in live-born infants. *Arch Gynecol Obstet*. 2007;276(5):491–498.

62. Malone FD. First trimester screening for aneuploidy. In: Callen PW, ed. *Ultrasonography in Obstetrics and Gynecology*. 5th ed. Philadelphia: Saunders Elsevier; 2008.

63. Yeo L, Vintzileos AM. The second trimeseter genetic sonogram. In: Callen PW, ed. *Ultrasonography in Obstetrics and Gynecology*. 5th ed. Philadelphia: Saunders Elsevier; 2008.

64. Yeo L, Vintzileos AM. The second trimester genetic sonogram. In: Callen PW, ed. *Ultrasonography in Obstetrics and Gynecology*. 5th ed. Philadelphia: Saunders Elsevier; 2008.

65. Ghi T, Simonazzi G, Perolo A, et al. Outcome of antenatally diagnosed intracranial hemorrhage: case series and review of the literature. *Ultrasound Obstet Gynecol*. 2003;22:121.

66. Ghi T, Pilu G, Falco P, et al. Prenatal diagnosis of open and closed spina bifida. *Ultrasound Obstet Gynecol*. 2006;28:899–903.

67. Mitchell LE. Epidemiology of neural tube defects. *Am J Med Genet C Semin Med Genet*. 2005;15;135(1):88–94.

68. Rasmussen SA, Chu SY, Kim SY, et al. Maternal obesity and risk of neural tube defects: a metaanalysis. *Am J Obstet Gynecol*. 2008;198(6):611–619.

68. Kibar Z, Torban E, McDearmid JR, et al. Mutations in VANGL1 associated with neural-tube defects. *N Engl J Med*. 2007;5;356(14):1432–1437.

69. Blaas HG, Eik-Nes SH, Isaksen CV. The detection of spina bifida before 10 gestational weeks using two- and three-dimensional ultrasound. *Ultrasound Obstet Gynecol*. 2000;16:25–29.

70. Chen CP. Prenatal diagnosis, fetal surgery, recurrence risk and differential diagnosis of neural tube defects. *Taiwan J Obstet Gynecol*. 2008;47(3):283–290.

71. Gonçalves LF, Kusanovic JP, Gotsch F, et al. The fetal musculoskeletal system. In: Callen PW, ed. *Ultrasonography in Obstetrics and Gynecology*. 5th ed. Philadelphia: Saunders Elsevier; 2008.

72. Feldstein VA, Harris RD, Machin GA. Ultrasound evaluation of the placenta and umbilical cord. In: Callen PW, ed. *Ultrasonography in Obstetrics and Gynecology*. 5th ed. Philadelphia: Saunders Elsevier; 2008.

73. Moise KJ. Ultrasound evaluation of hydrops fetalis. In: Callen PW, ed. *Ultrasonography in Obstetrics and Gynecology*. 5th ed. Philadelphia: Saunders Elsevier; 2008.

74. Bonilia-Musoles F, Machado LE, Raga F, et al. Prenatal diagnosis of sacrococcygeal teratomas by two- and three-dimensional ultrasound. *Ultrasound Obstet Gynecol*. 2002;19(2):200–205.

75. Choi SH. The role of fetal surgery in life threatening anomalies. *Yonsei Med J*. 2001;42(6):681–685.

76. Yoon H, Chung IS, Seol EY, et al. Development of the lip and palate in staged human embryos and early fetuses. *Yonsei Med J*. 2000;41(4):477–484.

77. The Visible Embryo. Available at: http://www.visemb .com/baby/index.html. Accessed June 2010.

78. Chiari Malformation Fact Sheet. National Neurological Disorders and Stroke. Avail www.ninds.nih.gov/disorders/chiari Accessed June 2010.

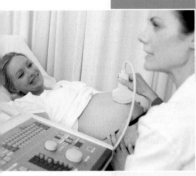

20 Ultrasound of the Normal Fetal Chest, Abdomen, and Pelvis

Robert G. Magner, Jr. and Cheryl A. Vance

OBJECTIVES

Determine fetal lie in relation to maternal anatomy

Discuss the difference between anatomic planes and Digital Imaging and Communications in Medicine (DICOM) and International Society of Ultrasound in Obstetrics and Gynecology (ISUOG) anatomic reference terms

Explain basic embryology for systems located within the thorax, abdomen, and pelvis

Recognize the sonographic appearance of normal chest, abdomen, and pelvic anatomy

Summarize the use of three-dimensional (3D) volumes in determining normal vs. abnormal anatomy

Identify male and female genitalia on the sonographic image

Describe the appearance of pseudoascites of the abdomen

KEY TERMS

amniotic fluid level | fetal lie | fetal position | anatomic position | ventral | cranial | caudal | dorsal | look direction | pseudoascites | VOCAL | oligohydramnios

GLOSSARY

3D imaging From a volume data set, static 3D images can display height, width, and depth of anatomy (three dimensions) from any orthogonal plane

4D imaging Adds motion to static 3D imaging, allowing for real-time 3D imaging of anatomy in motion

Anatomic position Body in the erect position with the palms forward and feet pointed forward

Aplasia Complete absence of a body part

Ascites Accumulation of fluid in the abdominal cavity

B-mode imaging "Brightness-mode" imaging displays anatomy in two dimensions on the display screen. The stronger the returning echo, the brighter the corresponding dot is on the display. Distance from the transducer face is displayed with the near-field anatomy on the top of the display and far-field anatomy at the bottom of the monitor display

Biliary atresia Congenital blockage or absence of the bile duct

Caliectasis Dilation of the renal calices

Cardiomegaly An enlarged heart

Caudal Toward the feet or tail end

Chorioamnionitis An inflammation of the fetal membranes (amnion/chorion) due to infection

Cranial Toward the head or cranium

Dorsal Toward the back or spine

Echogenic Generates echoes; brighter sonographically

Echogenicity Ability to generate echoes; the sonographic brightness or darkness

Echotexture Relative level of sonographic echogenicity of a structure

Fetal lie Position of the fetus in utero

Fetal presentation Term used to describe which portion of the fetus will deliver first

HASTE Half-Fourier acquisition single-shot turbo spine-echo; a fast spin method to obtain the MRI data set

Hematopoiesis Formation of blood cells

Hydronephrosis Dilation of the renal pelvices and calices, usually caused by obstruction

Hyperintense Areas of high intensity or increased brightness on the magnetic resonance imaging (MRI) image; equivalent to hyperechogenic

Hypoechoic Less echogenic or "darker" on a sonographic image

Hypointense Areas of low intensity or increased brightness on the MRI image; equivalent to hypoechogenic

Hypoplasia Underdevelopment or incomplete development of a body part

Isointense Areas of similar intensity or increased brightness on the MRI image; equivalent to isoechoic

IUGR (intrauterine growth restriction) Fetal weight below 10th percentile for gestational age

Longitudinal Along the length or long axis of the anatomy being imaged

Look direction Direction you are looking at a patient or structure, (i.e., anterior to posterior)

Myelomeningocele (spina bifida) Congenital disorder where the spinal cord does not close before birth

Osteogenesis imperfecta Genetic disorder causing extremely fragile bones

Parvovirus infection Congenital disorder caused by transplacental transmission of the parvovirus to the fetus, characterized by hydrops, ascites, ventriculomegaly, and other findings

Pulmonary hypoplasia Incomplete development of the lung tissue

Real-time imaging B-mode images are built onto the screen as the sound beam sweeps through the tissue

Transverse Along the axial cross-section or short axis of the anatomy being imaged

Trisomy Genetic abnormality where there is the presence of three copies of a particular chromosome

Ventral Toward the belly or front

VOCAL (virtual organ computer-aided analysis) Semiautomated process to calculate volume using a 3D data set

Sonography is the predominant imaging technique for the fetus. Diagnostic sonography has made a tremendous evolution over the last 50 years. In the 1960s, the fetus was assessed using B-mode scanners that produced a bistable (black and white) static image. By the early 1970s, gray-scale imaging became prominent, and by the late 1970s' real-time B-mode imaging appeared. Real-time imaging allowed the sonographer to track the moving fetus and make technical adjustments to enhance the image quality continuously throughout the exam. The 1980s brought 3D imaging and, by the late 1990s, real-time 3D (also known as 4D) had emerged. The 21st century has welcomed 3D/4D technology to simplify pathology diagnosis. Its uses range from multiplanar imaging to computer-aided diagnosis. High-resolution transducers have complimented the 3D/4D technology while enhancing the ability to visualize minute details within the growing fetus. This degree of detail visualization is critical when making decisions regarding care during and after the pregnancy.

Understanding and appreciating how the normal fetus appears sonographically leads to a greater awareness of variations that may help in the diagnosis of abnormalities. The ability to differentiate between subtle variations of normal permits the sonographer to achieve the sonographic diagnosis with confidence. Accurate prenatal diagnosis of abnormalities allows for parental counseling and, when necessary, fetal karyotyping, in utero fetal therapy, advanced delivery preparations, and appropriate antenatal follow-up. The information in this chapter will help the sonographer understand the normal sonographic anatomy of the normal fetal chest, abdomen, and pelvis.

SCANNING TECHNIQUES AND PRINCIPLES

Principles for the sonographic evaluation of the fetus are to a large extent similar to those used in evaluating newborn infants. When using B-mode imaging, the 3D anatomy is envisioned via 2D images from the transverse (transaxial), sagittal, and coronal planes. The following are considerations that may limit optimal fetal imaging.

AMNIOTIC FLUID LEVELS

Imaging the fetus sonographically requires an adequate amount of surrounding amniotic fluid to separate the fetus from the adjacent uterine wall. This is especially important in the evaluation of the skin surfaces of the thorax and abdomen or with 3D/4D data set acquisition. The fluid acts as a window for sonographic evaluation of internal and external fetal anatomy. Without sufficient fluid, anatomic interfaces become difficult, if not impossible, to visualize sonographically.

FETAL MOTION

Fetal position varies throughout the examination because of the natural movements of the fetus. During the first and second trimesters, the fetus has more room to move within the gestational sac. The sonographic evaluation may become more challenging as the fetus moves into different positions. Not only is it difficult for the examiner to capture the anatomy before the fetus moves, but shadowing from overlying structures also changes with each movement, causing additional imaging difficulties. Although the fetus has less room to move, third-trimester sonographic evaluation is also challenging. Later in the pregnancy, the fetus is evaluated in a flexed position because the uterus is smaller than the fetal length. In this instance, imaging the fetus may be challenging because the fetus may not move into a position that allows better sonographic visualization of the anatomy.

SCAN PLANES AND LABELING STANDARDS

When discussing the fetal position and scanning techniques, it is important to understand the terminology used to describe the various anatomical scan planes (Fig. 20-1). When referencing the maternal or fetal scan planes, sagittal refers to a vertical plane that divides the maternal or fetal body into sections. Transverse or axial refers to a vertical plane that divides the maternal or fetal body into unequal superior and inferior sections. Coronal references a vertical plane that divides the maternal or fetal body into anterior and posterior portions.

Two labeling standards exist to aid in both 2D and 3D imaging. One part of the Digital Imaging and Communications in Medicine (DICOM) standards outlines the anatomic position for the neonate or adult.[1] In standard anatomical position, the orientation superior and inferior correspond to the head and feet. The head end is referred to as the superior end, while the feet are referred to as the inferior end. Thus, the axis formed by joining the two is the superior-inferior axis or the axial

plane on the standard plane division of the body. These axis points become important when orienting with the 3D data set and image.

In medical imaging, the right and left sides of the patient are oriented as if we were facing the patient. When we display an image on a view box or monitor, it is as if the patient faces toward the clinician. Thus, the sagittal plane divides the right side of the patient, which is on the left side of the image. Following suit, the left side of the patient is on the right side of the image.

When dividing the body into anterior and posterior planes or the coronal plane, the back of the patient labeling becomes posterior while the front is anterior. If there is a combination of directions, then the labels combine the direction of the plane in the look direction. The look direction is simply how you are viewing the patient. For example, if you are in front of the patient looking toward the back, the look direction is anterior to posterior or AP.

The International Society of Ultrasound in Obstetrics and Gynecology (ISUOG) published a labeling standard for fetuses to standardize terminology and labeling between 2D and 3D imaging.[2] When viewing the fetus from the front, the term *cranial* references the skull, equating to superior in the DICOM labeling. Similarly, the term *caudal* refers toward the feet, and the *craniocaudal axis* runs between the head and feet of the fetus. This terminology is used in respect to the head and main body (trunk) and not when considering the limbs.

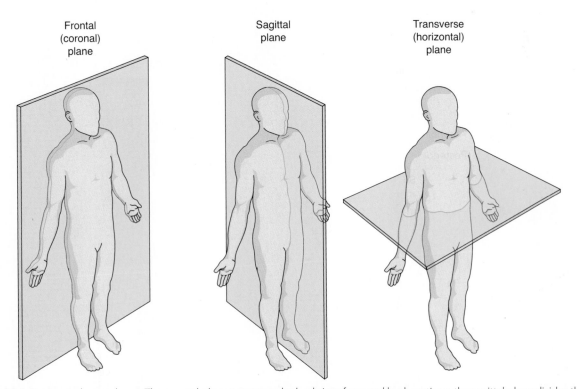

Frontal	Sagittal	Transverse
(coronal)	plane	(horizontal)
plane		plane

Figure 20-1 Anatomical scan planes. The coronal plane separates the body into front and back sections, the sagittal plane divides the body into right and left sections, and the transverse creates upper and lower portions.

The next plane is from the back (dorsal) to the abdomen (ventral). The *dorsoventral axis* forms by connecting the front to the back of the fetus. This term may be shortened to dorsoventral or DV.

As with anteroposterior, the terms *dorsal* and *ventral* are also used to describe relative positions along the dorsoventral axis. Thus, the fetal spine is dorsal to the cord insertion or the fetal heart is ventral to the spine. These axes become important when rotating the image/data set and maintaining fetal orientation (Table 20-1).

FETAL LIE

The examiner must be aware of the fetal orientation within the uterus. This is imperative when attempting to determine normal organ situs (i.e., fetal heart and

TABLE 20-1				
Anatomic Position Orientation				
	DICOM		**ISUOG**	
Anterior to posterior	**Su**perior		**Cr**anial	
	Inferior		**Ca**udal	
	Le**t**		**L**e**t**	
	Righ**t**		**R**igh**t**	
Lateral	**An**terior		**D**o**r**sal	
	Posterior		**V**e**n**tral	

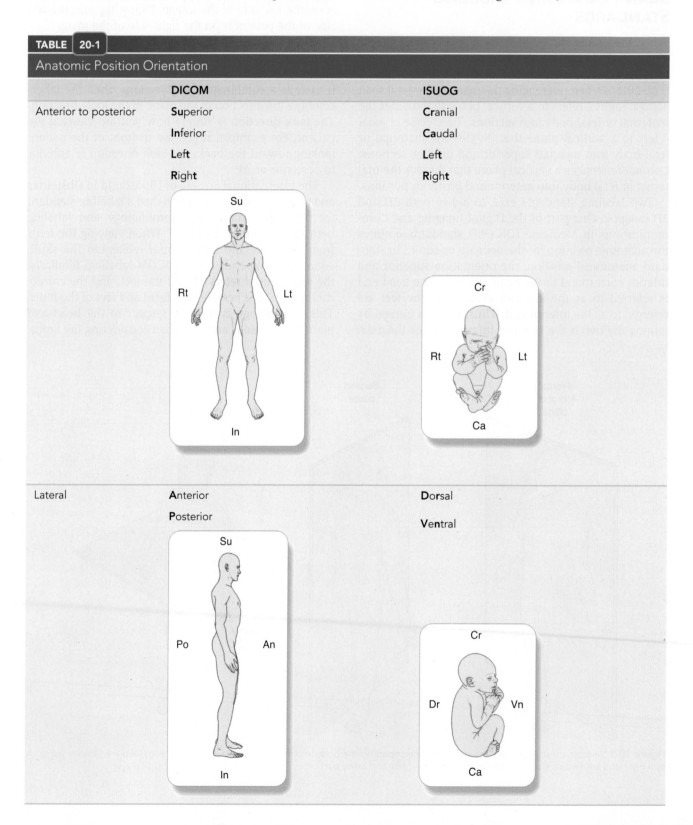

stomach on the fetal left side). A best practice is to use a dual display mode with one image demonstrating the stomach, then the second image demonstrating the heart (Fig. 20-2). This gives the interpreting physician confidence of heart/stomach situs. Bony elements cause shadowing that may obstruct the view of anatomy deep to the bones. Therefore, the spine is best visualized when the fetal spine is up (prone), whereas the abdominal organs and most of the heart structures are better visualized then the fetal spine is down (supine) or lateral.

To determine fetal lie, follow the transverse spine from head to rump, observing the location of the head and rump as the transducer is moved across the patient. Once the location of the head and rump is identified, fetal position can be determined (breech, vertex, transverse, or oblique). Next, determine how the fetus is lying within the gestational sac by identifying the transverse spine's location on the display monitor. If the transverse spine is toward the top of the monitor, the fetus is prone. If the transverse spine is toward the bottom of the monitor, the fetus is supine (Table 20-1).

When the fetus is vertex and the transverse spine is on the right of the monitor, the fetus is lying on its left side. When the fetus is breech and the transverse spine is on the right side of the monitor, the fetus is lying on its right side. When the fetus is vertex and the transverse spine is on the left side of the monitor, the fetus is lying on its right side. When the fetus is breech and the transverse spine is on the left side of the monitor, the fetus is lying on its left side (Table 20-2).

Imaging success depends on scanning technique. Higher frequency transducers produce increased resolution. Lower frequency transducers have increased penetration. Always use the highest frequency transducer that allows for proper depth penetration. Additionally,

one should keep the transducer's focal zones at or slightly below the anatomy of interest. Structures deep to the transducer's focal zones display with decreased resolution because of the tissue interaction with the sound.

Special techniques may be necessary to adequately visualize the fetus. These techniques include small corrections in transducer angulation, broad shifting of the transducer position along the maternal abdomen, altering the mother's position on the table, having the mother walk around the department, or, in unusual circumstances, postponing evaluation to another day. Endovaginal and less "invasive" translabial imaging may aid in the evaluation of fetal structures lying low within the maternal pelvis at the time of the ultrasound examination. These two techniques may also be used when maternal obesity or abdominal scarring obscures adequate fetal visualization.

FETAL PRESENTATION

The fetal presentation varies throughout the pregnancy and is described in terms of what fetal part is closest to the cervix. The term *vertex* refers to the topmost point of the skull. In obstetrics, the term vertex (also called cephalic) is used to indicate when the fetal head is down (toward the cervix), which is the normal presentation for birth. The fetus may be vertex facing toward the maternal back or vertex facing toward the maternal abdomen. Occasionally, the fetus does not move into the vertex position. When the fetus lies transverse in the maternal uterus, it is common practice to indicate the fetal presentation according to which side the fetal head is located in reference to the mother (e.g., "transverse fetal lie–head maternal left"). The term *breech* indicates that the fetal buttocks are down (toward the cervix). This is an abnormal presentation for birth and may require a cesarean delivery. There are several variations of breech. Complete breech refers to when the buttocks present first (toward the cervix) and both the hips and knees are flexed. Incomplete or "footling" breech indicates that the fetus has one or both feet down (toward the cervix), so its leg(s) are poised to deliver first. Frank breech indicates that the fetal buttocks present first (toward the cervix) and the hips are flexed so the legs are straight and completely drawn up toward the fetal chest. And finally, the fetus may lie in an oblique position. When the fetus lies obliquely, it's good practice for the examiner to indicate either vertex or breech oblique presentation plus which side the fetal head is lying (e.g., "breech oblique fetal lie–head maternal right")(Fig. 20-3).

THE THORAX

The thorax is surrounded by the spine and ribs and is separated from the abdominal cavity by the diaphragm (at the base of the lungs). When examining the thorax and its contents, start at the thoracic inlet at the base

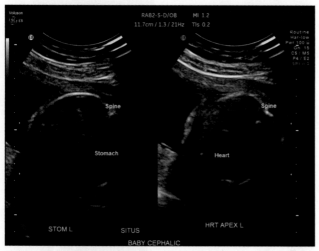

Figure 20-2 Dual display image demonstrating the stomach on the left side of the display and the heart on the right side of the display. Gives the interpreting physician confidence that the stomach and the heart are on the same side within the fetus.

TABLE 20-2

Fetal Position Based on Spine Location

	Position	Sonographic Image
Breech fetal position with the fetal spine toward the top of the monitor indicates a prone lie.	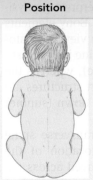	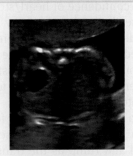
Vertex fetal position with the spine toward the top of the monitor indicates a prone lie.	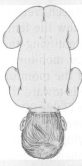	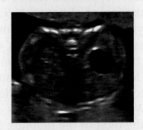
Breech fetal position with the spine toward the bottom of the monitor indicates a supine lie.	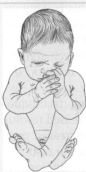	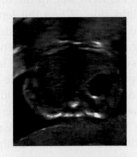
Vertex fetal position with the spine toward the bottom of the monitor indicates a supine lie.	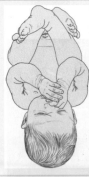	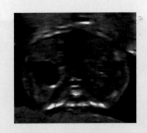
Vertex fetal position with the spine toward the right side of the monitor indicates the fetus is lying on its left side.	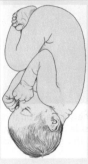	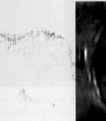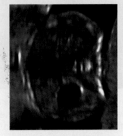

TABLE **20-2** *(continued)*

Fetal Position Based on Spine Location

	Position	Sonographic Image
Breech fetal position with the spine toward the right side of the monitor indicates the fetus is lying on its right side.		
The fetus is vertex and the transverse spine is on the left side of the monitor, therefore the fetus is lying on its right side.		
The fetus is breech and the transverse spine is on the left side of the monitor, therefore the fetus is lying on its left side.		

of the neck (the level of the clavicles) and continue through the diaphragm. As with most anatomy, transverse and longitudinal views are taken. The examiner should assess the fetal heart, the pulmonary echotexture, the diaphragm, the bony elements (for symmetry), and the chest size (in relation to the fetus in general and in relation to the fetal abdomen in particular). With additional effort, smaller structures such as the fetal trachea, thyroid, and esophagus may be visualized.

BONY ELEMENTS OF THE THORAX

The bony thorax consists of the clavicles, ribs, scapulae, vertebral bodies, and sternum. The bony thorax surrounds the lungs, heart, and mediastinum. In the early stages of pregnancy, only ossified portions of the fetal skeleton are imaged (seen as areas of increased echogenicity). Knowledge of the timing of ossification center development may help in determining gestational age. The clavicles ossify as early as 8 to 9 weeks, the ribs and

scapulae ossify beginning at 10 to 11 weeks, and ossification of the sternum begins between 21 and 27 weeks.[3] As the pregnancy progresses, more hypoechoic, purely cartilaginous structures may also be visualized.

The clavicles are seen as bright echoes at the junction of the fetal neck and thorax. Their hypoplasia or aplasia may be noted as part of several clinical syndromes. In the transverse plane, the clavicles should be symmetric. At times, especially in older fetuses, it may be difficult to image the clavicles in their entirety because of their natural curvature. Clavicular growth has a direct relationship to gestational age.[4]

Ribs appear as echogenic bands projecting in a fan-like pattern from the spine. It is difficult to image large portions of adjacent ribs because of their curvilinear shape. Use 3D techniques for better visualization of the ribs (Figs. 20-4 and 20-5). Assess the ribs for symmetry, as this is an indication of the correct scan plane for biometric measurements (e.g., thoracic and abdominal circumference [TC/AC]). Particularly thick or thin ribs

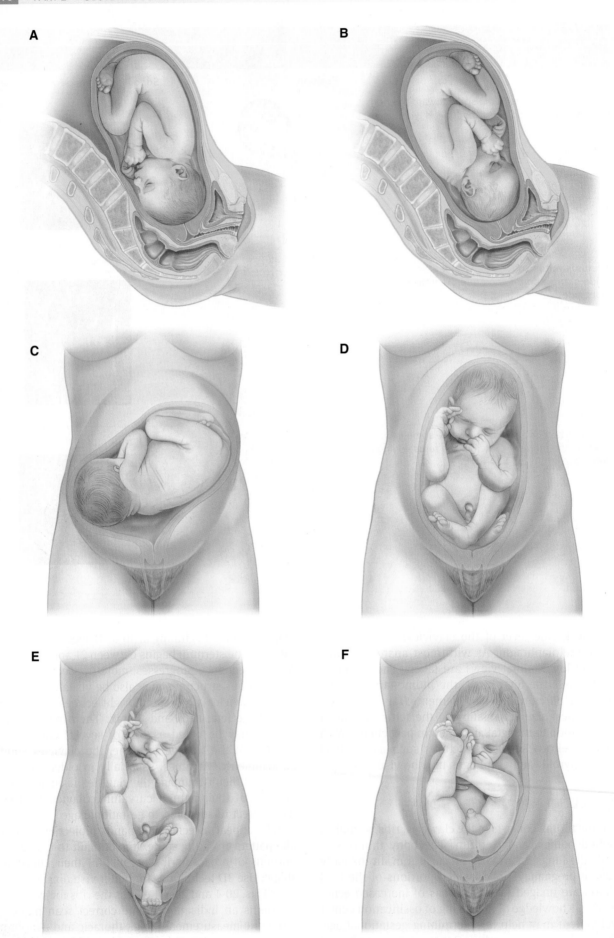

Figure 20-3 A–F: Fetal position variations.

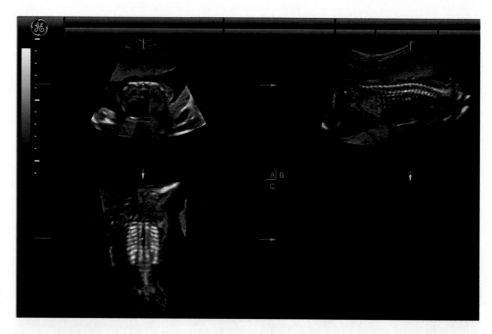

Figure 20-4 3D multiplanar image demonstrating the ribs in the bottom left display.

suggest abnormality (e.g., the ribs of a patient with osteogenesis imperfecta may be particularly thin).

The echogenic scapula images external to the ribs and surrounded by hypoechoic musculature. The typical scapula has a sonographic appearance of a Y or V shape, depending on the angle of insonation. 3D sonography is useful when assessing the scapula (Fig. 20-6).

Examine the vertebrae for convergence of the paired posterior ossified elements toward the nonossified spinous process and a single anterior element (Fig. 20-7). Evaluate the posterior skin surface to rule out the possibility of a break in the skin surface associated with myelomeningocele. The sternum is highly variable with respect to the development of its ossification centers.

SOFT TISSUE STRUCTURES OF THE CHEST

The muscles of the chest wall are hypoechoic and thin. They become somewhat more evident as the pregnancy progresses through the third trimester. The soft tissues may appear thick with generalized fetal edema or because of subcutaneous fat deposits in infants of diabetic mothers. Anterior chest wall masses consistent with fetal breasts under the influence of maternal hormone stimulation may be seen in fetuses of either sex.

CHEST BIOMETRY

Thoracic measurements may be taken in an attempt to assess gestational age or to rule out pulmonary hypoplasia. TC measurements (outer edge to outer edge) are obtained from a true transverse view just above the

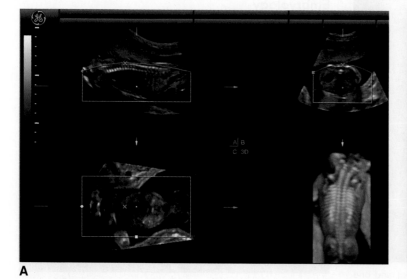

A

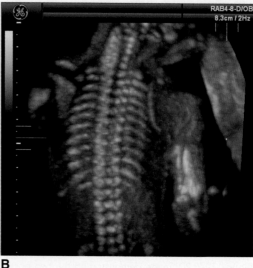

B

Figure 20-5 A: 3D multiplanar image demonstrating a rendered view of the ribs in the bottom right display. **B:** 3D image demonstrating the ribs using volume contrast imaging (*thick slice display*).

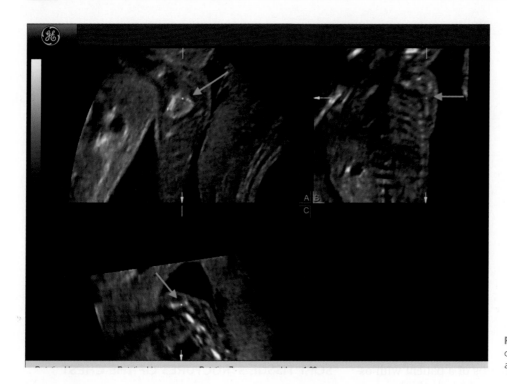

Figure 20-6 3D multiplanar image demonstrating the scapula (*green arrows*).

diaphragm at the level of the fetal heart (Fig. 20-8). A detailed explanation of the cardiothoracic ratio (CTR) technique can be found in Chapter 22.

Because the major components of the thorax are the heart and lungs, a significant decrease in lung volume, as found with pulmonary hypoplasia, should be reflected by TC measurements that are low for the patient's predicted gestational age. Many sonologists evaluate the TC by gestalt. A more exacting approach to evaluating a fetus for pulmonary hypoplasia would be analyzing the TC/AC ratio. Not all low TC/AC ratios are caused by pulmonary hypoplasia and may be the result of a small thorax, often

associated with various skeletal dysplasias. A normal TC also may be maintained in spite of pulmonary hypoplasia. Sonographic correlation of biometric measurements with the actual intrathoracic image is necessary for proper diagnosis. As a good rule of thumb in assessing the intrathoracic contents, a transverse view of the chest (at the level of the atrioventricular valves) should show the heart occupying about one-third of the thorax. If the heart (in the transverse view) appears to occupy more than its share of the thorax, pulmonary hypoplasia should be considered, as well as the more obvious possibility of cardiomegaly.

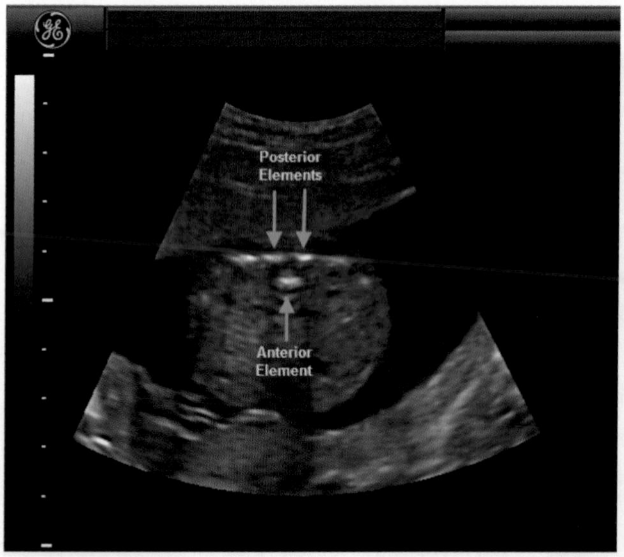

THE LUNGS

Embryology

Lung development occurs throughout gestation, resulting in the division of development into stages. These stages, embryonic, pseudoglandular, canalicular,

Figure 20-7 2D image demonstrating the two posterior and one anterior ossified elements of the spine (*green arrows*).

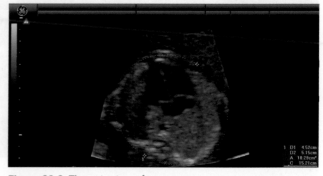

Figure 20-8 Thoracic circumference measurement.

terminal saccular, and alveolar, begin in the fourth week of gestation.

The lungs begin development in the embryo as a diverticulum extending from the tracheal bud. Once these develop into two outpouchings, the primary bronchial buds grow laterally into what will become the pleural cavity. In the fifth week, these buds join with the primitive trachea to form the bronchi. During the pseudoglandular period, the bronchi divide into secondary bronchi forming the lobar, segmental, and intersegmental branches. All the segmental bronchi form between the eighth and ninth week of gestation. At approximately the 16th to 28th week, during the canalicular period, vascularization and the terminal bronchioles increase in size. Because of the different development rates of the cranial and caudal lobes, the pseudoglandular and canalicular periods overlap. Respiration becomes possible during the 24th week because of some development of the terminal saccules. From 26 weeks to birth, during the terminal saccular period, there is continued development of the saccules and an increase in the ability of the lung to perform gas exchange. The alveolar period overlaps the terminal saccular from approximately 32 weeks to birth. During this time, the surfactant production increases, branching of the airways continues, and the blood–gas barrier thins (Fig. 20-9).[5,6]

Imaging Findings

Sonography

The lungs are separated from these abdominal organs by the diaphragm. Each lung may be compared to its counterpart. Normal fetal lungs have a homogeneous echotexture. Sagittal and coronal views allow the echogenicity of the lungs to be compared with that of the liver or spleen. Early in gestation, lung echogenicity is equal to or slightly less than that of the liver. As gestation progresses, lung echogenicity increases progressively until it is greater than that of the liver during gestation (Figs. 20-10 and 20-11).[7] Sonography is not reliable to indicate fetal lung maturity. It may be used to assess fetal maturity and gestational age when elective delivery later in pregnancy is considered. Amniocentesis remains the gold standard in accessing lung maturity.

Color and power Doppler imaging becomes helpful, as underdevelopment of the lungs results in decreased flow. Some studies have shown that detection of color flow within the lung supersedes the use of MRI for diagnosis (Fig. 20-12).[7]

The use of a 3D data set to obtain lung volumes became possible with the development of virtual organ computer-aided analysis (VOCAL). Several studies confirm the usefulness and interobserver reliability of obtaining the lung volume via a 3D data set.[8] The speed of the data acquisition becomes important in imaging the mobile fetus, and detection of the often irregular lung via VOCAL increases accuracy. The best acquisition plane for this volume is transverse imaging in a ventral to dorsal plane (Fig. 20-13).[8,9] For more information regarding VOCAL, refer to Chapter 32, "3D/4D Imaging in Obstetrics and Gynecology."

MRI

Fetal lung imaging with MRI helps in estimating the relative lung volume, as low volume increases fetal risk for pulmonary hypoplasia.[5] MRI fetal lung imaging has an advantage over sonography in the case of maternal obesity and oligohydramnios, when imaging becomes difficult with ultrasound.[10] The T1-weighted image (T2WI) obtained with a fast spin technique demonstrates the lungs as hypointense because of amniotic fluid (Fig. 20-14).[11]

THE DIAPHRAGM

Embryology

Development of the diaphragm completes at the end of week 8 with the fusion of the septum transversum, pleuroperitoneal membranes, dorsal mesentery of the esophagus, and muscular ingrowth from the lateral body walls.[5,6] Early in the gestation, at about 24 days, the septum transversum is close to the caudal end of the embryo. As the diaphragm develops and the embryo grows, the diaphragm moves closer to the caudal end of the embryo. At approximately 52 days, the diaphragm has become located in approximately midembryo (Fig. 20-15).[6]

Imaging Findings

Sonography

The diaphragm is seen as a thin, hypoechoic, dome-shaped muscular band separating the abdominal cavities from the thoracic's more echogenic lung tissues.[5,12] The sagittal plane displays the diaphragm's convex upper surface forming the floor of the thoracic cavity and its concave lower surface forming the roof of the abdominal cavity (Fig. 20-16). Imaging the diaphragm can help differentiate cystic intrathoracic masses of pulmonary origin from those that are of intra-abdominal origin. However, as with all curved structures, even when the fetus is positioned optimally, the entire structure may not be visualized and small defects may be missed. Fetal breathing may be detected by diaphragmatic motion when the pregnancy nears term.

MRI

The diaphragm images quite similar on the MRI as on the sonographic image. The dome-shaped muscular structure displays as a darker area located between the chest and abdominal organs (Fig. 20-17).

THE THYMUS

Embryology

Several balloonlike diverticula, pharyngeal pouches, give rise to structures of the mouth and upper chest. These four pouches result in multiple organs, however,

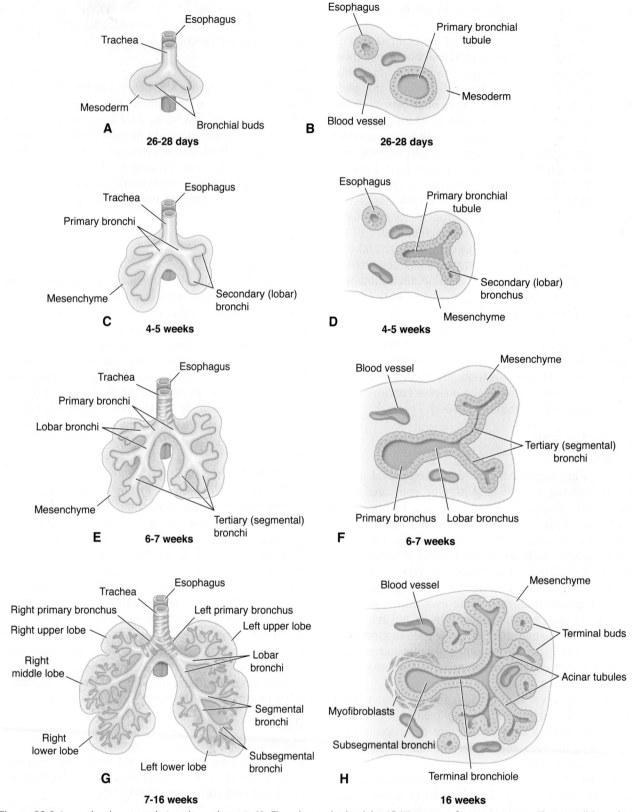

Figure 20-9 Lung development during the embryonic **(A–F)** and pseudoglandular **(G,H)** stages of organogenesis. The overall branching pattern of the primitive lung *(left panels)* results in the development of the bronchial tree. The histologic organization of the fetal lung becomes more complex as branching morphogenesis progresses through these stages *(right panels)*.

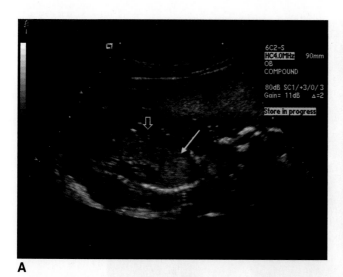

A

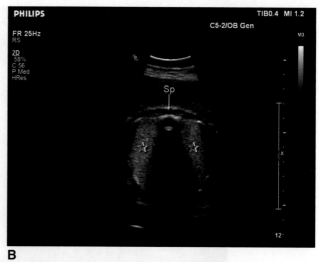

B

Figure 20-10 A: Sagittal plane looking from ventral to dorsal demonstrating the lung *(arrow)* seen early in gestation. The bowel *(open arrow)*, located below the domed hypoechoic diaphragm, has a less uniform appearance. **B:** The transverse image demonstrates the dorsal spine *(Sp)* at the top of the image with the lungs *(star)*. (Image **B** courtesy of Philips Medical Systems, Bothell, WA.)

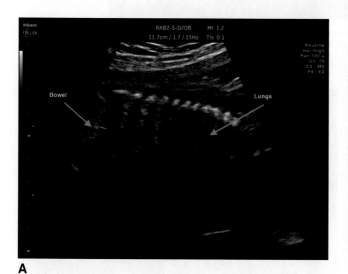

A

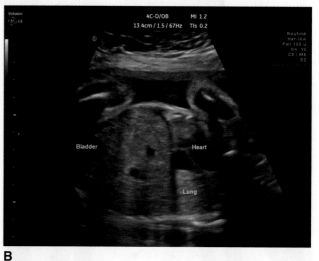

B

Figure 20-11 A: Fetal lungs are more hypoechoic earlier in gestation. **B:** Fetal lungs are more hyperechoic later in gestation.

Figure 20-12 Color Doppler image of lung vasculature helps rule out pulmonary agenesis. (Image courtesy of Philips Medical Systems, Bothell, WA.)

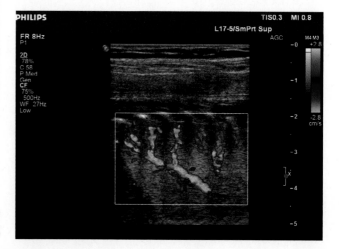

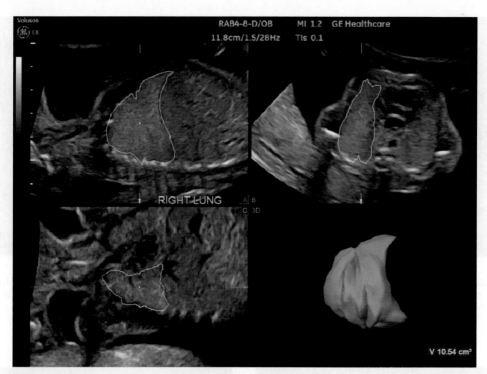

Figure 20-13 To perform a semiautomatic VOCAL measurement, trace the lung on all three multi-planar reconstruction (MPR) images and activate the volume. In this case, the estimated lung volume of the right lung is 10.54 cm³.

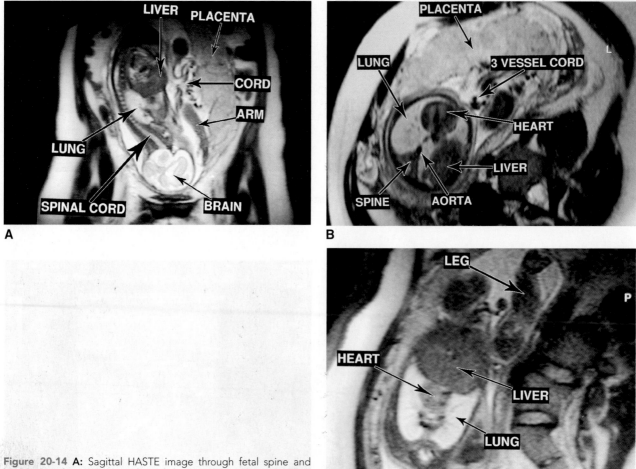

Figure 20-14 A: Sagittal HASTE image through fetal spine and body. **B:** Axial HASTE image through fetal thorax. **C:** Coronal HASTE image through fetal thorax.

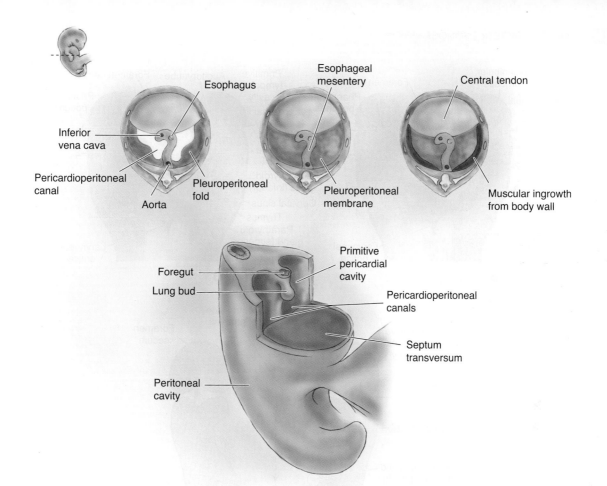

Figure 20-15 The diaphragm forms from the transverse septum, ingrowth of the pleuroperitoneal membrane from the lining of the cavity, a bit of dorsal mesentery of the foregut, and lastly, ingrowth of mesoderm from the body wall. The diaphragm is not a circular disc but a sheet of muscle that lies across the body over the liver and the stomach. The characteristic shape is due to migration in from the perimeter to give the central part more room to form a dome. Because it is formed from different sources, its sensory and motor supplies also come from separate sources. Motor fibers follow the transverse septum down from the head region (via the phrenic nerve of the cervical region), and sensory fibers come from both the phrenic and the same nerves that serve the body wall in this area (via intercostal nerves). (From Sadler T. *Langman's Medical Embryology.* 9th ed. Image Bank. Baltimore, MD: Lippincott Williams & Wilkins; 2003.)

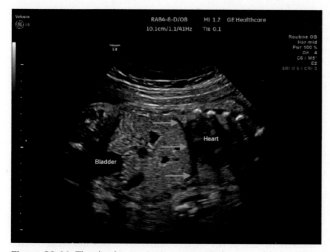

Figure 20-16 The diaphragm *(green arrows)* is the curved, hypoechoic structure separating the thoracic and abdominal cavities.

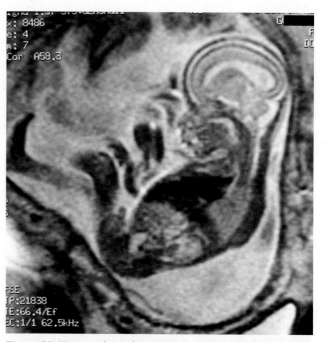

Figure 20-17 Large field of view T2-weighted sagittal image demonstrates the brain, chest, abdomen, and leg of a 20-week fetus.

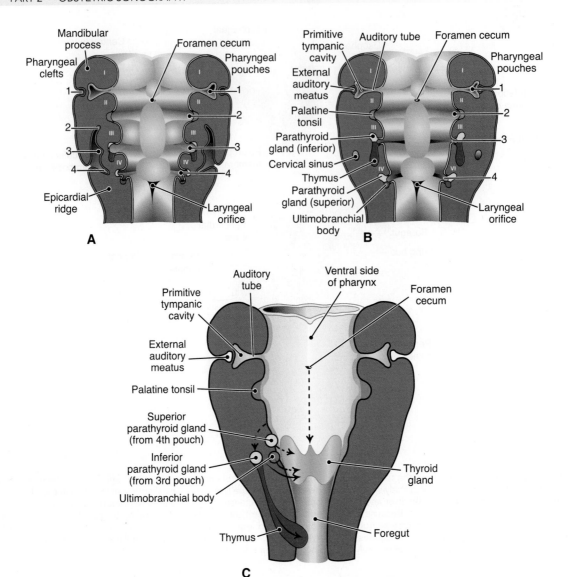

Figure 20-18 Coronal views of pharyngeal arch transformations. The first pouch hardly changes (**A**). It remains as a thin barrier between outside and inside—the tympanic membrane of the ear. On the inner side is the auditory tube, which is open to the throat, and on the outer side is the ear canal. The remaining clefts smooth over as a result of expansion and descent of the second arch, leaving the possibility of a trapped cyst or fistula in the connective tissue of the neck (**B**). The second pouch harbors a condensation of lymphatic tissue—the future tonsil (**C**). Parathyroid glands and critical immunologic tissue (the thymus gland) develop from involutions of the third and fourth pouches. From the midline of the ventral pharynx, the thyroid gland originates from the lining of the foramen cecum and descends external to the gut tube (**C**). (Adapted from Sadler TW. *Langman's Medical Embryology*. 10th ed. Baltimore, MD: Lippincott Williams & Wilkins; 2006. Fig. 16.10A & B, p. 263; Fig. 16.11, p. 264.)

only the third pharyngeal pouch contributes to the formation of the thymus (Fig. 20-18). The thymus descends from the superior mediastinum to its final location posterior to the sternum (Fig. 20-19).[6]

Imaging Findings

Sonography

The thymus is located posterior to the sternum at the level of the great vessels of the heart, anterior to the aorta and pulmonary artery.[13] It is a hypoechoic structure sonographically (Fig. 20-20). The thymus is rarely imaged in the routine targeted exam unless large pleural effusions are present.[14] Assessing the fetal thymus may be useful when determining intrauterine growth restriction (IUGR) and predicting chorioamnionitis.

MRI

The T2WI obtained with a fast-spin technique demonstrates the thymus as an intermediate signal.[11]

THE LARYNX

The larynx is located in the fetal neck anterior to the trachea at the level of the third to sixth cervical vertebrae (Fig. 20-21). The oropharynx and laryngeal pharynx are occasionally seen when they are filled with fluid (Fig. 20-22). Transverse scans through the upper neck are quite successful for visualizing the pharynx, but longitudinal coronal images display the anatomy to a greater advantage.[13] Laryngeal atresia or stenosis may be suspected with the presence of a persistently fluid-filled trachea.[12]

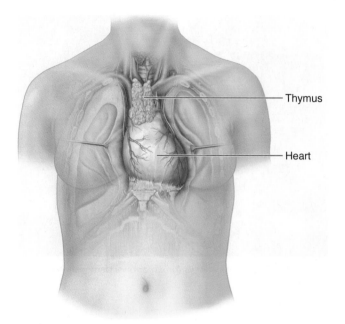

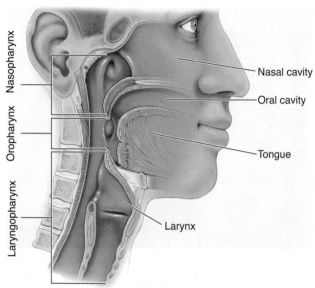

Figure 20-21 The larynx is located anterior to the trachea.

Figure 20-19 The thymus is located posterior to the sternum and anterior to the great vessels of the heart.

THE ABDOMEN

Early in the second trimester, the fetal abdominal organs have attained their normal adult position and structure. The liver, kidneys, and adrenal glands are readily identifiable. The anechoic gallbladder, stomach, and blood-filled large vessels make them readily distinguishable from surrounding organs. Visualization of the spleen is more variable, and the pancreas is seen far less often. Collapsed small bowel and, in the third trimester, fluid- or meconium-filled colon are often seen.

Assess the fetal abdomen in the transverse, coronal, and sagittal planes, using angular transducer manipulations to visualize the various organs. The transverse plane is used to visualize the spine, ensuring the posterior elements are parallel to each other and do not diverge or splay outward from the central vertebral body. The presence of an intact skin surface overlying the individual vertebral bodies is a helpful secondary sign to rule out myelomeningocele (spina bifida) (Fig. 20-23). Sufficient surrounding amniotic fluid and some distance from the uterine wall surface is needed to image the skin surface adequately. Images are recorded of the transverse view of the upper abdomen for AC measurements. This level usually demonstrates adequate views of the stomach and liver (Fig. 20-24). Continuing caudally down the abdomen, a transverse view is obtained to confirm the presence of two kidneys and to evaluate their anatomy (Fig. 20-25). A sagittal view of the thorax, abdomen, and pelvis allows evaluation of the relative size of the thorax and

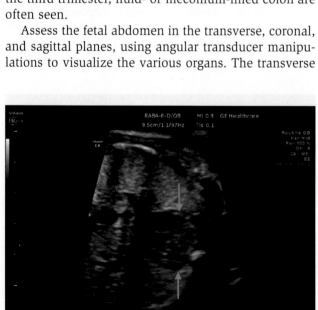

Figure 20-20 The thymus (between the *green arrows*) is more hypoechoic when compared to the surrounding tissues.

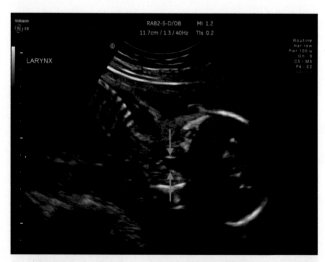

Figure 20-22 The oropharynx/laryngeal pharynx momentarily filled with fluid during fetal breathing/swallowing.

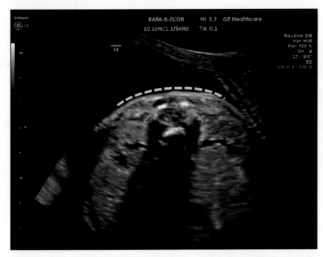

Figure 20-23 Transverse lumbar spine image demonstrating the parallel posterior elements *(green arrows)* and an intact skin surface overlying the spine *(yellow curved line).*

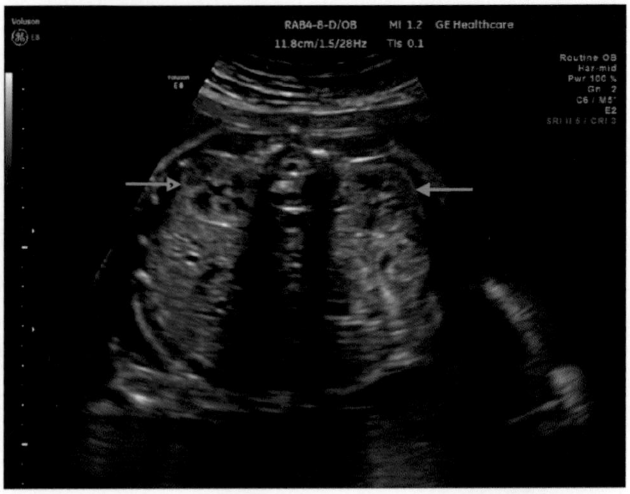

Figure 20-25 Bilateral kidneys *(green arrows)* demonstrated in the transverse plane.

abdomen, as well as the relation of umbilical vessel entry to the anterior abdominal wall. Umbilical vessel entry can also be readily noted on a transverse section of the abdomen taken at the level of the umbilicus. Both umbilical arteries traverse caudally from the abdominal insertion toward the fetal bladder (Fig. 20-26), while the umbilical vein courses cephalic into the left portal vein.

The abdomen and its contents are checked for congenital abnormalities on transverse, sagittal, and coronal views. While assessing the abdomen, evaluate the fetal body surface and orientation of the contained fetal structures. Right parasagittal views through the thorax and abdomen allow further comparison and evaluation of fetal lung and liver (Fig. 20-27A). Left parasagittal views denote the stomach and left kidney (Fig. 20-27B). Midline sagittal images allow evaluation

of the umbilicus in relation to the fetal anterior abdominal wall. The umbilical vein can be followed in its course from the anterior abdominal wall into the liver's left portal vein.

Transverse and, to a lesser extent, sagittal views can help determine the relationship of the abdominal organs (abdominal situs) to the intrathoracic organs, in particular, the position of the fetal heart and its apex. There is an increased incidence of anomalies among fetuses and children with partial situs inversus (i.e., with their cardiac apex on the opposite side of the body from the fetal stomach). Mirror imaging of the thoracic and abdominal contents, also known as situs inversus totalis (i.e., with the heart on the right side of the thorax and the abdominal organs transposed, with the spleen and stomach on the right and the liver and gallbladder on the left side), has only a minimal increased

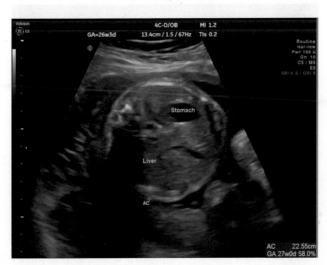

Figure 20-24 AC image demonstrating the stomach and liver.

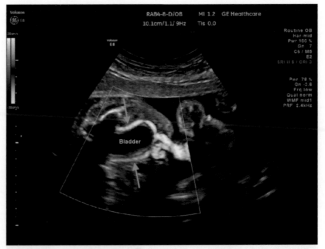

Figure 20-26 HD flow (directional power Doppler) demonstrating the two umbilical arteries *(green arrows)* coursing caudally along the fetal bladder.

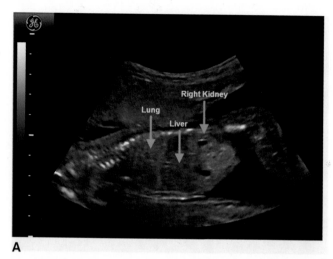

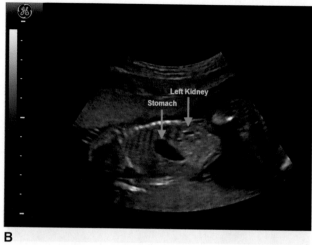

Figure 20-27 A: Sagittal view through the fetal right side demonstrating the lung, liver, and right kidney. **B:** Sagittal view through the fetal left side demonstrating the stomach and left kidney.

incidence of abnormalities. Therefore, it is important to determine the arrangement of these structures in the fetus. When in cephalic presentation, a fetus with normal abdominal situs should have its spine, stomach, and umbilical vein imaged in a clockwise manner on a transverse image. These structures would be in a counterclockwise arrangement when imaged on a transverse view of a fetus in breech presentation (Fig. 20-28). When the fetus is in a transverse lie, it is necessary to envision the lie of the fetus within the uterus, then determine the fetal stomach and heart's lie (should be on the fetal left side). If the organs are aligned this way, the situs is normal or, at the very least, there is situs inversus totalis, which, again, is cause for far less worry than partial situs inversus.

As with the thorax, anatomic evaluation of the abdomen depends on fetal position, fetal flexion, and

an adequate amount of surrounding amniotic fluid. Significant maternal body fat may limit fetal evaluation.

ABDOMINAL SOFT TISSUES

Sonographically, the abdominal wall displays an outer echogenic skin line and a deeper, 1- to 3-mm hypoechoic muscular layer. Occasionally, thin echogenic lines may be seen that represent fascial planes between the three main muscle groups (the internal oblique, transverse abdominal, and external oblique). The hypoechoic muscular layer is often referred to as *pseudoascites* and should not be confused with true ascites, which would have a more crescent shape (Fig. 20-29). When the fetal abdomen is flexed laterally, folds of fat may at times be visualized along the lateral skin line (Fig. 20-30).

UMBILICAL CORD AND ABDOMINAL VASCULATURE

The allantois, a caudal outpouching of the yolk sac (not visible sonographically), is involved in early blood production (Fig. 20-31). Its blood vessels eventually become the umbilical artery and veins. The umbilical cord consists of two umbilical arteries and one umbilical vein (Fig. 20-32). In 1% of singleton pregnancies, the right umbilical artery regresses or does not form, and there is a single umbilical artery.[15] A two-vessel cord is more common in twins than singletons.[15,16] Usually, a single umbilical artery is not significant, but it has been associated with gastrointestinal tract, renal, and cardiac abnormalities, as well as an increased incidence of trisomy.[12,16]

A major difference between fetal and adult abdominal anatomy is that the fetus has patent umbilical vessels and its ductus venosus acts as a conduit between the portal and systemic veins. The thin-walled single umbilical vein enters the anterior abdomen, taking a cephalad-oblique

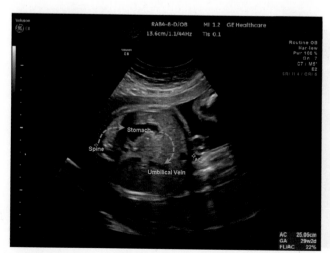

Figure 20-28 Fetus in cephalic presentation demonstrating fetal spine, stomach, and umbilical vein aligned in a clockwise (*green arrows*) arrangement.

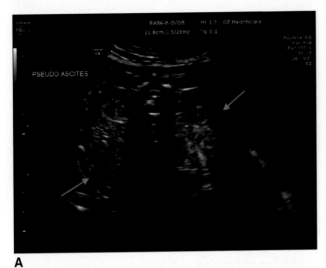

A

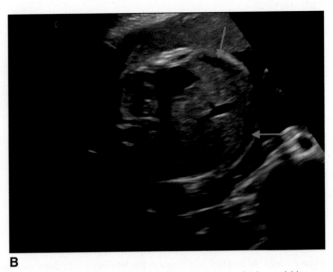

B

Figure 20-29 A,B: Hypoechoic pseudoascites (*green arrows*) are normal and should not be confused with true ascites, which would have a more crescent shape.

course and enters the left portal vein (Fig. 20-33). Some fetal blood flows from the left portal vein into the narrow channel of the ductus venosus, bypassing the liver and entering the systemic venous system by the left hepatic vein or inferior vena cava, but more typically, it flows medially into the right portal vein, perfusing the liver. After birth, the ductus venosus closes and is seen as an echogenic line in the fissure of the ligamentum venosum between the left and the caudate lobes.

The two umbilical arteries, which carry most of the fetal aortic blood to the placenta, can be followed caudad from the anterior abdominal wall cord insertion site (Fig. 20-34) to the internal iliac arteries, which are just lateral to the bladder. The vessels can be followed to their origin at the iliac artery bifurcation (Fig. 20-35). The abdominal aorta and inferior vena cava can often be seen throughout its course and is often an aid in noting the expected position of the kidneys on coronal views (Fig. 20-36).

BIOMETRY IN THE NORMAL ABDOMEN

Abdominal Circumference

The AC has proved to be a key and accurate measurement in the evaluation of gestational age and fetal weight and in ruling out asymmetric growth. Fetuses from diabetic mothers often have increased abdominal tissue and therefore a larger AC measurement than nondiabetic mothers. The AC should be measured in a true axial plane of the abdomen, demonstrating the transverse spine, left-sided stomach, and the umbilical vein entering into the left portal vein (Fig. 20-37). Measurements are made along the outer perimeter of the abdomen. Indications of proper positioning include a circular abdominal outline, equidistant left- and right-side rib echoes, and visualization of the three ossification centers of the vertebral body. A long segment of the intrahepatic portion of the umbilical vein, especially if it extends anteriorly, suggests an oblique

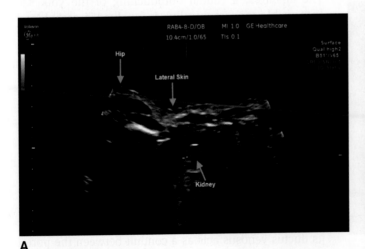

A

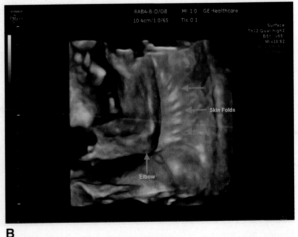

B

Figure 20-30 A: Normal lateral skin folds demonstrated when fetus flexes its abdomen. **B:** 3D rendered image demonstrating normal skin folds when the fetus flexes its abdomen.

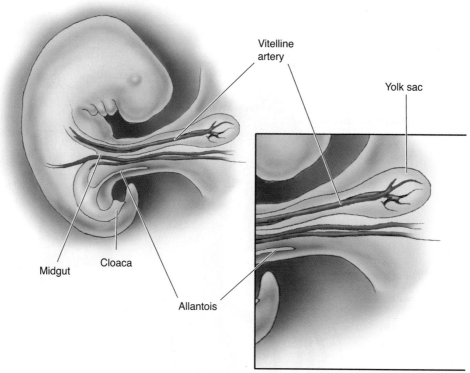

Vitelline artery

Yolk sac

Midgut

Cloaca

Allantois

Figure 20-31 Formation of the umbilical cord. The original yolk sac gets pinched off by lateral and longitudinal folding except for a dwindling pouch in the very center of the embryo. This is now called the *vitelline duct*, and it is a blind pouch that simply dangles there until the connecting stalk crashes into it during longitudinal folding, after which the vitelline duct and the blind pouch called the *allantois* incorporates with the connecting stalk as the umbilical cord. (Adapted from Sadler T. *Langman's Medical Embryology*. 9th ed. Image Bank. Baltimore, MD: Lippincott Williams & Wilkins; 2003.)

rather than a true axial view. Angulated views that include the lungs are not acceptable. A common error in AC measurements is measuring only to the boney structures (ribs/spine). The correct AC measurement should include the soft tissue surrounding the ribs/spine. The AC can be measured using an ellipse function or by measuring the circumference from the two diameters (e.g., transverse abdominal diameter and anterior-to-posterior abdominal diameter).

LIVER, GALLBLADDER, PANCREAS, AND SPLEEN

Embryology

The liver, gallbladder, ducts, and pancreas develop from the embryonic foregut. In the fourth week, an outgrowth develops on the caudal portion of the forgut. The hepatic diverticulum becomes the liver. The rapid growth of the liver from the 5th to 10th week results in the liver occupying most of the abdominal cavity. The second-trimester liver makes up 10% of the total weight, decreasing to 5% by term.[6,13] Functional lobes of the liver depend on the flow of oxygenated umbilical vein blood. In the 6th week, the bright red appearance of the liver is due to the start of hematopoiesis. Bile secretion begins in the 12th week.

The gallbladder forms from a caudal portion of the hepatic diverticulum. Ducts canalize through degeneration of epithelial cells, resulting in the tubular bile duct. After the 13th week, bile empties into the duodenum through the duct, resulting in the dark green color seen with meconium.

Concurrent development of the pancreas begins with development of two pancreatic buds. The dorsal

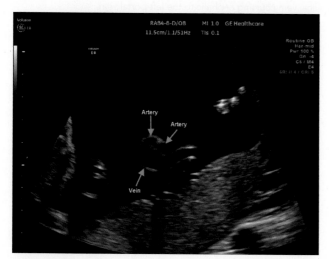

Figure 20-32 A transverse image of a normal umbilical cord demonstrating one umbilical vein and two smaller umbilical arteries.

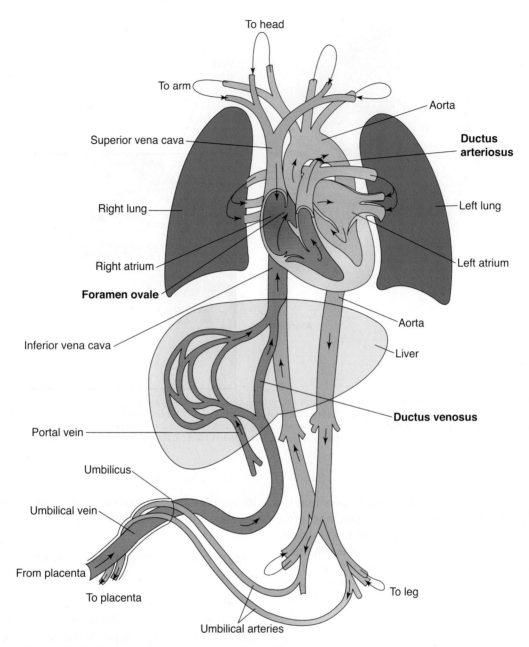

To head

To arm

Superior vena cava

Aorta

Ductus arteriosus

Right lung

Left lung

Right atrium

Left atrium

Foramen ovale

Inferior vena cava

Aorta

Liver

Ductus venosus

Portal vein

Umbilicus

Umbilical vein

From placenta

To leg

To placenta

Umbilical arteries

Figure 20-33 Diagram of fetal circulation showing umbilical vein coursing cephalic to the left portal vein.

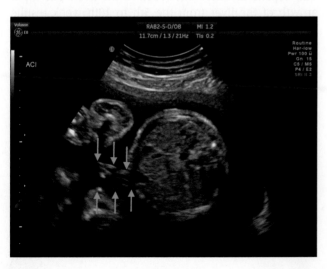

Figure 20-34 Transverse view of the abdominal umbilical cord (*green arrows*) insertion.

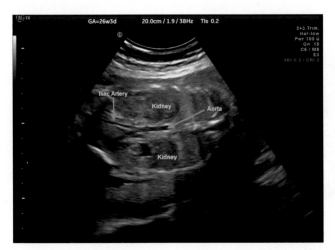

Figure 20-35 Coronal view demonstrating the aorta and iliac arteries.

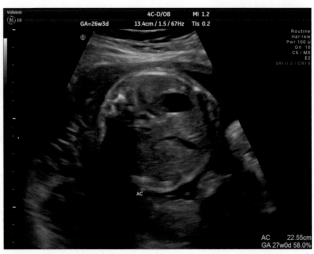

Figure 20-37 AC measured at the level of the transverse spine, stomach, and umbilical/portal vein using an ellipse measurement.

and ventral pancreatic buds develop, with the ventral forming the uncinate process and head of the pancreas. This portion of the pancreas follows the bowel rotation, placing the ventral bud in close proximity of the dorsal bud. These two portions fuse and the ducts fuse.

The spleen is part of the lymphatic system rather than the digestive; however, because of the concurrent development and rotation, the spleen is grouped with the digestive organs. The spleen develops during the fifth week of gestation as a lobulated organ located in the midline between the stomach and aorta. The organ contour smoothes before birth, occupying the characteristic left upper quadrant location after the midgut rotates and the liver moves into the right upper quadrant (Fig. 20-38).

Imaging Findings

Sonography

The fetal liver is a large, homogeneously echogenic organ occupying the right upper quadrant and crossing midline to the left. In an adult, the right lobe of the liver is much larger than the left lobe. In the fetus, the left lobe is as

large as or slightly larger than the right lobe. This may make it difficult to determine which side of the body is being imaged unless the fluid-filled, left-sided stomach is visible. The liver grows throughout pregnancy.

The gallbladder, in its position to the right of midline, separates the right lobe from the medial left lobe, as does the middle hepatic vein. Use color Doppler to differentiate the fluid-filled gallbladder (Fig. 20-39A) from the tubular intrahepatic portion of the umbilical vein (there should not be color flow in the gallbladder). Key differentiating points are the gallbladder's usually teardrop shape, its off-midline position (rather than midline), its extrahepatic location (posteroinferior to the liver), and the lack of communication between the gallbladder and vessels of the umbilical cord (Fig. 20-39B). Unlike the umbilical vein, the gallbladder does not reach the anterior abdominal wall. The gallbladder is passive in fetal life and does not respond to fat ingested by the mother. Absence of the gallbladder may be associated with several conditions, including biliary atresia.

The pancreas is rarely discretely imaged. Its echogenicity is similar to that of surrounding structures. Occasionally, the fluid-filled stomach and the location of the pancreas anterior to the splenic vein may aid in its identification (Fig. 20-40). Fetal pancreatic echogenicity is slightly greater than that of the liver.

The spleen is not always easily visualized. It is homogeneous and located posterior to the stomach and superior to the left kidney in the left upper abdomen. It is best seen on transverse scans. The spleen is similar in echogenicity to the kidney and slightly less echogenic than the liver (Fig. 20-41).

MRI

The T2WI demonstrates the liver and spleen as a dark structure, while the T2WI shows isointense organs. As with sonography, the gallbladder images as a cystic structure inferior to the liver[17] (Fig. 20-14).

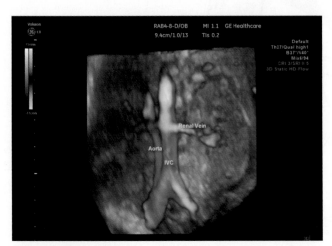

Figure 20-36 3D glass body rendering of the aorta and inferior vena cava and associated renal veins/arteries.

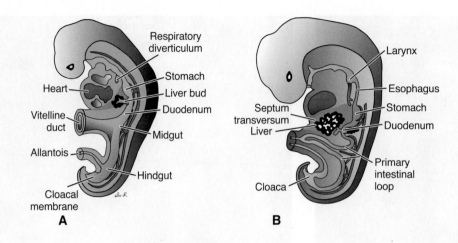

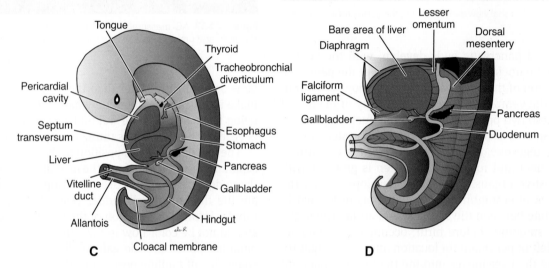

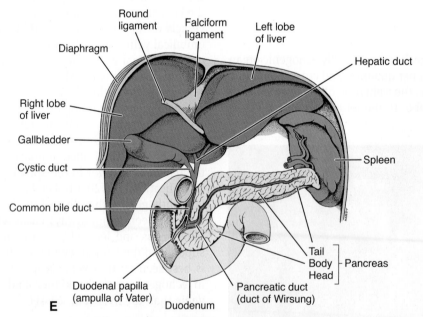

Figure 20-38 **A–B:** The accessory organs of digestion (liver, gallbladder, and pancreas) first emerge as buds of the foregut tube in the space provided by the ventral mesentery. **C–E:** As the organs enlarge and move, the foregut mesentery goes with them and persists in the same way that the dorsal mesentery does. (From Sadler TW. *Langman's Medical Embryology.* 10th ed. Baltimore, MD: Lippincott Williams & Wilkins; 2006. Figs. 14.14 and 14.15, p. 212; from *Stedman's Medical Dictionary.* 27th ed. Baltimore, MD: Lippincott Williams & Wilkins; 2000.)

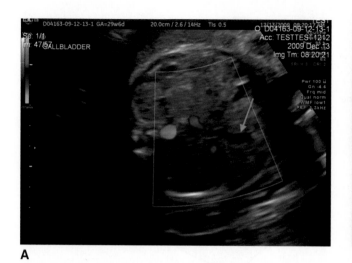
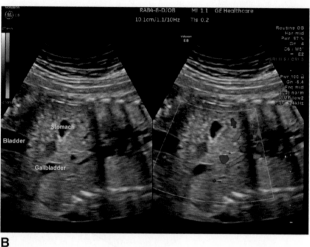

Figure 20-39 A: Transverse view of the fetal abdomen demonstrating no color flow in the gallbladder. **B:** Dual format of a coronal view of the fetal abdomen demonstrating no color flow in the gallbladder, stomach, and fetal bladder.

STOMACH AND BOWEL

Embryology

The stomach begins as a dilation of the stomach primorium site in the fourth week. The greater curvature of the stomach is the result of faster growth of the dorsal border. At the same time, the caudal portion of the foregut, splanchnic mesenchyme, and the cranial portion of the midgut begin to form the duodenum. During the fifth to sixth weeks, the duodenal lumen closes until degeneration of the epithelial cells resulting in the recanalized lumen at the end of the first trimester.[6]

In the first part of the sixth week, the midgut begins to elongate, forming a U-shaped gut loop, which creates the physiologic umbilical herniation imaged in the first trimester. This herniation, into the proximal portion of the umbilical cord, contains structures that will become the small intestine, most of the duodenum, cecum, appendix, ascending colon, and two-thirds of the transverse colon. The yolk stalk or vitelline duct provides communication between the midgut and yolk sac through the 10th week. At this stage, the liver and kidneys fill most of the abdomen, resulting in umbilical herniation of the rapidly growing midgut structures. In the latter portion of the first trimester, and after midgut loop rotation, the intestinal structures return to the abdomen (Fig. 20-42). This reduction of the physiologic midgut herniation results in positioning of the bowel in the locations found in the neonate and adult.[6]

Imaging Findings

Sonography

The stomach (Fig. 20-43A) images consistently in the second trimester because of variable filling of echo-free fluid. Because of the periodic filling and emptying of the stomach, an absent stomach requires further examination over time (several hours or on a follow-up examination). An absent stomach may be associated with

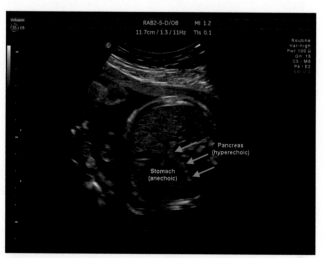

Figure 20-40 Fetal pancreas (*green arrows*) is demonstrated as slightly more echogenic than the surrounding anatomy.

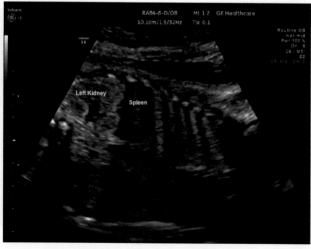

Figure 20-41 Fetal spleen and left kidney.

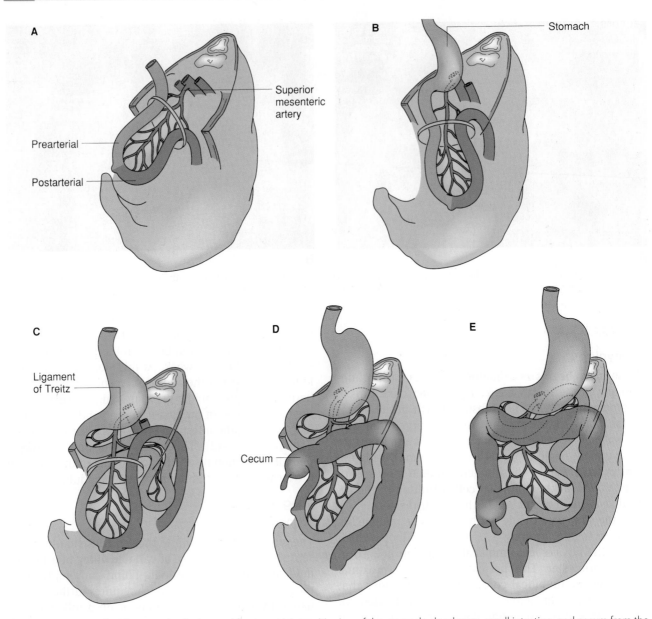

Figure 20-42 Normal midgut rotation is shown with appropriate positioning of the stomach, duodenum, small intestine, and cecum from the fifth gestational week **(A)** through completion by the 12th week **(E)**.

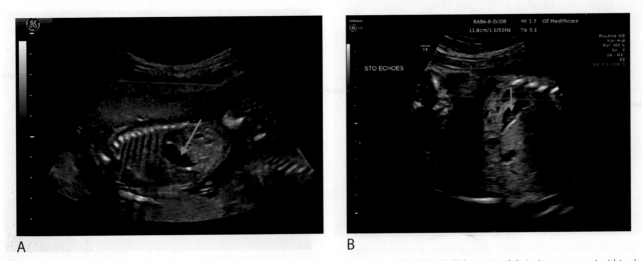

Figure 20-43 A: Sagittal view of the fetus demonstrating the anechoic stomach (*green arrow*). **B:** Echogenic debris (*green arrow*) within the fetal stomach.

abnormal outcomes. Echogenicity within the stomach fluid has been seen in cases of third-trimester placental abruption; this may represent swallowed blood or vernix (Fig. 20-43). The echogenicity within the stomach fluid is commonly seen in the second trimester and disappears on follow-up examinations.

Early in pregnancy, the midgut herniation images on the ventral portion of the embryo. This herniation is seen on the transverse image (Fig. 13-21A). Surface rendering of the embryo from the 3D data set also images the normal midgut herniation (Fig. 13-21B). By week 12, this normal herniation has been reduced and pathologic abdominal wall defects may be diagnosed thereafter. Before significant amounts of fluid enter it, the small bowel may appear as a heterogeneous, echogenic pseudomass without shadowing, occupying a substantial portion of the abdomen. It is more echogenic than the liver but typically less echogenic than bones. In the third trimester, the bowel becomes less echogenic and more sharply defined. The rate of fetal swallowing eventually overcomes the resorptive capacity of the stomach and proximal duodenum, allowing filling of the distal small bowel. Peristalsis may be seen in the small bowel that occupies the central abdomen. Normal fetal small bowel increases in diameter as gestational age increases.

The colon is a long, continuous, tubular structure with a hypoechoic lumen at the abdominal periphery (Fig. 20-44). Although it may be seen as early as the late second trimester, it is usually visualized more consistently in the third trimester. The transverse colon is seen most easily just caudad to the liver. The colon typically increases in diameter throughout the third trimester. It has far less peristalsis than the small bowel (Fig. 20-45). Meconium is composed of the materials the fetus ingests during its gestation (e.g., mucous, amniotic fluid, bile). It is less echogenic than the bowel wall and may be routinely noted in discrete portions of the colon. Sometimes, the normal colon with liquid meconium is mistaken for cysts, dilated bowel, and other anomalies.

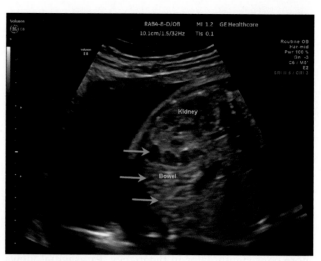

Figure 20-45 Transverse/oblique image demonstrating the fetal bowel (*green arrows*).

MRI

The MRI image demonstrates the stomach as a fluid signal intensity. The distal small intestine and colon images hyperintense on T2WI and hypointense on the T1WI because of the presence of amniotic fluid. The opposite is true in the presence on meconium.[17] Regardless of the type of MRI acquisition method, speed becomes important as the fetus seldom remains still for an extended period of time (Fig. 20-46).

GENITOURINARY SYSTEM

Embryology

The development of the genitourinary system is covered in detail in Chapter 2.

Imaging Findings

Sonography

Fetal urine becomes the primary source of amniotic fluid in the latter half of gestation.[13] The presence of oligohydramnios after 16 weeks' gestation raises suspicion for a malfunctioning genitourinary system because of

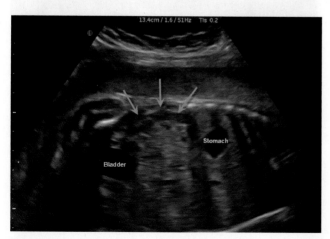

Figure 20-44 Parasagittal image demonstrating the colon (*green arrows*).

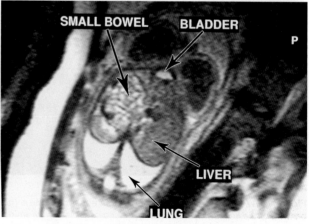

Figure 20-46 Coronal HASTE image through fetal abdomen.

a lack of urine production. Although the fetal kidneys may be imaged as early as 10 to 12 weeks' gestational age, the internal structures of the kidneys are not reliably assessed before 14 to 16 weeks. The lack of significant contrast between the kidneys and the nearby soft tissues decreases kidney identification early in gestation. Because of increased contrast resolution and a decrease in artifacts, newer sonographic equipment has improved visualization of the kidney anatomy. In the case of poor kidney visualization, the incorporation of color Doppler imaging aids in documentation of the renal arteries.

On transverse images, the kidneys are hypoechoic, ovoid masses on either side of the spine (Fig. 20-47A). Occasionally, the anechoic renal pelvis may be visualized. The echogenic center of renal sinus fat is noted more consistently later in pregnancy. Parasagittal views of each kidney show them to be paraspinous and bean-shaped. As in neonates, the normal hypoechoic medullary pyramids (Fig. 20-47B) may be seen arranged in anterior and posterior rows around the renal pelvis. They should not be mistaken for renal cysts. Kidney length ranges from 2 cm at 20 weeks to nearly 4 cm at term (Table 20-3). The renal pelvis is typically collapsed (i.e., not urine filled) and therefore is not imaged. If filled with urine, an anechoic renal pelvis may be noted (Fig. 20-48). This renal pelvic dilation is often evaluated by noting its anterior-to-posterior measurement. There is debate regarding how worrisome dilation is and how closely these fetuses should be monitored. Generally, allowances of 5 mm of pelvic dilation up to 20 weeks and 8 mm of pelvic dilation between 20 and 40 weeks.[18] This dilation may be related to transient fetal urinary reflux or obstruction of pelvic urine outflow from a fluid-filled fetal bladder. It is less worrisome if there is good bladder filling (evidence of at least one functioning and nonobstructed renal system) and normal amounts of amniotic fluid. Of key importance is the evaluation of this fetus

and its kidneys when it is a neonate. This is best performed at day 2 or 3 of life.

Another method to determine normalcy of the fetal kidneys is through the calculation of the renal volume. The formula traditionally used (length × width × height × 0.5233) often underestimates the actual volume.[19] 3D sonography has increased the accuracy of determining renal normalcy through the calculation of a volume. After obtaining a 3D data set of the fetal kidney, the use of the VOCAL technique allows for automatic volume calculation of the bean-shaped organ (Table 20-4)(Fig. 20-49).[19]

The adrenals are ovoid, triangular, or heart-shaped structures often imaged in the suprarenal area of the fetus. Adrenals may be imaged as early as the late first/early second trimester and are easiest to note in relation to the kidney on longitudinal images (Fig. 20-50A). On transverse view, the adrenals may resemble the shape of the kidney (Fig. 20-50B). This is particularly true in association with ipsilateral renal agenesis. There is an echogenic central medulla and a hypoechoic, thick outer cortex.

The fetal ureters are not normally visualized unless there is significant genitourinary system reflux or obstruction. The bladder (Fig. 20-51) is seen as an echo-free intrapelvic structure as early as 13 weeks' gestational age. It is circular to oblong. Wall thickness cannot be appreciated in the normal bladder without the presence of ascites. It is a dynamic structure whose size varies with the degree of filling. The fetus voids about once per hour. If the bladder fills, at least one functioning kidney is present. If no bladder is seen on examination, a repeat examination is performed. Occasionally, the bladder may appear distended when there is no pathologic process. When distended, normally or pathologically, the bladder rises out of the narrow pelvis and into the upper abdomen.

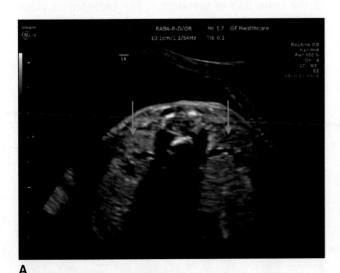

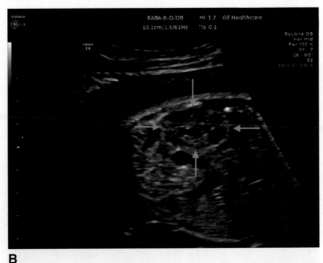

A   **B**

Figure 20-47 A: Transverse image of the bilateral fetal kidneys (*green arrows*). **B:** Sagittal image of the fetal kidney (*green arrows* outline the borders of the kidney). The normal hypoechoic medullary pyramids are visualized around the renal pelvis.

TABLE 20-3 Mean 2D Renal Lengths for Various Gestational Ages[21–23]		
Gestational Age (wk)	Mean Length (cm)	95%Confidence Interval (cm)
18	2.2	1.6–2.8
19	2.3	1.5–3.1
20	2.6	1.8–3.4
21	2.7	2.1–3.2
22	2.7	2.0–3.4
23	3.0	2.2–3.7
24	3.1	1.9–4.4
25	3.3	2.5–4.2
26	3.4	2.4–4.4
27	3.5	2.7–4.4
28	3.4	2.6–4.2
29	3.6	2.3–4.8
30	3.8	2.9–4.6
31	3.7	2.8–4.6
32	4.1	3.1–5.1
33	4.0	3.3–4.7
34	4.2	3.3–5.0
35	4.2	3.2–5.2
36	4.2	3.3–5.0
37	4.2	3.3–5.1
38	4.4	3.2–5.6
39	4.2	3.5–4.8
40	4.3	3.2–5.3
41	4.5	3.9–5.1

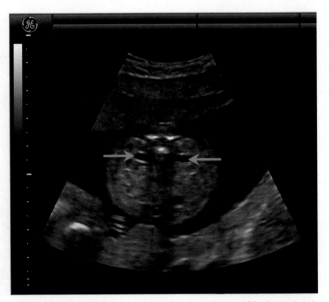

Figure 20-48 Transverse image of bilateral urine-filled renal pelvises (*green arrows*).

TABLE 20-4 Mean 3D Renal Volumes for Various Gestational Ages[19,24]				
Week	Left		Right	
	Mean Volume cm²	Min-Max	Mean Volume cm²	Min-Max
20	1.8	0.6–3.0	1.5	0.32–2.7
21	2.6	1.1–4.0	2.2	0.4–3.6
22	3.3	1.6–5.1	3.0	1.4–4.6
23	4.1	2.0–6.1	3.7	2.0–5.5
24	4.6	3.0–6.3	4.5	2.2–6.6
25	5.3	3.4–7.5	5.0	3.1–6.9
26	5.7	3.9–7.6	5.6	4.0–7.2
27	7.0	4.6–9.3	6.6	4.9–7.9
28	7.7	4.3–11.0	7.5	5.7–9.1
29	8.9	4.6–13.1	8.2	6.7–9.7
30	8.8	5.4–12.2	8.5	5.6–12.0
31	9.8	6.7–12.9	10.0	7.7–12.3
32	10.6	7.9–13.3	10.2	7.7–12.7
33	11.2	6.5–16.0	11.0	7.0–15.1
34	12.1	8.3–15.9	12.1	9.1–15.0
35	13.2	7.6–18.8	12.6	8.2–16.9
36	14.0	8.0–19.9	13.4	8.8–17.9
37	14.7	8.6–20.9	14.8	9.3–19.8
38	15.5	9.0–22.0	14.8	9.8–19.8
39	16.3	9.5–23.0	15.6	10.4–20.7
40	17.2	2.0–24.1	16.3	10.9–21.7

MRI

Most of the time, sonography images the fetal urinary tract; however, in cases of maternal body habitus, overlying bony structures, or oligohydramnios, the MRI exam helps with fetal renal imaging. In the case of inconclusive sonographic findings, MRI becomes the modality of choice. The urinary system, comprising the kidneys, renal pelvis, and bladder, images as fluid-filled structures on the T2WI (Fig. 20-52).[17]

THE PELVIS

The pelvis is a small structure in the fetus. Its sonographic image is made up predominantly of the bones of the pelvis, the pelvic muscles, and the bladder. The bony pelvis consists of echogenic iliac crests separated

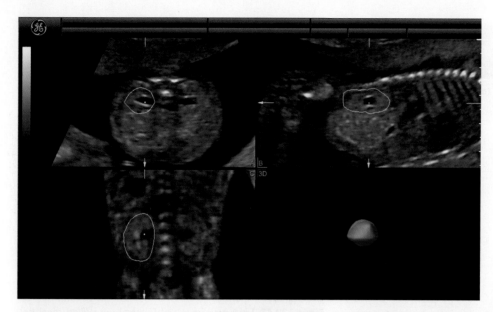

Figure 20-49 VOCAL tracing of a fetal kidney.

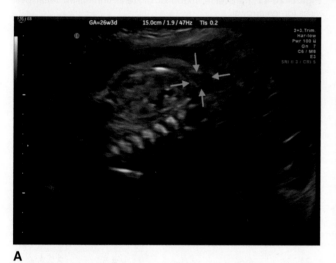

A

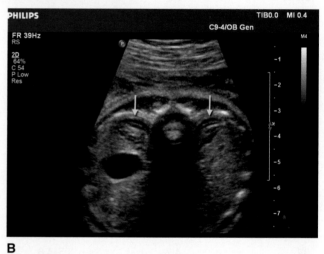

B

Figure 20-50 A: Longitudinal view of the left fetal kidney and adrenal (*green arrows* outline the adrenal). B: Transverse view of both adrenal glands (*yellow arrows*). (Image **B** courtesy of Philips Medical Systems, Bothell, WA.)

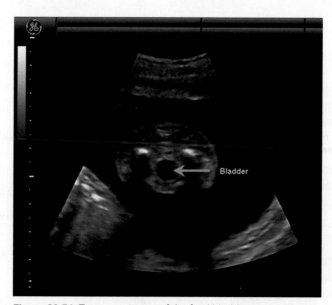

Figure 20-51 Transverse image of the fetal bladder (*green arrow*).

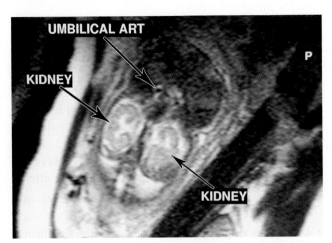

Figure 20-52 Coronal HASTE image through fetal kidneys.

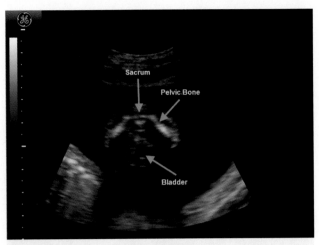

Figure 20-53 Fetal pelvis demonstrating sacral ossification centers, iliac bones, and normal soft tissue posterior to the sacrum.

from the echogenic sacrum by the hypoechoic sacroiliac joint (Fig. 20-53). Three ossification centers are noted along the sacrum. As in the craniocervical region, some soft tissue prominence may be noted in the lumbosacral region as hypoechoic density between skin and spine. Masses should not be seen. Thin fascial lines may separate the hypoechoic gluteal muscles. The ischium and pubis are noted as echogenic anterior densities, and often the echogenic, nonossified femoral head can be seen at the acetabular area.

GENITALS

Embryology

The development of the external genitalia is covered in detail in Chapter 2.

Imaging Findings

Sonography

The identification of fetal genitalia requires adequate visualization of the perineum. A crossed thigh can readily hide a scrotum. Gender identification is of clinical significance when suspecting X-linked inherited disorders, twin-to-twin transfusion, and other syndromes. Proof of different genitalia in twins can help prove dizygosity and rule out twin-to-twin transfusion syndrome and other problems associated with monozygotic twins. Rare intersex problems may be diagnosed if there is a discrepancy in karyotype gender from visualized genitals (e.g., testicular feminization syndrome, in which a fetus has a male karyotype and female genitalia).

In the male fetus, the penis and scrotum (Fig. 20-54) are readily visualized between the thighs. The sonographer must be aware of the possibility of a nearby umbilical cord simulating a penis. Voiding into the amniotic fluid may be seen. Erections are not unusual. In the third trimester, testicles have typically descended into the scrotum and are noted as echogenic structures.

In female fetuses (Fig. 20-55), the labia majora are noted as masses of moderate echogenicity off the perineum. A central linear echogenicity between them represents the labia minora. The normal ovaries, uterus, and vagina are not typically visualized in a normal fetus.

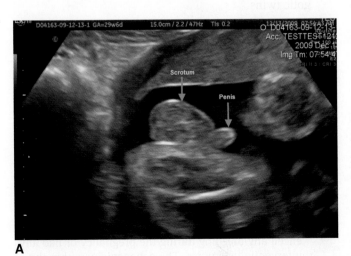

A

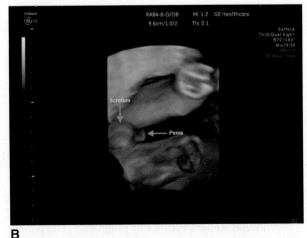

B

Figure 20-54 A: Fetal male genitalia imaged displaying the scrotum and penis. **B:** 3D rendered image of the male genitalia displaying the scrotum and penis.

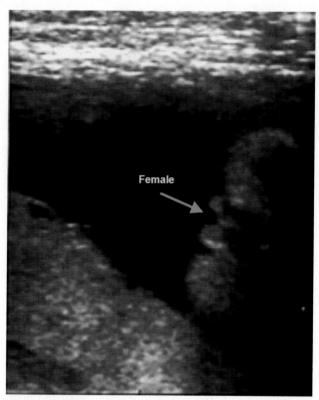

Figure 20-55 Female genitalia displaying the labia majora and labia minora.

SUMMARY

- In obstetrics, the term vertex or cephalic indicates when the fetal head is down toward the cervix.

- Complete breech refers to when the buttocks present first (toward the cervix) and both the hips and knees are flexed.

- Incomplete breech or "footling" breech indicates that the fetus has one or both feet down so its legs are poised to deliver first.

- Frank breech indicates that the fetal buttocks present first and that the hips are flexed so the legs are straight and completely drawn up toward the fetal chest.

- Obtain thoracic measurements from a true transverse view just above the diaphragm at the level of the fetal heart.

- Sonography is not reliable to indicate fetal lung maturity; amniocentesis remains the gold standard in this assessment.

- The thymus is located at the level of the great vessel of the heart, anterior to the aorta and pulmonary artery.

- The umbilical cord consists of one umbilical vein and two umbilical arteries.

- Usually, a single umbilical artery is not significant, but it has been associated with gastrointestinal tract, renal, and cardiac abnormalities as well as an increased incidence of trisomy.

- Measure the abdominal circumference in a true axial plane of the abdomen, demonstrating the transverse spine, left-sided stomach, and the umbilical vein entering into the left portal vein.

- Measurements are made along the outer perimeter of the abdomen.

- Absence of a visible stomach can be associated with abnormal outcomes; an absent stomach requires further examination over time.

- Echoes within the stomach can be associated with swallowed blood.

- By week 12, the small bowel should not be herniated within the base of the umbilical cord.

- The internal structures of the fetal kidneys are not reliably assessed before 14 to 16 weeks.

- Normal hypoechoic medullary pyramids should not be mistaken for renal cysts.

- Proof of different genitalia in twins can help prove dizygosity and rule out twin-to-twin transfusion syndrome and other problems associated with monozygotic twins.

Critical Thinking Questions

Case 1 Images:

1. A 36-year-old patient presented for a targeted ultrasound because of advanced maternal age. The exam was unremarkable with the exception of echoes appearing within the fetal stomach. The sonographer imaged the stomach echoes in both sagittal and transverse planes to ensure that they were not artifacts. Once the echoes were confirmed nonartifactual, the sonographer interrogated the patient to determine if she had experienced any bleeding or had any interventional studies during this pregnancy. The patient had amniocentesis last week but denied any bleeding with this pregnancy. What is the significance of the echoes visualized within the stomach?

ANSWER: Echogenic debris within the stomach is not an ominous sign. It is usually an idiopathic finding. The echogenic debris represents swallowed blood or vernix and may be associated with postinterventional exams such as amniocentesis and intrauterine transfusions. During obstetrical imaging, the stomach is documented for position, anomaly, and proper filling. If debris is visualized within the stomach, it is important to ask the patient if she has experienced any bleeding during the pregnancy or had any interventional studies. The echogenicity within the stomach fluid commonly disappears on follow-up examinations.

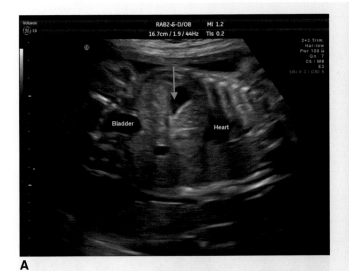

A

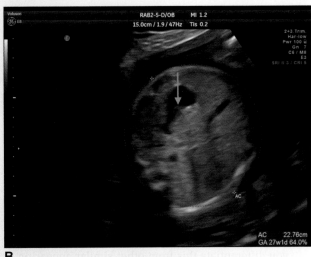

B

2. A patient arrives for a biophysical profile. The history reveals she has pregnancy-induced hypertension. The fetus measured 26 weeks 3 days and had normal breathing, tone, and movement. The four-pocket amniotic fluid index measured 12 cm. During the examination, the sonographer noticed that the right renal pelvis was prominent. The left renal pelvis measured 0.24 cm and the right renal pelvis measured 0.57 cm. The bladder appeared normal. The bladder emptied and began filling during the course of the biophysical profile. What are the normal parameters for the renal pelvis at this gestational age?

determine if there is pathologic urinary tract dilation. Transaxial and longitudinal images should be utilized to evaluate the kidneys. Measurements for renal pelvis enlargement are taken anteroposterior on the transaxial images. Pelviectasis is a common finding particularly in male fetuses and may be associated with posterior urethral valve obstruction. Caliectasis (dilation of the renal calices) in association with pelviectasis is an indication of hydronephrosis.

3. A patient presented for targeted exam with a prior history of IUGR. The gestational age by last exam is 26 weeks 3 days. Today's exam measures the fetus at 25 weeks 6 days. Describe the echogenicity of the bowel. What is the importance of this finding?

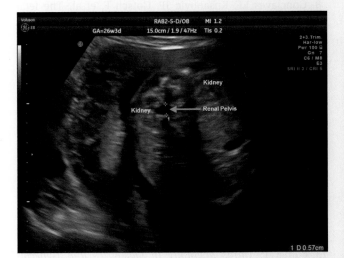

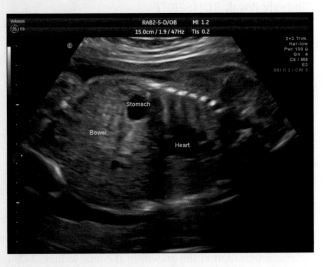

ANSWER: Imaging the fetal kidneys is a routine part of most standard obstetrical examinations. Pelviectasis, also known as pyelectasis, is the enlargement of the renal pelvis. Generally, allowances of 5 mm of pelvic dilation up to 20 weeks and 8 mm of pelvic dilation between 20 and 40 weeks.[18] This fetus was 26 weeks, so a renal pelvis measurement of 0.57 cm is within normal limits. When pelviectasis occurs, one should

ANSWER: The fetus measuring 4 days smaller than expected by previous exam, is well within normal limits. In this particular exam, there was a question concerning the bowel echogenicity. From the image, the echogenicity appears normal. Pseudoechogenic bowel is not an uncommon finding. Bowel is not considered

(continued)

"echogenic" unless it equals or exceeds the echogenicity of bones. There is an association with aneuploidy, cystic fibrosis, IUGR, cytomegalovirus, and postbleeding with absorption into the bowel.[20] Caution should be exercised when using high-frequency transducers. The bowel's echogenicity may appear increased when using higher frequencies. Changing to a lower frequency would decrease the likelihood of a pseudo increase in the bowel's echogenicity.

4. Patient presented with history of parvovirus exposure. The fetus was therefore being evaluated to rule out hydrops and any other potential associated anomalies. The fetus measured normal for gestational age. When the sonographer imaged the transverse kidneys, there appeared to be fluid in the abdomen. Discuss the probable cause of this finding. How can you differentiate this from other similar-appearing processes?

ANSWER: A fetus infected with parvovirus may display hydrops, ascites, and ventriculomegaly among other anomalies. When imaging a fetus for hydrops, one should include evaluations for ascites, plural effusions, pericardial effusion, placentamegaly, and polyhydramnios. The fetal abdomen is evaluated for

free fluid. On occasion, there is question of pseudoascites. When ascites is suspected, the area must be imaged in two orthogonal planes to eliminate possibility of pseudoascites. This fetus does not have ascites. The image demonstrates the common finding of pseudoascites.

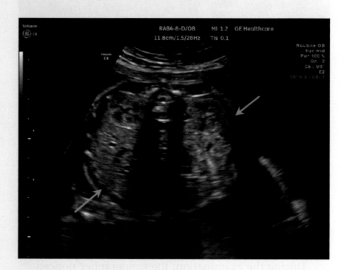

Acknowledgements: We would like to acknowledge the following for their support in this project and for their above and beyond help in obtaining images:

David Vance, MA
Sue Magner, RDMS
Mike Kammermeier, RDMS, RVT, RDC
Kimberly Royal, RDMS, RVT
Teresa Casto, RT, RDMS, RVT
Dawn Mulson RDMS RVT

Unless otherwise noted, sonographic images are compliments of GE Healthcare, Wauwatosa, WI.

REFERENCES

1. Digital Imaging and Communications in Medicine (DICOM) Part 3: Information Object Definitions. Available at: ftp://medical.nema.org/medical/dicom/2007/07_03pu.pdf. Accessed May 2010.

2. Merz E, Benoit B, Blaas HG, et al. Standardization of three-dimensional images in obstetrics and gynecology: consensus statement. *Ultrasound Obstet Gynecol.* 2007;29:697–703.

3. Bertagnoli L, Lalatta F, Gallicchio R, et al. Quantitative characterization of the growth of the fetal kidney. *J Clin Ultrasound.* 1983;11:349–356.

4. Sherer DM, Sokolovski M, Dalloul M, et al. Fetal clavicle length throughout gestation: a nomogram. *Ultrasound Obstet Gynecol.* 2006;27(3):306–310.

5. Wladimiroff JW, Cohen-Overbeek TE, Laudy JA. Ultrasound evaluation of the fetal thorax. In: *Ultrasonography in Obstetrics and Gynecology.* 5th ed. Philadelphia, PA: Sanders Elsevier; 2008.

6. Moore KL, Persaud TVN. *The Developing Human; Clinically Oriented Embryology.* 8th ed. Philadelphia, PA: Saunders; 2007.

7. Lee KA, Cho JY, Lee SM, et al. Prenatal diagnosis of bilateral pulmonary agenesis: a case report. *Korean J Radiol.* 2010; 11(1):119–122.

8. Gonclaves LF, Kusanovic JP, Gotsch F, et al. The fetal musculoskeletal system. In: *Ultrasonography in Obstetrics and Gynecology.* 5th ed. Philadelphia, PA: Sanders Elsevier; 2008.

9. Jani JC, Cannie M, Peralta CFA, et al. Lung volumes in fetuses with congenital diaphragmatic hernia: comparison of 3D US and MR imaging assessments. *Radiology.* 2007; 244:575–582.

10. Büsing KA, Kilian AK, Schaible T, et al. Fetal body volume at MR imaging to quantify total fetal lung volume: normal ranges. *Radiology.* 2008;246(2):553–561.

11. Shinmoto H, Kashima K, Yuasa Y, et al. MR imaging of non-CNS fetal abnormalities: a pictorial essay. *Radiographics.* 2000;20(5):1227–1243.

12. Rumack CM, Wilson SR, Charboneau JW, eds. *Diagnostic Ultrasound.* 3rd ed. St. Louis, MO: Elsevier Mosby; 2005.

13. Callen P. *Ultrasonography in Obstetrics and Gynecology.* 5th ed. San Francisco, CA: WB Saunders Company; 2008.

14. McGahan JP, Goldberg BB, eds. *Diagnostic Ultrasound.* 2nd ed. New York, NY: Informa Healthcare USA, Inc; 2008.

15. Heredia F, Jeanty P. Umbilical cord anomalies. Available at: http://www.sonoworld.com/Fetus/page.aspx?id=1149. Accessed April 2, 2010.

16. Doubilet PM, Benson CB. *Atlas of Ultrasound in Obstetrics and Gynecology: A Multimedia Reference.* Philadelphia, PA: Lippincott Williams & Wilkins; 2003.

17. Guo Y, Luo BN. The state of the art of fetal magnetic resonance imaging. *Chin Med J (Engl)*. 2006;119(15):1294–1299.

18. OBFOCUS. Fetal Pyelectasis (Pelviectasis). Available at: http://www.obfocus.com/high-risk/birthdefects/pyelectasis. htm. Accessed April 4, 2010.

19. Yu CH, Chang CH, Chang FM, et al. Fetal renal volume in normal gestation: a three-dimensional ultrasound study. *Ultrasound in Med & Biol*. 2000;26(8):1253–1256.

20. McNamara A, Levine D. Intraabdominal fetal echogenic masses: a practical guide to diagnosis and management (Abstract). *Radiographics*. 2005;25:533–645. Available at: http://radiographics.rsna.org/content/25/3/633.full. Accessed April 3, 2010.

21. Cohen HL, Cooper J, Eisenberg P, et al. Normal length of fetal kidneys: sonographic study in 397 obstetric patients. *Am J Roentgenol*. 1991;157:545–548.

22. Shin JS, Seo YS, Kim JH, et al. Nomogram of fetal renal growth expressed in length and parenchymal area derived from ultrasound imagines. *J Urol*. 2007;178:2150–2154.

23. Cannie M, Neirynck V, De Keyzer F, et al. Prenatal magnetic resonance imaging demonstrates linear growth of the human fetal kidneys during gestation. *J Urol*. 2007;178:1570–1574.

24. Tedesco GD, Bussamra L, Junior EA, et al. Reference range of fetal renal volume by three-dimensional ultrasonography using the vocal method. *Fetal Diagn Ther*. 2009;25:385–391.

21 Ultrasound of the Abnormal Fetal Chest, Abdomen, and Pelvis

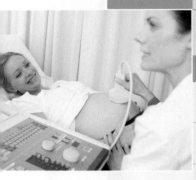

Gertrude Alfonsin Layton

OBJECTIVES

Differentiate intrathorax pathologies of a bronchogenic cyst, congenital cystic adenomatoid malformation, pulmonary sequestration, and a diaphragmatic hernia

Describe methods to use color Doppler to aid in identification of lung malformations, ventral wall defects, and Potter sequence renal malformations

Summarize immune and nonimmune fetal hydrops causes and sonographic appearance

Explain the sonographic identification of omphalocele, gastroschisis, and bladder exstrophy

Discuss bowel malformations of a midgut volvulus, duodenal atresia, and meconium ileus

Identify the causes, sonographic appearance, and consequences of fetal hydronephrosis

KEY TERMS

congenital multicystic adenomatoid malformation (CCAM) | pulmonary sequestration | bronchogenic cyst | pulmonary hypoplasia | immune fetal hydrops | nonimmune fetal hydrops | congenital diaphragmatic hernia (CDH) | omphalocele | gastroschisis | midgut volvulus | duodenal atresia | meconium ileus | renal agenesis | Potter sequence | prune belly syndrome | bladder exstrophy

GLOSSARY

Anasarca Generalized edema in the subcutaneous tissue

Bladder exstrophy Congenital anomaly where the bladder is outside the body through a ventral wall defect inferior to the umbilical cord

Bronchogenic cyst Solitary cyst within the lung

Congenital diaphragmatic hernia (CDH) Birth defect of the diaphragm that allows the abdominal contents to enter the chest

Congenital multicystic adenomatoid malformation (CCAM) Replacement of normal lung by nonfunctioning cystic lung tissue

Duodenal atresia Congenital absence or closing of the duodenal lumen.

Gastroschisis Membrane-free ventral wall defect with protrusion of abdominal contents lateral to the umbilical cord

Hemangioma Benign mass made up of blood vessels

Hirschsprung disease Congenital lack of nerves in the colon resulting in fecal impaction and a megacolon

Hydrops Accumulation of fluid in the fetal tissues, peritoneum, and pleural cavities due to either immune or nonimmune factors

Meconium ileus Bowel obstructed by mucus

Mediastinum Chest area lying between the lungs, which contains the heart, aorta, esophagus, trachea, and thymus

Midgut volvulus Bowel obstructed due to bowel twisting

Omphalocele Membrane-covered ventral wall defect containing abdominal contents involving the umbilical cord

Potter sequence This group of findings, also called Potter's syndrome or oligohydramnios sequence, includes renal conditions such as agenesis, obstructive processes and acquired or inherited cystic disease

Prune belly syndrome Congenital disorder of the urinary system resulting in the absence of the abdominal muscles

Pulmonary sequestration Noncommunicating lung tissue that lacks pulmonary blood supply

Renal agenesis Failure of renal development

Situs inversus Reversal of normal organ position

Upper GI Radiographic study using barium sulfate as a contrast agent to outline and fill the gastrointestinal tract

Knowledge of normal anatomy, embryology, biometry, and pathology, in combination with equipment advances, operator experience, and meticulous technique, allows for the superior diagnosis of abnormalities of the fetal thorax, abdomen, and pelvis. This chapter discusses some of these abnormalities and their diagnostic sonographic findings. Though not often used prenatally, complementary imaging such as radiography helps us understand sonographic findings and the underlying mechanism of anomalies of the chest, abdomen, and pelvis.

THORAX

Evaluation of the fetal thorax includes observation of overall size and symmetry of bony and soft tissue elements as discussed in Chapter 20. The normal intrathoracic contents consist of homogeneous, relatively symmetric lung parenchyma surrounding the central heart and mediastinum. Evaluation of the sonographic image for asymmetry, mass, mass effect, or mediastinal shift is essential in detecting possible intrathoracic pathology.

Routine observation of fetal breathing movements in the second and third trimester should be included, as well as the heart orientation. The heart lies with the apex oriented to the spleen in the midline left chest.[1] Careful imaging of the diaphragm in both sagittal and transverse planes helps exclude possible defects and abnormal locations of organs.

THE LUNGS

Normal fetal lungs have a symmetrically homogeneous appearance on the sonographic image as seen in Figure 20-10. Pleural effusions comprise half of all intrathoracic abnormalities noted on fetal examination.[2] Imaged intrathoracic masses, excluding congenital diaphragmatic hernias (CDH), are usually cystic, but they are at times solid and echogenic. These anomalies disrupt the homogeneity of the lung parenchyma or cause cardiac or mediastinal shifts.[1,2] The predominant cystic masses of the lung include the typically unilocular bronchogenic cyst and the multicystic cystic adenomatoid malformation (CCAM). Other reported masses include aortic aneurysm, pulmonary sequestration, congenital lobar emphysema, neurenteric cyst, bronchial atresia and, in rare instances, teratoma.[2]

Bronchogenic Cyst

Several cases of bronchogenic cyst have been diagnosed antenatally.[2,3] These cysts may be unilocular or multilocular and can displace mediastinal structures, although this is an uncommon finding in neonatal life. Bronchogenic cysts result from abnormal budding of the ventral diverticulum of the primitive foregut and are lined by epithelium similar to that of a normal bronchus and subsequently may contain cartilage, muscle, or mucus

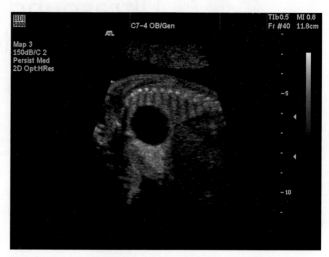

Figure 21-1 Anechoic bronchogenic cyst seen on a sagittal image. (Image courtesy of Philips Medical Systems, Bothell, WA.)

glands.[4] The cysts may be found within the lung parenchyma or mediastinum and often communicate directly with the trachea or main stem bronchi (Fig. 21-1).[2]

Congenital Cystic Adenomatoid Malformation

Excluding diaphragmatic hernias, congenital cystic adenomatoid malformation or CCAM is the most frequently identified mass in the fetal chest.[5] Accounting for 25% of congenital lung malformations,[6] this typically unilateral disorder involves either part of a lobe or more frequently an entire lobe.[2] It usually is found in the upper lobes and rarely includes the entire lung.[7] Involvement may also occur with equal frequency in both lungs. Histologic characterization demonstrates an adenomatoid increase in terminal respiratory elements, leading to the development of a pathologic mass consisting of multiple cysts of different sizes.[1,2,6]

There are three forms of CCAM:

- Type I consists of a single cyst or multiple large cysts measuring 2 to 10 cm in diameter with a trabeculated wall and, often, smaller cystic outpouchings. Broad, fibrous septa and mucin-producing cells may be responsible for areas of echogenicity within the mass and are unique to this subtype of CCAM.
- Type II is a mass effect made up of multiple, uniform-sized cysts 0.5 to 2 cm in diameter. These cysts resemble bronchioles.[6]
- Type III consists of multiple microscopic cysts measuring between 0.5 and 5.0 mm that, like the multiple small cysts of infantile polycystic kidney disease (PKD), present numerous reflecting surfaces to the ultrasound beam. Because these small cysts cannot be resolved individually, they appear as a single, solid, homogeneously echogenic mass.[1,6]

Patients with CCAM may have associated renal, cardiac, or gastrointestinal malformations (GI). These anomalies occur more commonly with type II CCAM. Fetuses

PATHOLOGY BOX 21-1

Congenital Cystic Adenomatoid Malformations[1,2,5,6]

Type	Histologic Findings	Sonographic Appearance	Differential Diagnoses
I	Single large cyst, usually 3–7 cm but at least 2 cm; trabeculated wall with smaller cystic outpouchings	Usually unilateral May involve a lung lobe or part of a lung lobe Rarely involves entire lung Can be bilateral Single large cyst with smaller cystic outpouchings visualized superior to the diaphragm in the fetal lung Can have echogenic areas within the cyst	Bronchogenic cyst Mediastinal mass Pleural and pericardial effusions Fluid-filled stomach and bowel in diaphragmatic hernia
II	Mass made up of multiple similar-sized cysts, 1.5 cm in diameter	Usually unilateral May involve a lung lobe or part of a lobe Rarely involves entire lung Can be bilateral Multiple similar-sized cysts seen in the fetal lung replacing normal lung parenchyma	Same as type I
III	Multiple small cysts (0.5–5 mm)	Cysts too small to be resolved sonographically appear as a single solid echogenic mass in the fetal lung	Pulmonary sequestration Rhabdomyoma Mediastinal teratoma Herniated liver, spleen, or rarely kidney

with CCAM may present with fetal hydrops, ascites, and polyhydramnios because of the compression placed on the lung. The CCAM lesion expansion results in a greater than normal increase in thoracic diameter as well as inversion of the diaphragm.[8] Stillbirth and premature labor are common among these fetuses. Patients with life-threatening intrauterine hydrops have the poorest prognosis. Fetuses whose lesions are imaged as cystic, types I and II, have a better prognosis than those with solid-appearing type III CCAM, which tends to be more extensive. Eighty percent of neonates who survive with CCAM present with respiratory distress at birth.[1,6] Patients can be asymptomatic and usually do well after surgical excision of these masses.[9,10]

Sonographic Imaging

The sonographic appearance of CCAM includes a unilateral pulmonary mass with one or more large cysts (type I), an echogenic mass containing small cysts (type II), or a homogeneous echogenic mass (type III). This process begins to develop in the first trimester; however, detection is not until the second trimester because of the size of the cysts. A large mass may result in a mediastinal shift and inversion of the diaphragm. Some fetuses demonstrate ascites, pleural effusion, and hydrops. Color Doppler imaging identifies arterial supply via the pulmonary vessels which is due to how the lungs develop in the embryo.[3] Identification of flow into the mass differentiates the CCAM from pulmonary sequestration[8] and diaphragmatic hernia. As with other lung masses, serial examinations have demonstrated a

significant decrease or the spontaneous resolution of CCAMs antenatally (Fig. 21-2).[1,2,6,8]

Other Imaging Modalities

The plain radiograph allows for diagnosis, with computed tomography (CT) used to clarify confusing cases (Fig. 21-3). CT has a higher accuracy rate for classification of the CCAM type (Fig. 21-4).[11] In the case of a suspected congenital malformation detected prenatally, magnetic resonance imaging (MRI) has a high rate of success. The multiple cysts seen with CCAM appear as a higher-intensity signal on the T2-weighted image. Pulmonary sequestration and CCAM have similar MRI appearances (Fig. 22-7).[12]

Differential Diagnosis

The differential diagnosis of type I and II lesions includes cystic lung and mediastinal masses as well as pleural and pericardial effusions. The differential diagnosis of the type III, solid-appearing CCAM includes pulmonary sequestration, rhabdomyoma, mediastinal teratoma, and herniated abdominal contents, which may include liver, spleen, or rarely kidney.[1,6] Noting the position of the fluid-filled stomach and any fluid-filled bowel, if present, can help differentiate between types I or II CCAM, in which the affected fetus has stomach and bowel in the normal subdiaphragmatic location and a fetus with a diaphragmatic hernia, in which the fluid-filled stomach and bowel are in an intrathoracic location, simulating CCAM.[1,6] CT is more accurate than sonography and radiography in classifying CCAM type.[1,6]

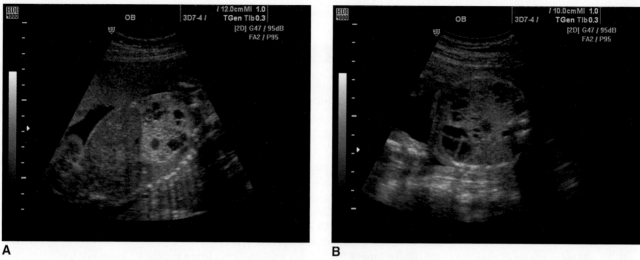

Figure 21-2 A: Sagittal view of the fetal chest with CCAM. **B:** Axial or transverse image of the same fetus demonstrating the cystic malformation of the lungs. (Images courtesy of Philips Medical Systems, Bothell, WA.)

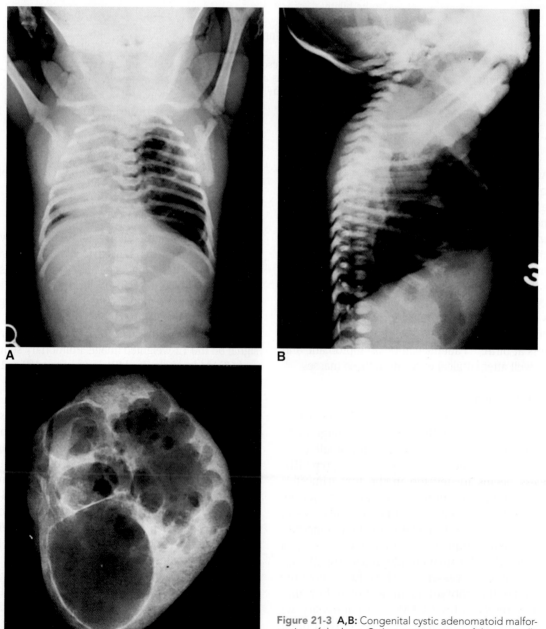

Figure 21-3 A,B: Congenital cystic adenomatoid malformation of the lung. **C:** A roentgenogram of the surgically resected specimen.

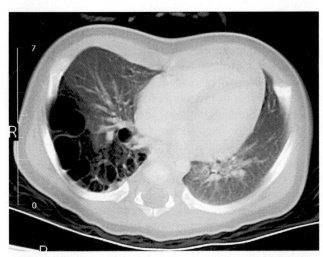

Figure 21-4 Transverse thoracic CT view of a newborn with CCAM.

Pulmonary Sequestration

A pulmonary sequestration is a solid, nonfunctioning mass of lung tissue contained within the pleural sac that lacks communication with the tracheobronchial tree and has a systemic arterial blood supply. This type of malformation accounts for approximately a quarter of lung lesions found in the prenatal exam and has a 4:1 male-to-female ratio.[13] The extralobar type either above or below the diaphragm has its own pleural sac and a systemic venous drainage.[1,13]

Sonographic Imaging

The lung mass of intralobar pulmonary sequestration is spherical, homogeneous, highly echogenic, and often found at the lung base or just inferior to the diaphragm (Fig. 21-5). A midline shift may occur in the presence of a large chest mass.[14] Color Doppler has been used to image the abnormal vascular supplies arising from the thoracic or abdominal aorta.[13,15] The determination of blood supply also aids in diagnosis as sequestration

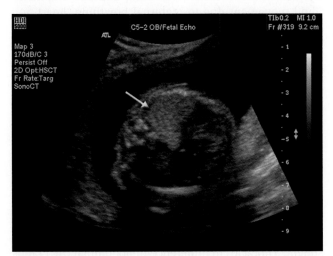

Figure 21-5 The echogenic homogeneous mass (arrow) within the posterior chest raises suspicion for pulmonary sequestration. (Image courtesy of Philips Medical Systems, Bothell, WA.)

PATHOLOGY BOX 21-2

Sonographic Appearance of Pulmonary Sequestration

Spherical mass
Homogeneous
Echogenic
Midline shift
Vascular supply from aorta

from CCAM, which has the arterial supply originating from the pulmonary artery. There is a localized, irreversible form of sequestration that may simulate the ultrasound image of types I and II CCAM.[16]

Other Imaging Modalities

Radiographs demonstrate a lack of airway communication with the lung tissue. This mass may appear as a cyst or infection with fluid levels. The mass effect may produce displacement of the bronchia on both the plain films and GI contrast studies.[14]

Sonography, the primary prenatal imaging modality for prenatal surveys, has limitations in differentiating and diagnosing pulmonary sequestration, often because of maternal obesity, lack of image contrast, a limited view field, and lack of sonographer skill. Thus, the MRI helps to eliminate many of these limitations for the prenatal exam. Fetal lungs image as homogeneous structures with a high T2 signal because of the amniotic fluid filling the lungs. In the case of pulmonary sequestration, the chest contains a well-defined mass with signal intensities higher than the normal lung but lower than amniotic fluid. MRI often is able to establish feeder vessels to the suspected sequestration (Fig. 22-7).[13,14]

Prognosis

Patients diagnosed with extralobar masses have a very favorable prognosis. Occasional cases have been noted to resolve spontaneously in utero.[13,17] These masses are associated with anomalies and fetal hydrops resulting in a poor prognosis.[1]

Differential Diagnosis

Differential diagnoses for this malformation depend on the type. Intralobar sequestration, which occurs within the pulmonary visceral pleura, may appear as a solid, fluid, or hemorrhagic mass. Atelectasis adjacent to the area often occurs, as well as cystic or emphysematous elements. The extralobar sequestration occurring below the diaphragm may mimic adrenal or abdominal organ masses.[14]

THE BONY THORAX AND ITS SOFT TISSUES

Some abnormalities that actually extend from the head and neck may be large or long enough to appear to involve the thorax. Inferior cephaloceles, a herniation of the meninges and brain through a defect in the calvarium,[1] and myelomeningocele, and a similar defect of the vertebral column, are predominantly cystic masses that may or may not contain echogenic brain or spinal cord. Upon elimination of an abnormality of the spine or calvarium, with a cystic mass in the region of the neck and upper thorax, the differential diagnosis must include fetal edema and cystic hygroma. Both of these abnormalities have an increased connection with karyotype abnormalities.[2,18]

Fetal edema may be limited to the neck but is more often associated with fetal hydrops and increased soft tissue thickness, forming a halo pattern around the neck, thorax, or abdomen. Nuchal area edema has been associated with nonimmune fetal hydrops, fetal demise, and some skeletal dysplasias.[2,19] The presence of abnormal and excessive skin or soft tissue in the nuchal area is a well-known clinical finding in many newborns with trisomy 21 (Down syndrome). Benacerraf and colleagues were the first to note this finding on antenatal ultrasound examination.[20] Gray and Crane showed that ultrasound screening for a nuchal fold thickness of 5 mm or greater (42% sensitivity) in the 14- to 18-week gestational age group and 6 mm or greater (83% sensitivity, positive predictive value of 1 in 38) in the 19- to 24-week gestational week group could be a more effective tool in diagnosing Down syndrome than the use of maternal age greater than 35 years (20% sensitivity) or low maternal serum alpha-fetoprotein levels (33% sensitivity).[21] Amniocentesis can certainly karyotype those fetuses with thick nuchal areas.[1,2]

Cystic hygromas, benign abnormalities of lymphatic origin occurring in 1 of every 6,000 pregnancies, are thought to be a result of a failure in the development of normal lymphatic venous communication. They are among the most common abnormalities seen in the first trimester.[1] The lymphatic sacs dilate, and sonographically, they appear as unilocular or multilocular cystic masses. Eighty percent of these originate at the posterolateral neck, and care must be taken to differentiate a cystic hygroma from nuchal skin thickening though they may occur simultaneously.[1] At least half of cystic hygromas are evident in antenatal life; 10% are bilateral.[6] They may be seen extending to or originating from the thorax or the mediastinum, as well as the axilla or groin.[22] Internal solid elements seen on the sonographic image probably represent surrounding connective tissue or hemangiomatous elements.[23]

The differentiation of cystic hygroma from the statistically less likely thoracic wall hemangioma is difficult. Large hemangiomas may be associated with cardiac dilatation because of the presence of arteriovenous shunting and increased blood return to the heart.[24] Cystic hygromas may spontaneously resolve before birth, possibly owing to further development of lymphatic channel communication with the venous system. This is thought by some to be the source of the webbed neck seen in patients with Turner syndrome, the most common abnormal fetal karyotype (XO) with cystic hygroma.[1,6] Cystic hygromas may also cause venous obstruction. In an affected fetus, ascites, pleural effusions, generalized edema, an enlarged edematous placenta, or cystic cutaneous lymphangiectasia may develop. The prognosis for such fetuses is poor.

In general, fetuses with cystic hygroma and hydrops succumb in utero or shortly after birth, but there have been reports of antenatal resolution of this finding.[25,26]

Other soft tissue masses involving the thorax are uncommon. Fetuses of diabetic mothers may exhibit soft tissue increases in the thorax based on subcutaneous fat deposition. Similar soft tissue increases may also be seen in patients with fetal anasarca or edema due to subcutaneous fluid. Another consideration is a teratoma with combined cystic and solid components. This mass may increase in size during pregnancy and become more echogenic or solid in appearance.[27] Hamartomas, a benign nonneoplastic overgrowth of the normal cellular elements of an affected area, often arise within a rib. They may have a disproportionately large intrathoracic component capable of displacing the fetal heart and causing respiratory insufficiency. Early diagnosis followed by complete resection in neonatal life is usually curative.[28]

The clavicles may be absent or hypoplastic in several syndromes, including cleidocranial dysplasia, Holt-Oram syndrome, and pyknodysostosis. Several skeletal syndromes and mucopolysaccharidoses demonstrate thick ribs, but diagnosis on prenatal ultrasound is often difficult. Any obvious narrowing of the fetal thorax in relation to the fetal abdomen should prompt the sonographer to rule out any skeletal dysplasias such as short-rib polydactyly syndrome, Jeune syndrome, and Ellis-Van Creveld syndrome.

PULMONARY HYPOPLASIA

The abnormal or lack of development of the lung (hypoplasia) is usually secondary to lung compression in utero. This is the result of numerous entities related to compression from intrathoracic masses but can also result from abdominal masses that restrict the downward movement of the diaphragm or have an intrathoracic component. The small thorax of several skeletal dysplasias is associated with lung underdevelopment. Fluid movement due to maternal breathing, heart and body motion on the chest wall is said to be necessary for normal lung development. In oligohydramnios, there is little fluid to transmit these movements and may be the cause of associated pulmonary hypoplasia.

Sonographic Imaging

Biometry allows for evaluation of the thorax for pulmonary hypoplasia and syndromes involving the size of the chest wall. Lung hypoplasia may be diagnosed by gestalt; a small chest cavity in relation to a larger abdominal cavity or a heart that occupies more than one-third of the thorax on a transverse view in a fetus without obvious cardiac disease suggests pulmonary hypoplasia.[2] Biometric methods for the evaluation of hypoplasia have been sought. Thoracic circumference-to-abdominal (AC) ratios have been most helpful. The normal ratio has a mean of 0.89, and measurements under 0.77 (>2 Standard Deviations below the norm) are considered abnormal

PATHOLOGY BOX 21-3

Causes of Pulmonary Hypoplasia

Intrathoracic masses that compress developing lung
  Pleural effusion
  Pulmonary cyst
  Teratoma
  Meningocele
  Hemangioma
Abdominal mass that prevents downward displacement of
    the diaphragm or compresses developing lung tissue
  Ascites
  Renal mass
  Diaphragmatic hernia and its contents
Oligohydramnios with a lack of transmitted fluid pulsation
    on the chest wall (said to be necessary for tracheobron-
    chial tree development)
  Bilateral renal agenesis or obstruction
  Bilateral ureteral obstruction
  Bladder outlet obstruction, usually urethral atresia
  Prolonged rupture of membranes
Small thorax as part of a skeletal dysplasia
  Thanatophoric dwarfism
  Jeune syndrome
  Ellis-Van Creveld syndrome
  Hypophosphatasia
  Cleidocranial dysostosis
  Metatropic dwarfism
  Campomelic dwarfism

and suggestive of lethal pulmonary hypoplasia.[1,2] The thorax-to-abdomen ratio is roughly 3 to 1 and measured around the bony component of the thorax.[29]

Prognosis

Prognosis is related to the degree of hypoplasia and is rarely the primary cause of inadequate lung growth.[2,6] Mortality is high in infants with pulmonary insufficiencies because of the lungs' inability to support extrauterine life.[30]

THE MEDIASTINUM

The mediastinum can be challenging to image clearly. Few clear-cut mediastinal masses image antenatally. These include extra pericardial and intrapericardial teratoma, enteric cyst, lymphangioma, thymic cyst, and mediastinal meningocele.[31,33] All may be associated with pleural effusion. Any shift of the mediastinum or heart during a survey of the fetal thorax should alert the sonographer for a possible mass. Compression on the esophagus by a mass could lead to polyhydramnios because of GI tract obstruction. Restriction of the trachea leads to pulmonary hypoplasia and respiratory distress postnatally. Mass impression on the vena cava may compromise blood return to the fetal heart and lead to the development of fetal hydrops.[2]

PLEURAL EFFUSION AND FETAL HYDROPS

Pleural effusion, also known as hydrothorax, is easily diagnosed using ultrasound. Any fluid in the pleural space of a fetus of any gestational age is abnormal.

Reported mortality is 50% and is highest when the pleural effusion is discovered before 33 weeks' gestation, is bilateral, or is associated with fetal hydrops.[2]

Sonographically, pleural effusions appear as hypoechoic areas on one or both sides of the chest, conforming to the shape of the chest cavity and its diaphragmatic contour. Large amounts of fluid may compress the lungs, resulting in pulmonary hyperplasia and displacement of the mediastinum and heart. Hydrothorax unrelated to hydrops usually has an extrathoracic cause, but an intrathoracic lesion such as CCAM plays an etiologic role. If large, the pleural effusion may flatten or evert the diaphragm.[2]

The underlying cause of pleural effusion and the degree of pulmonary hypoplasia affects fetal mortality. In the case of a fetus without lung abnormalities, an ultrasound-guided, mid-trimester thoracentesis removes pleural fluid.[20]

The typical isolated pleural effusion associated with respiratory distress in the newborn is a milky fluid consisting of lymph and fat (chylous), but these effusions appear just as anechoic as serous pleural effusions owing to the absence of large lipoproteins in the fetus.[2] An accumulation of lymph within the chest is referred to as a chylothorax. Most often unilateral and right sided, it occurs twice as often in male infants. This process has associations with congenital pulmonary lymphangiectasia, tracheoesophageal fistula, trisomy 21, and extralobar pulmonary sequestration.[33]

Pleural fluid may be an isolated finding, but more typically, it is part of other fetal pathologic processes. It is most often seen in association with fetal hydrops, a condition associated with excessive fluid accumulations within the fetal soft tissues and body cavities.[1,2] The two types of hydrops are immune and nonimmune.

Immune Fetal Hydrops

Erythroblastosis fetalis (severe anemia) or immune hydrops occurs in a fetus whose mother has been sensitized, usually in previous pregnancies, by a blood factor histoincompatibility, typically Rhesus (Rh) factor. Potentially any of myriad fetal red blood cell antigens can serve as sensitizing agents. An immune reaction occurs between maternal immunoglobulin G (IgG) and the fetal blood factor. This reaction leads to significant fetal morbidity and mortality, with a small amount of ascites or pericardial effusion representing early signs of impending decompensation. At one time, Rh incompatibility was the cause of 98% of all immune hydrops. The development of RhoGam to protect the Rh-negative mother from histoincompatibility reactions with a future Rh-positive fetus reduced this to about 55%.[2] The degree of fetal anemia can be determined through amniocentesis or cordocentesis. The same umbilical vessels allow for necessary blood transfusions in the fetus with a low hemoglobin level (Table 21-1).[1]

Nonimmune Fetal Hydrops

Nonimmune hydrops is a condition resulting from a variety of severe fetal diseases and is not associated with incompatibility of the fetal and maternal blood. This

	TABLE 21-1	
	Fetal Hydrops	

Type	Cause	Sonographic Features
Immune	Fetal anemia Rh incompatibility	

Nonimmune	Heart arrhythmias
	Intrauterine infection
	Chromosomal
	  anomalies
	Masses causing
	  venous obstruction
	Blood disorders
	Renal anomalies
	Maternal disease
		Anasarcia
		Pleural effusion
		Ascites
		Hepatomegaly
		Splenomegaly
		Thick placenta

usually fatal form of hydrops occurs in 1 in 1,500 to 1 in 4,000 births.[34] Sources include the following:

- Fetal cardiac arrhythmias or anomalies such as hypoplastic left heart and supraventricular tachycardia, the probable cause in many of the cases labeled idiopathic
- Intrauterine infection, the TORCH infections: *toxo*plasmosis, *r*ubella, *c*ytomegalovirus, *h*erpes
- Chromosomal abnormalities: Turner syndrome, trisomy 18 or 21
- Abdominal or pulmonary masses leading to venous obstruction: CCAM or neuroblastoma
- Congenital hematologic disorders: alpha-thalassemia, a common cause in Asia
- Renal abnormalities, congenital nephrosis
- Maternal origins such as diabetes and toxemia[1,2,6]

Sonographic Imaging

Regardless of the cause, hydrops has a specific presentation during the sonographic examination. The overaccumulation of fluid in fetal tissues results in skin thickening, pleural and pericardial effusion, ascites, hepatomegaly, and splenomegaly. The placenta thickens to greater than 4 cm because of severe fetal anemia. Before the development of frank hydrops, polyhydramnios is a warning sign of fetal distress. Suspicions are raised when at least two of these findings are present in a large for gestational age patient (Fig. 21-6).[34]

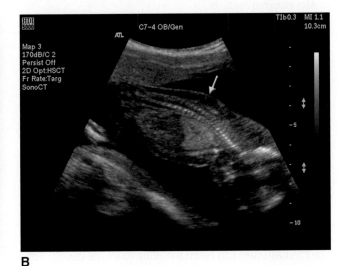

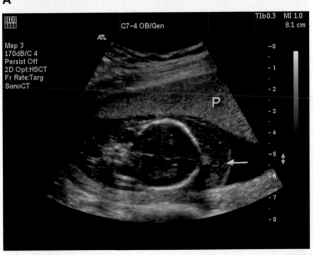

Figure 21-6 A: Sagittal image of the fetal chest and torso demonstrating pleural effusion (*P*) and ascites (*A*). Note the oligohydramnios and subcutaneous edema (anasarca). **B:** Another fetus demonstrating subcutaneous edema (*arrow*). **C:** Scalp edema (*arrow*) has a different appearance than the anteriorly located placenta (*P*). (Images courtesy of Philips Medical Systems, Bothell, WA.)

CONGENITAL DIAPHRAGMATIC HERNIA

Congenital diaphragmatic hernia (CDH) is a defect of the diaphragm that allows the contents of the abdomen to migrate into the thorax. CDH has an incidence of approximately 1 in 10,000 live births.[2] The origin of the hernia is the flawed formation or fusion of the diaphragm. This opening in the pleuroperitoneal membrane may result in several different diaphragmatic abnormalities:

- The posterolateral herniation through the foramen of Bochdalek, which accounts for over 90% of those found, usually on the left side[1,2,35]
- Retrosternal, anteromedial herniation through the foramen of Morgagni[35]
- Protrusion of the bowel through the diaphragm (eventration)
- Complete uncommon absence of a diaphragm[33,35]

Left-sided involvement is five times more common than right-sided involvement,[1,2,36] which may be because of the presence of the liver, whose mass is known to prevent cranial progression of the abdominal viscera into the thorax, thereby lessening symptoms and improving prognosis. CDH is unilateral 96% of the time and is found somewhat more commonly in male infants (Fig. 21-7).[2,30]

Rarely occurring are familial forms of CDH, reported in less than 2% of all cases.[35] Both autosomal dominant and autosomal recessive inheritance patterns have been documented.[35,37] These occur bilaterally in 20% of cases (a far greater incidence compared to the 3% incidence found among sporadic cases), and have a 2-to-1 male predominance and fewer associated anomalies.[2] One Finnish study showed a 2% recurrence risk of CDH among subsequent siblings.[38]

The majority cases of CDH have no known cause or related syndrome, with up to half occurring as an isolated defect.[35] In a fetus with congenital malformations of the diaphragm, the cause is a single or multiple chromosome anomalies. Though rarely inherited, clusters may occur in families in the form of a genetic syndrome or chromosomal anomaly.[35]

Sonographic Imaging

Early diagnosis is an important factor in the outcome and with the continued advances in sonographic detail resolution; several first-trimester cases have been reported using an endovaginal technique. The stomach, bowel, or other organs most often move into the chest via a posterior diaphragmatic defect. Peristalsis of the herniated small bowel and fluid-filled structures differ greatly from normal echogenic lung parenchyma. Cystic abnormalities of the lung can simulate CDH, and the sonographer must carefully survey the abdomen

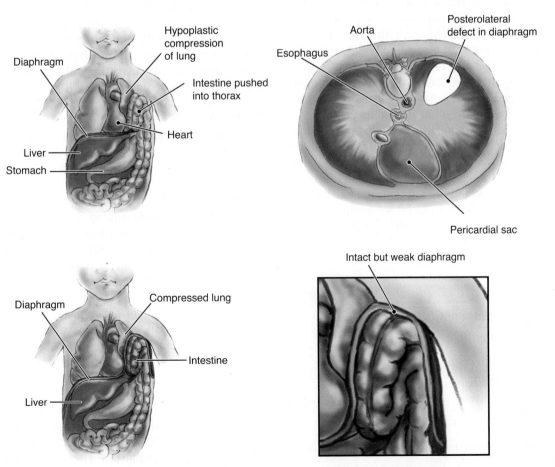

Figure 21-7 Congenital diaphragmatic hernia, typical (above) and variation (below).

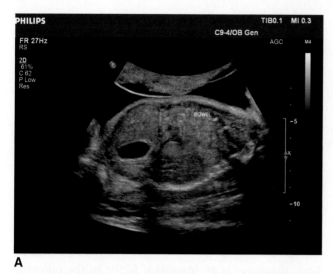 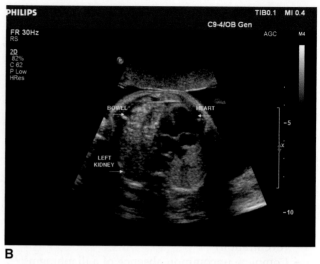

A

B

Figure 21-8 **A:** Sagittal image of a diaphragmatic hernia resulting in bowel within the chest. **B:** Axial or transverse view of the same fetus demonstrating the bowel to the left of the heart within the chest cavity. (Images courtesy of Philips Medical Systems, Bothell, WA.)

to confirm the absence of the stomach. The fetus with CDH often has a smaller than normal AC measurement. The heart and mediastinum shift away from the side of herniation. During fetal breathing, the abdominal organs may descend on the normal side and, paradoxically, ascend on the affected side. Other findings include polyhydramnios and pleural effusions. Polyhydramnios, in particular, is not a prognostically good sign; one series reported a 55% survival rate among patients with CDH without associated polyhydramnios but only 11% survival in cases with associated polyhydramnios. Patients with smaller diaphragmatic defects or herniations that occur later in gestation have a better prognosis. The left-sided hernia is easier to visualize because of the cystic nature of the stomach and its ectopic presence in the chest. The similar echogenicity of the liver and lung tissue can make the right-sided hernia more difficult to identify.[39] Color flow Doppler examination of the portal and umbilical veins aids in determination of position. Liver herniation seen with the CDH results in an abnormal location.[40] A careful sonographic search should be made of fetuses with CDH for other congenital anomalies (Fig. 21-8).[1,2,6]

PATHOLOGY BOX 21-4

Sonographic Findings of CDH

Stomach, bowel, or other abdominal organs within the chest
Peristalsis of structures within the chest
Small abdominal biometry
Descension and ascension of organs with fetal breathing
Pleural effusion
Polyhydramnios
Documentation of portal and umbilical vessels via color Doppler modes

---

Other Imaging Modalities

The radiograph of a neotate with a diaphragmatic hernia demonstrates air- and fluid-filled loops of bowel within the chest, usually the left side. This results in a mediastinal shift into the contralateral chest. If an orogastric tube is present, the position indicates the laterality of the mediastinal shift (Fig. 21-9).

The ability of MRI to differentiate internal fetal anatomy has resulted in an increase in its use to confirm the diagnosis of CDH. The fast spin-echo MRI data sets allow for calculation of lung volumes, which aid in determination of pulmonary hypoplasia, which directly relates to fetal outcomes (Fig. 21-10).

Differential Diagnosis

Anomalies mimicking CDH include CCAM, pulmonary sequestration, bronchogenic cyst, teratomas, or a neuroenteric cysts and bronchial atresia.

Prognosis

The pressure of the herniated abdominal contents on the pulmonary vessels and lungs, mimicking an intrathoracic mass, can lead to pulmonary hypoplasia. The hypoplasia may be bilateral despite a unilateral diaphragmatic lesion.[41] Overall mortality for CDH is 50% to 80%,[18] which includes a 35% rate of stillbirth. CDH is associated with major congenital anomalies of other body systems. Associated cardiovascular and central nervous system anomalies are the most lethal.[42]

The outcome of surgery and the degree of the diaphragmatic defect determines the prognosis for these children. Surgical intervention performed before fetal lung development is complete, usually by 24 weeks' gestation, can result in an improved prognosis by reducing pressure and avoiding development of significant pulmonary hypoplasia.[43] There is a direct relationship between the severity of the defect to the mortality

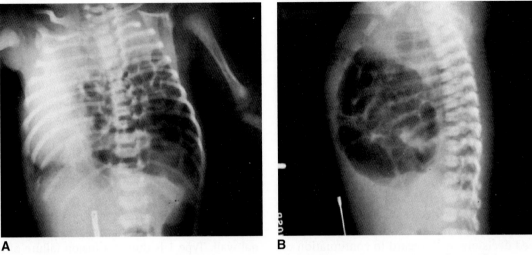

Figure 21-9 A,B: Congenital diaphragmatic hernia. There is herniation of small intestine, large intestine, and stomach (or parts thereof) into the left hemithorax. Note the air in the descending colon.

rate[39] and the location of the liver.[2] A liver within the abdomen shows over 90% survival rate.[2]

ABDOMEN

SCANNING TECHNIQUES

A general fetal abdominal survey begins with evaluation of the anterior abdominal wall to determine intactness. This is most important at the site of umbilical cord entry. While imaging the abdominal wall, be sure

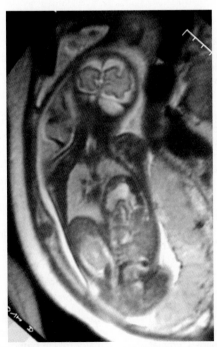

Figure 21-10 Congenital diaphragmatic hernia. Coronal T2-weighted image of a chest at 32 weeks' gestation demonstrates herniation of stomach, bowel, and spleen into the left hemithorax. There is minimal deviation of mediastinal structures with the right lung and left upper lobes expanded.

to rule out protrusions from the abdominal sidewalls. Thickened abdominal wall soft tissues is a finding noted not only in hydrops fetalis but also in the offspring of diabetic (type C) mothers.[9]

Abdominal situs is determined by noting the liver's position on the side opposite the cardiac apex. This is best accomplished by caudad and craniad angulations of the transducer in the transverse plane. Complete situs inversus (cardiac apex on right and liver on left) can be diagnosed only by meticulous attention to fetal position and visualized anatomy.[1,2] In cases of correct abdominal situs, transverse images of the abdomen show the spine, stomach, and umbilical vein in clockwise relation when the fetus is in cephalic presentation and counterclockwise when the fetus is breech.

Measurements of the AC assess conformity with accepted measurements for gestational age. Biometric evaluation of AC allows assessment of the nutritional status of the fetus. Asymmetric intrauterine growth retardation (representing 80% of all cases of IUGR) shows a smaller AC, owing to loss of glycogen stores in the liver and the resultant decrease in liver size; there is no associated decrease in head circumference (HC) or femur length (FL) measurements. HC/AC and FL/AC ratios also help determine IUGR.[1,2]

The remainder of the routine fetal abdominal survey includes evaluation of the transverse AC view for the presence of a fluid-filled stomach and assessment of the liver. A transverse view at the level of the kidneys may reveal renal obstruction. Coronal and longitudinal views may supplement the transverse views in further evaluating any area or organ of concern.

ABDOMINAL WALL DEFECTS

Ventral abdominal wall defects vary in type and complexity. The two most common types, omphalocele and gastroschisis, have been well evaluated by sonography. A common flaw is an umbilical hernia, with the linea alba defect and protruding bowel covered by skin and subcutaneous tissue. The distinguishing feature of an umbilical hernia versus an omphalocele is the position of the cord insertion.[1] Other rarer findings include the complex defects of cloaca or bladder exstrophy, ectopia cordis, amniotic band syndrome, and the limb–body wall complex. The development of the anterior abdominal wall is based on fusion of four ectomesodermal folds, a cephalic, a caudal, and a pair of lateral folds. Abdominal wall malformations are one of the sources of elevated alpha-fetoprotein levels in amniotic fluid or maternal serum. Knowledge of the actual defect and its associated abnormalities is necessary for making informed decisions with regard to continuation of pregnancy, method of delivery, and surgical treatment (Table 21-2).[1,2,6,30]

Omphalocele

The omphalocele is a midline defect occurring in 1 in 4,000 births. These are separated into two types by the mechanism of origin: those containing only bowel; and those containing organs, usually the liver, and bowel. A normal migration of the bowel into the umbilical cord occurs during embryologic development sometime between 8 and 12 weeks (Fig. 13-21). Occasionally, the bowel does not migrate back into the abdomen and remains in the extraembryonic coelom of the umbilical cord.[1,30] An omphalocele develops because body stalk persistence in an area normally occupied by abdominal wall. Type 1 is due to a fusion failure of the lateral

TABLE 21-2			
Anomalies Involving the Body Wall			
Type of Anomaly	**Description**	**Sonographic Appearance**	**Diagnostic Considerations**
Omphalocele	Herniation of abdominal viscera into the base of the umbilical cord; liver involvement common	Complex membrane-enclosed sac; midline anterior wall defect continuous with umbilical cord. Size varies with amount of involved viscera.	29%–66% association with other anomalies
Gastroschisis	Herniation of abdominal viscera through an off-midline defect in the abdominal wall, usually located just to the right of the umbilicus; liver involvement very unusual	Free-floating bowel loops not bound by a sac. Normal umbilical cord insertion.	Common: Associated gastrointestinal anomalies Rare: Anomalies of other systems
Umbilical cord hernia	Protrusion of a small amount of intestine at the umbilicus	Similar to omphalocele; covered by skin and subcutaneous tissue, usually less than 2–4 cm	Limited clinical significance Rare: Associated anomalies
Bladder exstrophy	Congenital failure of abdominal wall to develop over bladder; urinary bladder may be everted (inside may protrude through abdominal wall)	Variable: May see a fluid-filled intrapelvic portion of bladder with a contiguous extra-abdominal mass with echogenicity similar to that of soft tissue. More commonly, no fluid-filled intrapelvic bladder	Most common in boys; associated anomalies: • Gastrointestinal • Genitourinary • Musculoskeletal Must be differentiated from urachal cyst
Ectopic cordis	Defect of the lower sternum and anterior abdominal wall; heart protrudes into extrathoracic sac covered by skin or a thin membrane	Beating heart protrudes through anterior abdominal wall into amniotic fluid	Associated with: • Amniotic band syndrome • Craniofacial • Limb deformities • Omphalocele Very poor prognosis
Limb–body wall complex	Complex of anomalies including lateral body wall defects of thorax and abdomen with herniation of viscera; cranial, craniofacial, spinal, and limb anomalies common	Herniated viscera within a complex membrane-involved mass, severe scoliosis, cranial, and spinal defects	A severe form of amniotic band syndrome is thought to play a major role in pathogenesis; no genetic predisposition has been identified; not compatible with life

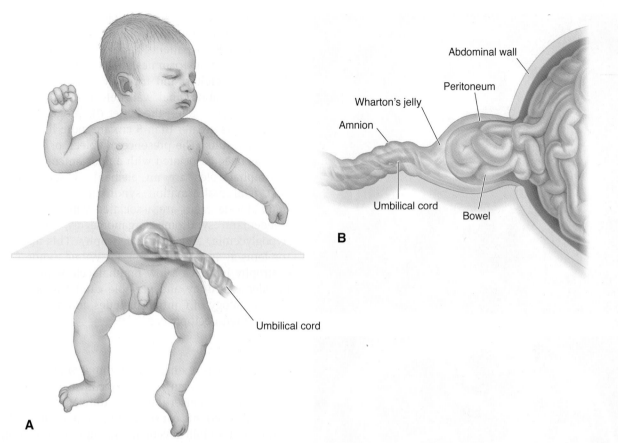

Figure 21-11 Typical features of the omphalocele with intracorporeal live on external examination **(A)** and on the cross-section view **(B)**.

ectomesodermal folds, whereas type 2 is the failure of the muscle, fascia, and skin to fuse.[2] The sonographer may find abdominal viscera and/or bowel protruding into the base of the umbilical cord. This defect can range anywhere in size from 2 to 10 cm and is always covered by a membrane and centrally located. The membrane is made up of amnion and peritoneum. There is often associated fetal ascites (Fig. 21-11).[2]

Sonographic Imaging

Proper imaging protocol to rule out an omphalocele requires evaluation of the anterior abdominal wall and noting the entry of the cord into an intact wall. Use of color Doppler helps document the umbilical cord vessels and the position of the abdominal organs and bowel. Because of the normal physiologic herniation of bowel into the umbilical cord, the clinician must be cautious about the diagnosis of omphalocele before 12 weeks' gestational age, by which time the physiologic event should have ended. A definitive first-trimester diagnosis is made by some imagers only if the omphalocele is larger than the abdomen itself.[2] Bowerman reported that an omphalocele may be suggested early in pregnancy, if the cord containing midgut has a maximal dimension of 7 mm or greater.[44] Occasionally, the antenatal evidence of a sac membrane enables an omphalocele to be differentiated from gastroschisis on the

postnatal examination of an infant whose sac ruptured during delivery (Fig. 21-12).

Other Imaging Modalities

MRI provides additional detail of the centrally located omphalocele defect. Herniation of the viscera into the thin-walled sac images well during the MRI exam. The

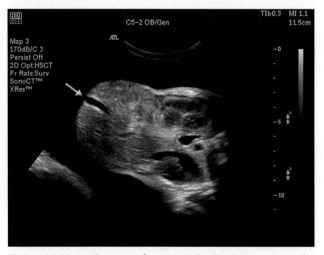

Figure 21-12 Axial image of an omphalocele demonstrating the central insertion of the umbilical vessels *(arrow)*. This defect has allowed the liver to extend into the sac. (Image courtesy of Philips Medical Systems, Bothell, WA.)

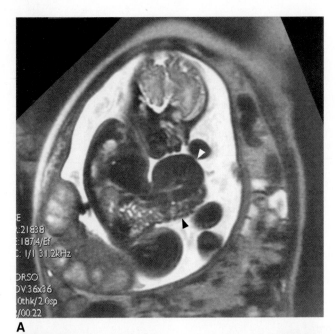

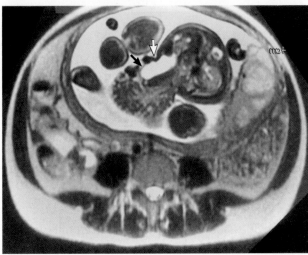

Figure 21-13 Omphalocele with extracorporeal liver at 35 weeks. **A:** MRI shows prolapse of the liver (*white arrowhead*) and small bowel loops (*black arrowhead*) into the omphalocele sac. **B:** An axial image shows prolapse of the stomach (*black arrow*) and colon (*white arrow*). (Reproduced with permission from Shinmoto H, Kashima K, Yuasa Y, et al. MR Imaging of non-CNS fetal abnormalities: a pictorial essay. *Radiographics*. 2000;20[5]:1227–1243.)

liver has a low signal intensity on the T2-weighted image (Fig. 21-13).[14]

Prognosis

Between 50% and 70% of omphaloceles are associated with other anomalies whose presence worsens the prognosis. Type 1 omphaloceles are more frequently associated with chromosomal and other abnormalities.[1,6,40] GI anomalies are found in 30% to 50% of cases—usually bowel malrotation, but sometimes atresia or stenosis of small bowel, bowel duplication, biliary atresia, tracheoesophageal fistula, and imperforate anus. Half of the anomalies are cardiovascular, including ventricular

and atrial septal defects, tetralogy of Fallot, pulmonary artery stenosis, and abnormalities of the great vessels. Forty to 60% of patients have a chromosomal abnormality, including trisomies 13, 18, and 21, as well as Turner, Klinefelter, and triploidy syndromes.[1,2,6,30] The smaller the abdominal wall defect and the fewer the associated anomalies, the better the prognosis. Fetuses with defects greater than 5 cm are more likely to have adverse results. The presence of spleen or heart in the sac has been associated with a poor outcome.[33]

Omphaloceles are an element of several significant fetal malformation syndromes. One-seventh of omphalocele cases are associated with the Beckwith-Wiedemann syndrome: organomegaly, macroglossia, hypoglycemia, and hemihypertrophy. This also places the fetus at an increased risk for Wilms tumor. Cloacal exstrophy involves a low omphalocele with cloacal or bladder exstrophy and variable caudal abnormalities. The pentalogy of Cantrell includes an omphalocele associated with ectopia cordis.[2,35]

Gastroschisis

Gastroschisis is a smaller abdominal wall defect, measuring from 2 to 4 cm, which typically occurs just to the right of the cord insertion and is unrelated to the umbilical cord. Theoretic causes include abnormal involution of the right umbilical vein and disruption of the omphalomesenteric artery.[1,2,30] Gastroschisis occurs once in every 3,000 pregnancies, usually in younger mothers.[2] Maternal use of vasoactive substances such as nicotine or cocaine increases the risk of fetal gastroschisis development.[43] Except for bowel malrotation and jejunal or ileal atresia, associated anomalies are probably related to vascular compromise of the malrotated bowel and are far less common than with omphalocele.[2,30]

Prenatal maternal serum screening reveals an increase in alpha-fetoprotein due to the direct contact of the bowel with the amniotic fluid. Though they can be elevated with an omphalocele, the values are much higher.[2]

The herniated viscera, usually comprising small or large bowel, are free-floating and not covered by a membrane (Fig. 21-14). This leads to the development of a fibrinous coating on the bowel, probably the result of chemical peritonitis produced by its contact with fetal urine in the amniotic fluid.[2] The liver is rarely present in this herniation. Although there is active debate over the method of delivery, most clinicians favor cesarean section to avoid further contamination of the uncovered, eviscerated bowel. During surgical repair, a Silastic covering protects the bowel and abdominal wall defect in the case of staged repairs.[45,46]

Sonographic Imaging

The omphalocele images as early as 14 to 16 weeks with ultrasound because of the free-floating loops of bowel within amniotic fluid. This defect results in a

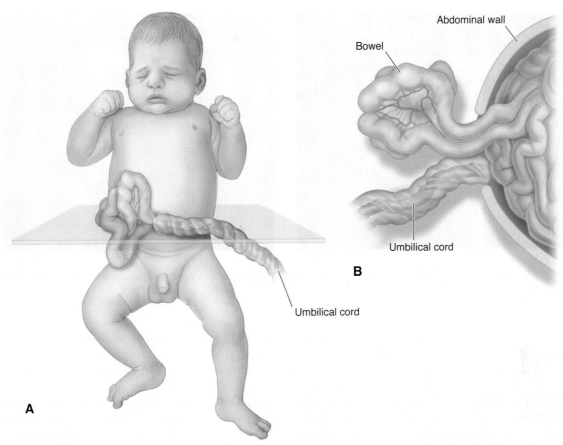

Figure 21-14 Typical features of gastroschisis shown on external examination (**A**) and on cross-sectional view (**B**).

right-sided cord insertion and a small AC because of the lack of internal organs. Sometimes the image may simulate that of an omphalocele, and the sonographer must rule out that possibility by proving that the mass is not associated with the umbilical cord. The free-floating bowel thickens as a result of chemical peritonitis, which occurs due to contact with the amniotic fluid. In approximately one-third of cases, oligohydramnios is present; however, polyhydramnios is also possible.[6] Color Doppler helps to confirm the course of the umbilical cord and vessels and to distinguish the bowel loops from the cord (Figs. 21-15 and 21-16).

Other Imaging Modalities

The MRI evaluation demonstrates bowel loop herniation through the periumbilical abdominal defect. The free-floating bowel images within the amniotic fluid and, as with ultrasound, demonstrate dilated, fluid-filled, thickened bowel (Fig. 21-17).[6,40]

Prognosis

Gastroschisis rarely occurs with other anomalies outside of bowel malformations increasing the survival rate.[40] The survival rates range from 85% to 95%.[40] This is a far better prognosis than that of a fetus with an omphalocele.

PERITONEUM AND ASCITES

Ascites represents fluid within the peritoneum. True fetal ascites is always abnormal. Depending on the amount, the fluid may collect in dependent portions of the fetus, for example, in the pelvis of a fetus in breech position. Large amounts can surround and shift intraperitoneal structures superiorly, inferiorly,

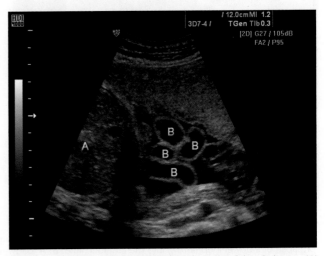

Figure 21-15 Bowel (*B*) floating in fluid outside of the abdomen (*A*) diagnosis a gastroschisis. (Image courtesy of Philips Medical Systems, Bothell, WA.)

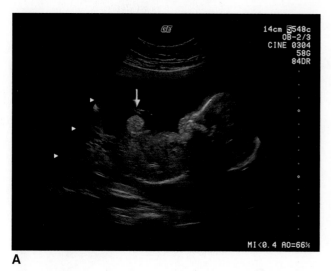
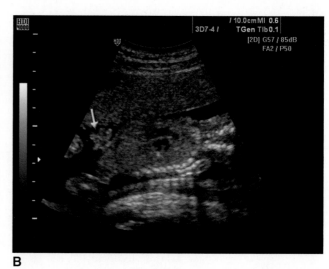

Figure 21-16 Compare the omphalocele on this sagittal image *(arrow)* **(A)** with an image of a gastroschisis **(B)**. (Image **A** courtesy of GE Healthcare, Wauwatosa, WI; image **B** courtesy of Philips Medical Systems, Bothell, WA.)

or laterally. Intraperitoneal fluid is seen best in the subhepatic space, flanks, and lower abdominal cavity or pelvis. The retroperitoneal structures such as the kidneys lie posterior to the free fluid. With patency of the processus vaginalis, ascitic fluid may extend into the scrotum as apparent hydroceles. In studies of intrauterine transfusions, the presence of at least 10 mL of intraperitoneal fluid at 22 weeks and 15 mL at 26 weeks is required before fetal ascites can be detected sonographically.[47]

Commonly noted in association with the multiple findings of fetal hydrops, fetal ascites may develop as an isolated finding in bowel perforation. Urinary ascites results from bladder outlet obstruction or renal forniceal rupture.[48] Heart failure, infections, tumors, and twin–twin transfusions are other sources. Sonography

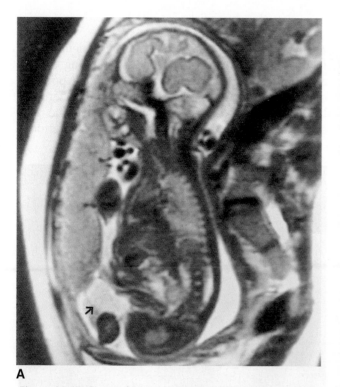
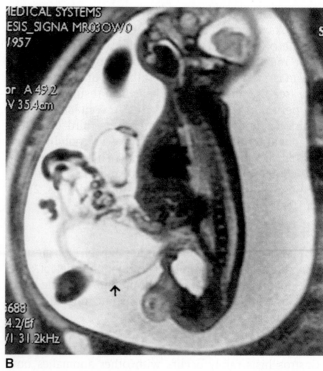

Figure 21-17 Gastroschisis in a 28-week-old fetus. **A:** A sagittal single-shot fast spin-echo MRI shows a midline abdominal wall defect and prolapse of a bowel loop *(arrow)* into the amniotic fluid. **B:** A follow-up sagittal MRI obtained 3 weeks later shows progressive change in the bowel prolapse; the markedly dilated small bowel loops are clearly identified *(arrow)*. Polyhydramnios has increased in volume. (Reproduced with permission from Shinmoto H, Kashima K, Yuasa Y, et al. MR imaging of non-CNS fetal abnormalities: a pictorial essay. *Radiographics.* 2000;20(5):1227–1243.)

typically demonstrates only 25% to 50% of the causes of ascites.[49]

If fetal ascites is detected, the sonographer must investigate further, looking for any bowel dilatation, a result of bowel obstruction, or dilatation of the pyelocaliceal system or bladder, indicating a genitourinary (GU) problem. Intra-abdominal cysts or peritoneal calcification can point to bowel perforation and resultant meconium peritonitis or pseudocyst formation.[2] Normal peristalsis is necessary to extrude meconium, so this phenomenon usually is not seen until the fifth month of fetal life.[2,6]

If sterile meconium associated with bowel perforation releases into the peritoneal cavity, an intense foreign body reaction occurs. Punctate echogenicities develop over time, owing to the resultant irritative peritonitis caused by meconium and its subsequent calcification. This calcification is most easily detected around the liver. Localized fibrotic reactions may cause walls to form around the areas of greatest meconium concentration within the peritoneum, forming meconium pseudocysts. These complex calcified masses may simulate retroperitoneal teratomas or calcified neuroblastomas. Other causes of peritoneal recess calcification include infections from TORCH (*to*xoplasmosis, *r*ubella, *cyto*megalovirus, *h*erpes) organisms.[1,2,6]

Pseudoascites

Chapter 20 discusses this phenomenon at length. Pseudoascites is a simulation of fluid that lies along the inner aspect of the anterior abdominal wall. The echo of the anterior abdominal wall and its subcutaneous tissue produces this hypoechoic band. Pseudoascites is a common observation in fetuses over 18 weeks' gestation.[1] The pseudoascites image is created by the hypoechoic quality of the abdominal wall musculature sandwiched between the highly echogenic subcutaneous and preperitoneal fat. Unlike true ascites, it does not outline parts of the falciform ligament or umbilical vein, and it does not surround other abdominal organs (Fig. 20-29).[1,2]

LIVER AND SPLEEN

The normal fetal liver has a homogeneous appearance. The fetal liver enlarges in association with immune or nonimmune hydrops. This is a result of increased production or red blood cells or hematopoiesis.[1] If the longest liver length to the right of the aorta on a coronal image increases more than 5 mm in a week, isoimmunization must be ruled out.[2,6] The umbilical vein is enlarged in hydrops and in association with placental chorioangioma. Macrosomic fetuses have large livers, as do the fetuses of diabetic mothers, whereas growth-retarded infants have small livers.[50]

Solitary liver cysts may develop because of interruption of the development of the intrahepatic biliary tree. A liver cyst as large as 10.5 cm has been reported.[7] The most common type of choledochal cyst is the cystic dilatation of the common bile duct, which may be seen in an intrahepatic or subhepatic location. Other types include multiple intrahepatic and extrahepatic cysts or a common bile duct diverticulum. Choledocal cysts may be mistaken for duodenal atresia or a defect of the stomach or bowel. These cysts usually lie in an anterior location, adjacent to the gallbladder.[1] Antenatal detection and early surgery during infancy may prevent some severe clinical consequences, especially the development of biliary cirrhosis and portal hypertension.[51,52]

Diffuse liver calcifications occur in fetuses with intrauterine infections, especially those caused by pathogens responsible for TORCH infections, and in particular toxoplasmosis and herpes simplex infection. There are also reported cases of fetal liver calcification due to ischemic, neoplastic, and idiopathic causes. Calcified portal thromboemboli have been reported on autopsy and plain films of newborn and stillborn infants. In a retrospective analysis of 25 fetuses with liver calcifications as their only imaged abnormality, prognosis was excellent, with 96% of the fetuses surviving (Fig. 21-18).[2]

Neonatal liver masses are unusual with the infantile hemangioendothelioma—the most common vascular tumor. This tumor has associations with hepatomegaly, anemia, or high-output congestive heart failure. Sonography has shown these masses to be of variable, mixed echogenicity in neonates. There are reports of the antenatal detection of liver hemangiomas,

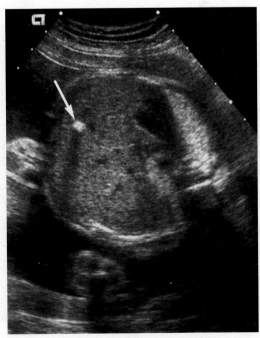

Figure 21-18 Intrahepatic calcification. Transverse view of the fetal abdomen reveals a calcification (*arrow*) with distal shadowing in the fetal liver.

as well as cases of focal nodular hyperplasia.[2,53–55] Hemangiomas are usually avascular when interrogated with color Doppler and, in some instances, contain calcifications.[56]

A gallstone in the fetus images as echogenic masses within the fetal gallbladder that may or may not demonstrate posterior shadowing. Similar to sonographically imaged gallstones discovered in neonates, the stones often resolve, possibly as a result of postnatal hydration or because of changes in bile metabolism.[56] In some cases, they may not be true gallstones but tumefactive sludge or thickened bile. The finding of sludge or gallstones is usually incidental and unrelated to fetal well-being. Those that have not resolved appear to be asymptomatic in neonatal life (Fig. 21-19).[23,29,57]

The formation of blood cells in the spleen (extramedullary hematopoiesis) or hydrops results in an enlarged spleen in the Rh and other isoimmunized fetuses. A significant correlation has been noted between the perimeter measurement of the spleen and fetal hemoglobin deficit, allowing spleen size to predict severe fetal anemia.[58] The spleen may also be enlarged in chronic infections such as toxoplasmosis, cytomegalovirus, rubella, and syphilis, as well as in inborn metabolic errors, such as Gaucher, Niemann-Pick, or Wolman disease.[35] The antenatal diagnosis of a congenital splenic cyst can be made if a cyst is noted in the left upper quadrant and can be separated from the imaged kidney and adrenal gland. Asplenia and polysplenia are associated with significant congenital heart disease, but the antenatal diagnosis of these entities is difficult.[10,59]

THE GASTROINTESTINAL TRACT

Esophagus

Rapid proliferation of the esophageal epithelium during the fetal embryonic period creates almost complete closure of the esophageal lumen. One infant in every 2,500 live births, predominantly male infants, may have a complication thought to be caused by this esophageal maldevelopment or by unequal partitioning of the foregut into the esophagus and trachea, resulting in esophageal atresia.[30] Several types are described. The most common consists of a proximal esophageal pouch, which communicates with the more distal GI tract through a fistula. The fistula follows a track between the tracheobronchial tree of the respiratory tract, usually at or near the tracheal bifurcation, and the distal esophagus and allows amniotic fluid to pass into the stomach. Communication with the more distal GI tract significantly reduces the number of fetuses that present with polyhydramnios because of impaired swallowing.

Polyhydramnios has been reported in 76% of affected fetuses but in only 8% of those with an associated fistula. Another helpful sign for the antenatal diagnosis of esophageal atresia is the absence of a fluid-filled stomach. A fetus with a tracheoesophageal fistula may have a stomach that is only partially filled with fluid, some of which can be the result of gastric secretions. If the esophagus is filled with swallowed amniotic fluid, the area of atresia may be visualized with ultrasound.[1] Serial scans that document polyhydramnios and nonvisualization of the stomach may be necessary to diagnose complete esophageal atresia.

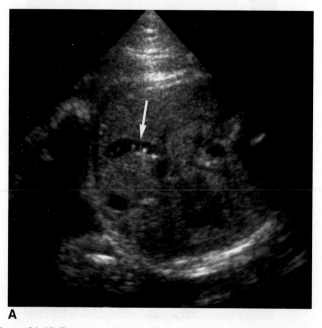

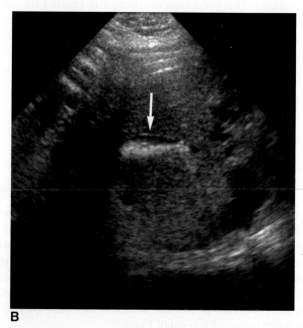

A **B**

Figure 21-19 Transient echogenic material in the gallbladder. Transverse views of two fetal abdomens demonstrate nonshadowing echogenic material in the fetal gallbladders (*arrows*), with (**A**) and without (**B**) the "comet-tail" artifact. Postnatal sonograms in both of these fetuses demonstrated normal gallbladders without stones or sludge.

Esophageal atresia is associated with Down syndrome and other chromosomal abnormalities and is part of the VACTERL association. Fetuses suspected of having esophageal atresia should be studied to note if any of these associated abnormalities are present.[6] The most common of these malformations is anorectal atresia.[1]

Stomach

A fluid-filled stomach noted in the left upper quadrant may allow the sonographer to image adjacent normal structures, such as the spleen, and rule out some other abnormalities, for example, abdominal situs inversus, diaphragmatic hernia, and obstruction of the upper GI tract. Oligohydramnios and the stress of nonimmune hydrops may result in physiologic absence of stomach fluid. However, absence of a stomach or the continuous imaging of an unusually small fetal stomach after 18 weeks' gestational age, with normal amniotic fluid levels is associated with a guarded prognosis. Long-term studies have identified GI tract anomalies, respiratory malformations, aneuploidies, and neuromuscular syndromes, as well as central nervous system and renal anomalies associated with prenatal stomach abscence.[60] Failure to identify the stomach on the prenatal sonogram raises suspicion for chromosomal abnormalities, however, 70% of the time the fetus has a normal karyotype.[2,60]

Duplications of Stomach and Bowel

Duplications can exist throughout the bowel, probably caused by errors of GI lumen recanalization, and in the stomach in particular, by errors in the development of normal inpouching of the longitudinal folds. Stomach duplication is the least common, although approximately 300 cases were reported in the literature through 2002.[61-65]

Diagnoses of antenatal duplications occur in all parts of the GI tract. They are typically echoless cystic structures, occasionally filled with echogenic hemorrhagic or inspissated material. The mucosal lining results in echogenic inner walls.[61-65]

SMALL BOWEL OBSTRUCTION

Causes of small bowel obstruction include the aforementioned intestinal duplications, as well as bowel atresia or stenosis, midgut volvulus and congenital peritoneal bands, internal hernias, and Hirschsprung disease when it involves the entire colon.[2]

Midgut Volvulus

A volvulus is an obstruction caused by the bowel twisting upon its blood supply.[2] The bowel attains its normal position and configuration after a 270-degree rotation, of which the first 180 degrees occurs in the extraembryonic coelom at the base of the umbilical cord during weeks 6 through 10. The remaining 90 degrees occurs within the fetal abdomen. If the small bowel fails to completely return to the abdominal cavity and rotate properly, the bowel may twist about the axis of the superior mesenteric artery, resulting in poor vascular flow distal to the point of obstruction or volvulus. This may also occur if the long mesenteric attachments that fix the bowel to the posterior abdominal wall fail to develop. Infarction results if this is not corrected surgically (Fig. 21-20).[2,30] Midgut volvulus is usually diagnosed in the first days of life; the infant may present with distention or obstruction, but, most typically, with bilious vomiting.

Sonographic Imaging

The sonographer may note, antenatally, a fluid-filled proximal duodenum with an arrowhead twist at the point of descending or transverse duodenal obstruction.[1,2] Mild polyhydramnios, an echogenic mass under the fetal liver, and slightly dilated bowel loops are other findings. Because of the twisting around the mesenteric vessels, the characteristic "whirlpool sign" images within the abdomen.[2] The color Doppler exam may also demonstrate the twisted vessels (Fig. 21-21).

Other Imaging Modalities

The upper GI is the gold standard for the midgut volvulus and malrotation. The sensitivity of radiography is as high as 95% with the barium study. Classic radiographic findings include obstruction leading to stomach and duodenal dilatation. The duodenojejunal junction moves inferior and anterior. The abnormal jejunual position contributes to findings of a dilated fluid-filled duodenum, proximal segment bowel obstruction, and mural edema. (Fig. 21-22).[66]

Duodenal Atresia

Duodenal atresia is the failure of the duodenum to change from a solid cord of tissue during development to a tube; it occurs in 1 in 10,000 births. There are three types of duodenal recanalization anomalies:

1. Duodenal diaphragm or web, resulting in stenosis
2. Solid cord with atresia
3. Segmental or partial absence of the duodenum[37]

The majority of atresias of the duodenum occur distal to the ampulla of Vater. The pancreatic and common bile duct join to form the hepatopancreatic ampulla, which is a major landmark marking the foregut to the midgut transition. It is at the halfway point of the second part of the duodenum. Pancreatic tissue may surround this second portion, causing obstruction or stenosis depending on the amount of pancreatic tissue. The annular pancreas is a secondary, not primary, cause of atresia or stenosis (Fig. 21-23).[37]

Jejunoileal or ileal atresia or stenosis occurs in 1 in 3,000 births. These small bowel atresias occur higher in the abdomen and demonstrate multiple cystic structures with associated hydramnios. Although small bowel obstructions may be caused by one long atresia or multiple, smaller-length areas of atresia, the antenatal ultrasound image typically shows only one area of

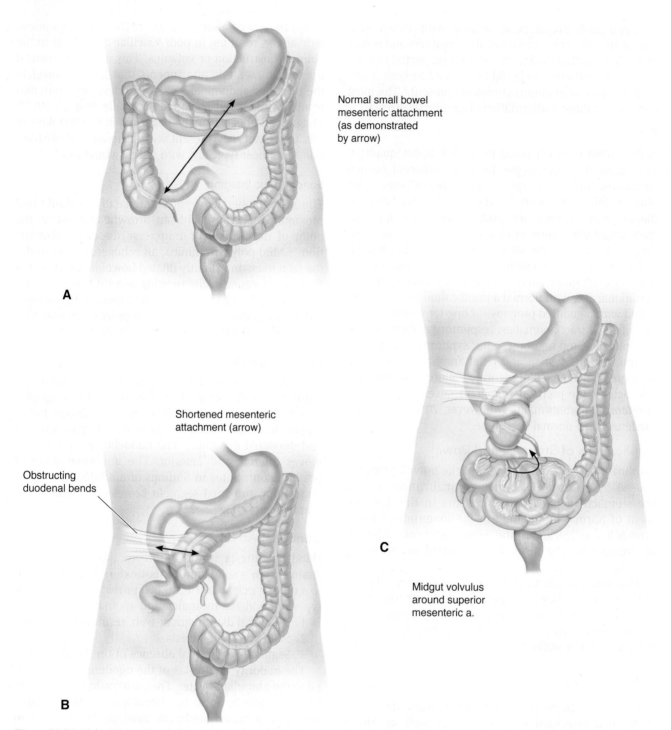

Normal small bowel mesenteric attachment (as demonstrated by arrow)

A

Shortened mesenteric attachment (arrow)

Obstructing duodenal bends

B

C

Midgut volvulus around superior mesenteric a.

Figure 21-20 Malrotation with volvulus. **A:** Normal small bowel mesenteric attachment (as demonstrated by the *arrow*). This prevents twisting of small bowel because of the broad fixation of the mesentery. **B:** Malrotation of colon with obstructing duodenal bands. **C:** Midgut volvulus around the superior mesenteric artery caused by the narrow base of the mesentery.

dilated fluid-filled loops proximal to the obstruction.[2] Smaller areas of jejunoileal atresia are more common, with the most common sites of involvement being the proximal jejunum or the distal ileum. Impairment of the antenatal blood supply is thought to be responsible or is a secondary result of volvulus or gastroschisis.[1] The polyhydramnios associated with proximal small bowel obstructive lesions is usually seen only in the third trimester. In distal obstructions, any increase in amniotic fluid occurs later and to a lesser degree. Of note, normal fluid-filled loops of bowel image in the third trimester.[1]

An extensive small bowel atresia, known as apple-peel or Christmas tree atresia, involves most of the small bowel distal to the obstruction. In this instance, the entire intestine may twist or wind around a fixed point

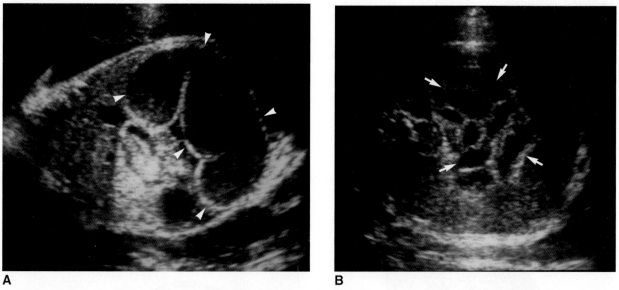

Figure 21-21 Volvulus. **A:** Oblique view of the fetal abdomen reveals markedly dilated loop of bowel *(arrowheads)*. **B:** Transverse section of the upper abdomen, superior to above this dilated loop, reveals multiple minimally dilated segments of bowel *(arrows)*. Based on this appearance, a diagnosis of volvulus was made prenatally and was confirmed after birth.

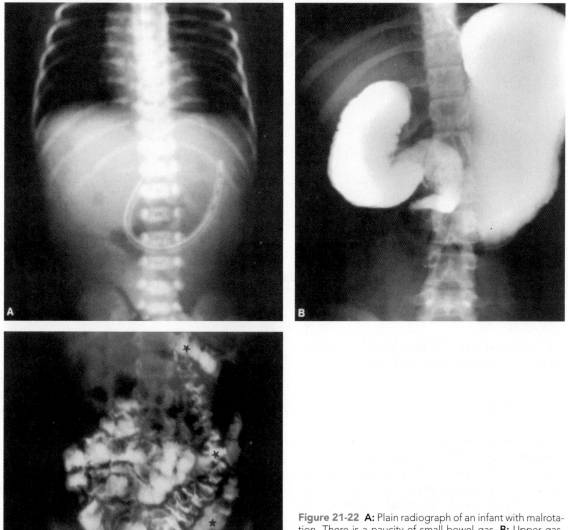

Figure 21-22 **A:** Plain radiograph of an infant with malrotation. There is a paucity of small bowel gas. **B:** Upper gastrointestinal contrast study demonstrating malrotation with midgut volvulus and duodenal obstruction. The position of the duodenojejunal junction is abnormal. **C:** Plain film showing a contrast-filled colon and cecum on the patient's left (asterisks). The entire small bowel is to the right of midline. These are typical radiographic findings of malrotation.

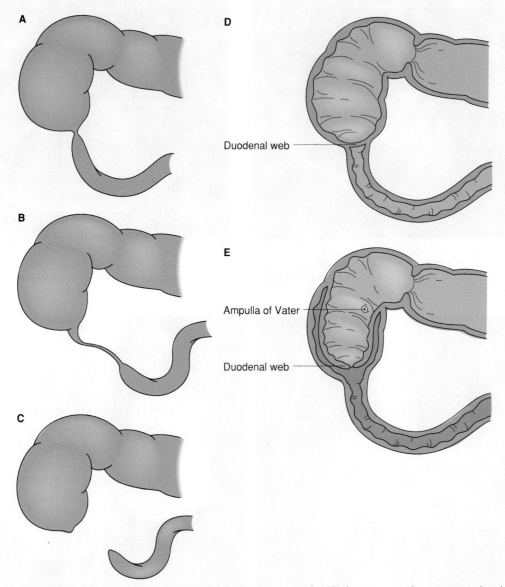

Figure 21-23 Anatomic forms of duodenal atresia **(A–C)** and webs **(D,E)**. In particular, **(E)** demonstrates the unique wind sock deformity. This lesion is important and potentially confusing because the point of obstruction is not at the apparent point of change in luminal diameter.

such as a congenital band or the ileocecal vessels.[67] Prompt diagnosis and treatment leads to an excellent prognosis.

Sonographic Imaging

Fluid filling the stomach and the duodenum at the site of obstruction creates the classic "double-bubble" image of duodenal atresia. The double-bubble image is nonspecific and can be seen in other entities, including duodenal stenosis, annular pancreas, anomalous peritoneal bands or Ladd bands, proximal jejunal atresia, bowel malrotation, and diaphragmatic hernia.[1,2] Affected fetuses often demonstrate symmetric growth retardation and, as with any high GI tract obstruction, many have polyhydramnios (Fig. 21-24).[1,2]

Duodenal atresia is most commonly associated with trisomy 21, occurring in as many as 22% to 30% of patients with some sort of duodenal obstruction.[37] Almost half of all duodenal atresia cases are associated with other anomalies. Associated malformations include cardiovascular anomalies, bowel malrotations, esophageal atresia, and tracheoesophageal fistula (Table 21-3).

Other Imaging Modalities

Radiographs demonstrate a double-bubble sign similar to the sonographic finding. This characteristic finding of duodenal atresia is due to the resultant obstruction. Bowel gas in the distal bowel indicates a stenosis (Fig. 21-25).

Differential Diagnosis

In the presence of the double-bubble sign, differential diagnoses include not only duodenal atresia but also an annular pancreas. Because of air in the stomach and

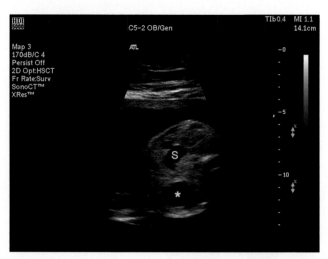

Figure 21-24 Transverse view of the fetal upper abdomen demonstrating the classic "double-bubble" sign representing the dilated stomach (S) and duodenum (star). (Image courtesy of Philips Medical Systems, Bothell, WA.)

duodenum, these spaces appear black or radiolucent on the radiograph. At times, it is difficult to differentiate between the two entities as they often coexist. In the absence of the second bubble, the suspicion of duodenal atresia increases. Other differentials include duodenal stenosis or a midgut volvulus.

Prognosis

Early neonatal surgery is associated with a good GI tract result.[1,2,6]

TABLE 21-3	
Fetal Hydrops	
Type	**Cause**
Midgut volvulus	Fluid-filled proximal duodenum
	Polyhydramnios
	Echogenic mass inferior to the liver
	Dilated bowel loops
	Whirlpool sign
	Twisted vessels with color Doppler
Duodenal atresia	Fluid-filled stomach and duodenum creating the double-bubble sign
	Symmetric intrauterine growth retardation
	Polyhydramnios
Muconium ileus	Dilated echogenic ileum
	Intraperitoneal fluid/ascites
	Possible pseudocyst
	Intra-abdominal calcifications
	Polyhydramnios
	Dilated small bowel
	Increased abdominal biometry
	Decreased bowel peristalsis

PATHOLOGY BOX 21-5

Prevalence of Anomalies Associated with Duodenal Atresia[1,2,6]

Anomaly	Prevalence (%)
Cardiovascular	20
Bowel malrotation	22–40
Trisomy 21	33
Symmetric growth retardation	50
Polyhydramnios	45
Esophageal atresia or tracheoesophageal fistula	7

Meconium Ileus

The third most common bowel obstruction in neonates is meconium ileus, most often due to cystic fibrosis.[1] This autosomal recessive[35] dysfunction of the exocrine and mucus-producing glands can present with dilated bowel loops in its early form. Cystic fibrosis most particularly affects the pancreas, biliary tract, intestines, and bronchi, with associated disturbances of mucus and electrolyte secretion. It is the most common lethal genetic condition among whites, occurring at an approximate frequency of 1 in 35,000 live births.[35] The small bowel obstruction of the distal ileus that fetuses with cystic fibrosis may have is a meconium impaction, the result of increased thickness and stickiness of the meconium and related poor motility of the bowel. Meconium ileus, like other causes of small bowel obstruction, can lead to bowel perforation and the complications and findings of meconium peritonitis.[2,6]

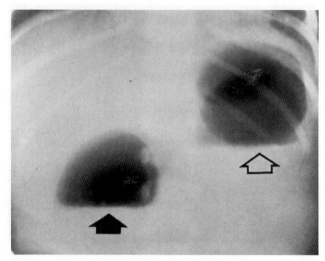

Figure 21-25 Duodenal atresia with double-bubble sign. The left bubble (open arrow) represents air in the stomach; the right bubble (solid arrow) reflects duodenal gas. There is no gas in the small or large bowel distal to the level of the complete obstruction.

Meconium peritonitis may result from meconium ileus and cystic fibrosis.[68] Meconium peritonitis occurs following rupture of the bowel, presenting with scattered calcifications throughout the peritoneum. These calcifications form from the response of foreign body giant cells and calcium deposits within inflamed tissue caused by sterile chemical peritonitis. The calcifications can usually be seen within 8 days of rupture, occurring in 86% of muconium peritonitis cases.[56] At least half of these perforations are thought to result from distal mechanical obstructions, whereas the remainder may be caused by viral infections such as cytomegalovirus or parvovirus B19.

Lack of bowel contents entering the large bowel can produce a microcolon. Associated bowel perforations, which often close before birth, may be the cause of ascites and meconium peritonitis.[2] Peristalsis, which in postnatal work may highlight bowel just proximal to a point of early obstruction, is not always easy to determine in antenatal small bowel evaluation. Functional causes of bowel dilatation may simulate obstruction, including the rare congenital chloridorrhea, with its profuse chloride diarrhea, dilated small bowel, and microcolon (Fig. 21-26).[2]

Sonographic Imaging

The meconium-impacted ileum becomes dilated, appearing echogenic on the sonographic image. If this bowel perforates because of the meconium overproduction, an inflammatory response occurs. With the initial perforation, free intraperitoneal fluid images with the development of a pseudocyst because of this chronic meconium peritonitis. Pseudocysts with a calcified rim or eggshell calcification may also form because of the chronic peritonitis.[1] In analyzing an area of increased echogenicity or possible calcification in the fetal

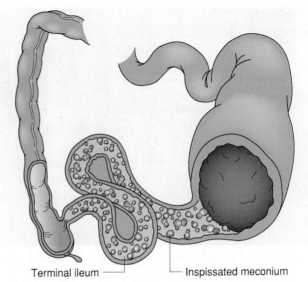

Figure 21-26 Meconium ileus causing obstruction of the terminal ileum from abnormally thick, inspissated meconium.

abdomen, consider that the increased echogenicity or calcification is neither in the organ parenchyma such as the liver nor within bowel lumen, but rather is on the peritoneal surface (Fig. 21-27).

Sonographic findings that should make the examiner suspect small bowel obstruction include:

- Polyhydramnios
- Disproportionately dilated proximal small bowel
- Failure to detect normal colon in late pregnancy
- Fetal ascites
- Peritoneal calcifications
- Decreased or absent peristalsis in dilated bowel loops noted over a period of time
- Large AC for gestational age

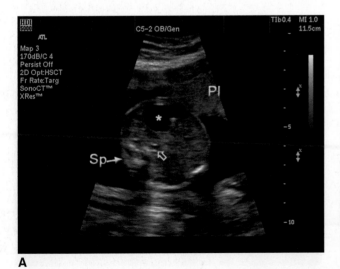

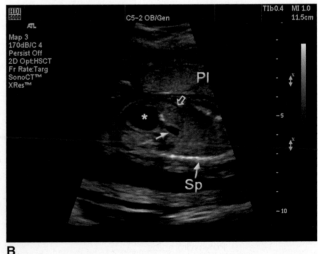

A **B**

Figure 21-27 A: A transverse image through the fetal abdomen demonstrating an anechoic meconium cyst (*star*). Use the aorta (*open arrow*), which lies slightly to the left of midline, to determine this cystic structure is on the left of the abdomen. **B:** A longitudinal image through the abdomen of the same fetus. The stomach (*solid arrow*) helps localize the cyst as a separate structure inferior to the left side of the hypoechoic diaphragm (*open arrow*). *Sp*, spine; *Pl*, placenta. (Image courtesy of Philips Medical Systems, Bothell, WA.)

Other Imaging Modalities

Usually not seen on a radiograph, meconium may appear as a mottled area within the abdomen in the first few days of life. More often the result of a rupture, meconium peritonitis appears as inflammation. Obstruction from the impacted meconium appears as multiple air-filled loops of bowel (Figs. 21-28 and 21-29).

Differential Diagnosis

Differential diagnoses include Hirschprung disease, bowel obstruction, meconium plug syndrome, and cystic fibrosis.[69,70]

Prognosis

Prior to 1970, patients with meconium ileus had poor outcomes; however, surgical improvements have resulted in very favorable outcomes.[70] In the case of cystic fibrosis as the cause for this finding, the prognosis mirrors the general cystic fibrosis morbidity and mortality rates.[70] Currently, prognosis is excellent for these patients.

LARGE BOWEL OBSTRUCTION

Obstructions of the colon or large bowel are more difficult to diagnose antenatally than are those of the small bowel, and they are not associated with increases in amniotic fluid. Normal colon tends to image only in the third trimester and is frequently observed without any obvious bowel peristalsis. The major causes of large bowel obstruction are imperforate anus, meconium ileus and Hirschsprung disease or megacolon, and aganglionosis of part of or the entire colon.

First described in 1886 by Danish physician Harold Hirschsprung, Hirschsprung disease is a functional disorder of the distal colon that results in perpetually contracted or tonic bowel. The colon does not relax because of the congenital absence of the neuroenteric ganglion cells in the mucosal layer of the bowel. These cells control the relaxation phase of peristalsis and consequently affect the movement of meconium resulting in a functional obstruction. Occurring more often in males, Hirschsprung disease usually affects a segment of bowel beginning at the distal portion.[6,67] Total colonic Hirschsprung disease is a particularly difficult diagnosis to make because of the lack of a normal segment of bowel for comparison.[1,2] Other entities may affect the motility of the fetal bowel and formation of a meconium plug, including maternal preeclampsia, maternal diabetes mellitus, maternal administration of magnesium sulfate, prematurity, sepsis, and hypothyroidism.[67]

A colon wall-to-wall diameter measurement varies with gestation age; however, a descending colon measurement greater than 20 mm in a preterm fetus is considered abnormal.[71] The fetal rectosigmoid colon, however, can reach a size of 2 to 3 cm when filled with meconium near term. An antenatal indication of Hirschsprung disease is a focal bowel dilatation proximal to the obstruction.

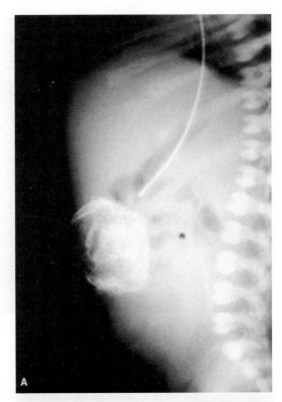

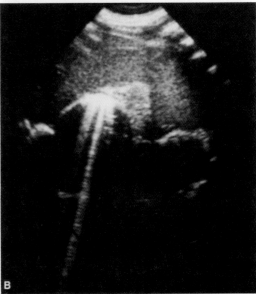

Figure 21-28 A: Plain film radiograph of calcified pseudocyst in complicated meconium ileus. **B:** In utero ultrasound demonstrating calcified pseudocyst.

ECHOGENIC BOWEL

The use of higher-frequency transducers in fetal ultrasound has resulted in the increase of echogenic bowel as a sonographic finding. It is reported to be the most common echogenic mass found in the fetal abdomen.[26] Clinical reports have noted that collapsed small bowel often appears as an echogenic nonshadowing mass in the lower abdomen and pelvis of normal fetuses. This is an especially common finding in the second trimester,

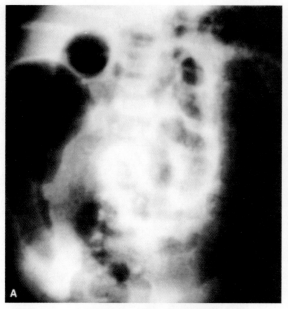 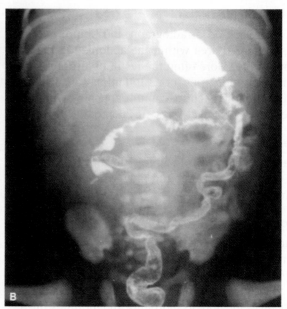

Figure 21-29 A. Plain radiograph of neonate with meconium ileus. **B:** Contrast enema in an infant with meconium ileus demonstrating an unused but intrinsically normal microcolon.

with approximately 50% of the reported cases resolving spontaneously.[56] However, it also can be a normal finding at other points in pregnancy, particularly the late third trimester because of the presence of meconium in the bowel.[2,6]

Several differential diagnoses with increased bowel echogenicity are as follows include

- Congenital fetal infections including cytomegalovirus
- Chromosomal abnormalities such as triploidy and trisomy 21, 18, or 13
- Mesenteric ischemia
- Meconium ileus with its hyperechoic intraluminal meconium
- Swallowed blood from intra-amniotic bleeding
- Intraluminal gas produced by bacteria associated with maternal amnionitis[1,2,6]

Exactly what represents increased echogenicity is highly subjective (Fig. 27-2). Certainly, bowel echogenicity greater than the echogenicity of nearby fetal bone has been commonly acclaimed as indicating greater risk for meconium ileus/cystic fibrosis and the pathologic processes associated with increased bowel echogenicity. Because of the increased association with fetal demise and IUGR, these fetuses should be followed closely.[2]

ENTERIC INCLUSION CYSTS

Enteric inclusion cysts are a rare finding but are more likely to be imaged with the increased resolution of sonographic equipment.[72] They may present as cystic or solid-appearing structures within the fetus. These cysts are formed by an inner epithelium of a respiratory or intestinal type and a two-layer smooth muscle wall. They

can be associated with other fetal abnormalities, especially of the spine or GI tract in 30% of cases. As many as 40% of enteric cysts involve the ileum and raise a possibility of small bowel obstruction.[56]

AMNIOTIC FLUID

Amniotic fluid is a dialysate of maternal serum, essential for the maintenance of an even fetal temperature and biochemical homeostasis. Its presence allows fetal movement and growth, and it is thought to be essential for the development of the tracheobronchial tree.[6] Typically anechoic, occasionally sonographers find echogenic material moving within the fluid. In one study of 19 fetuses with very echogenic amniotic fluid that soon after had a third-trimester amniocentesis, the echogenicity was caused by vernix caseosa in all but one case of fetal distress and intrauterine meconium passage.[72]

At 12 weeks' gestation, amniotic fluid volume averages 60 mL, increasing 20 to 25 mL per week until 16 weeks and then increasing 50 to 100 mL per week until 20 weeks. The mean fluid volume at 20 weeks is 500 mL. The fetus may contribute to amniotic fluid volume by fluid transfer across the fetal skin surfaces, including skin, cord, chorion, and amnion. Fetal urine production begins at 12 weeks, but the amount is insignificant until the 18th to 20th weeks of gestation. By the late third trimester, the fetus is producing approximately 450 mL of urine per day. Beyond 20 weeks, transudation of fluid across fetal surfaces is inadequate to maintain normal amniotic volume, and the fetus essentially modifies fluid volume and composition only by swallowing and urination.[1,2,6]

Normal amniotic fluid volume may be maintained by one functioning kidney and a nonobstructed GU tract. Oligohydramnios of fetal origin results from abnormality of the GU tract, usually bilateral renal agenesis, urethral atresia, or bilateral nonfunctional renal dysplasia. Oligohydramnios hinders fetal anatomy analysis because of the limitation of the fluid imaging window. The diagnosis of oligohydramnios is somewhat subjective and varies with fetal gestational age. Sonographically, the diagnosis is made by noting decreased fluid surrounding the fetus and crowding of fetal parts. Use of the amniotic fluid index (AFI) represents a more objective method of analyzing the fluid level. Uterine contractions compress the fetal abdomen, decreasing the surrounding amniotic fluid that may cause a pseudo-omphalocele.

GENITOURINARY SYSTEM

A routine second-trimester prenatal ultrasound may incidentally reveal abnormalities of the GU system. The identification of the fetal kidneys is possible by 22 weeks' gestation in 95% of patients scanned.[73] Fetal malformations are noted once in every 200 births and, of those, GU system anomalies are the most common. They account for about 30% of congenital abnormalities in the fetus. This early diagnosis not only allows for intervention, but also leads to controversial therapies for obstructive processes.[74] The amount of amniotic fluid observed has a direct correlation to the renal function of the fetus. Any unusual variation of the fluid volume should lead to careful assessment of the GU system. This survey includes visualization of the bladder and confirmation of renal arteries with color Doppler. By 9 weeks' gestational age, the kidneys should have attained their normal position and the blood supply established. A quarter of adults have more than two renal arteries on each side.[1]

The bladder, which may appear quite large in normal fetuses, images either on initial or during a diuretic enhanced follow-up examination in all fetuses older than 15 weeks. This finding helps to rule out bilateral renal dysfunction, bilateral renal, or ureteral obstruction. Fetal voiding decreases bladder size, thus eliminating bladder outlet obstruction with the finding of a large bladder. Bladder wall thickening, a sign of outlet obstruction, often caused by posterior uretheral valves (PUV), should be excluded. A dilated posterior urethra in a male fetus suggests obstruction, usually PUV.[1,2,6]

RENAL MALFORMATIONS

RENAL AGENESIS

Absence of one kidney, unilateral renal agenesis, occurs in 1 in 1,000 births and is considered very common.[75] Occurring in approximately 1 in 2,000 pregnancies, ectopic kidneys are found anywhere on the embryologic "migratory path." An ectopic kidney remaining in the pelvis appears as a mass in a female fetus.[1]

Asymmetry of renal tissue within or beyond the renal bed or an unusual kidney shape may be caused by a single horseshoe kidney, a duplicated system, a tumor, or fused or nonfused crossed renal ectopia.[1] Horseshoe kidneys are formed by the fusion of the lower poles and occur in 1 in 500 births. Seven percent of patients with Turner syndrome are diagnosed with a horseshoe kidney.[73] Crossed renal ectopia is found more frequently in male fetuses and affect the left kidney.[1] Renal function is usually normal in these incidences.

Bilateral renal agenesis, often considered the classic form of Potter sequence,[2] occurs at the rate of 1 to 3 cases per 10,000 live births, predominantly in male infants.[6] The reoccurrence rate in families is as high as 50% with autosomal dominant pattern and approximately 25% in autosomal recessive conditions.[6,35] Fetuses with bilateral renal agenesis have an increased incidence of other anomalies, especially involving the musculoskeletal system (in particular sirenomelia) and the cardiovascular system.[6] GI and central nervous system malformations are also difficult to confirm because of the lack of amniotic fluid. In the presence of an esophageal atresia or tracheoesophageal fistula, there may be an appearance of a normal amount of fluid.[1]

Sonographic Findings

The inability to locate a kidney during the prenatal exam raises suspicion for unilateral agenesis. This finding during sonographic exam should result in a search of the fetal abdomen from the pelvis to the renal fossa. In the case of the unilateral kidney, the size is larger than in a fetus with two kidneys because of compensatory mechanisms. Unilateral agenesis may not result in a change in amniotic fluid levels or bladder filling; however, with both kidneys absent, oligohydramnios and an empty bladder images.[8] In the presence of renal agenesis, the adrenal glands move into the renal fossa, assuming a position parallel to the spine.[6] See the adrenal section for a complete discussion of this finding. The adrenal gland may also enlarge imaging as a globular structure within the renal fossa.[2]

Severe oligohydramnios is usually noted between the 16th and 28th weeks of gestation in fetuses with bilateral renal agenesis. Bilateral renal agenesis results

---

PATHOLOGY BOX 21-6

Sonographic Findings with Renal Agenesis

Identification of one or both kidneys

Normal or oligohydramnios

Small thorax

Dolichocephaly

Absent bladder

Adrenal gland flattened in renal fossa

Absent renal arteries with color Doppler

in dolichocephaly and a small thorax due to oligohydramnios and the resultant uterine compression. Color Doppler visualizing the aorta and renal arteries is one method to confirm either unilateral or bilateral agenesis. The inability to image both the kidney and a renal artery helps diagnose this anomaly.

Other Imaging Modalities

If sonography is unable to provide a definitive diagnosis of renal agenesis, MRI may be of benefit.[2]

Differential Diagnosis

Other renal diseases to include with the finding of oligohydramnios include bilateral cystic kidney disease, bladder outlet obstruction, IUGR, and premature rupture of membranes.[6]

Prognosis

Bilateral renal agenesis is incompatible with life.[2,8] Individuals with one kidney, and no other coexisting malformations, have a normal life span.[2,6]

FETAL OBSTRUCTIVE UROPATHIES

Any blockage of urine flow in the urinary system results in a condition defined as an obstructive uropathy. The obstruction can occur anywhere along the tract: the ureter, bladder, or urethra.[75] Sonography allows for early detection of fetal hydronephrosis, the most common fetal anomaly.[1] The recognition of the dilated renal pelvis is important, because long-term obstruction can cause permanent damage to the kidneys (Table 21-4).

In some fetuses, the degree of pelvic dilatation has been noted to change, usually decrease, with fetal bladder emptying. This may be similar to the decrease or absence of renal pelvic dilatation seen in adults after the emptying of full bladders.[1] The postnatal confirmation of hydronephrosis should not be made within the first day or two of life because of neonatal dehydration and relatively low glomerular filtration rate of young infants, which may contribute to a falsely normal appearance of the newborn renal pelvis.[1,2,6]

A dilated renal pelvis can be caused by obstruction at any level of the urinary tract or by vesicoureteral reflux, or it can be related to prune belly syndrome.[8] On rare occasions, dilation can be caused by pressure from a pelvic mass. The finding of dilated renal pelvis raises suspicion for chromosomal anomalies.[2] The majority of kidneys with antenatal pyelectasis of less than 1 cm prove to be normal at birth. Many cases of antenatal GU tract dilatation are unrelated to either obstruction or vesicoureteral reflux in the neonate. As a result, serial sonograms to monitor the dilation have become common.

It is important to diagnose fetal hydronephrosis for a positive outcome. A grading system developed by the Society for Fetal Urology helps assess fetal hydronephrosis in relation to neonatal clinical outcome (Table 21-5).[33,34,43] The grades are also applied to various degrees of reflux as stated below:[32]

- Grade I- physiologic dilatation, ureter only
- Grade II- intermediate hydronephrosis, ureter renal pelvis, calyces without dilatation
- Grade III- intermediate hydronephrosis, dilatation of the ureter and/or dilated pelvis
- Grade IV- shape of calyces maintained but dilated, requires surgical intervention, renal pelvis greater than 1.5 cm
- Grade V- gross dilatation, requires surgical intervention, anteroposterior (AP) measurements of the renal pelvis greater than 1.5 cm[64]

Fifty percent of patients with intermediate hydronephrosis require postnatal surgical intervention. There is no standardized international classification or measurement technique; however, the Australasian Society for Ultrasound in Medicine uses the AP renal pelvic diameter correlating the size to gestational age. From 18 to 20 weeks, 4 mm is considered normal; 6 mm is considered normal at 32 weeks. Severe hydronephrosis is any gestation with greater than 10 mm of dilation (Fig. 21-30).[33]

Sonographic Imaging

After 24 weeks' gestation, it is common to see at least some dilatation of the central renal pelvis. The anechoic fluid is a sharp contrast to the normal echogenicity of the renal parenchyma. The renal pelvis may measure between 5 and 10 mm in AP diameter depending on gestational age and is often a transient finding.[1] Bilateral hydronephrosis is found in as many as 40% of cases, though only 5% of those require surgical intervention after birth.[73] Normal ureters are not imaged unless they are obstructed. Serial follow-up scans assess any

TABLE 21-4	
Etiologies of Hydronephrosis	
Type	**% of Occurrences**
Transient	48%
Physiologic	15%
Ureteropelvic junction (UPJ)	11%
Vesicoureteral reflux (VUR)	9%
Megaureter (obstructed or unobstructed)	4%
Multicystic dysplastic kidney	2%
Ureterocele	2%
Posterior urethral valves	1%
Other (ectopic ureter, prune belly, urachal cyst, and urethral atresia)	8%

Woodward M, Frank D. Postnatal management of antenatal hydronephrosis. *BJU International*. 2002;89(2):149–156.

TABLE 21-5		
Grading System for Fetal Hydronephrosis[64]		
Grade 0	Normal	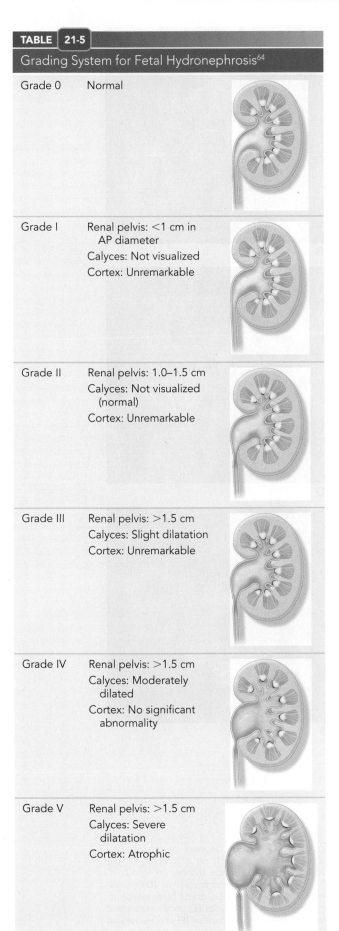
Grade I	Renal pelvis: <1 cm in AP diameter Calyces: Not visualized Cortex: Unremarkable	
Grade II	Renal pelvis: 1.0–1.5 cm Calyces: Not visualized (normal) Cortex: Unremarkable	
Grade III	Renal pelvis: >1.5 cm Calyces: Slight dilatation Cortex: Unremarkable	
Grade IV	Renal pelvis: >1.5 cm Calyces: Moderately dilated Cortex: No significant abnormality	
Grade V	Renal pelvis: >1.5 cm Calyces: Severe dilatation Cortex: Atrophic	

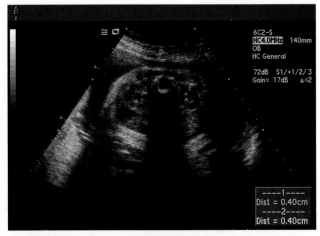

Figure 21-30 Transverse image of mildly dilated renal pelvis demonstrating the proper measurement method.

change in the AP measurement of the renal pelvis. With a persistent AP measurement of greater than 10 mm, 85% of fetuses have some sort of anatomic anomaly (Fig. 21-31).[75]

Complementary Imaging

The neonate with prenatally diagnosed hydronephrosis may need a voiding cystourethrogram (VCUG) to detect urinary reflux or ureteral abnormalities. An MRI provides images to aid in determination of anomalies causing the renal dilatation.[2]

Prognosis

The prognosis for fetuses with dilated renal pelvises depends on any coexisting malformations. There is a poor prognosis in fetuses with bilateral hydronephrosis, an obstructed bladder, low fluid, and resultant pulmonary hypoplasia.[2] Early diagnosis of renal obstruction and subsequent early pediatric surgery for correction is necessary to ensure future renal function.

CAUSES FOR HYDRONEPHROSIS

Ureteropelvic Junction Obstruction

The most common cause of congenital obstructive hydronephrosis is ureteropelvic junction (UPJ) obstruction, which occurs in 1 of every 2,000 newborns and is bilateral in almost one-third of cases. Bilateral involvement is usually asymmetric; severe bilateral involvement is unusual.[6]

UPJ obstruction occurs at the junction of the renal pelvis and the ureter. Several anatomic causes of UPJ are:
- Abnormal ureteral insertion
- Unusual shapes of the pyeloureteral outlet
- Ureteral valves
- Fibrous adhesions, bands, or kinks
- Aberrant lower pole vessels
- Absence of the longitudinal muscle essential to the excretion of urine from the kidney[1,75]

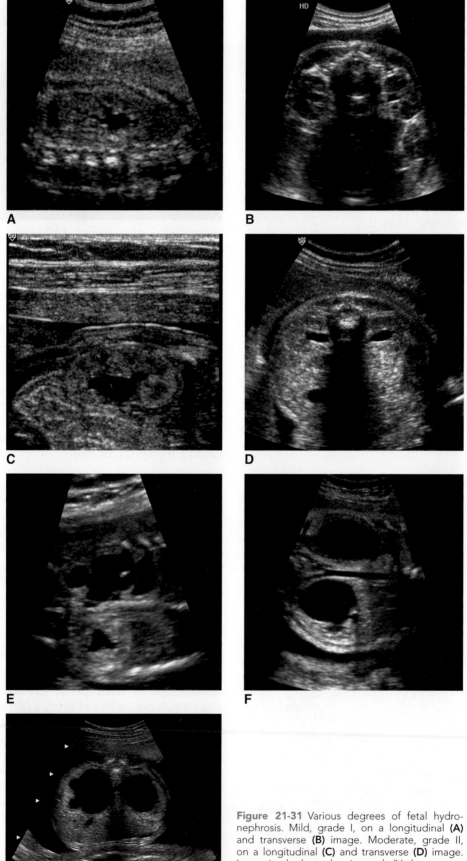

Figure 21-31 Various degrees of fetal hydronephrosis. Mild, grade I, on a longitudinal **(A)** and transverse **(B)** image. Moderate, grade II, on a longitudinal **(C)** and transverse **(D)** image. Increasing hydronephrosis, grade IV, demonstrating dilatation of the calyces **(E)** on a longitudinal image. A grade V on a coronal **(F)** and transverse **(G)** image.

Sonographic Imaging

Hydronephrosis without a hydroureter supports the diagnosis of UPJ obstruction.[8] Amniotic fluid levels are normal to increased.[6,8]

Ureterovesical Junction Obstruction

Ureterovesical junction obstruction is rare and noted by dilatation of the ureter to the level of the bladder. Megaureter can be classified as primary or secondary and is frequently idiopathic.[75] Primary megaureter can cause obstruction by lack of peristalsis in a focal portion of the distal ureter. A defect caused by fibrosis or stenotic ureteral valves can be the source of the megaureter.[1] Secondary megaureter is a result of an obstruction at another location, possibly from pressure of a vessel or mass.[1,75]

Occasionally, an antenatal observation of partial obstruction occurs in only one portion of a kidney. A common anomaly is renal duplication, consisting of two renal collecting system portions and their separate ureters. This may occur unilaterally or bilaterally. The upper pole of the duplicated kidney can appear cystlike because of obstruction. This is usually because of ectopic placement of its distal ureter and often is in association with an ectopic ureterocele. The lower portion, or moiety, frequently has associated vesicoureteral reflux that occasionally results in the appearance of pyelocalyceal dilatation. The prenatal diagnosis of a duplicated kidney system is often limited by the small size of the upper part and the changing size of the ureterocele owing to intravesical pressures. Ureteroceles found outside the bladder may simulate any pelvic cystic mass, including ovarian cyst, anterior meningocele, and hydrocolpos.

Sonographic Imaging

During the sonographic exam, the finding of a tortuous dilated ureter and renal pelvis raises suspicion for a ureterovesical junction obstruction. Unilateral obstruction demonstrates normal amniotic fluid levels with bilateral obstruction resulting in oligohydramnios.[6,8]

Posterior Urethral Valves

Posterior urethral valves may cause a distal urinary tract obstruction that may result in hydronephrosis, hydroureters, and dilation of the bladder.[1] Posterior urethral valve is a predominately male abnormality because of redundant membranous folds in the posterior urethra that lead to varying degrees of obstruction. Typically, there is a thick-walled, dilated bladder, and often an apparent dilated posterior urethra. If the obstructed urine refluxes with pressure into the renal pelvis, there may be forniceal rupture and the development of a perirenal urinoma or urinary ascites. These have been characterized as three different types of valves.[75]

- Type I—folds distal to the verumontanum, insert into lateral wall of urethra
- Type II—folds originate in the verumontanum, pass to the bladder neck, and divide into multiple membranes
- Type III—folds distal to verumontanum though not attached, small opening in diaphragm-like structure

The verumontanum is a landmark on the floor of the prostatic urethra near the entrance of the seminal vesicles.

Sonographic Imaging

Uretheral obstruction may result in low fluid levels and a thick-walled, dilated bladder. The urethra may be dilated with bilateral hydronephrosis and hydroureters.[8]

Bladder Outlet Obstruction

Any condition that blocks flow from the bladder is known as bladder outlet obstruction.[75] This type of obstruction is seen in patients with PUV, urethral atresia, and the caudal regression syndrome. In each case of bladder outlet obstruction, or megacystis, there may be retrograde filling and dilatation of bladder, ureters, and renal pelvis. The bladder wall proximal to an area of obstruction may become trabeculated and appear thickened.

Severe hydronephrosis is seen in about 15% of cases and may lead to Potter sequence. Another consideration should be megacystis-microcolon intestinal hypoperistalsis syndrome.[1] Complete urethral atresia is similar to severe PUV. The fetal urinary bladder changes in size as the fetus micturates into the abdominal cavity. If the bladder is not seen during an ultrasound examination, a recheck after 20 to 30 minutes demonstrates a filling bladder.[75]

PRUNE BELLY SYNDROME

This syndrome, also known as the urethral obstruction malformation complex,[1] presents with a triad of findings:

- Distention of the anterior abdominal wall
- Obstruction of the urinary tract
- Cryptorchidism[29]

The fetal abdomen can assume a particularly distended appearance from fetal ascites or an extremely dilated bladder, resulting in the characteristic laxity of the abdominal wall. The thorax is smaller in comparison, with hypoplastic lungs, and there is usually a degree of hydronephrosis observed along with oligohydramnios. Successful placement of a bladder shunt to drain the excess urine can result in reduced pressure, allowing development of the lungs and an improved prognosis.[1] Other sonographic findings include a large bladder with a thick wall, tortuous and dilated ureters, hydronephrosis, renal dysplasia, and a patent urachus. Associated anomalies include GI malformations, pulmonary hypoplasia due to oligohydramnios, and cardiac and skeletal malformations.

CYSTIC KIDNEY DISEASE (POTTERS SEQUENCE)

Polycystic kidney disease (PKD) is the result of a single gene mutation and is one of the most common renal disorders.[35] The autosomal dominant form has a higher incidence than the recessive form, affecting about half a million people in the United States. Affecting 1 in 500 to 1,000 individuals, the autosomal dominant form is more common than the recessive form.[35] Included in Potters sequence is multicystic renal dysplasia (MCRD), which is due to metanephros development failure and obstructive cystic dysplasia, which occurs as the result of a mechanical process.[6,30]

Osthanondh and Potter classified cystic dysplasias of the kidneys into four types:

- Type I- autosomal recessive polycystic kidney disease (ARPKD), also known as infantile polycystic kidney disease
- Type II- multicystic renal dysplastic disease (MCRD)
- Type III- autosomal dominant polycystic kidney disease (ADPKD), also known as adult polycystic kidney disease
- Type IV- obstructive cystic dysplastic disease[1,6,30]

Potter type I ARPKD affects both kidneys; its reported incidence is 2 cases in 100,000 births,[1] with a 25% recurrence rate in affected families. Saccular dilatations of the collecting tubules create multiple small cysts (typically 1 to 2 mm) that are too small to be resolved as cysts on sonography. The classic image is that of massively enlarged, homogeneously echogenic kidneys taking up most of the abdomen's space.[8] Unlike in other dysplasias, there is no increase in connective tissue within these kidneys. Affected fetuses tend to have severe oligohydramnios because of bilateral renal dysfunction, and the bladder is not imaged. Hypoplasia is the leading cause of neonatal death. Cases have been reported of kidneys later proven to have ARPKD that appeared normal on early antenatal scans, and abnormal only on scans in later pregnancy. Surviving children with PKD often have associated hepatic fibrosis, with a severity inversely related to the severity of their renal disease.[2,6]

Potter type II multicystic dysplastic disease is the most common of the cystic renal dysplasias. Some believe that MCKD results from early ureteropelvic atresia. Typically, MCKD is a unilateral finding and the amniotic fluid level is unaffected, allowing for normal lung development. Contralateral kidney anomalies are a common finding, as are contralateral UPJ obstructions. Bilateral MCKD occurs at 19% incidence in one study of contralateral MCKD or MCKD with contralateral renal agenesis (11%). There is a question of at least a partial genetic influence in this disorder, which has a 3% to 5% familial recurrence rate. The sonographic image (Fig. 28-22) consists of multiple, large anechoic cysts of variable size, the largest of which is *not* central, a more typical finding of hydronephrosis. The kidney may vary in size from small to normal to large, but the reniform shape is often absent. Increased echogenicity between the cysts is usually the result of connective tissue proliferation. The renal pelvis and proximal ureter are absent or atretic. Histologically, these kidneys typically consist of thick-walled cysts, small groups of tubules, and poorly formed glomeruli. Dysplastic kidneys occasionally

increase in size as a result of urine production by the few remaining nephrons. Many reports of disappearing MCDKs may, in part, be related to eventual cessation of any urine production.[2,6]

Potter type III ADPKD is rarely seen in antenatal life, though it may be diagnosed when there is a family history of polycystic kidneys.[1] Also known as adult PKD (APKD), this condition typically begins in adulthood and is often asymptomatic for years.[75] Case reports note cysts interspersed in the cortex and medulla of bilaterally enlarged kidneys. Small cysts may not be resolved, and the kidneys may appear only echogenic. Although Adult PKD is a bilateral disease, there may be asymmetry of involvement. The liver, pancreas, and occasionally, the spleen may also contain cysts. Amniotic fluid levels may be normal or decreased.[2,6]

Potter type IV obstructive cystic disease is thought to be secondary to an early obstruction of the GU tract. Usually seen in severe cases of PUV, it is commonly seen in association with the more severe obstruction of urethral atresia. It has been reported in the caudal regression syndrome with persistent cloaca and other obstructions. Focal and segmental dysplasia may be seen and are often caused by obstruction or atresia of one of the ureters extending from a duplicated kidney. Sonographic findings include significant oligohydramnios and moderately enlarged kidneys with small to medium capsular or peripheral parenchymal cysts. Other findings depend on the site and degree of obstruction. Chronic obstructions at or distal to the bladder may show bladder wall thickening and enlargement, as well as ureteral dilation and a tortuous ureteral course when there is obstruction along the course of the ureter.[6]

Several inherited syndromes have nonobstructive cystic renal dysplasia as part of their findings. These include Zellweger, Ehlers-Danlos, and von Hippel-Lindau syndromes. Meckel-Gruber syndrome is one such entity with renal cysts (usually as part of bilateral MCDK) associated with occipital encephalocele and polydactyly. It has a 25% recurrence rate in future pregnancies. Knowledge of the associated ultrasound findings of syndromes can aid in making a specific antenatal diagnoses. This is particularly true in assessing future pregnancies. Half of all patients with the VACTERL (*v*ertebral abnormalities, *a*nal atresia, *c*ardiac abnormalities, *t*racheo-*e*sophageal, *r*enal, and *l*imb [or *r*adius] abnormalities) association, one-third of those with trisomy 13, and one-tenth of those with trisomy 18 have associated renal cystic involvement.[1,2,6,35] For a summary of Potters sequence, see Table 28-1.

OTHER RENAL ANOMALIES AND FINDINGS

Tumors of the kidneys are unusual and should be questioned when the renal contour is distorted and without obvious renal parenchyma. Imaged as unilateral echogenic masses, fetal renal hamartomas or congenital mesoblastic nephromas are the most common renal neoplasms of the first few months of life. The enlarged but functioning kidneys associated with tyrosinosis, glycogen storage diseases, and other congenital metabolic disorders may simulate bilateral fetal renal tumors. Wilms tumor or nephroblastoma have also been identified.[75]

Renal vein thrombosis is a well-known entity in neonates that often presents with palpably enlarged kidneys and associated hematuria or varying degrees of renal failure. Theoretic etiologies include septicemia, maternal diabetes, prenatal steroid administration, and congenital renal defects. Linear echoes or densities within the kidneys suggest the pathognomonic intrarenal calcification within thrombosed renal vessels.[2,6]

ADRENAL GLANDS

The fetal adrenal gland, as previously mentioned, may assume a more circular shape and simulate a kidney in the presence of renal agenesis. The adrenal gland has also been described as appearing flat (Fig. 21-32) in other cases of fetal or neonatal renal agenesis or ectopia.[8] Anencephalic fetuses have small adrenal glands, allegedly because no adrenocorticotropic hormone is produced.[6] The adrenal gland is said to weigh less in the offspring of preeclamptic mothers and patients with antepartum hemorrhage.[2,6]

The diagnosis of congenital malignant neoplasms of the adrenal glands is very rare. Most of those discovered antenatally have been neuroblastomas, the most common extracranial solid malignancy of children. The sonographic patterns of those antenatally detected neuroblastomas have been nonspecific, with solid, mixed cystic and solid, and hyperechoic masses reported. The

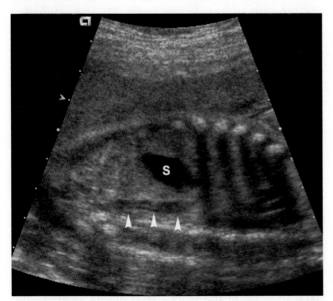

Figure 21-32 "Lying-down" adrenal gland in a renal fossa with an absent kidney. Left parasagittal view of the abdomen demonstrates the left adrenal gland (arrowheads) to be lying in a cephalocaudad orientation behind the stomas (S).

asymmetry of these masses from the contralateral adrenal gland may help differentiate them from enlargement due to fetal adrenal hemorrhage.[50]

PELVIS

The normal fetal pelvis is small, and masses within it typically extend into the abdomen. The only routinely visualized normal organ is the fluid-filled bladder. In the third trimester, the meconium-filled, echopenic, and tubular rectosigmoid may be noted. Echogenic fascial lines separate normal muscle groups. The two major groups of abnormality in this area are those of the female genital system, seen as pelvic masses that may extend beyond the pelvis and into the abdomen, and sacrococcygeal teratomas (SCT), noted as predominantly external masses with variable internal pelvic extension. A good check to determine that there is no external SCT is to look for symmetry of the soft tissues of the fetal rump without evidence of an associated mass.

PATENT URACHUS

The tube-like urachus connects the urinary bladder to the allantois. Early in fetal development, the patency is obliterated and the urachus becomes the median vesicular ligament, which extends from the bladder apex to the umbilicus.[1] Partial obliteration can lead to cystic masses between the bladder and umbilicus along the anterior abdominal wall. Three types of defects occur:

1. Urachal cyst: a cystic mass that forms along the duct's course but does not communicate with the bladder
2. Urachal sinus: a cystic mass that communicates with the anterior abdominal wall but not with the bladder
3. Partially patent urachus: a cystic tubular area communicating with the bladder but not the abdominal wall

Rarely, a complete communication between the bladder and anterior abdominal wall at the umbilicus occurs. This patent urachus is seen in 1 to 2.5 per 100,000 deliveries, twice as often in boys as in girls. The cystic mass extends from the bladder apex to the anterior abdominal wall at the umbilicus. The abnormality is limited and is not associated with other significant congenital abnormalities. In the case of an extra-abdominal mass, there must be differentiation from the more serious problem of bladder exstrophy (Fig. 21-33).[2,6]

BLADDER EXSTROPHY

Bladder exstrophy is a failure in development of a primitive streak of mesoderm in the allantoic extension of the cloacal membrane leading to variable presentations of bladder exstrophy, including split bony symphysis, divergent rectus muscles, and exteriorization of the bladder.[30] The bladder can appear as a solid anterior abdominal

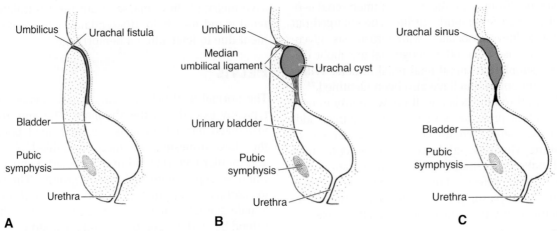

Figure 21-33 Urachal cysts and fistulas. The withered allantois does not always resorb itself into a fibrous cord (the urachus, or median umbilical ligament) between the bladder and umbilicus. If the urachus remains patent, fluid can weep out of the umbilicus through a fistula (**A**) or can be trapped as a cyst (**B**). The urachus also may form a sinus connection to the outside but not to the bladder (**C**). (From Sadler TW. *Langman's Essential Medical Embryology.* 10th ed. Baltimore, MD: Lippincott Williams & Wilkins; 2006. Fig. 7.6C-E, p. 77).

wall mass that may simulate an omphalocele. Bladder exstrophy occurs in 1 in 25,000 to 40,000 births, with a male prevalence of twice times that of females.[6] This serious anomaly is associated with other GU, GI, and musculoskeletal abnormalities. MRI helps confirm the diagnosis and assist in preoperative planning.

SONOGRAPHIC IMAGING

Bladder exstrophy demonstrates as a soft tissue mass extending from the lower anterior wall. It becomes important to differentiate this anomaly from an omphalocele or gastroschisis defect. In the case of bladder exstrophy, the soft tissue mass images inferior to the cord insertion because of the large infraumbilical defect.[8] Oligohydramnios may also be present because of the lack of fetal urination. Absence of the normal urinary bladder and the low insertion of the umbilical cord are other diagnostic criteria.[2,6]

PROGNOSIS

Correction of bladder exstrophy is achived through surgical closure and excision of the urinary defect.[6]

FETAL GENITALIA

HERMAPHRODITISM

Hermaphroditism is a rare condition that occurs when both male and female genitalia are present in the fetus. There are some mosaic karyotypes, but most fetuses are normal. The sonographer must be careful when determining fetal sex because other conditions can influence the appearance of the genitalia.[1]

MALE

Hypospadias is an incomplete fusion of the urogenital folds and is found in 1 in 300 births. The urethra can develop an abnormal opening along the ventral surface near the glans penis or at midpoint of the penis. This can also occur in females with a urethral meatus in the vagina.

Failure of the testes to complete the migratory descent into the scrotum via the inguinal canal is termed *cryptorchidism.*[1] It is the most common genital abnormality in children and can be unilateral or bilateral. Antenatal testicular torsion images similar to postnatal torsion. In the acute phase, the testis has a hypoechoic appearance and measures large when compared with the normal testis. As the torsion becomes chronic, the testis becomes small and may calcify.[2] This can be confirmed with color Doppler interrogation of the testicle.

Hydroceles

Fetal hydroceles are very common. A variable amount of fluid remaining from normal testicular descent into the scrotum surrounds the testes. This accumulation of serous fluid beneath the tunica vaginalis is normal. There are two types of hydroceles described[75]:

- Communicating: Continuous communication with the peritoneum and abdominal ascites allows for observable change in size of the hydrocele.
- Noncommunicating: These hydroceles do not increase in size and tend to be reabsorbed within the first 9 months of life.

Enlarging hydroceles indicate continued patency of the processus vaginalis, and increasing scrotal volume could be an indication of an inguinal hernia. Intrascrotal extension of meconium peritonitis may produce echogenic or calcified intrascrotal masses (Fig. 21-34).[2]

FEMALE

In the past, sonographers were unable to obtain antenatal imaging of the female fetal uterus, ovaries, and vagina. The increased detail resolution now allows imaging of the normal uterus in the close-to-term fetus (Fig. 7-1). Thus, modern imaging technology allows us

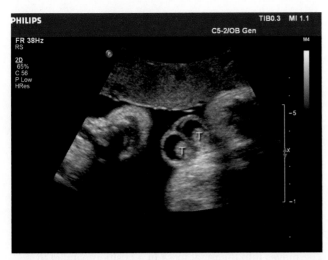

Figure 21-34 This view of the scrotum demonstrates the typical anechoic hydrocele appearance surrounding the testicle (*T*). (Image courtesy of Philips Medical Systems, Bothell, WA.)

to image the follicular cysts that result from the influence of maternal hormones.[8] Small follicular cysts not visualized on fetal examination are found in many autopsy specimens and are certainly a common finding in the ovaries of the neonate.[6]

Fetal ovarian cysts are noted infrequently and probably develop in response to maternal hormonal stimulation, hypothyroidism, toxemia, or diabetes.[2,6] Fetal ovarian cysts may be unilocular or multiseptate cystic masses that, when enlarged, may rise out of the pelvis and into the abdomen. Urachal cysts, enteric duplications, or mesenteric cysts may simulate these cystic masses. Bilateral multiseptate cystic pelvic masses in a female fetus suggest an ovarian origin.

Cystic ovaries are not of concern in the neonate and are often followed clinically when there are no symptoms. Surgeons will operate on a neonate with a cystic ovary on a pedicle because of the risk of torsion. Cystic ovaries with hemorrhage/fluid levels or those with contained

clot or multiple septations that suggest torsion has already occurred will also be surgically treated.[3] An ovarian mass on a pedicle can present in a high abdominal location, or in varying locations on follow-up examinations, thus obscuring its site of origin (Fig. 21-35).[2]

Hydrometrocolpos is the cystic dilation of the vagina and uterus resulting from the accumulation of fluid and mucus proximal to a point of obstruction. Hydrocolpos is the dilation of the vagina because of GI obstruction. Fetal development of these conditions is rare when compared with the incidence at puberty. This midline hypoechoic mass posterior to the bladder may occasionally compress the lower ureters, leading to hydronephrosis.[6] When the obstruction is caused by vaginal atresia or a vaginal membrane, there may be associated GU tract abnormalities.[2]

Associated findings with both of these conditions may make it difficult to separate the two entities. Polyhydramnios could be evident with ovarian cysts possibly due to obstruction of the small bowel. In the case of cystic rupture or retrograde uterine secretions due to hydrocolpos, ascites images in the abdomen.[6] Hydrocolpos is more likely to result in hydronephrosis; however, a large ovarian cyst may also have the same result.[6]

SUMMARY

- CCAM is the most frequently found mass within the fetal chest.

- To differentiate pulmonary sequestration from CCAM, use color Doppler to trace the origin of feeder vessels.

- Pulmonary hypoplasia is usually a secondary condition related to oligohydramnios found with renal anomalies.

- Fetal hydrops has the same sonographic appearance regardless of whether it is due to an immune or nonimmune condition.

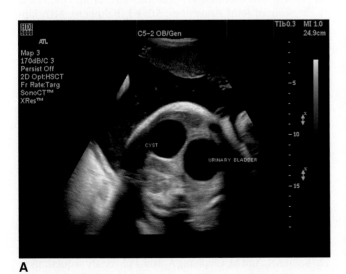

A

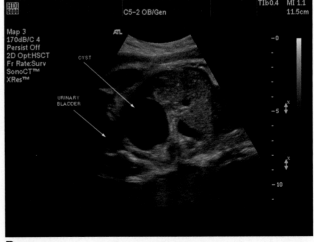

B

Figure 21-35 Unilocular fetal ovarian cyst on a transverse (**A**) and sagittal (**B**) plane. (Image courtesy of Philips Medical Systems, Bothell, WA.)

Critical Thinking Questions

1. During a routine antenatal exam for size and dates, the sonographer notes a soft tissue mass extending from the ventral abdominal wall. List the differentials and defining sonographic features for each.

   ANSWER: Differentials for this finding include an omphalocele, gastroschisis, and bladder exstrophy. The omphalocele has a membranous cover and the gastroschisis does not, which allows for the bowel to float freely in the amniotic fluid. Because of this contact with the fluid, chemical peritonitis may occur, resulting in thickened bowel loops. Bladder exstrophy is not as clear-cut, as it may image as a solid mass, somewhat similar to the omphalocele. A key finding is the insertion of the umbilical cord. Using either color or power Doppler modes, localize the umbilical cord in relation to the abdominal mass. The omphalocele has the cord inserting into the mass and usually into the underlying liver. In the case of the gastroschisis, the cord inserts to one side, usually the right. Finally, with bladder exstrophy, the umbilical cord may insert low; however, it is still superior to the mass.

2. What steps would the sonographer take during an exam when only a single kidney is found in the examined fetus? Discuss other sonographic findings you would expect with unilateral renal agenesis.

   ANSWER: In the event of finding only one kidney, the sonographer would search from the pelvis to the renal fossa for the kidney. In the early stages of development, the kidney forms in the pelvis and ascends into the renal fossa. This rise into the abdomen may cease at any level, resulting in a kidney anywhere along this path. If the kidney failed to form, the adrenal gland moves into the renal fossa in a position parallel to the spine. Other findings may be normal, such as the amniotic fluid levels, as the single kidney produces urine, helping to maintain the fluid levels. If the fetus has bilateral renal agenesis or a form of urinary output obstruction, we find oligohydramnios, head and chest compression, and possible limb clubbing.

- The spleen enlarges with immune fetal hydrops and infections.

- An omphalocele has a covering, whereas the gastroschisis demonstrated free-floating bowel within the amniotic fluid.

- The umbilical cord inserts into the omphalocele and to the side, usually the right, of the gastroschisis.

- Bladder exstrophy may demonstrate a mass similar to the omphalocele; however, this mass is inferior to the umbilical cord.

- Polyhydramnios is common with GI malformations.

- Oligohydramnios is common with renal malformations.

- Midgut volvulus is the twisting of bowel around the blood supply.

- The characteristic finding of duodenal atresias on both the radiograph and prenatal sonogram is called the double-bubble sign.

- The meconium ileus presents as a dilated, echogenic mass or structure on sonographic examination.

- Potter sequence includes renal agenesis, ADPKD and ARPKD, and acquired obstructive and multicystic kidney disease.

- Fetal hydronephrosis is a nonspecific finding of obstruction somewhere within the urinary system.

- In the event of renal agenesis, the adrenal gland moves into the renal fossa.

- Hydroceles are a common finding in the male fetus.

- Large ovarian cysts are hard to differentiate from hydrocolpos in the fetus.

REFERENCES

1. Hagan-Ansert S. *Textbook of Diagnostic Ultrasonography*. 7th ed. St. Louis, MO: Mosby Elsevier; 2011.
2. Callen P. *Ultrasonography in Obstetrics and Gynecology*. 5th ed. Philadelphia: Saunders Elsevier; 2007.
3. Bernasconi A, Yoo SJ, Golding F, et al. Etiology and outcome of prenatally detected paracardial cystic lesions: a case series and review of the literature. *Ultrasound Obstet Gynecol*. 2007;29(4):388–394.
4. Chen WS, Yeh GP, Tsai HD, et al. Prenatal diagnosis of congenital cystic adenomatoid malformations: evolution and outcome. *Taiwan J Obstet Gynecol*. 2009;48(3):278–281.
5. Hung JH, Shen SH, Guo WY, et al. Prenatal diagnosis of an extralobar pulmonary sequestration. *J Chin Med Assoc*. 2008;71(1):53–57.
6. Nyberg DA, McGahn JP, Pretorius DH, et al. *Diagnostic Imaging of Fetal Anomalies*. 5th ed. Baltimore, MD: Lippincott Williams & Wilkins; 2002.
7. Clifton MS, Goldstein RB, Slavotinek A, et al. Prenatal diagnosis of familial type I choledochal cyst. *Pediatrics*. 2006;117(3):e596–e600.
8. Brown SD, Estroff JA, Barnewoldt CE. Fetal MRI: prenatal MRI of the fetal body. *Applied Radiology*. 2004;33(2). http://www.medscape.com/viewarticle/470837_5. Accessed February 2011.
9. Kumar AN. Perinatal management of common neonatal thoracic lesions. *Indian J Pediatr*. 2008;75(9):931–937.
10. Cesko I, Hajdú J, Marton T, et al. Polysplenia and situs inversus in siblings. Case reports. *Fetal Diagn Ther*. 2001;16(1):1–3.
11. Dhingsa R, Coakley FV, Albanese CT, et al. Prenatal sonography and MRI imaging of pulmonary sequestreation. *AJR*. 2003;180:433–437.
12. Kahn AN, Aird M, Chiphang A, et al. Pulmonary sequestration imaging. eMedicine Web site. http://emedicine.medscape.com/article/412554-overview. Accessed February 2010.

13. Daltro P, Fricke BL, Kline-Fath BM, et al. Prenatal MRI of congenital abdominal and chest wall defects. *AJR.* 2005;185(3):1010–1016.

14. Reid JR. Midgut volvulus imaging: imaging. emedicine Web site. http://emedicine.medscape.com/article/411249-imaging. Accessed February 2011.

15. MacGillivray T, Harrison M, Goldstein R, et al. Disappearing fetal lung lesions. *J Pediatr Surg.* 1993;28(10):1321–1324.

16. Bowerman R. Sonography of fetal midgut herniation: normal size criteria and correlation with crown rump length. *J Ultrasound Med.* 1993;12:251–254.

17. Comstock C. Fetal masses: ultrasound diagnosis and evaluation. *Ultrasound Q.* 1988;6:229–256.

18. Colvin J, Bower C, Dickinson JE, et al. Outcomes of congenital diaphragmatic hernia: a population-based study in Western Australia. *Pediatrics.* 2005;116(3):e356–e363.

19. Baynam G, Kiraly-Borri C, Goldblatt J, et al. A recurrence of a hydrop lethal skeletal dysplasia showing similarity to Desbuquois dysplasia and a proposed new sign: the Upsilon sign. *Am J Med Genet A.* 2010;152A(4):966–969.

20. Benacerraf B, Brass V, Laboda L, et al. A sonographic sign for detection of Down syndrome. *Am J Obstet Gynecol.* 1985;151(8):1078–1079.

21. Gray D, Crane JP. Optimal nuchal skin-fold threshold based on gestational age for prenatal detection of Down syndrome. *Am J Obstet Gynecol.* 1994;171(5):1282–1286.

22. Nazir SA, Raza SA, Nazir S, et al. Challenges in the prenatal and post-natal diagnosis of mediastinal cystic hygroma: a case report. *J Med Case Reports.* 2008;2:256.

23. Chan KL, Tang MH, Tse HY, et al. Factors affecting outcomes of prenatally-diagnosed tumours. *Prenat Diagn.* 2002;22(5):437–443.

24. Senoh D, Hanaoka U, Tanaka Y, et al. Antenatal ultrasonographic features of fetal giant hemangiolymphangioma. *Ultrasound Obstet Gynecol.* 2001;17(3):252–254.

25. Perkins JA, Manning SC, Tempero RM, et al. Lymphatic malformations: review of current treatment. *Otolaryngol Head Neck Surg.* 2010;142(6):795.e1–803.e1.

26. Kiyota A, Tsukimori K, Yumoto Y, et al. Spontaneous resolution of cystic hygroma and hydrops in a fetus with Noonan's syndrome. *Fetal Diagn Ther.* 2008;24(4):499–502.

27. Comstock C. Fetal masses: ultrasound diagnosis and evaluation. *Ultrasound Q.* 1988;6:229–256.

28. Brar M, Cubberley D, Baty B, et al. Chest wall hamartoma in a fetus. *J Ultrasound Med.* 1988;7(4):217–220.

29. Fetal thorax normal measurements. wikiRadiography Web site. http://www.wikiradiography.com/page/Fetal+Thorax+Normal+Measurements. Accessed February 2011.

30. Lee KA, Cho JY, Lee SM, et al. Prenatal diagnosis of bilateral pulmonary agenesis: a case report. *Korean J Radiol.* 2010;11(1):119–122.

31. Comstock CH, Lee W, Bronsteen RA, et al. Fetal mediastinal lymphangiomas. *J Ultrasound Med.* 2008;27(1):145–148.

32. Takayasu H, Kitano Y, Kuroda T, et al. Successful management of a large fetal mediastinal teratoma complicated by hydrops fetalis. *J Pediatr Surg.* 2010;45(12):e21–e24.

33. Kim MJ, Cho JY. Prenatal ultrasonographic diagnosis of congenital diaphragmatic hernia at 11 weeks gestation. *JDMS.* 2000;17:286.

34. Bennett BH. Congenital diaphragmatic hernia. *JDMS.* 1991;7:81–84.

35. Sabbagha R, (Ed.). *Diagnostic Ultrasound Applied to Obstetrics and Gynecology.* 3rd ed. Philadelphia, PA: JB Lippincott; 1994.

36. Moore K, Persaud TVN. *The Developing Human: Clinically Oriented Embryology.* 7th ed. Philadelphia, PA: Saunders; 2002.

37. Springer SC, Glasser JG, Adamson WT, et al. Bowel obstruction in the newborn. http://emedicine.medscape.com/article/980360-overview. Accessed February 2011.

38. Genetics Home Reference. http://ghr.nlm.nih.gov/. Accessed February 2011.

39. Bejiqi RA, Retkoceri R, Bejiqi H. Echocardiographic measurements of normal fetal pulmonary artery and pulmonary branches and comparison on fetuses with congenital diaphragmatic hernia. *Med Arh.* 2010;64(6):365–367.

40. Foley PT, Sithasanan N, McEwing R, et al. Enteric duplications presenting as antenatally detected abdominal cysts: is delayed resection appropriate? *Journal of Pediatric Surgery.* 2003;38(12):1810–1813.

41. Butler N, Claireaux A. Congenital diaphragmatic hernia as a cause of perinatal mortality. *Lancet.* 1962;1(7231):659–663.

42. Norio R, Kaarininen H, Rapola J, et al. Familial congenital diaphragmatic defects: aspects of etiology, prenatal diagnosis and treatment. *Am J Med Genet.* 1984;17(2):471–483.

43. Mandell G. Imaging in duodenal atresia. http://emedicine.medscape.com/article/408582-overview. Accessed February 2011.

44. Kirk E, Wah R. Obstetric management of the fetus with omphalocele or gastroschisis: a review and report of one hundred and twelve cases. *Am J Obstet Gynecol.* 1983;146(5):512–518.

45. Lenke R, Hatch E Jr. Fetal gastroschisis: a preliminary report advocating the use of cesarean section. *Obstet Gynecol.* 1986;67(3):395–398.

46. Hashimoto B, Filly R, Callen P. Sonographic detection of fetal intraperitoneal fluid. *J Ultrasound Med.* 1986;5(4):203–204.

47. Mahony B, Callen P, Filly R. Fetal urethral obstruction: US evaluation. *Radiology.* 1985;157(1):221–224.

48. Brar M, Cubberley D, Baty B, et al. Chest wall hamartoma in a fetus. *J Ultrasound Med.* 1988;7(4):217–220.

49. Anderson NG, Notley E, Graham P, et al. Reproducibility of sonographic assessment of fetal liver length in diabetic pregnancies. *Ultrasound Obstet Gynecol.* 2008;31(5):529–534.

50. Chung W. Antenatal detection of hepatic cyst. *J Clin Ultrasound.* 1986;14:217–219.

51. Simchen MJ, Toi A, Bona M, et al. Fetal hepatic calcifications: prenatal diagnosis and outcome. *Am J Obstet Gynecol.* 2002;187(6):1617–1622.

52. Meirowitz NB, Guzman ER, Underberg-Davis SJ, et al. Hepatic hemangioendothelioma: prenatal sonographic findings and evolution of the lesion. *J Clin Ultrasound.* 2000;28(5):258–263.

53. Demir HA, Varan A, Akçören Z, et al. Focal nodular hyperplasia of the liver and elevated alpha fetoprotein level in an infant with isolated hemihyperplasia. *J Pediatr Hematol Oncol.* 2008;30(10):775–777.

54. Petrikovsky B, Cohen HL, Scimeca P, et al. Prenatal diagnosis of focal nodular hyperplasia of the liver. *Prenat Diagn.* 1994;14:406–409.

55. Tam PY, Angelides A. Perinatal detection of gallstones in siblings. *Am J Perinatol*. 2010;27(10):771–774.

56. Zalel Y, Perlitz Y, Gamzu R, et al. In-utero development of the fetal colon and rectum: sonographic evaluation. *Ultrasound Obstet Gynecol*. 2003;21(2):161–164.

57. Sumfest JM, Kolon TF, Rukstalis DB. Cryptorchidism. emedicine. http://emedicine.medscape.com/article/438378-overview. Accessed February 2011.

58. Boe NM, Rhee-Morris L, Towner D, et al. Prenatal diagnosis of omphalocele and left atrial isomerism (polysplenia) including complex congenital heart disease with ventricular noncompaction cardiomyopathy. *J Ultrasound Med*. 2008;27(7):1117–1121.

59. McKelvey A, Stanwell J, Smeulders N, et al. Persistent non-visualisation of the fetal stomach: diagnostic and prognostic implications. *Arch Dis Child Fetal Neonatal Ed*. 2010;95(6):F439–F442.

60. Bidwell J, Nelson A. Prenatal ultrasonic diagnosis of congenital duplication of the stomach. *J Ultrasound Med*. 1986;5(10):589–591.

61. Puligandla PS, Nguyen LT, St-Vil D, et al. Gastrointestinal duplications. *J Pediatr Surg*. 2003;38(5):740–744.

62. Karnak I, Ocal T, Senocak ME, et al. Alimentary tract duplications in children: report of 26 years' experience. *Turk J Pediatr*. 2000;42(2):118–125.

63. Bhat NA, Agarwala S, Mitra DK, et al. Duplications of the alimentary tract in children. *Trop Gastroenterol*. 2001;22(1):33–35.

64. Teklali Y, Kaddouri N, Barahioui M. Gastrointestinal system duplications in children (19 cases). *Arch Pediatr*. 2002;9(9):903–906.

65. McNamara A, Levine D. Intraabdominal fetal echogenic masses: a practical guide to diagnosis and management. *Radiographics*. 2005;25:633–645.

66. Brown D, Polger M, Clark P, et al. Very echogenic amniotic fluid: ultrasonography—amniocentesis correlation. *J Ultrasound Med*. 1994;13(2):95–97.

67. Johnson JA, Bush A, Buchdahl R. Does presenting with meconium ileus affect the prognosis of children with cystic fibrosis? *Pediatr Pulmonol*. 2010;45(10):951–958.

68. Doubilet PM, Benson CB. *Atas of Ultrasound in Obstetrics and Gynecology: A Multimedia Reference*. Baltimore, MD: Lippincott Williams & Wilkins; 2003.

69. Baun J. Fetal genitourinary system: anatomy and anomalies. www.jimbaun.com. Accessed February 2011.

70. Bowman E, Fraser S. Fetal hydronephrosis neonatal handbook. http://www.rch.org.au/nets/handbook/index.cfm?doc_id=626. Accessed February 2011.

71. Mandell G. Congenital cystic adenomatioid malformation. eMedicine. http://emedicine.medscape.com/article/407407-overview. Accessed Feruary 2011.

72. Rose A. Ultrasound Evaluation of the Fetal Genitourinary system. ;http://www.scribd.com/doc/2032598/Ultrasound Evaluation of the Fetal Genitourinary System. Accessed February 2011.

73. Hekmatnia A, McHugh K, Hiorns MP. Meconium ileus: imaging. emedicine Web site. http://emedicine.medscape.com/article/410845-imaging. Accessed February 2011.

74. Oliveria MCLA, Reis FJC, Monteiro APAF, et al. Effect of meconium ileus on the clinical prognosis of patients with cystic fibrosis. *Braz J Med Biol Res*. 2002;35(1):31–38.

75. Keays MA, Guerra LA, Mihill J, et al. Reliability assessment of Society for Fetal Urology ultrasound grading system for hydronephrosis. *J Urol*. 2008;180(4 suppl):1680–1682.

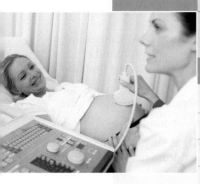

22 Fetal Echocardiography

Marium Holland and Joan M. Mastrobattista

OBJECTIVES

Summarize the embryonic development of the heart

Explain the differences in fetal and neonatal circulation

Describe the sonographic techniques for the basic fetal echocardiographic examination

List the five views used in the systematic examination of the fetal heart

Describe uses of a three-dimensional (3D) data set in imaging the fetal heart

Determine the presence of an arrhythmia from an M-mode tracing

Associate sonographic findings with cardiac abnormalities

KEY TERMS

four-chamber heart | left ventricular outflow tract (LVOT) | right ventricular outflow tract (RVOT) | three-vessel view | ductal arch | aortic arch | arrhythmia | ventricular septal defect (VSD) | atrial septal defect (ASD) | atrioventricular septal defects (AVSD) | hypoplastic left heart syndrome (HPLHS) | right ventricular hypoplasia | tricuspid atresia | coarctation of the aorta | tetralogy of Fallot | Ebstein's anomaly | transposition of the great arteries | truncus arteriosus | double outlet right ventricle (DORV) | rhabdomyoma

GLOSSARY

Akinetic Without motion

Arrhythmia Abnormal heart rate

Atrial septal defect (ASD) Abnormal opening between the right and left atrium

Atrioventricular septal defects (AVSD, aka endocardial cushion defect) Partial: ASD in the lower portion of the atrial septal defect without a ventricular defect; complete: a heart with both an ASD and VSD and a common valve

Atrioventricular valves (AV) Valves located between the atrium and ventricles

Bradyarrhythmia Slow heart rate

Coarctation of the aorta Narrowing of the aorta

Dextrocardia Apex of the heart points to the right

Double-outlet right ventricle (DORV) Both great arteries arise from the right ventricle with a VSD and pulmonary stenosis; the same process can occur with the left ventricle with associated AV and semilunar valve stenosis

Ductus venosus Connection between the umbilical vein and the inferior vena cava

Dyskinetic Impaired movement

Ebstein's anomaly Displacement of the tricuspid valve toward the apex of the heart resulting in tricuspid stenosis and/or regurgitation, atrialization of the right ventricle

Endocardial cushion Subset of cells found in the developing heart tube that will give rise to the heart's valves and septa critical to the proper formation of a four-chambered heart

Foramen ovale Opening between the atrium allowing for blood flow from the right to left during fetal life

Heart/thorax ratio (CTR) Calculation of the heart to chest size resulting in a ratio

Hypoplastic left heart syndrome (HPLHS) Underdevelopment of the left ventricle and aorta, stenosis or atresia of the aortic and/or mitral valves

Hydrops, nonimmune Accumulation of fluid in the chest and abdomen due to heart failure

Papillary muscles Muscular projections into the ventricles that anchor the cordae tendinae of the AV valves

Premature atrial contractions (PACs) Irregular extra contraction of the atria out of sync with the ventricles

Rhabdomyoma Common benign tumor found in either ventricle

Right ventricular hypoplasia (aka hypoplastic right heart) Underdevelopment of the right ventricle and hypoplasia of the tricuspid valve

Septum primum First section of the interatrial septum to form in the embryo

Supraventricular tachycardia (SVT) Fast irregular heartbeat that is not ventricular in origin; may originate from the atria, AV node, sinoatrial node, or as a result of a congenital syndrome such as Wolff-Parkinson-White syndrome

Tetralogy of Fallot Cyanotic heart malformation with a VSD, pulmonary stenosis, overriding aorta, right ventricular hypertrophy, pulmonary obstruction due to valvular stenosis

Transposition of the great arteries (TGA) Congenital heart malformation where the aorta arises from the right ventricle and the pulmonary artery arises from the left ventricle

Tricuspid atresia Congenital absence of the tricuspid valve

Truncus arteriosus Single artery spanning the ventricles

Ventricular septal defect (VSD) A single or multiple defect allowing oxygenated blood from the left ventricle to pass into the right ventricle

Improvement in sonographic technology has resulted in the evolution of a specialty focusing on the prenatal diagnosis of congenital heart disease. Fetal cardiac ultrasonography has evolved beyond obtaining only anatomic information in diagnosing congenital heart disease. Today, static images as well as cine loops, Doppler and 3D imaging enhance diagnostic capabilities in the fetal heart. This chapter contains information needed to perform a basic screening sonographic examination of the fetal heart.

EMBRYOLOGY

The cardiovascular system, which includes the heart, blood vessels, and blood cells, originates from the mesodermal germ layer. This system is one of the first to appear and function, with blood starting to circulate within the embryo by 3 weeks postconception (5 weeks gestational age), and cardiac motion can be observed with high-resolution imaging.[1]

The heart begins as a set of paired tubular structures known as the cardiogenic cords. These structures begin to fuse on the 22nd day of development to form the single heart tube. This slightly bent structure consists of an endocardial tube and myoepicardial mantle.[2] The cephalic portion of the tube then bends right and ventrally, while the caudal portion bends leftward, in a dorsocranial manner. This results in the formation of the atrioventricular loop. As the loop develops, a single common atrium is formed, descending into the pericardium along with the bilateral segments of the sinus venosus. The atrioventricular canal then forms, connecting the early atrium to the early ventricles (Fig. 22-1).[3]

At approximately 27 days, the endocardial cushions begin to develop, separating the atria and ventricles. By day 33 postconception, the mitral and tricuspid valves

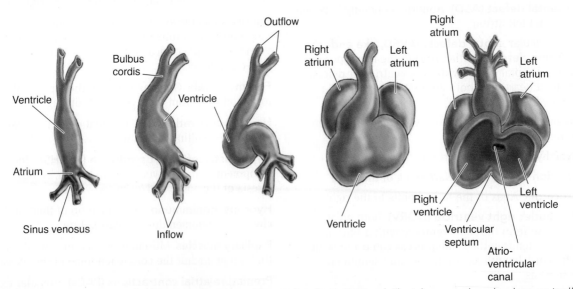

Figure 22-1 During its early stages, the heart is a tube with an input end and an output end. The tube expands and curls up on itself to stay contained in the mediastinum. Expansion of the heart tube takes the form of a small atrium and a large ventricle, with a constricted area between them. These early chambers play the obvious role of receiving blood (atrium), then pumping it vigorously onward through a contraction of the expanded ventricular muscle. Because we are air-breathing creatures, the heart tube soon divides itself into parallel right and left chambers to divert the incoming blood to the lungs before receiving it back again and pumping it through the aorta. (Adapted from Snell RS. *Clinical Anatomy.* 7th ed. Baltimore: Lippincott Williams & Wilkins; 2003.)

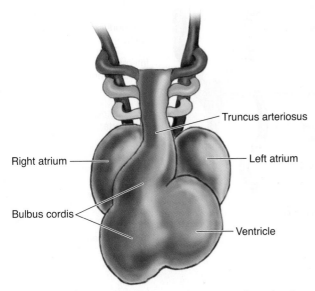

Figure 22-2 Fetal heart during the sixth and seventh weeks of gestation, demonstrating bulbus cordis, truncus arteriosus, ventricle, atria, and multiple aortic arches.

are formed, resulting from the ingrowths of the cushions. Concurrently, the ventricular septum begins to form as the primitive ventricles begin to dilate, causing the fusion of their medial walls. This process starts at the apex of the heart, with the muscular portion of the septum forming first, followed by the membranous portion. The septum primum also forms between the 25th and 28th day postconception, causing an initial division between the right and left portions of the atrium. Finally, the septum secundum is formed, though the foramen ovale remains to allow the right to left shunting until birth (Fig. 22-2).[3]

The great vessels (aorta and pulmonary arteries) arise from the common vessel of the truncus arteriosus. During the seventh week, the swellings in the truncus arteriousus form and twist around each other to form the aorticopulmonary septum. It is at this point that the vessels are divided into a pulmonary channel, contiguous with the right ventricle, and a systemic (aortic) channel, contiguous with the left ventricle. The pulmonic and aortic valves form at this time, as well (Fig. 22-3).[2,3]

The aortic and pulmonary arches themselves arise from a series of primitive aortic arches, which occur between 19 and 30 days postconception. The first two sets of aortic arches form and disappear without continuing as permanent structures. The third pair of aortic arches become the internal carotid arteries, and the fourth pair develop into the definitive aorta (left) and right subclavian artery. The fifth pair are vestigial and do not fully develop. The sixth and last pair of arches become the right and left pulmonary arteries (Fig. 22-4).[2,3]

CIRCULATION

By the beginning of the eighth week of gestation, the embryonic heart has completed its formation, and placental circulation has begun. Oxygenated blood enters the fetus's circulation from the placenta through the umbilical vein and travels to the hepatic circulation and the left portal vein. The majority of the blood from the umbilical vein is shunted into the ductus venosus, which bypasses the hepatic circulation and enters the inferior vena cava (IVC). The remainder of the blood flows through the hepatic circulation prior to entering the IVC through the hepatic veins.[1]

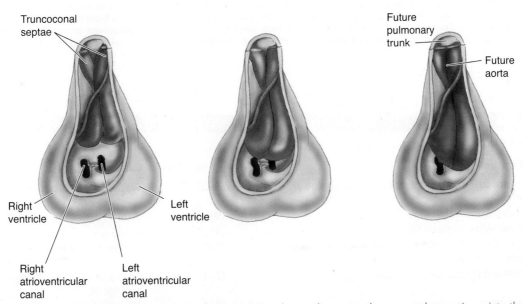

Figure 22-3 The outflow path from the heart also septates. Unlike the other cardiac septa, the septum that continues into the outflow tube spirals, which explains why the adult aorta appears to arise behind the pulmonary trunk but then arch forward, over it, and then behind it again. (From Sadler T. *Langman's Medical Embryology*. 9th ed. Image Bank. Baltimore: Lippincott Williams & Wilkins; 2003.)

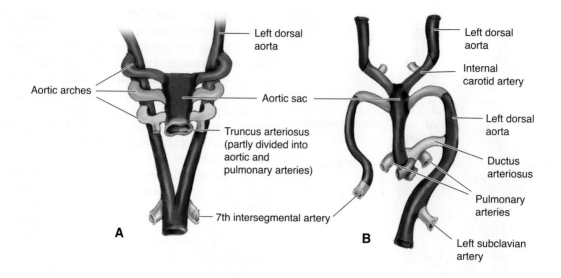

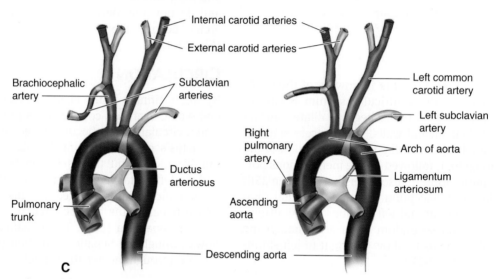

Figure 22-4 **A:** Aortic arches and dorsal aorta before transformation into the definitive vascular pattern. **B:** Aortic arches and dorsal aorta after the transformation. Broken lines, obliterated components. Note the patent ductus arteriosus and position of the seventh intersegmental artery on the left. **C:** The great arteries in the adult. Compare the distance between the place of origin of the left common carotid artery and the left subclavian in B and C. After disappearance of the distal part of the sixth aortic arch (the fifth arches never form completely), the right recurrent laryngeal nerve hooks around the right subclavian artery. On the left the nerve remains in place and hooks around the ligamentum arteriosum.

PATHOLOGY BOX 22-1

Embryology of the Heart[2,3,4,92]

Structure/Function	Development Day	Carnegie Stage
Cardiogenic cord fusion, contractions begin, heart has an "S" shape	19–23	Form in stage 9 and fuse in stage 10
Aortic and pulmonary arches	19–30	9–13
Endocardial cushions, septum primum	25–27	12–13
Mitral and tricuspid valves, right and left ventricles, conus cords, trucus ariousus	31–35	14; but may start as early as stage 12
Aortic and pulmonary channel separation	37–42	Begins at stage 16, completing in stage 18
Four-chamber heart	42–44	17
Majority of heart development ends	54–56	22

From the IVC, the blood enters the right atrium, where oxygenated blood is directed by the eustachian valve through the foramen ovale into the left atrium. The remainder, along with blood returning from the superior vena cava, passes through the tricuspid valve and enters the right ventricle. From the right ventricle, it passes through the semilunar pulmonic valve and into the pulmonary artery. As the fetus receives oxygenated blood from the maternal circulation, the majority of the blood that enters the pulmonary artery is diverted through the ductus arteriosus into the aorta and systemic circulation. The portion that continues through the pulmonary circulation is deposited into the left atrium by one of the four pulmonary veins.[1]

Blood in the left atrium, both that returning from the pulmonary circulation and that shunted through the foramen ovale, then travels through the mitral valve into the left ventricle. The contractions of the left ventricle then propel the blood through the aortic valve into the aorta. The more highly oxygenated portion of blood is shunted mainly to the cranial portion of the fetus via the brachiocephalic (subclavian and carotid) arteries arising from the proximal portion of the aortic arch. The remainder perfuses the distal portion of the fetus through the abdominal aorta and then returns to the placental circulation through the umbilical arteries (Fig. 22-5).[1]

SONOGRAPHIC TECHNIQUES AND BASIC ANATOMY

TIMING

Current suggestions are that the fetal cardiac exam be performed between 18 and 22 weeks of gestation.[1] However, the heart is still quite small at these gestational ages, and factors such as patient body habitus and fetal position may make it difficult to achieve a thorough exam. As the gestation progresses, there is increased attenuation due to the increasingly calcified fetal skull, ribs, spine, and limbs, which makes the examination increasingly difficult, despite the larger anatomy.[5] Examinations prior to 18 weeks, even if incomplete, may be of use in patients at extremely high risk of congenital heart disease to assess for major structural disease. However, several types of cardiac disease may not be recognized until later in gestation, and follow-up examinations should recommended.[6]

EQUIPMENT

Fetal echocardiography requires high- resolution equipment, with transducer frequencies ranging from 5 to 7 megahertz (MHz). The optimal frequency depends on factors such as gestational age and maternal body habitus. M-mode and Doppler (pulsed and color) and, increasingly, 3D capabilities should be available, as these

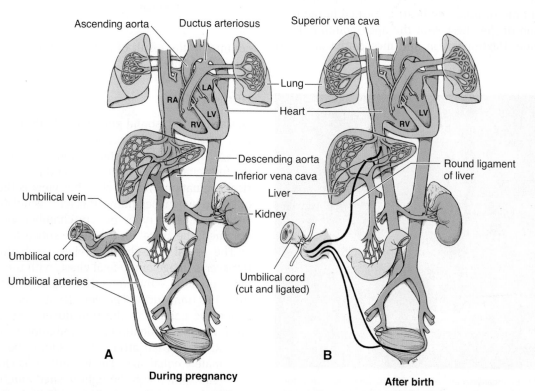

A **During pregnancy**   **B** **After birth**

Figure 22-5 Fetal circulation: **A:** during pregnancy, oxygen diffuses from the maternal circulation to the fetal circulation in the placenta; oxygenated blood (red) returns to fetus through umbilical vein; **(B)** after birth, umbilical cord is cut and blood is oxygenated as it passes through the lungs. *RA*, right atrium; *LA*, left atrium; *LV*, left ventricle; *RV*, right ventricle.

techniques allow for physiologic assessment of potential problems such as arrhythmias (M-mode) or septal defects and other anatomic malformations (Doppler).[5,8]

BASIC SONOGRAPHIC EVALUATION

The initial step in any examination should be the establishment of fetal presentation (breech, cephalic, transverse) and correct identification of the right and left sides of the fetus. Once fetal position is determined, the location and orientation of the heart can be evaluated.[5] In a cross-sectional view of the fetal chest, the heart should occupy the majority of the left side of the fetal chest with the apex pointing to the left. The normal angle of the heart should be 45 degrees to the left of midline, plus or minus 20 degrees. This orientation, called levocardia, should result in the left atrium located closest to the fetal spine, and the right ventricular wall closest to the anterior chest wall (Fig. 22-6).[1,9] While it is tempting to determine that the heart is on the "left" side of the fetal chest by examining other structures that should be on the left or right sides of the fetus (such as the stomach and the liver), this can lead to missed diagnoses as disorders of situs.

Levocardia is the normal position of the fetal heart. There are three abnormal positions of the fetal heart: dextrocardia, dextroposition, and mesocardia. Dextrocardia occurs when the heart is located in the right side of the chest with the apex also pointing to the right. Dextroposition refers to the heart being located in the right side of the chest but with the apex pointing to the left. In mesocardia, the heart is located in the middle portion of the chest with the apex pointing along the midline. Dextroposition and mesocardia are most

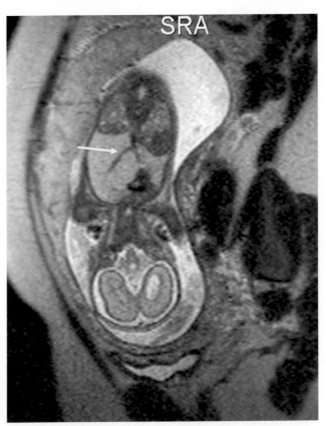

Figure 22-7 Coronal section of a fetal MRI of a 24-week fetus with a large left lung mass (bronchopulmonary sequestration). The left diaphragm is flattened and there is moderate dextroposition of the heart. A large vessel is seen coming from the low thoracic aorta *(arrow)*. The congenital cystic adenomatoid malformation volume ratio (CVR) was 1.96; however, hydrops did not develop and the baby "grew around" the mass.

commonly the result of a mass lesion in the left chest (Figs. 22-7 and 22-8).[9]

HEART VIEWS

Obstetrical ultrasound guidelines, both from the American Institute of Ultrasound in Medicine (AIUM) and American College of Obstetrics and Gynecology, include the four-chamber view as a standard part of any obstetrical evaluation.[5] A four-chamber view is the first view obtained when beginning the fetal echocardiographic evaluation. Two types of four-chamber views can be obtained, the apical view and the subcostal view.

The apical four-chamber view is obtained from a transverse image of the fetal chest, with the apex of the heart pointing either directly toward or directly away from the transducer. The ventricular and apical septa should be parallel to the transducer (Fig. 22-9). This view allows examination and evaluation of the:

* Right and left atria, which should be of approximately equal size. The left atrium is closest to the fetal spine, with the right located anteriorly
* Right and left ventricles, with the right ventricle appearing slightly larger than the left. This discrepancy is more pronounced later in gestational ages.

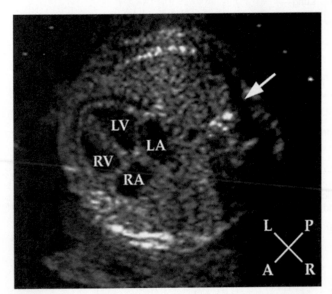

Figure 22-6 Echocardiogram of the normal fetal heart in a four-chamber view demonstrating the position of the heart and the cardiac chambers in a cross-section of the chest. *A*, anterior; *L*, left; *LA*, left atrium; *LV*, left ventricle; *P*, posterior; *R*, right; *RA*, right atrium; *RV*, right ventricle; arrow denotes the spine.

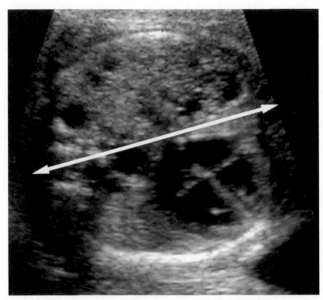

Figure 22-8 The heart is displaced from a more central position by the cystic adenomatoid malformation in the right side of the chest, but the normal 45-degree axis of the heart is preserved. The line from the fetal spine to the sternum normally should pass through the atria.

The right ventricle is located closest to the anterior chest wall, and contains the thick muscular moderator band, which runs from the interventricular septum to the free wall of the right ventricle[10]

- Mitral and tricuspid valves (atrioventricular valves) are located between the atria and the ventricles. The septal tricuspid leaflet inserts more apically than that of the mitral valve, giving the valves a slightly offset appearance
- Interventricular septum and interatrial septum are located between the atria and ventricles respectively. The ventricular septum should appear continuous, without any disruption. However, as the septum is parallel to the transducer beam, dropout may be

seen in the thin, membranous portion of the septum, causing the appearance of a septal defect.[11] If a defect is seen in this view, additional views of the ventricular septum should be obtained. The atrial septum should contain the normal opening of the foramen ovale. The foraminal flap should be visualized opening into the left atrium

- Two superior pulmonary veins should be seen entering into the left atrium.[1,12]

The subcostal four-chamber view is obtained by angling the transducer slightly cephalad from the apical view. As with the apical four-chamber view, the size and position of the atria and ventricles can be evaluated, as can the position of the tricuspid and mitral valves. This view is better for establishing the continuity of the interventricular septum, as the septum is no longer exactly parallel to the transducer, resulting in a thicker appearance to the septum and decreased signal dropout in the membranous portion.[11] Also, the subcostal view is typically used for M-mode views of the ventricles and Doppler interrogation of the AV valves.[1,13]

The outflow tracts are next evaluated. Long-axis views of the aorta can be obtained by angling the transducer toward the fetal right shoulder from the four-chamber view. This view should enable the examiner to confirm the continuity of the anterior wall of the aorta with the interventricular septum and the posterior wall of the aorta with the anterior leaflet of the mitral valve. If a ventricular septal defect is present, it should appear as a break in the continuity of the interventricular septum. The long-axis view of the pulmonary artery, or right ventricular outflow tract (RVOT), can be seen by angling the transducer further toward the fetal right shoulder while in the left ventricular outflow view (LVOT) (Fig. 22-10). Normally, the pulmonary artery courses cephalad, left and posterior from the right ventricle. Changing the transducer angulation

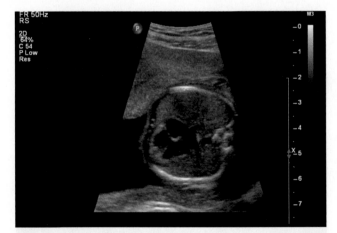

Figure 22-9 A sector image of the apical four-chamber view bisects the heart on a plane extending from the left hip to right shoulder of the fetus. In this image, the fetal head would be toward the sonographer with the feet away. The diagram and sonogram of the four-chamber heart illustrates anatomic position in relation to the fetal spine. (Image courtesy of Philips Medical Systems, Bothell, WA.)

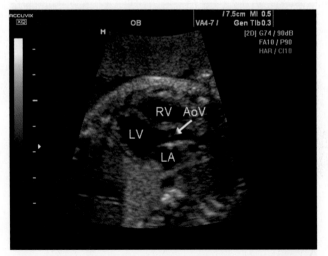

Figure 22-10 Sonogram demonstrating the LVOT of the fetal heart. *LA*, left atrium; *AoV*, aortic valve seen within the aortic root; *LV*, left ventricle; *RV*, right ventricle.

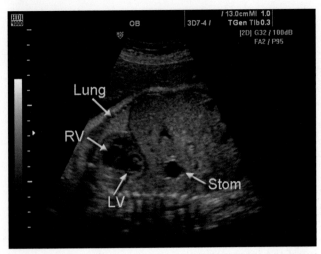

Figure 22-11 This short-axis of the ventricles is taken to the left of midline. The papillary muscles image as circular structures within the left ventricle. The hypoechoic diaphragm separates the chest and abdominal contents. This fetus is in a prone position with the head to the right of the image. *RV,* right ventricle; *LV,* left ventricle; *Stom,* stomach. (Image courtesy of Philips Medical Systems, Bothell, WA.)

Figure 22-12 Sonogram of the short axis view at the base of the heart often called the right ventricular outflow tract. The circular aorta demonstrates the valves and is at right angles to the pulmonary artery, an important relationship in this view. The tricuspid valve images between the RV and RA. *PA,* pulmonary artery; *RV,* right ventricle; *RA,* right atrium. (Image courtesy of Philips Medical Systems, Bothell, WA.)

and switching back and forth between the right and left long-axis outflow tract, views should show the aorta crossing anteriorly to the pulmonary artery. This confirms the normal orientation of the great vessels.

Continuing from the long-axis view of the pulmonary artery, further movement of the transducer to the right produces a sagittal view of the fetal chest and gives a short-axis view of the ventricles (Fig. 22-11). The moderator band should differentiate the right and left ventricles. This view can be used to measure the ventricular thickness and chamber size. Scanning up and down in this view along the interventricular septum may aid in the identification of ventricular septal defects.

In the short axis ventricular view, the transducer can be angled slightly toward the fetal left shoulder to give

the short-axis view of the great vessels (Fig. 22-12). Here, the aorta appears as a central circular structure encircled by the surrounding pulmonary artery. The aortic, pulmonary, and tricuspid valves are well visualized in this view, and the size of the aorta and pulmonary artery can be directly compared. The main pulmonary artery can be seen dividing into the right pulmonary artery and the ductus arteriosus as well.

Next, the aortic arch can be visualized by angling the transducer from the left shoulder to the right hemithorax while in a longitudinal view of the fetus (Fig. 22-13). Distinction between the aortic arch and the more caudal ductal arch is possible by identification of the head and neck vessels (brachiocephalic, left common carotid, and left subclavian artery), which arise from the superior

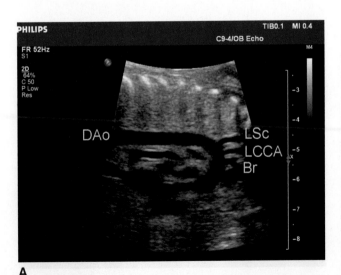

A

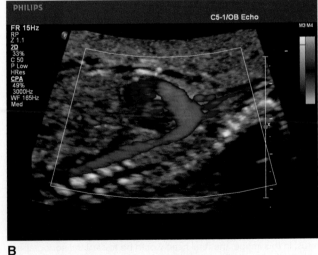

B

Figure 22-13 A: This fetus is in a prone position. Note the fetal aortic arch with the brachiocephalic or innominate (*Br*), left common carotid (*LCCA*), and left subclavian artery (*LSc*). *DAo,* descending aorta. **B:** Color Doppler image of the aortic arch with branches. This fetus is in a face up, prone position which allows for optimal imaging of heart structures. (Images courtesy of Philips Medical Systems, Bothell, WA.)

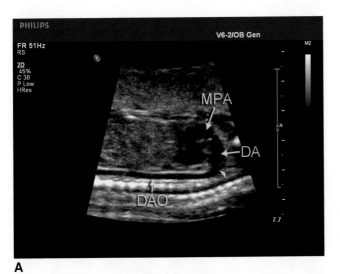

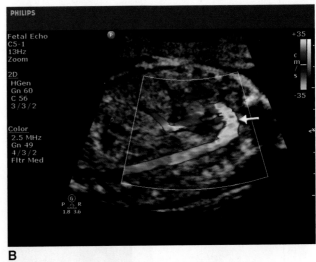

A   **B**

Figure 22-14 A: Sonogram of the ductal arch demonstrating the ductus arteriosus entering the descending aorta. The arrowhead indicates the ductus arteriosus insertion in the descending aorta. *MPA*, main pulmonary artery; *DA*, ductus arteriosus; *DAO*, descending arrow. **B:** Color Doppler image highlights the lack of branches from the aorta differentiating the ductal arch from the aortic arch. The aliasing of the color flow *(arrow)* in the DA is the result of normal flow changes due to the curvature of the vessel. (Images courtesy of Philips Medical Systems, Bothell, WA.)

aspect. Color Doppler may aid in the identification of these vessels. The arch is commonly said to have a "candy cane" appearance, in contrast to the more flattened "hockey stick" appearance of the ductal arch.[1,14] The ductal arch is seen by remaining in the longitudinal view, but rotating back to a straighter anterior-posterior view. It consists of the pulmonary artery, ductus arteriosus, and descending aorta (Fig. 22-14).

Finally, the three-vessel view may be useful in evaluating the size and location of the aorta, pulmonary artery, and superior vena cava (Fig. 22-15). To obtain this view, the apical four-chamber view is obtained, and the transducer is moved cephalad. From midline to lateral, the structures should be the superior vena cava, the aorta, and the pulmonary artery. The pulmonary artery appears somewhat elongated compared to the aorta and SVC, as it is being imaged at the level of the ductus arteriosus.[15] As with the short-axis view, direct side-by-side comparison can be made of the relative size of the aorta and pulmonary artery. Also, Doppler

---

PATHOLOGY BOX 22-2

Basic Protocol for 2D Fetal Echo imaging.[1,10,31,32]

	Normal	Abnormal
Upper abdomen with stomach	Check position of the aorta, spine, left sided stomach, IVC, and umbilical vein	Stomach or liver in abnormal position, polysplenia, aorta/IVC on same side, IVC interruption
Four-chamber	Check that the apex points 45 ± 20 degrees toward the stomach (left), heart fills approximately 1/3 of chest cavity, IVS, IAS, equal chamber size, CTR, foramen ovale flap opens into the LA, moderator band in the RV, thoracic aorta to the left of the spine, two atrioventricular valves, pulmonary veins entering the atria, papillary muscles in the LV, systolic function of the chambers	Incorrect heart position or axis, large heart, unequal chamber sizes, ventricular or atrial septal defects, apical displacement of the tricuspid valve, abnormal chamber or vessel connections
LVOT	Check the aorta and LV size, observe aortic valve movement, partial RV, descending aorta posterior to the LA, IVS and AoV continuity, Ao root and LA size approximately equal, aorta arising from the LV	Abnormal ventricular and vessel connections, VSD, aorta or pulmonary trunk overriding the IVS, abnormal size of ventricles or vessels
RVOT	Check aorta and main pulmonary arteries at right angles, three valve cusps in the aorta, pulmonary valve leaflets, PA originating from the RVOT, LA, descending aorta posterior to the LA	Outlet septum VSD, RVOT or aortic valve small/narrowed
3 Vessel	Check that the ductal and transverse aorta course in a "V" configuration, SVC at right angles to the aorta, PA and Ao to the left of the trachea, great vessel size approximately equal, color Doppler confirms same-direction flow	Enlarged vessels, differences in vessel sizes, unexpected vessel alignment, arrangement, or number, right-sided aorta, abnormal pulmonary artery course or origin, absent or small thymus

Basic Protocol for 2D Fetal Echo imaging.[1,10,31,32]

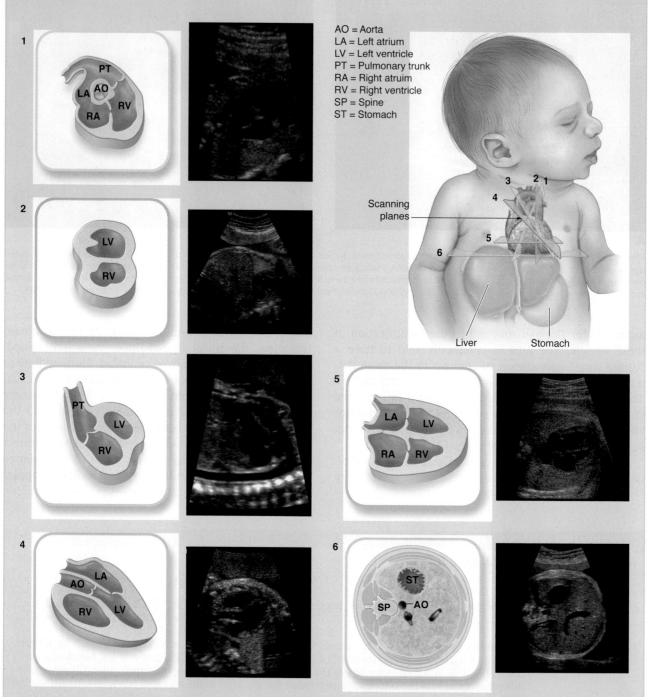

AO = Aorta
LA = Left atrium
LV = Left ventricle
PT = Pulmonary trunk
RA = Right atruim
RV = Right ventricle
SP = Spine
ST = Stomach

Basic views of the fetal heart. 1 - RVOT; 2 - Short axis of the ventricles; 3 - Ductal arch; 4 - LVOT; 5 - Four chamber; 6 - Upper abdomen.

PATHOLOGY BOX 22-3

Intracardiac Doppler Velocities (cm/sec) in the Normal Fetus

Parameter	Aorta	Main Pulmonary Artery	Mitral Valve	Tricuspid Valve
Maximum velocity	70 ± 3	60 ± 4	47 ± 4	51 ± 4
Mean velocity	18 ± 2	16 ± 2	11 ± 1	12 ± 1

(Modified from Reed KL, Meijboom EJ, Sahn DJ, et al. Cardiac Doppler flow velocities in human fetuses. *Circulation.* 1986; 73:41–46.)

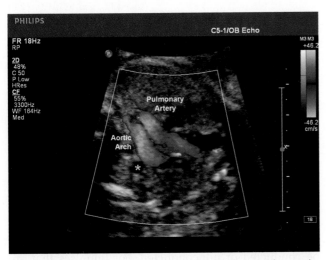

Figure 22-15 The axial color Doppler three-vessel view aids in evaluation of the pulmonary artery and aorta. To the right of the aorta, the superior vena cava (*star*) images as a circular structure. (Images courtesy of Philips Medical Systems, Bothell, WA.)

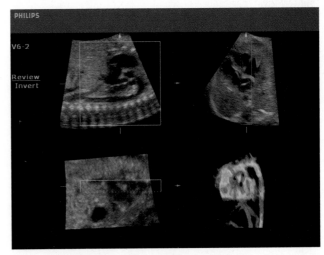

Figure 22-17 Postprocessing of MPR images 1, 2, and 3 removes the gray-scale data and inverts the anechoic chambers and ductal arch to create the IM image in the volume area. (Image courtesy of Philips Medical Systems, Bothell, WA.)

interrogation can be used in this view to confirm the proper directionality of blood flow in each vessel.

3D IMAGING AND THE FETAL HEART

A detailed explanation of the use of 3D and four-dimensional (4D) imaging on the fetal heart is beyond the scope of this chapter; however, a brief overview of available technology follows. One method, spatio-temporal image correlation (STIC), is an automated method of obtaining data. A discussion of STIC and the methods of the 3D data set acquisition and display can be found in Chapter 32.

The 3D data set allows for manipulation of the images displayed. Reconstruction of a sequential parallel display of two-dimensional (2D) images, similar to the CT or MRI display, is called tomographic ultrasound imaging (Fig. 22-16).[1,15] Matrix transducers allow for simultaneous imaging of the fetal heart on two planes (Fig. 32-9b).[18]

Postprocessing of the STIC black-and-white voxels allows for the display of the internal contours of the heart chambers and vessels.[16] Inversion mode (IM) is a process of analyzing tissue echogenicity and fluid areas within the volume. The reverse display of the white tissue and black, or color, results in a rendering of the chambers or flow. This method allows for display of both a volume of the chambers or display of the color flow within the chambers[15] and gives the user the ability to rotate the heart to view all areas (Figs. 22-17 to 22-19).[17]

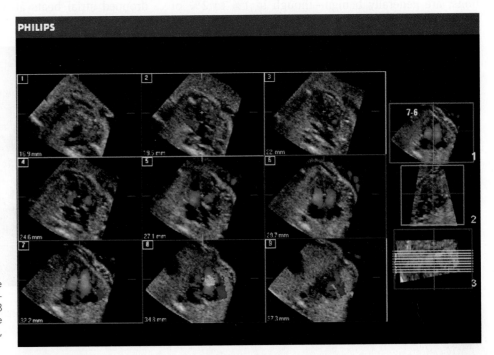

Figure 22-16 An example of the sequential display of a STIC acquisition. The MPR image labeled 3 indicated the slice location. (Image courtesy of Philips Medical Systems, Bothell, WA.)

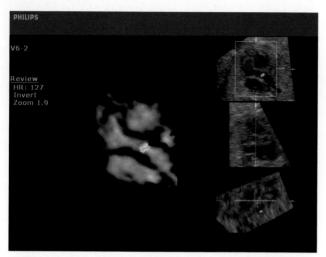

Figure 22-18 Color invert works on the same principle as gray scale; however, the color data helps to create the inverted image of the LVOT. (Image courtesy of Philips Medical Systems, Bothell, WA.)

Other methods of obtaining cardiac measurements include the use of stacked contours or VOCAL to obtain a volume of the fetal chambers (Fig. 22-20).[15,16]

THE ABNORMAL FETAL HEART

ARRHYTHMIAS

Fetal cardiac arrhythmias complicate up to 3% of pregnancies.[19] While the majority of arrhythmias are not clinically significant, sustained tachyarrhythmias or bradyarrhythmias can both have severe clinical consequences. Fetal heart rates greater than 180 beats per minute are referred to as tachyarrhythmias and those less than 100 beats per minute are bradyarrhythmias.[20] It is important to note, however, that the most commonly diagnosed arrhythmia, premature atrial contractions, are generally benign—though in 1% to 2% of

cases they can be associated with an underlying structural defect (Fig. 22-21).[21]

Arrhythmias are best assessed using M-Mode or motion mode imaging. Its high resolution and ability to correlate atrial and ventricular movements temporally allow for precise determination of the mechanics of a particular rhythm. M-mode imaging is performed by placing the cursor through one of the atria and one of the ventricles while in a four-chamber view. Alternatively, the short-axis view may be used, with the cursor placed between the left atrium and the aorta (Fig. 22-22).

Premature Atrial Contractions

Premature atrial contractions (PACs) are easily identified with M-mode (Fig. 22-23). The PAC may either be conducted or nonconducted. For impulses that are not conducted, an isolated deflection of the atrial wall is visualized without subsequent ventricular contraction, as the impulse was blocked by the AV note (image PAC nonconducted). For conducted PACs, a ventricular contraction follows the atrial contraction, but with a subsequent pause in the rhythm as the sinus node resets. Such PACs become clinically important when they occur in such timing as to cause entry into a sustained tachycardia. This appears to occur in approximately 2% to 3% of cases with frequent PACs.[22] Multiple blocked atrial beats with a slow ventricular rate are at higher risk for progression.[21] The presence of complex ectopy (couplets or triplets) also increases the risk.[1]

Tachyarrhythmias

Supraventricular tachycardia (SVT) is diagnosed when the heart rate is between 180 and 300 beats per minute with a 1:1 relationship on M-mode between the atrial and ventricular beats (image SVT). Atrial flutter is defined as an atrial rate between 300 and 400 beats, with dropped atrial beats at a set rate (image flutter). For

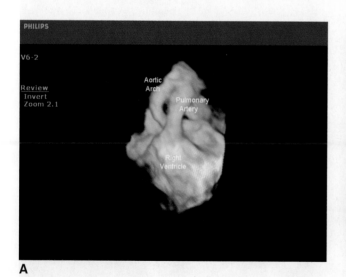

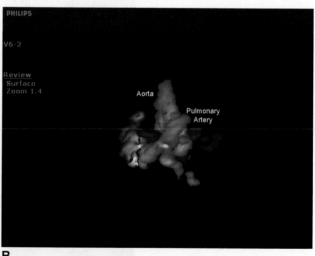

A   **B**

Figure 22-19 A: An IM image of the great vessels demonstrating the criss-cross pattern of normal vessels. **B:** Color invert image of the same anatomy. (Image courtesy of Philips Medical Systems, Bothell, WA.)

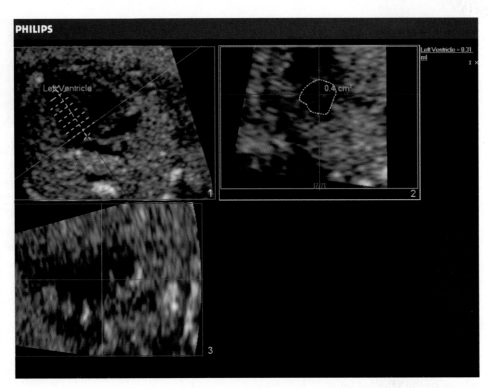

Figure 22-20 Demonstration of the auto stacked contours method of obtaining a left ventricular volume. In frame 1, the left ventricle length begins as a basis for the tracing. Plane 2 provides the cross-sectional measurements of the ventricle, which appear as the dotted lines perpendicular to the long axis on frame 1. (Image courtesy of Philips Medical Systems, Bothell, WA.)

example, in 2:1 flutter, two atrial beats occur for each ventricular rate. Thus, for an atrial rate of 300, the ventricular rate would be 150. Atrial fibrillation is extremely rare but would be seen with an atrial rate of greater than 400 without a set conduction pattern (Fig. 22-24).[22]

SVT is associated with structural cardiac lesions in up to 10% of cases, making detailed cardiac examination extremely important.[21] In the fetus without a structural lesion, restoration of a normal rate can be attempted using maternal medications. Common drugs used for this purpose in SVT include digoxin, amiodarone, flecainide, and sotalol. However, these drugs have significant side effects and must be administered carefully with maternal cardiac monitoring. For atrial

flutter, digoxin and sotalol are considered the agents of choice.[1,19,23] Fetuses that do not respond to medication are at risk for development of high-output heart failure and fetal nonimmune hydrops.

Bradyarrhythmias

Bradycardia is diagnosed when the heart rate is sustained below 100 beats per minute. The chief concern with bradycardias is that a type of heart block may be present. In its most severe form, complete heart block shows complete dissociation between the atrial and ventricular rates. Thus, the atrial rate will be normal (120 to 180 beats per minute) but there is a complete lack of conduction, leaving the ventricles to beat at

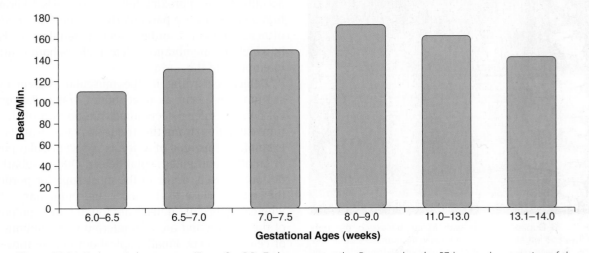

Figure 22-21 Embryonic heart rates. (From Cyr DR. Embryosonography. Presented at the 37th annual convention of the American Institute of Ultrasound in Medicine. Honolulu, Hawaii, 1993.)

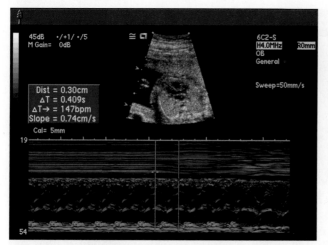

(**Figure 22-22** A normal M-mode tracing obtained thorough the aortic root.)

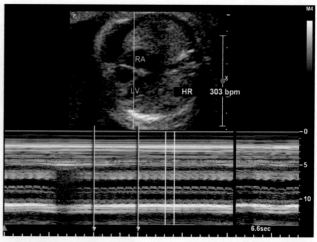

Figure 22-24 Duplex M-mode demonstrating a fetus with supraventricular tachycardia. The M-line is traversing the left (*LV*) and the right atrium (*RA*). On the M-mode, the arrows define a 1-second duration. (Image courtesy of University of Colorado Hospital.)

their inherent rate of around 70 beats per minute. Complete atrioventricular block is associated with the development of nonimmune hydrops and, depending on the gestational age, may necessitate delivery and external pacing of the affected fetus.

When bradyarrhythmia is noted, therefore, it is important to perform M-mode echocardiography. Careful examination of the atrial and ventricular rates allows differentiation of blocked PACs resulting in a bradyarrhythmia (most common in atrial bigeminy) versus complete heart block. Complete heart block in neonates is associated with either structural abnormalities such as congenitally corrected transposition of the great vessels or heterotaxy. In utero complete heart block may be seen with maternal autoimmune disease such as Sjögren's syndrome and the presence of elevated anti-Ro and anti-La antibodies.[24,25]

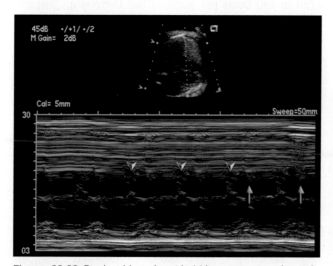

Figure 22-23 Duplex M-mode with M-line traversing the right atrium (RA) and left atrium (LA) in a fetus with premature atrial contractions. Arrowheads demonstrate normal atrial contractions and arrows depict the premature atrial beat. Images courtesy of Pamela M. Foy BS RDMS.

SEPTAL DEFECTS

Ventricular Septal Defects

Isolated ventricular septal defects (VSD) are the most common cardiac malformations, accounting for approximately 30% of cardiac abnormalities present in live births, with an incidence of 1% to 2%.[1] While the majority of VSDs occur in isolation, they also occur in complex cardiac lesions and in the setting of chromosomal disorders (40%).[1] Therefore, identification of VSD should trigger a detailed study to detect the presence of other, extracardiac, anomalies.

The interventricular septum functions to separate the right ventricular and left ventricular chambers and consists of both muscular and membranous portions. Presence of a defect in this region of the heart allows direct communication between the right and left ventricles. Defects can occur in either section of the septum, with membranous/perimembranous defects accounting for approximately 75% of VSDs.[26] Perimembranous lesions are particularly common in the setting of malalignment disorders, such as tetralogy of Fallot, in which the membranous defect allows both ventricles to empty into the aorta.[27]

Defects occurring in the muscular portion of the septum may occur as inlet, outlet, trabecular, or apical defects. Inlet defects affect the portion of the septum extending from the tricuspid valve leaflets; one example of this type of lesion is the ventricular portion of an atrioventricular septal defect. Outlet, subarterial, or conal defects occur in the most superior portion of the septum, close to the aortic and pulmonary valves, whereas trabecular defects are found in the midportion of the septum and are also referred to as midmuscular or central defects. Finally, apical defects are those that occur close to the apex of the heart, past the insertion point of the moderator band (Fig. 22-25C).[27]

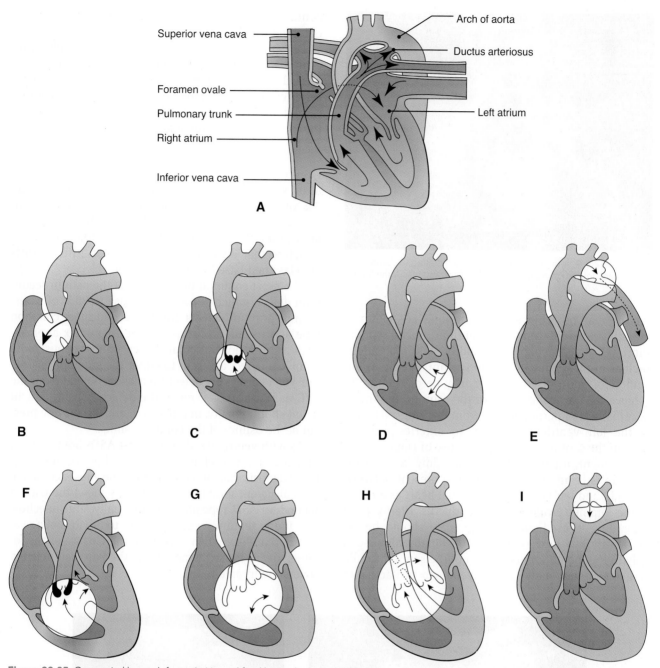

Figure 22-25 Congenital heart defects. **A:** Normal fetal heart showing the foramen ovale and ductus arteriosus. **B:** Persistence of the foramen ovale results in an atrial septal defect. **C:** Persistence of the ductus arteriosus (patent ductus arteriosus) forces blood back into the pulmonary artery. **D:** A ventricular septal defect. **E:** Coarctation of the aorta restricts outward blood flow in the aorta. **F:** Tetralogy of Fallot. This involves a VSD, dextroposition of the aorta, right ventricular outflow obstruction, and right ventricular hypertrophy. Blood is shunted from right to left. **G:** Endocardial cushion defects. Blood flows between the chambers of the heart. **H:** Transposition of the great vessels. The pulmonary artery is attached to the left side of the heart and the aorta to the right side. **I:** Patent ductus arteriosus. The high-pressure blood of the aorta is shunted back to the pulmonary artery.

In most cases, the four-chamber view is utilized for prenatal diagnosis of a VSD (Fig. 22-26). The highest resolution is generally achieved by use of a high-frequency transducer (5 to 7.5 MHz) with the direction of the beam perpendicular to the septum in the subcostal four-chamber view. A VSD appears as a dark, hypolucent area in the septum. A true VSD should be demonstrated in more than one plane, as the transducer is moved from the anterior to posterior aspects of the heart.[28,29] The "T sign" has been shown to be of assistance in differentiating true VSDs from signal dropout. In the "T sign," the anechoic area is bordered by a sharply defined hyperechoic portion of the septum.[30]

While the four-chamber view may be effective for the identification of inlet and trabecular defects, better views of the complete sweep of the interventricular

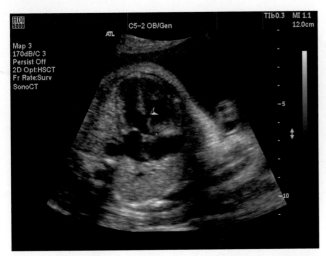

Figure 22-26 A four-chamber view demonstrating a large VSD (*arrowhead*).(Image courtesy of Philips Medical Systems, Bothell, WA.)

septum may be achieved by using long-axis views of the left and right ventricular outflow tracts and the short-axis biventricular view. Additionally, techniques such as in-plane viewing of the septum and the use of both color and pulsed Doppler may be of benefit. To achieve the "in-plane" view of the septum, the transducer is turned perpendicular from the long-axis view of the left ventricle, creating an anterior-posterior view of the septum.[1] Although the use of Doppler may be of benefit, it cannot demonstrate flow in all cases, as there is relatively equal pressure present between the right and left ventricle in the fetal heart as a result of the foramen ovale and patent ductus arteriosus. If color flow is used, the velocity scale should be set to identify low flow (Fig. 22-27).[36] Finally, flow seen only in the membranous portion of the septum (while in a 4-chamber view) is likely due to artifact, and

confirmation of the presence of a VSD needs to be obtained in other views.

Detection of VSDs has increased substantially in recent years. However, there are still substantial rates of missed diagnoses, with rates of 35% to 70% in some series examining diagnosis of isolated VSDs.[37,38] Current resolution limits of 1 to 2 millimeters (mm) still prevent the identification of small lesions.[34]

Atrial Septal Defects

Occurring in approximately 1 in 1,500 live births,[39] atrial septal defects (ASDs) account for approximately 7% of cardiac lesions.[40] They are the fifth most common congenital cardiac anomaly. As with the ventricular septum, the atrial septum is a musculomembranous structure that divides the right and left atrium. ASDs are classified based on their location.

The most common type of ASD is the ostium secundum defect, which accounts for close to 80% of cases. Ostium primum defects are the second most common type and usually occur as part of a complex anomaly such as an atrioventricular defect. Sinus venous ASDs involve a defect adjacent to either the superior or inferior vena cava. This defect then allows blood from the SVC or IVC to pass through the defect, causing a right to left shunt. Finally, in rare cases, an ASD may be present at the ostium of the coronary sinus.[41]

As with ventricular defects, most ASDs are best seen utilizing the four-chamber subcostal view; however, the diagnosis can be confused by the presence of the normal patent foramen ovale. In this view, the ostium secundum ASD appears as an unusually large anechoic area in the septum secundum close to the foramen ovale. Alternatively, when observing the closure of the foramen ovale, it may be noted that the flap insufficiently covers the foramen.

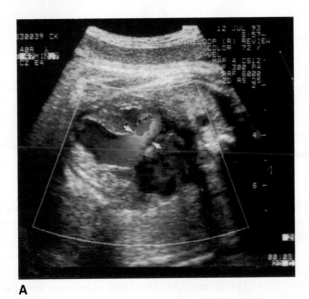

A

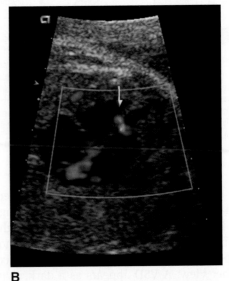

B

Figure 22-27 Color Doppler of a VSD demonstrates blood crossing from left to right through an interventricular septal defect (*arrow*). (Images courtesy of Pamela M. Foy BS RDMS.)

For the ostium primum ASD, the lower portion of the atrial septum immediately superior to the atrioventricular valves is absent. In some cases, a small area of thickened septum may be detected adjacent to the defect. In the normal fetal heart, the septal leaflet of the tricuspid valve inserts more apically than that of the anterior mitral valve leaflet. However, this offset is not apparent in an ostium primum defect; the leaflets appear to insert at the same level in an ostium primum defect. This same sonographic appearance is seen when the ostium primum defect occurs as part of the atrioventricular septal defect (Fig. 22-28).

Finally, while an attempt to utilize color flow in the setting of ASD may be made, its utility is limited in the diagnosis of small defects because of the normal turbulent flow occurring through the foramen ovale.

Although ASDs may occur in isolation, they are frequently associated with additional complex anomalies and may have significant prognostic implications. This is particularly true in conditions such as transposition of the great vessels and total anomalous pulmonary venous return, in which the presence of an ASD allows the only route for blood returning from the pulmonary circulation to enter the left side of the heart and thus the systemic circulation. Absence of an ASD in these cases results in a lethal anomaly when the foramen ovale closes at birth.[42] Chromosomal abnormalities are also relatively common in cases of ASD, as are

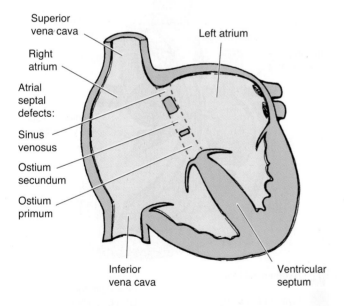

Figure 22-28 An atrial septal defect is an abnormal opening between the right and left atria. Basically, three types of abnormalities result from incorrect development of the atrial septum. An incompetent foramen ovale is the most common defect. The ostium secundum defect results from abnormal development of the septum secundum and causes an opening in the middle of the septum. Improper development of the septum primum produces an opening at the lower end of the septum known as an ostium primum defect, frequently involving the atrioventricular valves. In general, left-to-right shunting of blood occurs in all atrial septal defects.

syndromes such as Holt-Oram.[43] Thus, any diagnosis of ASD should trigger both an echocardiogram and detailed anatomy scan to identify concurrent extracardiac anomalies.

Atrioventricular Septal Defects

Atrioventricular septal defects (AVSD) encompass a range of cardiac malformations involving a combination of malformations of the interatrial septum (ostium primum ASD), interventricular septum (VSD), and the atrioventricular (tricuspid and mitral) valves. Also referred to as AV canal or endocardial cushion defects, AVSDs occur when the endocardial cushions of the heart fail to fuse properly. Accounting for approximately 3% of congenital heart diseases,[44,45] AVSDs are associated with a variety of syndromes and chromosomal abnormalities, including all three major trisomies (45% of heart lesions in trisomy 21 are AVSDs).[46] AVSDs can be classified into complete, intermediate, or partial defects.

Complete AVSDs consist of a large septal defect with both atrial and ventricular defects, and a common AV valve that connects both atria to the ventricles. The common AV valve consists of five leaflets. The anterosuperior and posteroinferior leaflets bridge the septal defects, and three lateral leaflets. Complete AV canals may be further subdivided on the basis of their chordal insertions (Fig. 22-25G).[47,48]

In partial AVSD, the mitral and tricuspid openings are separate, and the following findings are seen: (1) primum ASD, (2) VSD, (3) cleft anterior mitral leaflet, and (4) cleft septal tricuspid leaflet. Here, despite the presence of two separate valvular openings, the mitral and triscupid valves still appear to insert at the same level.[47,48]

The least common form of AVSD is the intermediate type. Here, the overall architecture is similar to that in a complete AVSD. However, the septal bridging leaflets are fused in an anteroposterior fashion. This results in division of the common valve into separate mitral and tricuspid orifices.[47,48]

Most AVSDs are large defects that are easily recognized in a subcostal or apical four-chamber view of the heart. In these views, a complete AVSD appears as a large, anechoic area encompassing the lower portion (primum) of the atrial septum, the upper portion of the ventricular septum, and the normal location of the mitral and tricuspid valves. As the transducer is moved back and forth in an anterior-posterior direction, the combined bridging leaflets of the common valve should come into view. These appear atypical on real-time sonographic evaluation both through the lack of the usual offset between the tricuspid and mitral valves and because of the fact that the valve motion is identical and continuous in both the right and left ventricles. Utilization of color Doppler confirms the communication among all cardiac chambers (Fig. 22-29).

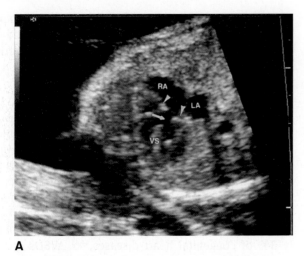

A

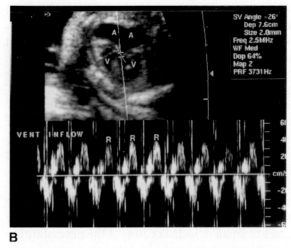

B

Figure 22-29 A: Four-chamber view demonstrating complete endocardial cushion defect *(arrow)*. *RA*, right atrium; *LA*, left atrium; *VS*, ventricular septum. Arrowheads point to common atrioventricular valve. **B:** Doppler interrogation of the common atrioventricular valve shows valve incompetence (regurgitation). *A*, atria; *V*, ventricles; *R*, regurgitation jets.

Partial and intermediate AVSDs are more difficult to identify, but the presence of both ASD and VSD should trigger the use of additional views of the tricuspid and mitral valves. The short-axis view can be used to image the atrioventricular junction. With complete AVSD, a large AV valve is seen; however, with the partial AVSD, right and left valvular openings are viewed. The mitral opening is triangular, as opposed to its normal elliptical form.

The aortic root should also be routinely visualized in cases of AVSD, as it normally lies within the annulus of the mitral and tricuspid valves. The position of the anterior septal leaflet commonly causes an anterior and superior displacement of the aortic root, with a subsequent narrowing of the left ventricular outflow tract. This "goose-neck" deformity can best be seen in a long-axis view of the left outflow tract.[48]

HYPOPLASTIC LEFT HEART

Hypoplastic left heart syndrome (HLHS) is the most severe left-sided obstructive lesion. The basic components of hypoplastic left heart include a hypoplastic left ventricle, aortic atresia, hypoplasia of the ascending aorta, mitral valve atresia and or hypoplasia, and in some cases a small left atrium. It is responsible for around 7% of congenital heart diseases[49] and is the most common cause of death from congenital heart disease in the neonatal period.

Although the severity of the abnormalities involved in the hypoplastic left heart syndrome frequently leads to easy diagnosis, it is important to realize that this lesion is often progressive, arising from an initial mitral stenosis with subsequent decreased development of the left ventricle and outflow tract. Therefore, in some cases, the characteristic sonographic findings may not be present until late in the second trimester. If the left-sided heart structures appear smaller than usual compared to

the right, or if there is any concern about the function of the mitral valve, imaging should be repeated later in gestation (Fig. 22-30).[49,50]

On sonographic examination, the hypoplastic left heart maintains its normal cardiac axis. The four-chamber subcostal view demonstrates a clear size discrepancy between the right and left ventricles. The moderator

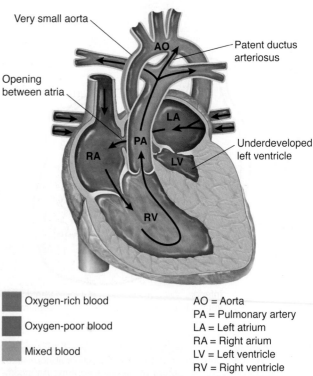

■ Oxygen-rich blood	AO = Aorta
	PA = Pulmonary artery
■ Oxygen-poor blood	LA = Left atrium
	RA = Right arium
■ Mixed blood	LV = Left ventricle
	RV = Right ventricle

Figure 22-30 In HLHS, blood returning into the left atrium via the pulmonary vein flows through an ASD, through the tricuspid valve, into the right ventricle and out of the heart via the pulmonary artery effectively bypassing the left ventricle. The flow into the right atrium from the SVC, IVC, and the added volume from the PV results in the large size. Flow through the ductus arteriosus provides flow to the fetal body.

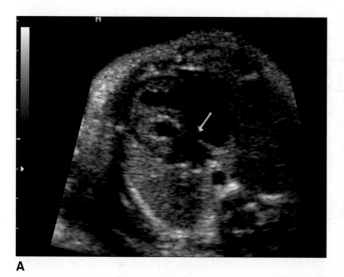

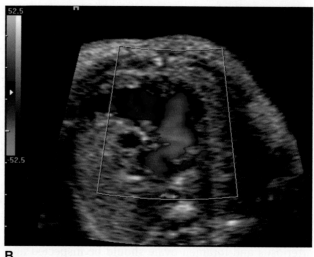

A   **B**

Figure 22-32 A: The ASD *(arrow)* allows pulmonary flow to cross from the left to the right atrium. Normal flow across the foramen ovale is from the right into the left atrium. **B:** The color Doppler image demonstrates flow toward the transducer from the left into the right atrium. Determination of flow direction is made through the use of the color bar located at the side of the image. Remember BART, blue away, red toward, which is the orientation on this image. (Images courtesy of Pamela M. Foy BS RDMS.)

band should be noted in the normal or enlarged right ventricle, to confirm that it is the left ventricle that is hypoplastic. Because of the left ventricular hypoplasia, the right ventricle actually forms the apex of the fetal heart (Fig. 22-31).

The degree of aortic atresia or hypoplasia can be assessed using the short-axis view of the right outflow tract or by inspection of the three-vessel view. In cases of atresia, the aorta may appear as a central echoluceny surrounded by the pulmonary outflow tracts. Hypoplasia can be diagnosed by comparing the diameter of the pulmonary outflow tracts circling the central aorta. Imaging of the aortic arch reveals the hypoplastic ascending aorta.[51]

As mentioned above, the mitral valve is generally stenotic or atretic in HLHS. The function of the mitral valve can be assessed in either the long-axis left outflow tract view or in the four-chamber view. If atretic, a membranous band may be apparent in place of valve leaflets. Pulsed and color Doppler may be of benefit in assessing blood flow through both the mitral and aortic valves. Also, as HLHS is a ductal dependent lesion, Doppler should be used to document the patency of both the ductus arteriosus and the foramen ovale (Fig. 22-32).[49]

M-mode examination should also be conducted to confirm the diagnosis. Diagnostic criteria include a left ventricular end-diastolic diameter of less than 9 mm with an aortic root diameter of less than 6 mm.[52]

In addition, HLHS can occur in conjunction with anomalous pulmonary venous return. To exclude this additional anomaly, connection of the pulmonary veins to the left atrium should be confirmed in the four-chamber view. Because of the mitral restriction, they may appear somewhat enlarged. Color Doppler may be of assistance in their identification.

RIGHT VENTRICULAR HYPOPLASIA (PULMONARY ATRESIA)

In contrast to HLHS, right ventricular hypoplasia is extremely uncommon, occurring in 0.1 to 0.4 in 10,000 live births.[1,54] When it occurs, it generally results from pulmonary atresia with an intact ventricular septum. Classification is based on the tripartite approach described by Goor and Lillehel, in which the right ventricle is partitioned into three separate areas: the inlet portion, including the tricuspid valve; an apical trabecular portion, which includes the area past the insertion of the tricuspid papillary muscles; and the infundibulum or conus, which encompasses the area surrounding the pulmonary valve. Using these regions, the partite

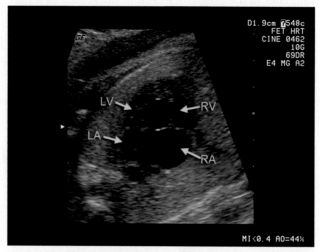

Figure 22-31 This four-chamber view demonstrates the large right atrium and ventricle. *RA*, right atrium; *RV*, right ventricle; *LA*, left atrium; *LV*, left ventricle. (Image courtesy of GE Healthcare, Wauwatosa, WI.)

system classifies lesions as tripartite (involving all regions), bipartite (with inlet and outlet components), or unipartite (consisting of an inlet lesion only).[1,55]

Right ventricular hypoplasia from pulmonary atresia can be diagnosed by identification of an unusually small right ventricle in either an apical or subcostal four-chamber view. Analysis of the tricuspid and pulmonary valves demonstrates patency of the tricuspid valve but may demonstrate regurgitation on Doppler views because of the downstream blockage. The long-axis view of the pulmonary artery or short-axis right outflow tract views show a small, hyperechoic pulmonary artery. Color or pulsed Doppler confirms the absence of blood flow. As with HLHS, right ventricular hypoplasia results in a ductal-dependent lesion; therefore, both the ductus arteriosus and foramen ovale should be inspected and documented to be patent.

Factors associated with poor prognosis include a tricuspid annulus less than 5 mm (>30 weeks gestation), a right ventricular:left ventricular ratio greater than 0.5, and absence of tricuspid regurgitation.[1] Although the aortic and mitral valves are usually normal in this setting, all cardiac anatomy should be carefully evaluated. It is not unusual to see left atrial/left ventricular enlargement, as in the absence of a restrictive foramen ovale there is a significant right to left shunt due to the lack of right ventricular and outflow tract development.

TRICUSPID ATRESIA

Tricuspid atresia, similar to pulmonary atresia, results in a right ventricular hypoplasia, in this case due to lack of inflow from the right atrium. As with the discussion of HLHS, this is a progressive lesion which tends to worsen as the pregnancy progresses, so any concern on an early ultrasound regarding the patency of the tricuspid valve should trigger repeat examination later in the pregnancy even in the setting of a relatively normal-appearing right ventricular size.[57] The

presence of a VSD may allow for a left to right shunt, which may preserve some of the right ventricular development (Fig. 22-33).

Sonographically, tricuspid atresia appears as a hyperechoic thickened valve, which when interrogated by Doppler imaging, shows no flow on either side of the valve. If a VSD is present, turbulent flow may be demonstrated across the ventricular septum, but such flow does not cross the atretic valve. In approximately 25% of cases, pulmonary atresia is also present.[53] Therefore, the pulmonary valve and artery should be carefully assessed as well, using short-axis right outflow tract views. If the pulmonary artery is normal or stenotic (rather than atretic), a VSD is necessary to supply blood flow for the pulmonary circulation. Therefore, the ventricular septum should be carefully inspected.

As with pulmonary atresia, a right to left shunt is essential after birth, therefore the foramen ovale should be carefully inspected for any restriction, as a restrictive foramen has significant postnatal prognostic implications. Also, the remainder of the cardiac structures including mitral and aortic valves is generally normal, but careful confirmation is nevertheless required. Some degree of left atrial and ventricular enlargement is expected in the presence of a normal foramen ovale; this enlargement can be followed throughout gestation and may have prognostic implications.

COARCTATION OF THE AORTA

Coarctation of the aorta refers to narrowing of the aorta along the aortic arch, resulting in outflow obstruction, with the degree of obstruction related to the degree of narrowing that occurs. The type of coarctation is described as preductal, ductal, or postductal using the position of the lesion in comparison to the ductus arteriosus as a reference. The majority of lesions are ductal or postductal; preductal lesions are generally associated with more complex cardiac lesions.[58] Generally

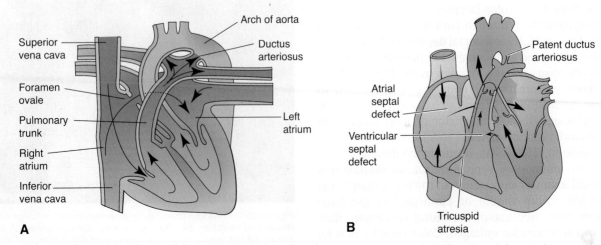

Figure 22-33 **A:** Normal heart. **B:** Tricuspid atresia. Note the small right ventricle and the large left ventricle.

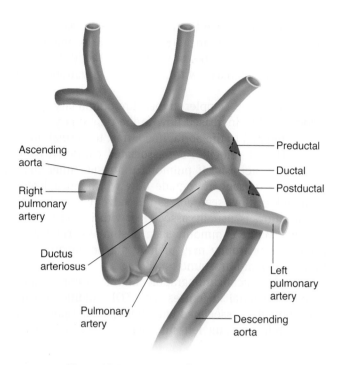

Figure 22-34 Locations of aortic coarctation.

coarctation results only in a narrowing of the aorta, though in severe cases a complete interruption may be present. Interrupted aortic arches are also classified based on the location of the lesion. Type A lesions occur just distal to the left subclavian; type B, between the left carotid and left subclavian; and type C between the innominate and left carotid.[59] Overall, coarctation accounts for approximately 7% of congenital heart disease.[60] Importantly, close to 70% of cases are associated with either additional vascular anomalies such as berry aneurysms or extracardiac anomalies (most commonly genitourinary) (Fig. 22-34).[61,62]

Coarctation remains one of the most difficult cardiac anomalies to diagnose prenatally. On the four-chamber view, right ventricular enlargement without visualization of other abnormalities should engender a high degree of suspicion, particularly in the second trimester. A series conducted by Hornberger et al. in 1994 demonstrated a ratio of right to left ventricular size of 2.25 in infants with coarctations compared to 1.25 for normal fetuses. Similarly, the ratio of the pulmonary artery diameter to that of the aorta was also enlarged, with affected fetuses' ratios approaching 2 and the unaffected ratio approximately 1.25. Thus, comparison of right to left ventricular size and pulmonary artery diameter to that of the aorta is beneficial.[63]

The aortic arch diameter should be evaluated for subtle signs of narrowing. This is best done in a sagittal view of the fetus in which the arch and length of the aorta are clearly demonstrated. Normative values based on gestational age are available for each segment of the aorta.[64,65] If an area of narrowing is visualized, Doppler imaging should be used to measure the postobstruction

velocity. In cases of obstruction, the velocity distal to the lesion is significantly higher (Fig. 22-35).

Finally, the structure of the aortic valve should be carefully evaluated using the short-axis right outflow tract view, as bicuspid aortic valve is associated with cases of coarctation.[66]

Diagnosis of interrupted aortic arch is more obvious. Sagittal views of the fetus in which the aortic arch is visible should allow for identification of the level of the lesion and hence proper classification. Doppler flow imaging may assist with determination of the subclavian, carotid, and innominate arteries in relation to the interruption. The short-axis right outflow view shows a hypoplastic ascending aorta and disproportionately small aortic root. Finally, in cases of an interrupted arch, a VSD is generally present.[67]

TETRALOGY OF FALLOT

One of the more common forms of congenital heart disease and the most common form of cyanotic heart disease, tetralogy of Fallot (TOF) occurs in approximately 1 in 3,600 live births, accounting for up to 7% of congenital heart disease (CHD). The four classic features of tetralogy are: (1) perimembranous (conal) ventricular septal defect; (2) overriding aorta, which encompasses the defect; (3) pulmonary stenosis or atresia; and 4) right ventricular hypertrophy (Fig. 22-25F).[1]

Sonographic identification of tetralogy generally begins with the identification of a perimembranous VSD seen in either the apical or subcostal four-chamber view. Color Doppler can be used to confirm the defect as previously described. Cranial rotation of the ultrasound transducer then obtains a five-chamber view, in which the aortic root can be seen to override the septal defect. Both the VSD and the aortic override can be further assessed in the long-axis view of the left ventricular outflow tract. Some confusion may arise

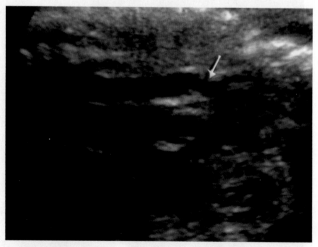

Figure 22-35 The aorta demonstrates a postductal coarctation (*arrow*) of the aorta. (Image courtesy of University of Colorado Hospital, Denver, CO.)

between an overriding aorta due to tetralogy versus a true double-outlet right ventricle (DORV); however, the use of the "50%" rule may be beneficial. If more than 50% of the aorta overrides the right ventricle, DORV is more likely.[1]

As would be suggested by the aortic override, dilation of the aortic root is a usual, though not absolute finding. Doppler views of the aortic valve may demonstrate regurgitation; if this is present, the degree of insufficiency should be monitored throughout the pregnancy.[70]

Next, the right ventricular outflow tract should be evaluated. Three types of pulmonary artery abnormality have been demonstrated in tetralogy: pulmonary stenosis, pulmonary atresia with a patent ductus, and pulmonary atresia with major aortopulmonary collaterals. This evaluation can be carried out using the short-axis right outflow tract views. If the pulmonary artery is present but small in diameter compared to the aortic root, this supports the diagnosis of TOF. Pulmonary

artery diameters have been shown to be between 40% and 55% smaller than aortic diameters in one series of third-trimester fetuses with TOF; the differences appeared to increase with increasing gestational age (Fig. 22-36).[71]

Use of pulsed Doppler to measure pulmonary artery velocity shows increased flow in the pulmonary artery (PA) compared to the aorta, in contrast to normal pregnancy. Higher velocities are associated with increasing degrees of stenosis. If pulmonary atresia rather than stenosis is present, retrograde flow will be visualized, with lack of flow seen across the valve itself. The retrograde flow is usually associated with increased turbulence. While commonly seen postnatally, right ventricular hypertrophy may or may not be apparent on initial prenatal ultrasound.

Complete echocardiographic and anatomic evaluation is essential in fetuses with TOF. Additional cardiac anomalies associated with TOF include right-sided aortic arch, aberrant left subclavian artery, and atrial

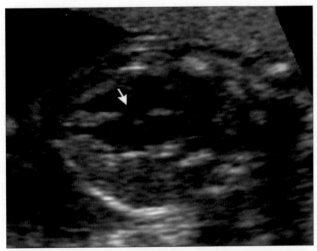

A

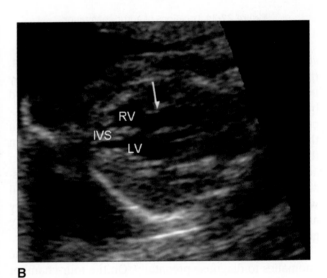

B

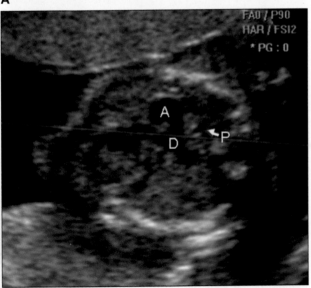

C

Figure 22-36 Tetralogy of Fallot. **A:** To obtain the best image of a VSD, image the IVS perpendicular to the transducer face. This VSD *(arrow)* is part of the TOF group of anomalies. (VSD, pulmonary stenosis, and overriding aorta). **B:** Long-axis view of the heart demonstrating the aorta overriding the intraventricular septum and VSD. *RV,* right ventricle; *LV,* left ventricle; *IVS,* interventricular septum. **C:** Long-axis view of the heart demonstrating a small pulmonary artery *(P)*. In the normal fetus, the aorta and pulmonary artery are approximately the same size. *A,* aorta; *DV,* ductus venosus. (Images courtesy of Pamela M. Foy BS RDMS.)

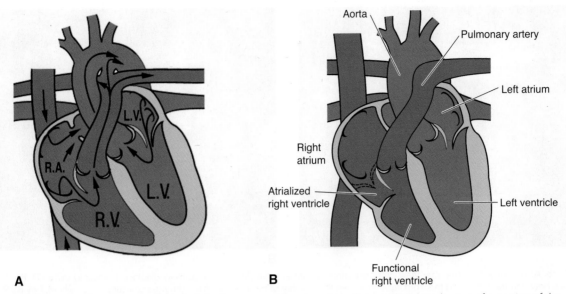

Figure 22-37 Ebstein's anomaly. Apical displacement of the tricuspid leaflets results in atrialization of a portion of the right ventricle. The functional right ventricle is small. An interatrial communication is usually present. (From Brickner ME, Hillis LD, Lange RA. Congenital heart disease in adults. *N Engl J Med.* 2000;342:340.)

septal or atrioventricular septal defects; extracardiac anomalies have included tracheoesophageal fistula, renal anomalies, clefts, and single umbilical artery. In addition, 12% of infants with TOF and 50% of fetuses diagnosed with TOF have chromosomal anomalies, most commonly DiGeorge syndrome and trisomy 21.[68]

EBSTEIN'S ANOMALY

In Ebstein's anomaly, the posterior and septal tricuspid valve leaflets are apically displaced from their normal location at the AV junction into the right ventricle. This results in an abnormally large right atrium and pathologically small right ventricle (Fig. 22-37). Complicating this issue, the aberrant leaflets of the tricuspid valve may be variably adherent to the ventricular wall, resulting in abnormally small mobile portions of the valve cusps. This, in turn, can lead to significant tricuspid regurgitation or, if the valves are essentially immobile, a functional tricuspid stenosis. The anterior leaflet remains correctly placed at the AV junction, and frequently appears enlarged and sail-like. The presence of tricuspid regurgitation or stenosis results in further right atrial enlargement.[72] Occurring in 3% to 7% of fetuses with cardiac disease, Ebstein's anomaly is unusual in that it frequently causes severe dysfunction in utero, including cardiomegaly, hydrops, and arrhythmias.[72] Because of this, the live birth rate is significantly lower, around 1 in 20,000. Maternal ingestion of lithium carbonate has been associated with a 28-fold increased risk of Ebstein's anomaly,[72] and it is associated with chromosomal abnormalities including trisomy 13, 18, and 21.[1,69]

Prenatal diagnosis of Ebstein's anomaly is usually straightforward. The key findings of right atrial enlargement with apical displacement of the tricuspid valve

are apparent on either apical or subcostal four-chamber views, and the degree of tricuspid regurgitation is easily measured with pulsed Doppler (Fig. 22-38). The unusual tethering of the tricuspid valve leaflets may be visualized on subcostal views as either thickening of the chordate or abnormal numbers of attachments (Fig. 22-39). Severe levorotation of the heart may be present because of the displacement caused by the enlarged right atrium. Right ventricular dilation may be present as well, with decreased wall thickness and/or dyskinesias. Finally, measurement of the offset between the septal leaflets of the mitral and tricuspid valves should be performed. The diagnostic offsets for fetuses with Ebstein's anomaly is anything greater than 8 mm.[73]

TRANSPOSITION OF THE GREAT ARTERIES

Transposition of the great arteries can be divided into two separate categories: complete transposition, or d-transposition, and congenitally corrected transposition, or l-transposition. The d- and l- are used to denote the location of the aorta in relation to the pulmonary artery, where d- denotes right and l- left. In both conditions, the pulmonary artery arises from the left ventricle and the aorta from the right ventricle; however, they are two distinct anomalies with widely divergent prognoses.[74]

In complete transposition, which encompasses the majority of infants with TGA, the connection between the atria and ventricles is concordant, meaning that the right atrium connects with the right ventricle, and the left atrium connects with the left ventricle. The aorta, however, comes off the right ventricle, causing deoxygenated blood to circulate systemically, and the pulmonary artery off the left ventricle. This results in systemic and pulmonary circulation that functions in parallel

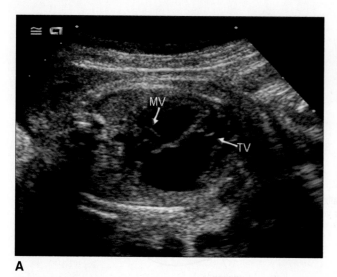
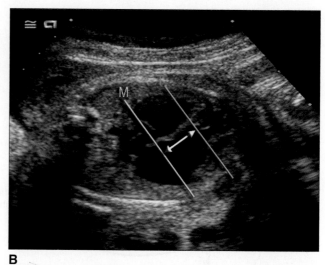

A   **B**

Figure 22-38 A: An apical four-chamber view demonstrating the mitral valve *(M)* and the apically displaced tricuspid valve *(T)*. **B:** Measuring the distance between the mitral and tricuspid valve indicates the severity of the inferior offset. (Images courtesy of Pamela M. Foy BS RDMS.)

rather than in sequence. Therefore, at least one avenue of mixing (such as ASD or VSD) must be present for oxygenated blood from the left ventricular (pulmonic) circulation to reach the right ventricular (systemic) circulation in order for life to be sustained until correction can be performed. This type of transposition has a higher incidence in males and accounts for 5% to 7% of all congenital heart disease in the fetal population (Fig. 22-25H).[75]

Key to the diagnosis of complete TGA is appropriate chamber identification. The atria are properly identified by their appendages and the foraminal flap, with the right atrial appendage appearing broad-based with

pectinate muscles and the left appendage long and narrow. The foraminal flap should be seen opening into the left atrium. The ventricles can be distinguished by valvular and muscular differences. The tricuspid valve (associated with the right ventricle) is inserted more apically than the mitral, and has distinct attachment to the interventricular septum. Also, the right ventricle contains the moderator band near the apex. The pulmonary artery and aorta can be distinguished by their branching patterns, where the pulmonary artery bifurcates into right and left branches in contrast to the aorta, which gives rise to the carotids, subclavians, and coronary arteries.[75]

Although prenatal diagnosis of complete TGA has been shown to improve outcomes, it remains one of the more difficult diagnoses. In complete transposition, the apical and subcostal four-chamber views are usually completely normal, as the relationship between the chambers is not altered. The key to diagnosis therefore rests on adequate visualization of the outflow tracts. In the short-axis view of the right outflow tract, the normal relationship of the pulmonary artery encircling the central aorta is lost, and the two vessels appear as either side-by-side circular structures or as parallel vessels (Fig. 22-40). In the long-axis views of the outflow tracts, the aorta and pulmonary artery are seen to run in parallel, without the normal crossing pattern. Upon closer inspection, the vessel arising from the right ventricle is seen to give rise to the head and neck vessels, whereas those arising from the left ventricle have the simple left and right branch pattern of the pulmonary artery. Color Doppler can be useful in demonstrating the branching patterns. Finally, on the three-vessel view normally obtained by angling the transducer cephalad from the four-chamber view, only two vessels, the aorta and superior vena cava, are identified.[75]

As was mentioned above, a channel for mixing is critical. Therefore, the ventricular septum should be

Figure 22-39 This subcostal four-chamber view demonstrates marked levorotation, a thickened tricuspid valve *(T)*, and an enlarged right atrium *(RA)* compressing the left atrium *(LA)*. *LV,* left ventricle; *RV,* right ventricle; *SP,* spine. (Image courtesy of University of Colorado Hospital.)

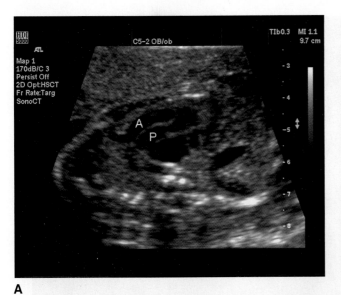

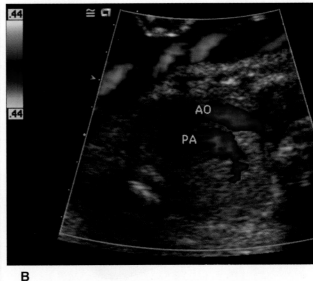

A **B**

Figure 22-40 **A:** This short axis view shows the aorta *(A)* and pulmonary *(P)* arteries arising from the heart in a parallel course. **B:** Color Doppler imaging helps in identification of the vessels, confirming flow direction in the aorta *(AO)* and pulmonary artery *(PA)*. (Image **A** courtesy of Philips Medical Systems, Bothell, WA. Image **B** courtesy of Pamela M. Foy BS, RDMS.)

carefully examined for a VSD, which is present in approximately 20% of cases. Left ventricular (i.e., pulmonary) outflow obstruction may be present as well. Extracardiac and chromosomal abnormalities are unusual, but careful evaluation is nonetheless warranted.

Congenitally corrected transposition (CCTGA or l-transposition) is extremely rare. In this syndrome, both the atrioventricular connections and the ventriculoarterial connections are discordant. Thus, the right atrium connects to the morphologic left ventricle, which is in turn connected to the pulmonary artery; the left atrium connects to the morphologic right ventricle, which in turn connects to the aorta. Typically the right and left atrium are present in their correct anatomic positions, but dextrocardia can be present in up to 20% of cases.[75]

As with complete TGA, diagnosis in CCTGA is dependent on correct identification of the chambers. In CCTGA, the moderator band and apically placed tricuspid valve is visualized connected to the left atrium rather than the right. The aorta and pulmonary arteries again exit in parallel. Finally, heart block may be present (Fig. 22-41).[25–26, 76–77]

TRUNCUS ARTERIOSUS

Truncus arteriosus is one of a group of rare conotruncal defects that account for approximately 1% of fetal cardiac lesions.[82] Here, the truncoconal ridges that normally divide the truncus arteriosus into aortic and pulmonary trunks fail to fuse, resulting in a single great vessel arising just above the interventricular septum. A VSD is uniformly present within the upper portion of the septum, just below the location of the truncus. A single valve is present either directly above the VSD or

above the right ventricle. The truncus receives blood from both the right and left ventricles and perfuses the pulmonary, systemic, and coronary systems. Associated cardiac anomalies include both valvular insufficiency or stenosis, absent ductus arteriosus (50% to 75%), and right-sided aortic arch (30%).[83] Truncus arteriosus can be further divided into type based on the origin and separation of the pulmonary arteries (Fig. 22-42).[80]

Diagnosis of truncus arteriosus is best made from the five-chamber view, in which a single vessel can be seen overriding a VSD. Although the VSD may be detected on inspection of either apical or subcostal views, it is sometimes missed, as the only abnormality on such views is the VSD. The long-axis view of the left ventricular outflow tract also produces the characteristic appearance of a single vessel overriding a VSD.

On the short-axis view of what would normally be the right outflow tract, the single truncal valve is seen. The normal encircling pulmonary artery is absent. The number of leaflets in the valve is variable, ranging from one to six, but a tricuspid configuration is most common.[81] Regurgitant flow is common, occurring in approximately 50% of cases, and can be readily seen with Doppler.[78] In some cases, the valve leaflets may appear thickened and stenotic. As the truncus is followed superiorly, it may be possible using color Doppler to identify the origin of the pulmonary arteries. As the ductus arteriosus is frequently absent, an attempt should be made to identify it.[79] Finally, the directionality and patency of the entire length of the aorta should be assessed. A right-sided aortic arch is present in up to 30% of patients, and an interrupted aortic arch has also been reported.[1]

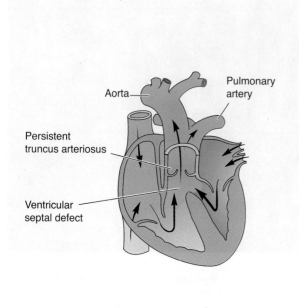

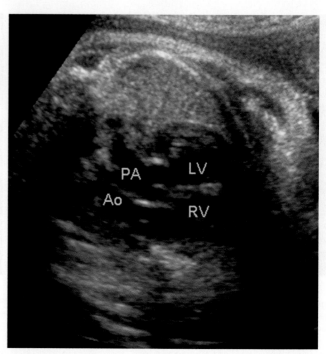

Figure 22-41 Persistent truncus arteriosus. The pulmonary artery originates from a common truncus **(A)**. The septum in the truncus and conus has failed to form. This abnormality is always accompanied by an interventricular septal defect. The four-chamber view demonstrates the aorta and pulmonary vessels originating from the opposite ventricles **(B)** than seen with the normal heart. The moderator band on the right aids in identification of the ventricles. (Image courtesy of University of Colorado Hospital, Denver, CO.)

DOUBLE-OUTLET RIGHT VENTRICLE

Double-outlet right ventricle (DORV) encompasses a group of disorders in which more than 50% of both the aortic root and pulmonary artery arise from the morphologic right ventricle, usually directly above a perimembranous VSD (Fig. 22-42). Several different classification schemes have been proposed on the basis of the exact relationship between the VSD to the

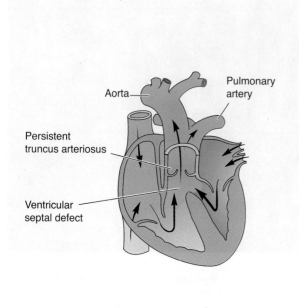

great arteries and the position of the great arteries at the level of the semilunar valves. Most commonly, the VSD is located below the aorta, with the aorta and pulmonary artery lateral to one another. However, many combinations are possible. Currently, four main types are accepted by the Society of Thoracic Surgeons:

1. VSD-type, in which there is DORV with a subaortic VSD
2. Fallot-type, DORV with subaortic or double committed VSD and pulmonary stenosis
3. TGA type, in which there is a DORV with a subpulmonary VSD
4. Noncommittal VSD-type, in which the VSD is remote from either great vessel[82] (Fig. 22-43)

Sonographic diagnosis can be difficult, and corrective strategies depend on correct identification of the abnormal connections. DORV may commonly be difficult to differentiate between conditions such as tetralogy (particularly the Fallot-type) or HLHS. The four-chamber views are generally normal in appearance, due to the fact that the VSD is typically anterior and thus may not be apparent on the apical or subcostal views. However, on the long-axis view of the aorta and/or pulmonary artery, a VSD can be visualized. In the most common side-by-side arrangement of the great vessels, the normal crossing of the pulmonary artery and aorta is lost, giving rise to parallel outflow tracts similar to those seen in TGA.

Once the diagnosis is made, pulsed Doppler evaluation should be used to confirm the patency of both the pulmonary artery and the aorta to rule out hypoplasia

Figure 22-42 An extended four-chamber view showing the common truncus great vessel, arising from both the right ventricle *(RV)* and left ventricle *(LV)*. This is consistent with truncus arteriosus *(TA)*. (Image courtesy of Pamela M. Foy BS, RDMS.)

Ao = Aorta
PT = Pulmonary trunk
IS = Infundibular septum
P = Posterior limbus

A = Anterior limbus
SMT = Trabecula septomarginalis
RV = Right ventricle
RA = Right atruim

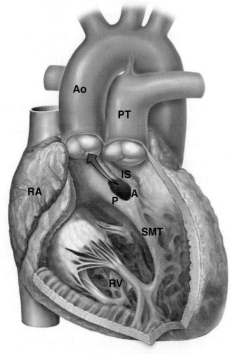

Subaortic VSD

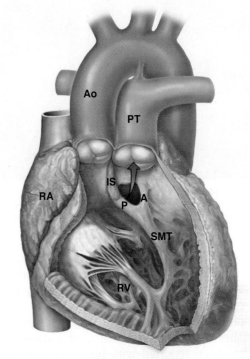

Subpulmonary VSD

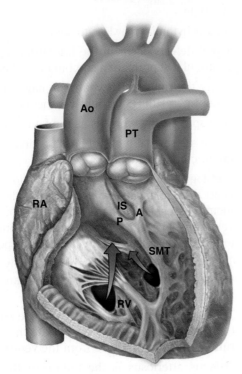

Noncommitted VSD

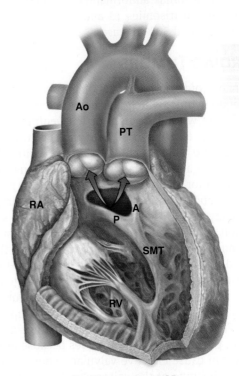

Doubly-committed VSD

Figure 22-43 Society of Thoracic Surgeons types of DORV.

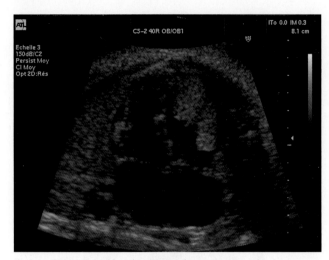

Figure 22-44 Four-chamber view demonstrating classic appearance of rhabdomyoma, which is located within the right ventricle. (Image courtesy of Philips Medical Systems, Bothell, WA.)

and coarctation. Also, the presence of separate mitral and tricuspid valves should be confirmed, as cases of large AVSDs have been reported where only one common valve is present.[1]

Additional cardiac (65% to 70%) and extracardiac anomalies (47%) are common, and a strong association has been reported with poorly controlled diabetes.[1] Chromosomal abnormalities including DiGeorge syndrome and trisomies 13 and 18 are also common, found in around 30% of cases.[85]

CARDIAC TUMORS

The most common prenatally diagnosed cardiac tumor is rhabdomyoma, which is usually noticed as an echogenic mass within the right or left ventricle or within the IVS. Up to 60% to 80% of patients with rhabdomyomas are subsequently diagnosed with tuberous sclerosis, so a careful family history and inspection of the patient for additional stigmata should be performed when rhabdomyoma is suspected.[90] The impact of rhabdomyomas is dependent on the number, size, and location of the tumors. Cardiac tumors can result in arrhythmias, most commonly supraventricular, therefore M-mode or pulsed Doppler should be used to document a normal heart rate or to evaluate any irregularity. In cases where SVT does occur, development of hydrops fetalis has been reported, and close follow-up is necessary. Finally, rhabdomyomas that obstruct mitral, tricuspid, pulmonary, or aortic valves because of their location can cause effective valvular stenosis. Therefore, Doppler imaging of the valves should be performed to document patency (Fig. 22-44).[88]

SUMMARY

- The heart begins beating at 3 weeks postconception.
- Cardiogenic cords, tubular structures, are the first sign of heart development.
- The atrioventricular loop forms as the tube bends.
- Endocardial cushions develop, separating the atria and ventricles, at approximately 27 days.
- In the seventh week, the truncus arteriosus forms, twisting into their proper location.
- Several sets of aortic arches form and regress.
- Fetal circulation has three bypasses: the ductus arteriosus, foramen ovale, and ductus venosus, which close at parturition.
- CHD is the most common malformation.
- CHD is associated with other structural anomalies and abnormal karyotypes.
- The best time to examine the fetal heart with ultrasound is between 18 and 22 weeks.
- The normal heart is at a 45-degree angle to the left of midline (levocardia).
- Dextrocardia, dextroposition, and mesocardia describe abnormal positions of the fetal heart.
- Obtain a minimum of five 2D views of the heart to determine normalcy.
- STIC is a 3D imaging mode specifically for use with fetal heart imaging.
- An M-mode helps detect heart rhythm anomalies when the M-line placement is through the atria and ventricle.
- Fetal arrhythmias may lead to nonimmune fetal hydrops.
- Septal defects occur in the interatrial septum, interventricular septum, or a combination of both (AVSD).
- Either the right or left ventricle may fail to develop, resulting in HPLHS or right ventricular hypoplasia.
- Tricuspid atresia worsens as the fetus matures.
- There are several types of aortic coarctation: preductal, ductal, postductal.
- Tetralogy of Fallot is the most common form of cyanotic heart disease and is the result of five defects: a perimembranous ventricular septal defect, outlet of conal ventricular defect, pulmonic stenosis, pulmonary artery hypoplasia, and right ventricular hypertrophy.
- The main findings in Ebstein's anomaly are an apically displaced tricuspid valve and a large, atrialized right ventricle.
- There are two types of TGA, complete and corrected transposition. Both types image with the great vessels running a parallel course from the ventricles.
- Truncus arteriosus is the failure of the embryonic truncus to separate into the aorta and pulmonary artery.
- DORV has more than 50% of the aortic root and pulmonary artery arising from the right ventricle.
- The rhabdomyoma is the most common solid, benign cardiac mass seen in the fetus and may be due to tuberous sclerosis and nonimmune fetal hydrops.

PATHOLOGY BOX 22-4

Outline of Fetal Congenital Heart Defects and Sonographic Appearances

Heart Defect	Sonographic Appearances
Atrioventricular septal defects/endocardial cushion defect	Dependent on type; includes various degrees of ostium primum ASD, VSD, common atrioventricular valve, anterior MV leaflet, cleft septal TV
Coarctation of the aorta	Possibly slight right ventricular enlargement. Possible turbulent descending aortic flow distal to ductus arteriosus entrance. Doppler/color may show reversed flow in ductus arteriosus in severe forms of coarctation
Double-outlet right ventricle	Dependent on type: 1. VSD-type, in which there is DORV with a subaortic VSD 2. Fallot-type, DORV with subaortic or double committed VSD and pulmonary stenosis 3. TGA-type, in which there is a DORV with a subpulmonary VSD 4. Noncommittal VSD-type, in which the VSD is remote from either great vessel
Ectopia cordis	Fetal heart is partially or totally outside fetal thorax, usually through sternal defect. Important to look for congenital heart disease, as well as other fetal abnormalities
Epstein's anomaly	Apically displaced TV, large RA, small RV, tricuspid regurgitation or stenosis, hydrops, arrhythmia, akinetic or dyskeinetic contraction of the right ventricle
Hypoplastic left heart	Small, hypertrophied LV, aortic atresia, hypoplasia of the ascending aorta, MV atresia or hypoplasia, small left atrium
Hypoplastic right heart/right ventricular hypoplasia	Pulmonary atresia, pulmonary valve fusion, small pulmonary annulus, ASD, underdeveloped right heart, small TV, increased right side of heart if no VSD present, large foramen ovale, nonvisualization of pulmonary artery in specific views (ant. four-chamber, short-axis). Careful duplex scanning may help in demonstrating no right ventricular outflow
Interrupted aortic arch	Slight increase in right ventricle size. Abnormally small ascending aorta. Doppler/color may show reversed flow in ductus arteriosus
Situs inversus	Important to be sure of left-right orientation of fetal heart in relation to fetal position. The fetal heart may appear normal. Abdominal structures may also be inversed
Tetralogy of Fallot	Perimembranous ventricular septal defect, pulmonic stenosis, pulmonary artery hypoplasia, right ventricular hypertrophy, overriding aorta, right sided aorta in 25% of cases
Total anomalous pulmonary venous return (TAPVR)	Several forms exist, very difficult diagnosis in utero. Important to follow pulmonary veins that may empty into right atrium or ventricle. Right chambers usually increase. Both great vessels appear normal.
Transposition of the great arteries	Dependent on type; Complete transposition: ventricular and atrial connection concordant; aorta originating from the RV; pulmonary artery originating from the LV; ASD or VSD CCTGA: RA connects to the LV; LA connects to the RV; LV connects to the pulmonary artery; RV connects to the aorta
Tricuspid atresia	RV hypoplasia, hyperechoic thickened valve, immobile valve, lack of flow through valve, VSD, pulmonary atresia, TGA
Truncus arteriosus	Single vessel overriding a VSD, single truncal valve, regurgitant flow, thickened stenotic valve, right-sided and/or interrupted aortic arch
Univentricular heart/univentricular atrioventricular connection	Two atria, one ventricle, one or two atrioventricular valves, associated with transposition of the great vessels, aortic arch interruption or coarctation, stenotic pulmonary artery
Valvular atresia	Chamber dilatation proximal to atretic valve. Contralateral dilatation if no VSD is present to decompress volume overload.

ASD, atrial septal defect; *VSD*, ventricular septal defect; *MV*, mitral valve; *TV*, tricuspid valve; *LV*, left ventricle; *RA*, right atrium; *RV*, right ventricle.

Critical Thinking Questions

1. A patient presents to your department for a routing 24-week obstetric exam. During the examination, a four-chamber view demonstrates a possible VSD. What techniques can the sonographer use to confirm or rule out this defect?

   ANSWER: The pseudoventricular septal defect occurs when the septum has a parallel angle of incidence to the sound beam. This echo dropout is due to the lack of available sound returning to the transducer. Since the angle of incidence is so important, the first thing to do is obtain an image with the IVS perpendicular to the beam or at a 90-degree angle of incidence. This image, taken from the same patient during the exam, confirms an intact IVS. Color or power Doppler image is another method to rule out a VSD.

2. The four-chamber heart image is one of the most important views to obtain in a routine OB exam. This image, taken during a 20-week study, provides an adequate view of the heart. What technique parameters would increase the detail and the diagnostic confidence of the four-chamber finding?

   ANSWER: Because of the high heart rate, a clear image of the fetal heart may be difficult to obtain. Decreasing the persistence helps catch the heart quickly, decreasing the sector width increases detail because of the increase in line density, using a read zoom eliminates extra data, and decreasing the dynamic range all help in obtaining the optimal heart image. This image, taken during an 18-week exam, utilizes these technique parameters.

3. A patient presents for her 22-week examination. The clinician was able to obtain Doppler heart tones in the office; however, the heart sounded different than expected. To date, the patient has had no complaints and the pregnancy has been uneventful. There is no family history of CHD and she has not taken any medication that might cause a heart defect. The following apical four-chamber heart view was obtained during the exam. What fetal structures help identify the chambers? What type of CHD does this image demonstrate? What modes and views can the sonographer obtain to aid in diagnosing the heart defect?

   ANSWER: To identify the heart chambers on an axial view, use the transverse thoracic spine as a reference. In closest proximity to the spine is the left atrium with the aorta located between the heart and spine. *Ao,* aorta; *SP,* spine; *LA,* left atrium.

   This apical four-chamber view demonstrates a small right ventricle, which is part of right ventricular hypoplasia from pulmonary atresia (aka hypoplastic right heart). The spectral Doppler examination of the tricuspid and pulmonary valves demonstrate TV patency, possibly with regurgitation due to the distal obstruction. A small hyperechoic pulmonary artery images on the RVOT and long-axis view. Color or pulsed Doppler then confirms the absence of blood flow through the pulmonary artery. (Image courtesy of University of Colorado Hospital.)

REFERENCES

1. Drose JA. Embryology and physiology of the fetal heart. In: Drose JA, ed. *Fetal Echocardiography.* 2nd ed. St. Louis: Saunders Elsevier; 2010.
2. Männer J, Thrane L, Norozi K, et al. High-resolution in vivo imaging of the cross-sectional deformations of contracting embryonic heart loops using optical coherence tomography. *Dev Dyn.* 2008;237(4):953–961.
3. Moore KL, Persaud TVN. *The Developing Human: Clinically Oriented Embryology.* St. Louis: Saunders Elsevier; 2007.
4. Drose JA. Embryology and physiology of the fetal heart. In: Drose JA, ed. *Fetal Echocardiography.* 2nd ed. St. Louis: Saunders Elsevier; 2010:1–14.
5. American Institute of Ultrasound in Medicine. AIUM Practice Guideline for the Performance of the Fetal Echocardiography. 2010.Available at: http://www.aium.org/publications/guidelines/fetalEcho.pdf. Accessed May 2010.
6. Li H, Wei J, Ma Y, et al. Prenatal diagnosis of congenital fetal heart abnormalities and clinical analysis. *J Zhejiang Univ Sci B.* 2005;6(9):903–906.
7. Allan LD. Cardiac anatomy screening: what is the best time for screening in pregnancy? *Curr Opin Obstet Gynecol.* 2003;15:143–146.
8. Acherman RJ, Evans WN, Luna CF, et al. Prenatal detection of congenital heart disease in Southern Nevada: the need for universal fetal cardiac evaluation. *J Ultrasound Med.* 2007;26(12):1715–1719.
9. Lapierre C, Déry J, Guérin R, et al. Segmental approach to imaging of congenital heart disease. *Radiographics.* 2010;30(2):397–411.
10. Zimbleman S, Sheikh A. Fetal echocardiography and the routine obstetric sonogram. *JDMS.* 2007;23:143–149.
11. Anteby EY, Shimonovitz S, Yagal S. Fetal echocardiography: the identification of two of the pulmonary veins from the four-chamber view during the second trimester of pregnancy. *Ultrasound Obstet Gynecol.* 1994;4:208–210.
12. Zielinsky P, Piccoli A Jr, Gus E, et al. Dynamics of the pulmonary venous flow in the fetus and its association with vascular diameter. *Circulation.* 2003;108(19):2377–2380.
13. Devore GR. The prenatal diagnosis of congenital heart disease – a practical approach for the fetal sonographer. *J Clin Ultrasound.* 1985;13:229–245.
14. Devore GR, Donnerstein RL, Kleinman CS, et al. Fetal echocardiography. I: Normal anatomy as determined by realtime-directed M-mode ultrasound. *Am J Obstet Gynecol.* 1982;144:249–290.

15. Espinoza J, Kusanovic JP, Gonçalves LF, et al. A novel algorithm for comprehensive fetal echocardiography using 4-dimensional ultrasonography and tomographic imaging. *J Ultrasound Med.* 2006;25(8):947–956.

16. Turan S, Turan O, Baschat AA. Three- and four-dimensional fetal echocardiography. *Fetal Diagn Ther.* 2009;25(4):361–372.

17. Kusanovic JP, Nien JK, Gonçalves LF, et al. The use of inversion mode and 3D manual segmentation in volume measurement of fetal fluid-filled structures: comparison with virtual organ computer-aided analysis (VOCAL™). *Ultrasound Obstet Gynecol.* 2008;31(2):177–186.

18. Benacerraf BR. Inversion mode display of 3D sonography: applications in obstetric and gynecologic imaging. *AJR.* 2006:187:874–965.

19. Acar P, Dulac Y, Taktak A, et al. Real-time three-dimensional fetal echocardiology using matrix transducer. *Prenatal Diagnosis.* 2005;25:370–375.

20. Villavicencio KL. Fetal arrhythmias. In: Drose JA, ed. *Fetal Echocardiography.* 2nd ed. St. Louis: Saunders Elsevier; 2010:306–323.

21. Simpson JM. Fetal arrhythmias. *Ultrasound Obstet Gynecol.* 2006;27:599–606.

22. Strasburger JF, Cuneo BF, Michon MM, et al. Amiodarone therapy for drug refractory fetal tachycardia. *Circulation.* 2004;109;375.

23. Simpson LL. Fetal supraventricular tachycardias: diagnosis and management. *Semin Perinatol.* 2000;24:360–372.

24. Fish F, Benson DJ. Disorders of cardiac rhythm and conduction. In: Allen HD, Gutgesell H, Clark EB, et al., eds. *Heart Disease in Infants, Children and Adolescents.* 6th ed. Philadelphia: Lippincott; 2001:482–533.

25. Armstrong WF, Ryan T. *Feigenbaum's Echocardiography.* 7th ed. Philadelphia: Lippincott Williams & Wilkins:2005.

26. Triendman JK, Walsh EP, Saul JP. Response of fetal tachycardia to transplacental procainamide. *Cardiol Young.* 1991;6:235.

27. Strasburger JF, Cuneo BF, Michon MM, et al. Amiodarone therapy for drug refractory fetal tachycardia. *Circulation.* 2004;109;375.

28. Simpson JM, Sharland GK. Fetal tachycardias: management and outcome of 127 consecutive cases. *Heart.* 1998;79:576.

29. Jaeggo ET, Hornberger LK, Smallhorn JF, et al. Prenatal diagnosis of complete atrioventricular block associated with structural heart disease: combined experience of two tertiary care centers and review of the literature. *Ultrasound Obstet Gynecol.* 2006;26:16–21.

30. Berg C, Geipel A, Kohl T, et al. Atrioventricular block detected in fetal life: associated anomalies and prognostic markers. *Ultrasound Obstet Gynecol.* 2005;26:4–15.

31. Mavroudis C, Backer CL, Idriss FS. Ventricular septal defect. In: Mavroudis C, Backer CL, eds. *Pediatric Cardiac Surgery.* 2nd ed. St. Louis: Mosby-Year Book; 1994:201–221.

32. Fontana RS, Edwards JE. Ventricular septal defect. In: Fontana RS, Edwards JE, eds. *Congenital Cardiac Disease. A review of 357 cases studied pathologically.* Philadelphia: WB Suanders; 1962:640–669.

33. Armstrong WF. Congenital heart disease. In: Feigenbaum H, ed. *Echocardiography.* 7th ed. Lippincott Williams & Wilkins; 2009.

34. Ramaciotti C, Vetter JV, Bornemeier RA, et al. Prevalence, relation to spontaneous closure and association of muscular ventricular septal defects with other cardiac defects. *J Thorac Cardiovasc Surg.* 1980;12:485–493.

35. Copel JA, Pilu G, Green J, et al. Fetal echocardiographic screening for congenital heart disease: the importance of the four-chamber view. *Am J Obstet Gynecol.* 1987;157:648–655.

36. Jaffe CC, Atkinson P, Raylor JKW. Physical parameters affecting the visibility of small ventricular septal defects using two-dimensional echocardiography. *Invest Radiol.* 1979;14:149–155.

37. Paladinni D, Russo M, Vassallo M, et al. The "in-plane" view of the inter-ventricular septum: a new approach to the characterization of ventricular septal defects in the fetus. *Prenat Diagn.* 2003;23:1052–1055.

38. Chao RC, Shih-Chu HE, Hsieh KS, et al. Fluctuation of interventricular shunting in a fetus with an isolated ventricular septal defect. *Am Heart J.* 1994;127:955–958.

39. Crawford DC, Chita SK, Allan LD. Prenatal detection of congenital heart disease: factors influencing obstetrical management and survival. *Am J Obstet Gynecol.* 1988;159:352–356.

40. Benacerraf BR, Pober BR, Sanders SP. Accuracy of fetal echocardiography. *Radiology.* 1987;165:847–849.

41. Samanek M. Children with congenital heart disease. Probability of natural survival. *Pediatr Cardiol.* 1992;13:152–158.

42. Hoffman JIE, Christianson MA. Children with congenital heart disease in a cohort of 19,502 births with long term followup. *Am J Cardiol.* 1978;42:641–647.

43. Fyler DC. Atrial septal defect secundum. In: Fyler DC, ed. *Nadas' Pediatric Cardiology.* Philadelphia: Hanley and Belfus; 1992:513–524.

44. VanMeter C, LeBlan JG, Culpepper WJ, et al. Partial anomalous pulmonary venous return. *Circulation.* 1990;82(5s):IV195–198.

45. Holt M, Oran S. Familial heart disease with skeletal malformations. *Br Heart J.* 1960;22:236–242.

46. Mitchell SC, Karones SB, Berendes HW. Congenital heart disease in 56,109 births: incidence and natural history. *Circulation.* 1971;43:323–332.

47. Drethen W, Peiper PG, van der Tuuk K, et al. Cardiac complications relating to pregnancy and recurrence of disease in the offspring of women with atrioventricular septal defects. *Eur Heart J.* 200;26:581–587.

48. Freeman SB, Taft LF, Dooley KJ, et al. Population-based study of congenital heart defects in Down syndrome. *Am J Med Genet.* 1998;80(3):213–217.

49. Calabro R, Limongelli G. Complete atrioventricular canal. *Orphanet J Rare Dis.* 2006;1:8.

50. Symth BC. Atrioventricular septal defects. In: Drose JA, ed. *Fetal Echocardiography.* 2nd ed. St. Louis: Saunders Elsevier; 2010:119–130.

51. Tongsong T, Sittiwangkul R, Khunamornpong S, et al. Prenatal sonographic features of isoloated hypoplastic left heart syndrome. *J Clin Ultrasound.* 2005;33:367–371.

52. Yagel S, Cohen S, Baruch M. First and early 2nd trimester fetal heart screening. *Curr Opin Obstet Gynecol.* 2007;109:376–383.

53. Todros T, Paladini D, Chiappa E, et al. Pulmonary stenosis and atresia with intact ventricular septum during prenatal life. *Ultrasound Obstet Gynecol.* 2003;21:228–233.

54. Goor DA, Lillehei CW. *Congenital Malformations of the Heart*. New York: Grune & Stratton; 1975.

55. Correa-Villasenor A, Cragan J, Kucik J, et al. The Metropolitan Atlanta Congenital Defects Program: 35 Years of Birth Defects Surveillance at the Centers for Disease Control and Prevention. *Birth Defects Res A Clin Mol Teratol*. 2003 Sep;67(9):617–624.

56. Lai YQ, Zhou QW, Wei H, et al. Intrapulmonary channel for one-stage correction of aortic arch obstruction. *Asian Cardiovasc Thorac Ann*. 2006;14(5):402–406.

57. Peterson RE, Levi DS, Williams RJ, et al. Echocardiographic predictors of outcome in fetuses with pulmonary atresia with intact ventricular septum. *J Am Soc Echocardiologr*. 2006;19:1393–1400.

58. Wald RM, Tham EB, McCrindle BW, et al. Outcome after prenatal diagnosis of tricuspid atresia: a multicenter experience. *Am Heart J*. 2007;153:772–778.

59. Allan LD, Chita SK, Anderson RH, et al. Coarctation of the aorta in prenatal life: an echocardiographic, anatomical and functional study. *Br Heart J*. 1988;59:356–360.

60. Hüdaoglu O, Kurul S, Cakmakci H, et al. Aorta coarctation presenting with intracranial aneurysm rupture. *J Paediatr Child Health*. 2006;42(7–8):477–479.

61. Rosenthal E. Coarctation of the aorta from fetus to adult: Curable disease process or lifelong disease process. *Heart Online*. Available at: http://heart.bmj.com/cgi/content/full/91/11/1495. Accessed October 23, 2011.

62. Vogel M, Vernon MM, McElhinney DB, et al. Fetal diagonis of interrupted aortic arch. *Am J Cardiol*. 2010;105(5):725–734.

63. Ferencz C, Rubin JD, McCarte RJ, et al. Cardiac and noncardiac malformations: observations in a population based study. *Teratology*. 1987;35:367–378.

64. Aboulhosn J, Child JS. Left ventricular outflow obstruction: subaortic stenosis, bicuspid aortic valve, supravalvar aortic stenosis, and coarctation of the aorta. *Circulation*. 2006;114:2412–2422.

65. Brown JW, Ruzmetov M, Okada Y, et al. Outcomes in patients with interrupted aortic arch and associated anomalies: a 20-year experience. *Eur J Cardiothorac Surg*. 2006;29(5):666–673.

66. Li H, Meng T, Shang T, et al. Fetal echocardiographic screening in twins for congenital heart diseases. *Chin Med J (Engl)*. 2007;120(16):1391–1394.

67. Bianchi DW, Cromblehome RM, D'Alton ME. Coarctation of the aorta. *Fetology*. 2000;46:365–369.

68. Moene RJ, Oppenheimer Dekker A, Wenink ACG. Relation between aortic arch hypoplasia of variable severity and central muscular ventricular septal defects. *Am J Cardiol*. 1981;48:111–116.

69. Poon LCY, Huggon IC, Zidere V, et al. Tetralogy of Fallot in the fetus in the current era. *Ultrasound Obstet Gynecol*. 2007;29:625–627.

70. Bolger DM. Tetralogy of Fallot. In: Drose JA, ed. *Fetal Echocardiography*. 2nd ed. St. Louis: Saunders-Elsevier; 2010:211–222.

71. Yacobi S, Ornoy A. Is lithium a real teratogen? What can we conclude from the prosepective versus retrospective studies? A review. *Isr J Psychiatry Relat Sci*. 2008;45(2):95–106.

72. Pinilla-Lozano M, Calzada MD, Lázaro-Aláez A. Prenatal diagnosis of Ebstein's anomaly. *Rev Esp Cardiol*. 2008;61(9):971.

73. Carlson BC. Prenatal diagnosis of congenitally corrected transposition of the great arteries. *JDMS*. 2007;23:153–156.

74. Martins P, Castela E. Transposition of the great arteries. *Orphanet J Rare Dis*. 2008;3(27):1750–1772.

75. Barbara DW, Edwards WD, Connolly HM, et al. Surgical pathology of 104 tricuspid valves (2000–2005) with classic right-sided Ebstein's malformation. *Cardiovasc Pathol*. 2008;17(3):166–171.

76. Warnes CA. Transposition of the great arteries. *Circulation*. 2006;114:2699–2709.

77. Vinals F, Ascenzo R, Poblete P, et al. Simple approach to prenatal diagnosis of transposition of the great arteries. *Ultrasound Obstet Gynecol*. 2006;28:22–25.

78. Rutledge JM, Nihill MR, Fraser CD, et al. Outcome of 121 patients with congenitally corrected transposition of the great arteries: ventricle to pulmonary artery connection. *Semin Thorac Cardiovassc Surg*. 1995;7:139–144.

79. Volpe P, Paladini D, Marasini M, et al. Common arterial trunk in the fetus: characteristics, associations and outcome in a multicentre series of 23 cases. *Heart*. 2003;89:1437–1441.

80. Allan LD, Crawford DC, Anderson RH. Spectrum of congenital heart disease detected echocardiographically in prenatal life. *Br Heart J*. 1984;54:523–526.

81. Artrip JH, Sauer H, Campbell DN, et al. Biventricular repair in double outlet right ventricle: surgical results based on the STS-EATCS International Nomenclature classification. *Eur J Cardiothorac Surg*. 2006;545–550.

82. Gedikbasi AG, Oztarhan KO, Gul AG, et al. Double outlet right ventricle: prenatal diagnosis and fetal outcome. *Ultrasound Obstet Gynecol*. 2007;30:598–599.

83. Ferencz C, Rubin JD, McCarter RJ. Congenital heart disease: prevalence at livebirth. The Baltimore-Washington Infant Study. *Am J Epidemiol*. 1985;121:31–36.

84. Paladini D, Sgalvo G, DeRobertis V, et al. Anatomy association and outcome of prenatally detected double-outlet right ventricle. *Ultrasound Obstet Gynecol*. 2007;30:408.

85. Uzun O, Wilson DG, Vuganic GM, et al. Cardiac tumors in children. *Orphan J Rare Dis*. 2007;2:1–4.

86. Lacey SR, Donofrio MT. Fetal cardiac tumors: prenatal diagnosis and outcome. *Pediatr Cardiol*. 2007;28:61–67.

23 Normal and Abnormal Fetal Limbs

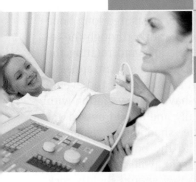

Molly Siemens

OBJECTIVES

Describe the normal sonographic appearance of the fetal skeletal system

Summarize measurement techniques of the fetal long bones

Evaluate limbs for abnormal size and appearance

Identify fetal skeletal abnormalities and their associated findings

Discuss differential diagnoses for pathology visualized

KEY TERMS

skeletal dysplasia | thanatophoric dysplasia | achondroplasia | achondrogenesis | short rib-polydactyly syndrome | asphyxiating thoracic dysplasia | Ellis-van Creveld syndrome | osteogenesis imperfecta | camptomelic dysplasia | congenital hypophosphatasia | dysostosis | polydactyly

GLOSSARY

Acromelia Shortening of the most distal portion of a fetal limb

Mesomelia Abnormal shortening of the middle portion of a limb

Micromelia Abnormally short limb

Platyspondyly Flattened vertebral bodies with a decreased distance between the endplates

Polydactyly Condition of having more than the normal number of digits on a hand or foot

Rhizomelia Shortening of the most proximal portion of a fetal limb

Syndactyly Fusion of soft tissue or bony segments of fetal digits

Talipes Abnormal position of the fetal foot and ankle

The routine ultrasound examination includes measurement of the fetal femur to determine gestational age (GA). Nonroutine measurements of other long bones, such as the humerus, also help to determine gestational age. When it becomes difficult to measure the femur or humerus, or if a skeletal abnormality is suspected, the radius, ulna, tibia, and fibula provide alternate dating measurements. Nomograms are available for most bones from the 12th week to term (see Appendixes).

In addition to dating the pregnancy, measurement and evaluation of fetal long bones documents their existence or absence and whether they are properly mineralized or formed, and also determines their position in relationship to the rest of the limb. In the presence of a suspected skeletal abnormality, the sonographer should obtain a detailed family history for any other genetically transmitted skeletal abnormalities. A detailed sonographic anatomic examination aids in diagnosis, as skeletal abnormalities are often characteristic of syndromes involving multiple organ systems.

This chapter contains information on normal and abnormal development, sonographic assessment of fetal limbs, and the most prevalent fetal limb malformations with their associated anomalies.

NORMAL FETAL LIMBS

ANATOMY

Fetal limb buds visualize as early as 8 weeks with endovaginal ultrasound, with the lower buds imaging before the upper buds.[1] Limbs fully develop and primary ossification centers image at 10 weeks. Movement of the limbs and terminal phalanges of the hands visualize at 11 weeks.[2] From 12 weeks on, the fetal long bones of the femur, humerus, radius, ulna, tibia, and fibula can be accurately measured through identification of their high-amplitude reflection with corresponding posterior shadowing. The high-amplitude reflection is generated by the calcium content of the bone (Fig. 23-1).

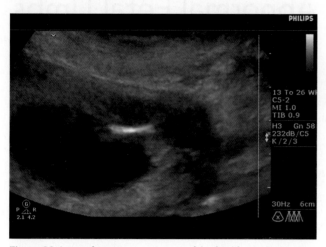

Figure 23-1 Late first–trimester image of the fetal femur. To increase the visualization of the femur, a decrease in dynamic range helps highlight the shades of white of the early ossified femur.

Secondary ossification centers, or epiphyses, can be visualized by ultrasound and are separated from the shaft of the fetal long bone by a layer of cartilage (Fig. 23-2). The distal femoral epiphysis, visible by 32 to 35 weeks, and the proximal tibial epiphysis, visible by 34 or 35 weeks, are the two most common secondary ossification centers visualized. The proximal humeral epiphysis may only be visualized at term. Visualization of these epiphyses aids in the determination of fetal maturity in late pregnancy.[3] Visualization of these structures before the expected time frame, however, should prompt the sonographer to further evaluate the fetus for possible abnormality.

The metacarpals and phalanges of the hands image in the second trimester, with ossification of the carpal bones occurring after birth. The phalanges of the foot and the talus, calcaneus, and pubis of the ankle also begin to ossify during the second trimester. The rest of the tarsal bones ossify after birth.

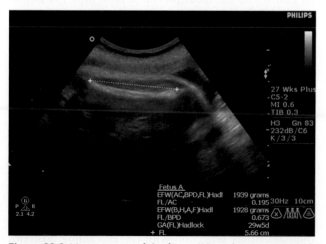

Figure 23-2 Measurement of the femur (29 weeks' gestation) with calipers placed at edge of hyperechoic shaft excluding diaphyses.

SONOGRAPHIC TECHNIQUE

The femur is the most commonly measured long bone and is identified by scanning inferiorly through the fetal thorax to the level of the bladder and rotating the transducer until the longest axis of the shaft appears. Normally the shaft is straight, symmetrical, and evenly ossified, but the contour may have slight variation with a straighter appearance laterally and a mild bowed appearance medially.[4] Acoustic shadowing visualized posterior and perpendicular to the bone verifies correctness of the scanning plane. To avoid measuring the bones of the calf, the sonographer should slightly rock the transducer back and forth to ensure that there is only a single bone in the same plane.

Measurements of the femur are taken when the transducer is perpendicular to the shaft to avoid artificially shortening the limb. Calipers are placed at opposite ends of the shaft from outer margin to outer margin, at the junction of bone and cartilage, excluding the femoral head and distal epiphyses (Figs. 23-2 and 16-10).[3,5] Measure the anterior-lying femur, as the artifactually bowed posterior femur results in an inaccurately short length. On average, the fetal femur grows approximately 3 millimeters (mm) per week from 14 to 27 weeks and slows to approximately 1 mm per week in the third trimester.[4] The accuracy of this measurement decreases with gestational age from +/− 1 week in the second trimester to +/− 3.5 weeks at term.[5] It has been shown that femoral length varies according to maternal height and weight.[6]

The humerus visualizes through lateral movement of the transducer from the fetal thorax or rotating the transducer from the level of the scapula until the longest axis of the bone appears. Rocking the transducer slightly back and forth guarantees the visualized bone is the humerus and not the radius or ulna. The humerus has a similar appearance to the femur: a straight, symmetrical, and evenly ossified shaft with posterior and perpendicular shadowing. Measurements of the humerus are taken when the transducer is perpendicular to the shaft and calipers are placed at opposite ends of the shaft (Fig. 16-11).[5]

Measurement of other long bones helps narrow the diagnosis of specific skeletal dysplasias, and nomograms exist for each of them. The tibia and fibula can be visualized by moving the transducer inferiorly down the leg from the femoral shaft (Fig. 23-3). The tibia is the thicker of the two bones and is oriented medially; the fibula lies laterally. To visualize the bones of the lower arm, move the transducer inferiorly down the arm from the humeral shaft. Both the distal radius and ulna should end at the same point, with the ulna being the longer of the two bones (Fig. 23-4).

Fetal hands and feet should be imaged to document their presence or absence. A normal appearance of the fetal hand includes unossified hypoechoic carpal

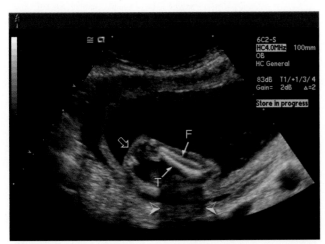

Figure 23-3 Normal alignment of tibia *(t)* and fibula *(f)* in the second trimester. The foot *(open arrow)* is in normal perpendicular alignment to the tibia and fibula. Note the posterior shadowing *(arrowheads)* which is a characteristic finding when imaging long bones.

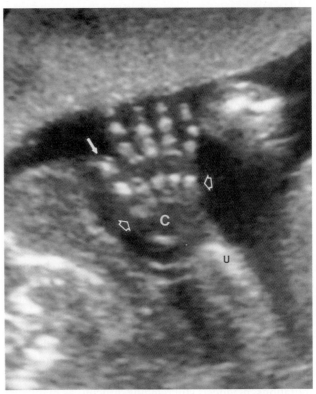

Figure 23-5 Hand demonstrating phalanges of the four fingers and thumb *(white arrow)* and the five metacarpals *(open arrows)*. *C,* carpus; *U,* ulna.

bones, five hyperechoic metacarpal bones, and five different independent digits of varying lengths, each with three ossified phalanges (except the thumb, which has two) (Fig. 23-5).[7] Slight flexion of the hand and wrist is normal, but the hand should always be observed in flexion and extension, as a consistently fixed position is abnormal.[7] A similar appearance of the foot should be identified, including the five tarsal bones and five independent digits, each with two phalanges (Fig. 23-6). Several studies have demonstrated that the fetal foot has a characteristic pattern of normal growth and can be used to accurately determine gestational age when other parameters are inaccurate because of other abnormal conditions.[8,9]

Multiple technical factors may inhibit the sonographer's ability to visualize fetal limbs. Oligohydramnios

results in poor overall resolution and a crowded fetus in which limbs are difficult to visualize. With polyhydramnios, the fetus can be very active or the limb may lie beyond the focal range of the transducer. Limbs located in the near field can be difficult to delineate. Having the patient change position, empty her bladder, or take a short walk can often improve visualization by

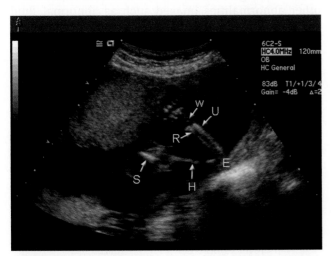

Figure 23-4 Normal alignment of the ulna *(U)* and radius *(R)*. The ulna extends farther into the elbow *(E)* than the radius; however, the radius and ulna end at the same point at the distal portion of the limb. Also note the contrast between the hyperechoic radius and ulna and the nonossified bones of the wrist *(w)*. *H,* humerus; *S,* scapula.

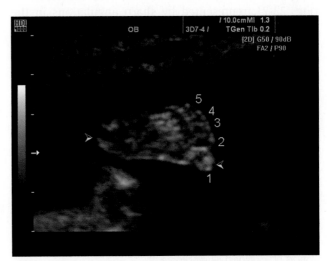

Figure 23-6 Second-trimester image of a foot demonstrating all five digits *(1 to 5)*. While this orientation is optimal for a heel-to-toe distance measurement *(arrowheads)*, this orientation can make it difficult to visualize individual digits or metatarsal bones. (Image courtesy of Philips Medical Systems, Bothell, WA.)

changing the fetal position. Patience is often the key in obtaining a good diagnostic scan.

ABNORMAL FETAL LIMBS

Skeletal dysplasia is the abnormal development of the cartilaginous and osseous tissues, resulting in bones that appear shortened, thin, or deformed, or that fail to form at all.[10] Fetuses with long bone measurements more than two standard deviations below normal require a detailed anatomic scan.[10] Some syndromes are uniformly lethal, and others are lethal in their more severe forms (Table 23-1).

While sonography is the most common method of identifying skeletal dysplasias, the diagnosis may be difficult to make because of their rarity[10] or similar findings.[11] Still others may not be severe enough to be demonstrated in utero. Diagnosis depends on many factors, such as the time frame in which the ultrasound exam was performed[10] or the presence of a family history of skeletal dysplasia.[12] A positive family history can help identify the skeletal dysplasia and determine the specific type, since many disorders inherit in an autosomal dominant or recessive fashion.[13] In new or spontaneous mutations, diagnosis still remains difficult, as many disorders have similar prenatal findings.[11]

SONOGRAPHIC TECHNIQUE

Skill, patience, and a complete and accurate patient history are the major ingredients for a thorough ultrasound examination, especially when there is suspicion of a skeletal dysplasia. When scanning an at-risk fetus, the sonographer should first document and image each limb that can be imaged. Long bones should be evaluated for bowing, which may result in a short-for-gestational age measurement, and for fractures (Fig. 23-7), represented by sharp angulations in the midshaft of the bone, which may also produce shorter-than-expected measurements. Care should be taken not to utilize measurements that include artificial

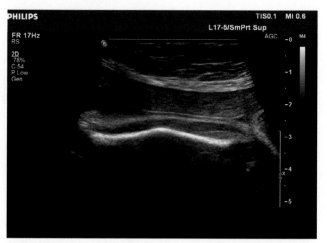

Figure 23-7 Fetal femur demonstrating midshaft bowing corresponding to a fracture. (Image courtesy of Philips Medical Systems, Bothell, WA.)

bowing of a limb or images that include shadowing from overlying fetal limbs that artificially shorten a long bone or create a gap that mimics a fracture. Abnormal skeletal mineralization may make the cranium or long bones difficult to visualize or make them appear thin or unevenly mineralized.[13]

The sonographer should determine the dominant type of limb shortening visualized. Short-limbed dysplasias are classified into four descriptive categories. In rhizomelia, only the proximal portion of the extremity is shortened (i.e., the humerus or femur). Mesomelia is the shortening of the middle or intermediate segment of an extremity (i.e., the radius, ulna, tibia, or fibula). Acromelia is the shortening of the distal portion of an extremity (i.e., the bones of the hands and feet). Micromelia is the shortening of an entire extremity (Table 23-2).[4]

In addition to documenting long bone appearance and length, the sonographer should capture any other abnormalities imaged such as abnormal fluid volumes, an abnormal number of digits, or any facial

TABLE 23-1
Lethal Skeletal Dysplasias
Achondrogenesis
Asphyxiating thoracic dysplasia*
Camptomelic dysplasia*
Ellis-van Creveld syndrome*
Homozygous achondroplasia
Hypophosphatasia*
Osteogenesis imperfecta Type II
Short rib-polydactyly syndrome
Thrombocytopenia-absent radius syndrome*
Thanatophoric dysplasia
VACTERL association*

*Mildly affected patients may survive.

TABLE 23-2	
Dominant Category of Limb Shortening in Skeletal Dysplasias	
Skeletal Dysplasia	**Dominant Category**
Achondrogenesis	Micromelia
Achondroplasia	Rhizomelia
Asphyxiating thoracic dysplasia	Mesomelia
Camptomelic dysplasia	Mesomelia, rhizomelia
Congenital hypophosphatasia	Micromelia
Ellis-van Creveld syndrome	Rhizomelia
Hypophosphatasia	Micromelia
Osteogenesis imperfecta	Micromelia
Short rib-polydactyly syndrome	Micromelia
Thanatophoric dysplasia	Micromelia

or cardiac defects.[13] Also evaluate the fetal skull for changes in shape. Craniosynostosis is a disorder defined as the premature fusion of one or more cranial sutures that can be found as an isolated incident caused by external forces such as premature descent into the maternal pelvic cavity,[14] or in many genetic syndromes and chromosomal disorders such as Apert's syndrome.[14] The most severe form of craniosynostosis is Kleeblattschadel or cloverleaf deformity and is associated with thanatophoric dysplasia.[15] Skull evaluation may also note micrognathia, an abnormally small lower jaw; abnormally shaped ears; or frontal bossing, an unusually prominent forehead (Fig. 23-8).[13]

Lethal skeletal dysplasias are often accompanied by pulmonary hypoplasia—a reduction in the number of lung cells, airways, and alveoli resulting in reduced lung volume and respiratory failure.[16,17] Pulmonary hypoplasia can be caused by pregnancy complications such as oligohydramnios or secondary to congenital disorders such as thanatophoric dysplasia and asphyxiating thoracic dysplasia.[13,16,17] Sonographically, pulmonary hypoplasia classically presents with a bell-shaped, narrow thorax.[17] The femur length/abdominal circumference (FL/AC) and the thoracic circumference/abdominal circumference (TC/AC) ratios can be utilized to rule out an abnormally small thorax. An FL/AC of less than 0.16 or a TC/AC of less than 0.79 indicate a hyperplastic thorax.[13,18,19]

Endovaginal ultrasound has allowed for earlier visualization of fetal limbs and limb abnormalities. First-trimester ultrasound can also help visualize an increased nuchal translucency, which is associated not only with chromosomal abnormalities but with certain cardiac defects and skeletal dysplasias.[2,20] Any abnormal findings can be verified with genetic amniocentesis if a genetically transmitted skeletal dysplasia

is suspected. Early detection of a lethal skeletal dysplasia gives parents the option of termination before viability. If parents choose to continue the pregnancy, it also allows physicians to prepare for mode of delivery (i.e., cesarean section if an abnormal skull shape is visualized) and possible delivery in a tertiary care center (Table 23-3).

TABLE 23-3	
Sonographic Findings in Skeletal Dysplasia	
Curved or bowed long bones	Camptomelic dysplasia
	Hypophosphatasia
	Osteogenesis imperfecta
	Thanatophoric dysplasia
Hypomineralization	Achondrogenesis
	Camptomelic dysplasia
	Hypophosphatasia
	Osteogenesis imperfecta
	Short rib-polydactyly syndrome
	Thanatophoric dysplasia
Narrow thorax	Achondrogenesis type I
	Achondroplasia
	Asphyxiating thoracic dysplasia
	Camptomelic dysplasia
	Short rib-polydactyly syndrome
	Thanatophoric dysplasia
Polydactyly	Asphyxiating thoracic dysplasia*
	Ellis-van Creveld syndrome
	Short rib-polydactyly syndrome
	VACTERL association*
Radial aplasia or hypoplasia	Holt-Oram syndrome
	Thrombocytopenia-absent radius syndrome
	VACTERL association
Bone fractures	Achondrogenesis
	Hypophosphatasia
	Osteogenesis imperfecta
Heart disease	Asphyxiating thoracic dysplasia
	Ellis-van Creveld syndrome
	Hold-Oram syndrome
	Short rib-polydactyly syndrome*
	VACTERL association*
Macrocephaly	Achondroplasia
	Camptomelic dysplasia*
	Thanatophoric dysplasia

*Does not occur in all cases

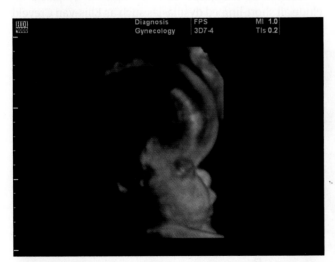

Figure 23-8 Three-dimensional rendering of the fetal profile demonstrating frontal bossing associated with craniosynostosis. (Image courtesy of Philips Medical Systems, Bothell, WA.)

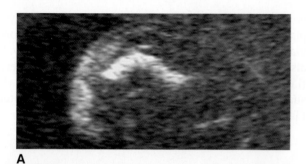

A

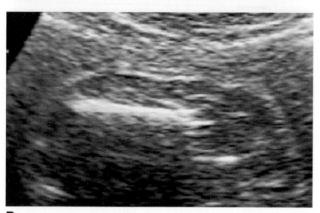

B

Figure 23-9 Thanatophoric dysplasia. Sonographic appearance of femur in type 1 **(A)** and type II **(B)**.

SKELETAL DYSPLASIAS

Skeletal dysplasias are complex disorders. Here we describe several of the more commonly seen dysplasias. Fetal sonography may or may not show some or all of these reported features. A thorough examination aids in the diagnosis of a general skeletal dysplasia and may on occasion even provide a definitive diagnosis.

THANATOPHORIC DYSPLASIA

Thanatophoric dysplasia (TD) is the most common form of lethal skeletal dysplasia,[13,19] occurring in 1 in

PATHOLOGY BOX 23-1

Anomalies Associated with Thanatophoric Dwarfism

Curved or bowed long bones
Hypomineralization
Macrocephaly
Frontal bossing
Narrow thorax

4,000 to 1 in 15,000 births.[21] *Thanatophoric* in Greek means "death bearing."[22] It occurs twice as often in males as in females.[23,24] Previously the etiology was unknown, but it is now believed to be transmitted in an autosomal dominant fashion by mutations of fibroblast growth factor receptor 3 (FGFR3).[22,24] The risk of recurrence is estimated at approximately 2%.[24] Parents of these fetuses are of normal stature.[21]

There are two types of TD. Type I is the most common type[22,] and is characterized by extreme rhizomelia (in most cases two standard deviations below the mean for gestational age), bowed long bones with a "telephone receiver" appearance (Fig. 23-9), normal trunk length, platyspondyly, and frontal bossing (prominent forehead) (Fig. 23-10). Type II is characterized by straighter long bones, taller vertebral bodies, and Kleeblattschadel (cloverleaf skull).[21,22,24] Other abnormalities observed with TD include a narrow thorax with a protruding abdomen—giving it a "champagne cork appearance"—horseshoe kidney, hydronephrosis, cardiac defects such as atrial septal defects, facial features such as hypertelorism, and imperforate anus.[21,22,24,25] Polyhydramnios is also associated with thanatophoric dysplasia and can lead to premature labor.[24] The prognosis for TD is poor, with most fetuses being stillborn or dying within hours after birth from respiratory failure from pulmonary hypoplasia.[21,22,24]

Differential diagnoses for thanatophoric dysplasia include all short-limbed dysplasias such as Ellis-van Creveld

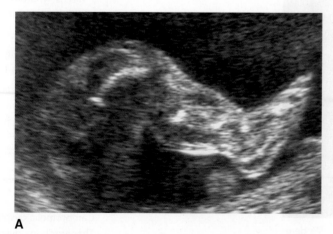

A

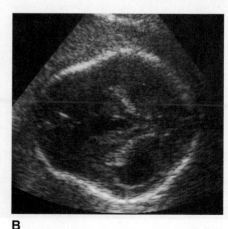

B

Figure 23-10 The two types of thanatophoric dysplasia. Type I **(A)** shows bowed femurs; type II **(B)** shows straight femora and a cloverleaf skull deformity.

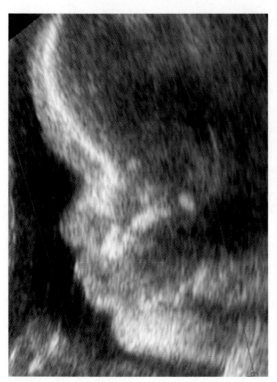

Figure 23-11 Facial profile of a 32-week gestational fetus with achondroplasia demonstrating frontal bossing.

syndrome, asphyxiating thoracic dysplasia, and short rib-polydactyly syndrome.[24,26] If type II TD is suspected, care should be taken to rule out syndromes that are associated with cloverleaf skull such as Apert syndrome.[24]

ACHONDROPLASIA

Achondroplasia is the most common nonlethal type of dwarfism[27] and occurs equally in males and females.[25] It is inherited in an autosomal dominant fashion caused by a spontaneous mutation in the FGFR3 gene.[25,28] Characteristic features are rhizomelic limb bowing, frontal bossing (Fig. 23-11) with a low nasal bridge, and a "trident" configuration of the hand (increased space between the third and fourth digits).[15,26,28] Macrocephaly and hydrocephaly may also be noted.[15,25] The prognosis for a child with achondroplasia is good; they can be expected to have normal intelligence and life expectancy with orthopedic problems being the only medical concern.[28] Differential diagnoses for achondroplasia include thanatophoric dysplasia, achondrogenesis, and osteogenesis imperfecta.[28]

PATHOLOGY BOX 23-2

Anomalies Associated With Achondroplasia

Macrocephaly
Hydrocephaly
Frontal bossing
Narrow thorax

PATHOLOGY BOX 23-3

Anomalies Associated With Achondrogenesis

Hypomineralization
Narrow thorax
Bone fractures
Micromelia
Micrognathia

ACHONDROGENESIS

Achondrogenesis is a rare and lethal skeletal dysplasia that can be separated into two different categories. Type I, or Parenti-Fraccaro, is autosomal recessive and characterized by extreme micromelia, a large head, short and thin ribs that may have fractures, and poor ossification of the skull, spine, and pelvic bones (Fig. 23-12).[29,30] Type II, or Langer-Saldino, is autosomal dominant and characterized by a prominent forehead, a flat face with micrognathia, the absence of rib fractures, and less severe mineralization of fetal bones and less severe micromelia.[29,30] Some fetuses may exhibit hydrops.[15] Achondrogenesis is lethal because of pulmonary hypoplasia.[29] Differential diagnoses include osteogenesis imperfecta type II and hypophosphatasia.[29]

SHORT RIB-POLYDACTYLY SYNDROME

This rare condition has an autosomal recessive transmission and no gender preference. It is characterized by micromelic dwarfism, short and horizontal ribs with a narrow thorax, and polydactyly (Fig. 23-13). Other findings can include syndactyly; cardiac, gastrointestinal, genital, and urogenital malformations; cleft lip and/or cleft palate; hydrops; and polyhydramnios. There are three types of short rib-polydactyly syndrome: Saldino-Noonan (type I), Majewski (type II), and Naumoff (type III). All three types are lethal, as affected fetuses die within a few hours after birth from pulmonary hypoplasia. The differential diagnoses include thanatophoric dysplasia, osteogenesis imperfecta, and camptomelic dysplasia.[25,31]

PATHOLOGY BOX 23-4

Anomalies Associated With Short Rib-Polydactyly Syndrome

Narrow thorax
Hypomineralization
Polycactyly/syndactyly
Gastrointestinal/genital/urogenital malformations
Cleft lip/palate

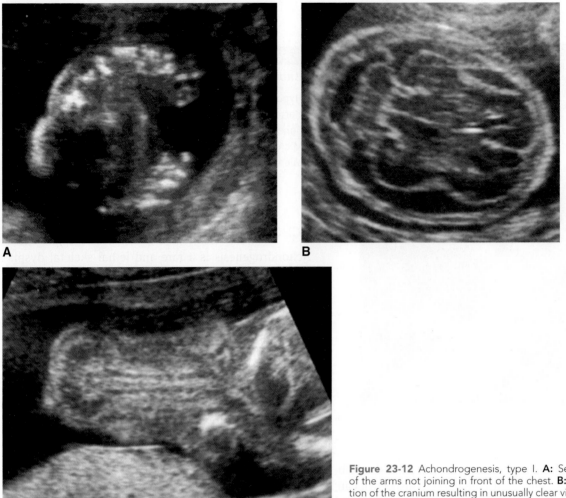

Figure 23-12 Achondrogenesis, type I. **A:** Severe micromelia of the arms not joining in front of the chest. **B:** Hypomineralization of the cranium resulting in unusually clear visualization of the brain. **C:** Longitudinal image of the spine demonstrating almost absent mineralization of the spine.

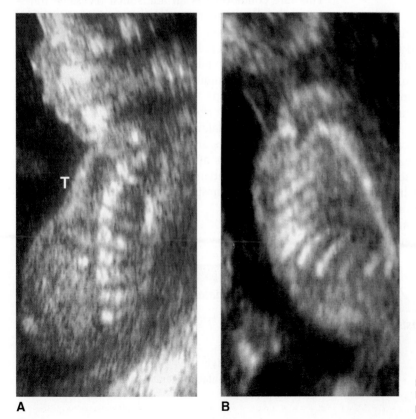

Figure 23-13 Short rib-polydactyly syndrome. **A:** Parasagittal image showing short ribs and a hypoplastic thorax (T). **B:** Normal fetus for comparison.

Anomalies Associated With Asphyxiating Thoracic Dysplasia

Narrow thorax
Polydactyly
Pelvic/renal anomalies

Anomalies Associated With Ellis-van Creveld Syndrome

Polydactyly
Short limbs
Narrow thorax
Heart malformations
Dysplastic nails/teeth
Abnormal upper lip

ASPHYXIATING THORACIC DYSPLASIA

Asphyxiating thoracic dysplasia, also known as Jeune syndrome, is a rare autosomal recessive disorder.[26,32,33] Patients with Jeune syndrome present with an extremely narrow thorax, rhizomelic limbs that are not as short as other similar dysplasias, polydactyly, and pelvic and renal anomalies.[25,32,33] Most cases are lethal because of pulmonary hypoplasia, but some patients have survived with the assistance of corrective surgical thoracic expansion. Some survivors later succumb to renal insufficiency because of associated renal anomalies.[33] The differential diagnosis for this disorder is Ellis-van Creveld syndrome.[32]

ELLIS-VAN CREVELD SYNDROME

Ellis-van Creveld Syndrome (EvC), also known as chondroectodermal dysplasia, is a rare autosomal recessive disorder that affects males and females equally but is frequently found in small communities where inbreeding may be prominent, such as those of the old-order Amish.[26,34] This dysplasia is characterized by short limbs, short ribs and a narrow thorax, polydactyly, dysplastic nails and teeth, abnormalities of the upper lip,

and congenital heart disease.[25,33,34] The prognosis for Ellis-van Creveld syndrome is good, with most affected patients living into adulthood. Any deaths from EvC are related to the presence of a cardiac abnormality, as death related to pulmonary hypoplasia is unusual for this dysplasia.[34] Differential diagnoses for EvC include asphyxiating thoracic dysplasia, short rib-polydactyly syndrome, achondrogenesis, and thanatophoric dysplasia.[26,34]

OSTEOGENESIS IMPERFECTA

Osteogenesis imperfecta (OI) is a rare, inheritable connective tissue disorder caused by defects in Type I collagen quality or quantity.[35] Type I collagen is found in skin, ligaments, tendons, and bone.[36,37] A defect in Type I collagen leads to the decreased mineralization of bone and bone fragility found in patients with OI.[13,26,37] OI is also characterized by long bone and rib fractures (Fig. 23-14), and extraskeletal abnormalities such as blue sclera and hearing impairment after birth.[35,38] OI has been classified into four different

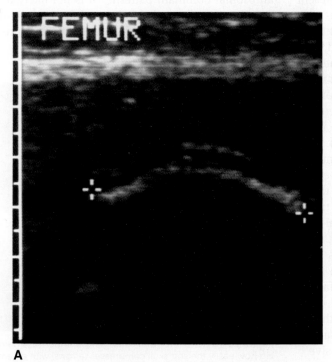

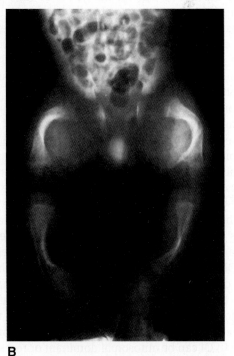

A **B**

Figure 23-14 Osteogenesis imperfecta type III. **A:** Longitudinal image of a fetal thigh at 38 weeks of gestation demonstrates a short, bowed femur *(cursors)*. **B:** Radiograph after delivery confirms the presence of short bowed femurs, tibia, and fibula bilaterally.

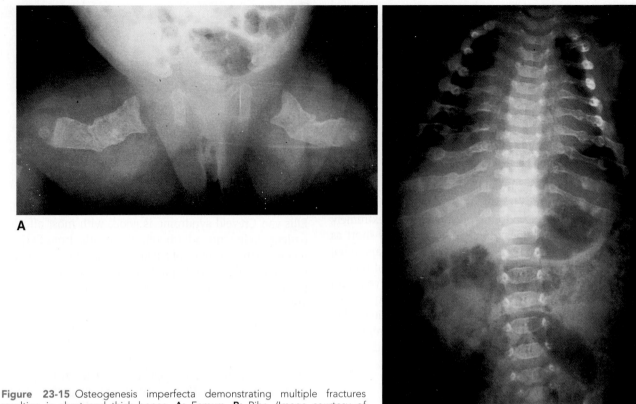

A

B

Figure 23-15 Osteogenesis imperfecta demonstrating multiple fractures resulting in short and thick bones. **A:** Femurs. **B:** Ribs. (Image courtesy of Alf Turner, MIR, BAppSc (Chiro), DACBR, Bournemouth, England.)

groups depending on genetic, radiographic, and clinical consideration.[36]

Type I OI is caused by abnormal decrease in the quantity of collagen produced[35] and is one of the milder forms of this disease.[36] It is transmitted in an autosomal dominant pattern.[37] Individuals with type I OI may present with femoral bowing sonographically in utero, but most fractures do not appear until after birth. These patients are usually of normal stature, and the prognosis is good.[36,37]

Type II OI is the most severe form and is inherited in an autosomal recessive fashion.[13,39] It is characterized sonographically by reduced echogenicity of the long bones, concave ribs resulting from rib fractures, and long bones that may appear thickened and angulated because of multiple fractures (Fig. 23-15).[25,26,39] The thorax may have a bell-shaped appearance and the skull lacks ossification (Fig. 23-16), making it easily compressible with even slight pressure from the transducer.[13,35,39] Another finding of type II OI is the transparent bone sign, in which the far side of the fetal long bone is visualized in addition to the near side. This appearance is nearly always observed in fetuses with lethal OI.[39] Prognosis for type II OI is poor, with most infants dying shortly after birth from pulmonary failure caused by multiple rib fractures.[28,36] Differential diagnoses for type II OI include achondrogenesis, thanatophoric dwarfism, and congenital hypophosphatasia.

Type III OI can be autosomal dominant or recessive.[37] While type III is less severe than type II in utero, infants

with type III can present with limb bowing in utero and multiple fractures at birth, leading to progressive bone deformities through adolescence.[36–38]

Type IV OI is the mildest form of this disease, as it does not present until later in life. It is inherited in an autosomal dominant pattern.[37] It is not likely to be detected prenatally, as bone deformities are mild and patients may only present with short stature or premature osteoporosis later in life.[37,38]

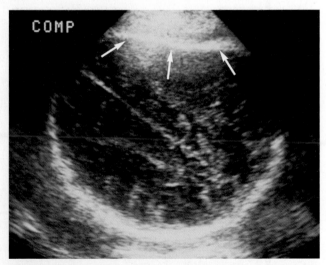

Figure 23-16 Term fetus with osteogenesis imperfecta demonstrating how easily the soft skull compresses (*arrows*) with external pressure. *COMP,* compression.

CAMPTOMELIC DYSPLASIA

Camptomelic dysplasia is a rare form of short limbed dwarfism transmitted in an autosomal dominant fashion caused by a mutation in the SOX9 gene, which plays a role in bone formation and testes development.[40,41]

It is characterized by short and bowed limbs, a short trunk, a large head, and a bell-shaped chest. Occasionally, it can present with hypoplastic scapulae (Fig. 23-17), cleft palate, micrognathia, pyelectasis, and hydrocephalus. Many different body systems can be harmfully affected, including the face, the heart, and the central nervous, respiratory, and genitourinary systems. Polyhydramnios may be visualized.[15,25,27,40] Prognosis for fetuses with camptomelic dysplasia is poor, as most die in utero or shortly after birth from respiratory complications caused by factors such as micrognathia and hypoplastic lungs.[40] Differential diagnoses for this disorder include thanatophoric dysplasia, congenital hypophosphatasia, and osteogenesis imperfecta.[40,41]

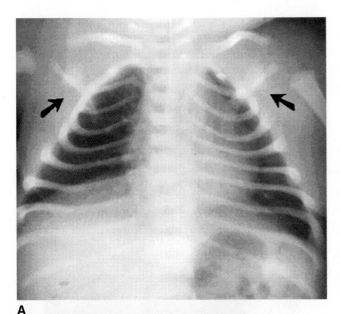

A

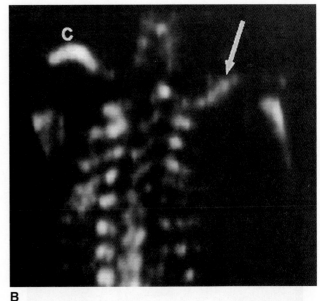

B

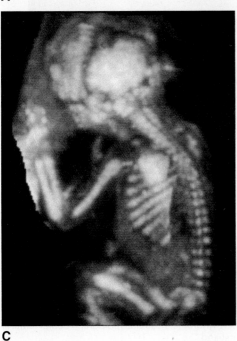

C

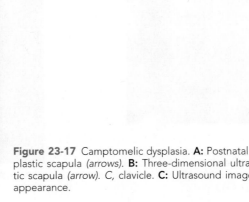

Figure 23-17 Camptomelic dysplasia. **A:** Postnatal radiograph demonstrating hypoplastic scapula *(arrows)*. **B:** Three-dimensional ultrasound image showing hypoplastic scapula *(arrow)*. *C,* clavicle. **C:** Ultrasound image demonstrating normal scapular appearance.

PATHOLOGY BOX 23-8

Anomalies Associated With Camptomelic Dysplasia

Curved or bowed long bones
Hypomineralization
Macrocephaly
Bell-shaped thorax
Micrognathia
Hydrocephalus
Cleft palate
Pyelectasis
Hypoplastic scapulae

PATHOLOGY BOX 23-9

Anomalies Associated With Congenital Hypophosphatasia

Hypomineralization
Curved or bowed long bones
Short bones

CONGENITAL HYPOPHOSPHATASIA

Congenital hypophosphatasia is a rare inherited disease of defective bone mineralization characterized by low or absent tissue-nonspecific alkaline phosphatase activity.[15,40,42] There are two types of congenital hypophosphatasia: type I is inherited as an autosomal recessive condition and can be detected prenatally; type II is inherited in an autosomal dominant fashion and is not detected until later in life.[15] A fetus with type I appears with an overall reduction in ossification (Fig. 23-18) and short, bent bones. The skull may be easily compressed and spurs may be visualized along the midshaft of long bones and at the knees and elbows.[15,25,42] Type I congenital hypophosphatasia is lethal. Differential diagnoses include osteogenesis type II and achondrogenesis.[42]

DYSOSTOSIS

Dysostosis is any condition characterized by abnormal ossification. Two of the more common sonographically visualized types include cleidocranial dysostosis and craniofacial dysostosis. Cleidocranial dysostosis is characterized by widening of the cranial fontanelles with an increase in the lateral aspect of the cranium. It is associated with absent or hypoplastic clavicles, spinal abnormalities, and hypoplastic middle and distal phalanges.[15]

Craniofacial dysostoses are commonly associated with craniosynostosis. One such dysostosis is Apert syndrome. It is characterized by craniosynostosis, midfacial hypoplasia (Fig. 28-11), and bilateral syndactyly.[43,44]

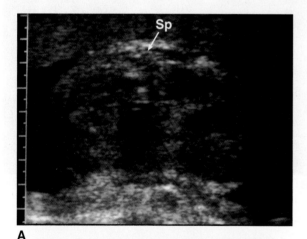

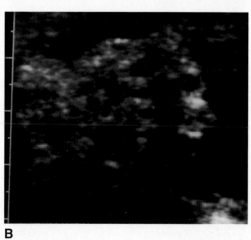

Figure 23-18 Hypophosphatasia. **A:** Transverse view of the spine and kidneys shows marked hypomineralization of the spine (*Sp*). **B:** Magnified view of hand showing marked hypomineralization. (Image courtesy of Glen Rouse, MD, CA.)

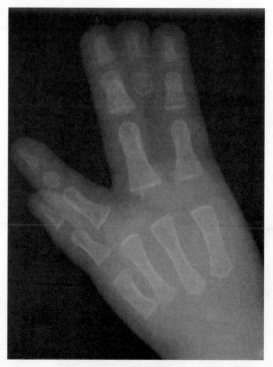

Figure 23-19 Apert syndrome. Postnatal radiograph demonstrating the typical "mitten hand."

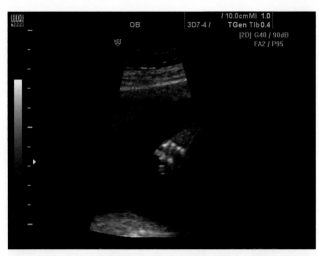

Figure 23-20 Clenched hand with overlapping fingers. (Image courtesy of Philips Medical Systems, Bothell, WA.)

Syndactyly of the four phalanges, excluding the thumb, is known as "mitten hand" (Fig. 23-19).[45] Other abnormalities include cardiac, genitourinary, and cerebral anomalies, of which corpus callosum abnormalities are the most common.[45,46] Apert syndrome is usually detected in the third trimester, as cranial sutures are best visualized at this stage and usually in conjunction with polyhydramnios, another classic finding.[45]

LIMB ABNORMALITIES

Individual limb abnormalities are often features of more complex genetic disorders or the result of other causes, including maternal teratogen exposure and amniotic band syndrome. Limb abnormalities are not life threatening in themselves. The prognosis for the fetus depends on whether other disorders are involved.

THE FETAL HAND

Hand anomalies encompass a large number of malformations from subtle defects to severe abnormalities; however, many hand anomalies are frequently missed during routine ultrasound evaluation. Examination of the fetal hands is best performed in the late first or mid-second trimester, as the fetus moves frequently and the hands are more often in an open position. The fetal hand should be evaluated for posture and the appearance and number

of digits visualized. For example, a persistently clenched hand with an overlapping index finger (Fig. 23-20) is strongly associated with trisomy 18, while a trident hand (three-pronged appearance) is characteristically found in achondroplasia (Fig. 23-21). If a major structural abnormality is found, the evaluation of the fetal hand can help in narrowing the differential diagnosis.[7]

POLYDACTYLY

Polydactyly is the presence of extra digits on the fetal hands or feet (Fig. 23-22).[47] It is one of the most common hand anomalies and may occur as an isolated finding or as part of a syndrome.[47,48] Polydactyly can be classified according to the location of the extra digit: pre-axial polydactyly affects the radial (thumb) side, postaxial polydactyly affects the ulnar (little finger) side, and central polydactyly affects the three central

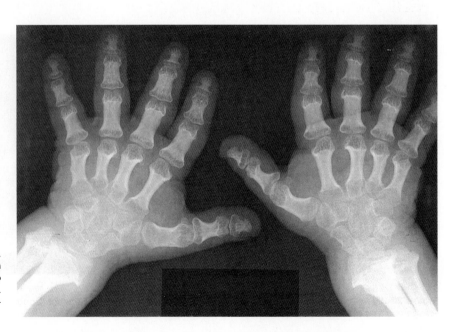

Figure 23-21 Achondroplasia. Trident hands. Observe the characteristic trident hand, with separation of the third and fourth digits. Also note that the fingers are all the same length. (Image courtesy of Bryan Hartley, MD, Melbourne, Australia.)

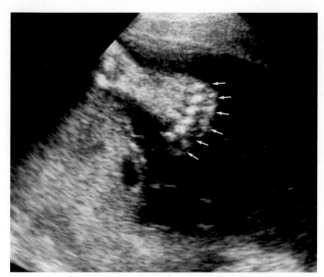

Figure 23-22 Polydactyly. Fetal foot with six phalanges *(small arrows)* forming six toes.

digits. Postaxial polydactyly (Fig. 23-23) is the most frequently encountered form, while central polydactyly is the least frequently visualized.[7] Polydactyly is found in many syndromes such as short rib-polydactyly syndrome, asphyxiating thoracic dysplasia, and aneuploidies such as trisomies 13, 18, and 21. Polydactyly can be visualized as early as 10 gestational weeks with endovaginal ultrasound.[48]

LIMB REDUCTION ABNORMALITY

Limb reduction is the congenital absence or incomplete development of one or more limbs or segments of limbs. The following terms are often used:

Aplasia: absence of a bone
Hypoplasia: incomplete development of a bone

Amelia: absence of one or more limbs (Fig. 23-24)
Hemimelia: absence of one or more extremities below the elbow or knee
Acheiria: absence of one or more hands
Apodia: absence of one or more feet
Adactyly: absence of one or more digits from the hands or feet
Phocomelia: absence of the proximal portion of an extremity with the hand or foot attached to the trunk
Meromelia: absence of part of a limb

Aplasia or hypoplasia of the radius is common in many different syndromes, including genetic syndromes, or may be caused by maternal exposure to illicit drugs or medications. Still others appear spontaneously. A hypoplastic radius would appear not to line up with the ulna at the distal end. An aplastic radius would not be present at all, and care would be needed to ensure that the single ulna is separate and different from the humerus. The hand of the affected limb would also be radially deviated, appearing as a club hand.[7]

HOLT-ORAM SYNDROME

Holt-Oram syndrome is an autosomal dominant syndrome characterized by skeletal and cardiac abnormalities. Skeletal defects mainly affect the upper limbs and include triphalangeal thumb (thumb includes three phalanges instead of the normal two), phocomelia, and radial ray defects. The most common cardiac defect is an atrial septal defect. Prognosis of this defect depends on the associated cardiac defects. Differential diagnosis includes thrombocytopenia-absent radius syndrome or VACTERL association and can mimic chromosomal abnormalities such as trisomies 18 and 13.[49-52]

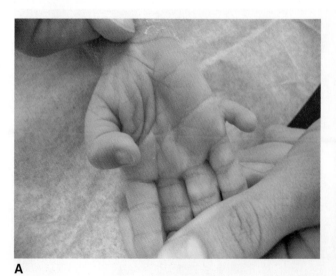

A

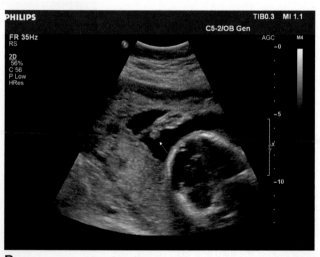

B

Figure 23-23 A: A newborn with postaxial fifth finger duplication of the right hand. (Courtesy of Paul S. Matz, MD.) **B:** Extra digit *(arrow).* (Image courtesy of Philips Medical Systems, Bothell, WA.)

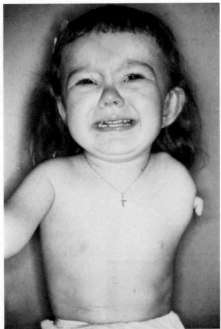
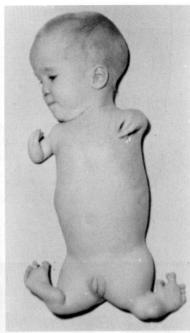

A   **B**

Figure 23-24 A: Child with unilateral amelia. **B:** Child with meromelia. An irregularly shaped bone attaches the hand to the trunk. Both infants were born to mothers who took thalidomide.

THROMBOCYTOPENIA-ABSENT RADIUS (TAR) SYNDROME

Thrombocytopenia-absent radius syndrome is an autosomal recessive disorder associated with decreased platelets. It is characterized by bilaterally absent radii but with five fully formed digits. Other abnormalities of the upper limbs may be present, and this condition is often associated with congenital heart disease. Prognosis is poor in many cases because of intracranial hemorrhage. Differential diagnoses for TAR include Holt-Oram syndrome and Roberts syndrome.[7,53]

VACTERL ASSOCIATION

VACTERL is an acronym for a combination of associated defects: *v*ertebral, *a*norectal, *c*ardiac, *t*racheoesophageal, *r*enal, and *l*imb abnormalities. To confirm this condition, at least three of the anomalies must be present. Polyhydramnios has been reported in affected fetuses. Prognosis depends on the severity of the associated anomalies. VACTERL can simulate many disorders such as trisomy 13, trisomy 18, and sirenomelia and can be triggered by a problem during embryogenesis including vascular insufficiency and chemical or pharmaceutical agents.[54,55]

CLUB FOOT

Club foot is a common birth defect characterized by the fetal foot being excessively medially deviated so that the bones of the foot lies in the same plane as the bone of the lower leg (Fig. 23-25). It can be an isolated finding or found as part of a syndrome. Clubfoot is commonly seen as a deformation caused by oligohydramnios or another condition that restricts fetal movement.[56,57] If a clubfoot is suspected, a thorough evaluation of all fetal anatomy should be performed to detect a chromosomal or syndromic abnormality. The suspected foot should also be re-evaluated at the end of the exam to determine if the abnormality is artifactual in nature.[56]

AMNIOTIC BAND SEQUENCE

Amniotic band sequence (ABS) is a group of fetal abnormalities that range from constriction rings and edema of the digits to multiple, complex anomalies of different portions of the fetal body.[58] The exact explanation of these bands is unknown but many theories have arisen as to their origin. Some postulate that the bands form after the rupture of the amnion early in the pregnancy; others have associated this condition with invasive procedures such as amniocentesis and chorionic villus sampling.[58,59] These bands may be recognized sonographically as a linear density that is attached from one uterine wall to another or from the uterine wall to a fetal part, or they may not be visualized at all. ABS can affect many different organ systems including cranial facial defects (anencephaly, cleft lip/palate), body wall defects (gastroschisis, omphalocele, ectopia cordis), and limb defects (amputation, clubfoot, lymphedema distal to a constriction ring) (Fig. 28-8).[59,60]

Amniotic sheets can be visualized prenatally and should not be confused with amniotic bands. Amniotic bands, also known as synechiae, are pre-existing bands of uterine tissue that become apparent as the uterine cavity fills with amniotic fluid. They are frequently associated with endometrial procedures (D&Cs) or intrauterine infections.[61] An amniotic sheet appears as

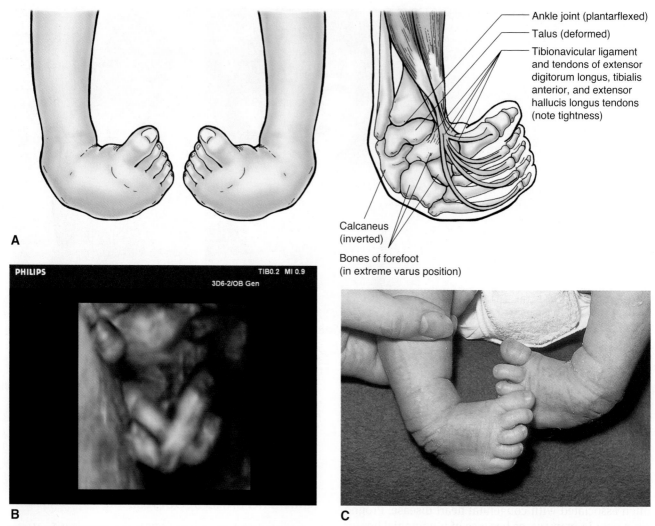

Ankle joint (plantarflexed)

Talus (deformed)

Tibionavicular ligament and tendons of extensor digitorum longus, tibialis anterior, and extensor hallucis longus tendons (note tightness)

Calcaneus (inverted)

Bones of forefoot (in extreme varus position)

Figure 23-25 Clubfoot. **A:** Artist's rendering of a clubfoot. **B:** Three-dimensional image of clubfoot. **C:** Postnatal image of a fetus with bilateral clubfoot.

a membranous pillar within the amniotic fluid and is characterized by a free edge that projects into the amniotic cavity. The fetus can move freely around this projection. While ultrasound is the modality of choice when searching for maternal/fetal complications associated with pregnancy, magnetic resonance imaging (MRI) can incorporate a wider field of view to more accurately diagnose amniotic sheets compared to amniotic bands.[60,62]

SIRENOMELIA

Sirenomelia, also known as "mermaid syndrome," is a rare and lethal abnormality that has been associated with maternal diabetes, monozygotic twinning, and maternal cocaine use.[63] It is characterized by the fusion of both lower extremities or a single lower extremity and renal agenesis that results in severe oligohydramnios (Fig. 23-26).[63,64] Sirenomelia is thought to result from an insult in early embryologic development, possibly by a vascular steal phenomenon—a persistent vessel from an early embryonic vascular system that diverts

blood flow, causing severe ischemia of the caudal portion of the fetus.[63,65,66] The prognosis for sirenomelia is generally poor because of renal agenesis.[65] The main differential diagnosis for sirenomelia is caudal regression syndrome, which is a partial or complete agenesis of the sacrum, the lumbar vertebrae, and the distal spinal cord, and lack of growth of the caudal region.[67,68]

MATERNAL CONDITIONS AND ASSOCIATED LIMB ABNORMALITIES

Obtaining a detailed and accurate medical and social history from the mother is very important. Maternal disease processes, medications, substance abuse, and exposure to radiation or industrial chemicals affect the environment of the developing fetus and may result in skeletal growth abnormalities.

Limb measurements below the 10th percentile may represent severe intrauterine growth restriction, fetal alcohol syndrome, illicit drug abuse, or a congenital or chromosomal anomaly. However, if both the mother and

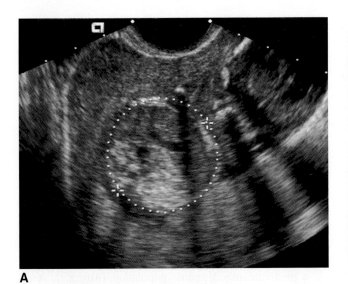

A

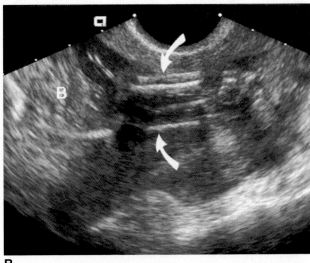

B

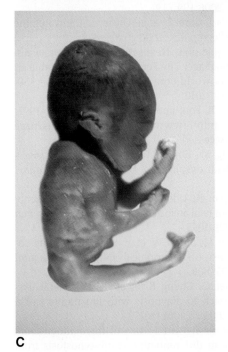

C

Figure 23-26 Sirenomelia. **A:** Transverse view of abdomen showing marked oligohydramnios second to renal agenesis. **B:** View of the lower legs showing the tibias and fibulas close to one another (*arrows*). Some cases show absence of one or more bones. **C:** Postnatal image of fetus with Sirenomelia.

father are short in stature, the fetus may simply be a normal, constitutionally small baby. Environmental factors such as oligohydramnios, uterine tumors, or Müllerian anomalies can deform limbs, while toxic agents can result in skeletal deformities. Mothers with insulin-dependent diabetes are at higher risk of having a fetus with caudal regression syndrome,[69] while craniosynostosis has been associated with mothers with hyperthyroidism.[70] Even medications that are intended to help can cause harm to the fetus. For example, pregnancies in which thalidomide (antinausea) was used resulted in fetuses with phocomelia,[7] while the use of warfarin (an anticoagulant) resulted in fetuses with craniosynostosis.[70]

Careful examination of the fetal skeleton is the first step in detecting a major abnormality. Early detection can give parents and physicians an opportunity to plan for delivery or interruption. Whenever a skeletal dysplasia is suspected, it is often recommended that the patient be referred to a tertiary sonographic laboratory for confirmation of the diagnosis.

SUMMARY

- Primary ossification centers of the limbs image as early as ten weeks.
- Long bone epiphysis visualizes by 35 weeks, helping in determination of fetal maturity.
- On average, the fetal femur grows 3 mm a week up to 27 weeks, slowing to 1 mm per week for the rest of gestation.
- Skeletal dysplasias occur with other, often fatal, fetal anomalies.

- TD has two forms and is universally fatal.
- The autosomal dominant achondroplasia results in an individual with a large head, bowed limbs, trident hands, and a low nasal bridge.
- The lethal achondrogenesis has two forms.
- All three types of the lethal short rib-polydactyly syndrome include findings of a narrow thorax, polydactyly, short, horizontal ribs, micromelic dwarfism, and pulmonary hypoplasia.
- A fetus with an extremely narrow thorax, rhizomelic limbs, polydactyly, and pelvic and renal anomalies describes asphyxiating thoracic dysplasia.
- Short limbs, short ribs and a narrow thorax, polydactyly, dysplastic nails and teeth, abnormalities of the upper lip, and congenital heart disease describe Ellis-van Creveld syndrome.
- Prenatal bone bowing and fractures describe characteristics of OI.
- Short and bowed limbs, a short trunk, a large head, and a bell-shaped chest describe a type of dwarfism called camptomelic dysplasia.
- The main characteristic of congenital hypophosphatasia is a lack of bone mineralization.
- Apert syndrome is a form of dysostosis.
- Fetal hand and feet malformations include extra or a reduction of fingers and clubbing.
- Syndromes that include limb abnormalities include Holt-Oram syndrome, thrombocytopenia-absent radius (TAR) syndrome, and VACTERL association.
- Amniotic band sequence results in amputation of limbs and digits if they extend through the amnion.
- Fusion of the lower extremities is the result of a vascular steal phenomenon and is part of sirenomelia.

Critical Thinking Questions

1. **Why is consistency and accuracy in measurements and anatomic surveys important when evaluating the fetal skeleton?**

   ANSWER: Some types of skeletal dysplasias become evident in the second or third trimester. Consistent measurement techniques are important to ensure proper monitoring of fetal limb growth.

2. **If the femur length is thought to be shorter than normal for gestational age, what other measurements should be taken/other anatomic structures looked at to help make the diagnosis of a skeletal dysplasia?**

   ANSWER: Measurement of the long bones, humerus, tibia/fibula, and radius/ulna aid in determining normalcy of the limbs.

REFERENCES

1. Monteagudo A, Dong R, Timor-Tritsch I. Fetal fibular hemimelia. *J Ultrasound Med.* 2006;25:533–537.
2. Fong K. Detection of fetal structural abnormalities with US during early pregnancy. *Radiographics.* 2004;24:157–174.
3. MacKenzie A, Stephenson C, Funai E. Prenatal assessment of gestational age. Online UpToDate (serial online). June 5, 2009.
4. Nyberg DA, McGahan JP, Pretorius DH, et al. *Diagnostic Imaging of Fetal Anomalies.* Philadelphia: Lippincott Williams & Wilkins; 2003.
5. Hearn-Stebbens B. Normal fetal growth assessment: a review of literature and current practice. *J Diagn Med Sonography.* 1995;11:176–187.
6. Agboola I, Sangihaghpeykar H, Zacharias N. Maternal-fetal characteristics and fetal femur diaphysis length in a predominantly Hispanic population (Abstract). *Am J Obstet Gynecol.* 2008;199:S191.
7. Rypens F, Dubois J, Garel L, et al. Obstetric US: watch the fetal hands. *Radiographics.* 2006;26:811–829.
8. Chatterjee M, Izquierdo L, Nevils B, et al. Fetal foot: evaluation of gestational age. The Fetus.net. 1994. Available at: http://www.sonoworld.com/Fetus/page.aspx?id = 350. Accessed April 19, 2010.
9. Furness M, Khor B. Foot anomalies. The Fetus.net. 1992. Available at: http://www.sonoworld.com/Fetus/page.aspx?id = 351. Accessed April 19, 2010.
10. Pantaleo J, Craig M, Ehman D. Hypochondrogenesis: a rare lethal skeletal dysplasia. *J Diagn Med Sonography.* 2001;17:354–357.
11. Luewan S, Sukpan K, Udomwan P, et al. Prenatal sonographic features of fetal atelosteogenesis type I. *J Ultrasound Med.* 2009;28:1091–1095.
12. Wax J, Carpenter M, Smith W, et al. Second trimester sonographic diagnosis of diastrophic dysplasia. *J Ultrasound Med.* 2003;22:805–808.
13. Dighe M, Fligner C, Cheng E, et al. Fetal skeletal dysplasia: an approach to diagnosis with illustrative cases. *Radiographics.* 2008;28:1061–1077.
14. Krakow D, Santulli T, Platt L. Use of three-dimensional ultrasonography in differentiating craniosynostosis from severe fetal molding. *J Ultrasound Med.* 2001;20:427–431.
15. Glass R, Fernbach S, Norton K, et al. The infant skull: a vault of information. *Radiographics.* 2004;24:507–522.
16. Gerards F, Twisk J, Fetter W, et al. Predicting pulmonary hypoplasia with 2- or 3-dimensional ultrasonography in complicated pregnancies. *Am J Obstet Gynecol.* 2008;198:140–142.
17. Green I, Grube G, Rouse G, et al. Sonographic detection of fetal and neonatal intrathoracic and pulmonary abnormalities: a review. *J Diagn Med Sonography.* 1990;5:270–278.
18. Rahemtulla A, McGillivray B, Wilson RD. Suspected skeletal dysplasias: femur length to abdominal circumference ratio can be used in ultrasonographic prediction of fetal outcome. *Am J Obstet Gynecol.* 1997; 177:864–869.
19. Parilla B, Leeth E, Kambich M, et al. Antenatal detection of skeletal dysplasias. *J Ultrasound Med.* 2003;22:255–258.
20. Souka A, Von Kaisenberg C, Hyett J, et al. Increased nuchal translucency with normal karyotype (Abstract). *Am J Obstet Gynecol.* 2005;192:1005–1021.

21. Schade Griffis W. Thanatophoric dysplasia: a case study. *J Diagn Med Sonography*. 1994;10:24–27.

22. Bircher A, Heredia F, Jeanty P. Thanatophoric dysplasia. The Fetus.net. 2002. Available at: http://www.sonoworld.com/Fetus/page.aspx?id = 1016. Accessed April 19, 2010.

23. Sallout B, D'Agostini D, Pretorius D. Prenatal diagnosis of spondylocostal dysostosis with 3-dimensional ultrasonography. *J Ultrasound Med*. 2006;25:539–543.

24. Jeanty P, Silva S. Thanatophoric dysplasia. The Fetus.net. 1999. Available at: http://www.sonoworld.com/Fetus/page.aspx?id = 381. Accessed April 19, 2010.

25. Burmagina Y, Kaloyanova E. Achondroplasia. The Fetus.net. 2008. Available at: http://www.sonoworld.com/Fetus/page.aspx?id = 2531. Accessed April 19, 2010.

26. Glass R, Norton K, Mitre S, et al. Pediatric ribs: a spectrum of abnormalities. *Radiographics*. 2002;22:87–104.

27. Cheema J, Grissom L, Harcke T. Radiographic characteristics of lower-extremity bowing in children. *Radiographics*. 2003;23:871–880.

28. Jeanty P, Silva S. Achondroplasia. The Fetus.net. 1999. Available at: http://www.sonoworld.com/Fetus/page.aspx?id = 323. Accessed April 19, 2010.

29. Jeanty P, Silva S. Achondrogenesis. The Fetus.net. 1999. Available at: http://www.sonoworld.com/Fetus/page.aspx?id = 321. Accessed April 19, 2010.

30. Thomas D, Lejeune R, Mortier G, et al. Achondrogenesis, Type II. The Fetus.net. 2003. Available at: http://www.sonoworld.com/Fetus/page.aspx?id = 1085. Accessed April 19, 2010.

31. Silva S, Jeanty P. Short rib polydactyly syndromes. The Fetus.net. 1999. Available at: http://www.sonoworld.com/Fetus/page.aspx?id = 372. Accessed April 19, 2010.

32. Jeanty P, Silva S. Asphyxiating thoracic dysplasia. The Fetus.net. 1999. Available at: http://www.sonoworld.com/Fetus/page.aspx?id = 335. Accessed April 19, 2010.

33. Sleurs E, Clavelli WA. Asphyxiating thoracic dystrophy. The Fetus.net. 2001. Available at: http://www.sonoworld.com/Fetus/page.aspx?id = 356. Accessed April 19, 2010.

34. Gardner S, Almon J, Barton L, et al. Ellis-van Creveld syndrome. *J Diagn Med Sonography*. 2006;22;111–116.

35. McEwing R, Alton K, Johnson J, et al. First-trimester diagnosis of osteogenesis imperfecta type II by three-dimensional sonography. *J Ultrasound Med*. 2003;22: 311–314.

36. Beary J, Chines A. Clinical features and diagnosis of osteogenesis imperfecta. Online UpToDate (serial online). January 25, 2010.

37. Jeanty P, Silva S. Osteogenesis Imperfecta. The Fetus.net. 1999. Available at: http://www.sonoworld.com/Fetus/page.aspx?id = 363. Accessed April 19, 2010.

38. Rauch F, Glorieux F. Osteogenesis imperfecta. *Lancet*. 2004;363:1377–1385.

39. Palmer T, Rouse G, Song A, et al. Transparent bone and concave ribs: additional sonographic features of lethal osteogenesis imperfecta. *J Diagnc Med Sonography*. 1998;14:246–250.

40. Eger K. Camptomelic dysplasia. *J Diagn Med Sonography*. 2005;21:343–349.

41. Jeanty P, Silva S. Camptomelic dysplasia. The Fetus.net. 2000. Available at: http://www.sonoworld.com/Fetus/page.aspx?id = 337. Accessed April 19, 2010.

42. Jeanty P, Silva S. Hypophosphatasia. The Fetus.net. 1999. Available at: http://www.sonoworld.com/Fetus/page.aspx?id = 355. Accessed April 19, 2010.

43. Suchet I. Apert syndrome. The Fetus.net. 2008. Available at: http://www.sonoworld.com/Fetus/page.aspx?id = 2559. Accessed April 19, 2010.

44. Jeanty P, Silva S. Apert syndrome. The Fetus.net. 2000. Available at: http://www.sonoworld.com/Fetus/page.aspx?id = 333. Accessed April 19, 2010.

45. Cuillier F, Dillon C, Lamaire P, et al. Apert syndrome: acrocephalosyndactyly. The Fetus.net. 2007; Available at: http://www.sonoworld.com/Fetus/page.aspx?id = 2095. Accessed April 19, 2010.

46. Lam H, Lo T, Lau E, et al. The use of 2- and 3-dimensional sonographic scans in the evaluation of cranial sutures. *J Ultrasound Med*. 2006;25:1481–1484.

47. Zun K, Kim MW, Choi HM. Crossed polydactyly prenatally diagnosed by 2- and 3-dimensional sonography. *J Ultrasound Med*. 2007;26:529–534.

48. Zimmer E, Bronshtein M. Fetal polydactyly diagnosis during early pregnancy: clinical applications (Abstract). *Am J Obstet Gynecol*. 2000.183:775.

49. Cuillier F, Broussin B, Malauzat A. Holt-Oram syndrome. The Fetus.net. 2003. Available at: http://www.sonoworld.com/Fetus/page.aspx?id = 1144. Accessed April 19, 2010.

50. Quiroga H, Ottolina Y. Holt-Oram syndrome, 5 patients in the same family. The Fetus.net. 2003. Available at: http://www.sonoworld.com/Fetus/page.aspx?id = 1228. Accessed April 19, 2010.

51. Manohar S, Karthikeyan MM, Vidya S. Holt-Oram syndrome. The Fetus.net. 2010. Available at: http://www.sonoworld.com/Fetus/page.aspx?id = 2767. Accessed April 19, 2010.

52. Jeanty P, Silva S. Holt-Oram syndrome. The Fetus.net. 1999. Available at: http://www.sonoworld.com/Fetus/page.aspx?id = 354. Accessed April 19, 2010.

53. Kalish RB, Moquete R, Chasen S. Accuracy of prenatal ultrasound diagnosis of isolated clubfoot in singletons vs. twins (Abstract). *Am J Obstet Gynecol*. 2008; 199:S190.

54. Weiner N. Prenatal ultrasound diagnosis of multiple fetal anomalies: VACTERL association. *J Diagn Med Sonography*. 2002;18:167–169.

55. Bates C, Guadette L, Myles I. A rare case of VACTERL and oculo-auriculo-vertebral spectrum complicated by oligohydramnios. *J Diagn Med Sonography*. 2003;19: 175–179.

56. Magriples U. Prenatal diagnosis of talipes equinovarus (clubfoot). Online UpToDate (serial online). February 9, 2010.

57. Mammen L, Benson C. Outcome of fetuses with clubfeet diagnosed by prenatal sonography. *J Ultrasound Med*. 2004;23:497–500.

58. Allen L, Silverman R, Nosovitch J, et al. Constriction rings and congenital amputations of the fingers and toes in a mild case of amniotic band syndrome. *J Diagn Med Sonography*. 2007;23:280–285.

59. Bodamer O. Amniotic band sequence. Online UpToDate (serial online). May 28, 2009.

60. Richardson SM, Gill K, Arcement L. Amniotic band syndrome. *J Diagn Med Sonography*. 1994;10:137–143.

61. Burton E. Serial evaluation of perinatal uterine synechiae versus amniotic bands. *J Diagn Med Sonography*. 2004; 20:51–56.

62. Kato K, Shiozawa T, Ashida T, et al. Prenatal diagnosis of amniotic sheets by magnetic resonance imaging. *Am J Obstet Gynecol*. 2005;193:881–884.

63. Heflin D. Sirenomelia in the first trimester. *J Diagn Med Sonography*. 2007;23:365–367.

64. Vijayaraghavan SB, Amudha AP. High-resolution sonographic diagnosis of sirenomelia. *J Ultrasound Medicine*. 2006;25:555–557.

65. Pinette MG, Hand M, Hun R, et al. Surviving sirenomelia. *J Ultrasound Med*. 2005;24:1555–1559.

66. Stroustrup Smith A, Grable I, Levine D. Case 66: caudal regression syndrome in the fetus of a diabetic mother. *Radiology*. 2004;230:229–233.

67. Diawara F, Camara M, Thera M, et al. Sonographic diagnosis of caudal regression syndrome. *J Diagn Med Sonography*. 2009;25:267–271.

68. Gonzalez-Quinter VH, Tolaymat L, Martin D, et al. Sonographic diagnosis of caudal regression in the first trimester of pregnancy. *J Ultrasound Med*. 2002;21:1175–1178.

69. Bacino C. Approach to congenital malformations. Online UpToDate (serial online). July 16, 2008.

70. Stahl S, Holier L, Cole P. Overview of craniosynostosis. Online UpToDate (serial online). May 6, 2009.

24 Doppler Ultrasound of the Normal Fetus

Tonya N. Brathwaite

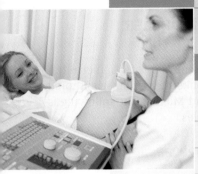

KEY TERMS

bioeffects | continuous-wave Doppler | pulsed-wave Doppler | aliasing | angle of insonation | pulse repetition frequency | mirror imaging artifact | color Doppler | color power Doppler | directional color power angio | S/D ratio | resistive index | pulsatility index

GLOSSARY

Aliasing Distortion of the spectral tracing due to a low sampling rate

Bioeffects Damage to tissue due to heat or cavitation produced by ultrasound

Brain sparing Increase of blood flow to the brain

Color Doppler Doppler data conversion into a directional velocity color overlay on the gray-scale image

Color power Doppler Doppler data conversion into a nondirectional amplitude color overlay on the gray-scale image

Continuous-wave Doppler Type of Doppler that continuously sends and receives signals

Circle of Willis Ring of arteries located at the base of the brain

Directional color power angio Combination of directional color Doppler and nondirectional amplitude color Doppler modes

Doppler effect Change in frequency due to an object moving toward or away from the detector

Mirror imaging artifact False reproduction of a structure next to a highly reflective interface

Nyquist limit Half the sampling frequency; aliasing occurs when the frequency exceeds this valueless limit

Pulsatility index Quantification of an arterial velocity waveform through the use of pulsatility

Pulse repetition frequency Number of cycles (frequency) of pulses per second

Pulsed-wave Doppler Type of Doppler in which the transmitting crystal sends a signal, listens for a return signal, and then sends another pulse of sound

Quantitative Numerical measurement

Qualitative Description of quality of components without a numerical component

Resistive index (aka Pourcelot ratio) Measure of the force needed to move blood through a vessel

S/D ratio Comparison of the systolic to diastolic flow to identify the resistance to flow

Supine hypotension Drop in blood pressure resulting from compression of the inferior vena cava due to pregnancy

Triphasic Three phases

Wharton's jelly Covering of the umbilical cord

HISTORY OF DOPPLER ULTRASOUND TECHNIQUE

In 1842, an Austrian professor of mathematics and geometry, Christian Andres Doppler, first described in detail the effect that now bears his name.[1] Doppler did not observe the effect of motion on sound frequencies but on shifts in light frequencies emitted from double stars.

Before the application of the Doppler effect to evaluate the vasculature, research of the circulatory system entailed surgery and radiology. In the 1930s, Barcroft and associates performed radiographic studies on fetal lambs and goats to establish the circulatory pathways.[2] Lind and Wegelius in 1954 used cardiographic techniques to describe the arterial and venous circulation in human fetuses and found it was similar to that of fetal sheep. Numerous other investigators reported on highly invasive procedures on pre-abortive fetuses.[3]

Satomura first described the clinical application of Doppler ultrasound technology in 1959.[4] The simplest type of Doppler is continuous wave (CW). Early CW transducers were not very specific because they were unable to distinguish whether flow moved toward or away from the transducer. The addition of spectrum analyzers and audible signals overcame this deficit, which allowed estimation of the frequency of the Doppler shift and the direction of flow.

Pulsed-wave (PW) Doppler adds information on the location of a moving target. Introduced in the late 1960s almost simultaneously by two independent laboratories, Baker in Washington studied transcutaneous blood flow measurements in humans,[5,6] whereas Peronneau and colleagues in France used their system initially on animals.[7,8] Duplex Doppler imaging—PW Doppler used in conjunction with two-dimensional ultrasound imaging—helps guide the Doppler sampling from the ultrasound vessel visualized.

Color flow mapping and color power Doppler provide color-coded flow direction and aid in vessel identification. Contrast agents, the most recent development, are increasing the signal strength to make imaging small vessels much easier.[9]

BIOEFFECTS

To date, Doppler and real-time ultrasound have not been associated with any ill effects to the fetus or mother. This assessment has been arrived at independently by every consensus group that has reviewed the literature and research findings in this area.

The U.S. Food and Drug Administration (FDA) guidelines state that there are no known risks associated with use of Doppler ultrasound at the recommended power levels. There are specific FDA guidelines for fetal ultrasound, including that the Doppler spatial peak-temporal average intensity (SPTA) be less than 94 mW/cm^2 in situ.[10] SPTA is a unit used to measure ultrasound energy intensity. Most commercial equipment uses variable acoustic power outputs between 1 and 46 mW/cm^2. The power output of a given Doppler unit should be known before it is used on a fetus.

THE PRINCIPLES OF DOPPLER ULTRASOUND

A complete discussion of the physics of Doppler ultrasound can be found in textbooks such as those authored by Kremkau,[11] Edelman,[12] and Miele.[13] The following is an overview of these principles.

CONTINUOUS-WAVE DOPPLER ULTRASOUND

The Doppler effect is a change in frequency resulting from motion of the sound source (Fig. 24-1). The Doppler effect has applications in everyday life, ranging from home burglar alarms to police radar detectors. In medicine, Doppler ultrasound is used to detect and measure blood velocity and flow.

Reflections of blood flow can be studied with two basic Doppler techniques. The simplest technique is CW Doppler; the other, PW, is discussed later. With CW Doppler, a single transducer has two separate piezoelectric crystals, one that continuously emits sound, and another that simultaneously receives it (Fig. 24-2). The frequency of the received echo is compared to the frequency of the transmitted echo to derive the Doppler shift.

Because the crystals are continuously emitting sound waves and receiving them, CW Doppler cannot identify the location of sound reflection. No imaging is available with this system, but it may be used in conjunction with real-time imaging to locate or confirm the vessel-sampling site.

CW is limited to the study of superficial vessels because it cannot discriminate between signals arising from different structures along the beam path, but it is

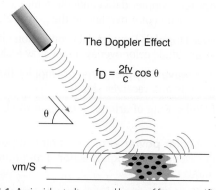

The Doppler Effect

$$f_D = \frac{2fv}{c} \cos\theta$$

Figure 24-1 An incident ultrasound beam of frequency (f) is scattered by moving red blood cells. As a result of the Doppler effect, the backscattered echo has a center of frequency that is higher by $f_D \cdot f_D = 2fv \cos\theta/c$, where f_D is the change in ultrasound frequency, also known as the Doppler shift frequency; f is the frequency of the incident ultrasound; v is the relative velocity between the target and the transducer; θ is the angle between the beam and the direction of the movement of the target; and c is the velocity of sound in the medium.

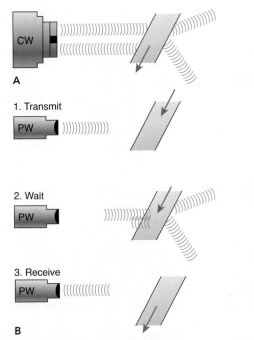

Figure 24-2 A: Continuous-wave (CW) Doppler transducer that continually transmits and receives reflections to and from the target. **B:** Pulsed-wave (PW) Doppler transducer (1) transmits a single pulse, and (2) waits for it to return. (3) The time it takes to return is determined by the depth of the target.

inexpensive, portable, and simple to operate. Because of CW limitations, PW Doppler is the preferred choice for obstetrics and gynecologic applications.

PULSED-WAVE DOPPLER

In PW Doppler, short bursts of ultrasound energy are emitted at regular intervals (see Fig. 24-2). The same piezoelectric crystal both sends and receives the signals, allowing for discrimination of range or depth. The depth of the target is calculated from the elapsed time between transmission of the pulse and reception of its echoes, assuming a constant speed of sound in tissues. With PW, a sample volume, which is a selected area to be studied, can be designated by manipulating the trackball or knob on the Doppler keyboard. This allows the operator to obtain a reading of a vessel at a certain depth through adjustment of the sample volume depth. The gate is the area inside the sample volume site. The gate or sample volume can be adjusted between 1 and 15 millimeters (mm) according to the size of the vessel being studied (Fig. 24-3).

Duplex Doppler sonography combines PW Doppler with real-time imaging, allowing the sampling of vessels at specific anatomic locations. Direct visualization

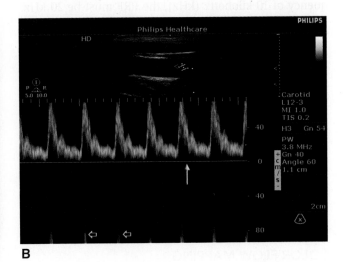

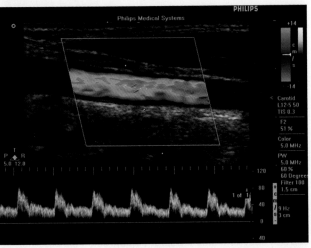

Figure 24-3 Duplex Doppler sonogram of the common carotid demonstrating aliasing. Note the wraparound of the systolic peaks *(open arrow)*. **A:** The area inside the opened gate is the sample volume site *(arrow)*. There are several methods to correct aliasing, such as selecting a different transducer frequency or, as in the case of this image, increase the scale *(box)*. **B:** This image also demonstrates aliasing; however, the artifact is due to an improper baseline location *(arrow)*. Peak systolic peaks *(open arrows)*. **C:** Correctly positioned baseline and scale selection. The yellow waveform is due to a color overlay called Chroma. (Images courtesy of Philips Medical Systems, Bothell, WA.)

of the vessel allows adjustment of insonation direction of the Doppler beam to obtain optimal waveforms with maximum velocities. Direct visualization also allows visualization during adjustment of the gate depth. For example, if no image is available to differentiate between them, an abnormal uterine artery waveform can produce the same Doppler signal as a normal common iliac artery waveform.

The angle of insonation is the angle at which the Doppler beam encounters or intersects the sampled vessel. Mirror imaging or other artifacts occur when the angle of insonation is close to 90 degrees. If this happens, the system cannot distinguish direction of flow and produces the same waveform above and below the baseline. The optimal angle for PW Doppler is 30 to 60 degrees.[11]

Aliasing is a phenomenon that occurs in PW systems when the pulse repetition frequency (PRF) is less than two times the Doppler shift frequency (see Fig. 24-3). This phenomenon does not occur with CW. This occurs during attempts to sample high-velocity blood flow. PRF is the number of pulses sent out by the transducer per second. The Nyquist limit is the minimum PRF required to register a frequency without aliasing.[14] This proves to be one-half the frequency. For example, to detect a frequency of 10 kilohertz (kHz), the PRF must be 20 kHz. The speed of sound in tissue basically limits the PRF. To avoid aliasing, increase the PRF, increase the angle of insonation, use a lower-frequency transducer, switch to CW (CW Doppler has no range resolution), or select a new ultrasonic window by using a shallower sample volume or using baseline shift for results that appear more pleasing to the eye.[12]

In a study by Mehalek and colleagues,[15] CW and PW flow velocity waveforms were compared using the patient as the control. The systolic-to-diastolic (S/D or A/B) ratios obtained with CW and PW Doppler systems were found to be comparable. Therefore, a laboratory can use either a CW or PW Doppler system effectively.

COLOR FLOW MAPPING

Color flow imaging involves the addition of color to overwrite the gray-scale ultrasound image to indicate movement such as blood flow. A bar of preselected colors displays on the left side of the ultrasound screen. As with CW and PW Doppler, the color bar has a baseline. The baseline on the color bar is the black line that separates the two main colors. This black line represents areas without Doppler shift. The color above this baseline indicates blood flow toward the transducer or positive Doppler shifts, and the color below the baseline indicates flow away from the transducer or negative Doppler shifts. Color flow mapping does not distinguish or code arteries versus veins; rather, it simply assigns color to flow toward or away from the transducer. Two arbitrary primary colors are selected and assigned to

differentiate blood flow. Typically, red is assigned for blood flow toward the transducer, and blue is assigned to blood flowing away. The colors can be changed by the operator. Once an appealing color scheme has been selected, the examiner should use the same combination of colors to ease the recognition of flow abnormalities. Positive velocities (when red is selected as the flow toward the transducer) can go from dark red to white or bright yellow. Negative velocities (when blue is selected as flow away from the transducer) can range from dark blue to white or light cyan. The color white is commonly used to represent an increase in blood velocity. Darker colors represent slower velocities. The color green represents flow disturbances. Turbulence is represented by a mixture of colors such as red, green, and blue (mosaic). Turbulent flow patterns are often associated with pathologies (Fig. 24-4).

The disadvantage of using color is that to obtain a high-quality color image, the gray-scale image is usually compromised or degraded, or vice versa. This is because the computer divides its processing time to generate one image into generating two separate images, one in gray scale and the other in color. Quality is therefore compromised. In addition, color flow is angle dependent, which means that color shadings become darker as the angle of insonation approaches 90 degrees. A tortuous vessel may change from red to blue even though it is the same vessel with constant flow. When the angle of insonation hits that same vessel, the area at 90 degrees to the beam has no color assigned and images as a black line. The optimal angle to sample with color flow is 30 to 60 degrees. Another potential error when using color is that flashes of color may be displayed by aberrant tissue motions. This produces frequency shifts and may result in confusing color displays. To avoid this, as with CW and PW Doppler, there is a "thump" filter, also known as a velocity or wall filter, built into every machine. A wall filter minimizes the flash artifacts by filtering out the low-level velocities without losing valuable information.

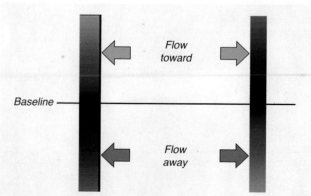

Figure 24-4 These two color bars demonstrate different colors for blood flow toward and away from the transducer. No matter the color selection, flow toward the transducer displays above the baseline and flow away from the transducer displays below the baseline.

COLOR POWER DOPPLER

Color power Doppler (CPD) is an addition to the Doppler evaluation family. It is also called energy mode or color angio.[12] CPD calculates the random noise in the CPD mode instead of the mean Doppler frequency shift. Random noise in the CPD mode is different from that in other Doppler modes, because the noise has a uniformly low power because of the standard signal-to-noise ratio. The color scale is calculated on the intensity, power, or amplitude of the signal, which displays indirectly the number of blood cells insonated by the Doppler beam. CPD is an alternate method for assessing low-flow velocities because they have a large number of reflectors moving at low velocities. On the unidirectional color map display, lower amplitude signals are darker and higher amplitude signals are lighter (Fig. 24-5).

There are some drawbacks to using CPD. Because the entire color scale is used, there is no differentiation in flow direction or speed. CPA is an amplitude mode color display showing the intensity of Doppler shifts. CPA is useful for showing slow or diminished flow because it is less angle dependent than color flow imaging.

Advantages over standard color Doppler are that CPD is angle independent and does not alias because the integral of the power spectrum is the same regardless of whether the signal wraps around. CPD also increases the usable dynamic range of the Doppler image because it extends the imaged flow down to the noise floor. CPD cannot distinguish blood flow reversal; it also cannot differentiate between arterial and venous blood flow.

CPD is extremely sensitive to low blood flow, which makes it very sensitive to motion artifacts. Power color Doppler is useful when the interventricular septum is oriented perpendicular to the ultrasound beam.[16] It is useful for identifying the presence or absence of blood

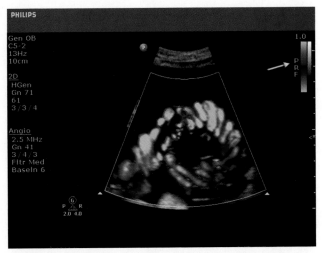

Figure 24-6 This DCPA image looks very similar to the color Doppler image. To tell the difference, look at the color bar (*arrow*) next to the image. Compare this bar to the color Doppler image and notice that there is a PRF but not a velocity (cm/s) value. (Image courtesy of Philips Medical Systems, Bothell, WA.)

flow within the arterial and ventricular chambers of the fetal heart, as well as the relationships of the right and left outflow tracts in difficult-to-image patients and fetuses. Power color Doppler has also been used to determine the number of umbilical arteries seen adjacent to the urinary bladder (Fig. 24-5).[16]

Another color Doppler mode, called directional color Doppler angio (DCPA) is a hybrid of color and CPA imaging. This mode displays both the power magnitude or amplitude of CPA and the direction of the flow velocity as in color. In DCPA mode, the signal brightness indicates the magnitude of the flow power. Bright signals have strong power; weak signals have a dark color. Hue, red or blue in most cases, indicates the direction of flow, toward or away from the transducer (Fig. 24-6). (S. Xuegong, personal communication, January 4, 2011).

ANALYSIS OF THE DOPPLER SIGNAL

Doppler ultrasound has many uses in examining the maternal-fetal circulation. Qualitative Doppler allows us to identify the direction of blood flow and detect flow disturbances such as stenosis or turbulence. More important, Doppler allows the sonographer to isolate

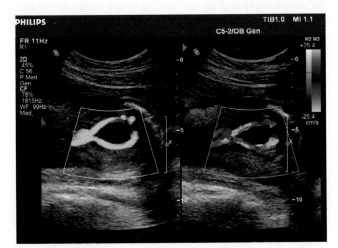

Figure 24-5 This dual image shows a color Doppler image of the two umbilical arteries lateral to the bladder (right). The left image demonstrates one type of CPA map of the same area. Notice the complete filling of the vessels. (Images courtesy of Philips Medical Systems, Bothell, WA.)

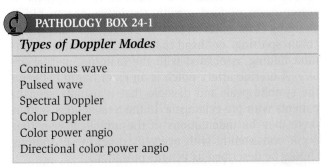

PATHOLOGY BOX 24-1

Types of Doppler Modes

Continuous wave
Pulsed wave
Spectral Doppler
Color Doppler
Color power angio
Directional color power angio

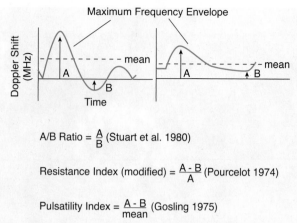

Figure 24-7 Diagram of Doppler waveform and the indices used to describe them. *A*, systole; *B*, diastole.

abnormal flow patterns that help to identify pregnancies at risk of poor fetal outcome. Quantitative flow measurements include blood velocity and flow. Qualitative measurements look at characteristics of the waveforms, which indirectly give an approximation of flow and resistance to flow. These include the S/D ratio,[17] the resistance index (RI),[18] and the pulsatility index (PI)[19] (Fig. 24-7). Waveform appearance is affected by cardiac contractility, blood viscosity, elasticity of the vessel wall, the peripheral resistance in the circulation, the distance of the sampling site from the heart, and the presence or absence of turbulence.[20]

INTERPRETATION OF WAVEFORMS

There are standard definitions used to report the Doppler findings pertaining to the obtained waveform. Most fetal and maternal vessels such as the uterine and arcuate arteries have ranges of normal previously established. The range may actually vary with the patient's gestational age. Any S/D, PI, or RI in those normal ranges should be reported as within normal limits. Report high flow ratios or flow indicating a slight resistance in the circulation. Absent end-diastolic velocity describes the absence of blood flow during the diastolic part of the cardiac cycle.

Flow extending below or under the Doppler baseline indicates reversal of flow. "Shunting" is a term used when blood flow in the fetal middle cerebral artery, normally a high-resistance circulation, is increased, resulting in low-resistance circulation. This happens in severe cases of fetal growth restriction due to blood shunting from other organs to protect the fetal brain, "brain sparring" or "head sparring." Notching is a common finding associated with the maternal uterine artery. A uterine artery notch is an extra bump between the systolic peak and diastole that is usually seen in patients with pre-eclampsia. In the fetal venous system there may be indentations in the umbilical vein that occur consistently with every diastole; these findings should be described as venous pulsations.

QUANTITATIVE DOPPLER INDICES

Quantitative Doppler can quantify flow disturbances, estimate absolute blood flow, assess vascular impedance, and help characterize tissue. Quantitative Doppler indices include velocity and flow measurements. Velocity is defined as the maximum Doppler shift over a cardiac cycle; flow is defined as the average velocity times the lumen area of a vessel. If the vessel is circular, the area can be determined from one diameter, whereas if it is an ellipse, two diameters are required.

Several potential errors are inherent in measuring fetal blood flow volume. One source of error is the inaccurate measurement of the angle of the vessel to the insonating ultrasonic beam. The estimate of velocity is strongly dependent on the magnitude of the angle. A linear-array transducer with a Doppler offset at a fixed angle gives an accurate measurement of the angle. If the insonating beam angle is two degrees, the error rate is 6%; increasing five degrees, there is a 15% velocity error rate, demonstrating the increases seen with an increased Doppler angle.[21] The need to measure the angle of insonation limits this method to vessels whose axis lies in the same plane for a few centimeters of their course. The intra-abdominal umbilical vein or the fetal descending aorta is suitable. Yet another error in estimating flow volume can arise in measuring the vessel diameter. Small measurement errors in vessels of small diameter create huge errors. For example, a 1-mm error in the measurement of an 8-mm vessel produces a 25% error variation in the flow calculation.[22] The diameter of vessels—especially the fetal aorta—may vary 20% over the cardiac cycle. The sample volume must embrace the entire lumen to ensure that it is uniformly insonated.

QUALITATIVE DOPPLER INDICES

Qualitative measurements of flow velocity waveforms are angle independent and are therefore easier to obtain. Flow samples taken from the fetus are mainly at the umbilical artery, middle cerebral artery (MCA), and the descending aorta. Indices used to determine normalcy include the S/D or A/B ratio, which uses the peak systolic, and end diastolic velocities. The PI is the systolic minus the diastolic divided by the mean of the maximum velocities. A fine formula, the RI uses the systolic minus the diastolic divided by the systolic velocities.[16]

CLINICAL APPLICATIONS
PLACENTAL CIRCULATION

Pregnancy places tremendous stress on the maternal circulation. Cardiac output increases in early pregnancy, reaching a peak of 30% to 50% above nonpregnant values at 20 to 24 weeks' gestation.[23] This increase in the maternal cardiac output is caused by the dramatic increase in uterine blood flow needed to satisfy the metabolic demands of the fetus. The maternal blood volume normally expands by approximately 40% to compensate for the slight drop in the mean arterial pressure.

In the placental circulation, blood enters the placenta from the fetus through the paired umbilical arteries. The blood distributes throughout the chorionic plate to the chorionic villi, where it passes through villous capillaries and drains into a network of veins that are parallel to the arteries. Exchange of oxygen, carbon dioxide, nutrients, and waste products occurs across the villous capillaries. The blood then returns to the fetus by way of the umbilical vein.

UMBILICAL CORD

The umbilical cord is the crucial intrauterine link between the fetal and the placental circulation. It is normally composed of two arteries and a single large vein, covered by amnion, and ensheathed in Wharton's jelly for protection.

The umbilical arteries are a single-layered intima of endothelial cells resting on a medium of smooth muscle cells. Fine elastic fibrils are scattered throughout the arterial walls. The umbilical vein consists of a thin intima and a well-defined internal elastic lamina. The medial subintimal smooth muscle fibers are arranged longitudinally.[24] The vessels arrange spirally to reduce torsion and knots that would occur if they were floating free. Doppler ultrasound can be used to determine adequacy of umbilical cord blood flow (Table 24-1).

TABLE 24-1	
Indications for the Fetal Doppler Exam	
Maternal disease	Hypertension (chronic or pregnancy-induced)
	Collagen vascular disease
	Renal disease
	Diabetes (classes B, C, R, F)
	Malnutrition
	Rh or Kell sensitization
	Anemia
Suspected IUGR	Estimated fetal weight <10th percentile
	Incorrect dates versus IUGR
	Unexplained oligohydramnios
Risk factors for IUGR	Previous IUGR infant
	Smoker >1 pack/day cigarettes
	Drug or alcohol ingestion
	Elevated maternal serum > fetoprotein
	Discordant growth of multiple gestations
Other	Umbilical cord anomaly
	Previous fetal demise
	Fetal chromosomal anomaly
	Inadequate placentation
	IUGR, intrauterine growth retardation

UTERINE VASCULATURE

The blood supply to the pregnant uterus is derived chiefly from the uterine arteries. The ovarian arteries also contribute, but to a lesser degree. The main uterine artery derived from the internal iliac artery branches off once it reaches the uterus to form the arcuate arteries. The main uterine arteries circle the anterior and posterior surfaces, forming anastomoses with the arcuate arteries on the opposite side (Fig. 6-11). The radial arteries branch off the arcuates and are directed into the uterine lumen to form the spiral arteries, which pass into the uterine decidua to feed the intervillous space.

Early in pregnancy, the trophoblast invades the spiral artery in the decidua to form lakes of maternal blood. At 16 to 24 weeks, the placental cytotrophoblasts invade the spiral arteries in the myometrium, eroding their walls and producing dilated vessels with low resistance. If this does not occur, the vessels remain constricted and exhibit increased resistance. This may place the patient at risk for pre-eclampsia and intrauterine growth restriction (IUGR). Early changes in uterine and arcuate artery blood flow can be detected and followed by serial Doppler flow studies.

SCANNING TECHNIQUE

CONTINUOUS-WAVE STUDY OF THE UMBILICAL ARTERY

Because CW Doppler systems are blind to the exact location of the Doppler signal, they are not routinely used in obstetrics. However, they may be used in conjunction with a real-time ultrasound system to aid in vessel identification. Real-time ultrasound may be useful for determining the origin of an abnormal signal, but each vessel has its own unique waveform and sound and can often be identified without real-time imaging.

The fetal umbilical artery and the maternal uterine and arcuate arteries are the vessels studied most commonly with CW Doppler. While the blood vessels are examined, the patient lies in a semirecumbent position to prevent supine hypotension.[25] To reduce Doppler scanning time, the umbilical cord can be identified with real-time sonography to guide the placement of the beam for Doppler scanning. It has been documented that arterial resistance is greater at the insertion of the umbilical cord into the fetal abdomen than at the placental cord insertion.[26] If the placental cord insertion cannot be identified, a free loop midcord is sampled. The angle of the transducer is manipulated slightly until a strong signal is obtained.

The signal should be sharp and easily distinguished. If the borders of the peak and troughs are not clear, the gain can be raised or lowered until a distinguishable signal is obtained. The normal waveform signal looks identical to the pulsed wave Doppler waveform (Fig. 24-8). Wall filters, which filter out low-level echoes, should be

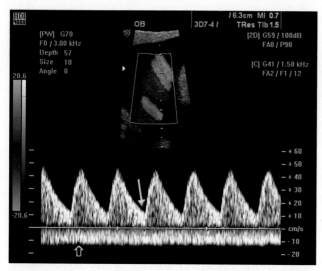

Figure 24-8 In the typical umbilical artery and vein waveform, the arterial blood flow is above the baseline. Note the clear systolic peaks of the artery with the arrow indicating the diastolic trough. Below the baseline is normal continuous venous flow (*open arrow*). Decreasing the sector width before entering the color mode increases image detail because of the increase in line density. After decreasing the sector size, the area of interest was then zoomed or magnified.

TABLE 24-2	
Comparison of Continuous and Pulsed Wave Doppler	
Continuous	**Pulsed**
Always transmitting and receiving with different crystals	Sends, listens, receives with each crystal
No image	Real-time image/tracing
Spectral tracing	Spectral tracing, color Doppler modes
No angle correction	Angle correction
No aliasing	Aliasing due to Nyquist limit Gate

set as low as possible. If the gain is lowered too much, the end-diastolic velocity may be falsely obliterated. The arterial signal should be visualized on one side of the baseline, with the steady nonpulsatile venous flow in the opposite direction. Because fetal breathing activity can alter flow ratios, it is good practice to wait until breathing stops.[25] Breathing can be identified either by an undulating venous Doppler signal or by fetal chest wall movements. Once three or four waveforms of equal height are obtained, the image is frozen while the necessary measurements are taken. A single waveform should never be used for quantitative assessment; rather, a number of sequential waveforms should be averaged to minimize beat-to-beat variation.[25]

Uterine Artery

To evaluate the maternal uterine or arcuate artery with CW Doppler, the transducer should be placed parauterine in the maternal iliac fossa. Slight medial and caudal angulation may be necessary to obtain the correct signal. Slight moves are made with the transducer until the much slower maternal pulse is audible. The normal uterine arterial waveform is distinct and should have sufficient diastolic blood flow (Fig. 27-4), whereas the iliac arteries have reversed or no end-diastolic flow. Abnormal uterine arteries can give a similar waveform to that of the internal iliac artery, so care must be exercised.

Arcuate arteries are located between the umbilicus and the iliac crest on the lateral side of the uterine fundus, although the exact location varies with gestational age. Having the patient lie in the semirecumbent position makes obtaining the signal quicker and easier. The

transducer can be angled medial until the proper signal is obtained (Table 24-2).

PULSED-WAVE DOPPLER

Umbilical Artery Waveforms

Imaging the umbilical artery with a duplex system is easy. The cord is located with the real-time transducer, a loop is identified at midcord or at the placental umbilical cord insertion,[26] and the Doppler cursor is dropped into the umbilical vessels. Because S/D, PI, and RI (also known as the Pourcelot ratio) are angle-independent measurements, it is not necessary to correct for the angle of insonation. The umbilical waveform should demonstrate clean peaks of equal height, and umbilical vein flow should be visible in the opposite direction (see Fig. 24-8).

Umbilical Vein Waveforms

Umbilical venous blood flows from the placenta, through the ductus venosus, into the inferior vena cava, across the right atrium, through the foramen ovale into the left atrium, and out the left ventricle. The rate of umbilical vein flow steadily increases with advancing gestational age and parallels fetal growth until approximately 37 weeks, after which there is a reduction. Animal studies have suggested that a major determinant of umbilical venous flow is resistance in the fetal–placental circulation.[27] Indik and Reed[28] showed that umbilical arterial flow returning to the placenta affects the flow velocity of the umbilical venous blood flow returning to the fetus, and vice versa. Umbilical venous flow should be constant and nonpulsatile (see Fig. 24-8), which means the diameter of the waveform should remain the same throughout the entire fetal cardiac cycle. When alterations in flow are noticed, it should be ascertained that the fetus is not breathing because this causes fluctuations in the flow. Umbilical vein pulsations have been associated with adverse fetal outcomes.[29] This is due to

TABLE 24-3

Pulsed Wave Spectral Appearance

Location	Sampling Location	Normal Waveform	Abnormal Waveform
Umbilical artery	Cord insertion—placenta and fetus; midcord	Low resistance above the baseline	High resistance with no or little end diastolic flow; possible flow reversal
Umbilical vein	Fetal abdomen; free floating cord	Constant; non-pulsatile	Flow fluctuation/pulsations
Uterine artery	Lateral to the uterus at the level of the external iliac artery	First trimester—Diastolic notch; second trimester—low resistance	Persistent notch after the first trimester
Fetal descending aorta	Level of the diaphragm	First trimester—absent end-diastolic flow; second/third trimester—diastolic flow	Increase in PI due to absent end-diastolic flow
Inferior vena cava	Entrance of the right atrium	Triphasic	Pulsatile
Ductus venosus	Midsagittal above the umbilical sinus; upper fetal abdomen	Triphasic; higher velocity than the IVC	Flow reversal increase
Middle cerebral artery	Anterior to the thalamus	High resistance decreases with fetal age	Marked decreased resistance; increase in flow volume
Internal carotid artery	Proximal or mid-internal carotid artery	Low resistance	Increased resistance

congestive heart failure. Umbilical vein pulsations are described as repetitive, persistent decreases in venous velocity that are coincident with the fetal cardiac cycle (see Fig. 24-8). There is an increase in the volume flow and velocity in the umbilical vein in severely anemic fetuses. For a summary of fetal pulsed wave appearances, see Table 24-3.

Uterine Waveforms

To image the uterine artery with PW Doppler, the external iliac artery is first visualized with real-time equipment. The external iliac artery most commonly appears in the maternal iliac fossa as a large, long vessel running parallel to the uterus. The uterine artery is seen branching around the external iliac artery and is located medial to the iliac artery but lateral to the uterus. The operator should try to identify the vessel first on real-time, to save actual Doppler time. If it is technically impossible to get good duplex images, the sonographer must search up and down the medial aspect of the external iliac artery until the proper signal is obtained (Fig 27-4). Color flow can aid in quick vessel identification.

In early pregnancy and in nonpregnant women, the uterine artery waveform has a notch at the beginning of the diastolic phase of the cardiac cycle. A true notch represents a deceleration of at least 50 Hz below the maximum diastolic velocities and rarely occurs after the 20th week of gestation. In nonpregnant women and in early pregnancy, the uterine artery waveform has a high pulsatility with reduced diastolic velocity. In the second trimester there is a decrease in impedance that continues until 24 weeks'

gestation.[30] One reason for this is the invasion in the myometrial portion of the spiral arteries, which occurs around 16 weeks' gestation.[30] The presence of a notch or persistently elevated ratios may imply that the pregnancy suffers from inadequate nutrition and oxygenation, which leads to pre-eclampsia and IUGR. Yet another explanation may be a maternal vasospasm causing increased resistance inside the vessel.

Fetal Descending Aorta

Most studies of fetal blood flow have evaluated volume flow and velocity in the aorta. In 1979, Gill used a modified eight-transducer water-path transducer to perform the first flow studies. He estimated that he achieved errors of less than 10%.[21]

Various investigators have used a linear-array transducer with a pulsed Doppler transducer at a fixed angle of 45 degrees. The fixed angle helps ensure that the angle of insonation of the Doppler beam is less than 60 degrees from the direction of flow of the red blood cells.[31] The fetal descending aorta and umbilical vein are the vessels most often studied with flow velocity. The descending aorta should be examined just above the level of the diaphragm. The transducer should be parallel to the aorta. The sample gate should be opened beyond the lumen walls, to ensure even insonation of the vessel (Fig. 24-9).

Gill[32] has shown that for low beam–flow angles, increasing the gate to exceed the lumen diameter compensates in part for the inadequate beam width.

The aortic flow velocity waveform shows rapid acceleration during systole. From peak systole to end-diastole

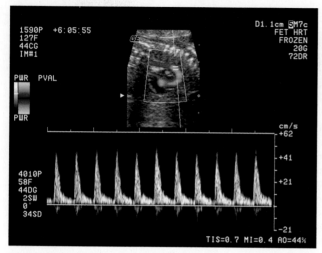

Figure 24-9 The normal waveform in the fetal descending aorta demonstrates a rapid deceleration from peak systole to end diastole. The color reference image uses CPA. (Sonographic image courtesy of GE Healthcare, Wauwatosa, WI.)

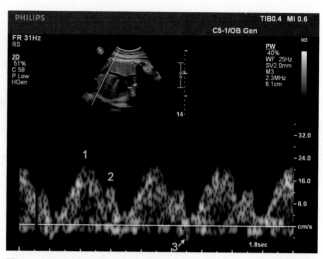

Figure 24-10 Normal triphasic flow seen in the IVS proximal to termination into the right atrium. To separate the waveform peaks, this image uses a faster sweep speed and has a decreased 2D reference image. *1*, systole; *2*, atrioventricular valves opening; *3*, late diastole reverse flow.

there is rapid deceleration. There is no reversal of flow during diastole in normal fetuses. At 12 to 13 weeks, there is absent end-diastolic blood flow. Diastolic flow gradually appears, suggesting a lowering of systemic vascular resistance. After 17 to 18 weeks, there is no significant decrease in the PI with advancing gestational age. The S/D, RI, and PI show little change in the third trimester, except for a slight increase in end-diastolic flow. The aortic blood flow velocity changes with increasing distance from the fetal heart.[33] This index is affected significantly by changes in the fetal heart rate and fetal behavioral state such as fetal breathing; therefore, sampling should not be done during these times. In growth-restricted fetuses, the PI is increased.[34] There is an adverse fetal outcome in fetuses with absent end-diastolic velocity compared to fetuses with normal blood flow.[35]

Inferior Vena Cava

In the fetal inferior vena cava (IVC), blood flows in three phases. This is demonstrated in the Doppler waveform. The first spike is consistent with systole because forward flow occurs when the atrium relaxes. During diastole, a second peak occurs as the atrioventricular valves open. The third phase is characterized by reverse flow during late diastole. In a healthy fetus there is a significant decrease of reverse flow as the gestational age advances.

The IVC Doppler sampling should be taken immediately distal to its widening, which is its entrance into the right atrium. This site allows a truer sample of the IVC to be taken without reverberation interference from the adjacent hepatic veins and ductus venosus (Fig. 24-10).

In a normal, healthy fetus, the highest peak and time–velocity integral occur during systole, followed by a smaller peak and time–velocity integral during diastole. The pulsatility of blood flow increases in fetal hypoxia.

Ductus Venosus

The fetal ductus venosus functions exclusively in the fetal circulation. It forms a shunt between the umbilical vein and the IVC, allowing blood to bypass the hepatic circulation (Fig. 24-11). Approximately 50% of umbilical blood flow passes through the ductus venosus; the remainder enters the hepatic-portal venous system and passes through the hepatic vasculature.[27] The fetal liver receives its blood supply not only from the umbilical vein, but also from the portal vein and hepatic artery. The umbilical venous blood flow contributes approximately 75% to 80% of total blood supply of the liver. The other 15% to 20% come from the

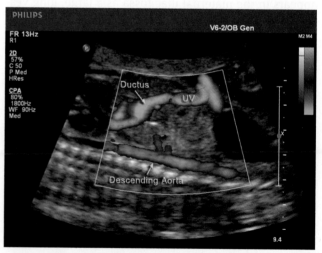

Figure 24-11 A DCPA sagittal image of the late first trimester fetal abdomen demonstrating the connection of the ductus and the umbilical vein *(UV)*. To determine the type of color mode used to obtain an image, check the color bar. This color bar lacks the velocity unit (cm/s), indicating that the color mode is DCPA. (Image courtesy of Philips Medical Systems, Bothell, WA.)

portal venous blood flow, and hepatic arterial blood flow from the aorta is about 4% to 5%.[27] The ductus venosus Doppler waveform should be sampled mid-sagitally immediately above the umbilical sinus or obliquely, transecting the upper fetal abdomen. The characteristic waveform has the classic triphasic pattern that is also seen in the IVC. The ductus venosus and IVC waveforms both have triphasic patterns but are differentiated from each other first by the location of the Doppler sampling site and second by the waveform architecture itself. The ductus venosus waveform has a high diastolic flow component, whereas the IVC does not. The waveform pattern has a systolic and early diastolic forward component with a late diastolic reverse component. Because the ductus venosus has a narrow lumen, it can demonstrate very high velocities. The average velocity in the ductus venosus is approximately three to four times higher than in the IVC and umbilical vein. Blood flow velocities in the ductus venosus increase with advancing gestational age (Fig. 24-12). When evaluating the waveform, the sonographer should look at the peak systolic velocity, minimum velocity during atrial contractions, and time-average velocity. There will be an increase in reversal of flow in diastole with fetal hypoxia or heart failure.

Cerebral Blood Flow

In a normal pregnancy, there is continuous forward flow in the fetal middle cerebral artery throughout the cardiac cycle. The middle cerebral artery (MCA) is the main lateral branch of the circle of Willis. This high-resistance circulation results in a high Doppler reading in a normal fetus, which is actually the opposite of the case in other fetal vessels. With fetal growth restriction, there is a marked increase in internal carotid resistance and a decrease in cerebral resistance.[36] This decrease in cerebral resistance results in a low Doppler ratio. Intrauterine

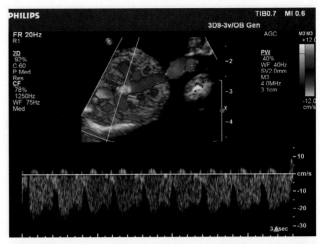

Figure 24-12 Ductus venosus blood flow pattern in a normal fetus with the characteristic triphasic pattern. The first spike represents ventricular systole, the second is a result of ventricular diastole, and the sudden dip coincides with atrial systole. Also notice that there is high forward flow throughout the entire cardiac cycle. (Image courtesy of Philips Medical Systems, Bothell, WA.)

asphyxia alters blood flow to the fetal organs and brain, which may ultimately cause brain damage.

To sample the middle cerebral artery, first obtain an image at the biparietal diameter level using duplex sonography. The middle cerebral artery appears anterior to the thalamus on either side of the midline. This is the level of bifurcation into the middle and anterior cerebral arteries (Fig. 24-13). In normal pregnancy, the middle cerebral S/D ratio and PI decrease with advancing gestational age, signifying decreasing resistance. In the face of IUGR and hypoxic stress (fetal anemia), a drop in the middle cerebral S/D ratio and PI signify a marked decrease in resistance, and perhaps increased blood flow to the brain. This is believed to be a brain-sparing effect (Fig. 24-14).

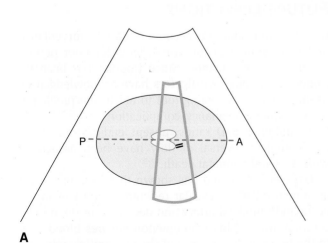

A

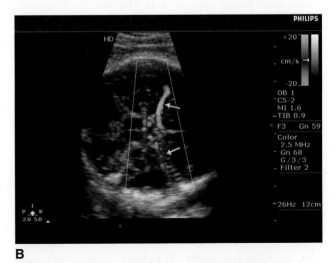

B

Figure 24-13 A: Diagrammatic representation and **(B)** sonographic representation of the Doppler sampling site for the middle cerebral arterial (MCA) waveform. Either vessel provides the appropriate waveform for measurement. Reducing the color Doppler region of interest (ROI) increases sensitivity because of the decreased sample area. A, anterior; P, posterior; MCA, arrows. (Image courtesy of Philips Medical Systems, Bothell, WA.)

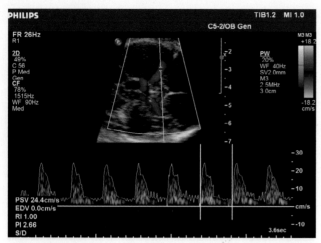

Figure 24-14 A normal fetal middle cerebral artery waveform. The fetal middle cerebral artery is normally a high-resistance circuit. Note the normally high systolic peaks and the low diastolic trough. In the face of fetal growth restriction or hypoxic stress, the fetal mechanism of brain sparing takes effect in an effort to protect and conserve the fetal brain, and blood shunts away from vital organs and is sent to the fetal brain, thereby creating a low-resistance circuit. (Image courtesy of Philips Medical Systems, Bothell, WA.)

FACTORS THAT AFFECT WAVEFORMS

Most investigators perform fetal Doppler studies with the patient supine or semirecumbent. According to Marsal and colleagues,[25] the patient should be semirecumbent to avoid supine hypotension. When fetal breathing occurs, flow patterns in the umbilical vein and artery are modulated. This is because the increase in tracheal or intrapleural pressure increases venous return to the heart. Fetal breathing may be associated with an irregular heart rate, owing to respiratory sinus arrhythmia. Doppler sampling should not be performed during episodes of fetal breathing movements.

Because fetal blood flow is affected by irregularities in the fetal heart rate pattern, Doppler examination should not be performed during episodes of fetal bradycardia or tachycardia. Normal waveforms are altered by changes in heart rate or rhythm. With extrasystolic beats, there is a lower peak and mean velocity. The first postextrasystolic beat shows an increase in blood velocity that does not fully compensate for the extrasystolic beat. Compensation does occur, however, over the next three or four beats.[37,25]

The influence of pharmacologic agents on uterine and fetal blood flow is variable and controversial. Joupilla and others have observed no major change in umbilical vein flow associated with the mother's smoking or being administered oxygen, caffeine, labetalol, alcohol, or anesthesia.[38–41,3] Medications that alter heart rate, such as β-mimetics (ritodrine, terbutaline) used for tocolysis, may lower Doppler S/D ratios in the fetal aorta and uterine artery, thus confusing interpretation of the waveforms.[42]

PATHOLOGY BOX 24-2

Factors Affecting the Spectral Waveform

Patient position
Fetal and/or maternal breathing
Fetal cardiac arrhythmias
Maternal ingestion of pharmacologic agents

IDENTIFYING PLACENTAL AND FETAL INSERTION

Investigators have noted the clinical significance of the effect of waveform sampling site on Doppler ratios. This is more pronounced in the fetal umbilical circulation than in the maternal uterine circulation. The uterine circulation is composed of multiple vessels that branch and are fed by collateral vessels, whereas the umbilical circulation consists of the umbilical cord itself. Because resistance to blood flow is greater at the fetal umbilical cord insertion than at the placental cord insertion,[26] it is important to obtain a fetal umbilical waveform sample as close to the placental cord insertion as possible (Fig. 24-15).

Several theories might explain the lower ratio at the placental cord insertion than at the fetal cord site. One is that the changes in arterial diameter or wall elasticity may alter the waveform. Another is that pressure changes across the fetal abdominal wall lead to changes in resistance. The third explanation is that the decrease in the ratio may be the result of dampening and attenuation of the propagated wave. If the sampling location is not known and ratios are high, the examiner should take multiple samples at different locations along the cord to see whether the results are consistent. The accuracy of Doppler measurements depends on consistent and uniform measurement techniques.

FUTURE DIRECTIONS

Doppler ultrasound has become routine in surveillance and management of the at-risk fetus for poor perinatal or neonatal outcome. Since Doppler has been introduced, various investigators have acknowledged its usefulness as a screening tool to aid in the prediction of subsequent pregnancy complications.[43–45,22,29,46] Very high umbilical S/D ratios, absent end-diastolic flow, and complete reversal of flow have been associated with fetal and neonatal death.[47–50]

Doppler ultrasound has shown that in fetuses with asymmetric IUGR, vascular resistance increases in the aorta and umbilical artery and decreases in the middle cerebral artery. This phenomenon ensures blood flow to the brain at the expense of the extremities, reinforcing the head-sparing theory. Increased vascular resistance is reflected by diminished or absent umbilical diastolic flow, leading to an increased S/D ratio or PI.

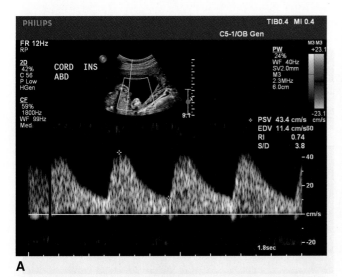

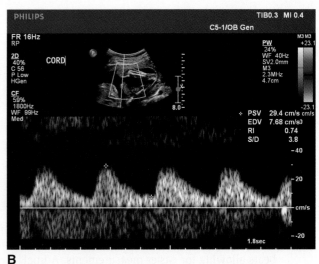

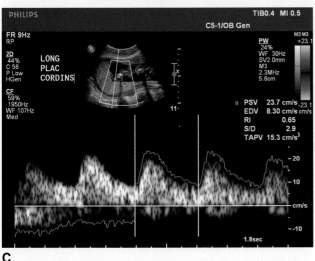

Figure 24-15 Normal duplex sonogram measurements demonstrate the differences in umbilical artery Doppler waveforms due to sampling site. **A,B:** At the abdominal insert and with a section of free-floating cord, the RI is 0.74 and the S/D ratio is 3.8. **C:** At the placental cord insertion, the RI is 0.65 and the S/D ratio is 2.9. These images use a faster sweep speed, allowing for visualization of the waveform. The automatic tracing decreases inter- and intraoperator measurement variation.

Extreme cases of elevated resistance causing absent or reversed umbilical end-diastolic flow velocity waveforms are associated with high rates of morbidity and mortality.[48]

It is just as important to evaluate the maternal vessels as it is to evaluate the fetal side of the circulation. Abnormal waveform readings can be early signs of a predisposing condition and should not be ignored.[30,51-53] The finding of an abnormal fetal or uterine waveform necessitates careful monitoring, which should include repeated Doppler examinations, growth scans, and tests of fetal well-being. These tests may be suggested to the attending obstetrician.

The advent of duplex Doppler sonography permits the sonographer to be very specific as to which vessels to study. Vessels from the umbilical cord to the intricate circle of Willis have been studied. Technology has now made it possible to study vessels with very low flow. Color flow mapping and color power Doppler have helped further our understanding of the complicated fetal circulatory pathways—not only of the vessels but of the organs they supply. It is anticipated that Doppler studies will help the clinician to take better care of the fetus and provide a noninvasive means of studying the pathophysiology of disease states.

SUMMARY

- The Doppler spatial peak-temporal average intensity (SPTA) should be less than 94 mW/cm² in situ.

- Continuous-wave transducers send and receive uninterrupted sound waves.

- Short bursts of ultrasound energy at regular intervals describes pulsed wave.

- Duplex imaging includes both 2D gray-scale imaging and a spectral tracing.

- Triplex imaging adds a color mode to the 2D gray-scale image and spectral tracing.

- The optimal angle of insonation for fetal Doppler is between 30 to 60 degrees.

- Aliasing with pulsed wave is due to exceeding the Nyquist limiting pulse repetition frequency.

Critical Thinking Questions

This umbilical Doppler image is from a third-trimester gestation. Critically analyze for the following:

1. Spectral tracing technique.

2. Measurements to determine normalcy.

3. Spectral waveform appearance.

4. ROI, sample gate, and angle correct position.

ANSWER:

1. A decrease in the overall gain would reduce the speckle seen surrounding the waveforms. Fetal heart rates are much higher, and reducing the sweep speed decreases the number of displayed beats allowing for easier measurements. A final adjustment would be to make the spectral tracing larger, as this is the area of interest.

2. Measurements vary to the lab protocol but include the S/D ratio, RI, and PI.

3. Both the artery and vein image on this tracing. On qualitative observation, the arterial tracing appears to have a higher resistance; however, only qualitative measurements would confirm this finding. The venous flow has a normal nonpulsatile appearance.

4. The ROI appears to be appropriately sized, as does the 2D reference image. The sample gate is within the umbilical artery; however, to reduce the venous component the sonographer can move or reduce the gate size. There is no need to angle correct, as the S/D ratio, RI, and PI are angle independent.

- Color modes are the translation of the Doppler signal into a color overlay on the gray-scale image.

- The S/D ratio, RI, and PI give an angle-dependent, quantitative measure to the spectral tracing.

- Resistance and waveform appearances differ depending on gestational age, location, and maternal factors

- Averaging of multiple Doppler measurements allows for higher accuracy of quantitative values.

REFERENCES

1. Doppler CJ. Uber das farbige Licht der Dopplersterne. *Abhand Lungen der Koniglishen Bohmischen Gesellschaft der Wissenchaften*. 1842;2:465.
2. Barcroft J, Flexner LB, McClurkin T. The output of the fetal heart in the goat. *J Physiol*. 1934;82(4):498–508.
3. Kirkinen P, Joupilla P, Koivula A, et al. The effect of caffeine on placental and fetal blood flow in human pregnancy. *Am J Obstet Gynecol*. 1983;147(8):939–942.
4. Satomura S. A study on examining the heart with ultrasonics: I. principles. II: instruments. *Jpn Circ J*. 1956;20:227.
5. Baker DW. Pulsed ultrasonic Doppler blood flow sensing. *IEEE Transsonics-Ultrasonics*. 1970;17:170–185.
6. Baker DW, Watkins D. A phase-coherent pulsed Doppler system for cardiovascular measurement. In: *Proceedings of the 20th Alliance for Engineering in Medicine and Biology*. Stockholm. 1967;27:2.
7. Peronneau P, Deloche A, Bui-Mong-Hung H, et al. Debitmetrie ultrasonore: developments et applications experimentales. *Eur Surg Res*. 1969;1:147.
8. Peronneau P, Hinglais H, Pellet M, et al. Velocimetre sanguin par effet Doppler a l'emission ultrasonore pulsáe. *L'onde Electrique*. 1970;59:369.
9. Schleif R. Ultrasound contrast agents. *Curr Opin Radiol*. 1991;3(2):198–207.
10. American Institute of Ultrasound in Medicine. Bioeffects Committee of the American Institute of Ultrasound in Medicine. *J Ultrasound in Med*. 2008;27:503–515.
11. Kremkau F. *Doppler Ultrasound*. 2nd ed. Philadelphia: WB Saunders; 1995.
12. Edelman SK. *Understanding Ultrasound Physics*. Canada: Knowledge Masters Inc.; 2005.
13. Miele Frank R. *Ultrasound Physics & Instrumentation*. 4th ed. USA: Davies Publishing; 2006.
14. Nyquist H. Certain topics in telegraph transmission theory. *Transactions of the American Institute of Electrical Engineering*. 1928;47:617–644.
15. Mehalek KE, Berkowitz GS, Chitkara U, et al. Comparison of continuous-wave and pulsed-wave S/D ratios of umbilical and uterine arteries. *Am J Obstet Gynecol*. 1988;72(4):603–606.
16. Nyberg D, McGahan J, Pretorius D, et al. *Diagnostic Imaging of Fetal Anomalies*. Philadelphia: Lippincott Williams & Wilkins; 2003.
17. Byun YJ, Kim HS, Yang JI, et al. Umbilical artery Doppler study as a predictive marker of perinatal outcome in preterm small for gestational age infants. *Yonsei Med J*. 2009;50(1):39–44. Epub 2009 Feb 24.
18. Misra VK, Hobel CJ, Sing CF. Placental blood flow and the risk of preterm delivery. *Placenta*. 2009;30(7):619–624. Epub 2009 May 21.

19. da Silva FC, de Sá RA, de Carvalho PR, et al. Doppler and birth weight Z score: predictors for adverse neonatal outcome in severe fetal compromise. *Cardiovasc Ultrasound.* 2007;5:15.

20. Hill M, Lande I, Grossman J. Duplex evaluation of fetoplacental and uteroplacental circulation. In: Grant EG, White EM, eds. *Duplex Sonography.* New York: Springer-Verlag; 1988.

21. Lui EY, Steinman AH, Cobbold RS, et al. Human factors as a source of error in peak Doppler velocity measurement. *J Vasc Surg.* 2005;42(5):972–979.

22. Chan F, Pun T, Lam C, et al. Pregnancy screening by uterine artery Doppler velocimetry: which criterion performs best? *Obstet Gynecol.* 1995;85(4):596–602.

23. Itzkovitz J. Maternal–fetal hemodynamics. In: Maulik D, McNellis D, eds. *Ultrasound Measurements of Maternal–Fetal Hemodynamics.* New York: Perinatology Press; 1987.

24. Lewis SH, Benirschke K. Placenta. In: Mills SE, ed. *Histology for Pathologists.* 2nd ed. Baltimore: Lippincott Williams & Wilkins; 2007.

25. Marsal K, Lindblad A, Lingman G, et al. Blood flow in the fetal descending aorta: intrinsic factors affecting movements and cardiac arrhythmias. *Ultrasound Med Biol.* 1984;10(3):339–348.

26. Mehalek K, Rosenberg J, Berkowitz GS, et al. Umbilical and uterine artery flow velocity wave forms: Effect of the sampling site on Doppler ratios. *J Ultrasound Med.* 1989;8(4):171–176.

27. Dawes GS. The umbilical circulation. *Am J Obstet Gynecol.* 1962;84:1634–1648.

28. Indik J, Reed KL. Variation and correlation in human fetal umbilical Doppler velocities with fetal breathing: Evidence of the cardiac placental connection. *Am J Obstet Gynecol.* 1990;163(6 Pt 1):1792–1796.

29. France RA. A review of fetal circulation and the segmental approach in fetal echocardiography. *JDMS.* 2006;22:29–39.

30. Campbell S, Cohen-Overbeek TE. Doppler investigation of the uteroplacental circulation during pregnancy. In: Maulick D, McNellis D, eds. *Doppler Ultrasound Measurement of Maternal-Fetal Hemodynamics.* New York: Perinatology Press; 1987.

31. Tonge HM, Wladimiroff JW, Noordam MJ, et al. Blood flow velocity wave forms in the descending fetal aorta: Comparison between normal and growth-retarded pregnancies. *Obstet Gynecol.* 1986;67(6):851–855.

32. Gill RW. Accuracy calculations for ultrasonic pulsed Doppler blood flow measurements. *Austral Phys Eng Sci Med.* 1982;5:51–57.

33. Lingman G, Marsál K. Fetal central blood circulation in the third trimester of normal pregnancy—a longitudal study. II. Aortic blood velocity waveform. *Early Hum Dev.* 1986;13(2):151–159.

34. Creasy R, Resnik R. *Maternal-Fetal Medicine Principles and Practice.* 3rd ed. Philadelphia: W.B. Saunders Company; 1994.

35. Callen P. *Ultrasonography in Obstetrics and Gynecology.* Philadelphia: W.B. Saunders; 2000.

36. Verburg BO, Jaddoe VW, Wladimiroff JW, et al. Fetal hemodynamic adaptive changes related to intrauterine growth: The generation R study. *Circulation.* 2008;117(5):649–659. Epub 2008 Jan 22.

37. Lingman G, Dahlstrom JA, Eik-Nes SH, et al. Hemodynamic evaluation of fetal heart arrhythmias. *Br J Obstet Gynaecol.* 1984;91:647.

38. Joupilla P, Kirkinen P, Eik-Nes S. Acute effect of maternal smoking on the human fetal blood flow. *Br J Obstet Gynaecol.* 1983;90:7.

39. Joupilla P, Kirkinen P, Koivula A, et al. The influence of maternal oxygen inhalation on placental and umbilical venous blood flow. *Eur J Obstet Gynecol Reprod Biol.* 1983;16(3):151–156.

40. Joupilla P, Kirkinen P, Koivula A, et al. Ritodrine infusion during late pregnancy: effects on fetal and placental blood flow, prostacyclin and thromboxane. *Am J Obstet Gynecol.* 1985;151(8):1028–1032.

41. Joupilla P, Kirkinen P, Koivula A, et al. Labetalol does not alter the placental and fetal blood flow or maternal prostanoids in pre-eclampsia. *Br J Obstet Gynaecol.* 1986;93:543–547.

42. Nimrod C, Davies D, Harder J, et al. Doppler evaluation of the impact of beta mimetic therapy on human fetal aortic and umbilical blood flow. In: *Proceedings of the Society of Perinatal Obstetricians.* Sixth Annual Meeting. San Antonio; February 1986.

43. Bewley S, Cooper D, Campbell S, et al. Doppler investigation of the uteroplacental blood flow resistance in the second trimester: A screening study for pre-eclampsia and intrauterine growth retardation. *Br J Obstet Gynaecol.* 1991;98:871–879.

44. Bower S, Bewley S, Campbell S. Improved prediction of pre-eclampsia by two stage screening of uterine arteries using the early diastolic notch and color Doppler imaging. *Obstet Gynecol.* 1993;82(1):78–83.

45. Bower S, Schuchter K, Campbell S. Doppler ultrasound screening as part of routine antenatal scanning: Prediction of pre-eclampsia and intrauterine growth retardation. *Br J Obstet Gynaecol.* 1993;100(11):989–994.

46. North RA, Ferrier C, Long D, et al. Uterine artery Doppler flow velocity wave forms in the second trimester for the prediction of pre-eclampsia and fetal growth retardation. *Obstet Gynecol.* 1994;83(3):378–386.

47. Berkowitz GS, Chitkara U, Rosenberg J, et al. Sonographic estimation of fetal weight and Doppler analysis of umbilical artery velocimetry in the prediction of intrauterine growth retardation: A prospective study. *Am J Obstet Gynecol.* 1988;158(5):1149–1153.

48. Mari G, Hanif F, Drennan K, et al. Staging of intrauterine growth-restricted fetuses. *J Ultrasoaund Med.* 2007;26(11):1469–1477.

49. Mihu CM, Susman S, Ciuca DR, et al. Aspects of placental morphogenesis and angiogenesis. *Rom J Morphol Embryol.* 2009;50(4):549–557.

50. Haws RA, Yakoob MY, Soomro T, et al. Reducing stillbirths: Screening and monitoring during pregnancy and labour. *BMC Pregnancy Childbirth.* 2009;(9 Suppl 1):S5. Review.

51. Fleisher A, Schulman H, Farmikides G, et al. Uterine artery velocimetry in pregnant women with hypertension. *Am J Obstet Gynecol.* 1986;154:806–813.

52. Jacobson SL, Imhof R, Manning N, et al. The value of Doppler assessment of the uteroplacental circulation in predicting pre-eclampsia or intrauterine growth retardation. *Am J Obstet Gynecol.* 1990;162:110–114.

53. Todros T, Ferrazz E, Arduini D, et al. Performance of Doppler ultrasonography as a screening test in low risk pregnancies: results of a multicentic study. *J Ultrasound Med.* 1995;14(5):343–348.

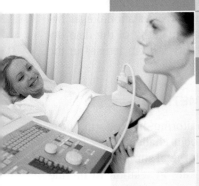

25 The Biophysical Profile

Meredith O. Cruz and Isabelle Wilkins

KEY TERMS

biophysical profile (BPP) | antepartum testing | antepartum surveillance | cardiotocographic | nonstress test (NST) | vibroacoustic stimulation | false positive | false negative | hypoxemia | oxytocin challenge test (OCT) | amniotic fluid volume (AFV) | amniotic fluid index (AFI)

GLOSSARY

Acidosis Blood pH below 7 resulting from an increase in hydrogen concentrations due to impaired blood supply to the fetus

Amniotic fluid index (AFI) Rough estimate of the fluid surrounding the fetus obtained through the measurement of four pockets of amniotic fluid, one from each of the abdominal quadrants

Amniotic fluid volume (AFV) Amount of fluid within the amniotic sac surrounding the fetus; the AFI is an estimate of this amount

Asphyxia Decrease in oxygen content of the blood accompanied by an increase in carbon dioxide

Biophysical profile (BPP) Monitoring of fetal activity to include breathing movements, discrete movements, tone, and fluid surrounding the fetus accompanied by an NST

Cardiotocographic (CTG) Technique of concurrently recording the fetal heartbeat and uterine contractions

False negative Incorrect negative test result when the state being tested is present. Example: The fetus reacts

during a BPP; however, there is fetal compromise due to acidosis

False positive Positive result when the state being tested is absent. Example: Nonreactive BPP due to fetal sleep cycles

Hypercapnia Abnormally high level of circulating carbon dioxide

Hypoxemia Reduced blood oxygen levels

Modified biophysical profile (mBPP) Prenatal testing including only the NST and AFI

nonstress test (NST)

Oligohydramnios Low fluid surrounding the fetus

Oxytocin challenge test (OCT) Intravenous injection of oxytocin causing the uterus to contract; monitoring of the fetal reaction to uterine contractions aims to determine how the fetus reacts to environmental stress

pH Measure of alkalinity or acidity of the blood: 7 is neutral, greater than 7 is alkaline, less than 7 is acidic

Direct observation of a patient is a vital part of the clinician's examination. In the last 100 years, the observation of in utero activity led to the scientific study of fetal movements and breathing. Ultrasound allows the direct observation of qualitative, as well as quantitative, aspects of fetal motor behavior throughout the course of pregnancy. The visualization of fetal activity in terms of the current status of that activity, as well as its development, has proven vital to the assessment of fetal condition. Clinical investigation demonstrates the presence of fetal physiologic processes. These parameters allow the clinician to determine the fetal risk for mortality and take appropriate action.

Maternal perception of fetal movements has been the main determinant in assessing fetal well-being throughout history. The first written record of fetal movement can be found in the Bible, where the twins of Rebecca "struggled together within her."[1] Studies evaluated fetal development through maternally perceived fetal movements in the second half of pregnancy. Studies of fetal movement timing demonstrated movement of delivered 20-week fetuses.[2,3] To this day, maternal perception of fetal movements is an important aspect of prenatal care and concern, as any decrease is a common reason for a visit to an obstetrical emergency center. Using maternally monitored fetal "kick counts" is an accepted and scientifically valid way of assessing fetal well-being in the third trimester.[4]

Real-time ultrasound has made it possible to observe the fetus in a noninvasive manner to evaluate its state of health. In 1980, Manning and colleagues developed the biophysical profile (BPP) for evaluation of fetal health and to identify those at risk.[5] The method described used five observations to determine fetal well-being: spontaneous breathing, overall body movements, tone, heart rate changes, and urine output measured through the amniotic fluid volume (AFV). The BPP has been shown to be very sensitive in predicting acute fetal compromise as well as identifying normally oxygenated fetuses.[6]

This chapter reviews the technical issues in performing a BPP, the principles of antenatal surveillance, and clinical application in the determination of fetal well-being. When properly used, careful interpretation of the BPP allows for informed diagnosis and development of management plans concerning the ongoing pregnancy and timely delivery of the fetus.

ANTEPARTUM TESTING

RATIONALE FOR PERFORMANCE

Antepartum testing is a method developed to detect fetal asphyxia. This has a wide application in high-risk pregnancies, particularly in fetuses at risk for in utero demise. In almost all circumstances, the testing is used to determine whether a fetus should be delivered or allowed to remain in utero. Therefore, this testing is only indicated in pregnancies in which delivery would be a reasonable option if the results of testing are worrisome. This also means that it is never used at early gestational ages before fetal viability, and the vast majority of the data describing the use and applicability is from fetuses in the latter part of the third trimester.

CARDIOTOCOGRAPHIC METHODS

Electronic fetal heart rate monitoring, in the form of the nonstress test (NST) or oxytocin challenge test (OCT), are frequently used methods for fetal surveillance. These tests monitor the fetal heart rate in relation to uterine contractions, either spontaneous (NST) or induced (OCT). Decelerations of the fetal heart rate late in the contraction cycle help identify fetal mortality risk. The negative test demonstrates normal fetal heart rates with three uterine contractions in a 10-minute period. However, the use of only the fetal heart rate for fetal health evaluation limits testing and results in high false-positive rates.[4] That is, a relatively high proportion of healthy fetuses have a nonreactive NST.[6]

The OCT has much lower rates of false positives and false negatives. However, this cumbersome test requires careful infusion of intravenous oxytocin and usually takes several hours to complete.[4]

THE BIOPHYSICAL PROFILE

The development of real-time ultrasound made it possible to perform noninvasive, in utero observations of the fetus to evaluate its state of health. The BPP provides a more complete evaluation of the state of fetal health and addresses parameters of fetal well-being other than heart rate. There is a lower false-positive rate than the NST and a comparably low false-negative rate to the OCT. For most obstetrical clinics and inpatient units, with the widespread availability of ultrasound scanning, the BPP is a good alternative form of testing to the two established forms using electronic fetal monitors.

FETAL BIOPHYSICAL COMPONENTS

The components of the fetal BPP include observations of fetal breathing movements, gross fetal body movements, fetal tone, amniotic fluid volume, and the NST during the same observation period. Except for the NST, all variables are recorded using real-time ultrasound. These variables are initiated and regulated by the fetal central nervous system (CNS), and it is thought that the presence of any given variable is indirect evidence of hypoxia or acidemia.[4]

FETAL BREATHING

Fetal breathing can be visualized by obtaining a longitudinal sectional view with a real-time scanner. These movements consist of spontaneous movement of the diaphragm in a caudad-cephalad direction, leading to

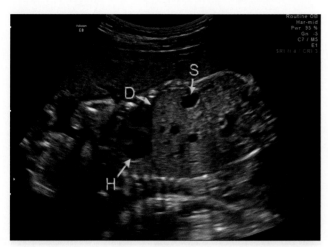

Figure 25-1 The sagittal plane through the chest and abdomen allows for observation of diaphragmatic movement as well as chest and abdominal changes. *S*, stomach; *H*, heart; *D*, diaphragm.

an inward movement of the anterior chest wall and a simultaneous outward movement of the anterior abdominal wall.[7] The suggested plane for assessing breathing movements can be seen in Figure 25-1. An alternate observation is the caudad-cephalad movement of the kidneys.[8] The presence of at least one episode of sustained fetal breathing of at least 30 seconds' duration (with breath-to-breath intervals of less than 6 seconds) within a 30-minute observation period is required to satisfy the breathing requirement of the BPP. Shorter breathing episodes fail to meet this criterion.

FETAL MOVEMENTS

Motor behavior of the fetus, including both fetal movements and breathing movements, has been demonstrated to be a normal fetal function throughout the course of pregnancy. Quickening is the first maternal perception of fetal movement and usually occurs between the 16th and 20th weeks of gestation.[8] The study of fetal movements in pregnancy is important in that they reflect the development of the fetal CNS. As such, fetal motor activity can be seen as a function controlled by the CNS and can reflect both the neural development and possible disturbances in the CNS.[9]

Gross fetal movements are considered present if three or more rolling movements of the trunk are observed within a 30-minute observation period (Fig. 25-2). Movements may be obtained via a longitudinal or transverse sectional view; however, a survey of gross fetal movements would likely be easier to observe in a view with the transducer along the longitudinal axis of the limbs. Other movements in this category that count include large limb movements, face and hand movements, and swallowing.[10]

FETAL TONE

Fetal tone is considered normal if at least one episode of extension of extremities with return to position of flexion, or extension of spine with return to position of flexion, is visualized in the 30-minute observation period.[9] As suggested with gross fetal movements, fetal tone can also be observed in any orientation as long as the extremities are well visualized (Fig. 25-3).

AMNIOTIC FLUID VOLUME

This parameter is a direct measure of the fetus and placenta, while the preceding observations related to the fetal CNS.[9] Quantification of the amniotic fluid volume (AFV) is an area of some variation in practice. The BPP was originally described with AFV determined by measurement of the largest vertical pocket of amniotic fluid; a pocket of 2 centimeters (cm) was considered adequate. Since that time, the standard for measuring AFV by ultrasound in general has changed, and the

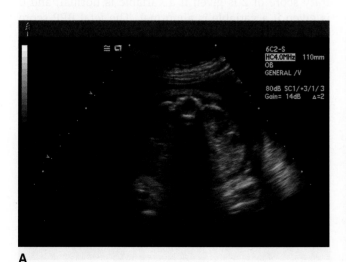

A

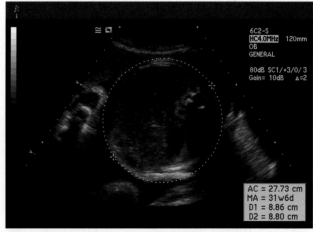

B

Figure 25-2 A: Image demonstrating the fetal abdomen at the level of the kidneys with the spine to the anterior maternal abdomen. **B:** The fetus rolled clockwise on this image taken at the level of the abdominal circumference level. This rolling movement occurred multiple times during the exam.

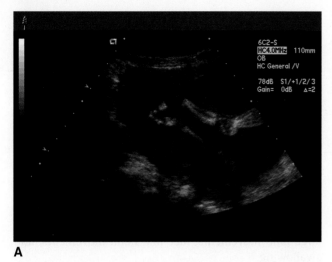

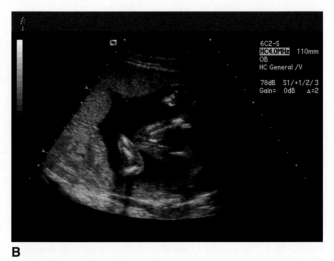

A   **B**

Figure 25-3 The right leg extended **(A)** and quickly flexed **(B)**.

amniotic fluid index (AFI) is commonly used throughout the third trimester to objectively assess this.

The AFI is determined by dividing the maternal abdomen into four quadrants, using the umbilicus and linea nigra as the horizontal and vertical reference points of division, respectively (Fig. 25-4). While holding the ultrasound transducer perpendicular to the floor (if the patient is supine), the vertical diameter of the largest pocket of amniotic fluid in each quadrant is identified and measured.[9] These measurements should be taken in cord loop–free pockets of amniotic fluid. These aspects of the measurement technique for AFV assessment are identical, whether measuring a single deepest pocket or the AFI. In the case of the AFI, the numbers from each quadrant are summed and the total reported (Fig. 25-5). The four quadrants should be obtained in sequence within a few minutes, so that the fluid does not shift from one to quadrant to another as the fetus moves.

This method was first suggested by Phelan, who suggested that an AFI of 5.0 cm or less is indicative of oligohydramnios.[10,11] The AFI has replaced measurement of the deepest vertical pocket of amniotic fluid in most practices, though either of these methods of amniotic fluid assessment may be used, and there is data to support each (Fig. 25-6).[12-14]

PUTTING IT ALL TOGETHER

SCORING

In general, measurements of the BPP parameters have been made as objective as possible to eliminate the possibility of any qualitative judgments in assessment of the fetus. Each biophysical variable is coded as normal whenever fixed criteria are reached, regardless of the duration of observation, up to a maximum of 30 minutes for the ultrasound variables, and up to 40 minutes when determining fetal heart rate reactivity. An arbitrary score of 2 is given if a variable is normal, and 0 is given if a variable is abnormal. The fetal BPP score is the result of adding each score of all five variables.

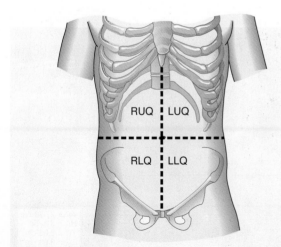

Figure 25-4 The linea nigra, a horizontal line extending from the sternum to the symphysis pubis, divides the abdomen into right and left sections. A perpendicular line bisecting the umbilicus designates the upper and lower halves of the abdomen. These two lines create the four quadrants used to measure the AFI.

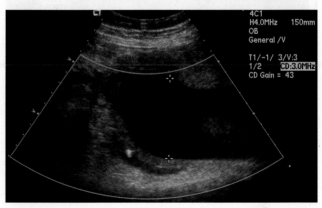

Figure 25-5 An example of a right upper quadrant horizontal measurement of a fluid pocket. The use of color Doppler ensures the pocket is free of cord.

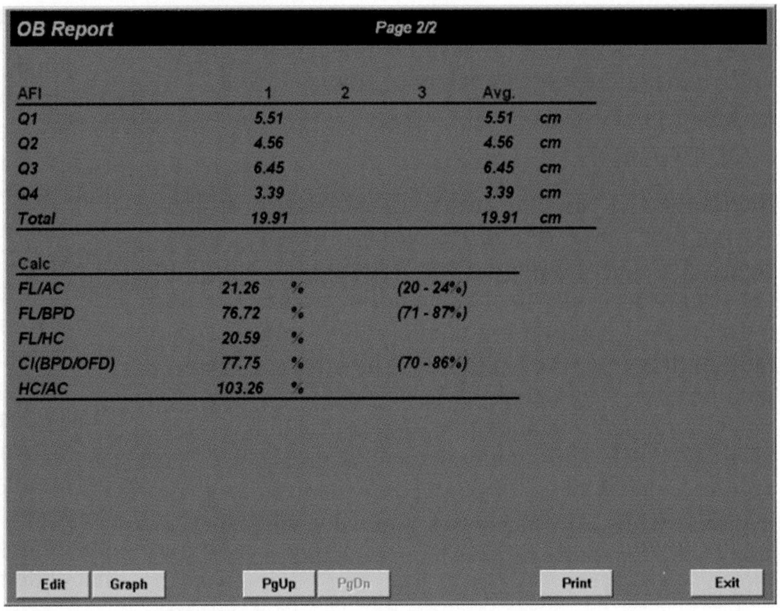

Figure 25-6 An example of an equipment-generated obstetric report for an AFI.

The characteristics of the BPP are summarized in Table 25-1.

The highest possible score obtainable is 10; the lowest score that can be observed when all the parameters are abnormal is 0.[4] A combined score of 8 or 10 is regarded as normal. An equivocal score of 6 indicates the need for further evaluation. For example, in the postterm fetus, this will usually prompt delivery. However, if this is not a preferred option in the clinical circumstances, further surveillance is usually ordered and the profile repeated within 24 hours. A score of 4, 2, or 0 is indicative of fetal compromise and mortality, resulting in consideration of delivery of the fetus.[4]

A deviation from this system applies in the case of oligohydramnios. Oligohydramnios should prompt further evaluation, even if the remaining biophysical parameters are reassuring.[4] At term, this will almost

TABLE 25-1		
Biophysical Profile Scoring		
Variable	**Score 2**	**Score 0**
Nonstress test (may be omitted without compromising validity if all four components of ultrasound are present)[41]	Presence of two or more fetal heart rate accelerations of at least 15 beats per minute lasting at least 15 seconds and associated with fetal movement in 40 minutes	No acceleration or less than two accelerations of the fetal heart rate in 40 minutes of observation
Fetal breathing movements	Presence of at least one episode of sustained fetal breathing of at least 30 seconds' duration within a 30-minute observation period	Absence of fetal breathing or the absence of an episode of breathing of at least 30 seconds' duration during a 30-minute observation period
Fetal movements	Three or more gross discrete body or limb movements in 30 minutes of observation	Two or less gross body movements in 30 minutes of observation
Fetal tone	One or more episodes of extension of a fetal extremity with return to flexion, or opening or closing of a hand	Extremities in position of extension or partial flexion. Spine in position of extension. Fetal movement not followed by return to flexion
Qualitative amniotic fluid volume	Largest vertical pocket of amniotic fluid ≥2 cm or amniotic fluid index ≥5	Largest vertical pocket of amniotic fluid <2 cm or AFI <4
Maximum score	10	
Minimum score		0

certainly prompt delivery, but in the preterm fetus, other surveillance may be instituted depending on the underlying fetal and maternal condition.

MODIFIED BPP

Alternatives to the BPP are the modified BPP or simply the BPP alone without the NST. As the BPP would score an 8 if all parameters are reassuring, the NST is not strictly necessary to obtain a normal score. Alternatively, many centers use a modified BPP (mBPP). The mBPP refers to an NST plus AFI. The rationale for this modification is that these two biophysical parameters reflect both acute fetal oxygenation and acid-base balance (NST) and chronic fetal oxygenation (AFV).[10] The NST is believed to be the first component affected by hypoxia, while AFV decreases gradually when perfusion to the brain and heart is increased and renal blood flow is reduced.[9,15]

The criteria for reactivity and amniotic fluid volume assessment when using an mBPP are similar to that of the BPP. If the mBPP is equivocal or positive (i.e., nonreactive NST or abnormal AFI), then the remainder of the BPP is performed. Multiple observational and retrospective studies exist that suggest that the mBPP has efficacy similar to the OCT and BPP, with perinatal morbidity and mortality comparing favorably.[10,16,17]

NONSTRESS TEST

DESCRIPTION AND DEFINITIONS

During a nonstress test, uterine contractions and fetal heart rate monitoring occurs through the use of a cardiotocometer and Doppler.[9] The patient presses a marker whenever she observes fetal movement. The cardiotocometer records a pattern of fetal heart rate; this includes both a baseline heart rate and any periodic changes, in particular accelerations or decelerations from the baseline rate.

A standard definition of a reactive NST is the occurrence of two accelerations within a 20-minute period. An acceleration is defined as an increase of the fetal heart rate over the baseline of at least 15 beats per minute and lasting at least 15 seconds associated with fetal movement (Fig. 25-7).[4,9]

As the occurrence of accelerations is in part a function of maturation of the fetal sympathetic nervous system, different criteria are used below 32 weeks of gestation. In that case, an acceleration is defined as an increase of fetal heart rate over the baseline of at least 10 beats per minute and lasting at least 10 seconds.[4]

In general, if the test is not reactive within 20 minutes, it is continued for one more 20-minute period. Failure to demonstrate a reactive pattern resulting from either lack of accelerations with movement or lack of fetal movement is termed a nonreactive NST.

FETAL STIMULATION

Although the reactive NST has been found to be a safe and reliable indicator of fetal well-being, a nonreactive NST is a less sensitive indicator of fetal compromise. Episodes of nonreactivity are often related to fetal behavioral state. One of the problems with antepartum fetal heart rate testing is the difficulty in separating healthy fetuses at rest from sick fetuses who are not moving because of asphyxia. In other words, the false-positive rate (where "positive" means a nonreactive test) is high, but the false-negative rate is quite low.

Some practitioners attempt to decrease this high false-positive rate by stimulating the fetus, theoretically, to "waken" it from its sleep state. Various attempts to stimulate the fetus have mixed success. These include the administration of orange juice to the mother before testing and manual manipulation of the maternal abdomen.[17]

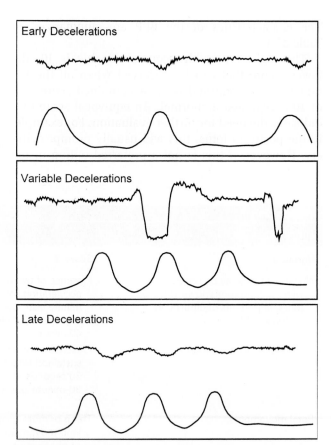

Figure 25-7 The bottom graph indicates uterine contractions; the top is the fetal heart rate. The top graph indicates a deceleration concurrent with the uterine contraction. Early decelerations are considered benign, and there are no adverse effects. The middle graph demonstrates random fetal heart decelerations, which are due to umbilical cord compression. As the umbilical vein compresses, venous return decreases, hypovolemia begins, and the fetal heart rate increases. On the bottom graph, the deceleration occurs after the uterine contraction. This pattern is the result of inadequate uteroplacental oxygen transfer during contractions. Note: Fetal heart rate acceleration result in the graph moving the opposite direction as the deceleration.[4]

In the same vein, vibroacoustic stimulation can be performed as an adjunct to improve the efficacy of antepartum fetal heart rate testing. On stimulation with sound, the fetus responds with a significant increase in fetal movements associated with a corresponding increase in basal fetal heart rate and fetal heart rate accelerations.[18,19] In practice, this stimulus is generated by an artificial larynx or a similar commercially produced device. When it is applied to the maternal abdomen, the well-oxygenated fetus reacts with a startle response.

Several studies have reported that the use of vibroacoustic stimulation results in a significant reduction in the number of nonreactive NSTs and a decrease in the time required for a reactive test to occur.[4] Reactivity achieved with stimulation has a predictive value equal to that of a spontaneously reactive NST. Vibroacoustic stimulation, however, can cause a decrease in fetal breathing movements that can persist for up to an hour after the stimulus.[20,21]

COMPONENTS OF BPP ACROSS GESTATIONAL AGE

FETAL MOVEMENTS

DeVries and associates examined qualitative aspects of the development of fetal movement and determined a specific sequence of emergence of the movements evident in all fetuses studied (Table 25-2).[22] All movements that could be identified in the term fetus were present by the age of 15 weeks. The morphologic appearance of movement patterns has little variance

TABLE 25-2					
Classification and Week of Onset of Fetal Movements					
DEVRIES, ET AL., 1982[27]		**BIRNHOLZ, ET AL., 1978[50]**		**IANNIRUBERTO AND TAJANI, 1981[51]**	
Week of onset	**Movements**	**Week of onset**	**Movements**	**Week of onset**	**Movements**
7	Just-discernible movements	7–16	Twitch	6–7	Vermicular movements
8	Startle extension General movements trunk and limbs	10–12	Independent limb movements	8–18	Jerky global flexion and extension
9	Hiccup Isolated arm or leg movement, independent movement of limbs Isolated retroflexion of head	14	Isolated rotation of head Isolated flexion of head Isolated extension of head	11–18	Jumps with change of lying position
9–10	Isolated rotation of head	12–16	Combined/repetitive simultaneous or serial movements of head, trunk, and limbs	12–13	Isolated or independent movements of limbs Head rotation Hands in contact with hand, face, or mouth
10	Breathing movements Isolated anteflexion of head Hand-face contact face or mouth Stretch Rotation of embryo	16	Hand–face contact	13–14	Breathing movements Opening of mouth Swallowing
10–11	Jaw movements	24	Probable thumb sucking Vigorous diaphragmatic excursions Sudden rhythmic diaphragm movements Respiratory	16	Global extension
11	Yawn				
12	Sucking and swallowing			22	Sudden rhythmic diaphragm movements

(Modified from DeVries JIP, Visser GH, Prechti HFR. Fetal mortality in the first half of pregnancy. *Clin Develop Med.* 1984;94:46–64.)

throughout pregnancy once these patterns emerge (Table 25-3).

As discerned from these studies, the earliest movement of the fetus can be appreciated as early as 6 weeks of gestation. By eight weeks, general movements of the limbs, trunk, and head can be identified. Concomitantly, a "startle" motion was seen in this period. Hiccups were observed by nine weeks of gestation. Fetal breathing movements, both regular and irregular in pattern, have been identified as early as 10 weeks as solitary movements or in combination with jaw opening or swallowing. Identification of rotation of the fetus, as well as active locomotion resulting in position change, is seen at 10 weeks.

Quantitatively, the very young fetus has been found gradually to increase the amount of time spent moving. By 11 weeks, the fetus moves approximately 21% to 30% of the time observed, with a wide range of activity demonstrated between individual fetuses.[23] An increased number of movements occur in the younger fetus; however, these movements have a shorter duration than movements observed at a later gestational age.[24]

Analysis of fetal movement patterns during the second half of pregnancy is characterized by a decrease in the number and incidence of movement as gestational age increases, as well as the association of typical fetal heart rate patterns with fetal movement.[24-28] These facets of movement can be related to the maturation of the CNS. Movement may have a diurnal pattern of motility. Twenty-four-hour observations of fetal movements have demonstrated that the 24- to 28-week fetus has an increase in the incidence of movement during the late night to early morning hours (11 p.m. to 8 a.m.).[24] The 30- to 40-week fetus, however, has a more limited diurnal pattern in which an increase of movement is seen only from 9 p.m. to 1 a.m.[27]

Correlation of fetal movements with fetal heart rate has been found as early as 20 to 22 weeks of gestation.[29] The interaction between movements and heart rate accelerations becomes more evident by 32 weeks' gestation. The number and amplitude of fetal heart rate accelerations associated with movements increase as the fetus approaches 32 weeks.[27] It appears, therefore, that as the fetus nears this gestational age, there is an increasing probability that an NST will be reactive. Before this gestational age, an apparently nonreactive NST may merely be a function of gestational age and therefore CNS immaturity.

TABLE 25-3

Classification of Fetal Movement Patterns

Movement	Description
Just-discernible movements	Slow and small shifting of the fetal contour, lasting from 0.5 to 2 seconds
Startle	Quick, generalized movement always initiated in limbs and sometimes spreading to neck and trunk. Flexion or extension of limbs usually of large amplitude, but can be small or just discernible. Movements last about 1 second
General movements	Whole-body movement without a distinctive pattern or sequence of body part movement
Hiccups	Consists of a jerky contraction of diaphragm; abrupt displacement of diaphragm, thorax, and abdomen
Breathing movements	"Inspiration" consists of fluent, simultaneous movement of diaphragm (caudal direction), leading to movements of thorax (inward) and abdomen (outward)
Isolated arm or leg movements	May be rapid or slow movements involving extension, flexion, external and internal rotation, or abduction and adduction of an extremity without movements in other body parts
Isolated retroflexion of the head	Displacement of the head can be small or large. Large movements may cause overextension of the fetal spine
Isolated rotation of the head	Head may turn from a midline position to one side and back; often associated with hand–face contact
Isolated anteflexion of the head	Carried out at a slow velocity. Occurs independently or with hand–face contact, with observable sucking
Sucking and swallowing	Rhythmic bursts of regular jaw opening and closing at rate of about one per second may be followed by swallowing. Swallowing consists of displacements of tongue or larynx
Hand–face contact	Hand slowly touches face and fingers frequently extend and flex
Stretch	Carried out at a slow speed. Consists of forceful extension of back, retroflexion of head, and external rotation and elevation of arms
Yawn	Prolonged wide opening of jaws, followed by quick closure, often with retroflexion of head and sometimes elevation of arms
Rotation of fetus	Rotation occurs around sagittal or transverse axis. Complex general moments change around transverse axis and include alternating leg movements. Leg movements with hip rotation or head followed by trunk around the longitudinal axis.

(DeVries JIP, Visser GHA, Prechtl HFR. The emergence of fetal behavior: I. qualitative aspects. *Early Hum Dev.* 1982;7:301–322.)

OTHER BIOPHYSICAL PARAMETERS

Fetal breathing movements are considered essential for fetal lung growth and for preparation for extra uterine breathing.[30] Fetal respiratory activity permits both the skeletal and neuromuscular development of the respiratory system to occur and enables the appropriate respiratory epithelial development of the gas-exchanging surfaces of the lung.[31]

Hiccups, also a diaphragmatic contraction, count as breathing movements if sustained for the requisite 30-second duration.[10] Fetal hiccups have been recognized as early as 9 weeks, and their incidence is noted to decrease as gestational age advances. These movements consist of a jerky contraction of the fetal diaphragm. On sonographic scans, hiccups are seen as an abrupt displacement of the diaphragm, thorax, and abdomen. They may occur as single events, but most frequently follow each other in regular succession.[10]

The earliest breathing movements involving regular movement of the diaphragm have been observed at 10 weeks' gestation, with a tendency for these movements to have a regular pattern. Fetal breathing at this gestational age may be observed alone or in combination with jaw opening or swallowing, as well as with general body movements.[29] The incidence of breathing increases with maturity of the fetus; however, it dramatically decreases during labor and up to 3 days before the initiation of labor.[32,33]

INTERPRETING THE BPP

FALSE POSITIVE AND NEGATIVE RESULTS

Misinterpretation of the BPP may have serious consequences in pregnancy. The greatest fear is assigning a reassuring score to a fetus that is hypoxic and could have benefited from more active intervention. On the other hand, a falsely worrisome score that results in the unnecessary delivery of a healthy fetus, perhaps preterm, who was not in need of intervention, is also problematic. One must be aware of a number of variables that may affect the BPP in order to avoid inappropriate interpretation of results, resulting in possible preterm delivery or discharging a patient with a falsely reassuring result.

It has been established that the biophysical activities that appear first during fetal life are the last to disappear in the presence of fetal asphyxia or intra-amniotic infection.[7] The first component of the BPP that becomes abnormal in the face of fetal hypoxia and acidemia is fetal heart rate reactivity, followed by fetal breathing. As fetal acidemia progresses, gross fetal body movements become absent followed by decreased fetal tone.[7] Therefore, one should be wary of a BPP in which the only abnormally scored parameter is tone, as this is likely an inaccurate finding.[7]

FACTORS AFFECTING SCORES

In addition to fetal acidemia, other factors may have an effect on fetal breathing. Breathing movements increase during periods of hypercapnia, but decrease with maternal hyperventilation.[7] During maternal hypoxemia, cessation of fetal respirations occurs.[7] Fetal breathing movements can be reduced in other circumstances, such as after operative manipulation or after the ingestion of sedatives and alcohol.[7]

Feeding a patient before an ultrasound examination has been suggested as a way of reducing false results, though this is not supported in clinical trials.[24,27] Cigarette smoking does not alter the incidence of fetal movements, though it does alter the pattern of movements, which should not affect the scoring.[34] Maternal caffeine use does not appear to have an effect on general fetal body movements.[35] A variety of fetal and maternal conditions affect amniotic fluid volume, including certain medications (e.g., indomethacin), maternal diabetes, and maternal dehydration.[36] The effects of magnesium sulfate have also been studied by multiple groups. Overall, investigators have found a decrease in fetal heart rate reactivity and fetal breathing movements but no change in fetal tone or amniotic fluid volume.[37–39]

PHYSIOLOGY

Because nervous tissue is highly dependent on adequate oxygenation, the presence or absence of these biophysical activities may reflect the state of fetal oxygenation. It has been theorized that an asphyxial insult, regardless

---

PATHOLOGY BOX 25-1

Patterns of Fetal Breathing Movements

Pattern	Characteristics of Patterns	Rate
Regular	Regular in rate and amplitude	40–60 breaths/min
Irregular	Observed in the fetus <26 wk gestational age; highly irregular in rate and amplitude	20–100 breaths/min
Irregular slow	Slow, large amplitude	6–20 breaths/min
Periodic accelerated	Crescendo–decrescendo changes in rate and amplitude	30–90 breaths/min
Hiccups	Irregular, intermittent, large-amplitude breaths; short duration of individual breaths	20–60 breaths/min

(Manning FM, Platt LD. Fetal breathing movements: antepartum monitoring of fetal condition. *Clin Obstet Gynecol*. 1979;6:335–349.)

of cause, elicits adaptive protective fetal responses that manifest as consistent changes in biophysical variables. With regard to short-term biophysical variables that reflect an acute fetal condition (heart rate reactivity, fetal movement, fetal breathing, and fetal tone), the fetal response to hypoxia is a suppression of some or all of these activities, which may in turn reduce fetal oxygen consumption.[7] Furthermore, fetal asphyxia induces redistribution of cardiac output toward essential fetal organs (brain, heart, and placenta) at the expense of the kidneys and lungs. A prolonged or repeated episode of hypoxia leads to a near cessation of perfusion of the fetal lung and kidney, resulting in decreased urine and lung fluid production and resultant oligohydramnios.[10]

Variations in sensitivity to hypoxemia of specific areas of the brain responsible for the initiation of biophysical activities results in a progressive loss of biophysical function. The biophysical activities that become active first in fetal development appear to be the last to disappear when asphyxia arrests all biophysical activities. In terms of development, the fetal tone center is the earliest to function during intrauterine life (7.5 to 8.5 weeks), followed by the fetal movement, fetal breathing movement, and heart rate reactivity centers.[40] Clinical studies have demonstrated that the NST results and fetal breathing movements are the first biophysical variables to become abnormal in the asphyxiated fetus, followed by fetal movements, and finally by fetal tone.[7] The absence of any one of these variables does not necessarily imply that the CNS is not intact and functioning. Because of the cyclic nature of many of these factors, absence of any one of the variables may reflect a sleep–rest state rather than a neurologic depression.[7]

CLINICAL APPLICATIONS

The fetal BPP is used primarily in patients with high-risk conditions. Initiation of testing is set at a gestational age identical to that used in other methods of fetal surveillance (the OCT and the NST)—that is, the gestational age at which the physician would be willing to intervene should an abnormal test be observed. The BPP is more easily interpreted at early gestational ages than the NST. The goals of fetal assessment are to identify fetuses that are well oxygenated or at risk for hypoxia and to enable appropriate intervention so that perinatal mortality and morbidity can be prevented or reduced.[4]

A number of prospective studies have reported on the BPP results of more than 26,000 high-risk patients, demonstrating that a significant exponential rise in perinatal morbidity and mortality occurs with decreasing profile scores.[42] Further, the value of the BPP in assessing the fetus at risk for asphyxia has been substantiated in a number of clinical studies that have revealed a strong relationship between the fetal BPP score and umbilical venous pH. Manning and colleagues compared fetal BPP scores with umbilical venous pH values and discovered that there was a highly significant linear correlation between BPP score and umbilical venous pH.[4] A score of 0 out of 10 was always associated with a pH less than 7.20, and a score of 8 or 10 was always found to be associated with a pH greater than 7.25. Further, the umbilical venous pH fell significantly as the BPP score fell.

Studies have been carried out on the usefulness of the BPP in specific high-risk conditions including twin gestations,[43] postdate pregnancy,[44] premature rupture of membranes,[45] diabetes mellitus,[36] and intrauterine growth restriction.[46] Studies by Lodeiro et al. have looked at the use of the BPP as an early predictor of fetal infection in patients with premature rupture of the membranes.[47] The absence of fetal breathing and a nonreactive NST were the first signs of impending infection, whereas decreased tone and fetal movement were late manifestations of this obstetric complication.

One unresolved issue has been the interval for testing. Most studies have used weekly testing, though more frequent intervals have been proposed for very high-risk situations or in cases in which there is a change in fetal or maternal status.[48,49]

SUMMARY

- Antepartum testing helps detect the presence of fetal asphyxia through observation of activity within a specified amount of time.
- Cardiotocographic methods of electronic fetal heart rate monitoring include the NST and OCT.
- The BPP is the direct observation of fetal activity (breathing, tone, movement) and an estimate of fluid volume (AFI).
- The fetus obtains a score of 0 (absent) or 2 (present) for each BPP parameter.
- The sagittal plane through the fetal chest, diaphragm, and abdomen provides the best visualization of fetal breathing.
- Sustained breathing movements and/or hiccups lasting 30 seconds within a 30-minute period has a score of 2.
- Three or more full body rolls, large limb movements, swallowing, and face and hand movements within the 30-minute test results in a score of 2 for fetal movements
- The extension and flexion of the spine or limbs within the 30-minute BPP results in a 2 for fetal tone
- A normal AFI for gestational age results in a score of 2
- A total of sonographically obtained BPP points equals 8
- The combination of a reactive NST and the normal BPP results in a score of 10
- Vibroacoustic stimulation, maternal movement, manual manipulation of the maternal abdomen, or ingestion of orange juice helps to awaken or stimulate a nonreactive fetus
- Fetal movements change with gestational age, oxygenation, maternal factors, and circadian rhythms

Critical Thinking Questions

1. A 25-year-old G3P2002 at 32 weeks gestational age with a history of chronic hypertension and on medication presents for antenatal testing. The NST is nonreactive, and a BPP is performed. The following is visualized: fetal breathing for 30 seconds, rolling of the fetal trunk, movement of three extremities, and opening and closing of the hand. The following image of fluid was obtained.

   • What is this patient's BPP score?
   • During the sonographic exam, what accompanying image/measurements would help in diagnosis?

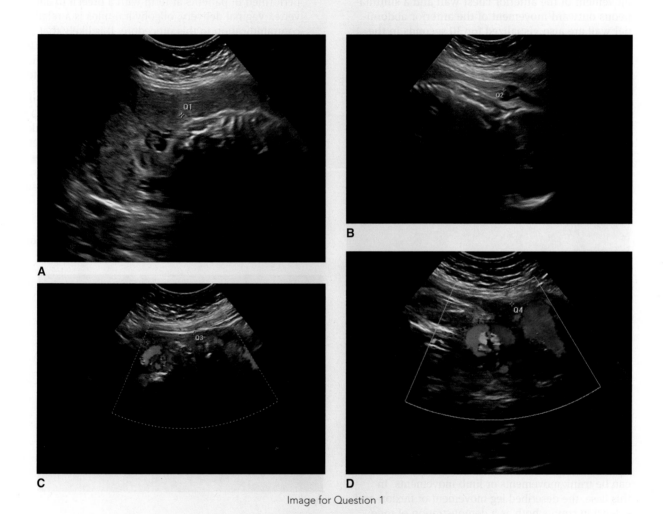

Image for Question 1

ANSWER: Quadrant one has a fluid measurement of 0.6 cm, quadrant two a measurement of 0.4 cm, and no fluid is seen in quadrants three and four, resulting in an AFI of 1.0 cm. Quadrant four appears to have adequate fluid, but on more careful imaging, it is found to be filled with loops of umbilical cord and therefore cannot be measured, resulting in a diagnosis of oligohydramnios. The patient received 2 points each for fetal breathing, fetal movements, and fetal tone for a score of 6. She received zero for amniotic fluid volume and NST, so her total score is 6/10.

Hypertension is associated with a variety of adverse outcomes, including IUGR, pre-eclampsia, indicated preterm delivery, abruption, and stillbirth. In a patient with a history of chronic hypertension and with newly diagnosed oligohydramnios, one would be worried about IUGR and therefore it would be important to measure growth in the fetus if it has not been done recently. Umbilical artery Doppler is a very useful tool in this clinical scenario, as an abnormal finding predicts perinatal morbidity and mortality in IUGR. In a fetus with growth restriction or abnormal Doppler values, the patient will need further evaluation and close monitoring, likely including an inpatient admission.

2. A 33-year-old G1P0 presents to antenatal testing at 41 weeks of gestation. Her prenatal care has been uncomplicated; she has no medical problems. An NST demonstrates moderate variability with one fetal acceleration in 20 minutes. A BPP visualized the following: one episode of rolling of the trunk, one episode of leg flexion, extension with return to flexion, and an AFI measuring 0.5 cm. An inward movement of the anterior chest wall and a simultaneous outward movement of the anterior abdominal wall are also visualized for 30 seconds in the following image. The fetus is noted to be in a breech presentation.

- What is the BPP score?
- How can determining the type of breech presentation help the clinician?

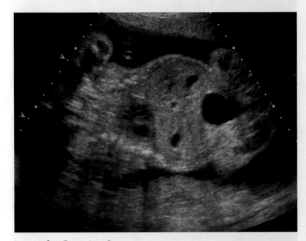

Image for Question 2

ANSWER: The image in this case demonstrates fetal breathing, which is adequate for the fetus to score 2 points. The fetal tone is also adequately seen with flexion and extension of a limb. Fetal movements can be trunk movements or limb movements. In this case, the described leg movement of flexion and extension counts both as a demonstration of tone and as a second fetal body movement. However, as only two movements are seen in 30 minutes, 0 points are awarded for fetal movements. There is not an adequate volume of amniotic fluid, so 0 points are awarded for this. In addition, interpretation of the NST describes one acceleration in 20 minutes, which is inadequate. The NST is nonreactive and is awarded 0 points. The biophysical score in this case is 4/10.

Postterm or postdate pregnancy is a high-risk situation, as perinatal morbidity and mortality increase after 40 weeks. The increase is modest until 42 weeks, when it becomes marked. Antenatal testing is therefore commonly ordered after 40 weeks, and delivery is usually recommended by 42 weeks. One of the key findings in postmaturity syndrome is oligohydramnios. Most obstetricians consider oligohydramnios is this setting as an absolute

indication for delivery, even if other testing is reassuring. In this case, the overall testing is NOT reassuring, so it is likely that she will be delivered expeditiously. The incidental finding of a breech presentation is important in planning the next step for this patient. The type of breech (e.g., frank vs. footling) may be useful to the delivering physician and is therefore useful to delineate. Although external cephalic version may be performed in patients at term with a breech to allow a vertex vaginal delivery, oligohydramnios is a relative contraindication to this procedure. It is likely that she will be scheduled for a cesarean delivery within a few hours. Therefore, notifying her physician before she leaves the unit is the single most important next step.

3. A 29-year-old G4 P1112 at 32 weeks of gestation is scheduled for a BPP because of Class C diabetes and a nonreactive NST. During the BPP frequent trunk movements are demonstrated, there is an open fetal hand, and no movements of the lower extremities are seen as demonstrated in the following figures. Fetal breathing movements for 60 seconds are visualized. The AFI is 26.2 cm.

- What is the BPP score?
- What additional images would help the clinician with this patient?

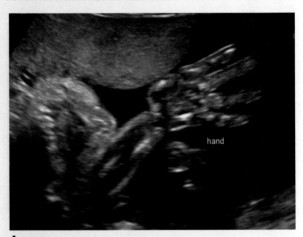

A

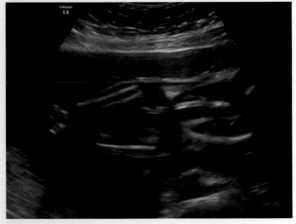

B

Image for Question 3

ANSWER: The fetus received 2 points for gross fetal movements, 2 points for fetal breathing, and 2 points for amniotic fluid volume. Although the amniotic fluid volume is abnormal, this is not reflected in the BPP scoring system and should be separately reported. The NST is nonreactive and receives 0 points. Finally, the fetal tone could not be demonstrated. This receives a score of 0. Therefore, the overall score for the BPP is 6/10. This is an unusual situation and should prompt careful attention to the findings. As the management algorithm for a score of 6 includes further evaluation, the unusual nature of these findings should be included in the overall assessment of the case.

Diabetes follows White's classification in pregnancy, and Class C indicates long-standing disease. These pregnancies are high risk for many adverse outcomes, including fetal anomalies, miscarriage, stillbirth, polyhydramnios, and macrosomia. The BPP results in this case are unusual, as absent fetal tone is a late finding in fetal asphyxia and usually occurs after the cessation of fetal movements and breathing. This leads one to suspect that there may be a different reason for the poor movement of the lower extremities. Polyhydramnios, which may be due to the maternal diabetes, also has associations with anomalies common in diabetes particularly of the CNS, neural tube defects, and cardiac anomalies. Sacral defects such as caudal regression syndrome are specific to diabetes but much less common. The next best step in management would be to perform a targeted scan, which would require a detailed look at the anatomy, as these findings are very worrisome for a fetal anomaly.

4. A patient is a 32-year-old G2 P1001 at 35 weeks of gestation, who presents to antenatal testing because of a history of mild pre-eclampsia. A BPP is performed, which demonstrates a single rotation of the spine and trunk (see image below), active movements of two extremities, flexion and extension of both the upper and lower extremities with return to flexion, more than 30 seconds of fetal breathing movements, and an AFI of 18.2 cm.

- How would you score this BPP?
- What interval of antenatal testing would the clinician request?
- Are biometric measurements obtained during each BPP? Why or why not?
- The patient presents to the emergency room later that evening for vaginal bleeding. An NST is performed and found to be nonreactive; therefore, a BPP is performed. Rolling of the trunk is seen once and there is flexion and extension of the right arm, 10 seconds of fetal breathing movements, and an AFI of 10.2 cm. You notice that the patient had an ultrasound earlier in the day where all four components of the BPP were visualized as above. What is the BPP for this exam?

ANSWER: The initial BPP score includes 2 points for breathing, 2 points for a normal amniotic fluid volume, 2 points for tone, and 2 points for fetal movements. Although an NST is not performed, a score of 8 has been attained and is as predictive of a good outcome as a score of 10. Therefore, it may be omitted. However, as it was not done, it is scored as a 0. Therefore, the BPP in this case is 8/10. Some centers, to distinguish a case such as this from a case in which the NST is nonreactive, score this as an 8/8.

As the testing is reassuring, the next step in management is to schedule repeat testing. It is not necessary to perform an NST, as the predictive value of the BPP would be unchanged. Testing intervals are generally weekly, with exceptions for unstable patients and those with certain specific diagnoses where it is felt that more frequent testing may be beneficial. These diagnoses include IUGR and poorly controlled pregestational diabetes. As this patient has mild pre-eclampsia, she is likely to be a good candidate for weekly testing. Umbilical artery Dopplers would only be considered if the fetus had IUGR. The obstetricians may well be moving toward delivery in her case as she gets to term.

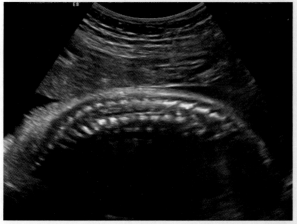

A

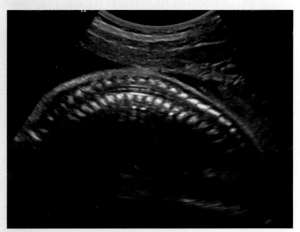

B

Biometric testing does not occur with each BPP because of lack of interval growth during the weekly cycle of observation. Usually BPD, HC, AC, and FL measurements occur every 3 to 4 weeks, depending on the interpreting physician's preference.

The fetal parameters are markedly different than earlier in the day. There is adequate tone demonstrated (although the description seems to indicate that the fetus barely meets criteria compared to the findings of the morning). The amniotic fluid index is still adequate. This is unsurprising, as this is a slowly changing parameter of fetal well-being in the absence of ruptured membranes. The other parameters are abnormal and score a 0. The BPP is therefore a 4/10 (+2 for AFV and tone). The patient now has a more severe manifestation of her original condition, or a new problem, but we cannot assume that the fetal condition is stable. Therefore, repeat testing, as ordered, is clearly indicated. The BPP is properly scored during one 30-minute period of observation. Therefore, the movements from the earlier BPP cannot be applied to the evaluation of the fetus in triage. Pre-eclampsia can be associated with placental abruption and with fetal demise. The new, lower, more worrisome score should be reported.

REFERENCES

1. Genesis 25:22 (English Standard Version).
2. Preyer WF. *Specielle Psiologie des Embryos: Untersuchungenuber die Lebenserscheimungenvor die Gebart*. Leipzig: Griegen, 1885.
3. Sontag LW. The significance of fetal environmental differences. *Am J Obstet Gynecol*. 1941;42:996.
4. Spong CY. Assessment of fetal well-being. In: Gibbs RS, Karian BY, Haney AF, Nygaard I, eds. *Danforth's Obstetrics and Gyenecology*. 10th ed. Philadelphia: Wolters Kluwer/Lippincott Williams & Wilkins; 2008.
5. Manning FA, Platt LD, Sipos L. Antepartum fetal evaluation: Development of a fetal biophysical profile. *Am J Obstet Gynecol*. 1980;136:787.
6. Alberry M, Soothill P. Management of fetal growth restriction. *Arch Dis Child Fetal Neonatal Ed*. 2007;92(1): F62–67.
7. Chavez MR, Oyelese Y, Vintizileos AM. Antepartum fetal assessment by ultrasonography: the fetal biophysical profile. In: Callen PW, ed. *Ultrasonography in Obstetrics and Gynecology*. 5th ed. Philadelphia: Saunders Elsevier; 2008.
8. Sorokin Y, Dierker LJ. Fetal Movement. *Clin Obstet Gynecol*. 1982 Dec;25(4):719–734.
9. Hagen-Ansert S. Fetal growth assessment by ultrasound. In: *Textbook of Diagnostic Ultrasonography*. Volume 2. 6th ed. St. Louis: Mosby; 2006.
10. Harman CR. Biophysical profile scoring. In: Rumack CM, Wilson SR, Charboneau JW, Johnson JM, eds. *Diagnostic Ultrasound*. 3rd ed. St. Louis: Elsevier Mosby; 2005.
11. Phelan JP, Smith CV, Broussard P, et al. Amniotic fluid volume assessment with the four-quadrant technique at 36–42 weeks' gestation. *J Reprod Med*. 1987;32:540–542.
12. Phelan JP, Ahn MO, Smith CV, et al. Amniotic fluid index measurements during pregnancy. *J Reprod Med*. 1987;32(8):601–604.
13. Dawes GS. Breathing before birth in animals and man. *N Engl J Med*. 1974;290(10):557–559.
14. American College of Obstetricians and Gynecologists. Antepartum Fetal Surveillance. Practice Bulletin #9: Oct 1999.
15. Ebrashy A, Azmy O, Ibrahim M, et al. Middle cerebral/umbilical artery resistance index ratio as sensitive parameter for fetal well-being and neonatal outcome in patients with preeclampsia: Case-control study. *Croat Med J*. 2005;46(5):821–825.
16. Williams KP, Farquharson DF, et al. Screening for fetal well-being in a high-risk pregnant population comparing the nonstress test with umbilical artery Doppler velocimetry: A randomized controlled clinical trial. *Am J Obstet Gynecol*. 2003;188(5):1366–1371.
17. Devoe LD. Antenatal fetal assessment: contraction stress test, nonstress test, vibroacoustic stimulation, amniotic fluid volume, biophysical profile, and modified biophysical profile—an overview. *Semin Perinatol*. 2008;32(4):247–252.
18. Petrović O, Finderle A, Prodan M, et al. Combination of vibroacoustic stimulation and acute variables of mFBP as a simple assessment method of low-risk fetuses. *J Matern Fetal Neonatal Med*. 2009;22(2):152–156.
19. Papadopoulos VG, Decavalas GO, Kondakis XG, et al. Vibroacoustic stimulation in abnormal biophysical profile: Verification of facilitation of fetal well-being. *Early Hum Dev*. 2007;83(3):191–197.
20. Olesen AG, Svare JA. Decreased fetal movements: Background, assessment, and clinical management. *Acta Obstet Gynecol Scand*. 2004;83(9):818–826.
21. Gagnon R, Hunse C, Carmichael L, et al. Effects of vibratory acoustic stimulation on human fetal breathing and gross fetal body movements near term. *Am J Obstet Gynecol*. 1986;155(6):1227–1230.
22. deVries JIP, Visser GH, Prechtl HFR. Fetal motility in the first half of pregnancy. *Clin Develop Med*. 1984;94:46–64.
23. Dierker LJ, Rosen MG, Pillay S, et al. The correlation between gestational age and fetal activity periods. *Biol Neonate*. 1982;42(1–2):66–72.
24. Natale R, Nasello-Paterson C, Connors G. Patterns of fetal breathing activity in the human fetus at 24 to 28 weeks of gestation. *Am J Obstet Gynecol*. 1988;158:317–321.
25. Patrick J, Campbell K, Carmichael L, et al. Patterns of gross fetal body movements over 24-hour observation intervals during the last 10 weeks of pregnancy. *Am J Obstet Gynecol*. 1982;142(4):363–371.
26. Prechtl HFR. Continuity and changes in early neural development. *Clin Develop Med*. 1984;94:1–15.
27. deVries JIP, Visser GHA, Mulder EJ, et al. Diurnal and other variations in fetal movement and heart rate patterns at 20–22 weeks. *Early Hum Dev*. 1987;15(6):333–348.
28. Cohn HE, Sacks EJ, Heymann MA, et al. Cardiovascular responses to hypoxemia and acidemia in fetal lambs. *Am J Obstet Gynecol*. 1974;120(6):817–824.

29. Connors G, Hunse C, Carmichael L, et al. The role of carbon dioxide in the generation of human fetal breathing movements. *Am J Obstet Gynecol.* 1988;158(2): 322–327.

30. Carmichael L, Campbell K, Patrick J. Fetal breathing, gross fetal body movements, and maternal fetal heart rates before spontaneous labor at term. *Am J Obstet Gynecol.* 1984;148:675–679.

31. Richardson B, Natale R, Patrick J. Human fetal breathing activity during electively induced labor at term. *Am J Obstet Gynecol.* 1979;133(3):247–255.

32. Vintzileos AM, Gaffney SE, Salinger LM, et al. The relationship between fetal biophysical profile and cord pH in patients undergoing cesarean section before the onset of labor. *Obstet Gynecol.* 1987;70(2):196–201.

33. Vintzileos AM, Fleming AD, Scorza WE, et al. Relationship between fetal biophysical activities and umbilical cord blood gas values. *Am J Obstet Gynecol.* 1991;165(3): 707–713.

34. Cowperthwaite B, Hains SM, Kisilevsky BS. Fetal behavior in smoking compared to non-smoking pregnant women. *Infant Behav Dev.* 2007;30(3):422–430.

35. McGowan J, Devoe LD, Searle N, Altman R. The effects of long- and short-term maternal caffeine ingestion on human fetal breathing and body movements in term gestation. *Am J Obstet Gynecol.* 1987;157:726–729.

36. Zisser H, Jovanovic L, Thorsell A, et al. The fidgety fetus hypothesis: fetal activity is an additional variable in determining birth weight of offspring of women with diabetes. *Diabetes Care.* 2006;29(1):63–67.

37. Darmstadt GL, Yakoob MY, Haws RA, et al. Reducing stillbirths: interventions during labour. *BMC Pregnancy Childbirth.* 2009;(9 Suppl 1):S6.

38. Manning FA, Snijders R, Harman CR, et al. Fetal biophysical profile score: VI. Correlation with antepartum umbilical venous fetal pH. *Am J Obstet Gynecol.* 1993; 169(4):755–763.

39. Platt LD, Eglinton GS, Sipos L, et al. Further experience with the fetal biophysical profile score. *Obstet Gynecol.* 1983;61(4):480–485.

40. Vintzileos AM, Campbell WA, Ingardia CJ, et al. The fetal biophysical profile and its predictive value. *Obstet Gynecol.* 1983;62:271–278.

41. Manning FA, Morrison MB, Harman CR, et al. Fetal assessment based on fetal biophysical profile scoring: Experience in 19,221 referred high risk pregnancies. *Am J Obstet Gynecol.* 1987; 157:880–884.

42. Manning FA, Harman CR, Morrison I, et al. Fetal assessment based on fetal biophysical profile scoring: IV. An analysis of perinatal morbidity and mortality. *Am J Obstet Gynecol.* 1990;162(3):703–709.

43. Devoe LD. Antenatal fetal assessment: Multifetal gestation—an overview. *Semin Perinatol.* 2008;32(4):281–287.

44. Bresadola M, Lo Mastro F, Arena V, et al. Prognostic value of biophysical profile score in post-date pregnancy. *Clin Exp Obstet Gynecol.* 1995;22(4):330–338.

45. Chauhan SP, Parker D, Shields D, et al. Sonographic estimate of birth weight among high-risk patients: Feasibility and factors influencing accuracy. *Am J Obstet Gynecol.* 2006;195(2):601–606.

46. Kaur S, Picconi JL, Chandha R, et al. Biophysical profile in the treatment of intrauterine growth-restricted fetuses who weigh <1000g. *Am J Obstet Gynecol.* 2008;199(3):264.e1–e4.

47. Lodeiro JG, Vintzileos AM, Feinstein SJ, et al. Fetal biophysical profile in twin gestations. *Obstet Gyncol.* 1986;67(6):824–827.

48. Habek D, Hodek B, Herman R, et al. Fetal biophysical profile and cerebro-umbilical ratio in assessment of perinatal outcome in growth-restricted fetuses. *Fetal Diagn Ther.* 2003;18(1):12–16.

49. Odibo AQ, Quinones JN, Lawrence-Cleary K, et al. What antepartum fetal test should guide the timing of delivery of the preterm growth-restricted fetus? A decision-analysis. *Am J Obstet Gyncecol.* 2004;191(4):1477.

50. Birnholz JC, Stephens JC, Faria M. Fetal movement patterns: A possible means of defining neurologic developmental milestones in utero. *AJR Am J Roentgenol.* 1978;130(3):537–540.

51. Ianniruberto A, Tajani E. Ultrasonographic study of fetal movements. *Semin Perinatol.* 1981;5(2):175–181.

26 Multiple Gestations

Julia A. Drose

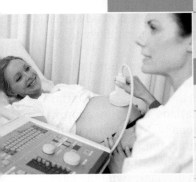

OBJECTIVES

List the types of twin gestations and how they occur

Describe the clinical and laboratory findings found with a multiple pregnancy

Summarize the sonographic criteria for determining chorionicity and amnionicity in the first, second, and third trimesters

Explain the differences and similarities of the sonographic examination between a singleton and a multiple pregnancy

Identify the process occurring with a vanishing twin, vasa previa, twin reversed arterial perfusion (TRAP) sequence, twin-to-twin transfusion syndrome (TTTS), and conjoined twins

Understand maternal and fetal complications that occur with multiple and higher-order pregnancies

KEY TERMS

multiple gestations | twins | triplets | twin peak sign | chorionicity | amnionicity | twin-to-twin transfusion syndrome | twin reversed arterial perfusion (TRAP) sequence | conjoined twins

GLOSSARY

Amnionicity Determination of the number of fetal amniotic membranes

Anembryonic Lack of an embryo

Biometry Measurements done on an embryo or fetus such as a crown-rump length (CRL) or biparietal diameter (BPD)

Chorionicity Determination of the number of chorionic membranes adjacent to the uterus

Dizygotic (DZ) Two zygotes as a result of the fertilization of two ovum

Follicle-stimulating hormone (FSH) Hormone that induces the growth of Graafian follicles

Gamete intrafallopian transfer (GIFT) Mixing of the ovum and sperm within the fallopian tubes allowing for fertilization within the woman's body

Hypervolemic Increase in circulating blood volume

Hysterotomy Surgical incision into the uterus (i.e., cesarean section)

Intracytoplasmic sperm injection (ICSI) Injection of a sperm into the oocyte

In vitro fertilization (IVF) Fertilization of the ovum outside the uterus

Macrosomic Large fetus that falls in the 90th percentile for weight

Monoamniotic One amnion

Monzygotic (MZ) One zygote

Morbidity Incidence of disease

Mortality Death rate due to a specific disease

Nonimmune hydrops Edema, accumulation of fluid in tissues and in the peritoneal cavity, and chest, in a fetus not affected by erythoblastosis fetalis

Oligohydramnios Low amniotic fluid levels

Plethoric Abundant

Polyhydramnios Too much amniotic fluid

Quadruplet Four

Thermocoagulation Use of heat to seal tissue

Zygote Fertilized ovum with 23 pairs of chromosomes

Multiple births have increased dramatically in the last decade, currently accounting for approximately 3% of all live births.[1-2] Two primary factors have contributed to this increase: delayed childbearing and increased utilization of assisted reproductive technologies (ART).[3] The risk of multiple births in naturally occurring pregnancies is known to increase with maternal age. Additionally, the need for utilizing ART also increases as women age.

The occurrence rate of triplet and higher-order multiple pregnancies also increased secondary to ART until the late 1990s, but has since begun to stabilize.[4-5]

This stabilization may be secondary to stricter guidelines regarding the number of embryos transferred during an in vitro fertilization (IVF) procedure.

Ultrasound plays an important role in monitoring multiple-gestation pregnancies, including determining amnionicity and chorionicity, identifying fetal anomalies, and evaluating growth throughout gestation. Ultrasound is also commonly used to guide various procedures that may be warranted when an in utero abnormality is detected in a multiple gestation.

CLINICAL INFORMATION

INCIDENCE

Between 1975 and 1998, the rate of twin births increased by 50% to 60% in the United States. The rate of triplet or higher-order multiple births increased by approximately 69%.[6] ART is responsible for the majority of this increase. This includes drug-induced ovulation stimulation as well as IVF procedures, including embryo transfer, intracytoplasmic sperm injection (ICSI), gamete intrafallopian transfer (GIFT), and oocyte donation. It is estimated that infertility treatments are responsible for 75% of triplet pregnancies that occur in the United States.[6]

The effect of ART is seen in both dizygotic and monoamniotic twining rates. Environmental factors affecting multiple gestation rates appear to influence only dizygotic twinning. Monozygotic twinning is relatively constant across populations and independent of other known contributing factors, such as maternal age, race, and heredity.

Multiple gestations, specifically dizygotic twinning, increases with maternal age. In studies conducted before the inception of ART, the rate of twins was reported to increase by 300% between the ages of 15 and 37 years.[7]

In 2006, Beemsterboer and colleagues published a study showing that this increase was due to an increase in follicle-stimulating hormone (FSH) concentration as women age. This increase in FSH resulted in an increased tendency toward multiple follicle development.[8] Since women have been delaying childbirth over the last two decades, advanced maternal age has become a more significant factor in multiple births.[6] It should also be born in mind that women of advanced maternal age are also the population most likely to utilize ART.

Race also plays a role in multiple gestation rates. In the United States, African Americans have the highest rate at 1/76 births and Asians the lowest at 1/92 births. Multiple gestations in Caucasians occur in approximately 1/86 births.[9] Internationally, Nigeria reports the highest rate of multiple gestations and Japan the lowest. The differences between racial and ethnic groups are due primarily to differences in dizygotic twinning rates. The rate of monozygotic twinning remains fairly constant throughout the world.[10]

Epidemiologic studies have shown spontaneously occurring monozygotic twinning to be heavily influenced by genetic factors, whereas spontaneous occurrence of dizygotic twining may result more from environmental influence.[10]

CLINICAL ASSOCIATIONS

A common reason for suspecting a multiple-gestation pregnancy is the physical finding of uterine size being larger than expected for gestational age. The differential diagnosis for this clinical presentation includes polyhydramnios, uterine fibroids, erroneous dates, macrosomic fetus or an extrauterine mass (i.e., ovarian). Physical examination may also prompt the diagnosis of a multiple gestation if two or more fetal heart tones are detected by auscultation or Doppler examination.

Laboratory values may indicate multiple gestations as well. A maternal serum α-fetoprotein (MSAFP) level of >2.5 Multiples of the Mean (MOM) is associated with a higher-order gestation approximately 10% of the time.[11] Other causes of an increased MSAFP include erroneous dating, fetal abnormalities such as an open neural tube defect or abdominal wall defect, and placental masses (i.e., choriocarcinoma).

ANATOMY AND PHYSIOLOGY

CLASSIFICATIONS

Two types of twinning occur. Thirty percent of all twins are monozygotic (MZ), in which a single ovum divides after fertilization. This type of event appears to be random and independent of most clinical and epidemiologic factors.[9] Nearly 70% of all twin gestations are dizygotic (DZ), the result of fertilization of two ova. DZ twinning is influenced by genetic factors, environmental factors, advanced maternal age, and the use of ART.

In pregnancy, the placental membranes are composed of two layers, the outer layer (chorion) and the inner layer (amnion). Three types of placentation or combination of placental membranes are possible with twin gestations. Since all DZ twins result from two separate fertilized ova, they are always going to have two

TABLE 26-1

Association of Placentation of Monozygotic Twins With Timing of Zygote Division

Stage of Zygote Division (days)	MZ Placentation	Approximate Frequency
3	DC/DA	25%
4–7	MC/DA	75%
8–13	MC/MA	1%
13+	Conjoined Twins	1/50,000– 1/100,000

placentas, thus two separate chorions (dichorionic) and two separate amnions (diamniotic).

The number of placentas, amnionicity, and chorionicity of a MZ twin pregnancy can vary, however, and is determined by the stage at which the single fertilized ovum (zygote) divides (Table 26-1). Division of the zygote prior to day 4 (Carnegie stages 1 and 2)[87] following fertilization results in adichorionic/diamniotic gestation, similar to all DZ twins. This occurs in approximately 25% of monozygotic twin pregnancies. When division occurs between 4 and 8 days (Carnegie stages 3–4),[87] only one placenta forms but there are two separate gestational sacs. Therefore, it is a monochorionic (one chorion)/diamniotic gestation. Almost 75% of MZ pregnancies are monochorionic/diamniotic. In less than 1% of cases, division occurs more than 8 days postfertilization. When this occurs, only one placenta with one gestational sac forms, thus a monochorionic/monoamniotic pregnancy results. Division of the zygote more than 13 days after fertilization is exceedingly rare, but if it occurs it will result in conjoined twins. All conjoined twins are monochorionic/monoamniotic (Fig. 26-1).[12]

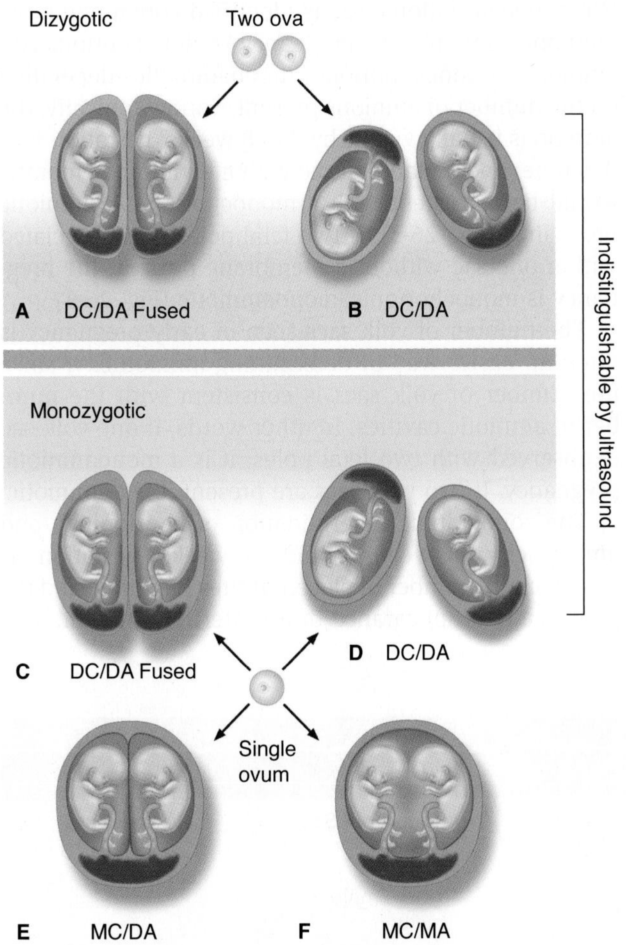

COMPLICATIONS

Multiple gestations in general are considered high-risk pregnancies, accounting for almost 10% of all perinatal morbidity and mortality.[13,14] Perinatal mortality in twins is four to six times higher than in singletons. Additionally, the morbidity rate is twice as high.

Preterm birth, intrauterine growth restriction, and fetal anomalies are all increased in multiple gestations. Twins and higher-order multiples may also develop unique abnormalities such as twin-twin transfusion syndrome (TTTS), twin reversed arterial perfusion (TRAP) sequence, and conjoined twinning.

Maternal complications associated with multiple gestations include an increased risk of pre-eclampsia,

Figure 26-1 Twin development.

PATHOLOGY BOX 26-1

Multiple Pregnancy

Risk Factors	Fetal Complications	Maternal Complications
Assisted reproductive technologies (ART) In vitro fertilization (IVF) Embryo transfer Intracytoplasmic sperm injection (ICSI) Gamete intrafallopian transfer (GIFT) Maternal age Race Family history of monozygotic twins	Increased morbidity and mortality Intrauterine growth restriction (IUGR) Birth weight under 2500 grams Delivery before 37 weeks Twin-twin transfusion syndrome (TTTS) Twin reversed arterial perfusion (TRAP) sequence Conjoined twinning Congenital malformations	Increased risk of: • Mortality • Pre-eclampsia • Hypertension • Placental abruption • Placenta previa • Postpartum hemorrhage • C-section

hypertension, placental abruption, placenta previa, and postpartum hemorrhage.[15]

The risk of abnormality or adverse outcome is also related to the type of twinning. Monozygotic twins are at higher risk than dizygotic twins.[14,16] Dichorionic twins have a reported perinatal mortality risk of 10%, whereas in monochorionic/diamniotic twins the risk is 25% and in monochorionic/monoamniotic gestations the risk increases to 50%. Congenital malformations occur two to three times more often in twins, particularly in monozygotic twins, than in singletons.[17,18] Abnormalities may involve the central nervous system, cardiovascular system, or the gastrointestinal system. An increase in mouth and palate anomalies has also been reported.

Genetically similar MZ twins are nearly 100% concordant for genetic defects (e.g., Down syndrome). The most common discordant genetic defect in an MZ twin pair is a normal fetus paired with one that has Turner syndrome (XO). MZ twins are only 2% to 10% concordant for isolated developmental defects.[19] Because DZ twins are not genetically identical, they have a very low concordance for both genetic and developmental abnormalities. For these reasons, sonography plays a crucial role in determining the type of twinning, the presence of abnormalities, and the monitoring of concordant growth.

SONOGRAPHIC ASSESSMENT

FIRST TRIMESTER

Sonographic determination of chorionicity and amnionicity is most accurate in the first trimester of pregnancy (Table 26-2). In the case of a suspected multiple gestation, an ultrasound examination, both transabdominal and endovaginal, is indicated.

Chorionicity can be determined in the first trimester, by counting the number of gestational sacs. If only one sac is visualized, the pregnancy is monochorionic. Two sacs would be consistent with a dichorionic pregnancy. However, prior to 7 weeks, accurately determining the number of gestational sacs or fetuses present may be challenging. Doubilet and Benson reported that 11% of dichorionic twin gestations were initially diagnosed as singletons on sonograms performed between 5 and 5.9 weeks gestation, as were 86% of monochorionic twin gestations. Additionally, 16% of higher-order

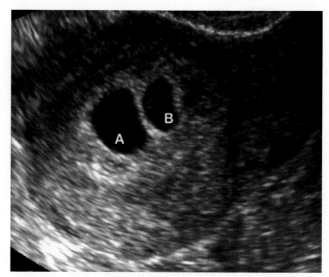

Figure 26-2 Early twin gestation showing two separate, distinct, gestational sacs (*A & B*)

multiples were undercounted. All but one of the undercounted cases was performed endovaginally.[20]

As stated, all dichorionic twin pregnancies must be diamniotic. Therefore, if two distinct gestational sacs are observed in early pregnancy, it is appropriate to classify the pregnancy as dichorionic/diamniotic (Fig. 26-2). When one gestational sac is identified containing more than one fetal pole, the pregnancy is monochorionic/diamniotic or monochorionic/monoamniotic, depending on the number of amnions present. Sonographically, the amnion is usually visible by 7 to 8 weeks' gestation.[21] At this time, one gestational sac with a dividing membrane would be consistent with a monochorionic/diamniotic pregnancy (Fig. 26-3). If two fetal poles are appreciated within one sac without a membrane present, the pregnancy is monochorionic/monoamniotic (Fig. 26-4).

The number of yolk sacs seen in early pregnancy is often an easier way of determining amnionicity, since the number of yolk sacs is consistent with the number of amniotic cavities. In other words, if one yolk sac is observed with two fetal poles, it is a monoamniotic pregnancy. If two yolk sacs are present it is diamniotic.

The sonographic determination of chorionicity and amnionicity, between 11 and 14 weeks' gestation, is based on the number of placental sites identified and the presence and appearance of an intertwin membrane.[22]

TABLE 26-2				
First Trimester Sonographic Criteria for Determination of Chorionicity/Amnionicity				
TYPE	# Gestational Sacs	# Amniotic Cavities	# Embryos/ Sac	# Yolk Sacs
DC/DA	2	2	1	2
MC,DA	1	2	1 per amniotic cavity	2
MC,MA	1	1	2	1

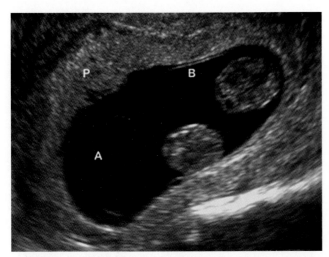

Figure 26-3 Early MC/DA twin gestation. One placenta is visualized (P), with each embryo in a separate amniotic sac (A & B).

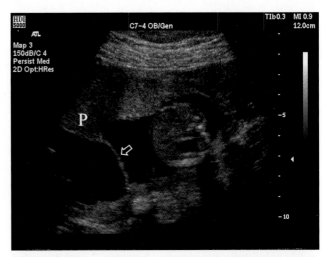

Figure 26-5 Twin peak sign in a first trimester DC/DA gestation. Placental tissue (P) is interjected between the two chorionic membranes. The thick amniotic membrane visualized between the fetuses (open arrow). (Image compliments of Philips Medical Systems, Bothell, WA)

If two separate placentas are identified, the pregnancy has to be dichorionic/diamniotic. If only one placenta is present, the pregnancy is monochorionic. Unfortunately, it is not always possible to determine sonographically if one visualized placenta mass is actually one placenta or two placentas that have become fused secondary to the proximity of implantation. In 1992, Finberg described the "twin peak sign," which refers to the presence of a triangular projection of placental tissue extending up into the base of the junction of two chorionic membranes (Fig. 26-5).[23] If only one chorionic membrane is present, thus one placenta, this triangular extension of placental tissue would not occur.

In 2002, Stenhouse and colleagues reported a 95% accuracy in determining chorionicity when utilizing the twin peak sign.[24] An additional paper in 2002 by Carroll and associates also described utilizing the number of placental sites and the shape of the junction between the membranes and the placenta to diagnose chorionicity.[22] They referred to the wedge-shaped junction (similar to the twin peak sign) formed by placental tissue extending into the base of the chorionic membranes as the "λ" or "lambda sign" and also described a "T-sign," which referred to the T-shaped junction formed when two amniotic membranes fused with one placenta, and therefore one chorionic membrane (Fig. 26-6). Their λ-sign was observed in 97% of dichorionic pregnancies and 0% of monochorionic pregnancies. The T-sign was seen in 100% of monochorionic gestations and in two where dichorionicity was confirmed postnatally.

Thickness of the intertwin membrane has also been described as a predictor of chorionicity. In dichorionic/diamniotic gestations, the membrane comprises two layers

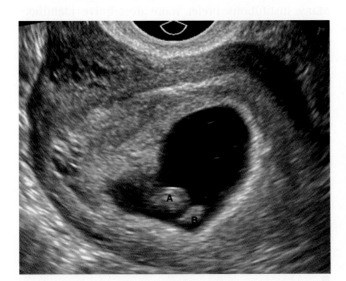

Figure 26-4 Early MC/MA twin gestation showing two fetuses with no intertwin membrane.

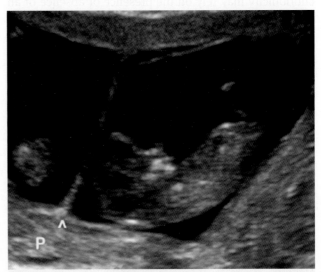

Figure 26-6 Early twin gestation showing the amniotic membranes (arrow head) abutting the placenta (P) to form a "T" sign in a MC/DA pregnancy.

of chorion and two layers of amnion. Sonographically it should appear thicker than the membrane present in a monochorionic/diamniotic membrane, which consists of only two layers of amnion with no interposing chorion.[21] Although an absolute definition of what constitutes a "thick" versus "thin" membrane has not been established, most reported criteria suggest a thick membrane indicating dichorionicity to be of at least 1.5 millimeters (mm) and a thin membrane reflective of monochorionicity as less than 1 mm.[25,26] In Carroll's 2002 paper, an intertwine membrane less than 1.5 mm accurately identified a monochorionic pregnancy in 94.3% of cases, while a membrane greater than 1.5 mm accurately identified a dichorionic pregnancy 94.3% of the time.[22] Bora and colleagues evaluated chorionicity and amnionicity in 67 viable twin pregnancies between 7 and 9 weeks' gestation, utilizing endovaginal ultrasound. Determination was correct in 97% of cases.[27] In 2008, Moon and associates reported 100% accuracy between 11 and 14 weeks' gestation.[28]

SECOND AND THIRD TRIMESTER

Identification of the number of placentas, and the presence and characteristics of an intertwin membrane, are also used in determining chorionicity and amnionicity in the second and third trimesters. Additionally, determining fetal gender can be useful. Twins of different genders are virtually always going to be dichorionic/diamniotic, since they originate from two separate ova and are thus dizygotic. If twins are of the same gender or if gender cannot be identified, chorionicity cannot be determined utilizing this criteria.

As with first-trimester pregnancies, if two discrete placentas can be identified on ultrasound, the pregnancy must be dichorionic/diamniotic (Fig. 26-7). If only one placental mass is observed, the determination of chorionicity may rely on the presence or absence of an intertwin membrane. When a membrane is visualized,

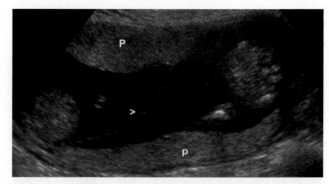

Figure 26-7 Second trimester DC/DA twin pregnancy in which two separate placentas (*P,p*) are visualized, along with an intertwin

the pregnancy is diamniotic. The membrane characteristics described previously can be utilized to aid in determination of chorionicity (Fig. 26-8). However, membrane thickness has been reported to be more reliable before 26 weeks' gestation, due to thinning of the membrane as pregnancy progresses.[29,30] When no membrane is identified, several possibilities exist, including a monoamniotic gestation (Fig. 26-9), a diamniotic gestation in which the membrane is not identified, or in rare cases a stuck twin associated with TTTS.

Sonographic assessment of multiple gestations should include:

- Number of fetuses
- Fetal lie
- Number of placentas
- Presence or absence of membranes
- Standard biometry/anatomy
- Qualitative assessment of amniotic fluid or maximal vertical pocket (MVP)
- Pulsed and/or color Doppler if indicated

By convention, the twin with the presenting part is labeled "Twin A." However, this may become problematic on subsequent exams because the presenting twin may not be the same from one examination to the next. Many institutions prefer more descriptive identifiers

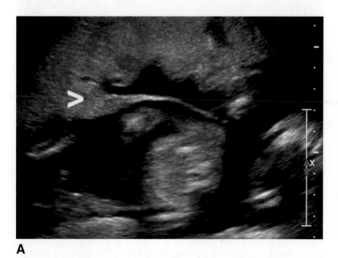

A

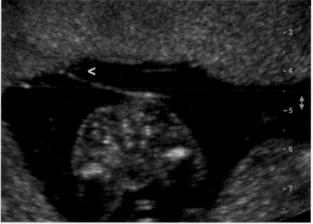

B

Figure 26-8 Twin peak sign in a second-trimester DC/DA twin gestation **(A)**. T-sign in a second-trimester MC/DA twin gestation **(B)**.

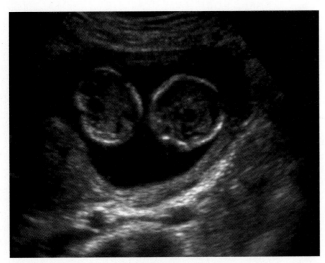

Figure 26-9 MC/MA second-trimester gestation showing both fetal heads without an intertwin membrane.

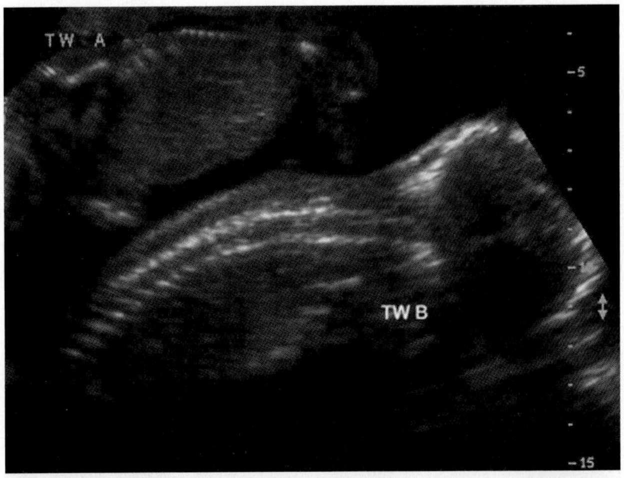

Figure 26-10 First-trimester twins showing a growth discrepancy between a smaller Twin A and a larger Twin B.

such as "right cephalic twin" or "left upper twin." If an abnormality is detected in one twin or if they are determined to be of opposite genders, identification from exam to exam, utilizing these characteristics, is usually straightforward.

The number of placentas, presence or absence of a dividing membrane, and characteristics of the membrane should then be evaluated to determine chorionicity and amnionicity. Some recent studies have advocated the use of three-dimensional (3D) technology in accessing membrane thickness, particularly if difficult to discern by two-dimensional (2D) ultrasound.[31]

Biometry and identification of fetal anatomy, as specified by the American Institute of Ultrasound in Medicine (AIUM), the American College of Radiology (ACR), or the American College of Obstetricians and Gynecologists (ACOG),[32–34] should then be performed on all fetuses, similar to evaluation of a singleton pregnancy.

The growth rate of fetuses in multiple gestation pregnancies is similar to singletons in early pregnancy.[21] Crown-rump length (CRL) measurements may vary slightly between fetuses in the same pregnancy. In that situation, averaging the CRLs may provide the most accurate dating of the pregnancy.[35] Significant discordance is defined as 5 or more days' difference between the CRLs and is usually associated with abnormalities of one or all fetuses (Fig. 26-10).[36] Bora and associates reported that a large intertwin CRL discrepancy in early pregnancy is associated with spontaneous reduction to a singleton pregnancy. They also suggested that the greater the intertwin discrepancy, the higher the likelihood of single fetal loss. In their cohort of 77 pregnancies, a discrepancy of <20% was frequently found in ongoing twins; when the discrepancy was greater than 20%, a single fetal loss was more common.[37]

Several authors have reported that the growth rates of normal multiples in the second and third trimesters also follow that of singleton pregnancies until around 30 weeks. After that time the biparital diameter (BPD) and abdominal circumference (AC) may start to lag behind singletons.[38–40] In triplet or higher-order gestations, biometric parameters may start to lag sooner in pregnancy, except for femur length, which seems to closely follow nomograms developed for singletons.[41]

Birth weights of multiple gestations are uniformly lower than in single fetuses. This reflects the growth lag that occurs later in gestation, as well as the fact that almost all multiple pregnancies deliver early. Growth discordance between twins is one of the most common problems encountered in multiple gestations (Fig. 26-11). Estimated fetal weight percentages that differ by more than 20% are usually considered discordant.[40]

Pulsed Doppler may play an important role in diagnosing and following growth restriction in the presence of discordance between twins (Fig. 26-12). An increased resistance to blood flow within the umbilical

---

PATHOLOGY BOX 26-2

Sonographic Determination of Chorionicity and Amnionicity

First Trimester	Second/Third Trimester
Chorionicity	**11 weeks to term**
• One sac = monochorionic	• Placental sites
• Two sacs = dichorionic	• Two placentas = dichorionic/diamniotic
Yolk sac number	• One placenta = monochorionic
• One yolk sac + two fetal poles = monoamniotic pregnancy	• Intertwin membrane
	• Dichorionic/Diamniotic = thick
• Two yolk sacs + two fetal poles = diamniotic	• Monochorionic/diamniotic = thin
	• Gender

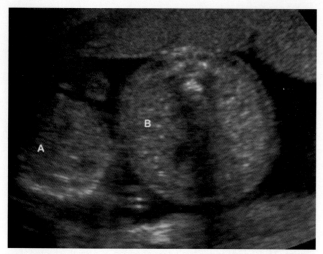

Figure 26-11 Growth discrepancy between fetal abdomens in a second-trimester twin gestation. Twin A's abdomen is markedly smaller than Twin B's.

arteries (UA) or a decreased resistance observed in the middle cerebral arteries (MCA) may occur in the setting of intrauterine growth restriction (IUGR). The various measurements utilized to quantify peak systolic velocities, resistive indices, and systolic to diastolic ratios are similar to those utilized in singleton pregnancies.

As with all pregnancies, amniotic fluid in twin pregnancies should be quantified.

When twins are diamniotic, the amount of amniotic fluid in each gestational sac should be assessed separately. This is usually most easily accomplished by measuring the MVP of fluid in each sac. In the setting of a monoamniotic gestation, either a MVP measurement or a four-quadrant amniotic fluid index (AFI) can be performed.

VANISHING TWIN

In 1986 Landy and associates described the "vanishing twin." They reported that in as many as 20% of twin gestations diagnosed in the first trimester, one twin would "vanish," resulting in a singleton birth.[42] In a study by Gindoff and coworkers,[43] 23 multiple pregnancies were identified in a total of 300 prospectively examined women. Three of the 21 women diagnosed as carrying early twin pregnancies ultimately delivered twins, and of the two remaining multiple gestations, one triplet pregnancy resulted in normal twins, and a quadruplet pregnancy resulted in a normal singleton birth. A "vanishing" second gestational sac may also occur when two sacs are identified early in pregnancy, but subsequent sonograms confirm only one fetus. One explanation for this phenomenon is that the nonviable gestation represented an anembryonic gestational sac, which is proposed to be the cause of 50% to 90% of early spontaneous abortions (Fig. 26-13).[44] Histopathologic examination of these anembryonic gestations reveals autosomal trisomies (52%), triploidies (20%), and monosomy X (15%), among other disorders. Slowed gestational sac growth early on can suggest the diagnosis of an anembryonic gestation, because a normal sac grows at a rate of approximately 0.12 centimeters (cm)/day, and a nonviable pregnancy grows at 0.025 cm/day. Later on, the nonviable gestational sac may begin to involute.

Sonographic criteria for this vanishing sac include a smaller gestational sac than expected for menstrual age, an irregular margin of the sac, and a crescent-shaped sac with an incomplete trophoblastic ring (Fig. 26-14).[43]

One prospective study of multiple-gestation pregnancies documented a group of cases in which twins were identified with fetal cardiac activity at first-trimester ultrasound, but subsequent scans revealed only a singleton pregnancy.[42] This occurred in approximately 21% of prospectively imaged twins. This rate of spontaneous

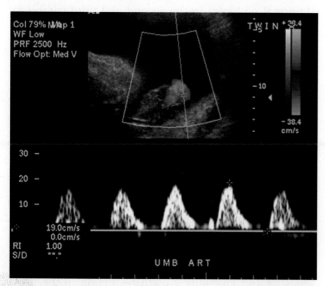

Figure 26-12 Abnormal umbilical artery Doppler waveform in a twin with IUGR. No diastolic flow is appreciated secondary to increased placental resistance, resulting in an abnormal resistive index of 100%.

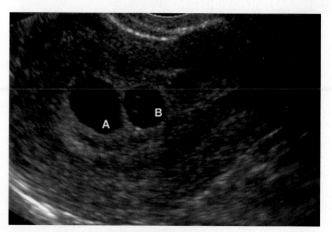

Figure 26-13 Longitudinal image showing two gestational sacs early in pregnancy. One containing a yolk sac (B) and one an embryonic sac (A).

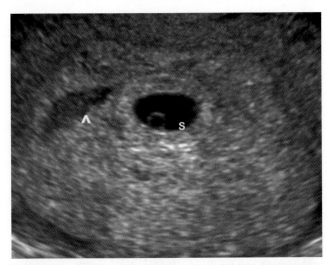

Figure 26-14 Transverse image showing a gestational sac containing a yolk sac *(S)* and a second irregular "saclike" area *(arrowhead)* consistent with an implantation bleed.

the gestation, the more time in which demise might occur), chorionicity of the pregnancy, and abnormal sonographic findings, such as subchorionic fluid, uterine fibroids, or discrepancy between sac sizes. Neither advanced maternal age nor ART appeared to have an effect on outcome.

If fetal loss occurs in the second or third trimester, or in the setting of a monozygotic twin gestation, the demised fetus may develop into a fetus papyraceus.[46] Instead of the usual complete decomposition and absorption of the fetus, the fetus papyraceus ("paperlike") is preserved in a distorted form (Fig. 26-15). In twins, a postulated cause of fetus papyraceus is transient polyhydramnios of one fetus in a monochorionic-diamniotic pregnancy exerting a lethal compressive effect on the other twin. Fetal papyraceus occurs in 1 of 12,000 live births, but is more common in the subgroup of twin gestations (1 in 184 twin births).[42]

TECHNICAL PITFALLS

Technical pitfalls exist in imaging multiple gestations. An important factor that should be borne in mind when determining whether there is a multiple-gestation pregnancy is that crescentic areas of implantation hemorrhage or amniotic-chorionic separation may be mistaken for second gestational sacs or nonviable pregnancies (Fig. 26-16). The distinction is usually obvious by the configuration of the fluid collections and the lack of a well-defined decidual rind in nongestational collections.

demise is actually similar to that of spontaneous singleton demise. Early fetal demise has not been associated with adverse outcome in the surviving twin.

A study by Benson and colleagues looked at first-trimester twin pregnancies to determine criteria for predicting pregnancy outcome with regard to number of live-born infants.[45] Of 137 patients evaluated, 110 (80.3%) had viable twins, 12 (8.8%) had 1 infant, and 15 (10.9%) had none. The criteria they found to be statistically significant included gestational age at the time of the ultrasound (the inference being that the earlier

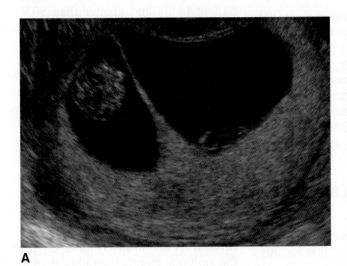

A

B

Figure 26-15 A: Twin pregnancy with a normal twin in the amniotic sac on the left and a fetal demise which resulted in a fetus papyraceus, on the right. **B:** Fetus papyraceus. One twin is larger, and the other has been compressed and mummified, hence the term papyraceus. Reprinted with permission from Stevenson RE, Hall, JG, Goodman RM (eds). Human Malformations and Related Anomalies. New York: Oxford University Press, 1993.

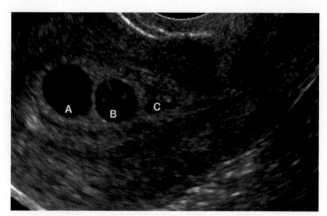

Figure 26-16 First-trimester ultrasound showing what appears to be three gestational sacs. However, sac "C" was actually an early subchorionic bleed.

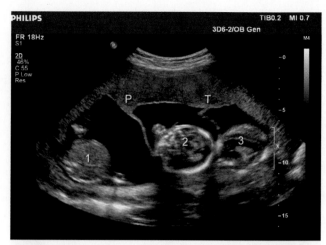

Figure 26-17 A triplet pregnancy demonstrating the placental twin peak sign (P) and the T sign (T). One abdomen (1) and two fetal heads (2, 3) confirm the triplet pregnancy. (Image compliments of Philips Medical Systems, Bothell, WA.).

Although it seems intuitively unlikely, late in pregnancy a second fetus may be completely overlooked because the nondependent fetus obscures the underlying one. This possibility should be considered if the visualized fetus is situated more anteriorly than would be expected and if there are more fetal parts in the image than seems appropriate. Later in pregnancy, owing to relative decreases in amniotic fluid with respect to the fetal volume, important areas of fetal anatomy may be hidden, and an effort must be made to evaluate obscured anatomy by scanning from multiple angles and with the mother in different positions.

HIGHER-ORDER MULTIPLE GESTATIONS

Although the average incidence of twins is 1 in 100 pregnancies, triplets occur in only approximately 1 in 7,600 pregnancies, and the spontaneous rates for quadruplet and quintuplet pregnancies are 1 in 729,000 and 1 in 65,610,000, respectively.[47] Interestingly, triplet pregnancies—and even quadruplet pregnancies—may be MZ. For example, 60% of triplet pregnancies are secondary to the fertilization of two ova, 30% arise from the fertilization of three ova, and 10% arise from the fertilization of a single ovum (Fig. 26-17).[48]

COMPLICATIONS OF MULTIPLE-GESTATION PREGNANCIES

Multiple gestations are at significantly increased risk of adverse fetal and maternal outcomes.[6,16,49] It is for this reason that all multiple gestations should be considered high-risk pregnancies and periodic monitoring by sonography is warranted.

MATERNAL COMPLICATIONS

Maternal complications include an increased mortality rate during pregnancy, delivery, and immediately postpartum that is three times higher than for a singleton

pregnancy.[6] This is usually the result of hypertension or postpartum hemorrhage. Maternal admission to an intensive care unit is also twice as high in these patients.[50] Except for an increased rate of cesarean section in advanced maternal age (AMA) twin pregnancies, age does not appear to be associated with an increased risk of adverse outcome.[51]

FETAL COMPLICATIONS

The primary risk factors for mortality and long-term morbidity in the fetus of a multiple gestation are premature delivery and low birth weight.[6] Approximately half of twins and greater than 90% of triplet pregnancies are born before 37 weeks' gestation or under 2,500 grams.[3,52]

Other risk factors in multiples are usually related to the type of chorionicity/amnionicity present. Monozygotic twins are associated with an increased risk of congenital anomalies.[13,16,19,24] Monochorionic twins, sharing a placenta, run the risk of abnormal anastomoses of arteries and veins developing. This puts them at risk for TTTS and TRAP sequence, as well as all of the sequalae associated with those processes.

VASA PREVIA

Vasa previa is defined as fetal vessels overlying the cervical os due to insertion of the umbilical cord into the amniotic membrane rather than the placenta.[3] It is a rare abnormality that is associated with fetal mortality due to rapid fetal exsanguinations at the time of membrane rupture. The occurrence rate in singleton pregnancies is reported as 1/2,500 pregnancies.[53] In a multiple pregnancy this rate rises to 2.5%.[6] ART has also been shown to increase the rate of vasa previa. Since many multiple gestations are often the result of ART, the higher rate observed in multiple gestations

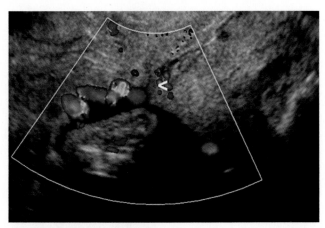

Figure 26-18 Endovaginal ultrasound utilizing color Doppler to show fetal vessels covering the internal cervical os *(arrowhead)* consistent with a vasa previa.

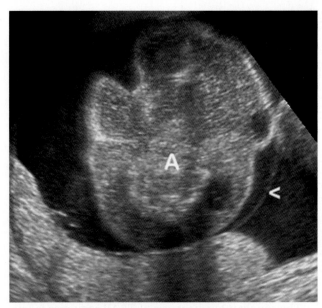

Figure 26-19 Amorphous acardiac fetus *(A)* coexisting with a normal fetus (not shown), consistent with TRAP sequence. The intertwin membrane *(arrowhead)* was visualized.

makes sense. Vigilant sonographic evaluation of the lower uterine segment, particularly in the setting of a low-lying placenta or a placenta previa, is therefore warranted when assessing a multiple gestation (Fig. 26-18).

TWIN REVERSED ARTERIAL PERFUSION SEQUENCE

TRAP sequence is also commonly referred to as acardiac twinning. It is a rare complication of monochorionic pregnancies, with a reported occurrence rate of 1/35,000 pregnancies and 0.3% of all monozygotic twin gestations.[54]

This abnormality is diagnosed by observing one normal twin, often referred to as the "pump" twin, and one amorphous twin without a well-defined cardiac structure, referred to as the "acardiac" twin (Fig. 26-19). The acardiac twin is hemodynamically dependent on the normal twin for all circulation. In this abnormality, arterial-to-arterial and venous-to-venous anastamoses occur on the surface of the shared placenta. This results in blood flow from the pump twin flowing to the placenta via its umbilical arteries, then entering the abnormal arterial-to-arterial connections and flowing in a retrograde fashion to the acardiac twin through the umbilical arteries. Since this blood flow has essentially not gone thorough the placenta, it is relatively deoxygenated and nutrient poor. The blood enters the acardiac twin via the hypogastric arteries and essentially perfuses only the caudal aspect of the fetus. This is why usually only the lower pelvis and extremities of the acardiac twin tend to develop. More cephalic structures, such as the head, upper body, and heart are either completely absent or severely maldeveloped.[21]

The blood returning from the acardiac twin flows back to the placenta via the umbilical vein. Color and/or spectral Doppler evaluation of the umbilical arteries and vein of the acardiac twin readily show this reversal of blood flow (Fig. 26-20). Chromosomal abnormalities have been reported in approximately 50% of acardiac twins.[55,56] Because of the altered hemodynamics, the pump twin carries a 50% risk of morbidity or mortality secondary to developing high-output congestive heart failure, nonimmune hydrops fetalis, and polyhydramnios.[57] This risk increases as the size of the acardiac twin increases. Therefore, several treatment options aimed at stopping perfusion of the acardiac twin have been attempted. These include open hysterotomy and selective delivery, as well as various methods of occluding blood flow, including bipolar, harmonic scalpel, thermal or laser coagulation, coil embolization, and radiofrequency ablation.[57] Holmes and colleagues reported a 73% survival rate of the pump, or normal, twin following thermocoagulation, whereas a survival rate of 92% was reported by Lee and associates following radiofrequency ablation of the umbilical cord.[57,58]

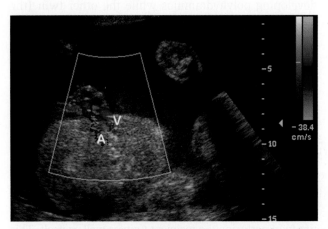

Figure 26-20 Color Doppler image showing retrograde flow of the umbilical artery *(A)* and vein *(V)* in an acardiac twin.

Twin Reversed Arterial Perfusion (TRAP) Sequence

Formation	Sonographic Findings
Monochorionic/ monoamniotic pregnancy	Retrograde umbilical artery flow to the acardiac twin
Twins	Only lower pelvis and extremities of acardiac twin form
• One normal	
• One acardiac	
Placental arterial-to-arterial and venous-to-venous anastomoses	Congestive heart failure in normal twin due to increased load
Acardiac twin supported by normal fetus via placental anastomoses	Nonimmune hydrops fetalis in acardiac twin
	Polyhydramnios

The sonographic diagnosis of TRAP sequence is fairly straightforward and has been made as early as 11 weeks' gestation.[56,59] A normal-appearing fetus, which may or may not show signs of hydrops, is observed in conjunction with a markedly malformed fetus with no discernible cardiac structures. It is not uncommon for the acardiac twin to enlarge as pregnancy progresses. Most twin gestations affected with TRAP sequence are monochorionic/monoamniotic. As stated, Doppler confirmation of reversal of flow in the umbilical cord of the acardiac twin confirms the diagnosis.

TWIN-TO-TWIN TRANSFUSION SYNDROME (TTTS)

TTTS occurs in monochorionic/diamniotic pregnancies. It results when arterial-to-venous anastomoses occur within the shared placenta. This results in returning blood from one fetus to be shunted directly to the other fetus, causing an imbalance of perfusion between the two fetuses.[40] When pregnancies are affected by TTTS, an imbalance in amniotic fluid occurs, resulting in one twin (the "recipient" twin) becoming larger and developing polyhydramnios while the other twin (the "donor" twin) is smaller and develops oligohydramnios. The lack of fluid in the amniotic sac of the donor twin can cause the intertwin membrane to encase this fetus, giving the appearance of a "stuck" twin.[21] When this occurs, the membrane may not be visualized at all, but the fetus appears immobile and in essence "stuck" to the uterine wall (Fig. 26-21). Sonographically, TTTS can be diagnosed in a twin pregnancy when the fetuses are noted to be monochorionic/diamniotic, of the same gender, with a weight discordance of 20% or greater, and having a major imbalance of amniotic fluid between the two amniotic sacs.

The hemodynamic alterations in TTTS result in the donor twin perfusing the recipient twin as well as itself. This in turn causes the donor twin to become growth restricted,

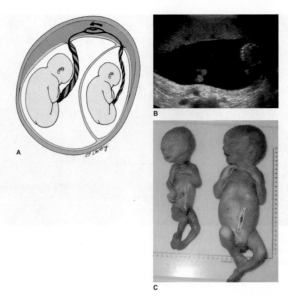

Figure 26-21 A: Twin-twin transfusion syndrome: Position of twins in the uterus with a schematic representation of the circulation problem that causes uncompensated arteriovenous shunting during twin-twin transfusion syndrome. **B:** Donor twin in a TTTS gestation, "stuck" to the uterine wall secondary to oligohydramnios and the intertwin membrane (not visualized) encasing it. **C:** Monozygotic twins with twin transfusion syndrome. Placental vascular anastomoses produced unbalanced blood flow to the two fetuses. Photo from Sadler T, PhD. *Langman's Medical Embryology*, 9th ed. Image Bank. Baltimore: Lippincott Williams & Wilkins, 2003.

hypovolemic, and anemic. Since the recipient twin is being perfused by the placenta as well as the donor twin, it becomes macrosomic, hypervolemic, and plethoric. Hydrops may develop in the recipient twin or, less commonly, the donor twin. Both twins are at increased risk of morbidity and mortality.[60] Cardiovascular manifestations are not uncommon in TTTS. The hypervolemic recipient twin may develop cardiomegaly, biventricular hypertrophy (Fig. 26-22), and tricuspid regurgitation (Fig. 26-23).[61–64]

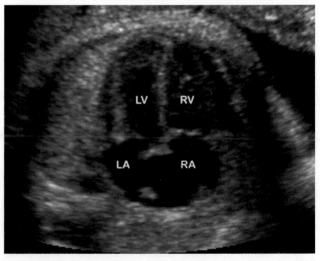

Figure 26-22 Thickened interventricular septum and heart walls of the right (*RV*) and left (*LV*) ventricles, consistent with concentric hypertrophy in the recipient twin of a TTTS pregnancy. *LA*, left atrium, *RA*, right atrium.

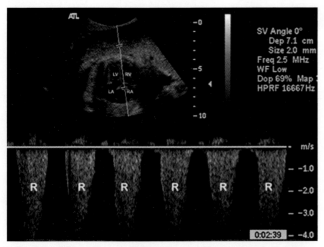

Figure 26-23 Spectral waveform showing massive tricuspid regurgitation (R) in the recipient twin of a TTTS pregnancy. *LA*, left atrium; *LV*, left ventricle; *RA*, right atrium; *RV*, right ventricle.

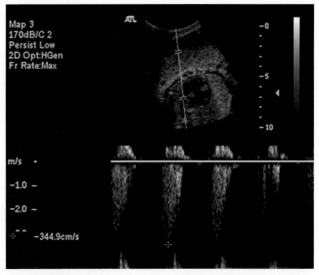

Figure 26-24 Elevated velocity through the pulmonary artery of a recipient twin in a TTTS pregnancy, consistent with pulmonary stenosis.

As cardiac dysfunction progresses throughout pregnancy, various types of cardiac abnormalities may develop. These are usually right-sided defects. including pulmonary stenosis or atresia, resulting from the hypertrophied ventricular heart walls and interventricular septum obstructing right ventricular outflow (Fig. 26-24). The hypovolemic donor twin is at significantly less risk of developing cardiac pathology; however, dilated cardiomyopathies and small pericardial effusions have been reported.[61,65] For these reasons, formal fetal echocardiography is warranted in the setting of TTTS.

Velamentous cord insertion, in which the cord inserts directly into the membranes instead of the placenta, has been associated with a greater than 50% risk of TTTS.[66]

TTTS can present at any time in pregnancy. The earlier the onset, the poorer the prognosis.[66] If left untreated, TTTS has a reported mortality rate for both twins of 60% to 100%.[66] Additionally, if one twin dies in utero, the surviving twin is at risk of developing multiorgan damage, specifically abnormalities of the brain, secondary to emboli from the deceased fetus. Adverse long-term neurologic deficits have also been reported in surviving infants.[67-68]

The prenatal sonographic diagnosis of TTTS relies on identification of a single placenta, same sex fetuses, a weight discordance of greater than 20% between the fetuses, and significant discrepancy in amniotic fluid volume. A "stuck" twin is usually observed. Quintero and associates developed a classification for accessing disease severity. In Stage I, oligohydramnios of the donor twin is present but a fetal bladder can be visualized. In Stage II the donor's bladder is no longer visualized. In Stage III, pulsed Doppler evaluation shows absent or reversed end-diastolic velocities of the donor's umbilical arteries, reversed flow in the ductus venosus, or pulsatile flow in the umbilical vein. TTTS is considered Stage IV if hydrops is present in the recipient twin and Stage V is when one or both fetuses have died in utero.[69]

In utero treatment of TTTS depends on the gestational age at the time of diagnosis. If diagnosed in early pregnancy, selective termination or termination of the entire pregnancy may be considered. In the second trimester, treatment options include serial reduction amniocentesis, septostomy of the amniotic membrane, and laser or radiofrequency ablation of the anastomoses.

Serial reduction amniocentesis involves removing fluid from the polyhydramniotic sac, returning it to a normal volume. The theory behind this treatment is that removing the excessive fluid decreases the pressure on

---

PATHOLOGY BOX 26-4

Twin-to-Twin Transfusion Syndrome (TTTS)

Formation	Sonographic Findings
Monochorionic/ diamniotic twins	Recipient twin
Arterial to venous anastomoses between placentas	• Polyhydramnios
	• Macrosomic
	• Hypervolemic
Flow shunting from one fetus to the other creating a perfusion imbalance	• Plethoric
	• Hydrops
	Donor twin
	• Oligohydramnios
	• Growth restricted
	• Hypovolemic
	• Anemic
	Same gender
	20% weight discordance
	Cardiovascular malformations
	Velamentous cord insertion

the oligohydramniotic sac and allows increased perfusion of that fetus. Since production of amniotic fluid is a continual process, serial fluid reductions are usually necessary.

Amniotic membrane septostomy involves inserting a needle through the dividing membrane, essentially creating a monoamniotic pregnancy to allow equalization of amniotic fluid. However, since monoamniotic pregnancies carry their own inherent risks, this procedure is not widely utilized.

Ablation of the placental anastomoses involves identifying the abnormal vessel connections within the placenta with a fetoscope and then ablating them with laser or radiofrequency technology. This procedure is usually done in conjunction with reduction amniocentesis.

All treatments carry risk and varying success rates have been reported, depending on sample size and the precise technique utilized.[70-74] In 2004, Senat and colleagues published a study comparing laser ablation and serial amnioreduction for treating TTTS between 15 and 26 weeks' gestation. They reported a 76% survival rate of either twin at 28 days of life for laser ablation versus a 56% survival rate when only serial amnioreduction was utilized. At 6 months of age, the survival rates were 76% and 51% respectively. The study also reported fewer neurologic sequelae in the laser ablation group.[75] Interestingly, the cardiac abnormalities associated with TTTS do not necessarily resolve or improve following any of the in utero therapies.[61,64,65]

CONJOINED TWINS

Conjoined twins occur in approximately 1 in 50,000 to 1 in 100,000 live births.[76] Conjoined twins are classified by the conjoined (shared) body area. Thoracopagus (joined at the thorax), omphalopagus (joined at the abdominal wall), or a combination of the two constitute approximately 70% of all conjoined twins. Other varieties include craniopagus (joined at the head), pygopagus (joined at the buttocks), ischiopagus (joined at the ischia), and cephalothoracopagus (Figs. 26-25 and 26; Table 26-3).[48,77,78]

Developmentally, conjoined twins arise from monochorionic/monoamniotic gestations with incomplete division of the embryo occurring after the 13th day of conception during Carnegie stage 5.[87] They are always of the same sex, and 70% are female. Sonographic findings in conjoined twins include lack of visualization of a separating membrane between the twins, inability to separate the fetal bodies or heads (Figs. 26-27 to 26-29) despite changes in fetal position, more than three vessels in a single umbilical cord, and complex fetal structural anomalies.[79] Polyhydramnios is more common in conjoined twins, occurring in approximately 50% of cases.[76] Most conjoined twins are born prematurely and approximately 40% are stillborn. Survival of conjoined twins is

PATHOLOGY BOX 26-5	
Conjoined Twins	
Formation	**Sonographic Findings**
Monochorionic|—monoamniotic gestation	Same sex (70% are female)
	Lack of visualization of a separating membrane
Incomplete embryonic division after 13th day (Carnegie stage 5)	Inability to separate the fetal bodies or heads despite positional changes
	More than three vessels in a single umbilical cord
	Complex fetal structural anomalies
	Polyhydramnios

ultimately dependent on the organs shared, particularly the heart. Seventy-five percent of thorocopagus twins share a heart and thus are not candidates for successful separation.[80] Sharing of brain tissue in craniopagus twins is also associated with poor outcomes. Conjoined twins can occur in higher-order gestations as well.[81]

3-Dimensional ultrasound (Fig. 26-30) or magnetic resonance imaging (MRI) may be a useful adjuncts to conventional ultrasound when attempting to determine the extent of organ involvement in conjoined twins.

Another form of abnormal twinning is the parasitic twin found within the abdomen of its sibling. This is referred to as fetus in fetu[82] and should not be confused with a teratoma. Although the distinction between parasitic twin and teratoma may be difficult, it is an important point to establish, because teratomas have a definite malignant potential, whereas the fetus in fetu is technically a hamartoma and entirely benign. Fetus in fetu occurs more commonly in the upper retroperitoneum, whereas teratomas usually arise in the lower abdomen, most commonly in the ovaries or the sacrococcygeal region. Also, there is usually radiographic or at least microscopic evidence of a vertebral column in a fetus in fetu.

MONOAMNIOTIC TWINS

Monoamniotic twins account for approximately 1% of all monozygotic twin gestations. This type of twining is at highest risk, with a mortality rate of approximately 50%.[21] Fetal death is usually the result of cord entanglement or preterm birth.

Congenital anomalies occur in monoamniotic twins in 20% of cases.[83] Monoamniotic twins may be diagnosed sonographically in the absence of an intertwin membrane; however, thin membranes may be present but difficult to visualize sonographically, so this is not always a reliable sign. Color and pulsed Doppler can be utilized to identify cord entanglement, which would confirm one amniotic cavity. Color Doppler can be utilized to identify multiple entangled vessels (Fig. 26-31), while pulsed Doppler should be able to document two

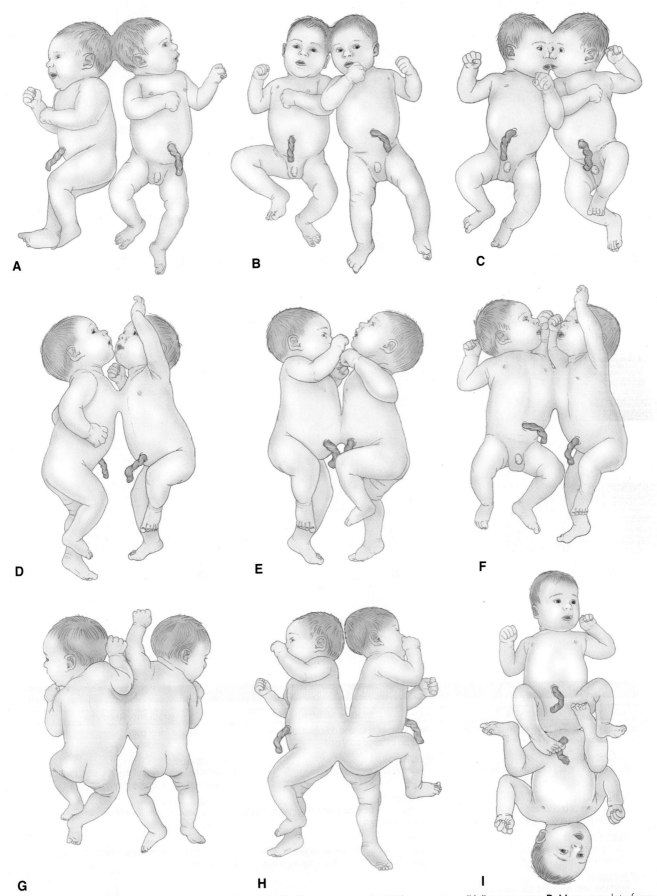

Figure 26-25 A: Possibilities for partial fusion of fetuses: **(A–C)** craniopagus; **(D–G)** thoracopagus; **(H–I)** pygopagus. **B:** More complete forms of conjoined twinning. (From Patten BM. *Human Embryology.* New York: McGraw-Hill; 1968). *(continued)*

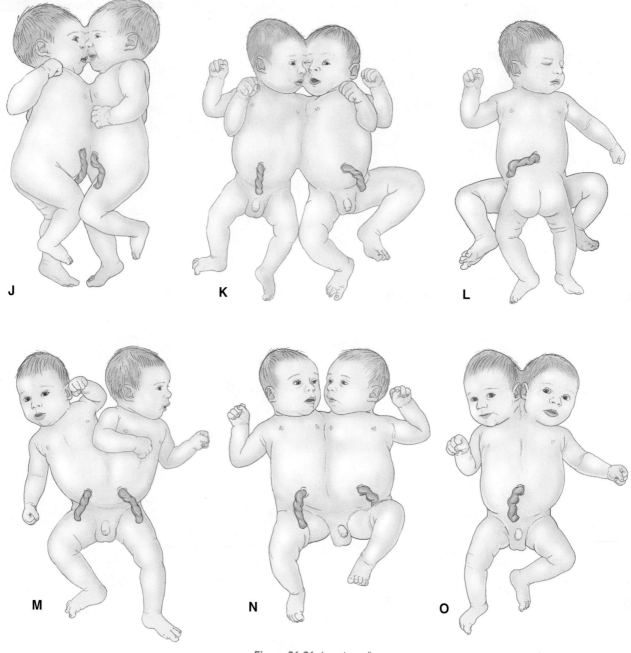

J   K   L

M   N   O

Figure 26-26 *(continued)*

classification of conjoined twins		
terata catadidyma	**terata anadidyma**	**terata anacatadidyma**
joined by lower part of body, or twins single in lower body and double in upper body	single in upper body and double in lower body, or joined by some body part	united at midpoint of body

a) pygopagus
   back to back, coccyx and sacrum joined
	a) cephalopagus
	   fused in the cranial vault
		a) thoracopagus
		   attached along part of thoracic wall; thoracic and abdominal organs may be abnormal

b) ischiopagus
   inferior parts of coccyx and sacrum fused; separate vertebral columns lying in same axis
	b) syncephalus
	   united at the face; may also be joined by thorax (cephalothoracopagus)
		b) omphalopagus
		   attached from umbilicus to xiphoid cartilage

c) dicephalus
   two separate heads on one body
	c) dipygus
	   single head, thorax, and/or abdomen; pelvis, external genitalia, and limbs are duplicate
		c) rachipagus
		   attached at the vertebral column above the sacrum

d) diprosopus two faces with one head and one body		

Table 26-3 Classification of conjoined twins.

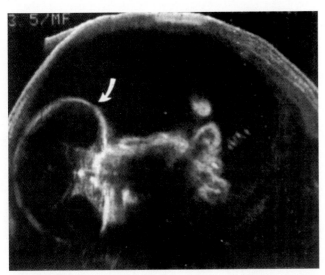

Figure 26-27 Transverse static scan showing fused crania (curved arrow) in cephalothoracoomphalopagus twins with grossly abnormal intracranial contents.

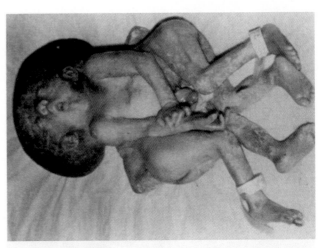

Figure 26-28 Fetuses with fusion of the heads, thoraces, and abdomen.

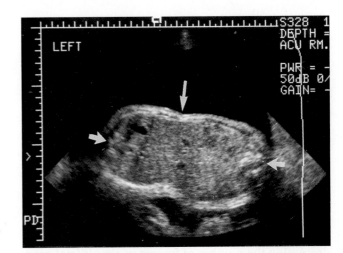

Figure 26-29 Transverse sonogram shows conjoining of twins across the anterior abdomen (long arrow). Two fetal spines (short arrows) image posteriorly.

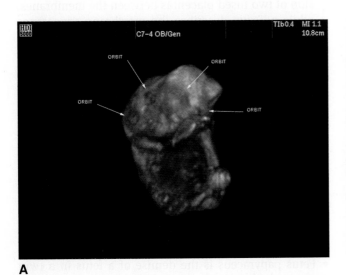

Figure 26-30 3D reconstruction of conjoined diprosopus twins that have two faces (A) one head, and one body. This rare configuration demonstrates two spines (B). (Image compliments of Philips Medical Systems, Bothell, WA.).

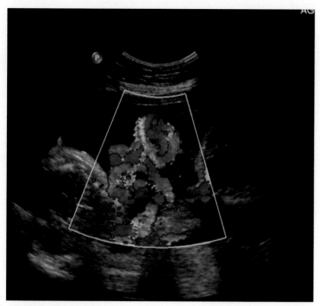

Figure 26-31 Color Doppler showing entangled umbilical cords in a MC/MA twin gestation.

separate heart rates. Cord entanglement is not always associated with a poor outcome. Rodis and colleagues reported a 100% live birth rate and 92% perinatal survival rate in 13 monoamniotic twin gestations diagnoses with cord entanglement.[84] Early delivery is often recommended in cases of monoamniotic twins.

SELECTIVE REDUCTION

Should serious complications occur or serious anomalies be detected in multiple gestations, selective termination may be offered to the parents as an option. In cases in which only one twin is affected with a serious chromosomal or congenital anomaly, or when decreasing the number of fetuses in a multifetal pregnancy might improve the perinatal result, selective termination of fetuses may be a reasonable alternative. This procedure usually involves the direct injection of potassium chloride into the fetal heart or umbilical vein of the designated twin. Selective termination should be performed only in dichorionic pregnancies.

If selective termination is performed on a monochorionic pregnancy or if spontaneous fetal demise occurs in a monochorionic pregnancy, the potential exists for a thromboembolic substance to be released from the dead twin, passing into the surviving twin, and causing intrauterine disseminated intravascular coagulation (DIC) with potential brain and multiorgan damage or death.[85] Because monozygotic twins are rarely discordant for genetic defects, selective termination in monozygotic pregnancies would involve cases of isolated congenital anomalies or would be performed to reduce the number of fetuses. The role of ultrasound in this procedure includes locating the appropriate fetus, guiding the needle for puncture, and monitoring the well-being of surviving fetuses. In a series of 100 patients undergoing selective reduction, a 4% loss rate of the entire pregnancy was reported.[86]

SUMMARY

- Multiple births increase because of delayed childbearing, race, genetics, environmental factors, and the use of ART.

- Clinical findings that raise suspicion for a multiple pregnancy are maternal LGA, finding multiple heart tones, and a MSAFP level of >2.5 MOM.

- Monozygotic twining is a random event of ovum division after fertilization.

- Dizygotic twinning is influenced by genetic factors, environmental factors, advanced maternal age, and the use of ART and is the result of two ova fertilization.

- Two placentas and membrane sets occur with dizygotic twin gestations, resulting in a dichorionic/diamniotic configuration.

- Monozygotic placentation and the number of membranes depends on timing of the division of the ovum with membrane configurations of dichorionic/diamniotic, monochorionic/dichorionic, monochorionic/monoamniotic.

- Complications of a multiple pregnancy include preterm birth, IUGR, fetal anomalies, fetal death, low birthweight, pre-eclampsia, placental abruption, hypertension, placenta previa, and postpartum hemorrhage.

- Number and chorionicity can be determined in the first trimester; however, as many as 20% of twin pregnancies result in a singleton delivery (vanishing twin).

- The twin peak sign is a lambda-shaped (λ) extension of two fused placentas between the membranes, while a T-sign describes the membrane appearance with one placenta and two amnions.

- Four layers of fetal membranes in a pregnancy before 26 weeks, two chorions and two amnions, are described as a thick membrane (~1.5 mm), while a thin membrane (<1 mm) has only two amnions.

- A gestational sac lacking fetal membranes is a monoamniotic pregnancy.

- Biometric measurements for twins mimic a singleton pregnancy until approximately 30 weeks, when growth may slow.

- An increased resistance to blood flow within the UAs or a decreased resistance observed in the MCAs may occur in the setting of IUGR with a multiple pregnancy.

- Fetus papyraceus is the demise of a fetus in a twin pregnancy, which results in the preservation of a paperlike fetus within the uterus.

Critical Thinking Questions

A twin pregnancy has the following findings:

- Fetus 1
  - Hydrops fetalis
  - Polyhydramnios
- Fetus 2
  - Only pelvis and lower extremities developed
- Single placenta
- Monochorionic membrane configuration

1. Name the syndrome described above.

2. What is the process that resulted in the findings for fetus 2?

3. How does this sequence differ from TTTS?

4. Describe how to differentiate the TTTS or TRAP syndrome from conjoined twins.

ANSWER 1: TRAP sequence or acardiac twinning

ANSWER 2: Due to the arterial-to-arterial and venous-to-venous anastomoses on the surface of the single placenta, blood flows from the pump twin (fetus 1) to the placenta via its umbilical arteries, then enters the abnormal arterial-to-arterial connections and flows in a retrograde fashion to the acardiac twin through it's umbilical arteries.

ANSWER 3: TTTS occurs in monochorionic/diamniotic pregnancies with arterial to venous anastomoses occurring within the shared placenta. There is also discordant growth and hydramnios between the fetuses.

ANSWER 4: Conjoined twins are always monochorionic/monochorionic pregnancies and have an attachment somewhere between the two fetuses, which is due to late division of the morula. During the sonographic examination the fetuses do not change position and appear to be joined at the area that failed to separate.

- The risk of vasa previa, defined as fetal vessels overlying the cervical os due to insertion of the umbilical cord into the amniotic membrane rather than the placenta, increases with multiple pregnancies and ART.

- Acardiac twinning or TRAP sequence is a complication seen in monozygotic twins when one twin's heart supports two fetuses through arterial-to-arterial and venous-to-venous anastamoses occurring on the surface of the shared placenta.

- The monochorionic/diamniotic twin gestation is at risk for development of TTTS in which a shared placenta develops arterial to venous anastomoses. The perfusion imbalance of the returning blood results in disparate fetal size, and fluid levels.

- Conjoined twins are the result of incomplete division of the embryo during the implantation stage occurring after day 13 (Carnegie stage 5).

REFERENCES

1. Egan JFX, Borgida AF. Multiple gestations: the importance of ultrasound. *Obstet Gynecol Clin North Am.* 2004;31(1):141–158.

2. Martin JA, Kung HC, Mathews TJ, et al. Annual summary of vital statistics: 2006. *Pediatrics.* 2008;121(4):788–801.

3. Gandhi M, Cleary-Goldman J, Ferrara L, et al. The association between vasa previa, multiple gestations, and assisted reproductive technology. *Am J Perinatol.* 2008;25(9):587–590.

4. Reynolds MA, Schieve LA, Martin JA, et al. Trends in multiple births conceived using assisted reproductive technology, United States, 1997–2000. *Pediatrics.* 2003;111(5 Part 2):1159–1162.

5. Collins J. Global epidemiology of multiple birth. *Reprod Biomed Online.* 2007;(15 Suppl 3):45–52.

6. Blondel B, Kaminski M. Trends in the occurrence, determinants, and consequences of multiple births. *Semin Perinatol.* 2002; 26(4):239–249.

7. Bortolus R, Parazzini F, Chatenoud L, et al. The epidemiology of multiple births. *Hum Reprod Update.* 1999;5(2):179–187.

8. Beemsterboer SN, Homburg R, Gorter NA, et al. The paradox of declining fertility but increasing twinning rates with advancing maternal age. *Hum Reprod.* 2006;21(6):1531–1532.

9. Crane JP. Sonographic evaluation of multiple pregnancy. *Semin Ultrasound CT MR.* 1984;5:144–156.

10. Bortolus R, Parazzini F, Chatenoud L, et al. The epidemiology of multiple births. *Hum Reprod Update.* 1999;5(2):179–187.

11. Pretorius DH, Budorick NE, Scioscia AL, et al. Twin pregnancies in the second trimester in women in an α-fetoprotein screening program: sonographic evaluation and outcome. *AJR Am J Roentgenol.* 1993;161(5):1007–1013.

12. Benirschke K, Kim C. Multiple pregnancy. *N Engl J Med.* 1973;288:1276–1284.

13. Ghai V, Vidyasagar D. Morbidity and mortality factors in twins. An epidemiologic approach. *Clin Perinatol.* 1988;15(1):123–140.

14. Naeye RI, Tafari N, Judge D, et al. Twins: Causes of perinatal death in 12 United States cities and one African city. *Am J Obstet Gynecol.* 1978;131(3):267–272.

15. Spellacy WN, Handler A, Ferre CD. A case-control study of 1253 twin pregnancies from a 1982–1987 perinatal data base. *Obstet Gynecol.* 1990;75(2):168–171.

16. Sherer DM. Adverse perinatal outcome of twin pregnancies according to chorionicity: Review of the literature. *Am J Perinatol.* 2001;18(1):23–37.

17. Kohl SG, Casey G. Twin gestation. *Mt Sinai J Med.* 1975;42(6):523–539.

18. Luke B, Keith LG. Monozygotic twinning as a congenital defect and congenital defects in monozygotic twins. *Fetal Diagn Ther.* 1990;5(2):61–69.

19. Newton ER. Antepartum care in multiple gestation. *Semin Perinatol.* 1986;10(1):19–29.

20. Doubilet PM, Benson CB. "Appearing twin": Undercounting of multiple gestations on early first trimester sonograms. *J Ultrasound Med.* 1998;17(4):199–203.

21. Barth RA, Crowe HC. Ultrasound evaluation of multifetal gestations. In: Callen PW, ed. *Ultrasonography in Obstetrics and Gynecology.* 4th ed. Philadelphia: W.B. Saunders Company; 2000:171–205.

22. Carroll SG, Soothill PW, Abdel-Fattah SA, et al. Prediction of chorionicity in twin pregnancies at 10–14 weeks of gestation. *BJOGl.* 2002;109(2):182–186.

23. Finberg HJ. The "twin-peak" sign: reliable evidence of dichorionic twinning. *J Ultrasound Med.* 1992;11(11):571–577.

24. Stenhouse E, Hardwick C, Maharaj S, et al. Chorionicity determination in twin pregnancies: how accurate are we? *Ultrasound Obstet Gynecol.* 2002;19(4):350–352.

25. Hertzberg BS, Kurtz AB, Choi HY, et al. Significance of membrane thickness in the sonographic evaluation of twin gestations. *AJR Am Roentgenol.* 1987;148(1):151–153.

26. Kurtz AB, Wapner RJ, Mata J, et al. Twin pregnancies: accuracy of first-trimester abdominal US in predicting chorionicity and amnionicity. *Radiology.* 1992;185(3):759–762.

27. Bora SA, Papageorghiou AT, Bottomley C, et al. Reliability of transvaginal ultrasonography at 7–9 weeks' gestation in the determination of chorionicity and amnionicity in twin pregnancies. *Ultrasound Obstet Gynecol.* 2008;32(5):618–621.

28. Moon MH, Park SY, Song MJ, et al. Diamniotic twin pregnancies with a single placental mass; prediction of chorionicity at 11–14 weeks of gestation. *Prenat Diagn.* 2008;28(11):1011–1015.

29. Townsend RR, Simpson GF, Filly RA. Membrane thickness in ultrasound prediction of chorionicity of twin gestations. *J Ultrasound Med.* 1988;7(6):327–332.

30. Hertzberg BS, Kurtz AV, Choi HY, et al. Significance of membrane thickness in the sonographic evaluation of twin gestations. *AJR Am J Roentgenol.* 1987;148(1):151–153.

31. Senat MV, Quarello E, Levaillant JM, et al. Determining chorionicity in twin gestations: three-dimensional (3D) multiplanar sonographic measurement of intra-amniotic membrane thickness. *Ultrasound Obstet Gynecol.* 2006;28(5):665–669.

32. American College of Obstetrics and Gynecology. Ultrasound in Pregnancy. *Practice Bulletin No. 101.* Washington, D.C. ACOG; February 2009.

33. American College of Radiology. ACR practice guideline for the performance of obstetrical ultrasound. Reston, VA. *ACR.* 2007;(25):1093–1101.

34. American Institute of Ultrasound in Medicine. American Institute of Ultrasound in Medicine guidelines for the performance of the antepartum obstetrical ultrasound examination. Rockville, MD. *AIUM;* 2007.

35. Saade GR, Gray G, Belfort MA, et al. Ultrasonographic measurement of crown-rump length in high-order multifetal pregnancies. *Ultrasound Obstet Gynecol.* 1998;11(6):438–444.

36. Weissman A, Achiron R, Lipitz S, et al. The first-trimester growth-discordant twin: An ominous prenatal finding. *Obstet Gynecol.* 1994;84(1):110–114.

37. Bora SA, Bourne T, Bottomley C, et al. Twin growth discrepancy in early pregnancy. *Ultrasound Obstet Gynecol.* 2009;34(1):38–42.

38. Ananth CV, Vintzileous AM, Shen-Schwarz S, et al. Standards of birth weight in twin gestations stratified by placental chorionicity. *Obstet Gynecol.* 1998;91(6):917–924.

39. Vintzileos AM, Rodis JF. Growth discordance in twins. In: Divon MY, ed. *Abnormal Fetal Growth: IUGR and Macrosomia.* New York, NY: Elsevier; 1995:289–299.

40. Divon MY, Weiner Z. Ultrasound in twin pregnancy. *Semin Perinatol.* 1995;19(5):404–412.

41. Weissman A, Jakobi P, Yoffe N, et al. Sonographic growth measurements in triplet pregnancies. *Obstet Gynecol.* 1990;75(3 Pt 1):324–328.

42. Landy HJ, Weiner S, Corson SL, et al. The "vanishing twin": Ultrasonographic assessment of fetal disappearance in the first trimester. *Am J Obstet Gynecol.* 1986;155(1):14–19.

43. Gindoff PR, Yeh MN, Jewelewicz R. The vanishing sac syndrome. Ultrasound evidence of pregnancy failure in multiple gestations, induced and spontaneous. *J Reprod Med.* 1986;31(5):322–325.

44. Bernard KG, Cooperberg PL. Sonographic differentiation between blighted ovum and early viable pregnancy. *AJR Am J Roentgenol.* 1985;144:597–602.

45. Benson CB, Doubilet PM, David V. Prognosis of first trimester twin pregnancies: Polychotomous logistic regression analysis. *Radiology.* 1994;192(3):765–768.

46. Gericke GS. Genetic and teratological considerations in the analysis of concordant and discordant abnormalities in twins. *S Afr Med J.* 1986;69(2):111–114.

47. Crane JP. Sonographic evaluation of multiple pregnancy. *Semin Ultrasound CT MR.* 1984;5:144–156.

48. Hartung RW, Yiu-Chiu V, Aschenbrener CA. Sonographic diagnosis of cephaloghoracopagus in a triplet pregnancy. *J Ultrasound Med.* 1984;3(3):139–141.

49. Monteagudo A, Roman AS. Ultrasound in multiple gestations: Twins and other multifetal pregnancies. *Clin Perinatol.* 2005;32(2):329–354.

50. Senat MV, Ancel PY. How does multiple pregnancy affect maternal mortality and morbidity? *Clin Obstet Gynecol.* 1998;41(1):79–83.

51. Fox NS, Rebarber A, Dunham SM, et al. Outcomes of multiple gestations with advanced maternal age. *J Matern Fetal and Neonatal Med.* 2009;22(7):593–596.

52. Blondel B, Kogan MD, Alexander GR, et al. The impact of the increasing number of multiple births on the rates of preterm birth and low birthweight, an international study. *Am J Publ Health.* 2002;92(8):1323–1330.

53. Oyelese Y, Catanzarite V, Perfumo F, et al. Vasa previa: the impact of prenatal diagnosis on outcomes. *Obstet Gynecol.* 2004;103(5 Pt 1):937–942.

54. Bornstein E, Monteagudo A, Dong R, et al. Detection of twin reversed arterial perfusion sequence at the time of first-trimester screening: the added value of 3-dimensional

volume and color Doppler sonography. *J Ultrasound Med.* 2008;27(7):1105–1109.

55. O'Neill JA Jr, Holcomb GWD, Schnaufer L, et al. Surgical experience with thirteen conjoined twins. *Ann Surg.* 1988;208(3):299–312.

56. Moore TR, Gale S, Benirschke K. Perinatal outcome of forty-nine pregnancies complicated by acardiac twinning. *Am J Obstet Gynecol.* 1990;163(3):907–912.

57. Lee H, Wagner AJ, Sy E, et al. Efficacy of radiofrequency ablation for twin-reversed arterial perfusion sequence. *Am J Obstet Gynecol.* 2007;196(5):459.e1–e4.

58. Holmes A, Jauniaux E, Rodeck C. Monopolar thermocoagulation in acardiac twinning. *BJOG.* 2001;108(9):1000–1002.

59. Stiller RJ, Romero R, Pace S, et al. Prenatal identification of twin reversed arterial perfusion syndrome in the first trimester. *Am J Obstet Gynecol.* 1989;160(5 Pt 1):1194–1196.

60. Bebbington M. Twin-to-twin transfusion syndrome: Current understanding of pathophysiology, in-utero therapy and impact for future development. *Semin Fetal Neonatal Med.* 2009. doi:10.10.16/j.siny2009.05.001.

61. Herberg U, Gross W, Bartmann P, et al. Long-term cardiac follow-up of severe twin-to-twin transfusion syndrome after intrauterine laser coagulation. *Heart.* 2005:1–16.

62. Bahtiyar MO, Dulay AT, Weeks BP, et al. Prevalence of congenital heart defects in monochorionic/diamniotic twin gestations: A systematic literature review. *J Ultrasound Med* 2007;26(11):1491–1498.

63. Campbell KH, Copel JA, Ozan Bahtiyar M. Congenital heart defects in twin gestations. *Minerva Ginecol.* 2009;61(3):239–244.

64. Pruetz JD, Chmait RH, Sklansky MS. Complete right heart flow reversal: Pathognomonic recipient twin circular shunt in twin-twin transfusion syndrome. *J Ultrasound Med.* 2009;28(8):1101–1106.

65. Barrea C, Alkazaleh F, Ryan G, et al. Prenatal cardiovascular manifestations in the twin-to-twin transfusion syndrome recipients and the impact of therapeutic amnioreduction. *Am J Obstet Gynecol.* 2005;192(3):892–902.

66. Cleary-Goldman J, D'Alton ME. Growth abnormalities and multiple gestations. *Semin Perinatol.* 2008;32(3):206–212.

67. Lopriore E, Nagel HT, Vandenbussche FP, et al. Long-term neurodevelopmental outcome in twin-to-twin transfusion syndrome. *Am J Obstet Gynecol.* 2003;189(5):1314–1319.

68. Dickinson JE, Duncombe GJ, Evans SF, et al. The long term neurologic outcome of children from pregnancies complicated by twin-to-twin transfusion syndrome. *BJOG.* 2005:112(1):63–68.

69. Quintero RA, Morales WJ, Allen MH, et al. Staging of twin-twin transfusion syndrome. *J Perinatol.* 1999;19:550–555.

70. Malone ED, D'Alton ME. Anomalies peculiar to multiple gestations. *Clin Perinatol.* 2000;27(4):1033–1046.

71. Johnson JR, Rossi KQ, O'Shaughnessy RW. Amnioreduction versus septostomy in twin-twin transfusion syndrome. *Am J Obstet Gynecol.* 2001;185(5):1044–1047.

72. Saade GR, Belfort MA, Berry Dl, et al. Amniotic septostomy for the treatment of twin oligohydramnios-polyhydramnios sequence. *Fetal Diagn Ther.* 1998;13(2):86–93.

73. Pistorius LR, Howarth GR. Failure of amniotic septostomy in the management of 3 subsequent cases of severe previable twin-twin transfusion syndrome. *Fetal Diagn Ther.* 1999;14(6):337–340.

74. Fox C, Kilby MD, Khan KS. Contemporary treatments for twin-twin transfusion syndrome. *Obstet Gynecol.* 2005;105(6):1469–1477.

75. Senat MV, Deprest J, Boulvain M, et al. Endoscopic laser surgery versus serial amnioreduction for severe twin-to-twin transfusion syndrome. *N Engl J Med.* 2004;351(2):136–144.

76. Strauss S, Tamarkin M, Engleberg S, et al. Prenatal sonographic appearance of diprosopus. *J Ultrasound Med.* 1987;6(2):93–95.

77. McLeod K, Tan PA, DeLange ME, et al. Conjoined twins in a triplet pregnancy: Sonographic findings. *JDMS.* 1988;4:9–12.

78. Wilson DA, Young GZ, Crumley CS. Antepartum ultrasonographic diagnosis of ischiopagus: A rare variety of conjoined twins. *J Ultrasound Med.* 1983;2:281–282.

79. Koontz WL, Layman L, Adams A, et al. Antenatal sonographic diagnosis of conjoined twins in a triplet pregnancy. *Am J Obstet Gynecol.* 1985;153(2):230–231.

80. Nichols BL, Blattner RJ, Rudolph AJ. General clinical management of thoracopagus twins. *Birth Defects.* 1967;3(1):38–51.

81. Hughey MJ, Olive DL. Routine ultrasound scanning for the detection and management of twin pregnancies. *J Reprod Med.* 1985;30(5):427–430.

82. Nocera RM, Davis M, Hayden CK, et al. Fetus-in-fetu. *AJR Am J Roentgenol.* 1982;138(4):762–764.

83. Lumme RH, Saarikoski SV. Monoamniotic twin pregnancy. *Acta Genet Med Gemellol (Roma).* 1986;35(1–2):99–105.

84. Rodis JF, McIlveen PF, Egan JF. Monoamniotic twins: Improved perinatal survival with accurate prenatal diagnosis and antenatal fetal surveillance. *Am J Obstet Gynecol.* 1997;177(5):1046–1049.

85. Redwine FO, Hays PM. Selective birth. *Semin Perinatol.* 1986;10(1):73–81.

86. Berkowitz RL, Stone JL, Eddleman KA. One hundred consecutive cases of selective termination of an abnormal fetus in a multifetal gestation. *Obstet Gynecol.* 1997;90(4):606–610.

87. Liveissues.net. The Carnegie Stages of Early Human Embryonic Development: chart of all 23 Stages, Detailed Descriptions of Stages 1–6. http://www.lifeissues.net/writers/irv/irv_123carnegiestages3.html Accessed 9/2009.

27 Intrauterine Growth Restriction (IUGR)

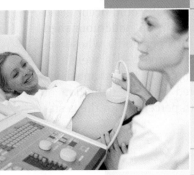

Michelle Kominiarek

OBJECTIVES

Define small for gestational age and symmetric and asymmetric IUGR

Summarize the adverse effects of intrauterine growth problems found in prenatal and postnatal life

Explain the different methods for identifying IUGR fetuses

List the two-dimensional (2D) and Doppler parameters that help in diagnosis and management of IUGR

Describe other methods of fetal assessment such as vibroacoustic stimulation (VAS) during an nonstress test (NST) or a biophysical profile (BPP) and contraction stress test (CST)

KEY TERMS

fetal growth restriction | intrauterine growth restriction (IUGR) | small for gestational age (SGA) | symmetrical IUGR | asymmetrical IUGR | nonstress test (NST) | biophysical profile (BPP) | pulsatility index (PI) | resistive index (RI) | systolic-diastolic (S/D) ratio | amniotic fluid index (AFI)

GLOSSARY

Acidemia Umbilical vessel pH less than 7.2

Aneuploidy Abnormal chromosome number

Biophysical profile (BPP) Combined observation of four separate fetal biophysical variables (fetal breathing movements, fetal body movement, fetal tone, amniotic fluid index) obtained via ultrasound

Brachycephaly Condition of having a short broad head

Contractions stress test (CST) Observation of the fetal heart rate response to three contractions that are felt by the mother in 10 minutes; also known as the oxytocin challenge test (OCT)

Dolichocephaly Condition of having a head with a long shape from the frontal to occipital bone

Doppler Noninvasive ultrasound test that measures blood flow

FASTER Study National Institute of Health (NIH) study that compared first-trimester β hCG/PAPP-A/NT with second-trimester screening methods

Hypoxemia Low oxygen blood level

Hypercapnia High levels of carbon dioxide

Idiopathic Without known cause

Intrauterine growth restriction (IUGR) Estimated fetal weight less than the 10th percentile for the gestational age

Low birth weight (LBW) Birth weight below 2,500 grams (g) or 5 lbs 8 oz

Macrosomic Weight greater than 4200 – 4500 grams

Morbidity Incidence of a specific disease in a population for a set amount of time

Nonstress test (NST) Method of assessing fetal well-being by observing the fetal heart rate response to fetal movement

Oligohydramnios Low amniotic fluid levels

Polyhydramnios High amniotic fluid levels

Preeclampsia Hypertension, and protein in the urine, occurring during pregnancy

Sensitivity The proportion of people who test positive for a disease who actually have the disease

Specificity The proportion of people who test negative for the disease who do not have the disease

Small for gestational age (SGA) Diagnosis used to describe an infant that is smaller than expected for the gestational age

Triploidy Having three complete sets of chromosomes

Trisomy Having three copies of a specific chromosome

Vibroacoustic stimulation (VAS) A noninvasive method of evoking a reactive NST in fetuses found to be in a low activity state via a device that emits vibration and sound

According to the Centers for Disease Control and Prevention, 4,265,555 infants were born in the United States in 2006.[1] Of these births, 8.3% had a low birth weight (LBW), and this is the highest number of LBW infants reported in four decades. In 2006, the infant mortality rate was 6.69 infant deaths per 1,000 live births.[2] Similarly, there were 6.22 stillbirths per 1,000 births in 2006. Although progress in perinatal care has resulted in increased survival for LBW infants, the rate of infant deaths attributed to prematurity/LBW was 113.5 per 100,000 live births in the United States in 2005.[3] A newborn's birth weight closely relates to risks for early death and long-term morbidity; infants born at the lowest weights have the highest mortality rates at one year of life.[2,4,5] Similarly, stillbirth rates decrease as fetal weight increases.[6] The majority of LBW infants are born prematurely (before 37 completed weeks of gestation); however, infants too small for their gestational age are likely a result of intrauterine growth restriction (IUGR). Reliable identification and treatment of these small infants before birth may greatly affect United States health care and its costs.

A fetus at risk for growth restriction is first identified by clinical and laboratory measures such as poor symphysis to fundal height growth, poor maternal weight gain, unexplained elevation in maternal serum alpha-fetoprotein (MSAFP), underlying maternal complication(s), or a history of IUGR in a prior pregnancy.[1] Prenatal sonography then evaluates the existence of a potential discrepancy between fetal size (as ascertained by sonography) and gestational age (as ascertained by the date of the last menstrual period or conception). Once this is established, sonography can assess interval growth and fetal well-being. Although several methods can identify IUGR fetuses, ultrasound seems to be the most accurate and sensitive.

DEFINITION OF IUGR

An electronic search of the Medline database (www .pubmed.com) for "intrauterine growth restriction" found over 14,000 articles on this subject. Despite the plethora of studies, there is still confusion about the definition and treatment of fetuses with IUGR. Consequently, the diagnosis is not always straightforward. The estimate of fetal weight (EFW) has served as the basis for assessment of normal fetal size and growth. IUGR has been defined in several ways, including an EFW below the 3rd, 5th, or 15th percentile for a population, two standard deviations (SD) below the mean for gestational age, or a weight decline of at least 10% between two weight estimates as determined by sonographic biometry.[7,8] A lagging abdominal circumference, defined as either below the 10th percentile, or two SD below the mean for gestational age, has also

defined IUGR.[8,9,10] EFW combined with physiologic or clinical parameters, ponderal indices below 10%, failure to achieve growth potential have also defined IUGR.[11] By this latter method, IUGR could occur at an EFW above the 10th percentile in an undernourished fetus that measures at the 15th percentile whose genetic composition would have predicted a weight at the 90th percentile, for example. In this chapter, we use the most widely accepted prenatal definition of IUGR: an EFW below the 10th percentile for the gestational age.

PREVALENCE

The prevalence of IUGR in the general population depends on the definition used. That is, if less-than-10th-percentile defines IUGR, then 10% of infants in a low-risk population will be affected; if one chooses less-than-third-percentile, 3% will be affected, and so on. However, in populations at risk, the prevalence increases. For example, women with hypertension or a previous growth-restricted infant have greater risks for IUGR, and the prevalence may be as high as 25% or more in these populations.[12]

ADVERSE EFFECTS

For fetuses identified as having IUGR, many clinical problems occur more commonly during perinatal life, childhood, and adulthood than in the normal population.

PATHOLOGY BOX 27-1

Pathology Associated With IUGR

Perinatal

Intrapartum fetal heart rate abnormalities
Hypoglycemia
Hypocalcemia
Meconium aspiration
Hypothermia
Complex hematologic problems (anemia, thrombocytopenia, polycythemia)
Necrotizing enterocolitis
Multisystem organ failure
Mortality

Childhood

Hypertension
Decreased intelligence and motor development
Poorer performance in school

Adult

Cardiovascular disease
Hypertension
Diabetes
Obesity

EFFECTS AND ASSOCIATIONS DURING PERINATAL LIFE

The perinatal period is the interval between the onset of fetal viability (~24 weeks) and the end of the neonatal period (~28 days after delivery). The fetus with poor intrauterine growth has a fivefold to tenfold increase in risk for perinatal mortality (~0.5% to 1% risk), compared with the normal size fetus (0.1%).[13] In addition, 26% of stillborn fetuses are small for gestational age,[14] and the risk for stillbirth is more pronounced with preterm IUGR.[15]

Fetal adaptations occur in response to an adverse environment such as IUGR. The responses are described in further detail below, but they include redistributions in blood flow such that nutrients and oxygen are directed to essential organs such as the brain. There is also a decrease in umbilical vein (UV) volume,[16] which leads to a greater diversion of the relatively nutrient- and oxygen-rich umbilical venous blood through the ductus venosus (DV) away from the liver and to the fetal heart. This blood then passes through the foramen ovale and enters the left side of the heart, where it is preferentially directed to the coronary and cerebral circulations.[17,18] Changes that occur later in the process include decreased cardiac output as a result of rising afterload (tension produced by a chamber of the heart in order to contract). As a result, the ability to handle preload (the pressure stretching the ventricle of the heart after passive filling of the ventricle and subsequent atrial contraction) significantly decreases, leading to an elevated central venous pressure (CVP). The final stage in the process of adaptation is decompensation with global heart dysfunction and dilatation.

Some immediate neonatal risks include meconium aspiration, hypoglycemia, electrolyte abnormalities, hematologic complications, and hypothermia.[19] These risks are even greater for preterm gestations. Several studies suggest that the intact survival rates are less than 50% for fetuses with IUGR at gestations under 28 weeks.[20,21,22]

EFFECTS DURING CHILDHOOD

Children who were growth restricted in utero have an increased risk for short- and long-term morbidity.[13] Physical, metabolic, and neurologic complications occur. Studies have also shown that IUGR infants born at term are at increased risk for having learning disabilities, behavioral problems, and worse performance in school than term, average for gestational age (AGA) children.[23] Neurologic damage can be seen as low scores on neurodevelopmental tests and reduced cognitive function.[8,25,26]

Children affected by IUGR have been found to have higher blood pressure compared with controls.[73] Most infants catch up on growth by 18 years, but fetuses that are below the 3rd percentile tend to have lower weights and shorter statures than their AGA counterparts. Preterm IUGR children are more likely to have neurodevelopmental abnormalities and cognitive impairment.[23,26]

EFFECTS IN ADULTHOOD

Advances in neonatal care have dramatically improved the survival of both IUGR and LBW infants. There is a long-term cost to restore normal growth in infancy and childhood. Adults who had IUGR are at a much higher risk for acquired heart disease, lipid abnormalities, and diabetes in later life.[27] Multiple studies have supported the Barker hypothesis, which states that the in utero environment leads to the fetal origins of adult disease that persist into infancy, childhood, and adulthood.[28,29] The intrauterine vascular changes become detrimental long term, resulting in hypertension, cerebral vascular accidents, diabetes, atherosclerosis, and obesity.[27,28,30] Although seemingly paradoxical, poor nutrition during fetal life, infancy, and early childhood alters gene expression and thereby establishes adult responses, with one of the end results being obesity.[31]

ETIOLOGY

Fetal growth abnormalities are thought to be idiopathic in half of the cases and multifactorial in the remainder. Some fetuses are constitutionally small because of genetic or racial influences.[32] It is difficult to discern the normal group from fetuses that are compromised by malnourishment, uteroplacental insufficiency, or other hemodynamic malady. Recent advances in prenatal Doppler interrogation are reducing the number of idiopathic cases by identifying the underlying causes of disease. However, the mechanisms that cause the poor growth are not well understood. Risk factors or etiologies of IUGR can be divided into three groups: maternal, fetal, and placental.

Of all the maternal factors, pre-eclampsia is associated with the most severe growth deficits.[33] Upon the diagnosis of IUGR there should be a thorough search for an etiology with a detailed exam of the fetal anatomy. Depending on the findings and clinical history, an evaluation for aneuploidy and infection might be indicated. Poor intrauterine growth and subsequent LBW are common features of many chromosomal abnormalities and in other fetuses with structural abnormalities.[35] The incidence of a chromosome abnormality in an infant of LBW is approximately 10%.[35] Many of these fetuses have multisystem malformations and altered body proportionality. Triploidy and trisomy 18 are the most common chromosomal defects associated with IUGR between 17 and 39 weeks.[35] When no sonographically identifiable malformation can be seen, the incidence of aneuploidy decreases. With severely impaired fetal growth, the risk of a chromosome abnormality is increased even more if there are abnormal amounts of amniotic fluid or there are abnormal

PATHOLOGY BOX 27-2

Risk Factors Associated With IUGR

Maternal

Low socioeconomic status/poor maternal nutrition (prepregnancy weight <50 kg)

Coexisting maternal disease, infection, or genetic disorder, including:
- Collagen vascular disease (i.e., systemic lupus erythematosus)
- Chronic and severe renal, cardiovascular, or respiratory diseases
- Hypertension and preeclampsia
- Diabetes

Antiphospholipid antibody syndrome

Inflammatory bowel disease

Lung disease

Sickle cell anemia

Maternal drug use/teratogenic exposure
- Alcohol
- Narcotics
- Nicotine
- Dilantin
- Propranolol
- Steroids
- Irradiation

Prior child of unexplained low birth weight

History of IUGR pregnancy

Preterm birth

High altitude

Fetal

Aneuploidy

Congenital infections (cytomegalovirus, varicella zoster)

Genetic syndromes

Congenital anomalies

Monochorionic twins

Twin-to-twin transfusion

Higher-order multiples

Placental

Placental mosaicism

Placental abruption

Placenta previa

Marginal or velamentous umbilical cord insertion

Placental neoplasms

Circumvillate placenta

Advanced placental grade

---

placentofetal Doppler indices.[36] Abnormal placental development is associated with poor placental function, and the chromosomally abnormal fetus has a chromosomally abnormal placenta. Therefore, the IUGR associated with the aneuploid (karyotypically abnormal) fetus may also be caused by primary placental insufficiency due to placental maldevelopment. Although most fetuses with perinatal-acquired infections such as herpes simplex virus, cytomegalovirus, rubella, and varicella zoster do not have ultrasound findings, head and central nervous system abnormalities (ventriculomegaly, intracranial calcifications, microcephaly, hydrancephaly), organomegaly (heart, liver, spleen), nonimmune hydrops, and parenchymal calcifications (i.e., liver) can occur.

IDENTIFICATION OF IUGR

WEIGHT-BASED THEORIES

As stated, the sonographic prediction of EFW forms the foundation for the identification of the small fetus and poor fetal growth. Table 27-1 lists birth weight percentiles from the 23rd to the 44th week of pregnancy. This table shows, for example, that LBW fetuses weigh less than approximately 2,510 g and 2,750 g at the 38th and 40th weeks of pregnancy, respectively. It should be noted that the birth weights listed in Table 27-1 are derived from pregnant women living at or near sea level. One of the original articles on growth curves and birth weights described Caucasian and Hispanic populations in Denver, Colorado.[37] Habitants of higher altitudes live in a chronic hypoxemic state, which results in lower birth weight. There is also a direct relationship between increasing altitude and lower birth weight, as determined by studies done in Denver, Colorado (altitude 1,600 m) and Leadville, Colorado (altitude 3,100 m), Tibet (altitude 3,658 m), and Peru.[38–40] Birth weight data from 15 areas in Peru located anywhere from sea level to 4,575 m showed that birth weight declines an average of 65 g for every additional 500 m in altitude above 2,000 m.[39] Pregnancy among inhabitants of Cerro de Pasco, Peru (altitude 4,370 m) was associated with 31% lower maternal cardiac output and 11% lower birth weight than observed in pregnant women residing at sea level (mean birth weight 2,935 and 3,290 g, respectively).[40] It is also important to note that there are several options available for determining birth weight percentile, including ones specific for preterm gestations.[36,41–44]

IUGR CATEGORIES

The traditional model for abnormal fetal growth defines two types of aberrant growth: symmetric and asymmetric IUGR. An asymmetrical growth pattern usually refers to a growth pattern where the abdominal circumference that lags greater than the biparietal diameter for the gestational age. Placental insufficiency is often presumed to be the etiology in these cases, whereas genetic disorders, aneuploidy, fetal infections, congenital malformations, and other syndromes account for symmetrical growth lag (all biometry measurements are small).

Not all clinicians or ultrasound units accept this division of IUGR types. A newer classification that

TABLE 27-1

Fetal Weight Percentiles Throughout Pregnancy

Gestational Age (Menstrual Weeks)	Smoothed Percentiles				
	10	25	50	75	90
23	370	460	550	690	990
24	420	530	640	780	1,080
25	490	630	740	890	1,180
26	570	730	860	1,020	1,320
27	660	840	990	1,160	1,470
28	770	980	1,150	1,350	1,660
29	890	1,100	1,310	1,530	1,890
30	1,030	1,260	1,460	1,710	2,100
31	1,180	1,410	1,630	1,880	2,290
32	1,310	1,570	1,810	2,090	2,500
33	1,480	1,720	2,010	2,280	2,690
34	1,670	1,910	2,220	2,510	2,880
35	1,870	2,130	2,430	2,730	3,090
36	2,190	2,470	2,650	2,950	3,290
37	2,310	2,580	2,870	3,160	3,470
38	2,510	2,770	3,030	3,320	3,610
39	2,680	2,910	3,170	3,470	3,750
40	2,750	3,010	3,280	3,590	3,870
41	2,800	3,070	3,360	3,680	3,980
42	2,830	3,110	3,410	3,740	4,060
43	2,840	3,110	3,420	3,780	4,100
44	2,790	3,050	3,390	3,770	4,110

Adapted from Brenner WE, Edelman DA, Hendricks CH: A standard of fetal growth for the United States of America. *Am J Obstet Gynecol.* 1976;126:555.

includes Doppler (discussed in subsequent sections in this chapter) and clinical parameters in addition to biometry allows for the classification of IUGR and also has some prognostic value for perinatal outcomes, i.e., worsening of stage is correlated with higher perinatal morbidity and mortality.[45] In this classification, fetuses in stage I have an abnormal umbilical artery or middle cerebral artery pulsatility index (PI). Those in stage II have an abnormal middle cerebral artery peak systolic velocity, absent or reversed umbilical artery diastolic flow, UV pulsations, and an abnormal DV PI. Fetuses in stage III have reversed flow at the DV or reversed flow at the UV, an abnormal tricuspid E wave (early ventricular filling)/A wave (late ventricular filling) ratio, and tricuspid regurgitation. Each stage is subdivided into either A (amniotic fluid index <5 cm) or B (amniotic fluid index >5 cm). This particular staging criteria included fetuses with an EFW below the 10th percentile but excluded those with structural anomalies, aneuploidy, or infection. The investigators in this study managed stage I fetuses as an outpatient, while both stage II and III were admitted to the hospital, stage II for observation and the majority of stage III for delivery. The rationale behind the

different categories and staging examples is that IUGR fetuses are not a homogeneous group and outcomes differ depending on IUGR etiology. Most ultrasound units have individualized practices regarding categorization of IUGR fetuses.

CALCULATING WEIGHT PERCENTILE

Doubilet and Benson originally described a "straightforward" approach to screen for IUGR by assessing for an EFW below the 10th percentile.[46] It is presented below in a modified version. Calculating the weight percentile requires three steps[47]:

1. Determination of gestational age from the first ultrasound examination, last menstrual period, or conception date. For every subsequent examination, calculate the gestational age by adding the number of weeks that have passed since the first examination. Biometry obtained at all subsequent examinations should never be used to redate the pregnancy.[48] This basic tenet of pregnancy dating cannot be overemphasized, especially in the screening and diagnosing of IUGR. The predictive error of ultrasound increases as

PATHOLOGY BOX 27-3

Fetal Growth Categories[8,88,118–124]

Type	Definition	Cause	Potential 2D Findings	Potential Doppler Findings
Symmetric IUGR*	All biometric parameters below 10%	Maternal infection; fetal chromosome anomalies or placental insufficiency occurring in the first trimester; maternal hypertension	BPD, AC, FL, HC measure small; normal BPD/AC ratio, possible oligohydramnios, estimated fetal weight below 10th percentile, grade III placenta	Increased RI, PI, S/D ratio in aorta, umbilical cord artery, and maternal uterine artery; reversed or absent umbilical cord artery flow; umbilical vein pulsations; decreased RI, PI, S/D ratio in MCA, reversed flow in the DV or UV; abnormal tricuspid E wave A wave ratio; tricuspid regurgitation
Asymmetric IUGR	Discordant biometric growth pattern	Normal growth in the first trimester; maternal, fetal, or placental disorders occurring in the second and third trimester; maternal hypertension	BPD/HC correlate with dates, AC/FL lag, BPD/AC ratio 2 standard deviations above the normal, possible oligohydramnios, estimated fetal weight below 10th percentile, grade III placenta	
Small for gestational age (SGA)	All biometric parameters below 10%	No known cause. May relate to parental habitus, and family history, normal maternal blood pressure	BPD, AC, FL, HC measure small; normal BPD/AC ratio; normal fluid, placenta appropriate for gestational age	Values may or may not change, usually normal

*Often considered a subset of the SGA category; however, there are different causes of the growth changes.

the gestation increases and is approximately ±5 days in the first, ±10 days in the second, and ±21 days in the third trimester. If ultrasound estimates of gestational age differ by a greater number, then redating is appropriate in most instances at the first ultrasound. It is also known that earlier sonographic biometry has a greater accuracy of gestational dating. The accuracy of measuring all biometric parameters decreases with advancing gestational age; femur length is least affected.[49] Of note, a study of over 17,000 patients between 8 and 16 weeks' gestation found ultrasound to be superior to LMP for estimation of gestational age.[50]

2. Estimate the fetal weight. There are multiple articles providing formulas or tables using various body parts in estimation of fetal weight.[51–53] The formulas were developed more than 25 years ago and are still used today. Schemes with two, three, or more measurements have been offered, including those using the biparietal diameter, head circumference, abdominal circumference, femur length, and humerus length (discussed in Chapter 16). A reasonable model for estimating fetal weight would include measurement of the fetal head, abdomen, and femur.[54] The use of multiple parameters has been shown to decrease both interobserver and intraobserver error. The

accuracy of the predicted EFW falls within 10% to 20% of the actual weight in 80% to 95% of cases.[54] The reliability of EFW predictions is not influenced by amniotic fluid amounts or maternal weight.[55]

Most of these formulas for EFW use the biparietal diameter (BPD), head circumference (HC), abdominal circumference (AC), or femur length (FL) measurements. Campbell et al., Ferrero et al., Hadlock et al., and Warsof et al. formulas used the FL and AC; Shepard et al. used BPD and FL; Hadlock et al., Hill et al., Woo et al., and Benson et al. used FL, AC, and BPD; Roberts et al. used FL, AC, BPD, and HC; and Sabbagha et al. used HC, AC, and FL (see Appendixes L, M, N).[9,10,14,15,20,32,41–44,46,47,52,53]

In this chapter, we discuss the three most popular formulas.

FORMULA BY SHEPARD AND COWORKERS[56]

This formula incorporates only BPD and AC. Its predictive error is high (±10% to 15%), and it is particularly accurate in small infants.[57] Although there have been several articles that validate the efficacy of this formula, it has two limiting factors. First, "normal" changes in head shape as pregnancy continues, or normal variants in head shape such as dolichocephaly and brachycephaly, can alter BPD measurements. Second, it does not use the HC and FL, considered by some as important measurements in determining weight. Despite these problems, many recommend this technique for estimating the fetal weight.[58]

FORMULA BY HADLOCK AND COWORKERS

This formula incorporates three basic measurements: HC, AC, and FL (Table 27-2).[57] With this approach, the two SD variation in the prediction of birth weight has been reduced.[59] However, the authors have reported a wide error (±19.4%) in estimating the size of fetuses that weigh less than 1,500 g. The formula has been found more accurate in fetuses over 2,500 g, and it does not consider the proportional contributions of HC and AC to birth weight. These contributions are known to be in a dynamic state of change. In other words, the HC/AC ratio normally changes throughout pregnancy and with some pathologic states. The following examples illustrate the dynamic differences that exist in the HC/AC ratios: (1) Before the 36th pregnancy week, the HC/AC ratio is greater than 1.0. (2) Following the 36th pregnancy week, the HC/AC ratio is less than 1.0. (3) In the macrosomic fetus, the HC/AC ratio is less than 1.0.

FORMULAS BY SABBAGHA AND COWORKERS

To account for the dynamic varying proportional contributions of the HC and the AC, these investigators derived three formulas, one from each of three fetal groups: large, appropriate, and small for gestational age. Each of the three formulas is targeted to a specific group of fetuses. All three targeted formulas incorporate the following four parameters: gestational age in weeks, HC, AC (multiplied by 2), and FL. The accuracy of the assigned gestational age should be within ±2 weeks and preferably decided by one of the following criteria: (1) early crown-rump length (CRL) or BPD (measurements obtained before 13 and 26 weeks' gestation, respectively); (2) known ovulation dates or certain last menstrual period; (3) confirmation of menstrual dates by early CRL or BPD, as defined in criterion 1; (4) the average of different dates estimated by early CRL and/or BPD, and FL, if the estimates do not differ from each other by more than a week; and (5) the average of different dates

provided by early CRL, and/or HC, or AC, and FL, again, if the estimates do not differ from each other by more than one week.

In estimating fetal weight by the targeted formulas, the percentile rank of the AC determines which of the three formulas should be employed. For example, if the AC is at least in the 90th percentile, the formula for the large-for-dates fetus is used. On the other hand, if the AC is average (between 10th and 90th percentile), the formula for the appropriate-for-dates fetus is used. Finally, if the AC is below the 5th percentile, the formula for the small-for-dates fetus is used.

In comparison to Hadlock's formula, the targeted formulas reduce the cumulative two SD variation by 8.4%. On the other hand, the cumulative absolute two SD variation of the targeted formulas is 12% versus 15.6% for Hadlock's formula, a reduction of 23%.[58] Of all studies that incorporate fetuses of low birth weight, the formulas by Sabbagha et al. have the lowest systematic errors (1.7% to 2.8%) and SD (8.1% to 9.1%).[51] It should be emphasized that the advantage of reducing the two SD variation achieved by the targeted formulas may be lost if gestational age cannot be determined within a range of ±2 weeks.

The format of deriving estimates of fetal weight by the sum of four variables allows the sonographer the choice of reading the estimated fetal weight directly from a concise chart or entering all three formulas into a computer for automatic calculation of the estimated fetal weight.

The weight percentile is calculated from the estimated weight and the gestational age. This is typically accomplished using a published table that reports normal weight for gestational age. Of particular importance is the determination about whether the fetal weight falls below the 10% percentile (Table 27-1). In the second trimester, the femur length is the most accurate measure of gestational age, followed by head circumference, biparietal diameter, and abdominal circumference.[60] However, the AC percentile has both the highest sensitivity and negative predictive value for the sonographic diagnosis of IUGR.

The formulas described above relate to fetal measurements in the second or third trimester. Previously, it has been assumed that fetal growth is uniform in the first trimester in all pregnancies. Some studies have described a link between abnormalities in first-trimester growth and the risk for subsequent adverse outcomes. In a retrospective review of 30,000 pregnancy records, a first-trimester CRL that was 2 to 6 days smaller than expected was associated with an increased risk (as compared with a normal or slightly larger than expected CRL) of a birth weight below 2,500 g (relative risk [RR] 1.8, 95% confidence interval [CI] 1.3 to 2.4), a birth weight below 2,500 g at term (RR 2.3, 95% CI 1.4 to

TABLE	27-2

Formula for Estimation of Fetal Weight

$$Log_{10}BW = 1.5662 - 0.0108(HC) + 0.0468(AC) + 0.171(FL) + 0.00034(HC)^2 - 0.003685(AC \times FL)$$

From Hadlock FP, Harrist RB, Sharman RS, et al. Estimation of fetal weight with the use of head, body, and femur measurements: A prospective study. *Am J Obstet Gynecol.* 1985;151:333–337.

3.8), and a birth weight below the 5th percentile for gestational age (RR 3.0, 95% CI 2.0 to 44).[61] Similarly, in a prospective study of 976 assisted reproduction pregnancies, increased size for gestation in the first trimester was associated with higher birth weight, and the risk of delivering an SGA infant decreased as the first-trimester fetal size increased.[62] This again highlights the greater accuracy of early ultrasound for pregnancy dating.

NON-WEIGHT BASED PARAMETERS

Several other biometric methods have been proposed to aid in the identification of IUGR. These include the brain's gyral patterns,[63] the transcerebellar diameter,[61,64] evidence of decreased adipose deposits,[19,65] foot length,[66] the imaging of the distal femoral epiphysis or proximal humeral epiphysis, ratios of the HC to the AC[67,68] or the AC to the FL,[67] amniotic fluid volumes (without premature rupture of membranes),[68] the presence of a Grade 3 placenta,[47] echogenic bowel,[69] volumes of intracranial structures,[70] femur volume[71] and humerus volume (Figs. 27-1–3).[72] For an independent technique to be clinically useful, it must have a high degree of sensitivity, specificity, and high predictive values. Unfortunately, no single sonographic parameter allows for the confident diagnosis of IUGR. The most accurate diagnosis is achieved by using multiple biometric and structural parameters.[46]

Advances in ultrasound technology have enabled modern ultrasound equipment to acquire, analyze, and display 3D ultrasound volumes. This has allowed further definition fetal structure as well as an investigation into its use for predicting EFW. Lee et al. used 3D ultrasound to calculate fractional limb volumes in the third trimester and developed a formula incorporating fractional thigh volume and AC that gave a slight but statistically significant improvement in EFW compared with traditional 2D ultrasound techniques.[73] This

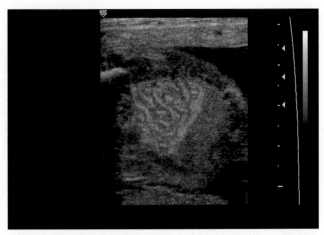

Figure 27-2 Echogenic bowel in the fetal abdomen. (Image courtesy of Philips Medical Systems, Bothell, WA.)

formula[73] and others[74,75] also show a slight improvement in measurement errors (6% to 7%) compared to 2D techniques. There have only been a few reports of 3D ultrasound in the LBW or IUGR fetus. Boito et al. described fetal brain/liver ratios (analogous to HC/AC ratios) measured by 3D ultrasound in 23 IUGR fetuses and compared these ratios with matched AGA fetuses. They found the ratio to be significantly elevated in 78% of the IUGR fetuses—the ratio in AGA fetuses was 3:1 compared to 5 to 7:1 in the IUGR fetuses.[148] Schild et al. reported 3D sonography in the EFW of smaller fetuses (greater than 1,600 g). With a formula involving the abdominal volume, HC, thigh volume, FL, and BPD, there was improvement in errors compared to the currently used formulas.[75] Although these studies show promise in improving the accuracy of EFW, the formulas have not been tested in large populations. In addition, 3D ultrasound techniques require technically sophisticated and expensive ultrasound equipment, special training and extra skills for examiners, and are more time

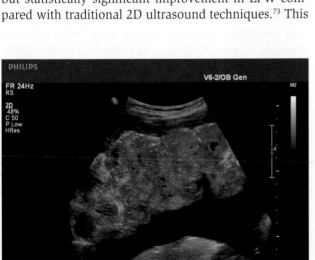

Figure 27-1 Grade III placenta with calcifications. (Image courtesy of Philips Medical Systems, Bothell, WA.)

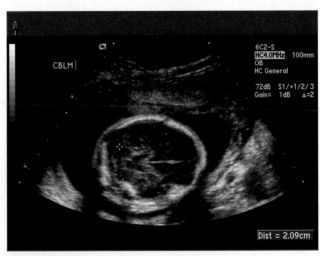

Figure 27-3 Measurement of the fetal cerebellum.

consuming compared to 2D ultrasound. Furthermore, whether or not 3D techniques significantly improve our ability to diagnose and manage IUGR has not been determined.

Magnetic resonance imaging (MRI) helps in pregnancy evaluation and can complement ultrasound studies. Though it is more commonly used for evaluation of fetal structure or placentation, several studies describe volume techniques to predict EFW. This includes Baker et al., who describe low systematic errors (0.4%) and SD (5.1%), and Uotila et al., who report a better correlation between MRI EFW (r = 0.95) and birth weight than ultrasound (r = 0.77).[76,77] Zaretsky et al. studied 80 pregnant patients at term and calculated EFW using both the Hadlock formula with ultrasound techniques and a volumetric formula, fetal weight = 0.12 + [0.031(volume in mL)] using MRI, which involved adding up the sum of the fetal areas from each MRI slice and converting it to fetal weight using the formula. These investigators concluded that MRI was significantly better than ultrasound in determining the EFW at term.[78] Whether or not MRI is equally accurate in early gestations or in IUGR fetuses has not been determined, but the volumetric equations with MRI may generate more accurate EFW compared to regression equations.

Whether or not to use individualized or customized fetal growth curves has been a matter of debate for several years. It is known that birth weight is related to maternal height and parity, paternal height, and fetal sex. In the United States, the populations are ethnically heterogeneous. With respect to IUGR, the use of customized growth charts based on maternal weight, height, ethnicity, and fetal gender may better predict perinatal morbidity.[6,15,32,79] An example of such a customized percentile calculator is available at www.gestation.net. In a retrospective analysis of a database from a multicentered ultrasound study in the United States, SGA defined by customized growth potential showed a higher risk for preterm labor, antepartum hemorrhage, pre-eclampsia, stillbirth, and early neonatal death.[80] More specifically, when they used maternal height, weight, parity, ethnicity, and fetal gender, 33% of the SGA group was small by customized percentiles, but not by population percentiles, and yet were associated with pregnancy complications. Importantly, the subgroup that was SGA by population percentiles but not by customized percentiles was not associated with any indicators of adverse outcome.[80] In summary, 17.4% of infants conventionally considered SGA were constitutionally small and the population standard missed one-third of infants that were small by customized standards. There are numerous birth weight curves, but no universally accepted national standard or agreement upon whether or not they should be used.[81]

Clinicians managing twins and other multiple gestations rely upon ultrasound to monitor fetal growth. It is normal for multiples to be smaller than singletons, but being smaller than singletons does not necessarily mean that multiples are pathologically growth restricted. Twins and triplets have different growth patterns compared to singletons. Twin growth is similar to that of singletons until 30 to 32 weeks and varies by chorionicity.[82,83] After 32 weeks, an asymmetric pattern of growth is more likely. A study of 2,477 triplets suggests that using singleton curves to diagnose growth restriction results in a higher false-positive rate than using triplet curves after 31 weeks of gestation; however, triplet curves are less sensitive.[84] There is some controversy in the literature as to the use of singleton growth curves for multiple gestations, and most ultrasound units individualize this practice.

CLINICAL PARAMETERS

Older studies have suggested using clinical parameters to improve predictability in cases of IUGR.[85] One particular approach allows the diagnosis of IUGR if the EFW corresponding to the gestational age, amniotic fluid volume, and maternal blood pressure status (Table 27-3) falls below the designated values. An EFW between these two groups of values is indeterminate for IUGR, whereas an EFW that falls in a higher zone of values excludes or "rules out" IUGR (with a similar high degree of confidence). Both the diagnosis and the exclusion of IUGR are 85% predictive.

FETAL GROWTH RATE

When IUGR is not diagnosed at term, then serial measurements at several points during the pregnancy are recommended so that longitudinal changes in growth can be shown.[46] Fetuses that are not constitutionally small grow at a slower rate than others. Growth assessment can be direct (monitoring the growth rate) or indirect (deviations from the expected size). Indirect assessment implies that the normal range of growth over time is known. This would allow for a computation of the growth rate by dividing the growth by the time interval. The growth rates for the BPD, AC, and FL are known.[86] Fetal growth is usually continuous and not sporadic. Because the technical capability of ultrasound limits the identification of growth problems, the recommended interval between ultrasound evaluations is approximately 3 weeks. Shorter intervals may increase the likelihood of a false-positive diagnosis of abnormal growth.[60]

FETAL PHYSIOLOGY

Fetal maladaptation syndrome (FMS) occurs when the fetus can no longer compensate physiologically in a stressful environment. One of the first sequelae of maladaptation is poor intrauterine fetal growth. Commonly,

TABLE 27-3

Critical Values for Estimated Fetal Weight for Diagnosing or Excluding IUGR Using the IUGR Score[25]

Gestational Age (weeks)	STATUS OF MATERNAL BLOOD PRESSURE AND AMNIOTIC FLUID VOLUME					
	Normal Blood Pressure			**Hypertension**		
	Norm/Poly	M-M Oligo	Sev Oligo	Norm/Poly	M-M Oligo	Sev Oligo
26	516–660	646–826	743–950	610–780	763–976	878–1,123
27	597–791	745–949	855–1,090	704–898	878–1,119	1009–1,285
28	693–877	859–1,087	982–1,244	813–1,030	1,008–1,276	1153–1,460
29	803–1,008	988–1,239	1,124–1,410	937–1,176	1,152–1,446	1312–1,646
30	931–1,155	1,132–1,405	1,281–1,589	1,078–1,337	1,311–1,627	1483–1,840
31	1,075–1,317	1,293–1,584	1,452–1,779	1,234–1,512	1,484–1,819	1667–2,042
32	1,235–1,493	1,468–1,774	1,635–1,976	1,404–1,698	1,670–2,018	1860–2,248
33	1,411–1,682	1,656–1,973	1,830–2,180	1,590–1,895	1,865–2,223	2061–2,456
34	1,600–1,880	1,853–2,177	2,031–2,386	1,785–2,098	2,067–2,429	2,266–2,662
35	1,798–2,083	2,055–2,382	2,236–2,590	1,987–2,302	2,272–2,633	2,471–2,863
36	1,997–2,285	2,257–2,593	2,437–2,789	2,189–2,504	2,474–2,830	2,671–3,056
37	2,192–2,479	2,452–2,774	2,631–2,976	2,383–2,696	2,666–3,016	2,861–3,236
38	2,371–2,658	2,631–2,949	2,807–3,147	2,563–2,872	2,843–3,186	3,034–3,400
39	2,526–2,812	2,785–3,101	2961–3,296	2,717–3,025	2,996–3,335	3,185–3,545
40	2,645–2,933	2,906–3,223	3083–3,419	2,838–3,147	3,118–3,458	3,307–3,668
41	2,717–3,013	2,985–3,310	3166–3,511	2,915–3,232	3,202–3,551	3,396–3,766
42	2,736–3,405	3,016–3,356	3205–3,567	2,942–3,274	3,243–3,609	3,447–3,836

For each pair, an EFW less than the lower value corresponds to an IUGR score of more than 60, allowing a confident diagnosis of IUGR (positive predictive value of 74%). An EFW value greater than the higher number corresponds with a score below 50, virtually excluding IUGR (negative predictive value of 97%). An EFW between the two values is equivocal (probability of IUGR is 13%).

NF, normal fluid; Poly, polyhydramnios; M-M, mild to moderate; Olig, oligohydramnios; Sev, severe

Modified from Doubilet PM. Benson CB. Sonographic evaluation of intrauterine growth retardation. *Am J Roentgenol*. 1995, 164:709–717.

this finding is followed by decreased amniotic fluid (from oliguria), abnormal umbilical arterial and venous Doppler assessment (reflecting declining cardiac output, increasing or decreasing vascular resistance in the fetus or placenta, or fetal hypoxia/acidemia with resultant arterial and venous cardiovascular adaptations), and pathologic fetal behavior (no movement or poor tone). Changes in fetal size/growth, developmental anatomy, physiology, and behavior have been observed to precede fetal compromise and eventual fetal death.[87] These changes can portend acute and chronic fetal deterioration. Several prenatal diagnostic techniques have been offered as predictors of poor growth. In this discussion, we focus on the sonographic tools used in the assessment of an IUGR fetus.

DOPPLER ASSESSMENT IN IUGR

In the fetus with IUGR, there is a normal redistribution of blood within the fetus and placenta. Doppler technology has had a significant impact on our ability to assess the physiologic status of the fetus. It can help in identifying changes in the fetal circulation at a time when other tests are normal and in so doing identify the truly hypoxic fetus. Interval changes

in Doppler values may be useful in determining the optimal time for delivery to reduce perinatal mortality and any subsequent complications. Common measurements of Doppler indices include the PI, resistive index (RI), and systolic-diastolic (S/D) ratio (Table 27-4).

During Doppler interrogation it is important to remember that fetal blood flow is influenced by cardiac contractility, the physical properties of the arterial

TABLE 27-4

Doppler Terminology

Term	Abbreviation	Calculation
Systolic-diastolic ratio	S/D ratio	Maximum velocity/ minimum velocity
Pulsatility index	PI	(Maximum – minimum velocity)/mean velocity
Resistance index	RI	(Maximum-minimum velocity)/maximum velocity
Peak systolic velocity	PSV	Maximum velocity (cm/s)

walls and the blood viscosity within, the size of small blood vessels, and the outflow impedance from the arterial tree.[8,88] Most reports regarding the interrogation of the fetal circulation use the PI because it is Doppler-angle independent. Furthermore, most literature on Doppler describes an analysis of three continuous waveforms that were selected from a group of 5 to 15 waveforms. Opinions that are more recent suggest that an assessment on one to three different occasions 5 to 10 minutes apart in the absence of fetal movement and breathing is more appropriate.[45] In each set, at least 10 to 15 waveforms should be obtained. If the waveform quality is adequate, the analysis can be performed either on the entire spectrum of waveforms or on three waveforms for each set. A grading system for results has also been proposed: normal, transitional, or abnormal.

Although Doppler interrogation has not been universally accepted for screening low-risk populations, it has been proven effective in the evaluation of high-risk pregnancies.[89] Several studies have shown that Doppler, specifically umbilical artery Doppler, is of value in identifying the physiologically compromised fetus, and equipment with pulsed Doppler capabilities should be available for high-risk pregnancies.[90]

UTERINE ARTERY DOPPLER

Normally, uterine vascular resistance decreases with advancing gestational age because of the changes in perfusion needs of the uterus. During the first 10 weeks of pregnancy, a persistent diastolic component of the uterine artery Doppler (utD) waveform is observed with an early diastolic notch, which is usually lost between 20 and 26 weeks.[91] The RI decreases from 0.8 to 0.63 between 8 and 17 weeks, and the PI decreases from 2.0 to 1.3 between 8 and 18 weeks' gestation.[92] In the normal pregnancy, this RI change is due to the development of the high-volume, low-resistance flow seen during pregnancy. These changes ensure adequate perfusion of the intervillous space via the spiral arteries of the mother. The placenta facilitates these changes to compensate for the growing embryonic nutritional needs. Higher ratios may suggest an abnormality and increasing resistance to flow (Fig. 27-4). In theory, an abnormal utD could detect an increase in placental vascular resistance, and this could predict which women are at risk for diseases like IUGR. An elevation of the RI or PI, or the persistence of a uterine artery diastolic notch, usually detects the presence of abnormally increased uteroplacental vascular resistance. In one review, an abnormal utD was a better predictor of pre-eclampsia than of IUGR after 16 weeks of gestation.[93] In this study, the best predictor of IUGR in high-risk patients was an increased RI. In a systematic review of 28 studies of utD, women with an abnormal utD had a likelihood

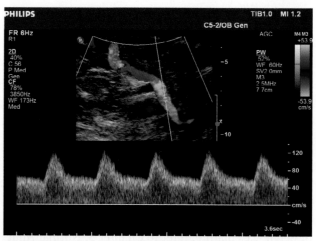

Figure 27-4 Normal uterine artery Doppler waveform. (Image courtesy of Philips Medical Systems, Bothell, WA.)

ratio (LR) of 3.6 (95% CI 3.2 to 4.0) for the development of IUGR and a negative result carried a 0.8 LR (95% CI 0.8 to 0.9).[94]

Early Pregnancy (12 to 13 weeks)

The PI of a utD waveform was analyzed in women of advanced maternal age (over 34 years) carrying fetuses between 12 and 13 weeks' gestation. Women with abnormally high values had higher risks of developing hypertensive disorders (four times normal), gestational diabetes (nine times normal), delivering SGA infants (twice normal), and having a preterm delivery (three times normal). PI values less than 1.24 were considered overtly normal, and greater than 1.67 was abnormal.[95,96] In pre-eclampsia, a prominent diastolic notch is seen in approximately 60% of cases.[97] In the FASTER study, a prospective trial of ultrasound and serum markers for aneuploidy in the first trimester, a utD RI value above the 75th percentile at 10 to 14 weeks predicted a 5.5-fold higher likelihood of subsequent IUGR.[97]

Early Second Trimester (16 to 20 weeks)

UtD interrogation during the second trimester can predict outcome in cases at risk for pregnancy-induced hypertension, IUGR, preterm delivery, gestational diabetes, and fetal asphyxia.[98-100] However, the value of routine screening for predicting pre-eclampsia and IUGR has yet to be accepted by all authors.[92]

Bromley and colleagues investigated the relationship between utD and the presence of uterine artery notching in terms of perinatal outcome.[101,102] In a population of women with elevated MSAFP test values, they found adverse outcomes in 13% without notching and 47% with Grade II notching. In this study, a grade I notch was an early diastolic drop, which was less severe than half of the total mid-diastolic frequency shift compared to a grade II notch, which indicated a drop in early diastole to less than half of the total diastolic frequency shift present during mid-diastole. Most studies use subjective criteria for the definition of a diastolic notch, but a drop of at least 50 cm/s from the maximum diastolic velocity is a reasonable criterion after 20 weeks.[93,103,104]

Although the utD literature continues to expand, it remains unclear when the assessment of utD should be done (at 16, 20, or 24 weeks of gestation) and which tool to use (uterine artery notch, PI, RI, or all of them). It is also unclear what constitutes an abnormal result—a single cutoff or percentile cutoffs.[45,92] They also have a low predictive value in a low-risk population.[105] Consequently, there are currently no practice standards for their use in obstetrics. For a detailed description of pelvic vasculature, refer to Chapter 5, Normal Anatomy of the Female Pelvis; for normal uterine Doppler parameters refer to Chapter 6, Doppler Evaluation of the Pelvis.

UMBILICAL ARTERIAL DOPPLER

Assessment of blood flow through the umbilical cord, primarily the umbilical artery, has been widely reported and is more uniformly accepted in practice compared to the utD.[106–108] The technique involves the analysis of a free umbilical cord loop with continuous or pulsed Doppler. Waveforms from the umbilical artery near the placenta usually have more end-diastolic flow than those near the cord insertion. In general, the umbilical artery circulation has a low impedance and the amount of end-diastolic flow increases with advancing gestation due to an increase in the number of tertiary stem villi as the placenta matures. Diseases that affect the small muscular arteries in the placental tertiary stem villi result in a progressive decrease in end-diastolic flow followed by absent (AEDF), then reversed flow in diastole (REDF) as the process worsens, resulting in an RI and PI value increase. Abnormally reduced diastolic flow velocities are predictive in identifying infants requiring early delivery and neonatal intensive care.[109,110]

Most studies focus on the findings of AEDF or REDF and the relationship between adverse outcomes (Figs. 27-5–6). This finding indicates increased placental resistance, which results in a higher risk of fetal demise.[111] The observation of AEDF may occur nearly 8 days before pathologic cardiotocographic findings are present.[6] The appearance of REDF is evidence

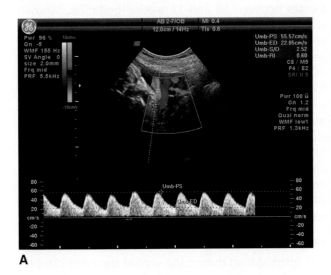

A

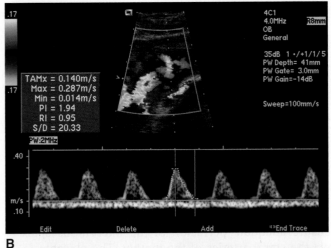

B

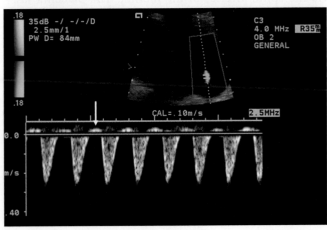

C

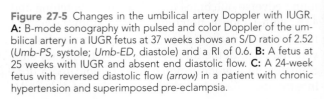

Figure 27-5 Changes in the umbilical artery Doppler with IUGR. **A:** B-mode sonography with pulsed and color Doppler of the umbilical artery in a IUGR fetus at 37 weeks shows an S/D ratio of 2.52 (*Umb-PS,* systole; *Umb-ED,* diastole) and a RI of 0.6. **B:** A fetus at 25 weeks with IUGR and absent end diastolic flow. **C:** A 24-week fetus with reversed diastolic flow *(arrow)* in a patient with chronic hypertension and superimposed pre-eclampsia.

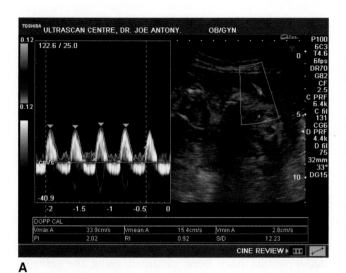
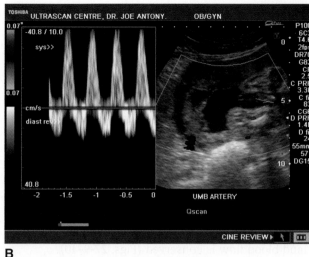

Figure 27-6 Color Doppler and spectral waveform imaging of the umbilical artery shows reversal of diastolic flow. This is an ominous sign of fetal compromise/hypoxia requiring further evaluation of the fetal middle cerebral artery and ductus venosus. The diastolic flow reversal in umbilical arteries signifies severe placental insufficiency and increased placental vascular resistance. (Image courtesy of Joe Antony, MD, Cochin, India. From the website at http://www.ultrasound-images.com/fetus-general.htm)

that (1) the lowest vascular resistance is in the fetal circulatory network rather than the placenta and (2) preplacental blood with low oxygen content from the descending aorta and pulmonary artery is being shifted toward the brain.[44] This is to be considered an alarming finding affecting obstetrical diagnosis and management. As a pathologic correlate, REDF can occur when 60% to 70% of the villous vascular tree is damaged.[107-109]

Although an association clearly exists, several investigators have tried to establish the applicability of umbilical artery Doppler (excluding absent diastolic flow) in the prediction of IUGR.[108] Fetuses with abnormal umbilical artery Doppler indices have only a twofold to fourfold risk of IUGR, compared with controls.[108,109] Although there is an increased risk of cesarean, preterm delivery, neonatal intensive care unit admission, assisted ventilation, and perinatal mortality, umb art Doppler has a low sensitivity in detecting IUGR so it is a poor screening tool in low risk population.[108,109] Conversely, a meta-analysis showed that Doppler sonography of the umbilical artery in high-risk pregnancies results in a significant reduction in intervention, reducing the odds of perinatal death.[112] In the setting of IUGR, umbilical artery Doppler can help stratify fetuses into low- and high-risk categories. For information on obtaining the umbilical cord Doppler, refer to Chapter 24, Doppler Ultrasound of the Normal Fetus.

MIDDLE CEREBRAL ARTERY DOPPLER

Prenatal interrogation of cerebral blood flow can be accomplished by assessing the common carotid artery, the internal carotid artery, or the anterior, middle, or cerebral arteries. The middle cerebral arteries (MCA) are major branches of the circle of Willis supplied by the internal carotid and vertebral arteries (Fig. 27-7). In contrast to the umbilical artery circulation, the MCA is part of a high-impedance vascular bed with lower end-diastolic velocities. There is continuous forward flow throughout the cardiac cycle in the MCA. The MCA is the most accessible cerebral vessel for Doppler studies and contains more than 80% of cerebral blood flow. This arterial system is best seen in a transverse plane of the fetal head obtained at the base of the skull. The appropriate sample site is from the proximal vessel soon after its origin at the internal carotid artery. This allows for measurement of the S/D ratio, RI,

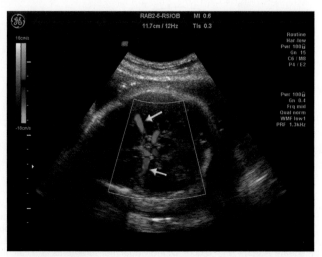

Figure 27-7 Color Doppler imaging allows easy identification of the two MCA (arrows). (Image courtesy of GE Healthcare, Wauwatosa, WI.)

PI, and peak systolic velocity (PSV). The flow velocity in the MCA is normally highly pulsatile, and the RI, PI, and S/D ratio increases up to 20 to 24 weeks' gestation and then decreases at term (Fig. 27-8).[113] In the normal fetus, the MCA-PSV increases with gestational age.[114] In fetal hypoxemia, there is a central redistribution of blood flow such that there is increased blood flow to the brain ("brain-sparing effect"), heart ("cardiac-sparing effect"), and adrenals.[115,116] MCA Doppler has been proven useful in detecting hypoxia associated with IUGR.[116] In fetuses with IUGR, the RIs in the MCA were increased because of the vasodilation seen in fetal adaptation to hypoxia.[117] It is thought that a hormonally mediated increase in fetal peripheral vascular resistance occurs so that cerebral, cardiac, and adrenal gland blood flow is conserved (Figs. 27-9–10).

Although better known in its application for fetal anemia assessment, the MCA-PSV has also been described in IUGR fetuses. In one cross-sectional review of 30 fetuses with IUGR, the MCA-PSV was the best parameter in the prediction of perinatal mortality (OR 14, 95% CI 1.4 to 130).[45] In anemic fetuses, the high MCA-PSV likely reflects an increased cardiac output and decreased blood viscosity, whereas in IUGR fetuses, the high MCA-PSV results from increased blood flow to the brain through increased cardiac output and placental resistance.

Early changes in fetuses with IUGR include an increased umbilical artery RI and decreased MCA RI. The MCA and umbilical artery Doppler are the best individual predictors of adverse fetal outcome. However, better results have been obtained using the ratio of

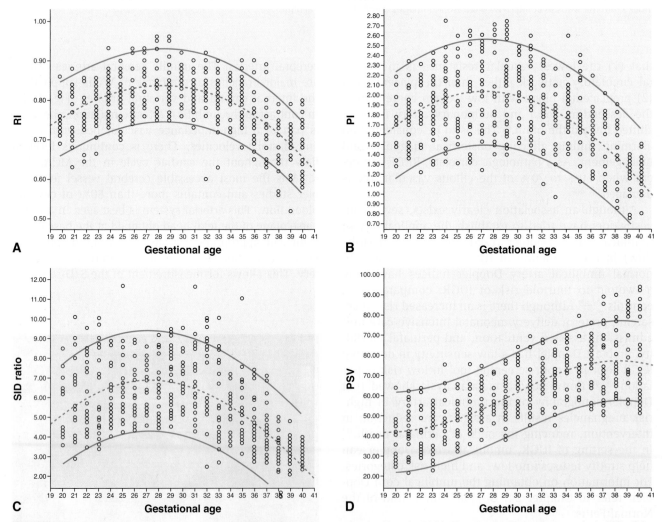

Figure 27-8 A: Individual measurements and calculated reference ranges for the RI in the MCA. The standard boundaries include 90% of the normal patient population (Cubic R square = 0.386, P = 0.000). **B:** Individual measurements and calculated reference ranges for the PI in the MCA. The standard boundaries include 90% of the normal patient population (Cubic R square = 0.340, P = 0.000). **C:** Individual measurements and calculated reference ranges for the S/D ratio in the MCA. The standard boundaries include 90% of the normal patient population (Cubic R square = 0.334, P = 0.000). **D:** Individual measurements and calculated reference ranges for the PSV in the MCA. The standard boundaries include 90% of the normal patient population (Cubic R square = 0.535, P = 0.000). (From Tarzamni MK, Nezami N, Sobhani N, Eshraghi N, Tarzamni M, Talebi Y. Nomograms of Iranian fetal middle cerebral artery Doppler waveforms and uniformity of their pattern with other populations' nomograms. *BMC Pregnancy Childbirth.* 2008 Nov 12;8:50.)

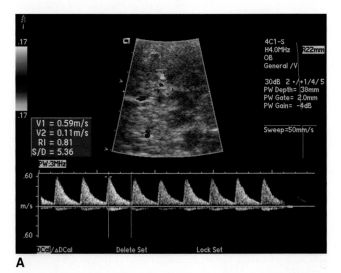

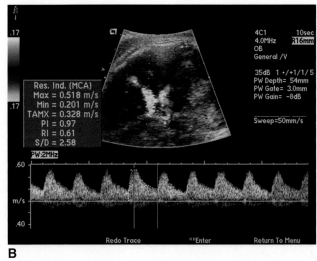

A   **B**

Figure 27-9 In hypoxia, the fetus will compensate by redistributing its cardiovascular load so that more blood is circulated to the fetal head (the brain-sparing effect), heart, and adrenal glands. Therefore, when compensating, the diastolic component of the MCA waveform will show increased flow. **A:** Transverse sonographic image of the fetal head in duplex mode (B-mode and pulsed Doppler) showing normal MCA flow at 35 weeks (RI 0.81, S/D ratio 5.36). This IUGR fetus is uncompromised. **B:** This transverse sonographic image of the fetal head at 37 weeks shows an increased diastolic component, consistent with circulatory redistribution in a compromised fetus (RI 0.61, S/D ratio 2.58).

these two values. The cerebroplacental ratio, or MCA/UA RI, is defined as the cerebral RI divided by the umbilical RI. A ratio above 1.0 indicates a normal perfusion pattern. Patients with pre-eclampsia and IUGR have been found to have lower values.[116] Fetuses with the low MCA/UA ratio were found to have decreased amniotic fluid, birth weights, and Apgar scores and an increased rate of morbidity and mortality.[112,116] Multiple studies validated findings when they reported that abnormal ratios were found in pregnancies with adverse outcomes.[112,116] For information on obtaining the MCA Doppler, refer to Chapter 24, Doppler Ultrasound of the Normal Fetus.

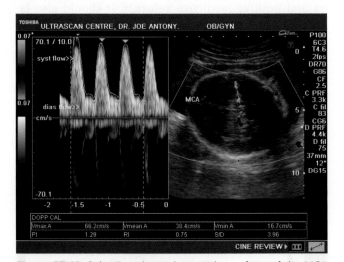

Figure 27-10 Color Doppler and spectral waveform of the MCA demonstrating the lowered cerebral vascular resistance due to the vasodilation seen with fetal hypoxia. (Image courtesy of Joe Antony, MD, Cochin, India. From the website at http://www.ultrasound-images.com/fetus-general.htm)

DUCTUS VENOSUS AND UMBILICAL VEIN DOPPLER

Venous waveforms of the DV and UV reflect the status of the right ventricle in the fetus. The DV is a regulator of oxygen to the fetus.[82] Half the oxygenated blood returning from the placenta is directed through the DV. This forms a preferential bloodstream through the foramen ovale to the left heart, into the aorta, and to the cranial vessels.[118] To obtain the DV waveform, the transverse view of the fetal abdomen at the same anatomic plane as the abdominal circumference is imaged and color flow Doppler is superimposed. The DV branches from the UV and, because of its narrow lumen, it has turbulent flow. This specific anatomy helps in identifying the waveform as well as the characteristic two-peaked DV waveform.[18] The first peak is the PSV and corresponds to the highest blood velocity in systole; it is followed by a period of decreased velocity (isovolumetric relaxation). The second peak corresponds to the rapid filling of the ventricles. The nadir is the "a-wave" and corresponds to atrial contraction.[18] Reversed flow (RF) during the a-wave is abnormal and often an ominous finding (Figs. 27-11).

Between 17 and 39 weeks, IUGR fetuses with normal chromosomes and no concomitant malformations can have reduced DV flows during atrial contraction.[119,120] This serious finding has been linked to a raised utD PI, REDV, or AEDF in the umbilical artery, and UV pulsations. During hypoxia, an increase in pressure in the UV occurs and more blood is shunted through the DV. In fetal compromise, as much as 70% of blood returning from the placenta is directed into the inferior vena cava through the DV.[122,124] It is also

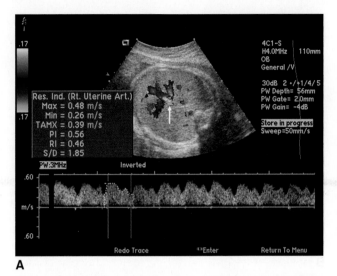

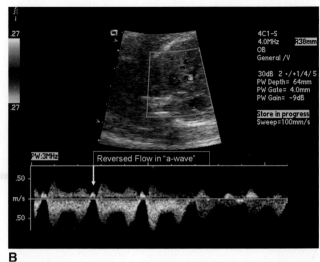

A   **B**

Figure 27-11 A: Normal DV waveform. **B:** This sonographic image of the DV shows an abnormal venous Doppler waveform in a fetus at 29 weeks with IUGR and oligohydramnios. This is a severely compromised fetus with reversed flow during the "a-wave."

important to consider gestational age when interpreting these results. After 27 weeks, an abnormal DV result is an important predictor of neonatal complications, whereas prior to 27 weeks the DV result may not be as useful in stratifying risk because the issues of prematurity predominate in these infants.[124] When the DV is assessed longitudinally in fetuses with IUGR, the progression follows 3 steps: (1) normal waveforms, (2) normal and abnormal waveforms, and (3) persistent abnormal waveforms.[45,122] A new index for the analysis of DV waveforms may better predict outcomes. The SIA index [(S-wave/(isovolumetric relaxation - a-wave)] for the analysis of DV waveforms may better predict outcomes compared with a-wave RF alone.[123] Based on the study by Piccione et al., a SIA index of 4.02 was associated with an almost certain perinatal death.

Increased pulsatility of the venous circulation reflects cardiac compromise from increased cardiac after-load (Fig. 27-12). UV pulsation is a common finding in the early, normal pregnancy and in association with fetal breathing. However, this phenomenon is associated with compromised fetal hemodynamics in the third trimester.[18,119] Thirty percent of cases with abnormal umD indices have umbilical vein pulsations (without breathing).[119] A biphasic or triphasic umbilical vein pulsation is an ominous finding.

For information on obtaining the ductus venosus and umbilical vein doppler waveform, refer to Chapter 24, Doppler Ultrasound of the Normal Fetus.

SUMMARY OF CLINICAL USE OF DOPPLER STUDIES IN OBSTETRICS

The preceding section described the techniques for obtaining Doppler studies, the vessels commonly studied in pregnancy, and selected outcomes with respect to

IUGR. The optimal testing protocol is controversial, but most reviews on the topic suggest incorporating MCA and venous Doppler with umbilical artery Doppler to provide the best prediction of acid-base status, risk of stillbirth, and anticipated rate of progression. Abnormal venous Doppler parameters are the strongest predictors of stillbirth. Even with severe arterial abnormalities such as AEDF or REDF, stillbirth primarily occurs in those fetuses with abnormal venous Doppler. This is further described in studies that report the sequential deterioration of IUGR fetuses and integrated testing algorithms.[125-127] Gestational age plays a role in these algorithms as well. Sequential deterioration of the hypoxemic fetus was rare after 34 weeks in one study.[128] Umbilical artery Doppler has the highest sensitivity and negative predictive value for poor perinatal outcome, but DV and UV parameters provide the best specificity and positive predictive values.[127] It should also be

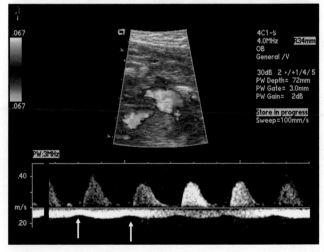

Figure 27-12 This is a spectral Doppler tracing of the umbilical cord of a 29 week fetus with IUGR. There are pulsations in the UV (*arrows*).

noted that significant variations in fetal adaptation to hypoxemia exist, and it is not always possible to predict outcomes.[129]

OTHER TOOLS IN THE ANTENATAL SURVEILLANCE OF THE IUGR FETUS

Similar to maternal diabetes, hypertension, postdatism, and a history of unexplained stillbirth, IUGR is thought to place the fetus at significant risk for fetal death and thus warrants close antepartum surveillance. Furthermore, IUGR is often an indicator of chronic fetal compromise and it may precede acute fetal deterioration and fetal death. Therefore, enhanced antenatal surveillance is needed to identify the fetus that is deteriorating. In this way, the most suitable time for delivering the affected fetus can be better determined. Once the diagnosis of IUGR is made, the exact mode of surveillance used by different clinical departments varies. Nonetheless, the usual modalities may include the biophysical profile (BPP), nonstress test (NST), or contraction stress test (CST). Importantly, when results of these tests are normal, they accurately predict fetal well-being. On the other hand, abnormal test results do not have a high correlation with poor outcome or fetal hypoxia; in other words, the false-positive rate of these tests is high.

BIOPHYSICAL PROFILE

The BPP is presented in detail in Chapter 25. In this discussion the reader is reminded that the BPP score is based on the evaluation of five biophysical functions: fetal breathing movement (FBM), fetal motion (FM), fetal tone (FT), amniotic fluid volume (AFV), and NST.[118,129,131,135] A score of two is assigned for each normal variable and a score of zero when the biophysical function is absent. All observations are made within an interval of 30 minutes.

The reactivity of the biophysical variables is dependent on an intact central nervous system (CNS). The reason for this is thought to relate to the "gradual hypoxia concept."[8] This concept has been formulated on the premise that (1) the later a neuroanatomic center develops, the more sensitive it is to the manifestations of acute hypoxia (the area of the fetal brain that regulates FT develops at 7 to 9 weeks, FM at 9 weeks, FBM at 20 to 21 weeks, and NST at 26 weeks to term), (2) FBM, FM, FT, and NST are acute biophysical parameters that represent the acute fetal condition, and (3) the amniotic fluid volume is a predictor of the chronic fetal condition. The BPP is a better predictor of normality than of abnormality (fetal hypoxia). First, the result is likely to be negative in 97.5% of tested fetuses, and the predictive value of a normal test is high.[8] It would be extremely unlikely for a preterm or term fetus to die within 7 days of a normal BPP result (8 or greater) or for a postterm fetus to die within 3 days. The

biophysical profile can be equivocal in 2% of fetuses. Under such circumstances, it should be repeated or a CST performed, depending on the management protocol of the particular institution.

Although the BPP is abnormal in only a small number (1%) of tested fetuses (value up to 4), the subsequent management of such fetuses is not uniform.[130,131] In some centers delivery may be indicated, particularly if the fetus has mature pulmonary indices. In other centers, a CST may be performed first to confirm fetal hypoxia or a continuous fetal biophysical survey may be observed for 2 to 3 hours before decisive action is taken. The rationale for the latter thinking is that absence of some biophysical functions may reflect normal periodicity rather than hypoxia. The absence of some biophysical functions for periods of 20 minutes to more than 2 hours can be normal. Absence of some biologic function may also be related to the time of testing or to maternal medication use. FBMs follow a circadian rhythm (i.e., appear more frequently at specific times), are more common 2 hours after meals, and can be suppressed by medication used to sedate the mother or treat her hypertension. The accuracy of the BPP is enhanced through testing 2 hours after a maternal meal, and discontinuance of medication known to depress the fetal CNS. With respect to IUGR and BPP, Vintzileos et al. have demonstrated that the four components of the BPP are affected at different levels of hypoxemia and acidemia. The first changes in fetal biophysical activity are loss of heat rate reactivity and fetal breathing. This is followed by decreased fetal tone and movement in association with more advanced acidemia, hypoxemia, and hypercapnia.

Two additional important components of the BPP are discussed below. It is important to emphasize that different institutions may employ different protocols for assessment. For example, one institution may consider weekly BPP assessments to evaluate the IUGR fetus, whereas another may use NST and AFI assessment; still others may use Doppler assessment in their "first line" of interrogation.

NONSTRESS TEST

Abnormal fetal heart rate patterns are thought to suggest heart failure and serve as an indirect measure of CNS integrity and function.[132] These patterns are thought to precede the development of hypoxia. A major advantage of the NST is its ease of performance and, consequently, it is the most common test used today. A drawback of the NST is that it is sensitive (most "abnormal" fetuses have abnormal results), but not very specific (most "abnormal" test results occur in normal fetuses). However, a normal NST (Fig. 27-13) has a good negative predictive value and thus remains an important part of antenatal assessment.[133] Normal fetuses may have an abnormal test result because of gestational immaturity, sleep cycles, or maternal sedation.

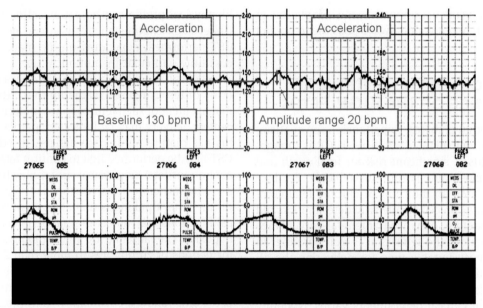

Figure 27-13 Bioelectric tracing shows a reactive nonstress test. The vertical line (y-axis) delineates the FHR per minute (30 bpm per cm of paper). The horizontal (x-axis) delineates time (3 cm/min). Note the following characteristics of a reactive test: (1) baseline between 120 and 160 bpm, (2) moderate variability, (3) no decelerations, and (4) two heart rate accelerations, each exceeding 15 bpm. A reactive test is normal.

Although NSTs are usually conducted by a nurse specialist, knowledge of the method of interpreting the test is important for sonographers. It involves computation of the baseline fetal heart rate (FHR) and any changes that occur in response to fetal movement. A normal (or reactive) test depends on detection of at least two FHR accelerations above the baseline. Normally, in a 20-minute period the FHR should accelerate by 15 beats per minute (bpm) for at least 15 seconds.[8] Indicators of well-being also include a baseline FHR falling between 120 and 160 bpm and absence of any decelerations; that is, decreases in the FHR below baseline. A normal or reactive result implies good fetal CNS integrity; that is, absence of asphyxia for 7 days in the preterm and term fetus and for 3 days in the postterm fetus.

An abnormal or nonreactive NST is defined by absence of fetal movements or by FHR accelerations less than 15 bpm. Additionally, the presence of spontaneous heart rate decelerations and/or loss of beat-to-beat heart rate variability (a characteristic of normal fetuses) may be associated with poor outcome. A nonreactive test correctly predicts fetal death (within 1 week of testing) in only 3% to 29% of cases. The reason may be partly related to the normal periodicity of fetal heart rates.

ASSESSMENT OF AMNIOTIC FLUID

Assessment of the amount of amniotic fluid is an important, albeit indeterminate, measure of the fetal condition. The amount of amniotic fluid is, at best, a weak predictor of perinatal morbidity and it needs to be used together with other biophysical parameters. Although decreased amounts of amniotic fluid can be the result of premature rupture of the membranes or renal anomalies, it can also occur as the result of decreased urine production from poor renal perfusion. Amniotic fluid is derived from fetal and maternal sources. The exchange occurs in two directions in three different sites with the importance and amount of fluid changing as the gestation progresses.[8,149-151]

SITE 1, MOTHER AND AMNIOTIC FLUID

The bidirectional flow takes place across the decidua and fetal membranes; at term, the normal net hourly exchange is approximately 135 milliliters (ml) in the direction of amniotic fluid. This transmembranous exchange occurs at the uterine wall and the amniotic-chorionic interface. Because of this exchange, we are able to increase the AFV by increasing maternal ingestion of water.

SITE 2, MOTHER AND FETUS

The bidirectional flow takes place across the intervillous space; at term, the normal net hourly exchange is approximately 50 to 90 ml in the direction of the fetus.

SITE 3, FETUS AND AMNIOTIC FLUID

The bidirectional intramembranous flow between the fetus and amniotic fluid mainly occurs through the respiratory, gastrointestinal, and urinary tracts, although some exchange occurs at the fetal skin, placental surface, and the umbilical cord. Fetal swallowing results in removal of amniotic fluid, whereas urination adds to the volume of fluid. The fetus swallows approximately half of the fluid produced via fetal urination. At term, the normal net hourly exchange is approximately 150 to 225 ml in the direction of the amniotic fluid compartment.

There are three methods of assessing the amounts of fluid in the amniotic cavity. First, quantitative methods were employed using the instillation of dye into the amniotic cavity and removal of the amniotic fluid. This was then titrated. The precise amount of amniotic fluid can then be determined, but this is not commonly practiced today. Second, semiquantitative methods were proposed, such as the maximum sonographically detectable vertical pocket of amniotic fluid or using the amniotic fluid index (or AFV, discussed in the following section). Last, subjective assessment using sonography by an experienced observer is highly predictive of oligohydramnios and polyhydramnios.

Of all the methods, the AFI is used most frequently for estimating AFV. Phelan and coworkers originally developed this ultrasound method, which allows quantification of normal AFV.[8] They divide the uterine cavity into four quadrants using two imaginary lines, one running transversely across the umbilicus and the other vertically using the linea nigra (Fig. 27-14). The vertical diameter of the largest pocket in each quadrant is measured and the sum of the four pockets is determined. This sum is called the AFI. The mean values (±2 SD) of the AFI throughout pregnancy are then determined (Fig. 27-15). In the third trimester of pregnancy, the two SD variation about the mean AFI is wide. Additionally, a progressive increase in the AFV is noted until the 28th to 30th week.

In the third trimester of pregnancy, oligohydramnios exists when (1) the diameter of the largest pocket of amniotic fluid is less than 3 cm (depending on the guidelines used),[8] (2) the AFI is less than 5 cm,[8] or (3) the experienced sonographer subjectively observes an overall paucity in AFV.

Using the subjective method of assessing AFV in a large unselected population of pregnant women, Philipson and coworkers showed that the prevalence of oligohydramnios is 3.9%.[134] The predictive value of oligohydramnios in the diagnosis of IUGR was only 19% to 40%.[134,135] The sensitivity of the test (i.e., presence of oligohydramnios) is also low, at 16%.[8] The fact that only 16% of all IUGR is associated with oligohydramnios may be related to the marked variation in AFV noted in different pregnancies. In other words, the AFV may be low in many normal pregnancies.

Phelan and colleagues showed that in postterm pregnancies with severe oligohydramnios (largest vertical fluid pocket less than 1 cm) the incidence of abnormal fetal heart tracings requiring cesarean section was 16.7%.[136] By comparison, in postterm pregnancies with normal AFV the incidence of abnormal fetal heart tracings requiring cesarean section was only 1.05%.[136] Thus, the presence of oligohydramnios in postterm pregnancy is an ominous finding and points to the need to deliver the fetus. Similarly, the presence of oligohydramnios in a fetus whose EFW is below the 10th percentile is predictive of poor outcome and is an indication for strict surveillance of the fetus so that the most appropriate time for delivery can be determined.

Some investigators argue that there is no need to spend a long time waiting to evaluate all the components of the BPP and that the results of both the NST and AFV suffice, also known as the modified BPP. The rationale: (1) a reactive NST implies that fetal motion is indeed present and indirectly tests for this important function of fetal motion; (2) an NST should always be part of the antenatal testing schema because it may show variable decelerations, a finding that may be missed completely if one relies only on the other four functions of the BPP; and (3) oligohydramnios may be a significant indicator of chronic hypoxia, particularly in the IUGR or postdate fetus, and should always be considered. Because specific management protocols are not universally accepted, the sonographer should follow the guidelines established by the institution.

OTHER METHODS OF ASSESSMENT

Two additional methods of assessment have also been used for fetal evaluation.. These are vibroacoustic stimulation (VAS) during an NST or a BPP and a contraction stress test (CST).

VAS is accomplished using an artificial larynx (EAL Bell Telephone) to generate an acoustic-vibratory stimulus lasting 2 to 5 seconds to stimulate a fetus to respond.[135] The average sound energy produced at 1 m of air equals 82 decibels (dB).[62,86] The frequency of the emitted sound is 80 hertz (Hz), with harmonics ranging from 20 to 9,000 Hz.[128] The artificial larynx is placed on the maternal abdomen over the fetal vertex and the fetal

---

PATHOLOGY BOX 27-4

Semiquantitative Measurements of Amniotic Fluid[8,47,118,135,136]

Measurement	Abbreviation	Definition	Technique
Amniotic fluid index	AFI	The sum of amniotic fluid measurements, which estimates the AFV	Measurement of a single pocket in each of the four uterine quadrants that is free of fetal parts or umbilical cord perpendicular to the table
Amniotic fluid volume	AFV	The total amount of amniotic fluid surrounding the fetus	

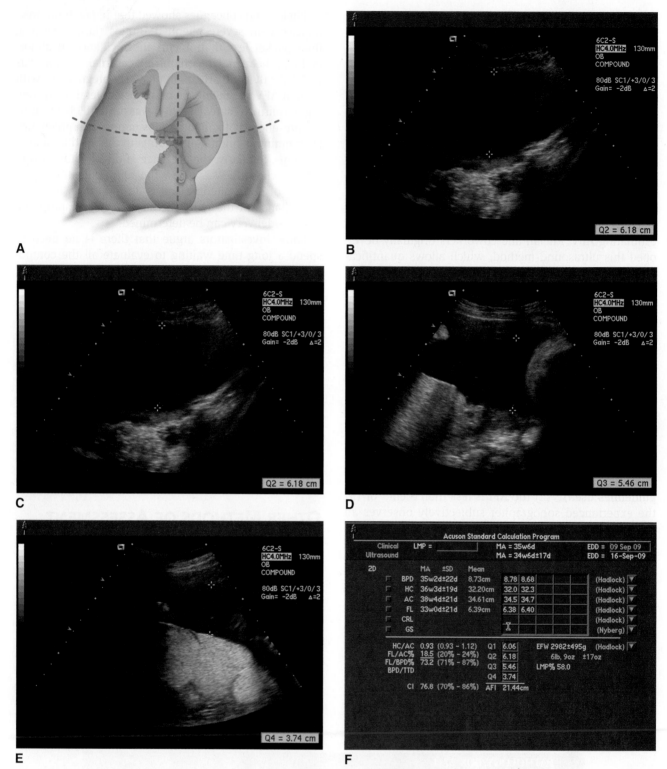

Figure 27-14 A: Diagram shows division of the pregnant abdomen into four quadrants for obtaining the AFI. **B-E:** Fluid pockets found in four different quadrants used in calculating the AFI **(F)**.

response is monitored. Investigators have studied the use of VAS in an effort to change the fetal behavioral state, evoke fetal heart rate accelerations and movements, and improve test specificity and efficiency. In one study, VAS improves the efficiency of the BPP by decreasing false-positive tests and improving test accuracy.[137]

The CST was one of the first forms of fetal surveillance and is the only modality that uses the principle of induced stress to reveal marginal placental insufficiency. During this procedure, the fetal heart rate is continuously monitored via cardiotography as an infusion of oxytocin is given to the patient to induce contractions.

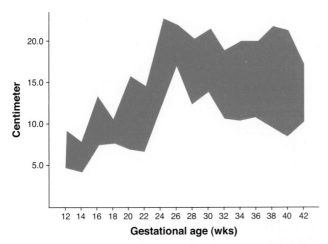

Figure 27-15 The blue area of the graph depicts the mean values (± 2 SD variation) of the AFI, from the 12th to the 42nd weeks of pregnancy. Note that at 40 weeks' gestation an AFI of 8 falls at a critical 2 SD level below the mean. (Reprinted with permission from Phelan JP, Ahn MO, Smith CV, et al: Amniotic fluid index measurements during the pregnancy. *Reprod Med.* 1987;32:602).

A hypoxic or compromised fetus will not tolerate the low intervillous blood flow and oxygen level caused by the stress of the induced uterine contractions. As a result, fetal myocardial hypoxia is manifested as repetitive, uniform, and late heart rate decelerations (decelerations that occur at the end of a uterine contraction). A negative CST is one that has no late fetal heart rate decelerations in the presence of three uterine contractions over a 10-minute period. The false positive rate is not as high as other tests (30% to 50%), but it has the lowest false-negative rate (0.3 stillbirths per 1,000 births).[136,137] The drawbacks to this test are that it is time consuming to perform, invasive, and expensive.

The concern with any diagnostic test is the false negative and false positive results that might prompt an early or late delivery. Failure to diagnose poor growth and associated IUGR bears considerable risk. Although the diagnosis of IUGR carries alarming concerns, the consequences of the misdiagnosis can be similarly alarming (Fig. 27-16). Ringa and coworkers studied the rate of preterm elective cesarean in pregnancies thought to have an EFW below 10%.[115] They reported in a series of almost 17,000 deliveries that 118 infants were falsely diagnosed as IUGR, and 13% of these had a needless elective cesarean. Their investigation illustrated the importance of supplemental tests to examine for fetal adaptation and decompensation to avoid unnecessary interventions.[115] A multicentered randomized trial, the Growth Restriction Intervention Trial (GRIT) evaluated differences between immediate versus delayed delivery in a population with IUGR.[147] More stillbirths occurred in the delayed group and more neonatal deaths occurred in the immediate delivery group. The issue of optimal timing of delivery remains unsolved.

When a fetus is identified as having IUGR, the fetus should be closely monitored for physiologic compromise

and properly delivered at an appropriate time. A typical pattern of fetal deterioration in IUGR is an early abnormal utD index (typical in women at risk for placental abnormality [i.e., elevated MSAFP] or pregnancy-induced hypertension), followed by abnormal fetal growth, abnormal umD and MCA Doppler values (or their ratio), abnormal UV pulsatility, and abnormal DV.

Any technique must be subjected to rigorous evaluation before its widespread acceptance. Although EFW, umD, and other antenatal testing approaches (NST, CST) are now accepted and have been proven effective for routine clinical management, other Doppler applications are undergoing further evaluation.

PROTOCOL FOR REPORTING ULTRASOUND FINDINGS

The sonographer in possession of the background information discussed in this chapter is in a position to present the comprehensive data to the referring physician. The challenge is to present it in an effective and practical way. The referring physician would like to have specific information regarding the following areas:

1. The assigned gestational age and the method used to assign this age. An example of important comments would be as follows:
   a. Dates are established by concurrence between the early ultrasound (before 26 weeks' gestation) and the menstrual dates, or menstrual dates are confirmed by known ovulation day.
   b. Dates are established by CRL.
2. The estimated fetal weight and the two SD variation of the formula used.
3. The birth weight percentile, as outlined in Table 27-1. For example, it should be stated that an EFW of 2,120 g at 36 weeks' gestation falls below the 10th percentile rank. The sonographer should specify which table was used.
4. The fetal growth pattern, once the diagnosis of IUGR is suspected (by an EFW below the 10th percentile). Other ultrasound data should be carefully examined and follow-up examinations are appropriate. The interval between these examinations should be agreed upon by the physician and the sonographer.
5. AFI/AFV. The sonographer should enter one or more of the following diagnostic criteria for oligohydramnios:
   a. Diagnosis of oligohydramnios is based on the subjective evaluation of AFV.
   b. Diagnosis of oligohydramnios is based on the largest vertical pocket of AF at less than 2 cm (depending on the accepted threshold for oligohydramnios in the ultrasound department).
   c. Diagnosis of oligohydramnios is based on an amniotic fluid index below 6 cm.

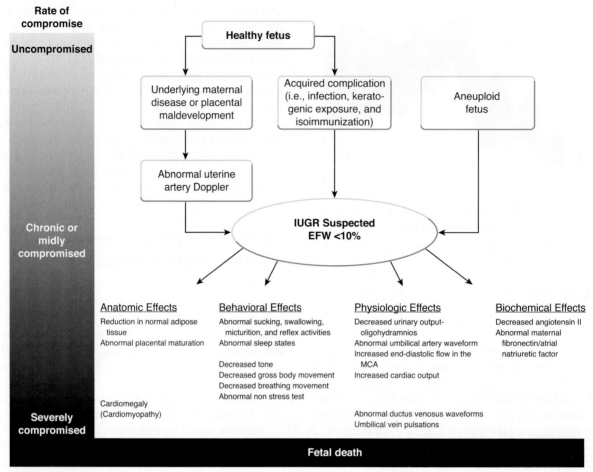

Figure 27-16 This algorithm shows the complexity of fetal deterioration. As the fetal condition evolves from health to death, many anatomic, behavioral, physiologic, and biochemical changes occur. The task of the prenatal diagnostician is to determine the risk and level of deterioration based on the sonographic variables.

6. Placental grade. A Grade III placenta may be associated with IUGR if it is noted before 36 weeks' gestation; this should be described.
7. BPP score. The biophysical profile score should be reported when requested. The results can be entered on one line, as in the following example: FBM = 0, FM = 2, FT = 2, AFV = 2, NST = 2; total score = 8.
8. Doppler velocimetry. Doppler assessment of the umbilical artery, MCA, and other vessels should be described in terms of the S/D ratio, PI, or RI (in accordance with your departmental policy) (see Chapter 24).

TREATMENT AND MANAGEMENT

A variety of treatment regimens have been considered for IUGR. Maternal bed rest, vitamin supplements and other antioxidants, aspirin, fish oil, hyperoxygenation, and hypervolumic hemodilution have been suggested, but none have shown significant promise in preventing or improving IUGR once diagnosed.[138-144]

The only scenario where intervention has shown a significant impact on fetal weight is smoking cessation. Smoking cessation and avoidance of smoking during pregnancy can increase birth weight.[145,146]

SUMMARY

- An IUGR fetus is defined as one that less than the 10th percentile for the gestational age
- Symmetric IUGR fetuses may be SGA; however, an SGA fetus does not necessarily mean IUGR is present
- Adverse effects of growth restriction occur both during the prenatal and postnatal life
- The cause of IUGR may be idiopathic or multifactorial
- Identification of growth-restricted fetuses is through estimated fetal weight, sonographic biometery, Doppler flow and amniotic fluid changes.
- Doppler parameters to aid in IUGR diagnosis include flow changes to the uterine artery, umbilical artery and vein, MCA, and the DV
- The five components of the BPP are an integral part of managing the IUGR fetus

Critical Thinking Questions 1

A 39-year-old gravida 2 para 0 presented at 24 weeks to the emergency department complaining of shortness of breath. She was found to have elevated blood pressures (170/120), pulmonary edema, and protein in her urine. Medications were given to control her blood pressure and help prevent seizures. Fetal monitoring demonstrated a normal baseline heart rate of 130 bpm, minimal variability, and late decelerations. A bedside fetal ultrasound showed a live fetus in breech presentation with an EFW of 500g with an AFI of 10.7cm.

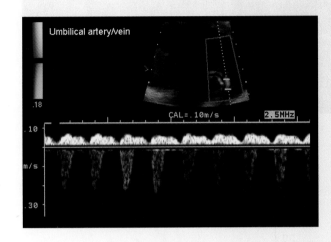
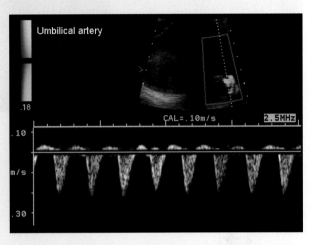

1. **What does her blood pressure and protein in her urine indicate?**

2. **Discuss the significance of the umbilical artery and vein findings.**

   ANSWER:

   Pre-eclampsia and hypertensive disorders are among the most common etiologies for IUGR. This case represents a severe form of maternal disease as well as severe manifestations in the fetus and neonate. Although several treatments have been proposed and studied (i.e. oxygen, vitamins, calcium, aspirin) there is no known method to prevent preeclampsia. The onset of seizures indicates a progression of maternal disease to eclampsia (toxemia) as discussed in chapter 29.

   I think this it is a good question, but if the chapter is about IUGR, then shouldn't the question make a comment about the EFW for the fetus? An EFW of 500g for a 24 weeker is probably not < 10th%

   When the Doppler studies of the fetus are viewed along a continuum with sequential changes occurring over time in the vascular system, the findings of abnormalities in the venous circulation in this case also represent fetal decompensation. The umbilical artery flow demonstrates reversed flow while the umbilical vein flow indicates pulsatile flow. Both are indicators of fetal compromise.

Critical Thinking Questions 2

A 21-year-old gravida 1 presented for prenatal care in the late second trimester. A fetal ultrasound at 28 weeks showed that the fetus was measuring at the 27th percentile with normal amniotic fluid. The fetal abdominal circumference measured at < 2.5th%, which prompted follow-up ultrasounds. Serial measurements indicated decreasing fetal growth – would be more specific here – i.e. dropped to the 10th% at 34 weeks,etc or refer to the graphs below. At 37 weeks the amniotic fluid index had decreased (6 cm) and the umbilical artery Doppler S/D ratio was increasing (this implies that it was measured previously and was presumably normal. I don't have the table of UA S/D ratios in front of me, but an S/D ratio of 2.8 at 37 weeks doesn't seem too elevated.

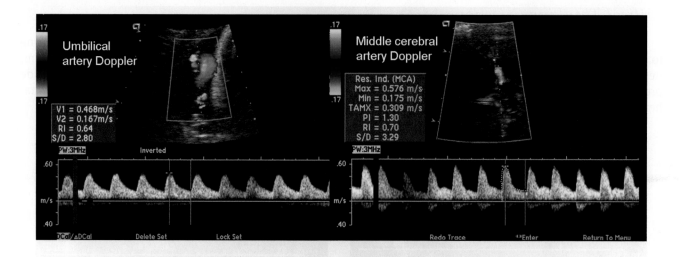

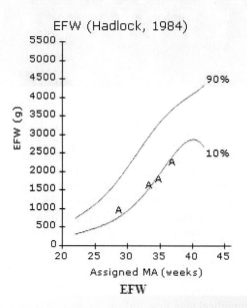

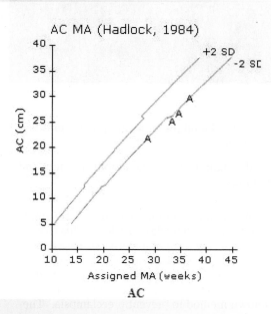

EFW

AC

1. Using the spectral Doppler images above, calculate the cerebroplacental ratio. What does this ratio indicate?

2. What do the AC and EFW charts indicate? Explain your answer.

The cerebroplacenal ratio is the middle cerebral artery RI divided by the umbilical RI. The right figure is an image of the middle cerebral artery Doppler where the RI = 0.70. The left figure is an image of the umbilical artery Doppler where the RI = 0.64. In this case; 0.7 / 0.64 = 1.09. Though still normal, the closeness to this value indicates development of IUGR. A value of 1.09 is considered elevated at 34 weeks. These two statements are contradictory – first sentence says it is normal, second says it is elevated. Can you pick results that are more clear-cut – i.e. clearly normal or clearly elevated.

These graphs demonstrate the estimated fetal weight ("A" values) based on the Hadlock formula with population growth percentiles (10th and 90th as denoted by the solid lines). The left diagram is a plot of the estimated fetal weight (EFW) in grams over weeks gestation. This showed progressively slowing fetal growth with a final value of the 5th percentile at 36 weeks. The right diagram is a plot of the abdominal circumference (AC) in centimeters over weeks gestation. These values were always less than two standard deviations below the mean. Both these graphs indicate progressing IUGR.

My interpretation of the graphs above is that the overall fetal growth was at the 10th% at 36 weeks (not 5th). The "A" touches the 10th% line. The abdominal circumference looks like it was mostly at the -2.5SD (not less).

REFERENCES

1. Martin JA, Hamilton BE, Sutton PD, Ventura SJ, et al. Births: Final data for 2006. National Vital Statistics Reports. 57(7). Hyattsville, MD: National Center for Health Statistics 2009.

2. Mathews TJ, MacDorman MF. Infant mortality statistics from the 2005 period linked birth/infant death data set. *Natl Vital Stat Rep*. 2008;57(2):1–32.

3. Mathews TJ, MaDorman MF. Infant mortality statistics from 2005 period linked birth/infant death data set. National Vital Statistics Reports. 57(2) Hyattsville, MD; National Center for Statistics 2008.

4. Fanaroff AA, Stoll BJ, Wright LL, et al. Trends in neonatal morbidity and mortality for very low birthweight infants. *Am J Obstet Gynecol*. 2007;196(2):147e1–e8.

5. Hack, M., Klein, N. K., and Taylor H. G. Long-Term Developmental Outcomes of Low Birth Weight Infants. *The Future of Children*, 5(1), 176-196.

6. Clausson B, Gardosi J, Francis A, et al. Perinatal outcome in SGA births defined by customized versus population-based birth weight standards. *BJOG*. 2001;108(8): 830–834.

7. Ananth CV, Vintzileos AM. Distinguishing pathological from constitutional small for gestational age births in population-based studies. *Early Hum Dev*. 2009;85(10): 653–658.

8. Abuhamad AZ. The role of Doppler ultrasound in obstetrics. In: *Ultrasonography in Obstetrics and Gynecology*. 5th ed. Philadelphia: Saunders Elsevier; 2008.

9. Miller J, Turan S. Baschat AA. Fetal growth restriction. *Sem Perinatol*. 2008;32(4):274–280.

10. Weine CP, Robinson D. The sonographic diagnosis of intrauterine growth retardation using the postnatal ponderal index and the crown heel length as standards of diagnosis. *Am J Perinatol*. 1989;6(4):380–383.

11. Basso O, Wilcox AJ, Weinberg CR. Birth weight and mortality: Causality or confounding? *Am J Epidemiol*. 2006;164(4):303–311.

12. Chatelain P. Children born with intra-uterine growth retardation (IUGR) or small for gestational age (SGA): Long term growth and metabolic consequences. *Endocr Regul*. 2000;34(1):33–36.

13. Mandruzzato G, Antsaklis A, Botet F, et al. Intrauterine restriction (IUGR). *J.Perinat Med*. 2008;36(4):277–281.

14. Morrison I, Olsen J. Weight-specific stillbirths and associated causes of death: An analysis of 765 stillbirths. *Am J Obstet Gynecol*. 1985;152(8):975–980.

15. McCowan LM, Harding JE, Stewart AW. Customized birthweight centiles predict SGA pregnancies with perinatal morbidity. *BJOG*. 2005;112(8):1026–1033.

16. Rigano S, Bozzo M, Ferrazzi E, et al. Early and persistent reduction in umbilical vein blood flow in the growth-restricted fetus: A longitudinal study. *Am J Obstet Gynecol*. 2001;185(4):834–838.

17. Bellotti M, Pennati G, DeGasperi C, et al. Simultaneous measurements of umbilical venous, fetal hepatic, and ductus venosus blood flow in growth-restricted human fetuses. *Am J Obstet Gynecol*. 2004;190(5):1347.

18. Kiserud T. The ductus venosus. *Semin Perinatol*. 2001;25:11.

19. Bernstein IM, Horbar JD, Badger GJ, et al. Morbidity and mortality among very low birth weight neonates with intrauterine growth restriction. The Vermont Oxford Network. *Am J Obstet Gynecol*. 2000;182:198.

20. Kamoji VM, Dorling JS, Manktelow BN, et al. Extremely growth-retarded infants: Is there a viability centile? *Pediatrics*. 2006;118(2):758–763.

21. Zelop CM, Richardson DK, Heffner LJ. Outcomes of severely abnormal umbilical artery Doppler velocimetry in structurally normal singleton fetuses. *Obstet Gynecol*. 1996;87(3):434–438.

22. Baschat AA, Cosmi E, Bilardo CM, et al. Predictors of neonatal outcome in early-onset placental dysfunction. *Am J Obstet Gynecol*. 2007;109(2 Pt 1):253–261.

23. Yanney M, Marlow M. Paediatric consequences of fetal growth restriction. *Semin Neonatol*. 2004;9:411.

24. Tideman E, Marsal K, Ley D. Cognitive function in young adults following intrauterine growth restriction with abnormal fetal aortic blood flow. *Ultrasound Obstet Gynecol*. 2007;29(6):614–618.

25. Upadhyay SK, Kant I, Singh TB, et al. Neurobehavioural assessment of newborns. *Electromyogr Clin Neurophysiol*. 2000;40(2):113–117.

26. McCarton CM, Wallace IF, Divon M, et al. Cognitive and neurologic development of the premature, small for gestational age infant through age 6: Comparison by birth weight and gestational age. *Pediatrics*. 1996;98 (6 Pt 1):1167.

27. Barker DJP. Adult consequences of fetal growth restriction. *Clin Obstet Gynecol*. 2006;49(2):270–283.

28. Barker DJ, Osmond C, Kajantie E, et al. Growth and chronic disease: Findings in the Helsinki Birth Cohort. *Ann Hum Biol*. 2009;36(5):445–458.

29. Dover GJ. The Barker hypothesis: How pediatricans will diagnose and prevent common adult-onset diseases. *Trans Am Clin Climatol Assoc*. 2009;120:199–207.

30. Sallout B, Walker M. The fetal origin of adult diseases. *J Obstet Gynaecol*. 2003;23(5):555.

31. Jackson AA. All that glitters. *Br Nutr Foundation Nutr Bull*. 2000;25:11–24.

32. Gardosi J. Fetal customized fetal growth standards: Rationale and clinical application. *Semin Perinatol*. 2004 Feb;28(1):33–40.

33. Spinillo A, Capuzzo E, Piazzi G, et al. Maternal high-risk factors and severity of growth deficit in small for gestational age infants. *Early Hum Dev*. 1994;38:35–43.

34. Haverkamp F, Wölfle J, Zerres K. et al. Growth retardation in Turner syndrome: Aneuploidy, rather than specific gene loss, may explain growth failure. *J Clin Endocrinol Metab*. 1999;84(12):4578–4582.

35. Mendilcioglu I, Ozcan M, Bagci G, et Al. Triploidy in a growth discordant twin pregnancy after intracytoplasmic sperm injection treatment. *Case Rep. Diagn Ther*. 2006;21(1):65–67.

36. Snijders RJM, Sherrod C, Gosden CM, et al. Fetal growth retardation: Associated malformations and chromosomal abnormalities. *Am J Obstet Gynecol*. 1993;168(2): 547–555.

37. Lubchenco LO, Hansman C, Dressler M, et al. Intrauterine growth as estimated from live born birth-weight data at 24 to 42 weeks of gestation. *Pediatrics*. 1963;32:793–800.

38. Moore LG, Young D, McCullough RE, et al. Tibetan protection from intrauterine growth restriction (IUGR) and reproductive loss at high altitude. *Am J Hum Biol*. 2001;13(5):635.

39. Mortola JP, Frappell PB, Aguero L, et al. Birth weight and altitude: a study in Peruvian communities. *J Pediatr.* 2000;136(3):324.

40. Kametas NA, McAuliffe F, Krampl E, et al. Maternal cardiac function during pregnancy at high altitude. *BJOG.* 2004;111(10):1051.

41. Burkhardt T, Schäffer L, Zimmermann R, et al. Newborn weight charts underestimate the incidence of low birth weight in preterm infants. *Am J Obstet Gynecol.* 2008;199(2):139.e1–e6.

42. Chitty LS, Altman DG, Henderson A, et al. Charts of fetal size: 2. Head measurements. *Br J Obstet Gynaecol.* 1994; 101(1):35–43.

43. Kurmanavicius J, Wright EM, Royston P, et al. Fetal ultrasound biometry: 1. Head reference values. *Br J Obstet Gynaecol.* 1999;106(2):126–135.

44. Salomon LJ, Duyme M, Crequat J, et al. French fetal biometry: Reference equations and comparison with other charts. *Ultrasound Obstet Gynecol.* 2006;28(2):193–198.

45. Mari G, Hanif F, Drennan F, et al. Staging of intrauterine growth-restricted fetuses. *J Ultrasound Med.* 2007; 26(11):1469–1477.

46. Doubilet PM, Benson CB. Sonographic evaluation of intrauterine growth retardation. *Am J Roentgenol.* 1995; 164(3):709–717.

47. Benson CB, Doubilet PM. Fetal measurements: Normal and abnormal growth. In: Rumack C, Charboneau W, Wilson S, eds. *Diagnostic Ultrasound.* St. Louis: Elsevier Mosby; 2005:1493–1526.

48. AIUM Practice Guideline for the Performance of Obstetric Ultrasound Examinations, 2007.

49. Ott WJ. Accurate gestational dating. *Obstet Gynecol.* 1985; 66(3):311–315.

50. Taipale P, Hiilesmaa V. Predicting delivery date by ultrasound and last menstrual period in early gestation. *Obstet Gynecol.* 2001;97:189–194.

51. Dudley NJ. A systematic review of the ultrasound estimation of fetal weight. *Ultrasound Obstet Gynecol.* 2005; 25(1):80–89.

52. Benson CB, Belville JS, Lentini JF, et al. Intrauterine growth retardation: Diagnosis based on multiple parameters—prospective study. *Radiology.* 1990;177(2):499–502.

53. Kurtz AB, Goldberg BB. Combined fetal head and body measurements. In: Kurtz AB, Goldberg BB, eds. *Obstetrical Measurements in Ultrasound: A Reference Manual.* Chicago: Year Book Medical Publishers; 1988:147.

54. Mladenović-Segedi L, Segedi D. Accuracy of ultrasonic fetal weight estimation using head and abdominal circumference and femur length. *Med Pregl.* 2005;58(11–12): 548–552.

55. Farrell T, Holmes R, Stone P. The effect of body mass index on three methods of fetal weight estimation. *BJOG.* 2002;109(6):651–657.

56. Shepard MJ, Richards VA, Berkowitz RL, et al. An evaluation of two equations for predicting fetal weight by ultrasound. *Am J Obstet Gynecol.* 1982;142:47.

57. Hadlock FP, Harrist RB, Sharman RS, et al. Estimation of fetal weight with the use of head, body, and femur measurements. *Am J Obstet Gynecol.* 1985;151(3):333–337.

58. Kurtz AB, Goldberg BB. Combined fetal head and body measurements. In: Kurtz AB, Goldberg BB, eds. *Obstetrical Measurements in Ultrasound: A Reference Manual.* Chicago: Year Book Medical Publishers; 1988:147.

59. Hadlock FP, Harrist RB, Carpenter RJ, et al. Sonographic estimation of fetal weight: The value of femur length in addition to head and abdomen measurements. *Radiology.* 1984;150(2):535–540.

60. Mongelli M, Yuxin NG, Biswas A, et al. Accuracy of ultrasound dating formulae in the late second trimester in pregnancies conceived with in-vitro fertilization. *Acta Radiol.* 2003;44(4):452–455.

61. Smith GC, Smith MF, McNay MB, et al. First-trimester growth and the risk of low birth weight. *N Engl J Med.* 1998;339(25):1817–1822.

62. Bukowski R, Smith GC, FASTER Research Consortium, et al. Fetal growth in early pregnancy and risk of delivering low birth weight infant: prospective cohort study. *BMJ.* 2007;334(7598):836.

63. Smith PA, Johansson D, Tzannatos C, et al. Prenatal measurement of the fetal cerebellum and cisterna cerebellomedullaris by ultrasound. *Prenat Diagn.* 1986;6(2):133.

64. Vinkesteijn AS, Mulder PG, Wladimiroff JW. Fetal transverse cerebellar diameter measurements in normal and reduced fetal growth. *Ultrasound Obstet Gynecol.* 2000; 15(1):47.

65. Chauhan S, West DJ, Scardo JA, et al. Antepartum detection of macrosomic fetus: Clinical versus sonographic, including soft-tissue measurements. *Obstet Gynecol.* 2000;95(5):639.

66. Hadlock FP, Deter RL, Harrist RB, Roecker E, Park SK. A date-independent predictor of intrauterine growth retardation: Femur length/abdominal circumference ratio. *Am J Roentgenol.* 1983; 141:979–984.

67. Hadlock FP, Harrist RB, Sharman RS, et al. Estimation of fetal weight with the use of head, body, and femur measurements: A prospective study. *Am J Obstet Gynecol.* 1985; 151:333–337.

68. Manning FA, Hill LM, Platt LD. Quantitative amniotic fluid volume determination by ultrasound antepartum detection of intrauterine growth retardation. *Am J Obstet Gynecol.* 1981;139:254–258.

69. Doubilet PM, Benson CB. Sonographic evaluation of intrauterine growth retardation. *Am J Roentgenol.* 1995;164(3): 709–717.

70. Bevavides-Serralde A, Hernandez-Andrade E, Ferna J, et al. Three-dimensional sonographic calculation of the volume of intracranial structures in growth-restricted and appropriate-for-gestational age fetuses. *Ultrasound Obstet Gynecol.* 2009;33(5):530–537.

71. Chang C, Tsai P, Yu C, et al. Prenatal detection of fetal growth restriction by fetal femur volume: Efficacy assessment using three-dimensional ultrasound. *Ultrasound Med Biol.* 2007;33(3):335–341.

72. Chang C, Yu C, Ko H, et al. Predicting fetal growth restriction by humerus volume: a three-dimensional ultrasound study. *Ultrasound Med Biol.* 2006;32(6):791–795.

73. Lee W, Deter RL, Ebersole JD, et al. Birth weight prediction by three-dimensional sonography. *J Ultrasound Med.* 2001;20(12):1283–1292.

74. Liang RI, Chang FM, Yao BL, et al. Predicting birth weight by fetal upper-arm volume with use of three dimensional sonography. *Am J Obstet Gynecol.* 1997;177(3): 632–636.

75. Schild RL, Fimmers R, Hansmann M. Fetal weight estimation by three-dimensional ultrasound. *Ultrasound Obstet Gynecol.* 2000;16(5):445–452.

76. Baker PN, Johnson IR, Gowland PA, et al. Fetal weight estimation by echo-planar magnetic resonance imaging. *Lancet.* 1994;343(8898):644–645.

77. Uotila J, Dastidar P, Heinonen T, et al. Magnetic resonance imaging compared to sonography in fetal weight and volume estimation in diabetic and normal pregnancy. *Acta Obstet Gynecol Scand.* 2000;79(4):255–259.

78. Zaretsky MV, Reichel TF, McIntire DD, et al. Comparison of magnetic resonance imaging to ultrasound in the estimation of birth weight at term. *Am J Obstet Gynecol.* 2003;189(4):1017–1020.

79. de Jong CL, Gardosi J, Dekker GA, et al. Application of a customised birthweight standard in the assessment of perinatal outcome in a high risk population. *Br J Obstet Gynaecol.* 1998;105(5):531–535.

80. Gardosi J, Francis A. Adverse pregnancy outcome and association with small for gestational age birthweight by customized and population based percentiles. *Am J Obstet Gynecol.* 2009;201(1):28.e1–e8.

81. Chauhan SP, Gupta LM, Hendrix NW, et al. Intrauterine growth restriction: comparison of American College of Obstetricians and Gynecologists practice bulletin with other national guidelines. *Am J Obstet Gynecol.* 2009;200(4):409.e1–e6.

82. Ananth CV, Demissie K, Hanley ML. Birth weight discordancy and adverse perinatal outcomes among twin gestations in the United States: the effect of placental abruption. *Am J Obstet Gynecol.* 2003;188(4):954.

83. Ananth CV, Vintzileos AM, Shen-Schwarz S, et al. Standards of birth weight in twin gestations stratified by placental chorionicity. *Obstet Gynecol.* 1998;91:917.

84. Shoshani M, Rhea DJ, Keith LG, et al. Comparison between singleton- and triplet-specific "growth" curves to detect growth restricted triplet infants. *J Perinat Med.* 2007;35(4):322.

85. Benson CB, Doubilet PM. Head-sparing in fetuses with intrauterine growth retardation: does it really occur? *Radiology.* 1986;161:75.

86. Nazarian LN, Halpern EJ, Kurtz AB, et al. Normal interval fetal growth rates based on obstetrical sonographic measurements. *J Ultrasound Med.* 1995;14(11):829–836.

87. Sinha SK, Donn SM. Fetal-to-neonatal maladaptation. *Semin Fetal Neonatal Med.* 2006;11(3):166–173.

88. Kahn BF, Hobbins JC, Galan HL. Intrauterine growth restriction. In: *Danforth's Obstetrics & Gynecology.* 10th ed. Philadelphia: Lippincott Williams & Wilkins; 2008.

89. McLeod L. How useful is uterine artery Doppler ultrasonography in predicting pre-eclampsia and intrauterine growth restriction? *CMAJ.* 2008;178(6):727–729.

90. Hoffman C, Galan HL. Assessing the 'at-risk' fetus: Doppler ultrasound. *Curr Opin Obstet Gynecol.* 2009;21(2):161–166.

91. Boukerrou M, Bresson S, Collinet P, et al. Factors associated with uterine artery Doppler anomalies in patients with preeclampsia. *Hypertens Pregnancy.* 2009 May;28(2):178–189.

92. Sciscione AC, Hayes EJ. Uterine artery Doppler flow studies in obstetric practice. *Am J Obstet Gynecol.* 2009;201(2):121–126.

93. Cnossen JS, Morris RK, ter Riet G, et al. Use of uterine artery Doppler sonography to predict pre-eclampsia and intrauterine growth restriction: a systematic review and bivariable meta-analysis. *CMAJ.* 2008;178(6):727–729.

94. Chien PF, Arnott N, Gordon A, et al. How useful is uterine artery Doppler flow velocimetry in the prediction of preeclampsia, intrauterine growth retardation and perinatal death? An overview. *BJOG.* 2000;107(2):196–208.

95. Melchiorre K, Leslie K, Prefumo F, et al. First-trimester uterine artery Doppler indices in the prediction of small-for-gestational age pregnancy and intrauterine growth restriction. *Ultrasound Obstet Gynecol.* 2009;33(5):524–529.

96. Carbillon L. First trimester uterine artery Doppler abnormalities predict subsequent intrauterine growth restriction. *Am J Obstet Gynecol.* 2006;195(6):e3.

97. Dugoff L, Lynch AM, Cioffi-Ragan D, et al. First trimester uterine artery Doppler abnormalities predict subsequent intrauterine growth restriction. *Am J Obstet Gynecol.* 2005;193(3 Pt 2):1208–1212.

98. Kwon HS, Kim YH, Park YW. Uterine artery Doppler velocimetry and maternal weight gain by the mid-second trimester for prediction of fetal growth restriction. *Acta Obstet Gynecol Scand.* 2008;87(12):1291–1295.

99. Audibert F, Benchimol Y, Benattar C, et al. Prediction of preeclampsia or intrauterine growth restriction by second trimester serum screening and uterine Doppler velocimetry. *Fetal Diagn Ther.* 2005;20(1):48–53.

100. Geipel A, Berg C, Germer U, et al. Doppler assessment of the uterine circulation in the second trimester in twin pregnancies: prediction of pre-eclampsia, fetal growth restriction and birth weight discordance. *Ultrasound Obstet Gynecol.* 2002;20(6):541–545.

101. Bromley B, Frigoletto FD, Harlow BL, et al. The role of Doppler velocimetry in the structurally normal second-trimester fetus with elevated levels of maternal serum alpha-fetoprotein. *Ultrasound Obstet Gynecol.* 1994;4:377–380.

102. Gramellini D, Piantelli G, Verrotti C, et al. Doppler velocimetry and non stress test in severe fetal growth restriction. *Clin Exp Obstet Gynecol.* 2001;28(1):33–39.

103. Valensise H, Vasapollo B, Gagliardi G, et al. Early and late preeclampsia: two different maternal hemodynamic states in the latent phase of the disease. *Hypertension.* 2008;52(5):873–880. Epub 2008 Sep 29.

104. Espinoza J, Romero R, Nien JK, et al. Identification of patients at risk for early onset and/or severe preeclampsia with the use of uterine artery Doppler velocimetry and placental growth factor. *Am J Obstet Gynecol.* 2007;196(4):326.e1–e13.

105. Papageorghiou AT, Yu CK, Bindra R, et al. Multicenter screening for pre-eclampsia and fetal growth restriction by transvaginal uterine artery Doppler at 23 weeks of gestation. *Ultrasound Obstet Gynecol.* 2001;18(5):441–449.

106. Predanic M, Perni SC. Antenatal assessment of discordant umbilical arteries in singleton pregnancies. *Croat Med J.* 2006;47(5):701–708.

107. Byun YJ, Kim HS, Yang JI et. al. Umbilical artery Doppler study as a predictive marker of perinatal outcome in preterm small for gestational age infants. *Yonsei Med J.* 2009;50(1):39–44. Epub 2009 Feb 24.

108. da Silva FC, de Sá RA, de Carvalho PR, et al. Doppler and birth weight Z score: predictors for adverse neonatal outcome in severe fetal compromise. *Cardiovasc Ultrasound*. 2007 20;5:15.

109. Malhotra N, Chanana C, Kumar S, Roy K, Sharma JB. Comparison of perinatal outcome of growth-restricted fetuses with normal and abnormal umbilical artery Doppler waveforms. *Indian J Med Sci*. 2006 Aug;60(8):311–317.

110. Seyam YS, Al-Mahmeid MS, Al-Tamimi HK. Umbilical artery Doppler flow velocimetry in intrauterine growth restriction and its relation to perinatal outcome. *Int J Gynaecol Obstet*. 200;77(2):131–137.

111. Verburg BO, Jaddoe VW, Wladimiroff JW, et al. Fetal hemodynamic adaptive changes related to intrauterine growth: the generation R study. *Circulation*. 2008;117(5):649–659. Epub 2008 Jan 22.

112. Yalti S, Oral O, Gürbüz B, et al. Ratio of middle cerebral to umbilical artery blood velocity in preeclamptic and hypertensive women in the prediction of poor perinatal outcome. *Indian J Med Res*. 2004;120(1):44–50.

113. Tarzamni MK, Nezami N, Gatreh-Samani F, et al. Doppler waveform indices of fetal middle cerebral artery in normal 20 to 40 weeks pregnancies. *Arch Iran Med*. 2009;12(1):29–34.

114. Tan KB, Fook-Chong SM, Lee SL, et al. Foetal peak systolic velocity in the middle cerebral artery: an Asian reference range. *Singapore Med J*. 2009;50(6):584–586.

115. Roza SJ, Steegers EA, Verburg BO, et al. What is spared by fetal brain-sparing? Fetal circulatory redistribution and behavioral problems in the general population. *Am J Epidemiol*. 2008;168(10):1145–1152.

116. Ebrashy A, Azmy O, Ibrahim M, et al. Middle cerebral/umbilical artery resistance index ratio as sensitive parameter for fetal well-being and neonatal outcome in patients with preeclampsia: case-control study. *Croat Med J*. 2005;46(5):821–825.

117. Alkazaleh F, Reister F, Kingdom JC. Doppler Assessment in Pregnancy. In: *Diagnostic Ultrasound*. 3rd ed. Volume 1. St. Louis: Elsevier; 2006.

118. Hagan-Ansert S. Fetal Growth Assessment by Ultrasound. In: *Textbook of Diagnostic Medical Ultrasonography*. 6th ed. Volume 2. St. Louis: Mosby; 2006:873–897.

119. Kiserud T, Eik-Nes SH, Blaas HG, et al. Ductus venosus blood velocity and the umbilical circulation in the seriously growth-retarded fetus. *Ultrasound Obstet Gynecol*. 1994;4(2):109–114.

120. Hecher K, Campbell S, Doyle P, et al. Assessment of fetal compromise by Doppler ultrasound investigation of the fetal circulation. Arterial, intracardiac, and venous blood flow velocity studies. *Circulation*. 1995;91(1):129–138.

121. Edelstone DI, Rudolph AM, Heymann MA. Liver and ductus venosus blood flows in fetal lambs in utero. *Circ Res*. 1978;42(3):426–433.

122. Picconi JL, Hanif F, Drennan K, et al. The transitional phase of ductus venosus reversed flow in severely premature IUGR fetuses. *Am J Perinatol*. 2008;25(4):199–203.

123. Picconi JL, Kruger M, Mari G. Ductus venosus SIA index and A-wave reversed flow in severely premature growth-restriction fetuses. *J Ultrasound Med*. 2008;27(9):1283–1289.

124. Baschat AA, Gembruch U, Weiner CP et al. Qualitative venous Doppler waveform analysis improves prediction of critical perinatal outcomes in premature growth-restricted fetuses. *Ultra Obstet Gynecol* 2003;22:240–245.

125. Hecher K, Bilardo CM, Stigter RH, et al. Monitoring of fetuses with intrauterine growth restriction: a longitudinal study. *Ultrasound Obstet Gynecol*. 2001;18(6):564–570.

126. Baschat AA, Gembruch U, Harman CR. The sequence of changes in Doppler and biophysical parameters as severe fetal growth restriction worsens. *Ultrasound Obstet Gynecol*. 2001;18(6):571–577.

127. Baschat AA: Integrated fetal testing in growth restriction: combining multi-vessel Doppler and biophysical parameters. *Ultrasound Obstet Gynecol*. 2003;21(1):1.

128. Harrington K, Thompson MO, Carpenter RG, et al. Doppler fetal circulation in pregnancies complicated by pre-eclampsia or delivery of a small for gestational age baby: 2. Longitudinal analysis. *Br J Obstet Gynaecol*. 1999;106(5):453–466.

129. Cosmi E, Ambrosini G, D'Antona D, et al. Doppler, cardiotocography, and biophysical profile changes in growth-restricted fetuses. *Obstet Gynecol*. 2005;106(6):1240–1245.

130. Voxman EG, Tran S, Wing DA. Low amniotic fluid index as a predictor of adverse perinatal outcome. *J Perinatol*. 2002;22(4):282–285.

131. Kennelly MM, Sturgiss SN. Management of small-for-gestational-age twins with absent/reversed end diastolic flow in the umbilical artery: outcome of a policy of daily biophysical profile (BPP). *Prenat Diagn*. 2007;27(1):77–80.

132. Read JA, Miller FC. Fetal heart rate acceleration in response to acoustic stimulation as a measure of fetal well-being. *Am J Obstet Gynecol*. 1977;129:512–519.

133. Pattison N, McCowan L. Cardiotocography for antepartum fetal assessment. *Cochrane Database Syst Rev*. 2000;(2):CD001068.

134. Philipson EH, Sokol RJ, Williams T. Oligohydramnios: clinical associations and predictive value for intrauterine growth retardation. *Am Obstet Gynecol*. 1983;146(3):271.

135. Khooshideh M, Izadi S, Shahriari A, Mirteymouri M. The predictive value of ultrasound assessment of amniotic fluid index, biophysical profile score, nonstress test and foetal movement chart for meconium-stained amniotic fluid in prolonged pregnancies. *J Pak Med Assoc*. 2009;59(7):471–474.

136. Phelan JP, Platt LD, Yeh SY, et al. The role of ultrasound assessment of amniotic fluid volume in the management of the postdate pregnancy. *Am J Obstet Gynecol*. 1985;151(3):304–308.

137. Papadopoulos VG, Decavalas GO, Kondakis XG, et al Vibroacoustic stimulation in abnormal biophysical profile: verification of facilitation of fetal well-being. *Early Hum Develop*. 2007;83(3):191–197.

138. Olsen SF, Secher NJ, Tabor A, et al. Randomised clinical trials of fish oil supplementation in high risk pregnancies. Fish oil trials in pregnancy (FOTIP) team. *BJOG*. 2000;107(3):382–395.

139. Askie LM, Duley L, Henderson-Smart DJ, et al. Antiplatelet agents for prevention of pre-eclampsia and its consequences: a systematic review and individual patient data meta-analysis. *BMC Pregnancy Childbirth*. 2005;5(1):7.

140. Makrides M, Duley L, Olsen SF. Marine oil, and other prostaglandin precursor, supplementation for pregnancy uncomplicated by pre-eclampsia or intrauterine growth restriction. *Cochrane Database Syst Rev*. 2006;(3):CD003402.

141. Hui L, Challis D. Diagnosis and management of fetal growth restriction: the role of fetal therapy. *Best Practice Res Clin Obstet Gynaecol*. 2008;22(1):139–158.

142. Duley L, Henderson-Smart DJ, Knight M, et al. Antiplatelet agents for preventing pre-eclampsia and its complications. *Cochrane Database Syst Rev*. 2004;(1):CD004659.

143. Goffinet F, Aboulker D, Paris-Llado, et al. Screening with a uterine Doppler in low risk pregnant women followed by low dose aspirin in women with abnormal results: a multicenter randomised controlled trial. *BJOG*. 2003;108(5):510–518.

144. Yu CK, Papageorghiou AT, Parra M, et al. Randomized control trial using low-dose aspirin in the prevention of preeclampsia in women with abnormal uterine artery Doppler at 23 weeks' gestation. *Ultrasound Obstet Gynecol*. 2003;22(3):233–239.

145. Lumley J, Oliver SS, Chamberlain C, et al. Interventions for promoting smoking cessation during pregnancy. *Cochrane Database Syst Rev*. 2004;(4):CD001055.

146. Dolan-Mullen P, Ramirez G, Groff JY. A meta-analysis of randomized trials of prenatal smoking cessation interventions. *Am J Obstet Gynecol*. 1994;171(5):1328–1334.

147. Whittle MJ, Hanretty KP, Primrose MH, Neilson JP. Screening for the compromised fetus: A randomized trial of umbilical artery velocimetry in unselected pregnancies. *Am J Obstet Gynecol*. 1994; 170:555–559.

148. Boito S, Struijk PC, Ursem NTC, et al. Fetal brain/liver volume ratio and umbilical volume flow parameters relative to normal and abnormal human development. *Ultrasound Obstet Gynecol*. 2003;21(3):256–261.

149. Callen PW. Amniotic fluid volume: its role in fetal health and disease. In: *Ultrasonography in Obstetrics and Gynecology*. 5th ed. Philadelphia: Saunders Elsevier, 2008.

150. Modena AB, Fieni S. Amniotic fluid dynamics. *Acta Biomed*. 2004;(75 Suppl 1):11–13.

151. Hutchinson DL, Gray MJ, Plentl AA, et al. The role of the fetus in the water exchange of the amniotic fluid in normal and hydramniotic patients. *J Clin Invest*. 1959;38(6):971.

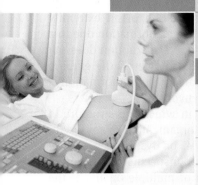

28 Patterns of Fetal Anomalies

John F. Trombly and Susan Raatz Stephenson

OBJECTIVES

Discuss patterns of anomalies using the terminology associated with each form.

Differentiate between mitosis and meiosis.

Compare structural and numerical abnormalities to a normal chromosome.

Describe autosomal dominant, autosomal recessive, X-linked, and multifactorial inheritance patterns.

Identify risk factors for chromosomal abnormality occurrence.

List the prenatal laboratory testing used to identify an abnormal embryo and/or fetus.

KEY TERMS

aneuploid | autosomal dominant | autosomal recessive | chromosome | deletion | deoxyribonucleic acid (DNA) | diploid | dysplasia | euploid | genes | genetic code | genetics | germ cells | haploid | inheritance | inhibin-A | Insertion | inversion | meiosis | mitosis | monosomy | multifactorial inheritance | nondisjunction | PAPP-A | somatic cells | syndrome | translocation | triploid | trisomy | unconjugated estriol | X-linked inheritance

GLOSSARY

Alpha-fetoprotein (AFP) Serum protein produced by the fetal yolk sac and liver that aids in detection of neural tube defects, ventral wall defects, skin disorders, and in rare cases, nephrosis

Analyte Any substance measured in a laboratory such as AFP, inhibin A, or human chorionic gonadotropin

Aneuploidy Abnormal number of chromosomes

Haploid Normal number of chromosomes in a cell

Heterogeneous disorder Mutations caused by multiple genes

Human chorionic gonadotropin (hCG) Hormone secreted by immature placenta

Inhibin A Protein secreted by the corpus luteum and placenta

Karyotype Arrangement of chromosomes by type, size, and morphology to determine normalcy

Mosaicism Presence of two different types of cell genotypes (karyotype) in an individual

Mitosis Division of a cell resulting in the normal haploid number

Meiosis Division of a cell in which there is a reduction, by half, in the normal haploid number of chromosomes

Multifactorial Involving several different factors

Pregnancy-associated plasma protein A (PAPP-A) Placental syncytiotrophoblastic hormone found in maternal blood serum

Pre-eclampsia Triad of hypertension, fluid retention (edema), and proteinuria occurring after 20 weeks' gestation

Quadruple screen Testing for maternal levels of AFP, unconjugated estriol, hCG, and inhibin A

Soft sonographic marker Nonspecific transient markers seen in normal and aneuploidy fetuses that have an increased incidence in the chromosomally abnormal fetus

Triple screen Testing for maternal levels of AFP, uE_3, and hCG

Unconjugated estriol (uE_3) Hormone produced by the syncytiotrophoblast

Vertical transmission From mother to child

Because of its ability to provide a detailed assessment of the fetal anatomy and accurately identify anomalies, sonography has become an adjunct to laboratory testing. This chapter contains information of inheritance patterns and categorization of developmental or acquired anomalies to include malformation, deformation, disruption, and dysplasia.

PATTERNS OF ANOMALIES

Sonography has proven to be an effective tool in the evaluation of the developing fetus and the detection of anomalies throughout pregnancy. Structural anomalies of the fetus may be solitary findings or they may be seen in multiples or patterns. A grouping or pattern of findings may represent a syndrome, an association, or a sequence. These terms describe the manner in which the findings are related.

- Syndrome. A pattern of multiple anomalies related to a single causative factor or pathology.[1,2,3] A trisomy would be considered a syndrome because of the multiple malformations found that are due to a chromosomal anomaly.[2]
- Association. A pattern of multiple anomalies seen in numerous individuals that is not related to a single causative factor or pathology.[1,2] With an association, finding one malformation leads to searching for others that are known to occur together. These are not part of a sequence or syndrome.[3]
- Sequence. A pattern of multiple anomalies that results from an initial single anomaly.[1,2] A sequence may be the result of a malformation, deformation, or disruption.[1]

Anomalies affecting the developing embryo or fetus are typically divided into four categories: malformation, deformation, disruption, and dysplasia.[3]

- Malformation. An anomaly, either single or multiple, in which the structure or tissue is abnormal from the beginning.[1,2] Clefting of the lip or palate is an example of a malformation. If a fetus has a primary birth defect, such as spina bifida, that results in other defects, hydrocephalus or club foot, the term malformation sequence[2] is used.
- Deformation. An anomaly that is either intrinsic or extrinsic in origin. When structure or tissue is acted upon by outside forces resulting in an abnormal shape or position, this is considered an extrinsic deformation.[1,2] Clubbing of the extremities caused by oligohydramnios is an example of a deformation. An intrinsic deformation is the result of a fetal malformation.[1] In the case of a renal malformation where the fetus fails to urinate, oligohydramnios develops, resulting in bilateral club foot.
- Disruption. An anomaly in which the structure or tissue, previously normal, breaks down as a result of some type of insult to the developmental process.[1,2] Intrinsic, extrinsic, and vascular insults

result in a disruption of development.[1] An example of disruption is amputation of an extremity due to amniotic bands or a malformation due to a teratogen such as rubella.[2,3] A disruption does not have a genetic component; however, the embryo can have a predisposition to the malformation if outside factors become involved.[2]

- Dysplasia. An anomaly in which the structure of tissue lacks the normal organization of cells.[2] Abnormal cell development, or dyshistogenesis, results in dysplasia.[2] This nonspecific process often results in malformation of multiple organs at the cellular level.[2] Congenital ectodermal dysplasia is an example of this type of anomaly.

The prenatal sonographic examination allows for detailed assessment of the fetal anatomy and an accurate identification of numerous anomalies. The examiner acts like a detective gathering clues at the scene of a crime. Once all the evidence is accumulated, a comparison of the findings with established patterns (syndromes, associations, or sequences) leads to a specific diagnosis in many instances.

GENETICS

Genetics is the study of heredity in living organisms. Genes, which are responsible for heredity, are made up of segments of deoxyribonucleic acid (DNA). Chromosomes contain the genes, and the cell nuclei contain the chromosomes. The arrangement of DNA in the genes is what gives us the genetic code. Replication of the genetic code results in transmission of traits and characteristics from one generation to the next (Fig. 28-1). This set of instructions contains the instructions for the formation and development of the tissue and structures that become the human body.

CHROMOSOMES

There are basically two groups of cells in the human body, germ cells (gametes) and somatic cells (everything else). Germ cells or gametes are the cells responsible for reproduction, the sperm and the egg. They contain 23 chromosomes, or one set. This set is termed haploid and consists of 22 autosomes and 1 sex chromosome, either an X or a Y. Somatic cells contain 23 pairs of chromosomes, 22 pairs of autosomes and 2 sex chromosomes, and are referred to as diploid.

Somatic cells replicate through the process called mitosis, which produces two daughter cells that contain the same genetic information as the original cell (46 chromosomes) as seen in Figure 28-1. A specialized process of cell replication called meiosis occurs in germ cells and produces four daughter cells that are haploid, containing 23 chromosomes (Fig. 28-2). Errors that occur during meiosis may result in differences in the number of chromosomes in each daughter cell, or in structural abnormalities in the chromosomes.

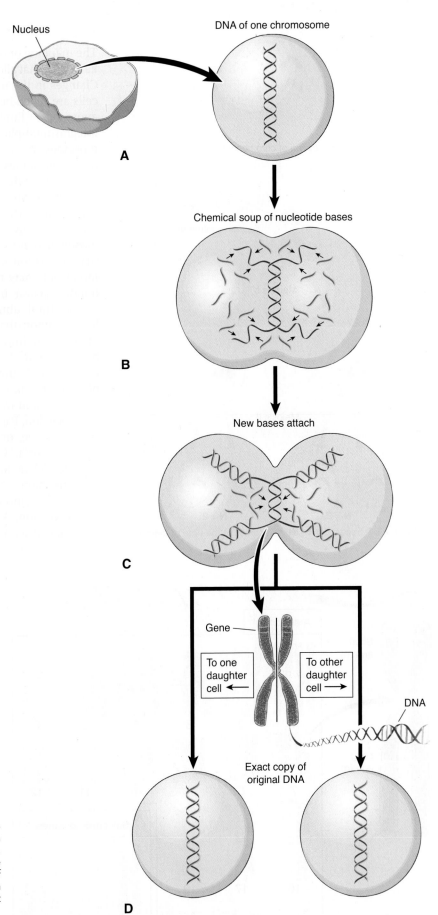

Figure 28-1 DNA replication. **A:** DNA before division. **B:** DNA begins to unravel, with each strand attracting new nucleotide bases. **C:** Cell division continues as new nucleotide bases attach to each strand to form a coil of new DNA. **D:** Cell division is complete. Each new cell contains an exact copy of the parent chromosome's DNA.

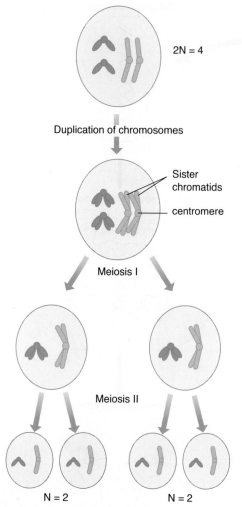

Figure 28-2 Separation of chromosomes at the time of meiosis.

CHROMOSOMAL ABNORMALITIES

The mapping of chromosomes from a sample results in a karyotype that allows counting of the numbers (Fig. 28-3). Changes in the number of chromosomes present in the cells are called heteroploidy and are considered numeric anomalies.[1,2] Euploidy is the condition in which there are integral multiples of the haploid number (23) of chromosomes. An example is triploidy, in which there are 69 chromosomes in the cell (3 × 23).[2] Aneuploidy is the condition in which there is a departure from the euploid number of chromosomes.[1] Having one extra chromosome in a set (trisomy) or missing a chromosome from a set (monosomy) are examples of aneuploidy.[2] This chromosomal nondisjunction occurs during meiosis.[2] Most trisomies result from maternal nondisjunction, whereas monosomy may result from either maternal or paternal nondisjunction, increasing with maternal age.[2]

Structural abnormalities of the chromosomes are less common than numerical abnormalities and most often result from breakage of the chromosome.[2] This breakage may be caused by exposure to factors such as drugs, radiation, viruses, or chemical agents.[2] Examples of structural abnormalities are deletion, insertion, inversion, and translocation.

- Deletion. Part of the chromosome may be lost during breakage, or in rare instances a ring chromosome may form.[2] Cri du chat syndrome is the result of partial deletion from the short arm of chromosome 5.[2]
- Insertion. The addition of genetic information to the chromosome, which occurs during meiosis.
- Inversion. A part of the chromosome may be rearranged within itself.[2] This does not result in a loss

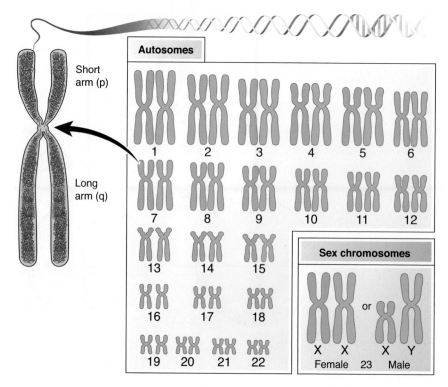

Figure 28-3 A set of normal chromosomes (karyotype). There are 46 total chromosomes, of which 44 are autosomes (pairs 1–22 in the figure; non-sex chromosomes) and two are sex chromosomes (pair 23 in the figure; two X chromosomes for a female, or one X and one Y for a male). The shorthand for a female is 46,XX and for a male 46,XY. In each pair, one is from the male (blue) and one is from the female (pink parent). Genes are short segments of DNA and are located either on the short **(p)** arm of the chromosome above the waist or the long **(q)** arm below it.

of genetic information and often does not result in abnormalities in the parent; however, this chromosomal anomaly can be found in offspring.[2]

- Translocation. During breakage a piece of one chromosome may be transferred to a different chromosome.[1] Translocations do not always cause abnormalities and are considered balanced translocation carriers (Fig. 28-4).[2]

Teratogens, agents that produce congenital malformations, come in many forms. Infection and drugs, considered environmental teratogens, mimic genetic defects.[2] Because of the embryonic sensitivity to teratogens, up to 10%[2] of congenital anomalies trace to these environmental causes. Two examples of environmental teratogens are fetal rubella syndrome, responsible for blindness and deafness, and fetal alcohol syndrome.

INHERITANCE

The transmission of the genetic code from parents to offspring is inheritance. Genetic code that influences structure, tissue, traits, and characteristics may be passed on to successive generations through several modes of transmission: autosomal dominant, autosomal recessive, X-linked, and multifactorial.

- Autosomal dominant. Conditions associated with the 22 non-sex chromosome are termed autosomal. In autosomal dominant transmission, one parent has the trait or condition, and this parent's genetic contribution "dominates" the genes from the other parent. When one parent has the dominant gene, there is a 50% chance each child will inherit the trait or condition (Fig. 28-5).[1]
- Autosomal recessive. Each parent carries the gene associated with the trait or condition but is not affected. Each child has a 25% chance of having the condition, a 50% chance of becoming a carrier, and a 25% chance of not inheriting the gene (Fig. 28-6).[1]
- X-linked. Conditions associated with genes located on the X chromosome may be dominant or recessive.[1] Recessive conditions are more common than dominant, with a preponderance in males.[1] Color-blindness is an example of an X-linked recessive disorder (Fig. 28-7).
- Multifactorial. Conditions may occur as a result of both genetic and nongenetic causes, and though they recur in families, there is no identifiable pattern of transmission. Cardiac defects, neural tube defects, and facial clefting are examples of multifactorial inheritance.

RISK FACTORS

A number of factors are known to increase the risk for the occurrence of chromosomal abnormalities. Some are readily identifiable, such as maternal age and a previous pregnancy with a chromosomal abnormality. Trisomy 21 occurs in newborns of 35-year-old women at a rate of 1 in 385, and women who have had a previous pregnancy with trisomy have a risk of recurrence up to eight times

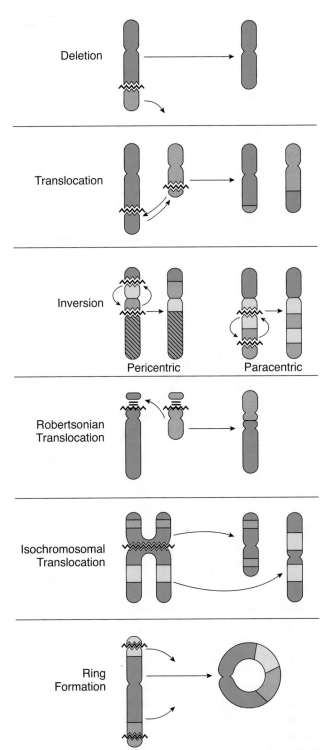

Figure 28-4 Structural abnormalities of human chromosomes. The deletion of a portion of a chromosome leads to the loss of genetic material and a shortened chromosome. A reciprocal translocation involves breaks on two nonhomologous chromosomes, with exchange of the acentric segments. An inversion requires two breaks in a single chromosome. If the breaks are on opposite sides of the centromere, the inversion is pericentric, whereas it is paracentric if the breaks are on the same arm. A robertsonian translocation occurs when two nonhomologous acrocentric chromosomes break near their centromeres, after which the long arms fuse to form one large metacentric chromosome. Isochromosomes arise from faulty centromere division, which leads to duplication of the long arm (iso q) and deletion of the short arm, or the reverse (iso p). Ring chromosomes involve breaks of both telomeric portions of a chromosome, deletion of the acentric fragments, and fusion of the remaining centric portion.

Autosomal dominant gene inheritance
Example: Familial hypercholesterolemia

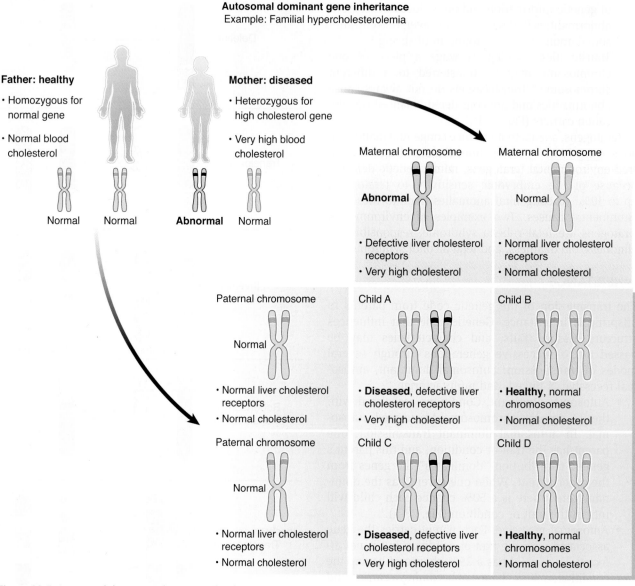

Figure 28-5 Autosomal dominant inheritance. The dominant gene is present in one affected, unhealthy (diseased) parent. Half of the children will be affected.

greater for maternal age. Certain ethnic groups are at increased risk for many Mendelian disorders. Sickle cell disease is more prevalent among individuals of African, Middle Eastern, Caribbean, Mediterranean, and Latin American descent. A history of early pregnancy loss and advanced paternal age are also associated with an increased risk of chromosomal abnormalities.

PRENATAL SCREENING

Medical screening procedures are valuable tools that allow health care providers to identify individuals at increased risk for a variety of diseases and conditions. Prenatal screening becomes beneficial for pregnant patients with personal or clinical risk factors that increase the possibility of genetic anomalies. Several biochemical and ultrasound markers aid in risk assessment for both disease and structural anomalies. The development of

maternal serum alpha-fetoprotein (MSAFP) testing in the 1980s established the value of prenatal screening. Today, prenatal screening is considered an effective test for aneuploidy. It is important to remember that screening does not confirm or rule out the presence of disease, but simply evaluates the risk relative to the general population.

FIRST TRIMESTER

In the first trimester, screening is useful in assessing the risk for trisomies 13, 18, and 21. Blood tests that measure the amount of human chorionic gonadotropin (hCG) and pregnancy-associated plasma protein A (PAPP-A), and sonographic evaluation of the nuchal region of the fetus, have all been shown to be effective in the identification of aneuploidy. Specifically, increases in hCG and decreases in PAPP-A, along with increased nuchal translucency (NT) measurements, have been associated with trisomy

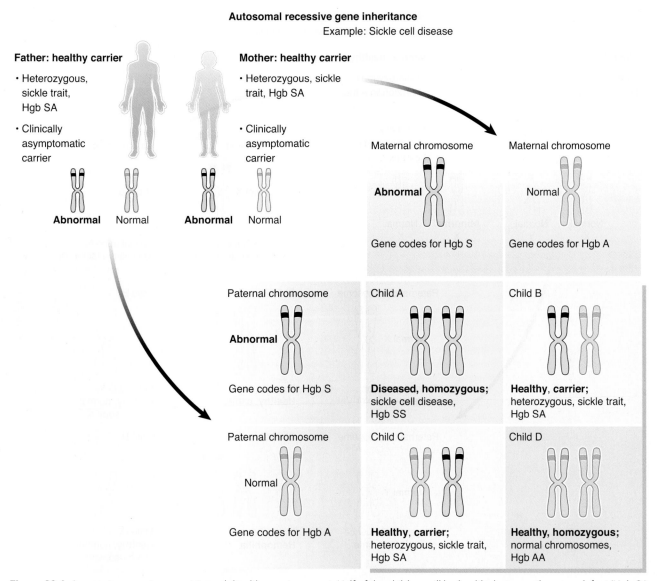

Autosomal recessive gene inheritance
Example: Sickle cell disease

Father: healthy carrier
- Heterozygous, sickle trait, Hgb SA
- Clinically asymptomatic carrier

Mother: healthy carrier
- Heterozygous, sickle trait, Hgb SA
- Clinically asymptomatic carrier

Abnormal   Normal   **Abnormal**   Normal

Maternal chromosome

Abnormal

Gene codes for Hgb S

Maternal chromosome

Normal

Gene codes for Hgb A

Paternal chromosome

Abnormal

Gene codes for Hgb S

Child A

Diseased, homozygous; sickle cell disease, Hgb SS

Child B

Healthy, carrier; heterozygous, sickle trait, Hgb SA

Paternal chromosome

Normal

Gene codes for Hgb A

Child C

Healthy, carrier; heterozygous, sickle trait, Hgb SA

Child D

Healthy, homozygous; normal chromosomes, Hgb AA

Figure 28-6 A recessive gene is present in each healthy, carrier parent. Half of the children will be healthy but carry the gene defect (Hgb SA, sickle cell trait); one-fourth will be genetically and clinically normal (Hgb AA); and one-fourth will have sickle cell disease (Hgb SS).

21 (Down syndrome). When used in combination in the first trimester (10 to 14 weeks), these three markers yield an 82% to 87% detection rate of trisomy 21.

SECOND TRIMESTER

Women who did not undergo screening in the first trimester should be offered biochemical screening in the second trimester, between 15 and 20 weeks. In the second trimester, four biochemical markers are used: MSAFP, hCG, unconjugated estriol (uE_3), and inhibin A.[1]

Unconjugated estriol is one of two syncytiotrophoblastic hormones used in prenatal screening. The fetal adrenal gland and liver synthesize the hormone and the placenta deconjugates the hormone. Fetal malformations disrupting the normal process result in unconjugated estriol in the maternal bloodstream.[1] HCG, also secreted by the syncytiotrophoblast, relates to the placental maturity.[1]

Each marker behaves differently. In trisomy 21, levels of MSAFP and uE_3 are low and levels of hCG and inhibin A are elevated.[1,16] Levels of uE_3, AFP, and hCG markers are low, AFP is high, and inhibin A shows no change in patients with trisomy 18.[1,16] The triple screen produces detection rates of 70%. The addition of inhibin A (the quad screen), which is increased in trisomy 21, improves the detection rate to 80%.[1] Regardless of the trimester or screening strategy used, these tests are an essential component of modern prenatal care. Women identified to be at increased risk can receive genetic counseling and be offered appropriate diagnostic tests.

PRENATAL DIAGNOSTIC PROCEDURES

Once increased risk for aneuploidy is established, diagnostic procedures may be performed to evaluate the genetic makeup of the fetus. Several procedures are

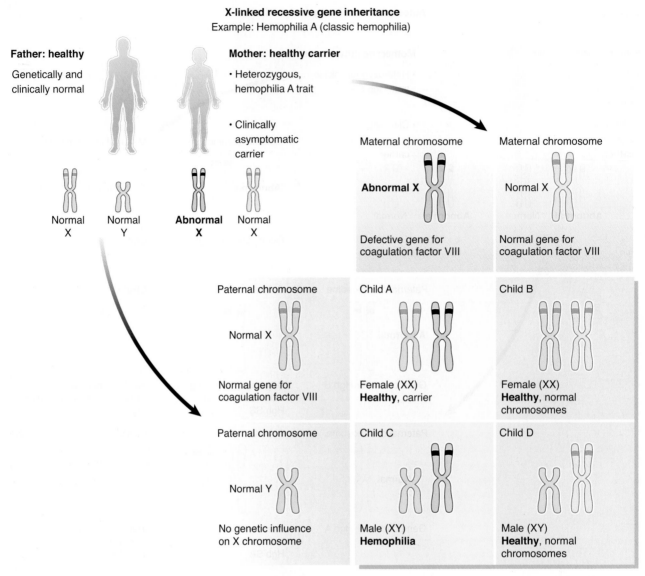

Figure 28-7 X-linked recessive gene inheritance. Example: Classic hemophilia (hemophilia A). The defective gene on the X chromosome is expressed in males only because the Y chromosome contains no matching normal gene (allele) to offset the effect of the defective X gene.

available, each with their own advantages and risks: amniocentesis, chorionic villus sampling, and umbilical blood sampling. These are discussed in greater detail in Chapter 31.

SYNDROMES, SEQUENCES, AND ASSOCIATIONS

Patterns of anomalies recognized in humans are categorized by type and often named after the individual or individuals who first described or identified the pattern. Today there are well over 10,000 recognized syndromes. As the understanding of the human genome grows, so too will the understanding of the nature of fetal anomalies. The syndromes, sequences, and associations presented here are just a sampling, chosen primarily because they have sonographically identifiable findings.

AICARDI SYNDROME

Description

Aicardi syndrome is a rare condition, with only a few thousand cases reported worldwide.[20,21] Syndrome frequency is unknown and shows no ethnic propensity.[20] Diagnosis of this syndrome is made through determining the presence of agenesis of the corpus callosum, chorioretinal lacunae, and infantile spasms.[34] Incidence rate varies with geography, with approximately a 1 per 100,000 occurrence.[34]

Lab Values

There are no specific maternal serum markers for Aicardi syndrome. The only method to ensure correct diagnosis is through amniocentesis, chorionic villi sampling, or percutaneous umbilical blood sampling (PUBS).[20]

Genetics

Aicardi syndrome occurs mainly in females.[21] Even though the syndrome is considered to have an autosomal recessive inheritance pattern,[20] the fact that it occurs in females classifies the syndrome as an X-linked dominant inheritance pattern.[21,34] New autosomal dominant mutations are also possible.[20]

The four genes known responsible for this mutation are TREX1, RNASEH2B, RNASEH2C, and RNASEH2A.[20,21] There has been a finding of Aicardi syndrome with a normal chromosomal karyotype, which suggested a disease-induced cause for the syndrome.[20]

Sonographic Findings

Agenesis of the corpus callosum is the most common finding.[3,22] Also seen are microcephaly, porencephalic cysts, microphthalmia, choroid plexus papilloma, Dandy–Walker malformation, dysgenesis of the corpus callosum, brain calcifications, brain asymmetry of gyri and sulci, and scoliosis.[3,16,20,21]

Prognosis

In 20% of cases, diagnosis of this syndrome is made through neonatal testing for elevated liver enzymes, thrombocytopenia, neurologic findings, and the presence of hepatosplenomegaly.[20] Affected individuals have moderate to severe mental deficiency,[3,21] seizures, and blindness.[20,21] Mortality is high in the first few years.[3,34]

AMNIOTIC BAND SEQUENCE

Description

Amniotic band sequence, or constriction band syndrome, begins with the rupture of the amnion and subsequently results in the entrapment of fetal parts.[22] The amnion constricts the growing fetal anatomy, leading to disruption and often amputation of the entangled part.[3] Most cases of amniotic band sequence are idiopathic, although in rare instances trauma is the cause. The incidence has a wide range of about 1 in 1,200 to 1 in 15,000[22] live births with a male to female ratio 1:1.[3]

Lab Values

No maternal or fetal laboratory values aid in diagnosis of this condition.

Genetics

Not known,[3,16] as the gene presentation of the fetus is karyotypically normal.[16] Associated with epidermolysis bullosa and Ehlers-Danlos syndrome.[3]

Sonographic Findings

Severity becomes dependent on when the fetus became entrapped by the amnion.[16] The presence of amniotic bands or sheets alone does not indicate amniotic band sequence. The entanglement of fetal structures or the obvious disruption of an extremity or other fetal part by bands or sheets is indicative of the sequence (Fig. 28-8).[3,16] Several studies link abnormalities such as holoprosencephaly, cerebellar dysplasia, heterotopia, and cardiac and renal

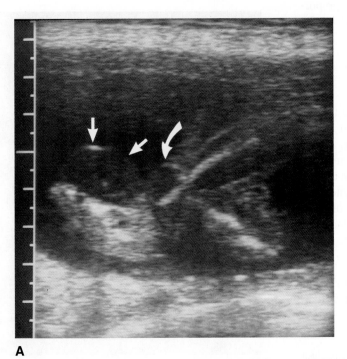
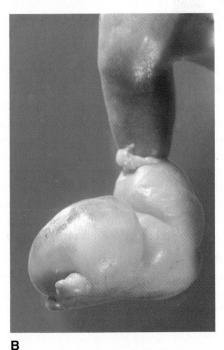

A   **B**

Figure 28-8 Amniotic band syndrome. **A:** Marked swelling and edema of the foot are evident *(arrows)*. A constriction band of the leg is suggested *(curved arrow)*. **B:** The pathologic photograph correlates with ultrasound findings, showing marked edema of the foot and lower leg secondary to constriction by amniotic band.

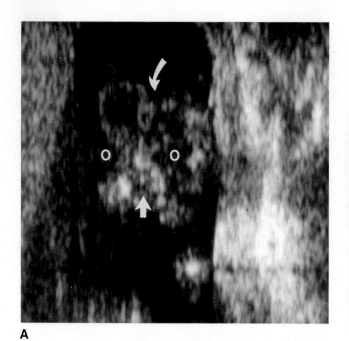

A

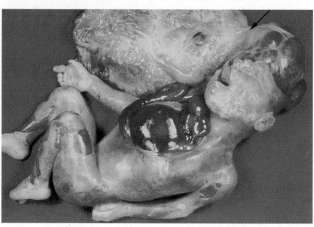

B

Figure 28-9 Amniotic band syndrome. **A:** A coronal scan of the face and head shows exencephaly with eviscerated brain *(curved arrow)*. A facial cleft *(straight arrow)* is also evident. *O,* orbits. **B:** A pathologic photograph of a similar case shows exencephaly, a ventral wall defect, and an amniotic band extending through the mouth.

abnormalities; however, a fetus with these abnormalities may have normal amnion.[3] Monozygotic twins are affected more than dizygotic twins.[3] Uterine synechiae or septations may mimic; however, these do not adhere to the fetus.[3]

Prognosis

Outcomes vary widely depending upon the nature and degree of entanglement, from minor disability associated with hands or fingers affected to death if large portions of the fetal head or torso are entrapped in the amnion (Fig. 28-9).[3]

APERT SYNDROME

Description

Apert syndrome is a rare condition (1 in 65,000 to 1 in 200,000)[3,16,21] characterized by premature fusion of the skull bones.[21] A form of acrocephalosyndactyly, it was first described in 1906.[3,16] Craniosynostosis is the main characteristic of Apert syndrome, which results in changes of head and face shape (Fig. 28-10).[21] Apert syndrome is part of a group of syndromes that contain craniosynostosis as a finding, along with Muenke, Crouzon, Jackson-Weiss, Pfeiffer, and Beare-Stevenson syndrome.[16]

Lab Values

There are no specific maternal serum markers for Apert syndrome. In the presence of an open spinal defect, MSAFP may be elevated.

Genetics

FGFR2 gene mutations result in Apert syndrome.[16,21] A protein produced by this gene performs multiple functions, one of which is the initiation of bone development

cells during embryogenesis. Lack of this protein results in the premature fusion of the skull, hand, and foot bones.[21] Since only one copy of the gene is necessary for development of Apert syndrome, it is considered to be autosomal dominant.[3,16,21] This malformation occurs sporadically and has associations with advanced

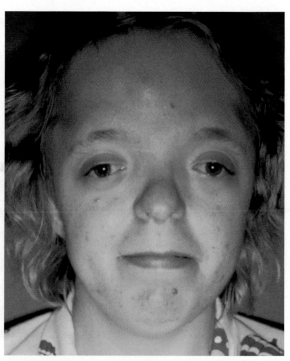

Figure 28-10 Typical facies of Apert syndrome. Note antimongoloid slanting of the palpebral fissures, exophthalmos, hypertelorism, oxycephaly, and midfacial hypoplasia.

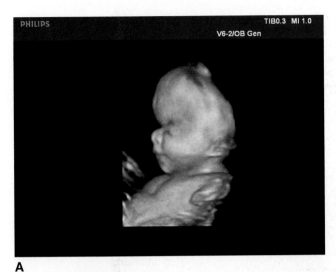
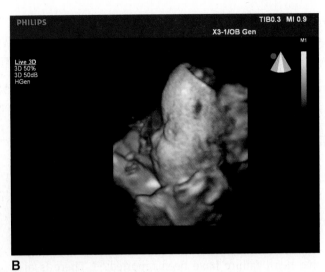

Figure 28-11 Apert syndrome. **A:** This surface-rendered 3D construction demonstrates a bulging forehead and upper facial sinking. **B:** Proptosis, bulging of the eyes, is seen in this surface rendering. (Image courtesy of Philips Medical Systems, Bothell, WA.)

paternal age.[3] When a parent carries the gene there is a 50% recurrence rate;[3] however, most cases are new.[16]

Sonographic Findings

Prominent or bulging forehead and increased cephalic index raise suspicion for craniosynostosis (Fig. 28-11).[3,16] The premature fusion of the skull results in sinking of the midface, wide-set eyes, and maxillary underdevelopment.[21] Other cranial findings include hypertelorism, agenesis of the corpus callosum, and ventriculomegaly.[3,16] Syndactyly and digit fusion is also frequently seen in Apert syndrome.[16,21]

Prognosis

Early surgery is often indicated to relieve increased intracranial pressure. Apert syndrome is often associated with varying degrees of mental deficiency related to the intracranial anomalies.[16]

BECKWITH-WEIDEMANN SYNDROME

Description

Beckwith-Weidemann syndrome (BWS) is an overgrowth disorder affecting 1 in 10,000 live births.[3] Diagnosis is made through five findings: macroglossia, anterior wall defects, hypoglycemia at birth, macrosomia, and hemihpyperplasia.[23,24]

Lab Values

In the fetus with BWS that has an omphalocele, there is an elevation of the maternal alpha-fetoprotein (AFP) 50% of the time.[16]

Genetics

Although most cases are sporadic with normal karotypes, 10% to 15% are autosomal dominant in nature and demonstrate translocations, inversions, and/or duplications

---

PATHOLOGY BOX 28-1

Pathologic and Clinical Features of Apert Syndrome

Central nervous system	Craniosynostosis with acrocephaly/turricephaly
	Agenesis/hypoplasia of corpus callosum
	Hydrocephalus
	Cephalocele
	Spina bifida
	Cerebral atrophy/hypoplasia of the white matter
	Gyral abnormalities, heterotopic gray matter
Extremities	Brachydactyly
	Broad thumbs
	Elbow/joint radiohumeral synostosis
	Hypoplastic or absent humerus
	Polysyndactyly of fingers (mitten hands)
	Polydactyly of toes
Facial	Cleft palate
	Hypertelorism
	Prominent eyes/proptosis
	Prominent forehead (frontal bossing)
	Malar hypoplasia
	Depressed nasal bridge with parrot-beaked nose
Cardiac anomalies	Pulmonic stenosis
	Overriding aorta
	Ventricular septal defects
Genitourinary	Hydronephrosis

Reproduced with permission from McKusick VA, ed. Online Mendelian inheritance in man. http://www.ncbi.nlm.nih.gov/omim/. McKusick-Nathans Institute for Genetic Medicine, Johns Hopkins University (Baltimore, MD) and National Center for Biotechnology Information, National Library of Medicine (Bethesda, MD), 2000.

of chromosome 11. Assisted reproduction techniques have shown to increase the incidence of BWS. These fetuses and neonates demonstrate the structural malformations of BWS but do not have the genetic causes.

Sonographic Findings

Macroglossia[3] is the classic sonographic finding in BWS,[2] as with trisomy 21; however, the combination of macrosomia and macroglossia raises concern for BWS.[16] Other findings include macrosomia, omphalocele, enlarged kidneys, cardiomegaly, and polyhydramnios (Fig. 28-12).[2,16,24] Normal karyotype is common with a fetus demonstrating an omphalocele-containing liver.[16]

Prognosis

Infant mortality rates as high as 21% due to congestive heart failure have been reported.[3,16] There is also an increased risk for pediatric neoplasia such as Wilms' tumor, hepatoblastoma, adrenal corticocarcinoma, neuroblastoma, and rhabdomyosarcoma.[16,24]

CAUDAL REGRESSION SYNDROME

Description

Caudal regression syndrome, also known as caudal dysplasia sequence, was previously thought to be related to sirenomelia.[10] They are now felt to represent two distinct anomalies. The cause of this disorder is unknown, though 16% have been associated with diabetic mothers.[3,9] Caudal defects vary from incomplete development of the sacrum and lumbar vertebrae to sacral agenesis and disruption of the distal spinal cord.

Sonographic Findings

See Chapter 19 for a detailed description of the sonographic features of caudal regression syndrome.

Lab Values

Open spinal defects and some types of teratomas, both which may be seen in this condition, may result in an increase in MSAFP.

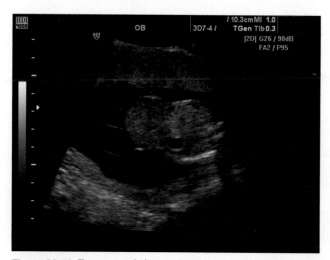

Figure 28-12 Transverse abdomen demonstrating an omphalocele. (Image courtesy of Philips Medical Systems, Bothell, WA.)

PATHOLOGY BOX 28-2

Pathologic and Clinical Features of Beckwith-Wiedemann Syndrome

Growth	Macrosomia
	Hemihypertrophy
Craniofacial	Metopic ridge
	Large fontanel
	Prominent occiput
	Coarse facial features
	Prominent eyes
	Linear earlobe creases
	Posterior helical indentations
	Macroglossia
Abdomen	Omphalocele
	Hepatomegaly
	Pancreatic hyperplasia
	Hepatoblastoma
	Adrenal carcinoma
Metabolic	Neonatal hypoglycemia
Hormonal	Adrenocortical cytomegaly
	Pituitary amphophil hyperplasia
Genitourinary	Renal medullary dysplasia
	Large kidneys
	Overgrowth of external genitalia
	Cryptorchidism
	Wilms' tumor
	Gonadoblastoma
Cardiovascular	Cardiomyopathy
	Cardiomegaly

Reproduced with permission from McKusick VA, ed. Online Mendelian inheritance in man. http://www.ncbi.nlm.nih.gov/omim/. McKusick-Nathans Institute for Genetic Medicine, Johns Hopkins University (Baltimore, MD) and National Center for Biotechnology Information, National Library of Medicine (Bethesda, MD), 2000.

Genetics

This autosomal-dominant trait, which has an association with an anterior meningocele, presacral teratoma, and anorectal anomalies, is often referred to as the Currarino triad.[27,28] A specific genetic cause had not been established; however, the syndrome has been linked to deletions in the 6q25.3, 7q36, and HLBX9 gene.[21,27,28]

Prognosis

How well the individual functions depends on the termination level and spinal stability. Medical problems include bladder and bowel incontinence, recurrent urinary tract infections, renal impairment, vesicourethral dysfunction, and the development of a neurogenic bladder.[29,30]

CHARGE SYNDROME

Description

Previously an association, CHARGE is a collection of rare malformations now recognized as a syndrome. The pattern of anomalies includes colobomatous malformation, heart defects, atresia choanae, retardation (mental and growth deficiencies), genital hypoplasia, and ear anomalies.[3,16] Occurrence rate for CHARGE is from 1 in 8,500 to 1 in 10,000 individuals.[21]

Two types of characteristics help identify CHARGE syndrome. Major characteristics specific to this syndrome include the coloboma (80% to 90%),[31] which is a hole in a structure of the eye. The coloboma affects eyesight, with the severity depending on the location and whether it affects one or both eyes. Eyes may be small, as may also be the nasal passages. Cranial nerve anomalies result in swallowing difficulties, and facial paralysis, diminished smell, and some degree of hearing loss are common due to abnormal function. Almost all individuals have ear anomalies that include abnormal shape of the external and internal structures.[21,31]

Other defects, often referred to as minor defects, are nonspecific to CHARGE syndrome and may not be readily identifiable at birth. These include heart defects and cleft lip and palate. Over half of individuals demonstrate hypogonadotropic hypogonadism of external genitalia resulting in delayed puberty. A tracheal esophageal (TE) fistula may also exist. Facial features include asymmetry and a square shape.[21,31]

Lab Values

As stated, in the fetus with an omphalocele there is an elevation of the maternal AFP.[16]

Genetics

This syndrome is usually a male dominated, new mutation[3] resulting from a short, nonfunctional protein produced by the CHD7 gene.[22,31] The remaining cases have no link to CHD7,[21] with some demonstrating a translocation, deletion, or rearrangement on chromosome 8.[3,31] This is inheritable from a parent,[21] with the severity increasing in the offspring.[32]

Sonographic Findings

Cardiac anomalies are the most likely finding to be seen in the prenatal period. Tetralogy of Fallot, double-outlet right ventricle with an artrioventricular canal, ventricular septal defect, atrial septal defect, and right-sided and interrupted aortic arch have all been observed with CHARGE syndrome.[3,16,31] Growth deficiencies are not usually observed in the prenatal period. Other occasional findings include micrognathia, cleft lip, cleft palate, renal anomalies, omphalocele, TE fistula, polydactyly, hemivertebrae, and hypertelorism (Fig. 28-13).[31]

Prognosis

Death in the perinatal period may occur as a result of cardiac anomalies, TE fistula, or choanal atresia.[31] Decreased growth and developmental delay appear in the first six months of life.[21] Cognitive function varies with most patients exhibiting some degree of mental deficiency.[21,31]

GOLDENHAR SYNDROME

Description

Also known as oculo-auriculo-vertebral syndrome,[3] Goldenhar syndrome is a rare condition documented in 1952 by Goldenhar but first recorded in 1845.[34] It is characterized by incomplete development of the ear, nose, soft palate, lip, and mandible on one side of the body.[16] This is a result of the first and second brachial arch developing abnormally in the embryo.[35] Because of the 85%[36] occurrence of ipsilateral underdevelopment of the external ear and face, these are considered the defining features of the syndrome; however, bilateral malformations may also occur.[35,36] Common associated anomalies of the spine include scoliosis, hemivertebrae, and cervical fusion.[36] This syndrome occurs between 1 in 3,000 and 1 in 50,000,[3,16] with a male-to-female ratio of 3:2.[35,36]

Lab Values

Routine maternal serum testing would not specifically diagnose Goldenhar syndrome; however, some cases of the syndrome occur with an occipital meningoencephalocele,[37] which could result in an increased AFP level.[16]

Figure 28-13 CHARGE (coloboma of the eye, heart defects, atresia of the choanae, retarded mental and growth development, genital anomalies, and ear anomalies) association. **A:** An axial image of the fetal head at 19 weeks shows mild cerebral ventricular dilation (11 mm). **B:** A follow-up exam at 36 weeks shows resolution of the ventricular dilatation and marked polyhydramnios, nonvisible stomach, and growth restriction. At birth, the infant was found to have the CHARGE association with choanal atresia, colobomas, and genital anomalies.

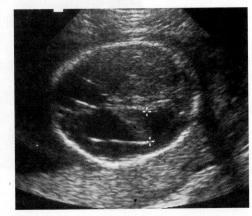

A

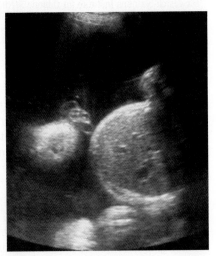

B

Pathologic and Clinical Features of CHARGE Association

Growth	Short stature
	Growth delay
Central nervous system/ neurologic	Dandy-Walker malformation
	Holoprosencephaly
	Mental retardation
	Deafness
Cardiovascular	Tetralogy of Fallot
	Double-outlet right ventricle
	Atrial septal defect
Craniofacial	Choanal atresia/stenosis
	Cleft lip/palate
	Ear abnormalities, deafness, abnormal auditory ossicles
	Vestibular dysfunction
	Temporal bone malformation
	Ocular abnormalities, colobomas
	Microcephaly
	Micrognathia
Gastrointestinal	Esophageal atresia/stenosis
	TE fistula
	Anal atresia, stenosis
	Omphalocele
Genitourinary	Central hypogonadism
	Cryptorchidism
	Horseshoe kidney
	Hydronephrosis
Hormonal	Hypopituitarism
	Hypothyroidism
	Parathyroid hypoplasia
	Growth hormone deficiency

CHARGE, coloboma of the eye, heart defects, atresia of the choanae, retarded mental and growth development, genital and ear anomalies.

Reproduced with permission from McKusick VA, ed. Online Mendelian inheritance in man. http://www.ncbi.nlm.nih.gov/omim/. McKusick-Nathans Institute for Genetic Medicine, Johns Hopkins University (Baltimore, MD) and National Center for Biotechnology Information, National Library of Medicine (Bethesda, MD), 2000.

Genetics

This syndrome has a sporadic pattern and the genetics are unknown, but there has been an association with mosaic trisomy 22[16] and it is thought to be a combination of multifactorial inheritance combined with environmental factors.[35]

Sonographic Findings

Facial anomalies such as asymmetry, cleft lip, cleft palate, and microphthalmia are frequent findings.[3,16] Hemivertebrae or scoliosis is common. Cardiac defects such as ventricular septal defects, tetralogy of Fallot, and coarctation of the aorta—along with renal anomalies, ureteropelvic junction obstruction, and multicystic dysplastic kidney—are occasional findings (Fig. 28-14).[3,16,36] A study by Monni et al. demonstrated a thickened nuchal lucency in an embryo that had a neonatal diagnosis of Goldenhar syndrome (Fig. 28-15).[38]

Prognosis

Most structural abnormalities are surgically correctable; however, the severity may lead to respiratory and feeding problems.[16] Affected individuals often suffer mental deficiency[3] but have a normal life span.[35]

HOLT-ORAM SYNDROME

Description

Also known as cardiac-limb syndrome, Holt-Oram syndrome (HOS) was first described by Holt and Oram in 1960. It is characterized by anomalies of the upper limbs and the heart[21] and has an incidence of approximately 1 in 100,000 live births.[21]

Lab Values

There are no known lab values diagnostic of HOS.

Genetics

HOS is an autosomal dominant mutation resulting from T-box (TBX) gene[3] on chromosome 12.[16,21] This gene, specifically TBX5, produces instructions for the creation of the T-box protein, which attaches to other genes aiding in organ formation.[21] In embryogenesis the T-box proteins help in development of the upper limbs and heart through activation of genes that form these body parts.[21] Since this protein also helps form the conduction system of the heart, its absence results in the abnormal rhythms seen with the syndrome.[21] Transmission of this syndrome is 100%.[16] Most cases are new mutations.[21]

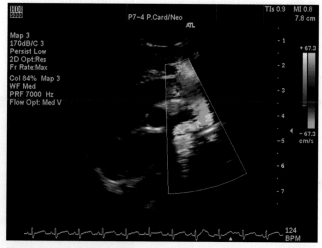

Figure 28-14 Color Doppler image demonstrating postductal coarctation of the aorta in a pediatric patient. (Image courtesy of Philips Medical Systems, Bothell, WA.)

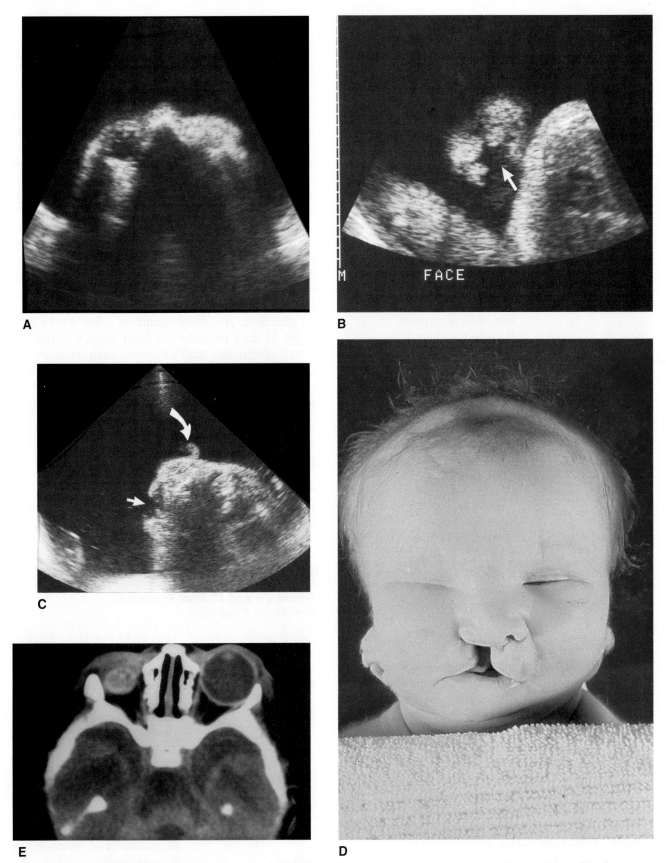

Figure 28-15 Goldenhar syndrome. **A:** An axial view through the orbits shows unilateral anophthalmia. **B:** Coronal view of the face shows unilateral cleft lip/palate *(arrow)*. **C:** Transverse view of the face shows cleft *(arrow)* and ipsilateral abnormal ear *(curved arrow)*. **D:** Postmortem photograph confirms the ultrasound findings. **E:** A postnatal computed tomographic image of another infant with Goldenhar syndrome shows anopthalmia.

PATHOLOGY BOX 28-4

Pathologic and Clinical Features of Goldenhar Syndrome

Central nervous system/neurologic	Lipoma of the corpus callosum
	Hydrocephalus
Cardiovascular	Cardiac defects
Craniofacial	Unilateral ear abnormalities
	Unilateral cleft lip/palate
	Preauricular tags, sinuses
	External auditory canal atresia
	Microtia
	Facial asymmetry, hemifacial microsomia
	Epibulbar dermoid
	Upper eyelid coloboma
	Microphthalmos, anophthalmia
	Macrostomia
	Mandibular hypoplasia
Skeletal	Vertebral anomalies
	Acro-osteolysis of terminal phalanges
Gastrointestinal	Anal atresia
	Situs abnormalities
	Biliary atresia
	Esophageal atresia
	TE fistula
Genitourinary	Ectopic and or fused kidneys
	Renal agenesis
	Ureteropelvic junction obstruction
	Multicystic kidney

Reproduced with permission from McKusick VA, ed. Online Mendelian inheritance in man. http://www.ncbi.nlm.nih.gov/omim/. McKusick-Nathans Institute for Genetic Medicine, Johns Hopkins University (Baltimore, MD) and National Center for Biotechnology Information, National Library of Medicine (Bethesda, MD), 2000.

Sonographic Findings

The most common sonographic findings are those affecting the upper extremities and the heart. Hand anomalies such as syndactyly (particularly between the thumb and index finger), clinodactyly, brachydactyly, and thumb anomalies are common.[3,21] The malformations may be asymmetric, with the left side more severely affected. Defects of the radius, ulna, humerus, clavicle, scapula, and sternum may also be seen. Common observable cardiac anomalies include atrial septal and ventricular septal defects, bradycardia, and fibrillation, though one-third may have other types of defects.[3,21] Occasional anomalies include hypertelorism, vertebral anomalies, and polydactyly.

Prognosis

The prognosis is dependent on the severity of the malformation.[1] Individuals may be affected with cardiac conduction defects which may worsen with time.[3]

LIMB-BODY WALL COMPLEX

Description

Limb-body wall complex (LBWC) is a collection of ventral wall and limb defects. Two types of LBWC identified in the literature separate fetuses with and without craniofacial defects. Those with the defect demonstrate an encephalocele or exencephaly with a facial cleft and an adhesion of the amnion between the placenta and cranial defect. The second type demonstrates a short cord, intact amnion, and extra embryonic coelom persistence, as well as urogenital malformations, anal atresia, and a meningocele in the lumbosacral region.[39]

These malformations depend on the time of pregnancy when the amnion ruptures and subsequent attachment of the embryo occurs. If the rupture occurs around 5 weeks, the embryo demonstrates anencephaly, asymmetric encephaloceles, and unique facial clefts, with the placenta attaching to the head and abdomen. A rupture occurring a few weeks later results in limb reduction or limb abnormalities and thoraco-abdominal malformations such as scoliosis. At the end of the first trimester and later, ruptures involve the limbs, resulting in hypoplasias, malformations, and amputation.[40] Reported incidence varies widely from 1 in 7,000 to 1 in 42,000.[16,43]

Lab Values

Elevated MSAPF is seen in the second trimester.[16]

Genetics

This complex is sporadic with an unknown etiology and no known genetic correlation.[16]

PATHOLOGY BOX 28-5

Pathologic and Clinical Features of Holt-Oram Syndrome

Cardiovascular	Atrial septal defect
	Ventricular septal defect
	Hypoplastic left heart syndrome
Thorax	Absent pectoralis major muscle
	Pectus excavatum or carinatum
Skeletal	Vertebral anomalies
	Thoracic scoliosis
	Absent thumb
	Bifid thumb
	Triphalangeal thumb
	Carpal bone anomalies
	Upper extremity phocomelia
	Radial-ulnar anomalies
	Asymmetric involvement
Hormonal	Hypopituitarism
	Hypothyroidism
	Parathyroid hypoplasia
	Growth hormone deficiency

Sonographic Findings

The fetus appears "stuck" or tethered to the placenta or uterus, with ventral wall defects, facial clefts, severe kyphoscoliosis, and limb anomalies (Fig. 28-16).[16,40]

Prognosis

LBWC is lethal.[16,39]

MECKEL-GRUBER SYNDROME

Description

Meckel-Gruber syndrome is rare and characterized by renal dysplasia, limb anomalies, and encephalocele.[16] It occurs in 0.07 to 0.7 in 10,000 births, except in Finland, where the reported incidence is 1.1 in 10,000.[3] There is a 1:1 ratio in males to females.[40]

Lab Values

There are no specific lab values to identify this syndrome; however, the presence of an encephalocele or other spinal defect could result in a high AFP.

Genetics

This disorder has a link to multiple chromosomes and is autosomal recessive.[3,21,40] Chromosome 17q22[16] contains the Meckel syndrome type 1 (MKS1) gene, which produces the protein required for primary cilium development of the ciliated epithelial cells.[21] Defects of MKS1 result in central nervous system anomalies, usually an encephalocele, cysts, and hepatic ductal dysplasia, plus polydactaly.[21] Other genes linked to this syndrome include CC2D2A, TMEM67, RPGRIP1L, and 11q.[16,21,40]

Sonographic Findings

Enlarged, echogenic kidneys due to polycystic disease, polydactyly, and an occipital encephalocele[3] are the classic findings of Meckel-Gruber syndrome.[16] Oligohydramnios

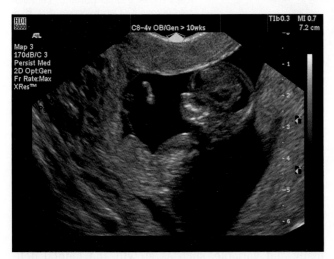

Figure 28-16 This sagittal image of a fetus with LBW complex demonstrates the tethering seen with this group of malformations. (Image courtesy of Philips Medical Systems, Bothell, WA.)

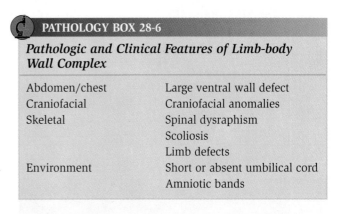

PATHOLOGY BOX 28-6

Pathologic and Clinical Features of Limb-body Wall Complex

Abdomen/chest	Large ventral wall defect
Craniofacial	Craniofacial anomalies
Skeletal	Spinal dysraphism
	Scoliosis
	Limb defects
Environment	Short or absent umbilical cord
	Amniotic bands

is a often seen as a result of inadequate urine production. Postaxial polydactyly may also be observed, as well as Dandy–Walker syndrome (Fig. 28-17).[16]

Prognosis

Affected individuals seldom survive more than a few days because of renal malformations.[3,16]

MONOSOMY X (TURNER OR XO SYNDROME)

Description

Turner syndrome, also known as monosomy X (45 XO), results from the absence of one of the two sex chromosomes.[1,3] Although it is seen in 1 in 8,000 live births,[2] 98% of monosomy X conceptions result in miscarriage[45]; it accounts for 10% of all spontaneous abortions.[3] Incidence is higher in individuals of Japanese descent.[3] The missing sex chromosome is more likely to be from the paternal contribution. Unlike Noonan syndrome, which has similar findings, Turner syndrome only affects females.

Lab Values

Turner syndrome has been found associated with an elevated maternal β hCG and inhibin in the presence of nonimmune fetal hydrops.[3,16] In the absence of hydrops, estriol is markedly decreased and the AFP and inhibin are low.[16]

Genetics

The cause of monosomy X is a sporadic event of a nondisjunction error occurring at gametogenesis.[3,16,21] Three-quarters of the cases trace to the sperm due to a missing X chromosome resulting in a genetic profile of one X, from the mother, and the O from the father.[2] Half of the Turner individual have a 45, X karyotype.[2]

There has been a link to the SHOX or short-stature homeobox gene. The X chromosome carries the SHOX gene, with normal individuals having two SHOX genes, whereas a Turner has only one. This gene produces the SHOX protein and, with only one

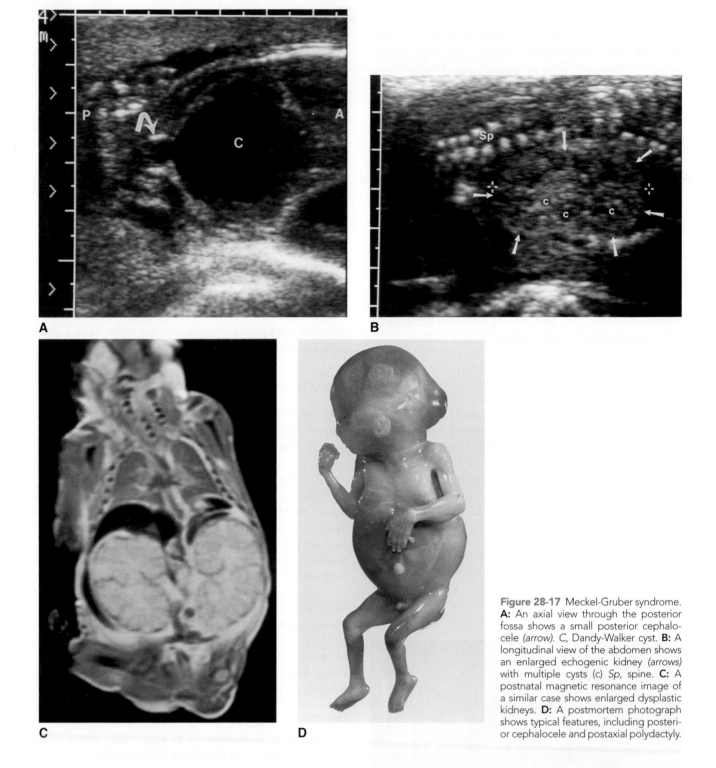

Figure 28-17 Meckel-Gruber syndrome. **A:** An axial view through the posterior fossa shows a small posterior cephalocele *(arrow)*. *C*, Dandy-Walker cyst. **B:** A longitudinal view of the abdomen shows an enlarged echogenic kidney *(arrows)* with multiple cysts *(c)* *Sp*, spine. **C:** A postnatal magnetic resonance image of a similar case shows enlarged dysplastic kidneys. **D:** A postmortem photograph shows typical features, including posterior cephalocele and postaxial polydactyly.

gene, the Turner female has only half of the needed protein for development of normal height and skeleton (Fig. 28-18).[21,41]

Sonographic Findings

The classic sonographic finding of Turner syndrome is a cystic hygroma (Fig. 28-19).[3] Renal anomalies related to morphogenesis, such as horseshoe kidney, may also be seen, as well as heart defects, coarctation of aorta,

hydrops, short c-spine, increased nuchal translucency, brachycephaly, hydramnios, and growth retardation.[1,3,16,21,41]

Prognosis

In live-born affected individuals, the abnormalities are many and variable, such as growth and mental deficiencies, congenital lymphedema, ovarian dysgenesis, and renal and cardiac malformations.[3]

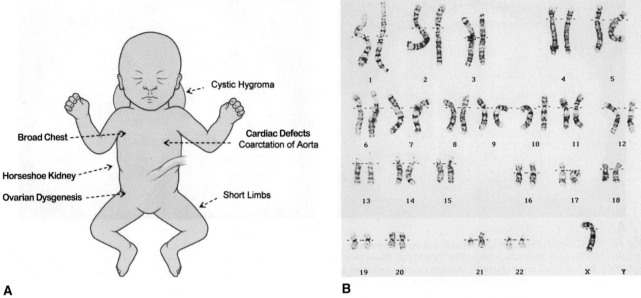

A

B

Figure 28-18 Turner syndrome (45, X). **A:** Common features. **B:** Karyotype showing 45, X.

NOONAN SYNDROME

Description

Phenotypically, the Noonan individual demonstrates hypertelorism, downward slanting eyes, and posteriorly rotated and low-set ears. The short stature, neck webbing, and cardiac anomalies result in comparisons to Turner syndrome.[42] This developmental disorder results in a short individual with heart defects, skeletal malformations, bleeding problems, and eye abnormalities. Occurrence rate is between 1 in 1,000 and 1 in 2,500 births.[21,42]

Lab Values

No lab values specific to Noonan syndrome have been identified.

Genetics

Noonan syndrome is an autosomal dominant[16] condition affecting males and females equally. This syndrome follows a sporadic occurrence because of mutations on chromosome 12.[3,42]

Sonographic Findings

The finding of cystic hygroma[3,16] is similar to Turner syndrome; however, the identification of male genitalia differentiates Noonan syndrome from Turner syndrome. Cardiac anomalies such as pulmonary valve stenosis, atrial septal defects, and ventricular septal defects are frequently seen.[3] Low set ears have also been reported (Fig. 28-20).[3]

Figure 28-19 Sagittal plane through the head and torso of a Turner syndrome fetus demonstrates bilateral cystic hygromas (arrows). These regress, resulting in the typical webbed appearance of the neck. (Image courtesy of Philips Medical Systems, Bothell, WA.)

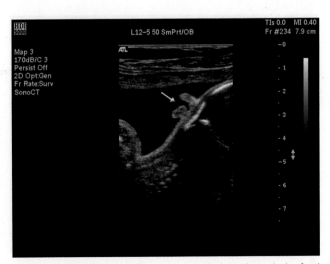

Figure 28-20 An image taken on a coronal plane through the fetal head demonstrates a malformed low-set ear (arrow). (Image courtesy of Philips Medical Systems, Bothell, WA.)

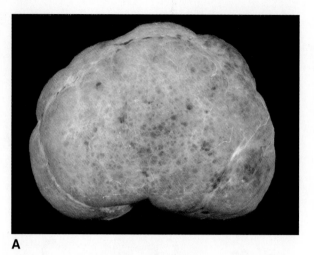

A

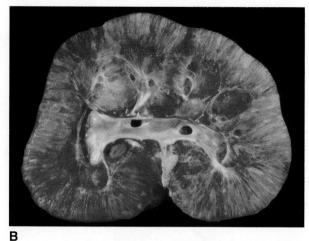

B

Figure 28-21 Gross pathology of neonatal autosomal recessive polycystic kidney disease (ARPKD). Left nephrectomy from a 10-week-old girl. **A:** The kidney is markedly enlarged (weight 745 g). Multiple small cysts are seen through the capsule. Lines of fetal kidney lobulation are apparent. **B:** The renal parenchyma is uniformly cystic, replaced by fusiform cysts that occupy the entire cortex and the medulla. (Courtesy Dr. Ashley Hill, Department of Pathology and Immunology, Washington University, St. Louis, MO.)

Prognosis

The range of effects varies. Two-thirds of individuals have heart defects, and males are sterile because of cryptorchidism.[21] Developmental delays are common.[16]

POTTER SEQUENCE

Description

The pattern of malformations associated with Potter sequence traces its cause to oligiohydramnios,[13] which in turn traces its cause to any number of abnormalities. Oligiohydramnios may be caused by renal anomalies (bilateral renal agenesis, multicystic dysplastic kidneys, genitourinary obstruction), amniotic leakage, or placental anomalies. The diminished amniotic fluid volume impairs normal development of fetal structures and results

in deformities of the extremities, abnormal appearance of facial features (Potter's facies), and pulmonary hypoplasia (Figs. 28-21–22).[2,48] A summary of the types and characteristics of Potter sequence can be found in Table 28-1.

PTERYGIUM SYNDROME

Description

There are four forms of this syndrome, which may be lethal or nonlethal depending on the type.[17,18] This syndrome has a characteristic webbing, called pterygia, in the joints.[16] Neck webbing, often called pterygium colli, also occurs.[3,16] Arthrogryposis, the permanent fixation of a joint in a contracted position, is a characteristic feature of all forms of pterygium syndrome.[16,18,21,65,66] These contractions result in decreased fetal movement.[18,21,65,66]

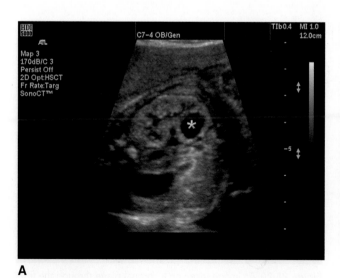

A

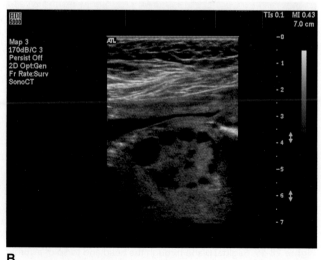

B

Figure 28-22 A cyst (star) located in the lower pole of the right kidney raises suspicion for ARPKD. (Image courtesy of Philips Medical Systems, Bothell, WA.)

TABLE 28-1

Potter Sequence[2,14,16,48,49]

Form	Type	Incidence	Lab	Genetics/Cause	Fetal Sonographic Features	Prognosis
Classic	Bilateral renal agenesis (BRA)	1 in 4,000-10,000 births, occurs with a male to female ratio of 3:1	None	Unknown	Absence of both kidneys, severe oligohydramnios in the second and third trimester, bladder may visualize up to 16 weeks, pulmonary hypoplasia, enlarged adrenal glands fill renal fossa, "lying down" adrenal sign, lack of renal arteries with color-flow Doppler, wide set eyes, receding chin	Fatal
Type I	Autosomal recessive (infantile) polycystic renal disease (ARPKD)	1 in 20,000-50,000 live births	Fetal karyotyping via amniocentesis or CVS	Autosomal recessive, chromosome 6p (PKHD1)	Symmetric enlargement of both kidneys, increased echogenicity, small or absent bladder, oligohydramnios	High fetal and neonatal mortality
Type II	Multicystic renal dysplasia (MCKD)	1 in 3,000 live births, 2/3 unilateral, male predominance	Fetal karyotyping via amniocentesis or CVS	None. Due to nephrogenesis disruptions	Multiple cysts of varying size, oligohydramnios	Good outcome with one normal kidney. Multiple anomalies results in a poor prognosis
Type III	Autosomal dominant (adult) polycystic renal disease (ADPKD)	1 in 1,000 live births	Fetal karyotyping via amniocentesis or CVS	Autosomal dominant, Mutation in chromosome 16 telomere (PKD1); small number caused by chromosome 4 (PKD2) anomalies	Symmetric enlargement of both kidneys, increased echogenicity, indistinct or accentuated corticomedullary junction, usually bilateral, oligohydramnios	Large portion die in the first year, hypertension by 12 months, renal failure by 36 months
Type IV	Obstructive cystic dysplasia	1 in 8,000 live births, bilateral dysplasia in 40%	Fetal karyotyping via amniocentesis or CVS	Due to early renal obstruction	Small echogenic kidneys, cortical cysts, hydronephrosis, severe bladder outlet obstruction, "keyhole" bladder, thick-walled bladder, severe oligohydramnios	Bilateral disease has a poor prognosis; unilateral dependent on normalcy and coexisting anomalies

PATHOLOGY BOX 28-7

Pterygium Syndrome[3,16,17,18,21,60,61]

	Incidence	Lab	Genetics	Sonographic Findings	Prognosis
Lethal multiple pterygium syndrome	Unknown	None specific	Mendelian disorder, autosomal recessive, X-linked genes; CHRND, CHRNA1, CHRNG, PIP5K1C, GLE1	First trimester; thickened nuchal lucency extending to the entire body, hydrops, cystic hygroma. Second trimester; multiple pterygia, IUGR, polyhydramnios, craniofacial/ocular anomalies, short forearms, pulmonary hypoplasia, scoliosis, fractures, hypoplastic lungs, spinal fusion, low-set ears	Lethal
Multiple pterygium syndrome (Escobar syndrome/ nonlethal arthrygryposis multiplex congenita)	Unknown	None specific	Mendelian disorder, autosomal recessive genes; IRF6, CHRND, CHRNA1, CHRNG, PIP5K1C, GLE1	Extremity contractures, pterygia, micrognathia, camptodactyly, syndactyly, rocker bottom feet, vertical clubfoot, abnormal genitalia, microcephaly, low-set ears, cleft palate/lip, spinal fusion, ocular hypertelorism, diaphragmatic hernia	Normal intelligence
Popliteal pterygium syndrome non-lethal type	1 in 300,000	None specific	Autosomal dominant genes; IRF6, CHRNG	Cleft lip/palate, popliteal pterygium, missing teeth, syndactyly, malformed genitalia, spina bifida occulta, clubfoot	Normal intelligence, delayed language development, learning disability
Popliteal pterygium syndrome, lethal type	Unknown	None specific	Autosomal recessive IRF6, CHRNG	Popliteal pterygium, synostosis, digital hypoplasia, syndactyly, cleft lip/palate, hypoplastic nose	Lethal

TRIPLOIDY

Description

Triploidy is the presence of a complete extra set of chromosomes.[1,21] The condition is thought to occur in 2% of conceptions and most result in miscarriage.[44] The incidence rate is 1 in 2,500 live births.[16] Only 3% of fetuses affected with triploidy (specifically 69 XYY, XXX, or XXY)[45] survive.

Lab Values

First-trimester screening demonstrates an elevation in the MSAFP and hCG and low PAPP-A.[47] In the second trimester the hCG may be low due to small placenta,[44] low estriol, with a low or normal AFP.[47] A central nervous system or ventral wall defect would result in an increased AFP.[16] In the case of a partial mole, inhibin A values increase.[16]

Genetics

Ninety percent of triploidy pregnancies are due to two sperm fertilizing one egg (diandry) or from an extra chromosome set from the mother (digyny)[16,44] Over half of triploidy fertilizations due to dual sperm result in a miscarriage, whereas maternal triploidy predominates in live births (Fig. 28-23).[44]

Sonographic Findings

Affected embryos and fetuses demonstrate multiple anomalies depending on which parent provided the extra set of chromosomes. In the event of the extra chromosomes coming from the father, a large, hydropic placenta with a small symmetrical IUGR fetus is often seen.[16,44] The placenta for this triploidy configuration is considered a partial hydatiform mole.[44] If the mother contributed the extra chromosomes, the opposite occurs: a fetus with asymmetric IUGR and a small placenta.[16,45] In the first trimester, nuchal thickening can be seen.[16] Structural anomalies frequently seen in a fetus with triploidy include hypertelorism, hydrocephalus, holoprosencephaly, micrognathia, syndactyly, clubfoot, atrial septal defects, adrenal hypoplasia, and ventricular septal defects (Fig. 28-24).[1,16,44]

Prognosis

Rarely do neonates survive beyond the first two months,[44] and none survive past the first year.[47]

TRISOMY 13 (PATAU SYNDROME)

Description

Trisomy 13 is a chromosomal condition that results in a pattern of malformations that cause a high rate of both intrauterine and neonatal death.[43] Patau syndrome

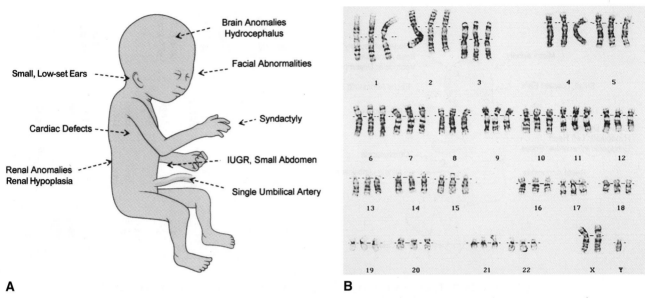

A

B

Figure 28-23 Cells with an additional set of chromosomes are considered triploid, resulting in a chromosome count of 69.

has a prevalence of 1 in 5,000 to 16,000 live births.[15,16] Advanced maternal age increases the probability of this malformation occurring.[21]

Lab Values

Maternal triple screening in the second trimester is not of benefit; however, the quadruple screen does show some benefit. An increase in the inhibin levels correlates with the presence of trisomy 13.[16] The AFP increases in the presence of a central nervous system or ventral wall defect.[16] In the first trimester the β hCG and PAPP-A are reduced.[16]

Genetics

The extra set of chromosomes disrupt normal embryonic development, causing the characteristic malformations seen with trisomy 13.[21] This is a chromosomal

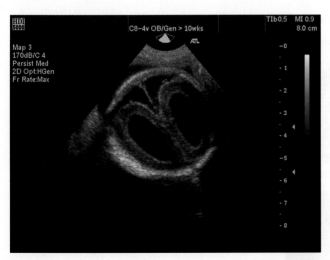

Figure 28-24 Dilated ventricles indicate the presence of hydrocephalus. (Image courtesy of Philips Medical Systems, Bothell, WA.)

PATHOLOGY BOX 28-8

Typical Pathologic and Clinical Features of Triploidy

Growth	Severe growth delay
	Head-abdomen discordance with small abdominal circumference hypotonia
Central nervous system/ neurologic	Holoprosencephaly
	Hydrocephalus
	Agenesis of the corpus callosum
	Myelomeningocele
Cardiovascular	Cardiac defects
Craniofacial	Microphthalmos
	Hypertelorism
	Colobomas
	Facial asymmetry
	Low-set, malformed ears
	Cleft lip/palate
	Micrognathia
	Nuchal thickening/increased nuchal translucency/cystic hygroma
Skeletal	Syndactyly, especially third and fourth digits
	Clubfeet
Gastrointestinal	Omphalocele
	Umbilical hernia
Genitourinary	Cystic dysplasia
	Hydronephrosis
	Renal hypoplasia
	Adrenal hypoplasia
	Hypospadias
	Cryptorchidism

Reproduced with permission from McKusick VA, ed. Online Mendelian inheritance in man. http://www.ncbi.nlm.nih.gov/omim/. McKusick-Nathans Institute for Genetic Medicine, Johns Hopkins University (Baltimore, MD) and National Center for Biotechnology Information, National Library of Medicine (Bethesda, MD), 2000.

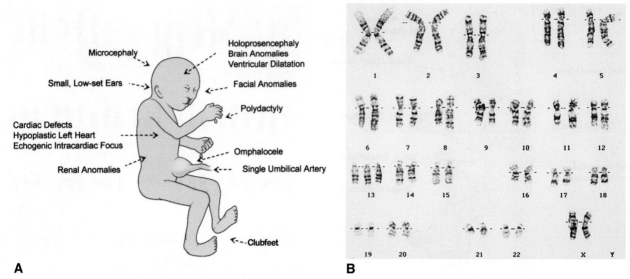

Figure 28-25 Trisomy 13. **A:** Common features. **B:** Karyotype showing trisomy 13.

anomaly of nondisjunction, mosaicism, or translocation resulting from an extra chromosome in the 13th set (trisomy 13).[16,21] The nondisjunction of the chromosomes occurs with meiosis and is a random, noninheritable event.[21] Translocation of the gene occurs early in embryonic development or during gamete production, which results in an extra inheritable 13th chromosome. A full translocation results in the full spectrum of malformations; however, it is possible to have a translocation.[21] The clinical presentation in these individuals depends on which portion of the chromosome translocates. A mosaic trisomy 13 is a person with the extra chromosome in some of his or her cells. The presentation of clinical signs of this form of trisomy 13 depends on which and how many cells have the abnormal number. (Fig. 28-25).[21]

Sonographic Findings

Common findings seen sonographically in individuals with Patau syndrome include cleft lip, cleft palate, ventricular septal defects, holoprosencephaly, microcephaly, micrognathia, polydactyly, and single umbilical artery[1,15,16,21] Other anomalies less frequently associated with Patau syndrome include omphalocele, syndactyly,

Trisomy 13

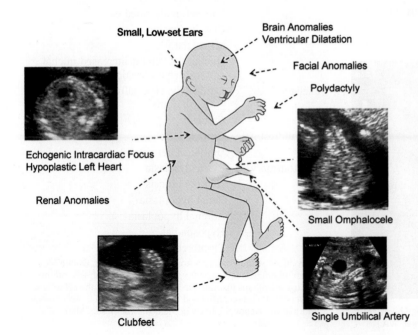

Figure 28-26 Sonographic markers or subtle abnormalities of trisomy 13. This does not include major abnormalities such as holoprosencephaly, cleft lip/palate, cardiac defects, and renal anomalies.

clubfoot (talipes), renal anomalies, agenesis of the corpus callosum, cerebellar hypoplasia, and meningomyelocele (Fig. 28-26).[1,16] In the first trimester, nuchal thickening can be seen.[16]

Prognosis

The median survival for Patau syndrome is two and a half days, and 82% of affected individuals die within the first month of life.[15,21]

TRISOMY 18 (EDWARD SYNDROME)

Description

Trisomy 18 was first described in 1960. It occurs in 1 in 3,000 conceptions and is seen in 1 in 5–8,000 live births,[15,21] making it the second most common of the trisomies that carry to term. Affected individuals are predominantly female, demonstrating a 3:1 prevalence[16,21] due to the higher mortality rate of male fetuses with trisomy 18.[16] Maternal age increases the chances of conceiving a child with trisomy 18.[21]

Lab Values

Using any combination of markers (AFP, estriol, free α hCG, free β hCG, estradiol, and human placental lactogen) results in a high detection rate.[16] The triple screen, which includes unconjugated estriol, hCG, and AFP, return with low values.[15,16] Inhibin A does not increase detection rates; however, it has been found that PAPP-A is one of the more discriminating tests for trisomy 18.[16] During the first trimester, free beta hCG and PAPP-A are reduced.[16]

Genetics

Chromosomal anomaly of nondisjunction, mosaicism, translocation[16] occurs in a manner similar to trisomy 13.[21] The noninheritable anomaly occurs during meiosis, whereas the inheritable form is due to translocation of the 18th chromosome (Fig. 28-27).[21]

Sonographic Findings

A majority of affected fetuses demonstrate micrognathia and microcephaly.[21] In particular, a prominent occiput creates the appearance of a "strawberry"-shaped skull. Cardiac anomalies (atrial and ventricular septal defects) and clenching of the hands are also seen in a majority of individuals.[1,21] Other frequent findings include cleft lip and cleft palate, syndactyly, omphalocele, rocker-bottom feet, clubfoot, renal anomalies, congenital diaphragmatic hernia, cerebellar hypoplasia, and meningomyelocele.[1,16] Occasional findings include hypertelorism and choroid plexus cysts.[1] The findings of small for gestational age or IUGR is due to decreased analytes, suggesting placental hormone secretion and/or synthesis and hydramnios (Fig. 28-28).[16] In the first trimester, nuchal thickening can be seen, greater than with trisomy 21 (Fig. 28-29).[16]

Prognosis

Outcomes are poor for affected individuals. The survival rate is low, with only 50% living to 2 months, and only 5% to 10% surviving 1 year.[16,21] The median lifespan is 5 to 15 days.

TRISOMY 21 (DOWN SYNDROME)

Description

The most common pattern of malformation in man,[43] this syndrome was first described by John Langdon Down in 1866. This chromosomal abnormality results in an individual with intellectual disabilities,

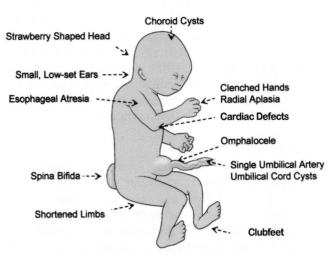

A

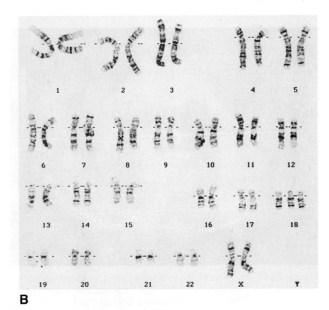

B

Figure 28-27 Trisomy 18. **A:** Common features. **B:** Karyotype showing trisomy 18.

Trisomy 18

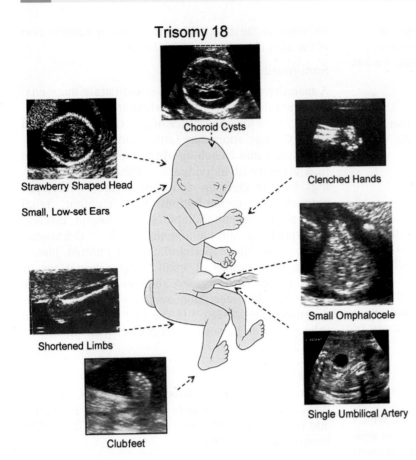

Choroid Cysts

Strawberry Shaped Head

Small, Low-set Ears

Clenched Hands

Small Omphalocele

Single Umbilical Artery

Shortened Limbs

Clubfeet

Figure 28-28 Sonographic markers or subtle abnormalities of trisomy 18. This does not include major abnormalities such as cardiac defects, cystic hygroma, radial aplasia, spina bifida, esophageal atresia, or cerebellar anomalies.

characteristic facial appearances, and neonatal hypotonia. Approximately half of fetuses with trisomy 21 have accompanying heart and gastric anomalies.[21] Attributed to the presence of an extra chromosome in the 21st set, trisomy 21 is seen in approximately 1 in 800 births, with an increase of incidence with advanced maternal age.[1,21]

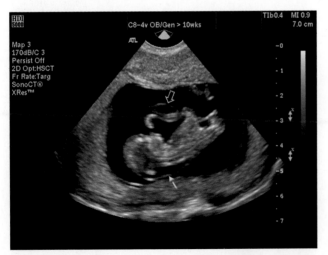

Figure 28-29 An 11-week fetus demonstrating an abnormally thick nuchal lucency (*arrow*) and an umbilical cord cyst (*open arrow*). (Image courtesy of Philips Medical Systems, Bothell, WA.)

Lab Values

There is no one test that identifies a trisomy 21 fetus. The highest detection rates occur with a combination of laboratory tests and sonography. Unconjugated estriol, PAPP-A, and AFP are known to be low, whereas hCG and inhibin A show elevated values (Table 28-2).[16]

Genetics

Maternal nondisjunction accounts for 95% of cases, with an increasing incidence with increasing maternal age. The remainder are the result of mosaicism (2%) or translocation (3%).[16,21] Trisomy 21 usually is a random event and cannot be inherited in the classic and mosaic form. If the syndrome is due to a translocation, the individual may not show signs but has an increased risk of having children with Down syndrome (Fig. 28-30).[21]

Sonographic Findings

Down syndrome has been extensively studied sonographically. There are several strategies for using sonography to evaluate and score the findings associated with Down syndrome, with the aim of achieving a sonographic diagnosis of the condition (Fig. 28-31). The common structural defects and soft sonographic markers associated with aneuploidy are listed in Table 28-3.

TABLE 28-2

Analyte and Sonographic Markers in the Most Common Aneuploidies in the Second Trimester[1,16,47,52–59]

Anomaly	hCG/β hCG	AFP	uE3	Inhibin A	PAPP-A	NT
Trisomy 21	↑	↓	↓	↑	↓	↑
Trisomy 18	↓	↓	↓	Normal	↓	↑
Trisomy 13	Normal	Small ↑	Normal	Normal	↓	↑
Turner syndrome	↑ with hydrops	Small ↓	Small ↓	↓	↓	↑
Other sex aneuploidies	Normal or ↑	Normal or ↑	Normal	NA	NA	↑
Triploidy Type 1	↑	Normal or ↑	↓	↓	Mildly ↓	↑
Triploidy Type 2	↓	↓	↓	NA	↓	Normal

HCG, Human chorionic gonadotropin; AFP, alpha-fetoprotein; uE₃, Unconjugated estriol; PAPP-A, pregnancy-associated plasma protein A; NT, nuchal translucency; NA, not available
↑ – increased
↓ – decreased

Prognosis

Most affected individuals have varying degrees of mental deficiency and hypotonia.[16,21] Mortality is often associated with cardiac defects. The median life span for affected individuals is 49 years.

VATER/VACTERL ASSOCIATION

Description

VATER association is a collection of anomalies that include vertebral defects, anal atresia, tracheoesophageal (TE) fistula, and renal anomalies.[16] The current term, VACTERL, includes vertebral defects, anorectal atresia, cardiac anomalies, TE fistula, and renal and limb anomalies.[16] Both terms are used, demonstrating the difficulty in defining this group of malformations. The pattern of anomalies may occur in an otherwise normal child, or they may be seen in individuals affected by a chromosomal abnormality. This uncommon defect has an unknown incidence (Fig. 28-32).[16]

Lab Values

There is no one specific lab test that would identify a fetus with VATER/VACTERL association. An occipital encephalocele or open spinal defect would result in an elevated AFP.

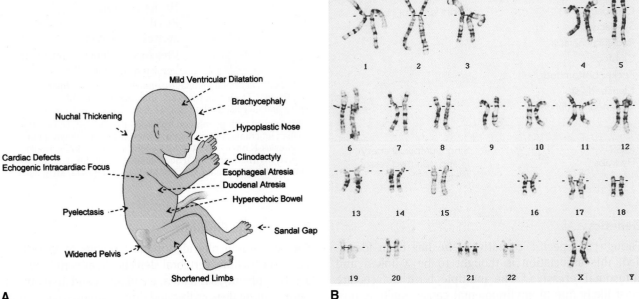

A Common features of trisomy 21

Mild Ventricular Dilatation
Brachycephaly
Nuchal Thickening
Hypoplastic Nose
Cardiac Defects
Echogenic Intracardiac Focus
Clinodactyly
Esophageal Atresia
Duodenal Atresia
Hyperechoic Bowel
Pyelectasis
Sandal Gap
Widened Pelvis
Shortened Limbs

B Karyotype showing trisomy 21

Figure 28-30 A: Common features of trisomy 21. **B:** Karyotype showing trisomy 21.

TABLE 28-3

Trisomy 21 Findings[1,15,16,47,50]

Structural Defects	Soft Markers
Brain/Head/Neck	
Ventriculomegaly	Choroid plexus cysts
Holoprosencephaly	Nuchal fold thickening
Hyper/hypotelorism	Hypoplastic or absent
Cleft palate/lip	nasal bone
Micrognathia	
Low-set ears	
Small ear	
Macroglossia	
Cystic hygroma	
Microcephaly	
Dysgenesis of the corpus callosum	
Shortened frontal lobe	
Heart	
Ventricular septal defect	Echogenic cardiac focus
Atrioventricular canal defect	
Endocardial cushion defect	
Hypoplastic left heart syndrome	
Tetralogy of Fallot	
Abdomen	
Third trimester esophageal and duodenal atresias	Echogenic bowel renal pyelectasis ≥4
Small bowel obstruction	
Diaphragmatic hernia	
Omphalocele	
Hydronephrosis	
Renal agenesis	
Dysplastic renal disease	
Widened pelvic angle	
Musculoskeletal	
Clinodactyly	Short femur or humerus
Syndactyly	
Radial ray aplasia	
Clubfoot	
Rocker bottom foot	
Clenched fist	
Widened sandal gap	
Other	
IUGR	Single umbilical artery and vein (two vessel cord)
Hydrops	

PATHOLOGY BOX 28-9

Pathologic and Clinical Features of VATER/VACTERL Syndrome

Growth	Growth Delay
Central nervous system/neurologic	Spinal dysraphia
	Occipital encephalocele
	Hydrocephalus
Cardiovascular	Ventricular septal defect
	Patent ductus arteriosus
	Tetralogy of Fallot
	Transposition of the great arteries
	Single umbilical artery
Craniofacial	Cleft lip/palate
Respiratory/chest	Choanal atresia
	Laryngeal stenosis
	Tracheal agenesis
	Rib anomalies
	Sternal anomalies
Skeletal	Vertebral anomalies
	Scoliosis
	Radial aplasia
	Radial hypoplasia
	Radioulnar synostosis
	Preaxial polydactyly
	Vertebral abnormalities (fusion, hemivertebrae)
	Absent or hypoplastic thumbs
	Syndactyly
	Triphalangeal thumb
Gastrointestinal	TE fistula
	Esophageal atresia
	Anal atresia
Genitourinary	Hypospadias
	Renal aplasia
	Renal dysplasia
	Hydronephrosis
	Renal ectopia
	Vesicoureteral reflux
	Ureteropelvic junction obstruction
	Persistent urachus

VACTERL, vertebral anomalies, anorectal atresia, cardiac anomalies, TE fistula, renal and limb anomalies; VATER, vertebral defects, anal atresia, TE fistula, and renal anomalies.

Reproduced with permission from McKusick VA, ed. Online Mendelian inheritance in man. http://www.ncbi.nlm.nih.gov/omim/. McKusick-Nathans Institute for Genetic Medicine, Johns Hopkins University (Baltimore, MD) and National Center for Biotechnology Information, National Library of Medicine (Bethesda, MD), 2000.

Genetics

Though no specific causative gene has been identified, this association is thought to be X-linked and autosomal-recessive.[3] The multiple birth defects are most likely due to environmental causes such as progesterone-estrogen, BCP[2], lead exposure, and maternal diabetes.[2,16]

Sonographic Findings

The sonographically identifiable findings of VATER association include vertebral defects (hemivertebrae, spinal dysraphism), TE fistula, esophageal and anal atresia, cardiac anomalies, radius and thumb abnormalities, limb dysplasia, preaxial polydactyly, and renal anomalies.[3,16] Affected individuals may also have growth deficiencies.

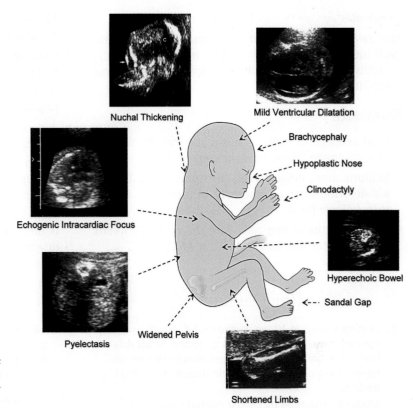

Figure 28-31 Common sonographic markers of trisomy 21. This does not include major structural defects such as cardiac defects, cystic hygroma, or duodenal atresia.

Nuchal Thickening

Mild Ventricular Dilatation

Brachycephaly

Hypoplastic Nose

Clinodactyly

Echogenic Intracardiac Focus

Hyperechoic Bowel

Sandal Gap

Widened Pelvis

Pyelectasis

Shortened Limbs

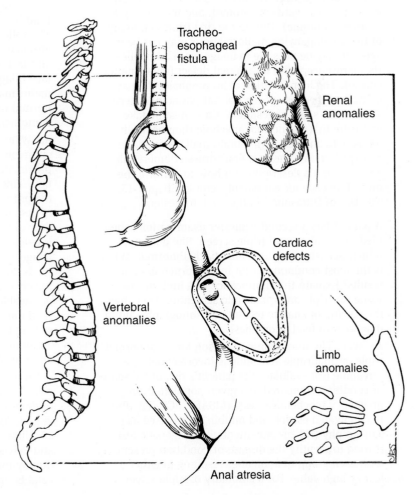

Tracheo-esophageal fistula

Renal anomalies

Cardiac defects

Vertebral anomalies

Limb anomalies

Anal atresia

Figure 28-32 The VACTERL association: vertebral anomalies, anal atresia, cardiac defects, TE fistula, renal and limb anomalies.

Prognosis

The severity and type of malformations determine each individual's prognosis.[16] The majority of affected individuals do well with surgical correction and rehabilitation.

SUMMARY

- Fetal anomaly classification is made through the use of a syndrome, association, or sequence.

- Malformation, deformation, disruption, and dysplasia describe how an anomaly influences a fetus's morphologic form.

- Mitosis results in two cells with the normal haploid number of chromosomes (46XX or 46XY).

- Meiosis results in two cells with half the normal haploid number of chromosomes (23X or 23Y).

- Chromosomal anomalies may be due to deletion, insertion, inversion, or translocation.

- A genetic trait inherited in the presence of a gene, regardless of sex, is an autosomal dominant trait.

- A genetic trait expressed in an individual requiring two genes is considered autosomal recessive.

- When a mother carries a gene that expresses itself in a male child, this is considered an X-linked chromosome.

- Prenatal testing for detection of fetal abnormalities is done through a combination of the triple screen, quadruple screen, and ultrasound.

Critical Thinking Questions

1. During a routine 10-week size and dates, the nuchal lucency measures larger than expected. With this finding, what additional images should the sonographer obtain? List the possible differentials for this finding.

   ANSWER: Although increased nuchal translucency is often tied to trisomy 21 (Down syndrome), it is also associated with trisomy 13 (Patau syndrome), trisomy 18 (Edwards syndrome), and monosomy X (Turner syndrome). During the first trimester, many of the accompanying malformations may not be imaged. It may be possible to image brain anomalies (holoprosencephaly) or a spinal defect (myelomeningocele). The identification of an omphalocele may be difficult because of the normal physiologic hernia seen at this stage of gestation. Care must be taken to ensure that the normal anechoic rhombencephalon is not confused with a brain malformation. For an explanation of normal first-trimester embryonic anatomy and a description on how to perform the nuchal lucency measurement, refer to Chapter 13, The Use of Ultrasound in the First Trimester.

2. A patient has a second-trimester examination scheduled for an abnormal triple screen. She does not remember which values came back abnormal. What is the most common reason for abnormal analyte results? Explain the significance of a high or low value for triple and quadruple screening. How does the pairing of analyte testing and sonography aid in diagnosis of fetal anomalies?

   ANSWER: The most common reason for an abnormal triple or quadruple screening is incorrect dates. A screening test evaluates the patient's risk of a disease or condition compared to a given population. In pregnancy biochemical tests (MSAFP, hCG, PAAP-A, unconjugated estriol, and inhibin A) are used as is sonography (NT measurements). A diagnostic test is used to identify the disease or condition present, with each group of anomalies resulting in either a low or high value. For a summary of triple screen test results, refer to Table 28-3. Sonography can identify structural abnormalities with a high degree of accuracy and can also identify certain chromosomal conditions with a high degree of confidence.

3. A patient had a routine size and dates sonographic exam at 18 weeks. At that time, several fetal structures were not imaged well, including the fetal kidneys. The imaged anatomy, placental location, and fluid level appeared normal for the gestational age. The follow-up exam, done at 30 weeks, revealed the absence of kidneys, a male fetus, oligohydramnios, and lack of renal artery flow. The fetal profile and face images appeared abnormal. Identify the type of malformation. Explain why the fluid level appeared normal in the first trimester and the follow-up exam demonstrated oligohydramnios.

   ANSWER: Fetal kidneys begin development early in embryonic life. By the end of the first trimester, at approximately 9 weeks, the kidneys begin urine formation. This continues throughout fetal life, becoming the primary source of amniotic fluid after 16 weeks of gestation. In the first trimester, fetal functions add little to the amniotic volume within the amnion. This is evidenced in the failed pregnancy when we fail to image an embryo. At this stage, the fluid within the sac is due to production by the placenta. At approximately 4 months, the fetal skin keratinizes, ending the permeable barrier that allows exchange of amniotic fluid into and out of the fetus via diffusion. In the second half of a pregnancy, the primary sources of amniotic fluid are the fetal kidneys and lungs. This is an example of a classic case of Potter's sequence.

   For a description of development of normal kidneys, refer to Chapter 2, Embryonic Development of the Female Genital System. For the normal sonographic appearance of fetal kidneys, refer to Chapter 20, Ultrasound of the Normal Fetal Chest, Abdomen, and Pelvis. An explanation of amniotic fluid production by the placenta can be found in Chapter 17, The Fetal Environment.

REFERENCES

1. Norton ME. Genetics and prenatal diagnosis. In: Callen P, ed. *Ultrasonography in Obstetrics and Gynecology*. 5th ed. Philadelphia: Saunders Elsevier; 2008.

2. Moore KL, Persaud TVN. *The Developing Human*. 8th ed. Philadelphia: Saunders; 2008.

3. Leite JM, Granese R, Jeanty P, et al. Fetal syndromes. In: Callen P, ed. *Ultrasonography in Obstetrics and Gynecology*. 5th ed. Philadelphia: Saunders Elsevier; 2008.

4. Sauerbrei EE. The fetal spine. In Callen P, ed. *Ultrasonography in Obstetrics and Gynecology*. 5th ed. Philadelphia: Saunders Elsevier; 2008.

5. Sicuranza GB, Steinberg P, Figueroa R. Arnold-Chiari malformation in a pregnant woman. *Obstetrics Gynecology*. 2003;102(5 Pt 2):1191–1194.

6. Chiari Malformation Fact Sheet. National Institute of Neurological Disorders and Stroke. http://www.ninds.nih.gov/disorders/chiari/detail_chiari.htm. Accessed June 2010.

7. Blencowe H, Cousens S, Modell B, et al. Folic acid to reduce neonatal mortality from neural tube disorders. *Int J Epidemiol*. 2010;(39 Suppl 1):i110–i121.

8. Callen AL, Filly RA. Supratentorial abnormalities in the Chiari II malformation, I: the ventricular "point". *J Ultrasound Med*. 2008;27(1):33–38.

9. Peregrine E, Pandya P. Structural anomalies in the first trimester. In: Rumack CM, Wilson SR, Charboneau JW, Johnson JM, eds. *Diagnostic Ultrasound*. 3rd ed. St. Louis: Elsevier Mosby; 2005.

10. Smith AS, Grable I, Levine D. Case 66: caudal regression syndrome in the fetus of a diabetic mother. *Radiology*. 2004;230(1):229–233.

11. Cameron M, Moran P. Prenatal screening and diagnosis of neural tube defects. *Prenat Diagn*. 2009;29:402–411.

12. Rumack CM, Drose JA. Neonatal and infant brain imaging. In: Rumack CM, Wilson SR, Charboneau JW, Johnson JM, eds. *Diagnostic Ultrasound*. 3rd ed. St. Louis: Elsevier Mosby; 2005.

13. Blaas HG, Eriksson AG, Salvesen KA, et al. Brains and faces in holoprosencephaly: pre and postnatal description of 30 cases. *Ultrasound Obstet Gynecol*. 2002;19(1):24.

14. Avni FE, Maugey-Laulom B, Cassart M, et al. The fetal genitorurinary tract. In: Callen P, ed. *Ultrasonography in Obstetrics and Gynecology*. 5th ed. Philadelphia: Saunders Elsevier; 2008.

15. Yeo L, Vintzileos AM. The second trimester genetic sonogram. In Callen P, ed. *Ultrasonography in Obstetrics and Gynecology*. 5th ed. Philadelphia: Saunders Elsevier; 2008.

16. Nyberg DA, McGahan JP, Pretorius DH, et al. *Diagnostic Imaging of Fetal Anomalies*. Philadelphia: Lippincott Williams & Wilkins; 2003.

17. *Multiple Pterygium Syndrome, Lethal Type*. Online Mendelian Inheritance in Man. http://www.ncbi.nlm.nih.gov/omim/253290. Accessed July 2010.

18. *Multiple Pterygium Syndrome, Escobar Variant*. Online Mendelian Inheritance in Man. http://www.ncbi.nlm.nih.gov/omim/265000. Accessed July 2010.

19. Newell ML, Borja MC, Peckham C, et al. Height, weight, and growth in children born to mothers with HIV-1 in Europe. *Pediatrics*. 2003;111(1): e52–e60.

20. Aicardi J, Crow YJ, Stephenson JBP. Aicardi-Goutières syndrome. In: Pagon RA, Bird TC, Dolan CR, Stephens K, eds. *GeneReviews* [Internet]. Seattle (WA): University of Washington, Seattle; 1993–2005 [updated 2008 Apr 17].

21. National Library of Medicine. Genetics Home Reference. August 1, 2011. http://ghr.nlm.nih.gov/. Accessed August 4, 2011.

22. Paladini D, Foglia S, Sglavo G, et al. Congenital constriction band of the upper arm: the role of three-dimensional ultrasound in diagnosis, counseling and multidisciplinary consultation. *Ultrasound Obstet Gynecol*. 2004;23(5):520–522.

23. Narea Matamala G, Fernández Toro Mde L, Villalabeitía Ugarte E, et al. Beckwith Wiedemann syndrome: presentation of a case report. *Med Oral Patol Oral Cir Bucal*. 2008;13(10):E640–E643.

24. Ortiz-Neira CL, Traubici J, Alan D, et al. Sonographic assessment of renal growth in patients with Beckwith-Wiedemann syndrome: the Beckwith-Wiedemann syndrome renal nomogram. *Clinics (Sao Paulo)*. 2009;64(1):41–44.

25. Amor DJ, Halliday J. A review of known imprinting syndromes and their association with assisted reproduction technologies. *Hum Reprod*. 2008;23(12):2826–2834.

26. Owen MC, Segars Jr JH. Imprinting disorders and assisted reproductive technology. *Semin Reprod Med*. 2009; 27(5):417–428.

27. Titomanlio L, Giurgea I, Sachs P, et al. A locus for sacral/anorectal malformations maps to 6q25.3 in a 0.3 Mb interval region. *Eur J Hum Genet*. 2006;14(8):971–974.

28. Pavone P, Ruggieri M, Lombardo I, et al. Microcephaly, sensorieural deafness and Currarino triad with duplication-deletion of distal 7q. *Eur J Pediatr*. 2010;169(4):475–481.

29. Samartis D, Shen FH. Caudal regression syndrome. *Ann Acad Med Singapore*. 2008;37(5):446.

30. Wilmhurst JM, Kelly R, Borzyskowski MB. Presentation and outcome of sacral agenesis: 20 years' experience. *Dev Med Child Neurol*. 1999;41(12):806–812.

31. Lalani SR, Hefner MA, Belmont JW, et al. CHARGE Syndrome. *GENEREVIEWS*. http://www.ncbi.nlm.nih.gov/bookshelf/br.fcgi?book = gene&part = charge. Accessed July 2010.

32. *Charge Syndrome*. Online Mendelian Inheritance in Man. http://www.ncbi.nlm.nih.gov/omim/214800. Accessed July 2010.

33. Global Measles and Rubella Laboratory Network. January 2004–June 2005. Center for Disease Control MMWR Weekly. 2005;54(43):1100–1104. http://www.cdc.gov/mmwr/preview/mmwrhtml/mm5443a3.htm. Accessed July 2010.

34. Kroner BL, Preiss LR, Ardini MA, et al. New incidence, prevalence and survival of Aicardi syndrome from 408 cases. *J Child Neurol*. 2008;23(5):531–535.

35. Vinay C, Reddy RS, Uloopi KS, et al. Craniofacial features in Goldenhar syndrome. *J Indian Soc Pedod Prev Dent*. 2009;27(2):121–124.

36. Mehta B, Nayak C, Savant S, et al. Goldenhar syndrome with unusual features. *Indian J Dermatol Venereol Leprol*. 2008;74(3):254–256.

37. Kita D, Munemoto S, Ueno Y, et al. Goldenhar's syndrome associated with occipital meningoencephalocele—case report. *Neurol Med Chir (Tokyo)*. 2002;42(8):354–355.

38. Monni G, Zoppi MA, Ibba RM, et al. Nuchal translucency in multiple pregnancies. *Croat Med J*. 2000;41(3):266–269.

39. Prasun P, Behera BK, Pradhan M. Limb body wall complex. *Indian J Pathol Microbiol*. 2008;51(2):255–256.

40. *Meckel Syndrome*. Online Mendelian Inheritance in Man. http://www.ncbi.nlm.nih.gov/omim/249000. Accessed July 2010.

41. Kannan TP, Azman BZ, Ahmad Tarmizi AB, et al. Turner syndrome diagnoses in northeastern Malaysia. *Singapore Med J.* 2008;49(5):400–404.

42. *Noonan Syndrome.* Online Mendelian Inheritance in Man. http://www.ncbi.nlm.nih.gov/omim/163950. Accessed July 2010.

43. Sieroszewski P, Perenc M, Basaa-Budecka E, et al. Ultrasound diagnostic schema for the determination of increased risk for chromosomal fetal aneuploidies in the first half of pregnancy. *J Appl Genet.* 2006;47(2):177–185.

44. McFadden DE, Robinson WP. Phenotype of triploid embryos. *J Med Genet.* 2006;43(7):609–612.

45. *Chromosomes in cells – Human Molecular Genetics.* NCBI Bookshelf. http://www.ncbi.nlm.nih.gov/bookshelf/br.fcgi?book=hmg&part=A196#bottom. Accessed July 2010.

46. Tsiga A, Dimopoulou D, Voyiatzis N, et al. Long survival in a 69, XXX triploid infant in Greece. *Genet Mol Res.* 2005;4(4):755–759.

47. *Birth defect risk factor series: Triploidy.* Texas Department of State Health Services Birth Defects Epidemiology and Surveillance. http://www.dshs.state.tx.us/birthdefects/risk/risk24-triploidy.shtm. Accessed July 2010.

48. Liapis H, Winyard PJ. Cystic diseases and development kidney defects. In: *Heptinstall's Pathology of the Kidney.* 6th ed. Philadelphia: Wolters Klewer Health/Lippincott Williams & Wilkins; 2007.

49. Fong KW, Maxwell CV, Ryan G. The fetal urogenital tract. In: Rumack CM, Wilson SR, Charboneau JW, Johnson JM, eds. *Diagnostic Ultrasound.* 3rd ed. St. Louis: Elsevier Mosby; 2005.

50. Raniga S, Desai PD, Parikh H. Ultrasonograhic soft markers of aneuploidy in second trimester: are we lost? *MedGenMed.* 2006;8(1):9.

51. Shaw-Smith C. Oesophageal atresia, tracheo-oesophageal fistula, and the VACTERL association: review of genetics and epidemiology. *J Med Genet.* 2006;43(7):545–554.

52. Malone FD. First trimester screening for aneupleudy. In: Callen P, ed. *Ultrasonography in Obstetrics and Gynecology.* 5th ed. Philadelphia: Saunders Elsevier; 2008.

53. Lambert-Messerlian GM, Saller DN Jr, Tumber MB, et al. Second-trimester maternal serum inhibin A levels in fetal trisomy 18 and Turner syndrome with and without hydrops. *Prenat Diagn.* 1998;18(10):1061–1067.

54. Souter VL, Nyberg DA. Sonographic screening for fetal aneuploidy: first trimester. *J Ultrasound Med.* 2001;20(7):775–790.

55. Watanabe H, Hamada H, Yamada N, et al. Second-trimester maternal pregnancy-associated plasma protein a and inhibin a levels in fetal trisomies. *Fetal Diagn Ther.* 2002;17(3):137–141.

56. Akolekar R, Pérez Penco JM, Skyfta E, et al. Maternal serum placental protein 13 at eleven to thirteen weeks in chromosomally abnormal pregnancies. *Fetal Diagn Ther.* 2010;27(2):72–77.

57. Barsoom MJ, McEntaffer A, Fleming A, et al. Marked abnormal quadruple screen in a patient with severe preeclapsia at 20 weeks with a triploid fetus. *J Matern Fetal Neonatal Med.* 2006;19(7):443–444.

58. Barken SS, Skibsted L, Jensen LN, et. al. Diagnosis and prediction of parental origin of triploidies by fetal nuchal translucency and maternal serum free beta-hCG and PAPP-A at 11–14 weeks of gestation. *Acta Obstet Gynecol Scand.* 2008;87(9):975–978.

59. Huang T, Alberman E, Wald N, et al. Triploidy identified through second-trimester screening. *Prenat Diagn.* 2005;25(3);229–233.

60. *Popliteal Pterygium Syndrome.* PPS. Online Mendelian Inheritance in Man. http://www.ncbi.nlm.nih.gov/omim/119500. Accessed July 2010.

61. *Popliteal Pterygium Syndrome, Lethal Type.* Online Mendelian Inheritance in Man. http://www.ncbi.nlm.nih.gov/omim/263650. Accessed July 2010.

29 Effects of Maternal Disease on Pregnancy

Tammy Stearns

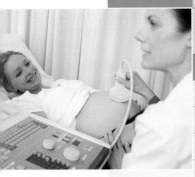

OBJECTIVES

List the maternal infections associated with the acronym TORCH

Explain maternal and fetal complications associated with maternal and gestational diabetes

Describe pregnancy-induced hypertension

Discuss the fetal associations with essential hypertension

Identify the differences between eclampsia and pre-eclampsia

KEY TERMS

congenital malaria | TORCH | toxoplasmosis | nonimmune fetal hydrops | immune fetal hydrops | rubella | diabetes mellitus | gestational diabetes | macrosomia | phenylketonuria | Rh isoimmunization | erythroblastosis fetalis | sickle cell disease | thalassemia | toxemia | eclampsia | pre-eclampsia | HELLP | thrombophilia | systemic lupus erythematosus | teratogenesis | fetal alcohol syndrome

GLOSSARY

Cytomegalovirus (CMV) Any of a group of herpesviruses that enlarge epithelial cells and can cause birth defects; can affect humans with impaired immunological systems

Diabetes mellitus Diabetes caused by a relative or absolute deficiency of insulin and characterized by polyuria

Eclampsia Coma and seizures in second and third trimester following pre-eclampsia

Epstein-Barr virus Herpesvirus that causes infectious mononucleosis

Essential hypertension Maternal high blood pressure that was diagnosed prior to pregnancy

Germ line Ovum or sperm (germ cells) that has genetic material that passes to offspring

Gestational diabetes (aka gestational diabetes mellitus, GDM) Condition in which women without previously diagnosed diabetes exhibit high blood glucose levels during pregnancy

Human immunodeficiency virus (HIV) Human immunodeficiency virus that progresses into AIDS (Acquired Immune Deficiency Syndrome)

Hyperparathyroidism Excessive secretion of parathyroid hormone resulting in abnormally high levels of calcium in the blood; can affect many systems of the body (especially causing bone resorption and osteoporosis)

Hyperthyroidism Overactive thyroid gland; pathologically excessive production of thyroid hormones or the condition resulting from excessive production of thyroid hormones

Hypothyroidism Underactive thyroid gland; a glandular disorder resulting from insufficient production of thyroid hormones

Influenza Acute febrile highly contagious viral disease

Intrauterine growth restriction (IUGR) Usually, fetal weight below the tenth percentile for a given gestational age

Nonimmune hydrops Accumulation of fluid in fetal tissues in the form of ascites, pleural fluid, and skin edema resulting from factors other than a fetomaternal blood group incompatibility

Parvovirus B-19 Erythema infectiosum or fifth disease; spread via the upper respiratory tract, this virus affects children more strongly than adults

Phenylketonuria Genetic disorder of metabolism; lack of the enzyme needed to turn phenylalanine into tyrosine, which results in an accumulation of phenylalanine in the body fluids, which causes various degrees of mental deficiency

Pinocytosis A mechanism by which cells ingest extracellular fluid contents

Rh isoimmunization Development of immunities to Rh-positive blood antigens from a fetus by an RH-negative woman

Rubella (aka German measles) Contagious viral disease that is a milder form of measles lasting 3 or 4 days

Sickle cell anemia Congenital form of anemia occurring mostly in blacks; characterized by crescent-shaped blood cells

Systemic lupus erythematosus Inflammatory disease of connective tissue with variable features including fever, weakness, fatigability, joint pains, and skin lesions on the face, neck, or arms

Thalassemia Inherited form of anemia caused by faulty synthesis of hemoglobin

Thrombophilias Thrombophilia or hypercoagulability is the propensity to develop thrombosis (blood clots) because of a coagulation abnormality

TORCH includes toxoplasmosis, other viruses (syphilis, varicella-zoster, parvovirus B19), rubella, cytomegalovirus, and herpes infections

Toxemia (aka pre-eclampsia) Abnormal condition of pregnancy characterized by hypertension, edema, and protein in the urine

Toxoplasmosis Parasitic infection transmitted to humans from undercooked meat or contact with cat feces

Varicella-zoster infection Chickenpox infection

Maternal disease places a pregnancy at risk because of the possibility of early zygote or embryonic destruction or the development of major malformations and fetal death. The mechanisms through which maternal diseases affect the fetus vary; however, it has been clearly established that the placenta plays a crucial role in preventing or facilitating the transmission process.[1,2]

The major physiologic function of the placenta is to exchange gas, nutrients, and waste products between the maternal and fetal circulations. Various methods help complete this process, including diffusion, active transport, and pinocytosis. For example, blood gases move or diffuse speedily and easily across the placenta from maternal to fetal circulation, but larger molecules, such as carbohydrates, must be assisted or actively transported across the placental membranes. Some substances, usually larger molecules, cannot cross the placenta and are thus effectively barred from entering the fetal circulation by the "placental barrier." This barrier prevents the mixing of the maternal and fetal circulations. Nevertheless, a variety of substances and agents move across this barrier, harming the developing fetus. Examples include infectious agents, drugs, and antibodies.

Indirect harm occurs to a fetus through placental injury caused by maternal diseases. Maternal vascular disease, such as hypertension, decreases uteroplacental blood flow, compromising placental nutrient function. Intrauterine growth restriction (IUGR) is a common finding with uteroplacental compromise.

Sonography has a valuable role in evaluating pregnancies complicated by maternal disease through fetal screening for malformations and IUGR. In addition, sonography allows assessment of placental maturation and amniotic fluid volume, and it provides pregnancy dating for cesarean section planning. In diagnostic procedures such as amniocentesis and percutaneous umbilical blood sampling (PUBS) of the umbilical vein, ultrasound allows for real-time needle guidance (Fig. 29-1).[3,4]

Doppler imaging provides sonformation about fetoplacental circulation. Evaluation is through measurement of the umbilical flow velocity and, less frequently, the uterine artery. The systolic-to-distolic (S/D) ratio calculation allows for a quantitative value indicating either a normal or abnormal state (Fig. 29-2).[5] Doppler velocity waveform monitoring of the umbilical artery is a useful indicator of fetal well-being. Normally, as pregnancy progresses, diastolic flow increases, representing reduced resistance to flow. Premature rupture of membranes (PROM), toxemia, IUGR, sickle cell disease, and diabetes mellitus result in a high S/D ratio, indicating increased vascular resistance.[3,6,7]

In this chapter, we discuss some of the more commonly encountered maternal diseases and conditions that adversely affect fetal outcome. These include infectious disease, endocrine and metabolic disorders, hematologic disorders, toxemia, drug addiction, and malnutrition. Included is a discussion of the specific role of sonography in these various situations.

INFECTIONS

Fetal infection from maternal disease occurs any time during gestation, resulting in a variety of clinical outcomes. Maternal infection, even before conception, may also have an adverse effect on future pregnancies.

The extent of fetal damage depends on several factors, such as agent virulence and transmission route. The gestational age is also of major importance, as the development stage determines fetal susceptibility to the teratogen. Organogenesis occurs during the first trimester, making the fetus susceptible to malformations, but infection can occur before conception, before implantation, after implantation, and in the puerperium.[8]

Infection before conception has been studied in mouse systems by researchers using retroviruses. Results demonstrated that viruses can infect the embryo, integrate into the germ line, and cause disease in future generations.

Maternal reproductive tract infections occur before and during pregnancy. The genital tract and circulation provide the transmission routes. The zona pellucida

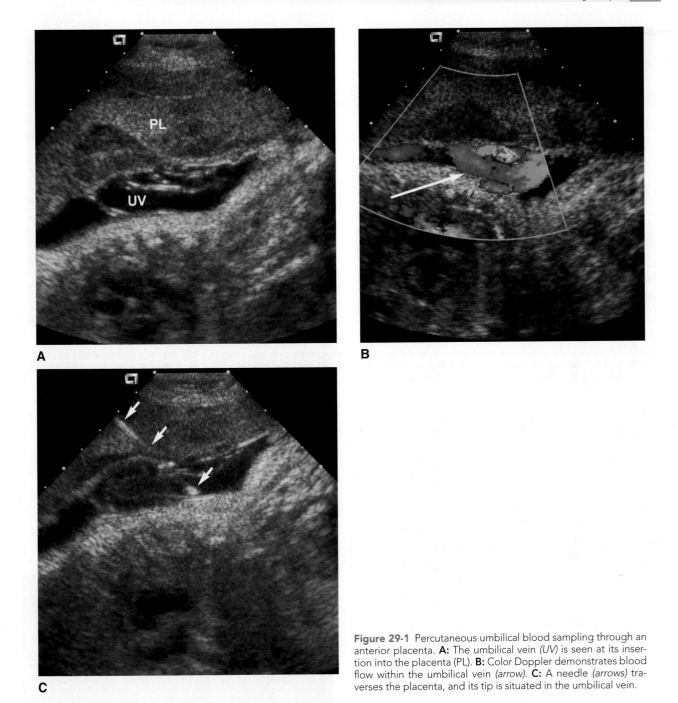

Figure 29-1 Percutaneous umbilical blood sampling through an anterior placenta. **A:** The umbilical vein *(UV)* is seen at its insertion into the placenta (PL). **B:** Color Doppler demonstrates blood flow within the umbilical vein *(arrow)*. **C:** A needle *(arrows)* traverses the placenta, and its tip is situated in the umbilical vein.

prevents the majority of teratogens from damaging the zygote or embryo.

Infection after implantation, particularly during organogenesis, accounts for the largest number of adverse fetal effects. The disruption of normal development at this stage leads to serious fetal abnormalities. Maternal infections result in viremia, bacteremia, or parasitemia, which then spread to the placenta through a hematogenous route. Organisms cross the placenta, enter the fetal circulation, and spread throughout the fetus's body. Fetal harm occurs as these agents destroy parenchymal cells and blood vessels. Growth patterns change and autoimmune responses occur because

of replication in fetal tissue. Maternal immunization reduces fetal damage.

VIRAL INFECTION

The majority of women of childbearing age in the United States show serologic evidence of past varicella-zoster (chickenpox) infection. Three outcomes have been described in pregnancies infected with the varicella virus: congenital abnormalities, postnatal newborn disease ranging from benign to fatal, and zoster (shingles), which may appear months or years after birth.[9] Congenital abnormalities, identified as early as 1947, include IUGR,

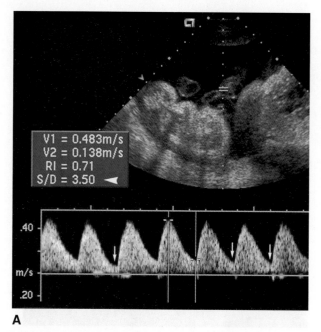
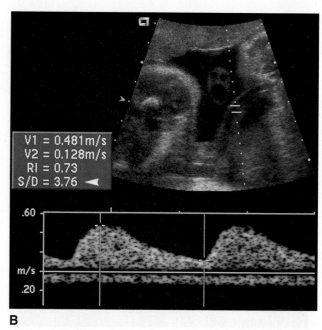

Figure 29-2 Diminished umbilical artery diastolic flow: **(A)** Spectral Doppler of the umbilical artery in a 35-week fetus demonstrates diminished diastolic flow (*arrows*) with an elevated systolic/diastolic (S/D) ratio of 3.5. **B:** Umbilical artery Doppler of another 35-week fetus demonstrates elevated S/D ratio of 3.76 because of diminished diastolic flow.

limb aplasia, microphthalmia, and brain calcifications.[3] Viral transmission to the fetus during weeks 8 to 20 result in the observation of these anomalies.

A common childhood viral infection, Epstein-Barr virus (EBV), does not occur often during pregnancy. In one study, only 7 of more than 10,000 pregnant women tested positive.[10,11] EBV infection, which causes mononucleosis, has been linked to spontaneous abortions, stillbirths, low-birth-weight infants, congenital heart anomalies, and microphthalmia (Fig. 29-3).[11–13] Questions continue in relation to the validity of these associations, requiring further research to determine the extent of the correlation between EBV and fetal congenital abnormalities. Some studies suggest that EBV does not represent a major teratogenic assault on the fetus.[11]

The evidence linking influenza virus to adverse pregnancy outcome has been inconsistent. Early reports of congenital malformation of the heart and central nervous system[59] remain unsupported by later studies. The indirect teratogenic effect of maternal influenza infection during pregnancy may be lessened by the use of appropriate medications to alleviate the accompanied symptoms, such as high body temperature.

Most cases of human immunodeficiency virus (HIV) (the agent of acquired immunodeficiency syndrome) infection in children result from transmission from mother to infant, which occurs near or at parturition. Factors affecting this transmission include the total number of maternal HIV particles, the effectiveness of the maternal and fetal immune response, and the integrity of the placental barrier.[15] In utero, effects of HIV on the fetus may lead to prematurity, IUGR, hepatomegaly, and lymphadenopathy.[8,16]

BACTERIAL INFECTION

Gonorrhea has been reported by Handsfield and colleagues[38] as a cause of increased prematurity, prolonged rupture of fetal membranes, chorioamnionitis, sepsis,

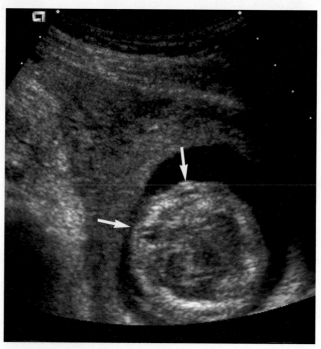

Figure 29-3 Microphthalimia. Axial image of the head at the level of the eyes demonstrates very small orbits (*arrows*).

and IUGR. Gonococcal infections in neonates can result in meningitis and arthritis. Syphilis and gonorrhea can be treated successfully with penicillin or with other antibiotics in the allergic patient.[18]

Lyme disease, transmitted by deerborne ticks, has become a cause of increasing concern in the northeast United States. There has also been a heightened awareness of the risk of contracting this infection elsewhere in the United States and in Europe. One large investigation has neither ruled out nor been able to discover specific abnormalities associated with an untreated infection.[19]

Urinary tract infections (UTIs) represent a common medical complication of pregnancy. Improper management results in adverse effects to both mother and fetus. UTIs include asymptomatic bacteriuria, acute cystitis, and acute pyelonephritis. Asymptomatic bacterial infection has been implicated as a cause in premature delivery and low birth weight, although some studies do not support this finding.[20] Pyelonephritis in pregnancy has been associated with low birth weight, increased perinatal mortality, anemia, toxemia, and premature rupture of membranes (PROM).[9] Mental and motor development of children of pyelonephrotic mothers has been found to be impaired. Patients with UTIs during pregnancy should be treated with antibiotics and monitored by frequent urine cultures.

PARASITIC INFECTION

Parasitic infection during pregnancy may not always pose a risk to the fetus or mother. Several factors determine the clinical manifestations of parasitic disease: the life cycle in the human host, the quantity and location of the parasite, and the host-parasite interaction. Fetal threat occurs when parasites penetrate and invade the host's viscera. These organisms may directly penetrate and infect the uterus and placenta or infect the fetus through fetomaternal circulation. Moreover, they are clearly a threat to both mother and fetus if they multiply within the human host. Two common human parasitic diseases include toxoplasmosis and malaria.

The incidence of congenital malaria increases in immune mothers residing in areas with a high incidence of the disease.[21] Maternal malaria promotes placental insufficiency, causing IUGR, low birth weight, abortion, and stillbirth.[21] Antiparasitic drug therapy successfully manages toxoplasmosis and malaria infections during pregnancy, but some medications are potential teratogens.

TORCH

Perinatal infections account for 2% to 3% of all congenital anomalies.[22] TORCH includes some of the common maternal infections associated with fetal congenital anomalies, such as toxoplasmosis, other viruses (syphilis, varicella-zoster, parvovirus B19), rubella, cytomegalovirus (CMV), and herpes. Nonimmune hydrops and/or intracranial calcifications also raise concern for congenital anomalies (Fig. 29-4).

Toxoplasmosis is a parasitic infection that is typically transmitted through undercooked or raw meat (lamb or pork) that is contaminated with cysts or through food or contaminated water. The obstetrical patient is to be advised not to handle cat litter during the pregnancy because of the risk of contracting the parasite. In the United States, the incidence of congenital toxoplasmosis is approximately 1 per 1,000 live births.[23]

The obstetrical patient is typically asymptomatic; however, 15% to 17% of maternal infection in the first trimester (7th to 14th week) results in transmission hematogenously via the placenta to the fetus and may cause anomalies. Of the 15% to 17% infected, only 10% have a severe infection. The severe infection presents as central nervous symptom anomalies (such as hydrocephalus, microcephaly, intracranial calcifications, seizures, and mental retardation), ascites, and hepatosplenomegaly in the fetus and neonate. Toxoplasmosis occurring early in pregnancy is less frequently transmitted to the fetus than is infection acquired during the last trimester. In early pregnancy, the small placenta usually protects the fetus from parasites. In late pregnancy, this barrier is not as effective, owing to the expanded maternoplacental interface and the aging placenta. Fetal effects are usually devastating.

The "others" in TORCH represents syphilis, varicella-zoster, and parvovirus B19. Infections with syphilis early in pregnancy may result in spontaneous abortion. Congenital disease due to later exposure increases the risk of stillbirths and neonatal mortality. Late-pregnancy syphilis infection may not show clinical signs of congenital syphilis for 2 to 4 weeks.[9] Hepatosplenomegaly, hyperbilirubinemia, evidence of hemolysis, and generalized lymphadenopathy characterize syphilis infection in the neonate.

Fetal contamination with the maternal chickenpox infection results in fetal varicella-zoster. Maternal infection at any time in the pregnancy exposes the fetus to a high risk of placental transmission. The risk for fetal anomalies, however, is at its highest in the first and second trimesters. Third-trimester exposure has a greater risk for varicella-zoster development during the neonatal period. Sonographic evidence of contamination of the varicella-zoster virus includes fetal demise, IUGR, abnormal positions of the hands and limbs, nonimmune hydrops, polyhydramnios, microcephaly, ventriculomegaly, and hyperechogenic hepatic foci (Fig. 29-5).

The development of an acute parvovirus B19, or fifth disease, infection during pregnancy can cause

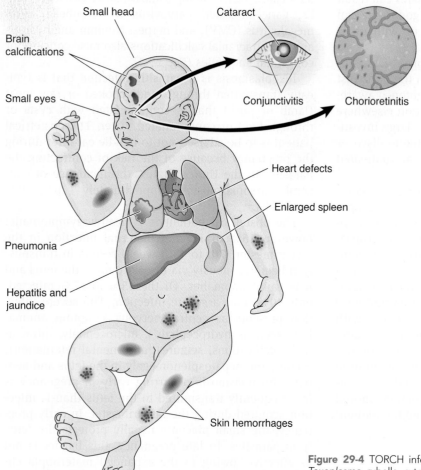

Figure 29-4 TORCH infections. Fetuses infected in the first trimester by *Toxoplasma*, rubella, cytomegalovirus, herpesvirus, or other microbes have similar clinical findings as those illustrated in this figure.

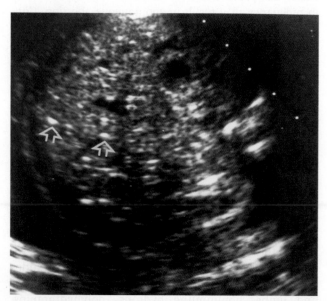

Figure 29-5 Varicella. A transverse view of the abdomen at 24 weeks demonstrates multiple hyperechoic foci within the liver *(arrows)*. A small rim of ascites is also evident. Maternal infection occurred at 16 weeks. (Reproduced with permission from Pretorius DH, Hayward I, Jones KL, et al. Sonographic evaluation of pregnancies with maternal varicella infection. *J Ultrasound Med.* 1992;11:459–463.)

pregnancy complications ranging from early pregnancy loss to nonimmune hydrops. Over 95% of fetal complications (fetal hydrops and death) occur within 12 weeks following acute parvovirus B19 (B19) infection in pregnancy.[24] Infection with parvovirus B19, which is different than the one that infects cats and dogs, can cause several serious complications in the fetus, such as fetal anemia, neurologic anomalies, nonimmune fetal hydrops (hydrops fetalis), and fetal death. Prevention of fetal complications is through early diagnosis and treatment. In the event of maternal infection, an anatomic survey and measurement of the peak systolic flow velocity of the middle cerebral artery are sensitive noninvasive procedures to diagnose fetal anemia and nonimmune hydrops (Fig. 29-6).[25]

Rubella (aka German or three-day measles) was one of the first recognized maternal infections that resulted in fetal anomalies.[26] Occurring in 3% to 5% of pregnancies, rubella causes malformations with first-trimester exposure.[26] The syndrome consists of cataracts, cardiac defects, and deafness.[10] Earlier exposure to the rubella virus increases the severity of the congenital defects.[8]

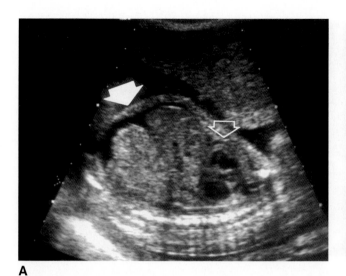

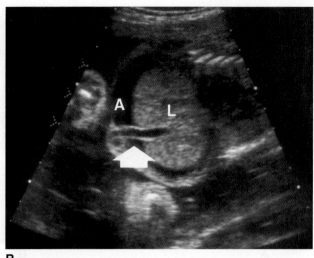

A

B

Figure 29-6 Parvovirus. **A:** A coronal image of the abdomen at 23 weeks' estimated gestational age shows ascites (*solid arrow*) and pericardial effusion (*open arrows*). **B:** A second coronal image demonstrates the umbilical vein (*arrow*) suspended within ascites (*A*). By 27 weeks, the hydrops resolved. Mother had a positive immunoglobin M titer for parvovirus and a history of a rash during the first trimester of pregnancy. *L*, liver.

Nonspecific malformations found in the rubella-exposed fetus include IUGR, cardiac and great vessel abnormalities, microcephaly, microphthalmos, hepatosplenomegaly, and osteopathy (Fig 29-7).[8,27,28]

The human herpesviruses (CMV, herpes hominis types I and II [herpes simplex viruses], varicella-zoster virus, and EBV) infect most people at some time during life. The viruses usually remain latent in the body but may reactivate periodically and produce disease.

Gestational herpesvirus infections reach the embryo or fetus through the placenta by ascending through the cervix or through fetal contact with the birth canal during vaginal delivery. CMV is the most common known cause of congenital infections in humans. Reports indicate that 6% of infants infected in utero contract the disease.[9] Features of CMV disease in neonates include hepatosplenomegaly, jaundice, thrombocytopenia, chorioretinitis, cerebral calcifications, and microcephaly (Fig. 29-8). Other reported associated congenital defects and findings include inguinal hernia, anomalies of the first branchial arch, and central nervous system anomalies. Other possible antenatal findings include ascites, splenomegaly, IUGR, hydrocephaly, and polyhydramnios.[23,29]

There is a high rate of transmission of the herpes simplex virus infection to the neonate.[30] There is a close connection between an increase in spontaneous abortions and stillbirths with a primary infection during the first half of pregnancy.[6] Associated congenital malformations include microcephaly, hydranencephaly, intracranial calcifications, microphthalmia, and hepatosplenomegaly. The presence of the virus in the maternal genital tract at the time of delivery indicates the need for a cesarean section because of the high neonatal infection rate with a vaginal delivery. A majority of the infants are born prematurely.

Sonography plays a unique role in the assessment of fetal growth and well-being during maternal infection. Fetal growth assessment allows for the comparison of head and abdominal size along with sequential study of the fetal growth. Diagnosis of IUGR occurs with fetal weight below the tenth percentile for gestational age. However, through sequential assessments, the fetal well-being can be assessed by comparing the estimated fetal weight. A combination of a sloped forehead and an abnormal cephalic index help diagnose microcephaly. Assessment of the amniotic fluid by estimation and/or amniotic fluid index (AFI) provides information concerning the amount of amniotic fluid. Polyhydramnios is a typical finding when a maternal infection has crossed the placenta.

Aside from sonographic measurements, the overall fetal well-being may be assessed by evaluating the fetal structures. CMV infection and toxoplasmosis commonly result in periventricular calcifications. These image as echogenic calcifications adjacent to the dilated ventricular wall. Maternal infections often result in nonimmune hydrops. Accumulation of interstitial fluid in any two of the pleural, peritoneal, and pericardial tissues along with the fetal soft tissue indicates nonimmune hydrops. This also has an association with the maternal infection crossing the placenta to the fetus.

Ultrasound has a useful role in evaluating fetuses exposed to infectious diseases. For example, fetal echocardiography helps exclude heart abnormalities in patients exposed to CMV and rubella. Serial biometry acquired during ultrasound exams helps determine the presence of IUGR due to a bacterial infection. Accurate sonographic dating allows for correct timing of a cesarean delivery for fetuses infected by viruses such as herpes.

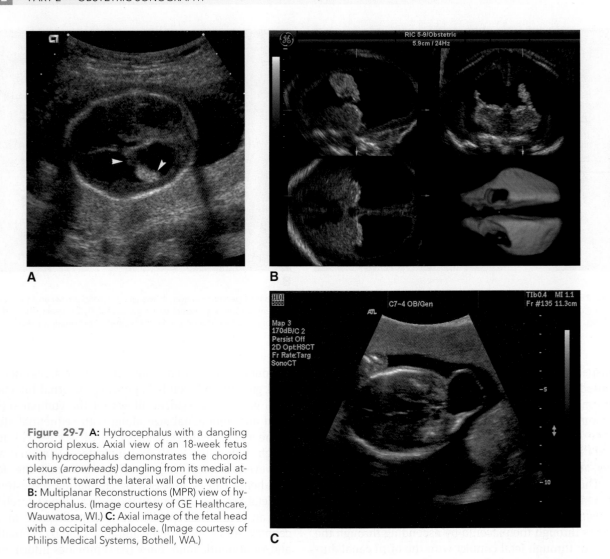

A

B

C

Figure 29-7 A: Hydrocephalus with a dangling choroid plexus. Axial view of an 18-week fetus with hydrocephalus demonstrates the choroid plexus *(arrowheads)* dangling from its medial attachment toward the lateral wall of the ventricle. **B:** Multiplanar Reconstructions (MPR) view of hydrocephalus. (Image courtesy of GE Healthcare, Wauwatosa, WI.) **C:** Axial image of the fetal head with a occipital cephalocele. (Image courtesy of Philips Medical Systems, Bothell, WA.)

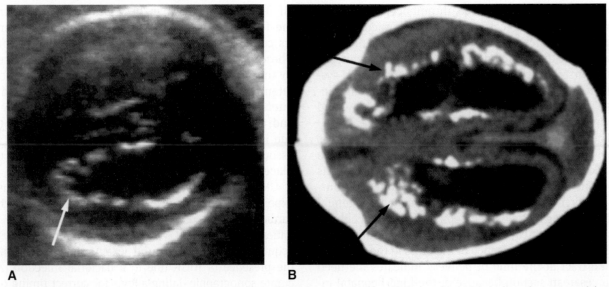

A   **B**

Figure 29-8 Cytomegalovirus. **A:** Transverse view of the head shows ventricular dilation and periventricular echogenic nodules *(arrow).* **B:** Computed tomography scan (oriented to correspond with ultrasound image) after birth confirms hydrocephalus and marked periventricular calcifications *(arrows).* (Courtesy of Luis Izquierdo, MD, Miami, FL.)

TORCH	Sonographic signs
Toxoplasmosis **O**ther (Syphilis, varicella-zoster, parvovirus B19) **R**ubella **C**ytomegalovirus **H**erpes	Hepatosplenomegaly, hydrocephalus, hydranencephaly, microcephaly, intracranial calcifications, ascites, IUGR, fetal demise, non-immune fetal hydrops, polyhydramnios, abnormal hand and limb position, ventriculomegaly, hyperechoic hepatic foci, increased S/D ratio of the middle cerebral artery, cardiac and great vessel anomalies

ENDOCRINE AND METABOLIC DISORDERS

DIABETES MELLITUS

Diabetes mellitus is perhaps the most common maternal disorder the obstetric sonographer encounters. It has been estimated that it occurs in 1 of every 324 to 350 pregnancies in the United States.[1] The condition is a disorder of carbohydrate metabolism related to insulin deficiency and characterized by hyperglycemia.

Diabetes mellitus is classified as type I (insulin dependent; formerly known as juvenile-onset diabetes), type II (noninsulin dependent; formerly known as adult-onset diabetes), and other, or secondary, diabetes. Causes of secondary diabetes include pancreatic disease or pancreatectomy, hormones, drugs, or chemicals, and certain genetic syndromes. Additional classes of diabetes mellitus include impaired glucose tolerance and gestational diabetes, a condition manifested only during pregnancy.[31]

The association between diabetes mellitus and fetal congenital anomalies was recognized as early as 1885. Today, the frequency of anomalies among offspring of diabetic mothers is estimated at 5% to 10%, with a 15% to 20% spontaneous abortion rate.[32] The explanation for congenital malformations seen with diabetes is that the high blood sugar levels (hyperglycemia) result in disruption of embryonic organogenesis. Early diabetes control has been found to reduce the incidence of congenital malformations and spontaneous miscarrages.[33]

Congenital anomalies in infants of diabetic mothers include skeletal, central nervous system, cardiac, renal, and gastrointestinal types (Fig. 29-9).[34] In addition, a single umbilical artery (SUA) occurs in about 6.4% of diabetic mothers' pregnancies (Fig. 29-10). Various malformations occur with an SUA, including cardiac and great vessel anomalies, pulmonary hypoplasia, genitourinary tract anomalies, vertebral anomalies, talipes equinovarus (clubfoot), inguinal hernias, and polydactyly (Fig. 29-11).[32] The finding of an SUA, therefore, warrants a thorough examination of the fetus to exclude these malformations. In addition to malformations, fetuses of diabetic mothers may also experience growth disturbance problems such as IUGR or macrosomia (increased body tissues and fat). Growth retardation of a fetus of a mother with severe diabetes is attributed to uteroplacental vascular insufficiency, which results in fewer nutrients being transferred to the fetus. Fetal hyperinsulinemia is thought to be responsible for the development of macrosomia, as continuous maternal hyperglycemia gains access to the fetal circulatory system. Macrosomia is a fetal weight in excess of 4,500 grams

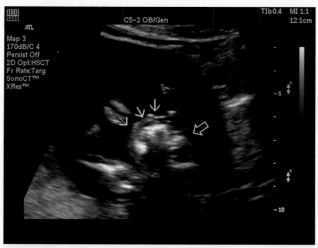

A

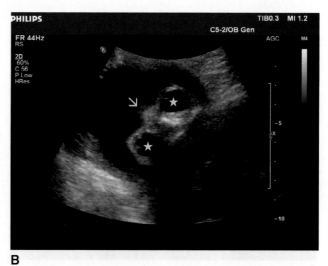

B

Figure 29-9 Anencephaly. **A:** Longitudinal sonogram demonstrates the fetal trunk and the facial structures (*solid arrows*). No cranial vault is discerned (*open arrow*). **B:** Sonographic section of the fetal orbits in a semiaxial plane. Note the nasal bridge (*arrow*) separating the echopenic globes of the eyes (*star*). (Images courtesy of Philips Medical Systems, Bothell, WA.)

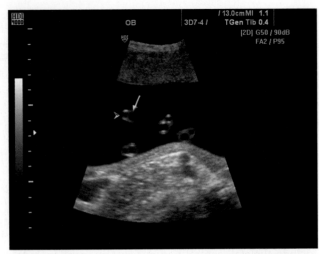

Figure 29-10 Cross-section of a two-vessel umbilical cord. Transverse image of free-floating cord demonstrates two vessels, the larger one is the umbilical vein (*arrow*) and the smaller is the single umbilical artery (*arrowhead*). (Images courtesy of Philips Medical Systems, Bothell, WA.)

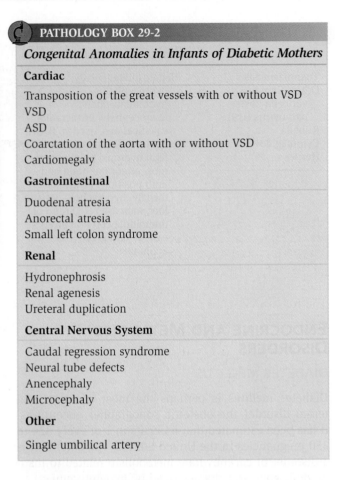

PATHOLOGY BOX 29-2

Congenital Anomalies in Infants of Diabetic Mothers

Cardiac

Transposition of the great vessels with or without VSD
VSD
ASD
Coarctation of the aorta with or without VSD
Cardiomegaly

Gastrointestinal

Duodenal atresia
Anorectal atresia
Small left colon syndrome

Renal

Hydronephrosis
Renal agenesis
Ureteral duplication

Central Nervous System

Caudal regression syndrome
Neural tube defects
Anencephaly
Microcephaly

Other

Single umbilical artery

(9 pounds 9 ounces) or a birth weight above the 90th percentile for gestational age.[35] This predisposes the fetus to complications such as stillbirth and intrapartum trauma.[36] Risk factors for fetal macrosomia include gestational diabetes, Type I or Type II diabetes, multiparity, advanced maternal age, excessive maternal weight gain and/or obesity, postterm delivery, and a previous history of having a large for gestational age (LGA) fetus.

Several growth parameters can be examined with ultrasound to monitor the diabetic mother's pregnancy. These include the biparietal diameter, the abdominal circumference, and the estimated fetal weight. Recent studies have confirmed that appropriately performed abdominal circumference measurements by ultrasonography in the third trimester is the best way of predicting neonatal weight, whereas biparietal diameter and chest

circumference are unreliable or poor predictors.[37] Excessive amniotic fluid defined as greater than or equal to 60th percentile for gestational age has recently been associated with macrosomia.[38] Diagnostic confidence for macrosomia increases in the presence of an increased abdominal circumference and excessive amniotic fluid. Less commonly used parameters are chest size determination and the assessment of fetal breathing movements.[39,40]

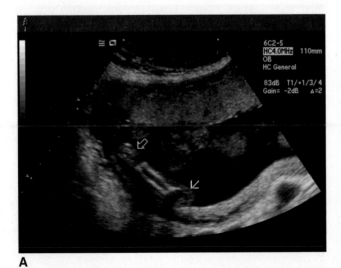

A

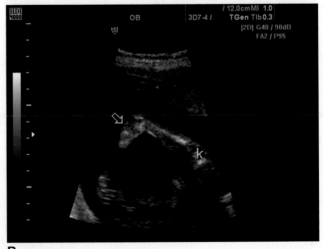

B

Figure 29-11 Normal and clubfoot. **A:** The normal leg and foot lies on a straight plane from the knee (*solid arrow*) to the foot (*open arrows*). **B:** A clubfoot (*open arrows*) deviates at right angles to the leg. *K*, knee. (Image courtesy of Philips Medical Systems, Bothell, WA.)

In the sonographic evaluation of the diabetic mother's pregnancy, it is recommended that an initial first-trimester examination be done to establish dates. An anatomic survey between 18 and 22 weeks allows screening for neural tube defects, caudal regression syndrome (with variable agenesis of the lower spinal segments, variable fusion of the lower extremities, and variable absence of the long bones), and cardiac defects and can exclude other gross malformations.[32] Follow-up examinations should then be done every 4 to 6 weeks for fetal growth and estimated weight. Placental enlargement occurs due to the chronic hyperglycemia seen with diabetes. Macrosomic and growth-restricted fetuses should be examined more frequently. Umbilical artery flow tracings, specifically high-resistance Doppler velocity patterns, have also proven significant.[7]

With a macrosomic fetus, the risk of maternal and fetal complications increases. The pregnancy is at risk for spontaneous abortion, polyhydramnios, and placentomegaly. Fetal risk includes congenital cardiovascular, renal, and gastrointestinal malformations, caudal regression syndrome, neural tube defects, shoulder dystocia, bony fractures, encephalopathy, and brachial plexus injury. The maternal complications include increased risks of hemorrhage, rectal and vaginal lacerations, and an increase in cesarean delivery. In addition, both maternal and perinatal morbidity and mortality increase in relation to increasing fetal birth weight,[34] highlighting the importance of diagnosing macrosomia.

Gestational diabetes—diabetes that occurs only during pregnancy—affects about 7% of all pregnant women.[41] It usually begins in the fifth or sixth month of pregnancy (weeks 24 and 28), disappearing shortly after delivery.[42] Historical risk factors for this condition include a previous stillbirth, a baby with congenital anomalies, a previous macrosomic infant, or a family history of diabetes.[43] Gestational diabetes affects the fetus similarly to pregestational diabetes; however, a later onset decreases the risk of malformations due to organogenesis disruption. Clinical symptoms may lag behind maternal metabolic changes, so there is no certainty that the fetus has gone through organogenesis unaffected, regardless of diagnosis timing. A common-sense approach, such as examining all fetuses whose mothers manifested symptoms before 24 weeks' gestation, is best.

A glucose tolerance test, performed between weeks 24 and 28, is the preferred diagnostic method. The glucose tolerance test involves drinking a glucose solution and checking the glucose level after an hour. A normal glucose level is less than 140 mg/dl. A higher glucose level requires a 3-hour glucose tolerance test. The diagnosis of gestational diabetes is made when two or more high glucose levels during the 3-hour glucose test occur.[44]

Sonographically, the gestational diabetic patient's pregnancy is at risk for macrosomia, polyhydramnios, placentomegaly, and all of the associated complications with each.

HYPERTHYROIDISM

Hyperthyroidism, also known as thyrotoxicosis, occurs in approximately 0.1% to 0.4% of pregnancies.[45] The additional thyroid stimulation produces thyroxine, disrupting normal cell development and causing a significant increase in the incidence of low-birth-weight infants and a slight increase in the neonatal mortality rate.

The most common cause of clinical hyperthyroidism is Graves' disease (toxic diffuse goiter), Plummer's disease (toxic nodular goiter), trophoblastic tumors, and hydatidiform mole.[46]

HYPOTHYROIDISM

The incidence of hypothyroidism is very low in pregnant women since the absence of normal hormone stimulation makes conception unlikely. There is a high rate of stillbirths in women who become pregnant.[47]

HYPERPARATHYROIDISM

The incidence of hyperparathyroidism in pregnancy is very low. The most common cause is parathyroid adenoma. There is an increase in prematurity, spontaneous abortions, fetal demise in late pregnancy, and hypocalcemia and tetany in newborns.[48]

PHENYLKETONURIA

Phenylketonuria (PKU) is an inherited, autosomal recessive disease that results in increased phenylalanine in the blood. The individual's diet provides this amino acid through the ingestion of protein (milk, eggs), and some artificial sweeteners such as aspartame.[49] The occurrence in the United States of this condition is 1 in 10,000–15,000 newborns. Due to newborn screening, the majority of PKU cases receive prompt treatment, resulting in few severe cases.

A woman who is not following a low-phenylalanine, low-protein diet develops potentially toxic levels of metabolic products. High levels of prenatal phenylalanine exposure result in an increased risk of spontaneous abortion, microcephaly, mental retardation, congenital heart disease, low birth weight, and behavioral problems.[35,49] To avoid fetal complications, dietary restriction of phenylalanine begins before conception. Maternal dietary adjustments reinstated after inception of pregnancy have been unsuccessful in preventing abnormalities.

HEMATOLOGIC DISORDERS

RH ISOIMMUNIZATION

Rh isoimmunization refers to the development of maternal antibodies to the surface antigens on fetal red blood cells. The maternal antibodies perceive the fetal antigens as foreign invaders, and they attempt to attack and destroy them. Erythroblastosis fetalis, a condition characterized by rapid destruction of fetal red blood cells and hepatosplenomegaly, may occur when an Rh-positive fetus is carried by an Rh-negative mother who has been sensitized to Rh antigen in a previous pregnancy (Fig. 29-12).[9] In its most severe form, a fluid overload condition known as immune hydrops fetalis

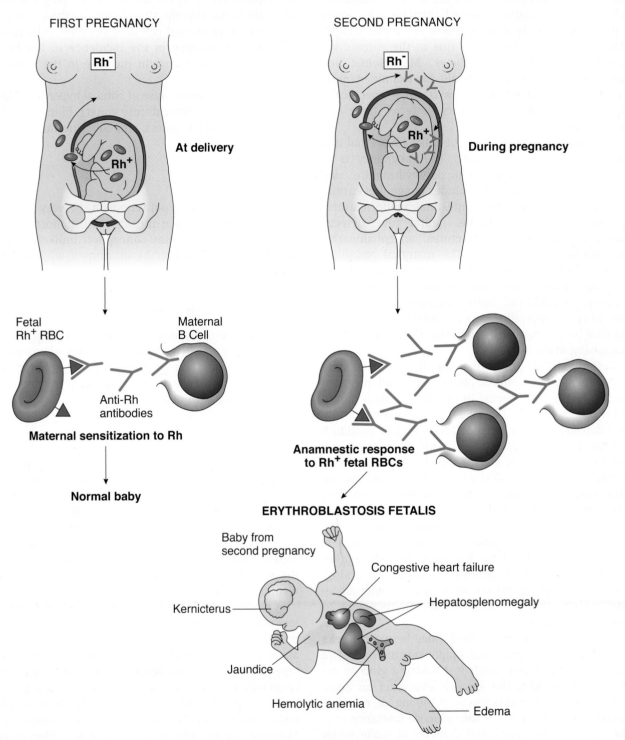

Figure 29-12 Pathogenesis of erythroblastosis fetalis due to maternal-fetal Rh incompatibility. Immunization of the Rh-negative mother with Rh-positive erythrocytes in the first pregnancy leads to the formation of anti-Rh antibodies of the IgG type. These antibodies cross the placenta and damage the Rh-positive fetus in subsequent pregnancies.

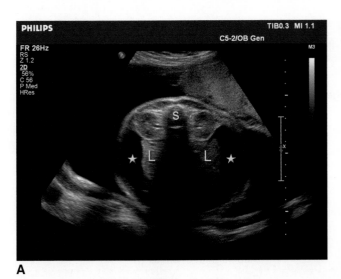

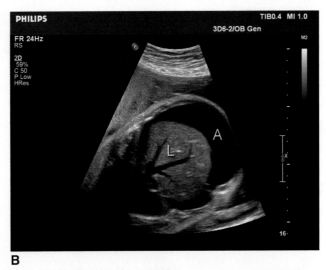

A

B

Figure 29-13 Hydrops fetalis. **A:** Transverse image of the fetal chest with the spine anterior *(s)*. Pleural fluid *(star)* surrounds the lungs (L). **B:** Axial image of the fetal abdomen demonstrating ascites *(A)* around the liver *(L)*. (Image courtesy of Philips Medical Systems, Bothell, WA.)

results (Fig. 29-13). With the introduction of preventive maternal immunologic blocking treatment, RhoGAM, clinical Rh isoimmunization to the Rh factor is much less common. However, isoimmunization due to major blood type (ABO) maternofetal incompatibility occasionally occurs.

Amniocentesis is an important procedure for monitoring the bilirubin concentration in amniotic fluid, as hemolytic disease severity directly relates to fluid bilirubin levels. The ultrasound exam aids in detecting extrafetal and intrafetal fluid changes and monitoring fetal growth. The establishment of accurate dates becomes essential for amniocentesis timing, delivery planning, and real-time observation of needle placement for the PUBS procedure (Fig. 29-14). Obtaining a direct sample of fetal blood from the cord allows for determination of antibody titers to help determine fetal prognosis. Blood transfusions into the umbilical vein at the placental insertion or into the fetal peritoneum has a high rate of success in treating isoimmunized pregnancies.[50,51]

Doppler ultrasound is also helpful in assessing the well-being of potentially affected fetuses. As the fetal hemoglobin decreases vascular resistance increases resulting in an increased S/D ratio.[52-54]

Hydrops can be caused by factors other than isoimmunization. This nonimmunologic hydrops may be caused by over 40 conditions.[14,55] Most commonly, nonimmunologic hydrops may result from fetal problems such as cardiovascular conditions (hypoplastic left heart, dysrhythmias), infections (toxoplasmosis, herpes simplex), obstructive vascular problems (umbilical vein thrombosis), pulmonary diseases (cystic adenomatoid malformation), neoplasms (neuroblastoma, teratoma), chromosomal anomalies (trisomy 18 or 21), and congenital nephrosis. Maternal causes include diabetes mellitus and toxemia.[56]

The ultrasound findings associated with hydrops include polyhydramnios, fetal ascites, pleural and pericardial effusions, fetal anasarca (subcutaneous edema with skin thickness greater than 5 millimeters [mm]), abnormally thickened placenta (greater than 6 centimeters [cm]), fetal hepatosplenomegaly and cardiomegaly, and umbilical vein dilatation.[7,9,33,55] The sonographically detectable structural anomalies associated with fetal hydrops are numerous and varied (Table 29-1).

SICKLE CELL DISEASE

Sickle cell disease, also called sickle cell anemia, is an inherited disorder that affects people from families originating in Africa, Central or South America, the Caribbean islands, Mediterranean countries, India, and Saudi Arabia.[49] In the United States, individuals of African descent have the highest incidence rate.[49] African Americans can expect a 1 in 500 chance of

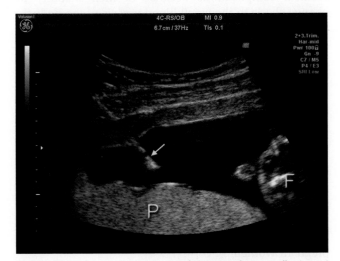

Figure 29-14 Sonographic image of the sampling needle *(arrow)* during an amniocentesis. The needle tip appears large because of reverberation artifact while the anechoic break is due to refraction. *P,* placenta; *F,* fetus. (Image courtesy of GE Healthcare, Wauwatosa, WI.)

TABLE 29-1

Sonographic Structural Anomalies Associated with Immune and Nonimmune Hydrops Fetalis

Structure	Sonographic Finding	Abnormality
Head	Intracranial mass, associated with congestive heart failure and microcephaly	Arteriovenous malformation, vein of Galen aneurysm, cytomegalovirus, or toxoplasmosis infection
Neck	Cystic neck masses	Lymphatic dysplasias
Thorax	Poorly contracting heart	Congestive heart failure
	Pericardial effusion, tachycardia	Cardiac anomaly
	Asystole	Demise
	Mediastinal mass	Tumor
	Chest mass	Cystic adenomatoid malformation
	Small thorax	Dwarfism
	Cystic masses crossing diaphragm	Diaphragmatic hernias
Abdomen	Tubular sonolucent structures	Gastrointestinal obstruction, atresia, or vovulus
	Abdominal masses	Tumors, neurofibromatosis
Retroperitoneum	Retroperitoneal mass	Neurogenic mass
	Hydronephrotic kidney	Hydronephrosis, posterior urethral valves
Extremities	Short arms, legs	Dwarfism
	Contractures	Arthrogryposis
	Fractures	Osteogenesis imperfecta
Placenta	Thick placenta	Infection, extramedullary hematopoiesis, anemia
Amniotic cavity	Number of fetuses, relative size, amniotic membrane	Twin-to-twin transfusion
		Single umbilical artery
	Umbilical cord anomalies	Umbilical cord torsion

(Adapted from Fleischer AC, Killam AP, Boehm FH, et al. Hydrops fetalis: Sonographic evaluation and clinical implications. *Radiology.* 1981;141:163–168.)

inheriting this condition, and Hispanic Americans have a 1 in 1,000 to 1,400 chance.[49]

Sickle cell disease affects the hemoglobin molecule in the blood. This is the blood component responsible for transporting oxygen to the body. The normal blood cell has a flexible round shape, but in this condition blood cells take on a rigid, sickle-shaped appearance. This shape change is due to a gene mutation on the hemoglobin beta (HBB) gene, which provides instructions for the production of beta-globin. A mutation in the

HBB gene results in low production of beta-globin, thus resulting in the characteristic sickle-shaped blood cell. The abnormally shaped cells die prematurely, leading to anemia. These inflexible, sickle-shaped cells cause medical complications because of their inability to change shape in the small blood vessels of the body.[49]

Incidences of spontaneous abortion, prematurity, stillbirth, and perinatal morbidity and mortality increase with sickle cell disease.[57] Other findings include short femurs and low birth weight.[58]

Sonographic follow-up in these fetuses checks for growth retardation and increased placental resistance to umbilical and uterine artery flow. Spectral Doppler helps with monitoring through the use of the S/D velocity ratio. The critical point for the S/D ratio value in the umbilical and uterine arteries is 3.0 or higher in a fetus of 30 weeks' gestation or greater. The same study recorded abnormal flow in at least one of these arteries, with abnormal flow in 88% of pregnant women with sickle cell disease, compared to 4% to 7% in normal pregnant women.[59]

Management of sickle cell patients during pregnancy includes dietary supplementation of iron and folic acid.[60,61] Prophylactic transfusions have been reported

PATHOLOGY BOX 29-3

Sonographic Findings in an Rh Isoimmunized Pregnancy

Hepatosplenomegaly

Immune fetal hydrops (ascites, pleural and pericardial fluid, anasarca)

Increased S/D ratios

Polyhydramnios

Thick placenta

Cardiomegaly

Umbilical vein dilation

to improve both maternal and fetal morbidity and mortality, although this procedure carries the risk of bloodborne infection and the formation of alloantibodies that may affect future transfusions.[62]

THALASSEMIA

Thalassemia has been cited as one of the most common maternal autosomal recessive genetic abnormalities associated with pregnancy worldwide.[49,63] Referred to as beta thalassemia, the characteristic finding of this blood disorder is a reduction the hemoglobin production. The lack of hemoglobin, the oxygen carrier in the blood, results in anemia. There are two forms of beta thalassemia the more severe form, thalassemia major (Cooley's anemia) and thalassemia intermidia.[49] Individuals from Mediterranean countries, North Africa, the Middle East, India, Central Asia, and Southeast Asia have the highest incidence of thalassemia.[49]

Mutations from the same gene (HBB) responsible for sickle cell disease also result in beta thalassemia. The reduced amount of beta-globin, beta-plus (B$^+$ or B^0), results in the lack of hemoglobin that disrupts red blood cell development. Due to the oxygen shortage, blood cells fail to mature, leading to organ damage and lack of growth due to oxygen deprivation.[49]

Thalassemia often shortens the life span of an affected person because of the iron overload that develops from the necessary multiple transfusions.[49] Most women with thalassemia major die before reaching reproductive age. In cases of successful pregnancy, effects on the fetus range from nonimmune hydrops and death to no effect at all.[41,63,64]

TOXEMIA AND HYPERTENSION

Toxemia (pre-eclampsia) of pregnancy is a third trimester disease characterized by maternal edema, hypertension, proteinuria, and central nervous system irritability. The disease has been classified into two stages, pre-eclampsia and eclampsia. Hypertension with proteinuria and/or edema marks pre-eclampsia. In the eclamptic stage, when one or more convulsions occur, there is a significant increase of maternal and fetal mortality.[48] Pre-eclampsia affects less than 1.5% of all pregnancies, but when it develops before 36 weeks' gestation, a prenatal mortality rate as high as 20% has been reported. The disorder has been found to occur most commonly in young primigravidas and in older multiparas. Although the etiology of pre-eclampsia remains unclear, immunologic, hormonal, and nutritional factors are thought to be responsible. It has been postulated that the reduction in prostaglandin synthesis seen in pre-eclamptic patients promotes placental vascular disease and decreased uteroplacental blood flow. Low birth weight, fetal distress, and placental abruption are all associated with toxemia.[66] Treatment of this condition depends on the severity of the disease. Antihypertensive drugs can be used to control blood pressure, and in severe disease anticonvulsant medication is prescribed for seizures. Immediate delivery of the fetus is indicated in most cases of toxemia (Fig. 29-15).

Of the patients that are diagnosed with pre-eclampsia, 2% to 12% are affected by the HELLP syndrome. HELLP is an abbreviation of the main findings; <u>h</u>emolysis, <u>e</u>levated <u>l</u>iver enzymes, and <u>l</u>ow <u>p</u>latelets. Estimated to occur in less than 1%[49,67] of the general population, HELLP rarely occurs until the third trimester,[49]

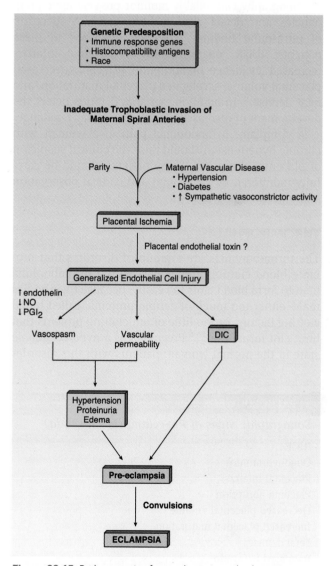

Figure 29-15 Pathogenesis of pre-eclampsia and eclampsia.

with about one-third developing the syndrome within 2 days after delivery.[67] HELLP occurs more in women of African descent[68] and in nulliparous white women[49] with pre-eclampsia and a family history.[28] The cause of this syndrome is poorly understood, with theories linking development to abnormal placental function, impairment of placental vascular perfusion, and oxidative stress resulting in maternal vascular changes.[49] In half the cases, maternal symptoms include right upper quadrant pain, nausea and vomiting, general malaise, visual symptoms, hypertension, proteinuria, excessive weight gain, and generalized edema similar to pre-eclampsia findings.[67]

Hypertension during pregnancy may also occur without the development of toxemia. Hypertension preceding or persisting after pregnancy is diagnosed as essential hypertension, whereas hypertension that occurs during pregnancy and disappears after parturition is considered to be pregnancy-induced hypertension. Hypertension during pregnancy, regardless of the type, always poses a risk to both mother and fetus.

Sonography can reliably monitor pre-eclamptic pregnancies and detect abnormalities early. A spectrum of ultrasound findings has been described in these patients: IUGR, oligohydramnios, placental infarcts, increased incidence of abruption placenta, decreased placental volume, accelerated placental maturation, and fetal demise.[15] In addition, serial S/D ratios detect the development of increased placental vascular resistance.

A complaint of abdominal pain in a woman with chronic hypertension should raise the clinical suspicion of placental abruption. These patients should be carefully monitored by ultrasound and clinical observation and placed on bedrest.

THROMBOPHILIAS

The thrombophilias are a group of disorders that promote blood clotting. Individuals with a thrombophilia tend to form blood clots too easily, because their bodies make either too much of certain proteins, called blood clotting factors, or too little of anticlotting proteins that limit clot formation.[49,70] Pregnancy is a hypercoaguable state in the normal woman; patients with this disorder also encounter pregnancy complications such as repeated late first-trimester miscarriages, stillbirth, placental abruption, IUGR, and maternal deep vein thrombosis (DVT). The most common acquired thrombophilia is antiphospholipid syndrome (APS). APS contributes to 10% to 20% of repeated spontaneous abortions and is also related to pre-eclampsia, IUGR, and premature delivery.[71]

SYSTEMIC LUPUS ERYTHEMATOSUS

Systemic lupus erythematosus is a multisystem autoimmune disease that is not uncommon in women, particularly in the childbearing years. Fetal effects may be caused by the transfer of autoantibodies across the placenta or indirectly as a result of the lack of maternal well-being. Pregnancy disorders that have been reported with this disease include fetal death, recurrent abortion, growth retardation, and toxemia.[72] Best fetal outcomes are obtained when pregnancies are planned for time periods when disease activity has been well controlled by small doses of steroids and aspirin.

DRUG USE AND NUTRITIONAL DISORDERS

Drug use during pregnancy affects outcomes by promoting fetal addiction, teratogenesis, altered uteroplacental blood flow, or IUGR.[9] This teratogenic effect depends on several factors, including the drug, its dosage, time of exposure, host susceptibility, genetic differences in the host, and interactions with other agents in the environment.[8] In general, in the early period of gestation, teratogens affect organs that develop first, such as the heart.

Although many drugs and chemicals have been sporadically associated with various fetal malformations, only a few are proven teratogens (Table 29-2). Some, unfortunately, are important medications, such as Coumadin (warfarin), whose use during pregnancy must be restricted.

Drugs used abusively include alcohol, amphetamines, barbiturates, and narcotics (heroin, methadone, and cocaine). Effects associated with these agents show a variety of fetal effects, ranging from mild to severe. In other than proven teratogens, the main effect appears to be IUGR as a result of poor nutrition associated with drug use.

Excessive consumption of alcohol, a known teratogen, during pregnancy can result in the fetal alcohol syndrome (FAS). This syndrome is part of an adverse outcome spectrum known as fetal alcohol spectrum disorder.[28] It is estimated that 11% of pregnant women are problem drinkers and about 5% to 10% of their offspring demonstrate full-blown FAS. Fetal alcohol syndrome is the leading cause of mental retardation in

---

PATHOLOGY BOX 29-5

Sonographic Signs of Pre-eclampsia (Toxemia)

IUGR
Oligohydramnios
Placental infarcts
Placenta abruption
Decreased placental volume
Increased placental maturation
Fetal demise
Increased S/D ratio

TABLE 29-2

TABLE 29-2
Teratogens and Their Fetal Effects[8,26,55,88]

Teratogen	Fetal Effects
Aminopterin	Meningoencephalocele, hydrocephalus, clubfoot, hypoplasia of fibula
Antithyroid drugs	Polydactyly, goiter
Azathioprine	Pulmonary valvular stenosis
Alcohol	IUGR, microcephaly, developmental delay, characteristic facies, ventricular septal defect, tetralogy of Fallot, aortic coarctation, cleft palate, meningomyelocele, hydrocephalus
Aspirin	Gastroschisis, premature closure of the ductus arteriosus
Carbon monoxide	Cerebral atrophy, hydrocephalus, cleft lip
Cigarettes	Oral clefts, IUGR
Cocaine	Placenta abruption, prematurity, fetal death, low birth weight, microcephaly, abnormal limbs, urinary tract malformations, poor neurodevelopmental performance, prune belly
Warfarin	Microcephaly, hypoplasia and calcific stippling of the epiphyses, cardiac malformations, hypertelorism, cleft palate or lip, growth retardation, developmental delay, eye defects, hearing loss, central nervous system defects
Cyclophosphamide	Tetralogy of Fallot, syndactyly, missing digits
Daunorubicin	Anencephaly, cardiac defects
Ethanol	Microcephaly, cardiac defects, growth retardation
Heparin	Absence of thumbs
Ibuprofen	Gastroschisis, premature closure of the ductus arteriosus
Methotrexate	Oxycephaly, absence of frontal bone, dextrocardia, growth retardation, micrognathia, low ears, maxillary hypoplasia, short limbs, talipes equinovarus, IUGR, microcephaly
Methyl mercury	Microcephaly, head asymmetry, cerebral atrophy, spacicity, blindness
Phenytoin	Microcephaly, cardiac malformations, hypertelorism, cleft palate or lip, growth retardation, bradycardia
Polychlorinated biphenyls	Growth retardation
Procarbazine	Cerebral hemorrhage
Radiation	Microcephaly
Retinoic acid	Congenital heart malformations, spine malformations, limb reduction, duodenal stenosis or atresia, pyloric stenosis, microtia
Thalidomide	Congenital heart malformations, spine malformations, limb reduction, duodenal stenosis or atresia, pyloric stenosis, microtia, phocomelia, polydactyly, syndactyly, oligodactyly, external ear defects, capillary hemangiomas of the face, cranial nerve VI and VII palsies, renal, gallbladder, spleen and appendix agenesis, clubfoot, extra toes
Trimethadione	Microcephaly, cardiac defects, clubfoot, esophageal atresia, growth deficiency, facial clefting, micrognathia
Valproic acid	Meningomyelocele, microcephaly, growth deficiency, tetralogy of Fallot, oral cleft, narrow bifrontal diameter, high forehead, epicanthal folds, infraorbital creases, telecanthus, low nasal bridge, short nose with inverted nares, midfacial hypoplasia, long philtrum, think vermillion border, small mouth, long digits, hyperconvex fingernails, cleft lip

the West, affecting as many as 2 cases in 1,000 live births.[28,68,73]

It has been established that there is no safe level of alcohol consumption during pregnancy. While most of the characteristics of the syndrome relate to cognitive and functional disabilities, some structural and growth anomalies occur in the fetal period.[28] This syndrome includes features of gross physical retardation, central nervous system dysfunction, and facial dysmorphology, including microcephaly and microphthalmia. Additional effects of alcohol include cardiac anomalies (such as ventricular septal defect), increased risk of infections,

TABLE 29-3

Sonographic Findings in Fetuses of Mothers with Disease[26,55]

Maternal Disease	Sonographic and Associated Findings
Viral Infection	
Cytomegalovirus	Microcephaly, hydrocephaly, cardiac abnormality, IUGR, hepatosplenomegaly, ascites, polyhydramnios, nonimmune hydrops, intracranial calcifications, linear striations of basal ganglia, echogenic bowel, chorioretinitis, seizures, blindness, optic atrophy
Herpes simplex	Microcephaly, hydranencephaly, intracranial calcifications, microphthalmia, hepatosplenomegaly, nonimmune hydrops, echogenic bowel
Varicella-zoster	IUGR, limb aplasia, microphthalmia, intracranial calcifications, hyperechoic liver foci, nonimmune hydrops, hypoplastic limbs, ventriculomegaly, microcephaly, cataracts, echogenic bowel
Epstein-Barr	Cardiac, IUGR, microphthalmia
Rubella	Microcephaly, hydrocephaly, cephalocele, agenesis of the corpus callosum, cataracts, abnormal long bones, septal defects, pulmonic stenosis
Influenza	Cardiac anomalies
Human immunodeficiency virus	IUGR, hepatomegaly
Bacterial Infection	
Syphilis	Hydrocephaly, iniencephaly, thick placenta, hydrops, osteitis, fetal demise, non immune hydrops, hepatosplenomegaly, bowel dilatation, IUGR
Gonorrhea	IUGR, oligohydramnios
Urinary tract infection	IUGR, oligohydramnios
Parasitic Infection	
Toxoplasmosis	IUGR, hydrocephaly, microcephaly, intracranial calcification, agenesis of the corpus callosum, hepatosplenomegaly, nonimmune hydrops, ventriculomegaly, hyperechogenic liver foci, placentomegaly
Malaria	IUGR
Endocrine and Metabolic	
Diabetes mellitus	Thickened placenta
Hyperthyroidism	IUGR
Hypothyroidism	Fetal demise, goiter
Hyperparathyroidism	Fetal demise, goiter
Phenylketonuria	Microcephaly, cardiac disease
Hematologic	
Isoimmunization	Pleural and pericardial effusion, ascites, skin thickening, polyhydramnios (immune fetal hydrops)
Sickle cell disease	Short femurs, IUGR
Thalassemia	Nonimmune fetal hydrops
Toxemia	IUGR, oligohydramnios, abruptio placentae, decreased placental volume, early placental maturation, fetal demise
Malnutrition	IUGR, oligohydramnios, decreased placental volume, intrauterine growth retardation

placental abruption, amnionitis, stillbirth, sudden infant death, and spontaneous abortion.[69,73] The role of street drugs (amphetamines, barbiturates, narcotics) in the development of congenital anomalies has been difficult to define because of complicating factors such as drug potency and purity, multiple drug use, and the high incidence of perinatal infection and malnutrition among drug abusers.[74] Amphetamines have been implicated as a cause of cleft palate and IUGR. Barbiturate use has been reported to carry an increased risk for cardiac anomalies as well as cleft lip and palate.[75]

The major effects of narcotics are drug dependency in both mother and fetus, and IUGR. In addition, cocaine use has an associated risk of abruptio placentae, genitourinary malformations, limb reduction anomalies, and cardiac defects.[76–78] Nicotine and caffeine have also been associated with adverse fetal outcome. Nicotine use has been linked to an increased risk of spontaneous abortion, perinatal mortality, placenta previa, preterm delivery, and low birth weight.[79,80] Excessive maternal caffeine consumption (100 mg/day) shows an increased rate of spontaneous abortion.[81]

Closely associated with drug abuse is the problem of malnutrition. Drug abuse commonly leads to neglect of personal care, including nutrition. Mild degrees of maternal malnutrition result in an increase in prematurity, low birth weight, and IUGR.[82] Maternal starvation in early gestation has been reported to be associated with central nervous system abnormalities (spina bifida and hydrocephalus). In later gestation, it can result in IUGR.

Obesity is the most common nutritional disorder in developed countries. This is defined as body mass index greater than 30.[83] Three major antenatal complications of moderate obesity are hypertension, pre-eclampsia, and gestational diabetes.[16,84,85] Massive obesity is a major technical problem with prenatal sonographic imaging and cesarean section.

Sonography has an important role in evaluating fetuses of drug-addicted, malnourished, and obese mothers. A considerable number of fetal structural anomalies can be detected in fetuses exposed to teratogenic agents. Careful sonography with high-resolution equipment helps rule out malformations such as hydrocephalus, limb reduction defects, and cardiac anomalies as early as 17 to 18 weeks of gestation. Serial scans monitor fetal growth patterns, allowing detection of IUGR or macrosomia. Pregnancies of malnourished or obese patients who require cesarean section can be dated accurately with sonography for correct planning of this procedure.

OTHER MATERNAL DISORDERS

Women with cyanotic congenital heart disease have pregnancies with a higher incidence of premature births, IUGR, and abortions.[86,87] The incidence of congenital heart disease in these infants is also somewhat higher than that in the normal population (Table 29-3).

SUMMARY

- The effect of viral, bacterial, or parasitic infections on the fetus depend on the gestational age of the fetus.
- TORCH is a grouping of five maternal infections related to congenital anomalies.
- Maternal diabetes, either type I or II, results in an increased incidence of fetal anomalies.
- Decreased fetal blood hemoglobin results in an increase in the S/D ratio.
- Because of hormonal imbalances, women with hyperthyroidism, hypothyroidism, hyperparathyroidism, and phenylketonuria rarely carry a pregnancy to term.
- Rh isoimmunization occurs when a mother is Rh negative blood type and the fetus is Rh positive blood type.
- Mixing of maternal Rh negative and Rh positive blood at parturition of either a term or aborted pregnancy can result in Rh isoimmunization.
- Rh isoimmunization increases the risk of immune fetal hydrops.

Critical Thinking Questions

1. A 38-year-old, Rh negative, G2P1 patient presents for her obstetric exam. During the pregnancy, she has gained 35 pounds and developed high blood pressure and gestational diabetes. Her previous child was normal with an Rh positive blood type and she is Rh antibody positive. A previous exam demonstrated a singleton pregnancy with a normal anatomic survey and an anterior placenta. Describe the expected appearance of the placenta. Explain the mechanism of the placental sonographic findings. How would these maternal conditions affect the fetus?

ANSWER: The placenta in a patient with gestational diabetes and high blood pressure has an increased chance of developing into a hydropic placenta. Findings include a placenta greater than 6 cm because of fluid overload. The placental findings are due to high-output cardiac failure in the fetus as a result of immune fetal hydrops. The fetal hydrops is probably due to an Rh sensitivity, which results in a placenta with a ground glass appearance and a fetus with abdominal ascites, pleural effusion, and generalized edema. For more information on the placenta, see Chapter 18.

2. A 40-year-old patient presents to the department with newly diagnosed gestational diabetes. She is a G7 P5A1 and has gained 60 pounds with this pregnancy. Two of her previous children had a birth weight in excess of 10 pounds. Findings identified during the sonographic examination include polyhydramnios, large abdominal circumference, an increase in the S/D umbilical cord ratio, and a placenta measuring 7 cm in anterioposterior (AP) dimension. Explain the two forms of growth disturbances seen in a mother with diabetes. What type of diabetes-linked growth disturbance would be expected in this patient? Explain your answer.

ANSWER: The fetus can either demonstrate IUGR or macrosomia. In the case of growth retardation, maternal diabetes is due to uteroplacental insufficiency resulting in a decrease of nutrient transference from the mother to the fetus. Macrosomic fetuses, weighing more than 4,500 grams, present with an increased weight and size is due to the continued high sugar levels (hyperglycemia) in the fetal blood system. In the described patient, a macrosomic fetus would be the expected finding because of the maternal age, excessive weight gain, and previous history of LGA children.

- Sickle cell disease and thalassemia are blood conditions resulting in anemia in the fetus and mother.

- Toxemia, or pre-eclampsia, is a grouping of symptoms that include hypertension, proteinuria, and edema.

- Eclampsia occurs upon the manifestation of seizures in the pre-eclampsia patient.

- Thrombophilias are a genetic form of hypercoagulability.

- Systemic lupus erythematosus is an autoimmune disease that increases the risk of fetal death, recurrent miscarriage, IUGR, and toxemia.

- Many prescription, illegal, and over-the-counter (OTC) drugs raise the chance of congenital anomalies in the fetus.

- Cyanotic heart disease results in premature birth, IUGR, and miscarriages, possibly due to the lower oxygen content in maternal circulation.

REFERENCES

1. Benson RC, Pernoll M. *Handbook of Obstetrics and Gynecology.* 10th ed. New York: McGraw-Hill Professional; 2001.

2. Kahn BF, Hobbins JC, Galan HL. Intrauterine growth restriction. In: Gibbs RS, Karlan BY, Haney HF, Ingrid Nygaard, eds. *Danforth's Obstetrics and Gynecology.* 10th ed. Baltimore: Wolters Kluwer Lippincott Williams & Wilkins; 2003:199.

3. Doubilet PM, Benson CB. *Atlas of Ultrasound in Obstetrics and Gynecology.* Lippincott Williams & Wilkins. Philadelphia; 2003.

4. Dugoff L. Prenatal diagnosis. In: Gibbs RS, Karlan BY, Haney HF, Ingrid Nygaard. *Danforth's Obstetrics and Gynecology.* 10th ed. Baltimore: Wolters Kluwer Lippincott Williams & Wilkins; 2003:119.

5. Dicke JM, Heuttner P, Yan S, et al. Umbilical artery Doppler indices in small for gestational age fetuses: correlation with adverse outcomes and placental abnormalities. *J Ultrasound Med.* 2009;28(12):1603–1610.

6. Sciscione Ad, Hayes EJ. Uterine artery Doppler flow studies in obstetric practice. *Am J Obstet Gynecol.* 2009; 201(2):121–126.

7. To WW, Mok CK. Fetal umbilical arterial and venous Doppler measurements in gestational diabetic and non-diabetic pregnancies near term. *J Maternal Fetal Neonatal Med.* 2009;22(12):1176–82.

8. Ferris TF. Toxemia and hypertension. In: Burrow GM, Ferris TF, eds. *Medical Co mplications During Pregnancy.* 3rd ed. Philadelphia: WB Saunders; 1988.

9. Burrow GN, Duffy T, Copel J. eds. *Medical Complication During Pregnancy.* 6th ed. Philadelphia: WB Saunders; 2004.

10. Avgil M, Diav-Citrin O, Shechtman S, et al. Epstein-Barr virus infection in pregnancy? A prospective controlled study. *Reproductive Toxicology.* 2008;25(4):468–471.

11. Avgil M, Ornoy A. Herpes simplex virus and Epstein-Barr virus infections in pregnancy: consequences of neonatal or intrauterine infection. *Reprod Toxicol.* May 2006;21(4):436–445.

12. Gibson CS, Goldwater PN, MacLennan AH, et al. Fetal exposure to herpesviruses may be associated with pregnancy-induced hypertensive disorders and preterm birth in a Caucasian population. *BJOG.* 2008;115(4):492–500.

13. Icarf J, Didier J, Dalens M, et al. Prospective study of EBV infection during pregnancy. *Biomedicine.* 1981;34:160.

14. Perlin BM, Pomerance JJ, Schifrin BS. Nonimmunologic hydrops fetalis. *Obstet Gynecol.* 1981;57:584–588.

15. Carroll B. Ultrasound features of preeclampsia. *J Clin Ultrasound.* 1980;8:483–488.

16. Temmerman M, Chomba EN, Ndinya-Achola J, et al. Maternal human immunodeficiency virus-1 infection and pregnancy outcome. *Obstet Gynecol.* 1994;83(4): 495–501.

17. Handsfield HH, Hodson WA, Holmes KK. Neonatal gonococcal infections: 1. Orogastric contamination with *Neisseria gonorrhoeae. JAMA.* 1973;225:697.

18. Strobino BA, Williams CL, Abid S, et al. Lyme disease and pregnancy outcome: A prospective study of two thousand prenatal patients. *Am J Obstet Gynecol.* 1993;169 (2 Pt 1):367–374.

19. Simpson ML, Graziano EP, Lupo VR, et al. Bacterial infections during pregnancy. In: Burrow GN, Ferris TF, eds. *Medical Complications During Pregnancy.* 3rd ed. Philadelphia: WB Saunders; 1988.

20. Sweet RL. Bacteriuria and pyelonephritis during pregnancy. *Semin Perinatol.* 1977;1:25.

21. Lee RV. Parasites and pregnancy: The problems of malaria and toxoplasmosis. *Clin Perinatol.* 1988;15(2):351–363.

22. Stegmann BJ, Carey JC. TORCH infections. Toxoplasmosis, other (syphilis, varicella-zoster, parvovirus B19), rubella, cytomegalovirus (CMV) and herpes infections. *Curr Womens Health Rep.* Aug 2002;2(4):253–258.

23. Rorman E, Zamir C, Rilkis I, Ben-David H. Congenital toxoplasmosis-prenatal aspects of *Toxoplasma gondii* infection. *Reprod Toxicol.* May 2006;1(4):458–472.

24. Enders M, Schalasta G, Baisch C, et al. Human parvovirus B19 infection during pregnancy—value of modern molecular and serological diagnostics. *J Clin Virol.* April 2006;5(4):400–406.

25. De Jong EP, De Haan TR, Kroes AC, et al. Parvovirus B19 infection in pregnancy. *J Clin Virol.* May 2006;36(1):1–7.

26. Freij BJ, South M, Sever JL. Maternal rubella and the congenital rubella syndrome. *Clin Perinatol.* 1988;15:247–257.

27. Eliezer S, Ester F, Ehud W, et al. Fetal splenomegaly: Ultrasound diagnosis of cytomegalovirus infection: A case report. *J Clin Ultrasound.* 1984;12:520–521.

28. Romero R, Chervenak FA, Berkowitz RL, et al. Intrauterine fetal tachypnea. *Am J Obstet Gynecol.* 1982;144:356–357.

29. Price JM, Fisch AE, Jacobson J. Ultrasound findings in fetal cytomegalovirus infection. *J Clin Ultrasound.* 1978;6:268.

30. Nahmias AJ, Josey WE, Naib WE, et al. Perinatal risk associated with maternal genital herpes simplex virus infection. *Am J Obstet Gynecol.* 1971;110:825–837.

31. National Diabetes Data Group. Classification and diagnosis of diabetes mellitus and other categories of glucose intolerance. *Diabetes.* 1979;28(12):1039.

32. Reece AE, Hobbins JC. Ultrasonography and diabetes mellitus in pregnancy. In: Sanders RC, James AE Jr, eds. *Ultrasonography in Obstetrics and Gynecology.* 3rd ed. Norwalk, CT: Appleton-Century-Crofts; 1985.

33. Pedersen J, Molsted-Pedersen L, Andersen B. Assessors of fetal perinatal mortality in diabetic pregnancy: Analysis of 1,332 pregnancies in the Copenhagen series 1946–1972. *Diabetes*. 1974;23(4):302.

34. Golditch IM, Kirkman K. The large fetus: Management and outcome. *Obstet Gynecol*. 1978;52:26–30.

35. Lenke RR, Levy HC. Maternal pheylketonuria and hyper-phenylalaninemia: An international survey of the outcome of untreated and treated pregnancies. *N Engl J Med*. 1980;303:1202.

36. Wladimiroff JW, Bloemsma CA, Wallenburg HCS. Ultrasonic diagnosis of the large-for-dates infant. *Obstet Gynecol*. 1978; 52:285–288.

37. Loetworawanit R, Chittacharoen A, Sututvoravut, S. Intrapartum fetal abdominal circumference by ultrasonography for predicting fetal macrosomia. *J Med Assoc Thai*. 2006;(Suppl 4):S60–S64.

38. Hackmon R, Bornstein E, Ferber A, et al. Combined analysis with amniotic fluid index and estimated fetal weight for prediction of severe macrosomia at birth. *Am J Obstet Gynecol*. Apr 2007;196(4):333.e1–e4.

39. Campbell S, Wilkin D. Ultrasonic measurement of fetal abdomen circumference in the estimation of fetal weight. *Br J Obstet Gynaecol*. 1975;82:689.

40. Grandjean SH, Saraman MF, DeMouzo J, et al. Detection of gestational diabetes by means of excessive fetal growth. *Am J Obstet Gynecol*. 1980;138:790–792.

41. Houchang D, Modanlou ND, Komatsu G, et al. Large-for-gestational-age neonates: Anthropometric reasons for shoulder dystocia. *Obstet Gynecol*. 1982;60:417–423.

42. Boney CM, Verma A, Tucker R, et al. Metabolic syndrome in childhood: association with birth weight, maternal obesity, and gestational diabetes mellitus. *Pediatrics*. Mar 2005;115(3):e290–e296.

43. Olson C. *Diagnosis and Management of Diabetes Mellitus*. 2nd ed. New York: Raven Press; 1985:181.

44. Hanna FW, Peters JR. Screening for gestational diabetes; past, present and future. *Diabetic Medicine*. May 2002;19(5):351–358.

45. Burrow GN. Thyroid diseases. In: Burrow GN, Ferris TF, eds. *Medical Complications During Pregnancy*. 3rd ed. Philadelphia: WB Saunders; 1988.

46. Fleischer AC, Killam AP, Boehm FH, et al. Hydrops fetalis: Sonographic evaluation and clinical implications. *Radiology*. 1981;141:163–168.

47. Creasy RK, Resnick R. *Maternal-fetal medicine: principles and practice*. Philadelphia: WB Saunders; 1984:926.

48. Kelton JG, Cruickshauk M. Hematologic disorders of pregnancy. In: Burrows GN, Ferris TF, eds. *Medical Complications During Pregnancy*. 3rd ed. Philadelphia: WB Saunders; 1988.

49. Genetics Home Reference. Berkowitz RL, Chitkara U, Goldberg JD, et al. Intravascular transfusion in utero: The percutaneous approach. *Am J Obstet Gynecol*. 1986;154:622–623. Accessed at http://ghr.nlm.nih.gov/50. Accessed on 10/2010.

50. Seeds JW, Watson AB. Ultrasound-guided fetal intravascular transfusion in severe rhesus immunization. *Am J Obstet Gynecol*. 1986;154:1105–1107.

51. Gill RW. Doppler assessment in obstetrics and fetal physiology. *Clin Diagn Ultrasound*. 1984;13:131–147.

52. Warren PS, Gill RW, Fisher CC. Doppler flow studies in rhesus isoimmunization. *Semin Perinatol*. 1987;11:375.

53. Weiner S, Bolognese RJ, Librizzi DO. Ultrasound in the evaluation and management of the isoimmunized pregnancy. *J Clin Ultrasound*. 1981;9:315–323.

54. Etches PC, Lemons JA. Nonimmune hydrops fetalis: Report of 22 cases including three siblings. *Pediatrics*. 1979;64:326–332.

55. Queenan JT, O'Brien GD. Diagnostic ultrasound in erythroblastosis fetalis. In: Sanders RC, James AE Jr, eds. *Ultrasonography in Obstetrics and Gynecology*. 3rd ed. Norwalk, CT: Appleton-Century-Crofts; 1985.

56. Serjeant GR. Sickle haemoglobin and pregnancy. *Br Med J*. 1983;287:628.

57. Roopnarinesingh S, Ramsewaks S. Decreased birth weight and femur length in fetuses of patients with the sickle-cell trait. *Obstet Gynecol*. 1986;68:46–48.

58. Anyaegbunam A, Langer O, Brustman L, et al. The application of uterine and umbilical artery velocimetry to the antenatal supervision of pregnancies complicated by maternal disease. *Am J Obstet Gynecol*. 1988;159: 544–547.

59. Desforges JF, Warth J. The management of sickle cell disease in pregnancy. *Clin Perinatol*. 1974;1:385–394.

60. Lindenbaum J, Klipstein FA. Folic acid deficiency in sickle cell anemia. *N Engl J Med*. 1963;269:875.

61. Morrison JC, Blake PG, Reed CD. Therapy for the pregnant patient with sickle hemoglobinopathies: A national focus. *Am J Obstet Gynecol*. 1982;144:268–269.

62. White JM, Richards B, Byrne M, et al. Thalassemia trait and pregnancy. *J Clin Pathol*. 1985;38:810.

63. Guy G, Coady DJ, Jansen V, et al. Alpha-thalassemia hydrops fetalis: Clinical and ultrasonographic considerations. *Am J Obstet Gynecol*. 1985;153:500–504.

64. Moore KL, Persaud TVN. *The Developing Human: Clinically Oriented Embryology*. Philadelphia: Saunders; 2003.

65. De Reu PA, Smits LJ, Oosterbaan HP, et al. Value of a single early third trimester fetal biometry for the prediction of birth weight deviations in a low risk population. *J Perinat Med*. May 2008;36(4):324–9.

66. Wall RE. Nutritional problems during pregnancy. In: Abrams RS, Waxler P eds. *Medical Care of the Pregnant Patient*. Boston: Little, Brown; 1983.

67. Sibai BM, Abdella TM, Anderson DG. Pregnancy outcome in 211 patients with mild chronic hypertension. *Obstet Gynecol*. 1983;61:571–576.

68. Rodgers BD, Lee RV. Drug abuse. In: Burrow GN, Ferris TF, eds. *Medical Complications During Pregnancy*. 3rd ed. Philadelphia: WB Saunders; 1988.

69. Robertson L, Wu O, Langhorne P, et al. Thrombophilia in pregnancy: a systemic review. *British Journal of Hematology*. Nov 2005;132(2):171–196.

70. Carp H, Dirnfeld M, Dor J, et al. ART in recurrent miscarriage: preimplantation genetic diagnosis/screening or surrogacy? *Human Reproduction*. July 2004;19(7): 1502–1505.

71. Ramsey-Goldman R, Kutzer LH, Guziick D, et al. Previous pregnancy outcome is an important determinant of subsequent pregnancy outcome in women with systemic lupus erythematosus. *Am J Reprod Immunol*. 1992;28:195–198.

72. Gray R, Mukherjee R, Rutter M. Alcohol consumption during pregnancy and its effects on neurodevelopment: What is known and what remains uncertain. *Addiction*. 2009;104(8):1270–1273.

73. Beckman DA, Brent RL. Mechanism of known environmental teratogens: Drugs and chemicals. *Clin Perinatol.* 1986;13:649–687.

74. Wladimiroff JW, Stewart PA, Reuss A, et al. The role of ultrasound in the early diagnosis of fetal structural defects following maternal anticonvulsant therapy. *Ultrasound Med Biol.* 1988;14:657–660.

75. Chasnoff IJ, Burns WJ, Schnolls, H et al. Cocaine use in pregnancy. *N Engl J Med.* 1985;313:666.

76. Chavez GF, Mulinare J, Cordero JF. Maternal cocaine use and the risk for genitourinary tract defects: An epidemiologic approach. *Am J Hum Genet.* 1988;43(Suppl):A43.

77. Cherukuri R, Minkoff H, Feldman J, et al. A cohort study of alkaloidal cocaine ("crack") in pregnancy. *Obstet Gynecol.* 1988;72:147–151.

78. Di Franza JR, Lew RA. Effect of maternal cigarette smoking on pregnancy complications and sudden infant death syndrome. *J Fam Pract.* 1995;40:385–394.

79. Meyer MB, Tonascia JA. Maternal smoking, pregnancy complications and perinatal mortality. *Am J Obstet Gynecol.* 1977;128:494–502.

80. Srisuphan W, Braken MB. Caffeine consumption during pregnancy and association with late spontaneous abortion. *Am J Obstet Gynecol.* 1986;154:14–20.

81. Landon MB, Gabbe SG, Mullen JL. Total parenteral nutrition during pregnancy. *Clin Perinatol.* 1986;13:57–72.

82. Treharne L. Obesity in pregnancy. *British Medical Journal.* 1984;4:127–138.

83. Rosett HL, Weinger L. *Alcohol and the Fetus: A Clinical Perspective.* New York: Oxford University Press; 1984.

84. Ruges S, Anderson T. Obstetric risks in obesity: An analysis of the literature. *Obstet Gynecol Surv.* 1985; 40:57.

85. Niebyl JR. Genetics and teratology, drug use in pregnancy. In: Pitkin R, Zlatnik F, eds. *1984 Year Book of Obstetrics and Gynecology.* Chicago: Year Book Medical Publishers; 1984.

86. Presbitero P, Somerville J, Stone S, et al. Pregnancy in cyanotic congenital heart disease: Outcome of mother and fetus. *Circulation.* 1994;89:2673–2676.

87. Koren A, Edwards MB, Miskin M. Antenatal sonography of fetal malformation associated with drugs and chemicals: A guide. *Am J Obstet Gynecol.* 1987;156:79–85.

30 The Postpartum Uterus

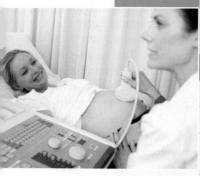

Dea Shatterly

OBJECTIVES

Describe changes in the uterus, ovaries, and ligaments after delivery

Explain normal postpartum physiology

Recognize the sonographic appearance of the normal and abnormal postpartum uterus

Differentiate between placenta accreta, increta, and percreta

Identify causes and sonographic appearance of puerperal infections

Summarize postpartum ovarian vein thrombophlebitis findings

List cesarean section complications

KEY TERMS

puerperium | puerperal infection | postpartum ovarian vein thrombophlebitis | placental accreta | placental increta | placental percreta | retained products of conception | uterine atony | endometritis

GLOSSARY

Atony Lack of normal muscle tone

Chorioamnionitis Inflammation of the amnion and chorion due to a bacterial infection

Coagulopathy Defect in the body's clotting mechanism resulting in bleeding

Decidua basalis Portion of the uterine lining that forms the maternal portion of the placenta

Emboli Moving particle, such as thrombosis or air, within the bloodstream

Hematoma Collection of blood outside the vessels

Hysterectomy Removal of the uterus

Involution Reduction of an organ to its normal appearance and size

Intravenous pyelogram (IVP) Radiographic images of the kidneys, ureters, and bladder after injection of a radiopaque dye

Nephrolithiasis Stones within the kidney

Thrombophlebitis Formation of a blood clot due to inflammation

Venogram Radiographic examination of the vein performed after injection of a radiopaque contrast medium

The postpartum period may also be called the puerperium. This is the period of time extending from immediately following the expulsion of the placenta and uterine contents to 6 to 8 weeks after birth or whenever the uterus regains its prenatal shape.[1] There are several reasons to perform a sonogram of the uterus in this period, with the most common being (1) postpartum hemorrhage; (2) searching for causes of puerperal infection; (3) evaluation for postpartum ovarian vein thrombophlebitis, and (4) complications arising from cesarean section such as hematomas and abscesses at the site of incision.

NORMAL POSTPARTUM ANATOMY AND PHYSIOLOGY

Physiologic and biochemical changes occur in the postpartum period because of the withdrawal of pregnancy-induced hormones. This causes the uterus to return or involute back to its prepregnancy state. Discontinuance of lactation results in ovulation and menstruation resuming.

Immediately after delivery, the uterus is heavy and bulky. Contraction and involution results in the uterus resuming the prepregnancy shape and position into the pelvic area between the symphysis pubis and the umbilicus. Except in cases of difficult or assisted delivery, such as forceps or large infant size, this involution typically occurs within 1 week of delivery. Sonography is not usually used during the puerperium period unless there are extenuating circumstances such as excessive bleeding, pain, or C-section deliveries. Bimanual exams or external exams done by the clinician can usually determine if the uterus has returned to the prepregnancy state.

SCANNING TECHNIQUES

When selecting a transducer, the sonographer needs to select the one with the highest frequency possible while still penetrating the structures and tissues beneath the skin surface to elicit adequate resolution. In most facilities, the transducer used most frequently is a curvilinear or vector-shaped transducer in the 2.5 to 5 megahertz (MHz) range. If needed, an endovaginal transducer can also be used with frequencies typically ranging from 5 to 8 MHz. Imaging of the pelvic structures requires a full bladder using the transabdominal approach. The bladder also pushes the gaseous bowel structures superior to the uterus. By adjusting the overall gain and time gain compensation (TGC), the sonographer adjusts brightness differences resulting from tissue attenuation or bladder enhancement. A thorough examination of the uterus includes the ovaries and other pelvic structures from both longitudinal and transverse planes from the transabdominal approach. Endovaginally, the pelvic organs can be studied on the sagittal and coronal planes. The combination of these imaging techniques provides an overall picture of the pelvic structures. A translabial or transperineal approach with sterile gel and a 2.5 to 5 MHz transducer visualizes the incision area of C-section patients who cannot tolerate transabdominal imaging. For these types of imaging, place the patient in the same position as for an endovaginal exam, placing the transducer adjacent to the labia.

It is also essential to remember to use a lighter pressure than when imaging the nongravid uterus, as a heavier pressure compresses the uterus, "thinning" the anteroposterior (AP) size and increasing the transverse dimension. Remember that these patients may have pelvic pain or tenderness, so the sonographer needs to keep patient comfort and pain tolerance in mind.

SONOGRAPHIC APPEARANCE OF NORMAL POSTPARTUM ANATOMY

Because of the enlarged nature of the postpartum uterus, bimanual or external exams may be inadequate to evaluate the uterus. Sonography provides dependable measurements of the uterus and ovaries along with any other pathology during initial and follow-up exams.

The postpartum uterus assumes various shapes during its involution to its nongravid state. It is common

to image the internal os on day one as partially open and ill-defined as it continues to close following delivery. The myometrium should be homogenous and pretty well delineated with measurements from 7 to 10 centimeters (cm) in total thickness. Due to uterine hypervascularity during pregnancy, it is common to visualize myometrial vessels in the postpartum two-dimensional (2D) and Doppler exam. The endometrium is thickened initially (up to 13 millimeters [mm] by some reports), but it should decrease to a normal thickness (3 to 8 mm) by the end of the postpartum period.[1] Free fluid in the endometrial cavity is a common finding, as blood and other substances slough off from the uterine cavity following birth.[1] These should not measure greater than 1.2 to 1.4 cm.

The uterus in longitudinal/sagittal imaging can measure from 14 to 25 cm as it shrinks to its prenatal size. If imaging in the very early stages of the postpartum period, the uterus may need to be measured in increments and added up to get a total length. The transverse/coronal width of the uterus can range from 7 to 14 cm. These measurements need to be done at a right angle to the longitudinal or sagittal plane where measurements were taken. There are several causes of erroneous measurements. These include (1) heavy external pressure during transabdominal imaging; (2) differing measurement sites; (3) uterine contractions; and (4) the amount of bladder distention that can affect the distance between the uterine fundus and the internal os (Fig. 30-1).

The adnexal ligaments of the postpartum patient are typically flaccid immediately following delivery, usually returning to their pregravid states within a month. It is important to recognize the broad ligament as a normal structure and not pathology. The ovaries should remain the same during pregnancy except for a few more cysts in the first trimester. As such, they should be imaged and recognized readily in the postpartum period.

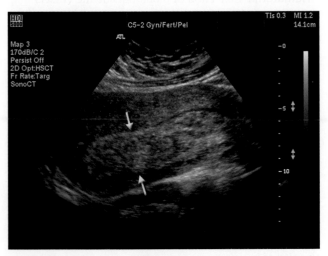

Figure 30-1 This postpartum uterus demonstrates a thick endometrium (arrows) within a large bulky uterus. (Image courtesy of Philips Medical Systems, Bothell, WA.)

Ranges of Normal Sonographic Postpartum Measurements[21-26]

Structure	Dimensions (centimeters)
Anteroposterior thickness	
Endometrium	0.4–1.3
Myometrium	3.0–6.5
Uterus	7.0–10.0
Length (sagittal measurement)	14.5–25.0
Width (transverse measurement)	7.0–14.0

POSTPARTUM HEMORRHAGE

The definition of postpartum hemorrhage is a blood loss of greater than 500 milliliters (ml) during the third stage of labor or immediately afterward in a vaginal delivery.[12] The cesarean delivery requires greater than a 1,000 ml loss to classify as having postpartum hemorrhage.[12] There are several causes of postpartum hemorrhage. The most common are conditions where the placenta has failed to attach properly to the myometrium of the uterus. Three terms describing the depth of the placental penetration are:

- Placenta accreta—Occurs when the placenta adheres to the myometrium of the uterus instead of the endometrium. Patients with a history of prior cesarean section[3] or women with other conditions causing uterine scarring are at increased risk for placenta accreta. According to Rumack, over 30%[2] of placenta accretas are associated with placenta previa.[3] This condition is not always found with sonography, especially if the defect is small (Fig. 30-2).
- Placenta increta—Occurs when the placenta invades the myometrium of the uterus further than is seen with accreta.[3]

- Placenta percreta—Occurs when the placenta completely penetrates the uterine myometrium and extends into the uterine serosa.[3]

All of these conditions are due to problems with the decidua basalis—either complete or partial absence of it.[8] Sonography helps identify the multiple intraplacental lakes that are indicators of placental invasion of the myometrium.[3,8] These are thought to be caused by atypical blood flow due to the abnormal decidua basalis. Rarely, antepartum rupture of the uterus occurs causing emergency delivery and hysterectomy.

Acute hemorrhage is severe bleeding immediately following delivery—usually resulting in emergency hysterectomy.[8] Delayed hemorrhage is bleeding that occurs over several days to a few weeks in the postpartum period. All of the following are associated with postpartum hemorrhage: decreased hematocrit, hypotension, hysterectomy, renal failure, shock, and sometimes death.

PUERPERAL INFECTION

Puerperal infection is any infection in the postpartum period characterized by a temperature over 100.4°F/38°C on any two successive days after the first 24 hours postpartum.[4] Uterine tenderness (not "afterpains") is usually the first sign of infection.[6] Other signs and symptoms include chills, headache, malaise, and anorexia.[4] The uterus is typically soft, tender, and large. Lochia, or vaginal discharge, may be diminished or it may be profuse and odorous.[4] Most puerperal infections are urinary tract infections, but they can also be breast infections, thrombophlebitis, or endometritis.

Endometritis is defined as infection of the endometrium—usually caused by migration of normal vaginal flora, which may result in postpartum bleeding.[13] Other causes include premature rupture of membranes, retained products of conception and prolonged

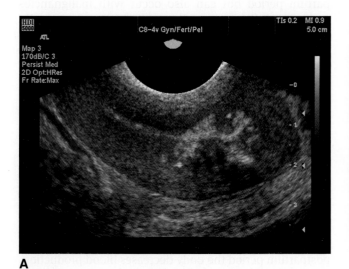
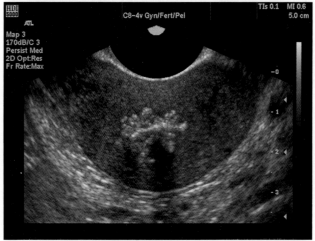

A   **B**

Figure 30-2 Uterine accreta. **A:** Sagittal, midline endovaginal image of early pregnancy accreta. **B:** Transverse image of the same uterus. (Image courtesy of Philips Medical Systems, Bothell, WA.)

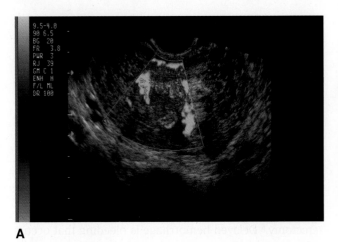

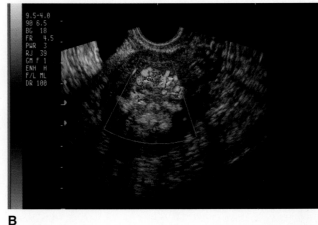

A

B

Figure 30-3 A: A placental polyp and associated vascular supply. Hysteroscopic resection was successful with resumption of normal menstruation. **B:** Another placental polyp.

labor.[4] Vaginal delivery after a C-section increases the incidence of endometritis.[4,5] The sonographic appearance of endometritis is that of a thick, irregular endometrium that may have fluid in the endocervical canal.[5] Some reports have also noted gas in the endometrial canal; however, up to 3 weeks postpartum, some gas in the endocervical canal is a normal finding.[1,5]

Another reason for postpartum hemorrhage is retained products of conception (RPOC).[5,12] This condition is characterized by incomplete expulsion of miscellaneous products of conception during labor and delivery. Retained products of conception can also cause infection. The sonographic appearance is that of a highly echogenic mass in the endometrial canal.[2] Remnants of placental tissue, called a placental polyp, are due to incomplete placental expulsion from the uterus (Fig. 30-3).[20] A heterogeneous mass may contain necrotic tissue, clot, or infection.[5] Endometritis

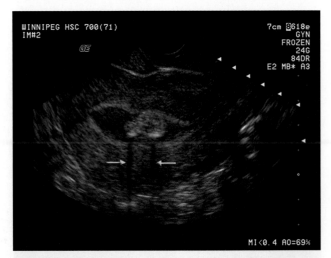

Figure 30-4 This is an image of a patient after an elective termination. Retained products of conception image as a hyperechoic mass within an irregularly shaped uterus. Artifacts *(arrows)*, possibly due to air, create a characteristic comet-tail type artifact. (Image courtesy of GE Healthcare, Wauwatosa, WI.)

and RPOC have very similar appearances sonographically (Fig. 30-4).

Uterine atony is one of the most frequent causes of postpartum hemorrhage.[9,10,12] Atony is when the uterus fails to reach pregravid tone and becomes flaccid and unable to hold its shape. A woman has an increased risk of developing atony with a multifetal pregnancy, macrosomy, prolonged labor, more than five term pregnancies, rapid labor, polyhydramnios, and chorioamnionitis.[12] Coagulopathy is also common in the postpartum period. Clotting is the natural reaction to bleeding; however, when the clot dislodges, hemorrhage occurs at the adherence site.

POSTPARTUM OVARIAN VEIN THROMBOPHLEBITIS

Thrombophlebitis by definition is the inflammation of a vein caused by a thrombus found in the lumen of the vessel. Postpartum ovarian vein thrombophlebitis (POVT) is a rare condition found typically in the postpartum period but can also occur with malignancies and pelvic inflammatory disease.[14] This rare, potentially life-threatening complication has a reported incidence from 1:600 to 1:2,000, with an increased number following cesarean deliveries.[14,16,17] The pathogenesis of POVT relates to Virchow's triad: (1) hypercoagulability of blood during pregnancy and the postpartum period; (2) venous stasis; and (3) venous wall damage as a result of uterus expansion and contraction.[7,15]

The majority of cases of POVT involve the right ovarian vein (80% to 90% in some literature).[5,15] This is thought to be due to the acute angle at which the right ovarian vein enters the IVC. Retrograde flow in the left ovarian vein reduces the spread of infection from the uterus.[5,15] The vein enlarges during pregnancy to accommodate the increased amount of blood flow. During the postpartum period the body decreases blood production, resulting in venous stasis. Incompetent valves in the ovarian vein is a possible cause for this venous stasis.

SYMPTOMS

Because the symptoms of POVT are similar to those of other disease processes, it can be difficult to diagnose based on clinical manifestations alone. The most common signs and symptoms of POVT include pelvic pain, fever, and right-sided pelvic mass.[11,17] One possible cause is the spread of bacterial infections from the uterus. Less commonly, the patient may experience nausea, vomiting, flank pain, groin pain, or even bowel ileus. Typically, the patient experiences these symptoms during the first 48 to 96 hours following delivery.[16]

DIAGNOSIS

The diagnosis of POVT has improved dramatically with the availability of computed tomography (CT), magnetic resonance imaging (MRI), and sonography.[17] Prior to the increased availability of these modalities, POVT was commonly diagnosed with intravenous pylograms (IVP) or venograms. Because of its ability to demonstrate the entire ovarian vein, CT is the preferred diagnostic method for POVT.[11,14] Sonographically, POVT images as a dilated anechoic to hypoechoic tubular structure extending superiorly from the adnexa (Figs. 30-5 and 6-19).[18] A typical finding is a lack of a color or spectral Doppler signal; however, echogenic thrombus in the lumen confirms the presence of thrombus.[18] Extension into the inferior vena cava (IVC) indicates propagation of the clot.[17] The thrombus also may image as a mass between the uterus and the psoas muscles, but the most common site for POVT is where the IVC and the right ovarian vein meet. Differential diagnosis of POVT includes appendicitis, fibroids, nephrolithiasis, ovarian torsion, and tubo-ovarian abscess requiring demonstration of thrombus in the ovarian vein to prove POVT.[14-17]

TREATMENT

Treatment of POVT is usually through intravenous (IV) therapy of anticoagulants such as heparin and blood thinners like warfarin.[18] Some patients benefit from IVC filters to keep the embolus from traveling into the heart or lungs and causing pulmonary emboli or death. Follow-up imaging studies help in monitoring thrombus resolution. Antibiotics may also be given.[14-17]

CESAREAN SECTION COMPLICATIONS

The Centers for Disease Control and Prevention (CDC) reported that, in 2007, cesarean section deliveries accounted for up to 31.8% of all deliveries in the United States, increasing by 50% in the last decade. Traditionally, the incision was performed vertically or longitudinally along the long axis of the uterus.[5] In an effort to increase vaginal deliveries following cesarean sections, most facilities are now employing a transverse incision. This incision may be anechoic to hypoechoic sonographically, depending on how the local tissue reacts to the surgery. Common complications of cesarean sections are hematomas at the site of incision and infection.[5]

HEMATOMAS

During a cesarean section, the surgeon typically incises the peritoneum between the urinary bladder and the uterus to access the lower uterine segment. This potential space is referred to as the bladder flap and is the site of most hematomas found after cesarean sections.[5] Hematomas occur when there is bleeding at the site of incision and the body has not reabsorbed the blood. Hematomas found in the bladder flap region are sonographically anechoic with ill-defined borders[5] that range in size from very small (less than 1 cm) to very large (greater than 15 cm). Sometimes, these appear as complex masses because of the blood components clotting or internal septations or debris within the hematoma.[19] A high-frequency transducer is sometimes needed to adequately visualize the structure and internal components completely (Fig. 30-6).

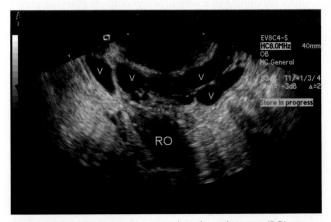

Figure 30-5 Varicosities (v) surrounding the right ovary (RO).

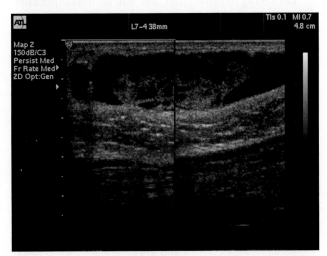

Figure 30-6 Dual image demonstrating the complex appearance of a resolving hematoma. (Image courtesy of Philips Medical Systems, Bothell, WA.)

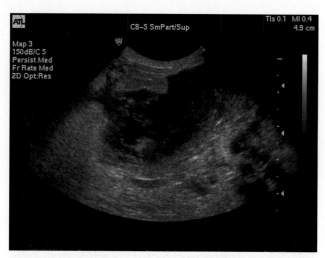

Figure 30-7 Complex appearance of a postsurgical abscess. (Image courtesy of Philips Medical Systems, Bothell, WA.)

INFECTIONS

Infections following cesarean sections may be caused by factors such as long operation time, endometritis, contamination of amniotic fluid entering the incision, and pre-existing infections. Any time a patient presents with fever following a cesarean section, infection must always be a suspicion. Infections can develop in the abdominal wall or uterine wall following cesarean section. Abscesses may also develop along the incision line. These complications may have a variety of appearances, including anechoic, cystic, complex, and with or without definite margins. CT may help give a better overall appearance to help with diagnosis (Fig.30-7).

Critical Thinking Question

A patient presents to the department 2 weeks after delivering her first child. She had an uncomplicated pregnancy and delivery. Her complaints are of bleeding, low-grade fever, and general malaise. On clinical exam she complained of a tender uterus. The pregnancy test was negative and there was no evidence of infection on her urinalysis. List the differentials for the patient's signs and symptoms. What sonographic findings would aid in establishing a diagnosis?

ANSWER: The patient's complaints and clinical findings could fit with endometritis, RPOC, or uterine atony. Endometritis and RPOC both demonstrate a thick, irregular endometrium. Uterine atony usually occurs with a history of multiple gestations, prolonged labor, or prenatal infection. This patient is a primigravida with a normal pregnancy, so this is the least likely cause of her problems. Due to the similarity between endometritis and RPOC, it is difficult to separate these two entities during the sonographic exam.

SUMMARY

- Placenta accreta, increta, and percreta are abnormal placental penetration of the myometrium, which may lead to postpartum bleeding.
- Endometritis is an infection of the endometrium that may extend to the myometrium and parametrial tissues.
- RPOC and endometritis have a similar sonographic appearance.
- Failure of the uterus to contract (atony) can lead to hemorrhage.
- POVT occurs more often in the right ovarian vein
- Hematomas and infection are two complications of a cesarean section.

REFERENCES

1. Poder L. Ultrasound evaluation of the uterus. In: Callen PW, ed. *Ultrasonography in Obstetrics and Gynecology*. 5th ed. Philadelphia: Saunders Elsevier; 2008.
2. Alkazaleh F, Viero S, Kingdom J. Sonographic evaluation of the placenta. In: Rumack CM, Wilson SR, Charboneau JW, Johnson JM, eds. *Diagnostic Ultrasound*. 3rd ed. Elsevier; 2005.
3. Feldstein VA, Harris RD, Machin GA. Ultrasound evaluation of the placenta and umbilical cord. In: Callen PW, ed. *Ultrasonography in Obstetrics and Gynecology*. 5th ed. Philadelphia: Saunders Elsevier; 2008.
4. Davies JK, Gibbs RS. Obstetric and perinatal infections. In Gibbs RS, Karlan BY, Haney AF, Nygaard I, eds. *Danforth's Obstetrics and Gynecology*. 10th ed. Baltimore: Wolters Klewer | Lippincott Williams & Wilkins; 2008.
5. Salem S, Wilson SR. Gyneoclogic ultrasound. In Rumack CM, Wilson SR, Charboneau JW, eds. *Diagnostic Ultrasound*. 3rd ed. Elsevier; 2005.
6. Osborne NG. Infections of the uterus. In: Baggish MS, Valle RF, Guedj H, eds. *Hysteroscopy - Visual Perspectives of Uterine Anatomy, Physiology and Pathology*. 3rd ed. Baltimore: Wolters Klewer | Lippincott Williams & Wilkins; 2007.
7. Singh RS, Galt SW. The role of ultrasound in the management of extremity diseaese. In: Zwiebel WJ, Pellerito JS, eds. *Introduction to Vascular Ultrasonography*. 5th ed. New York, Elsevier Saunders; 2005.
8. Yi KW, Oh MJ, Seo TS, et al. Prophylactic hypogastric artery ballooning in a patient with complete placenta previa and increta. *J Korean Med Sci*. 2010;25(4):651–655.
9. Bodelon C, Bernabe-Ortiz A, Schiff MA, et al. Factors associated with peripartum hysterectomy. *Obstet Gynecol*. 2009;114(1):115–123.
10 Baudo F, Caimi TM, Mostarda G, et al. Critical bleeding in pregnancy: a novel therapeutic approach to bleeding. *Minerva Anesthesiol*. 2006;72(6):389–393.
11. Karaosmanoglu D, Karcaaltincaba M, Karcaaltincaba D, et al. MDCT of the ovarian vein: normal anatomy and pathology. *AJR Am J Roentgenol*. 2009;192(1):295–299.
12. Postpartum Hemorrhage. *Merck Manual*. http://www.merck.com/mmpe/sec18/ch264/ch264h.html. Accessed July 2010.
13. Puerperal Endometritis. *Merck Manual*. http://www.merck.com/mmpe/sec18/ch265/ch265c.html. Accessed July 2010.

14. Chellman-Jeffers MR. Ovarian Vein Thrombosis. *WebMD*. http://emedicine.medscape.com/article/404364-overview. Accessed July 2010.

15. Takach TJ, Cervera RD, Gregoric ID. Ovarian vein and caval thrombosis. *Tex Heart Inst J*. 2005;32(4):579–582.

16. Prieto-Nieto MI, Perez-Robledo JP, Rodriguez-Montes JA, et al. Acute appendicitis-like symptoms as initial presentation of ovarian vein thrombosis. *Annuals of Vascular Surgery*. 2004;18(4):481–483.

17. Al-toma A, Heggelman BGF, Kramer MHH. Postpartum ovarian vein thrombosis: report of a case and review of literature. *Neth J Med*. 2003;61(10):334–336.

18. Akinbiyi AA, Nguyen R, Katz M. Postpartum ovarian vein thrombosis: two cases and review of literature. *Case Reports Med*. 2009. http://www.hindawi.com/journals/crm/2009/101367.html. Accessed July 2010.

19. Baker ME, Bowie JD, Killam AP. Sonography of post-cesarean-section bladder-flap hematoma. *AJR*. 1985;144: 757–759.

20. Yi JG, Choi SE, S YK, et al. Placental polyp: sonographic findings. *AJR*. 1993;161:345–346.

21. Defoort P, Benijts G, Thiery M, et al. Ultrasound assessment of puerperal uterine involution. *Eur J Obstet Gynecol Reprod Biol*. 1978;8:95–97.

22. Land JA, Stoot JE, Evers JL. Puerperal ultrasonic hysterography. *Gynecol Obstet Invest*. 1984;18:165–168.

23. Lavery JP, Shaw LA. Sonography of the puerperal uterus. *J Ultrasound Med*. 1989;8:481–486.

24. Rodeck CH, Newton JR. Study of the uterine cavity by ultrasound in the early puerperium. *Br J Obstet Gynaecol*. 1976;83:795–801.

25. VanRees D, Bernstine RL, Crawford W. Involution of the postpartum uterus: An ultrasonic study. *J Clin Ultrasound*. 1981;9:55–57.

26. Wachsberg RH, Kurtz AB, Levine CD, et al. Realtime ultrasonographic analysis of the normal postpartum uterus: Technique, variability, and measurements. *J Ultrasound Med*. 1994;13:215–221.

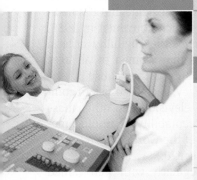

31 Interventional Ultrasound

Sanja Plavsic Kupesic

OBJECTIVES

Define amniocentesis, chorionic villi sampling (CVS), and percutaneous umbilical blood sampling (PUBS)

List the indications for amniocentesis, CVS, fetal tissue sampling, and endovaginal procedures

Determine the correct gestational age to perform a genetic amniocentesis or CVS sampling

Describe the procedure for performing amniocentesis and CVS

Summarize the procedure for performing an amniocentesis or pregnancy reduction with a multifetal pregnancy

Explain the differences between a transcervical and transabdominal technique of CVS

List invasive procedures that obtain tissue or blood samples from the fetus

Recall ultrasound-guided endovaginal invasive procedures

KEY TERMS

amniocentesis | chorionic villus sampling | percutaneous umbilical blood sampling (PUBS) | coelocentesis | cordocentesis | fetal therapy | mutifetal

GLOSSARY

Advanced maternal age (AMA) Woman 35 years of age or older

Amniocentesis Sampling of amniotic fluid

Chorionic villus sampling (CVS) Sampling of chorionic villus of the placenta

Coelocentesis Early sampling of the exocoelomic cavity fluid via placenta free areas

Mutifetal More than one fetus

Percutaneous umbilical blood sampling (PUBS, aka cordocentesis) Sampling of fetal blood via the umbilical cord

Petri dish Round dish used to culture fetal tissue or cells

Transcervical Through the cervix

Amniocentesis and chorionic villus sampling (CVS), the two most common clinical techniques for obtaining living fetal cells or fetal cell products from the pregnant uterus for prenatal diagnosis, are heavily dependent on the use of ultrasound. Percutaneous umbilical blood sampling (PUBS), also known as cordocentesis,[1] is another technique requiring the use of ultrasound to obtain fetal cells, but this technique carries a much higher procedure-related risk than either amniocentesis or CVS. PUBS is performed by carefully inserting a long, fine-gauged needle under ultrasound guidance through the skin, subcutaneous tissues, peritoneum, uterus, and amniotic sac of the mother's abdomen and tapping

one of the fetal umbilical vessels directly for microliter amounts of fetal blood to analyze. This procedure has a higher risk for complications and is therefore reserved for special indications and special analyses such as in later-stage pregnancies needing chemical assays or rapid blood cell cultures for chromosome studies requiring fetal blood.

The ever-increasing number of genetic disorders now diagnosed prenatally, particularly using DNA technology, has brought amniocentesis and CVS into the realm of everyday medical practice. Patient awareness of the invasive procedure benefits and limitations, as well as the complication rates, becomes imperative. Genetic counseling sessions provide the opportunity to impart this information to the patients and their families.

Genetic counseling has been described as a communication process by which the occurrence and the risk of recurrence of a genetic disorder within a family is discussed.[2] In fact, it is more than this: the genetic counselor provides the patient or the family with current relevant facts concerning a genetic disorder, including the risks involved in diagnosis and the available treatment options.[2,3]

Manipulations of the pregnant uterus and the developing fetus are highly charged emotional issues with moral and ethical overtones that need to be addressed with each patient. Thorough discussion of the procedures and patient questions meet the current standards of care in prenatal medical diagnosis. A team approach becomes useful, usually involving not only the obstetrician but also a genetic counselor, a sonographer, and appropriate surgical and medical specialists.

AMNIOCENTESIS

"Amniocentesis," derived from Greek, means "puncture of the amniotic sac." The amnion and the chorion, the two major membranous structures surrounding and protecting the developing fetus within the uterus throughout pregnancy, develop from the same fertilized ovum, as does the fetus. Birth signals the end of the placenta and membrane functions, resulting in expulsion of the tissues.

HISTORY

In 1881, Lamble and Schatz first described the amniocentesis procedure as a method for relieving intrauterine pressure resulting from abnormal accumulation of amniotic fluid.[4,5] Parvey, who was one of the first to report successful management of acute hydramnios with abdominal puncture, credits Bumm as the first to have attempted this procedure, as early as 1900.[6,7] Objections to the blind insertion of a needle into the pregnant uterus included possible injury to the fetus, damage to the placenta, uterine hemorrhage, infection, and interruption of the pregnancy. These objections were apparently sufficient to discourage further progress until Bevis showed that certain characteristics of amniotic fluid had diagnostic and prognostic value for hemolytic disease of the newborn.[8] Walker and later Liley were able to demonstrate the relative safety of the procedure by performing serial amnioceteses on one patient without incident.[9,10] Sonographic guidance now images the amniocentesis needle during the procedure, eliminating previously encountered complications of the procedure; however, some inherent risks remain.

Advanced maternal age (AMA) or a history of a child with a specific birth defect originally resulted in the recommendation to perform a prenatal diagnostic amniocentesis. However, the President's Commission for Study of Ethical Problems in Medicine and Biomedical and Behavioral Science, which convened in 1983, recommended reexamination of the eligibility criteria for genetic amniocentesis so that women of all ages might benefit from this procedure, if they chose.[11]

Increased diagnostic accuracy, decreased risk of complications, and publicity on television and other mass media have increased the acceptability of amniocentesis among most populations of the world. The reported risk of complications has been 0.5%, and in centers performing this procedure regularly with well-trained personnel, the actual procedure-related complication rate is less than 3 per 1,000 procedures.[12]

The number of requests for amniocentesis and for CVS has escalated significantly during the last decade, with the advent of newer DNA technology and the identification of an increasing number of chromosomal disorders detectable by molecular genetics methods.

INDICATIONS FOR AMNIOCENTESIS

Maternal age-related chromosome abnormality risk increases after the age of 35, commonly resulting in the performance of the genetic amniocentesis. This category accounts for 65% to 80% of requests for prenatal diagnosis.[13,14] Women whose maternal serum alpha-fetoprotein (MSAFP) screening results are either elevated or decreased below the median values for the general population comprise the second largest group of requests, accounting for 10% to 15% of the total. Leek and colleagues in 1972 first described the association between abnormally high levels of MSAFP and neural tube defects, whereas MSAFP values below the mean levels for a given gestational age have been associated with an increased risk for fetal chromosomal trisomy.[15,16]

Alpha-fetoprotein (AFP) is a serum protein found normally in the fetal circulatory system and produced by the fetal liver. Circulatory obstruction of amniotic fluid results in protein accumulation in the amniotic fluid, which subsequently appears as an increase in maternal blood serum. Other conditions associated with MSAFP elevations include multiple pregnancy, fetal demise, and a number of other fetal abnormalities.[17] MSAFP levels, as well as amniotic fluid AFP levels, change at different stages of gestation. The AFP level evaluation includes normalization in relation to the specific gestational age. An MSAFP value in excess of 2.5 times the mean for that gestational age is suspect. The currently accepted protocol for screening recommends an ultrasound examination to confirm gestational age and to determine the presence or absence of multiple pregnancies or other ultrasound-detectable abnormalities. The failure to determine correctly the gestational age may lead to incorrect interpretation of the MSAFP results. Careful ultrasound examination discloses neural tube

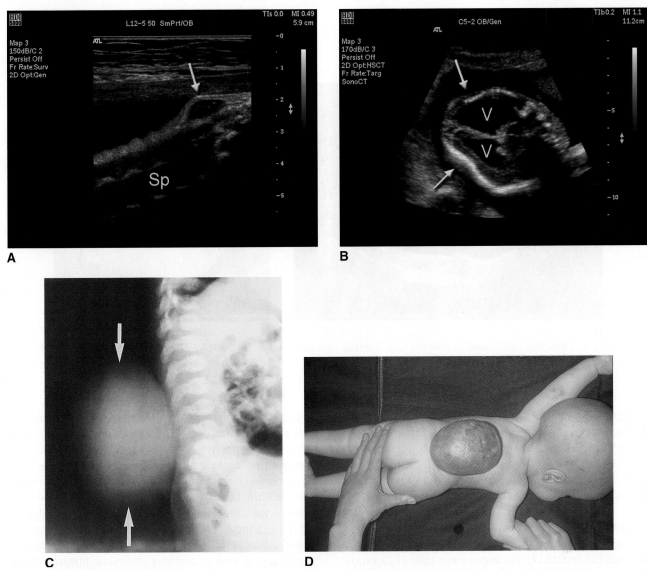

Figure 31-1 The patient presenting with a markedly elevated level of serum alpha-fetoprotein often leads to a sonographic examination of the fetus. **A:** Possible malformations include a myelomeningocele (*arrow*) extending posteriorly from the spine (Sp), in addition to (**B**) ventricularmegaly (V), and a positive "lemon" sign of the fetal skull (*arrows*). **C:** Radiographs demonstrate a soft tissue mass extending (*arrows*). **D:** A meningomyelocele. (Images A & B courtesy of Philips Medical Systems, Bothell, WA.)

defects as the cause for MSAFP elevation in almost all cases (Figs. 31-1–2).

A varying but steadily growing number of well-informed patients, who are at no specific risk category but are overly concerned about the possibility of an abnormal pregnancy outcome, is asking to be tested. Maternal anxiety has therefore become a recognized indication for prenatal genetic diagnosis regardless of maternal age.

Women who have delivered children with chromosomal defects or metabolic disorders in the past are also recommended for genetic amniocentesis. More than 100 metabolic disorders and an escalating number of DNA fetal defects are now detectable biochemically during the course of the prenatal period. The recurrence risks of genetic abnormalities depend on the mode of inheritance. The chances for recurrence range from less than 1% in the case of a previous child with a chromosomal defect not found in the parents to 25% in the case of an autosomal recessive biochemical defect such as Tay-Sachs disease or cystic fibrosis to 50% (for male children) in X-linked muscular dystrophy.

TIMING OF AMNIOCENTESIS

The optimal time to perform the genetic amniocentesis is between the 14th and 20th gestational weeks. Adequate fluid volume allows for obtaining useful samples with minimal threat to the fetus, and sufficient numbers of viable amniocytes are present to obtain a timely result. Furthermore, the sonographic fetal anatomy has increased definition at this gestational age, permitting easier detection of abnormalities.

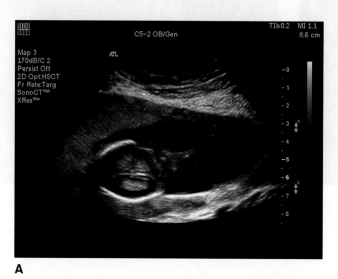

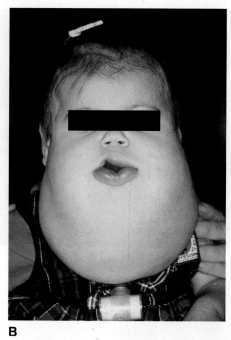

A   **B**

Figure 31-2 A: Cystic hygroma extending from the posterior fetal neck identified on sonographic examination. (Image courtesy of Philips Medical Systems, Bothell, WA.) **B:.** A large, soft cervical mass (cystic hygroma) in a 9-month-old. Tracheostomy was placed at birth. (Image courtesy of Ellen Deutsch, MD.)

Prenatal diagnosis attempts to obtain results as early in pregnancy as possible, but performing amniocentesis earlier than 14 weeks has been shown to significantly increase the risk for pregnancy loss.[18] Technically, amniocentesis can be safely performed at any time in the second and third trimesters; the deadline is related more closely to individual state legal restrictions for pregnancy termination than to any other factor.

The amniocentesis for determining fetal maturity is through the lecithin to sphingomyelin ratio (L/S ratio). The severity of erythroblastosis (by optical density measurements of the amniotic fluid) is another measurement obtained during this stage of pregnancy. The problems of amniocenteses performed after 20 weeks increase because of cell culture difficulties, resulting in an unsuccessful procedure. Because of this problem, it is not recommended to perform an amniocentesis in the late second or third trimesters.

The legal limit for elective termination of pregnancy is determined by each country, and even by state (United States) or province (Canada), varying from 12 to 24 weeks of gestation. The timing of genetic amniocentesis must therefore allow for completion of all laboratory testing, permitting the option of legal pregnancy termination to those who might choose this alternative for a nonlethal birth defect. The average waiting period for the results (i.e., detecting abnormalities in chromosome number such as trisomy 21 [Down syndrome], chromosome monosomy such as Turner syndrome, or chromosome structural rearrangements, translocations, deletions, insertions, etc.) is 7 to 10 days. In some cases, 3 weeks may be required to grow a sufficient number

of cells to obtain a result. Biochemical (enzyme) defects such as galactosemia, Gaucher disease, Niemann-Pick disease, phenylketonuria, and Tay-Sachs disease, to name just a few, are usually diagnosed sooner than chromosome culture analyses can be completed. Diagnosis within hours after specimen collection became possible with the advent of molecular probes for detecting DNA defects. This procedure helps in the diagnosis of many biochemical defects such as those mentioned previously, as well as diseases like cystic fibrosis, Duchenne muscular dystrophy, Prader-Willi syndrome, and the hemoglobinopathies.

To deal with problems of terminating pregnancies that have gone beyond the legal limit, particularly when a malformed fetus is an issue, many institutions have appointed ethics committees to evaluate each situation individually. The committee is composed of nonprofessionals, clergy, nonmedical, and medical professionals. They hear the evidence, evaluate the case, and make recommendations regarding these critical issues. In some cases, the legal abortion of the anencephalic fetus has occurred after 28 weeks of pregnancy.[19]

PROCEDURE FOR ULTRASOUND-GUIDED AMNIOCENTESIS

After genetic counseling and completion of the informed consent process, ideally done days or weeks before the performance of the procedure, scheduling of a simultaneous ultrasound and amniocentesis occurs. Amniocentesis is an outpatient procedure and is performed in the ultrasound laboratory in accordance with

PATHOLOGY BOX 31-1

Indications for Invasive Procedures

Procedure

Amniocentesis/CVS	AMA
	Elevated MSAFP
	History of birth defects
	Maternal metabolic disorders
	Parental genetic disorder carrier
	Abnormal sonographic finding
Fetal	Blood sampling (PUBS, intrahepatic vein sampling)
	• Rh sensitization
	• RBC disorders
	• Hemoglobinopathies
	• Platelet disorders
	• Intrauterine congenital infections
	• Thyroid disease
	• Hydrops of unknown origin
	• Fetal blood grouping
	• Rapid karyotyping
	Transfusion therapy
	• Blood transfusion
	• Drug infusion
	• FFTS/TTTS laser treatment
	Tissue sampling
	• Liver
	• Skin
	• Muscle
	Multifetal pregnancy reduction
Endovaginal	Oocyte retrieval
	Ovarian cyst aspiration
	Pelvis mass biopsy
	Abscess drainage
	Culdocentesis
	Local treatment of ectopic pregnancy
	Embryo transfer
	Tubal catheterization
	Hysterosonography/HSG
	IUCD position
	Radiotherapy planning and monitoring

the guidelines published by the American Institute of Ultrasound in Medicine (AIUM).[20]

The sonographer should obtain the following information before performance of the amniocentesis:

1. Number of fetuses, fetal position, and viability
2. Amniotic fluid volume (normal, decreased, or increased)
3. Placental location
4. Gestational age, by use of the following measurements: biparietal diameter, femur length, abdominal circumference, head circumference, and binocular (interorbital) distance
5. Assessment of the following anatomic structures: the cerebral ventricles, fetal heart (four-chamber view), stomach, urinary bladder, umbilical cord insertion, number of cord vessels, kidneys, spinal column, and limbs
6. Location of the optimal fluid pocket for amniocentesis
7. Evaluation of the fetal heart rate before and after the procedure

The procedure begins with draping of the operative site with sterile towels. Observation of strict sterile precautions reduces infection-related complications after amniocentesis. The ultrasound transducer is coated with regular transmission gel and held by an assistant as the physician covers the transducer with a sterile plastic bag.[21] Under sonographic visualization, a 3.5-inch long, 20-gauge, sterile, disposable spinal needle with a stylet is used to enter the amniotic sac. The sonographic image allows visualization of needle progress through the tissue layers. The beveled tip of the needle images as a bright spot on the ultrasound screen, described as a "flare."[22] The amniocentesis site is thus documented with an image. During the insertion procedure, exercise extra caution while directing the needle tip into the amniotic sac. It must be remembered that the ultrasound image of the needle position can be grossly distorted, due to refraction and reverberation artifacts, when viewed through fluid versus solid tissue interfaces.[22] Ultrasound monitoring and amniocentesis can be performed simultaneously by the same operator (Figs. 30-3–4).

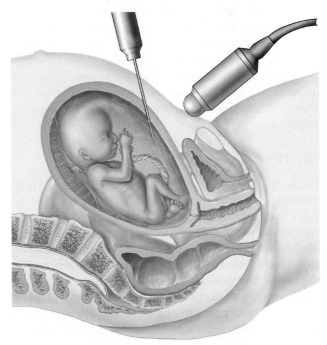

Figure 31-3 A genetic amniocentesis is usually performed at around 14 to 20 weeks, obtaining amniotic fluid, which contains fetal cells. Insertion of the amniocentesis needle is under direct ultrasonic guidance.

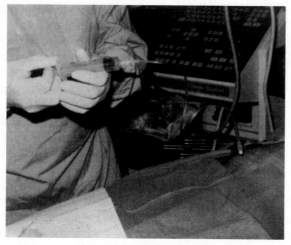

Figure 31-4 Amniotic fluid specimen is withdrawn under sterile conditions with a sterile plastic catheter attached at one end to the amniocentesis needle and to a 20-ml syringe at the other.

To avoid contaminating the specimen with maternal cells, discard the first few drops of fluid after removal of the stylet.[23,24] The Luer-lock needle hub provides an attachment location to the 20-inch length of sterile, flexible extension tubing. The opposite end of the tubing attaches to a sterile 20-milliliter (ml) syringe. The extension tubing provides greater ease and stability for amniotic fluid aspiration; alternatively, the syringe may attach to the needle hub without the use of tubing. Approximately 20 to 30 ml of amniotic fluid is withdrawn and transferred into a sterile, properly labeled, conical tube for transport to the laboratory. After aspiration of the fluid sample, the needle is withdrawn. Before patient discharge, there is a final check of the fetal heart.

Maternal injection of 300 milligrams (mg) of anti-D IgG immediately after amniocentesis of the Coombs test negative Rh-negative mother prevents sensitization, which occurs with a Rh-positive fetus.

Centrifugation separates the amniocytes from the amniotic fluid. A fluid assay detects AFP or other biochemical substances, and the cell cultures are used for karyotyping.

MULTIPLE PREGNANCIES

Ultrasound helps establish the gestational age, verify viability, and note the number and location of the fetuses and placentas and also identifies the presence of a membrane separating fetal compartments. In the event of diamniotic twins, each sac is identified sonographically and labeled A or B according to its position in the mother's abdomen. The easily identified membrane seen separating diamniotic twin sacs helps in planning the strategy for tapping each sac. Though a twin pregnancy, each fetus's biometric evaluation mirrors a singleton exam.

After removing the amniotic fluid from the first sac (twin A), an injection of 1 to 2 ml of indigo carmine

dye into sac A colors the fluid a bluish tint. A second amniocentesis is performed on twin B. Blue-stained fluid withdrawn from the second sac indicates that either a communication exists between the sacs, such as occurs with monoamniotic twins, or that the first sac was reentered. Direct simultaneous visualization of the inserted needle's progress with ultrasound helps to avoid reentry. Sampling of both fetal sacs is successful in approximately 88% of twin pregnancies. If there are triplets, repeat the "blue dye procedure" once more after successful tapping of the second sac.

CHORIONIC VILLUS SAMPLING

CVS is one of the more recently developed techniques for safe, effective sampling of first-trimester living trophoblastic tissue needed for genetic diagnosis. The tissue sampling allows the use of increasing number of tests for biochemical and molecular disorders of the fetus, as well as for fetal chromosomal abnormalities. The trophoblast, the tissue actually sampled, is one of the extraembryonic structures that develop from the fertilized egg, becoming the placenta as the pregnancy progresses.

HISTORY

In the pre-ultrasound era, the earliest investigators[25,26] passed a rigid endoscope called a hysteroscope through the uterine cervix to obtain trophoblastic tissue for analysis. Chinese physicians used a metal cannula with no ultrasound guidance to aspirate tissue for sex determination.[27] Kazy and colleagues[28] were the first to use ultrasound to guide a flexible biopsy forceps into the uterus to obtain tissue under direct vision. An Italian group[29,30] deserves most of the credit for defining the risks and benefits of the procedure and for demonstrating the value of CVS in biochemical fetal tissue diagnoses. Their results served to popularize the method and to stimulate further investigation of this procedure (Fig. 31-5).

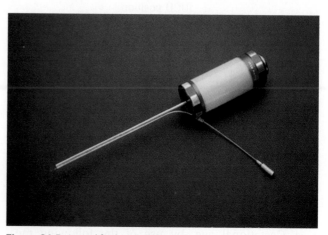

Figure 31-5 A modified contact hysteroscope with a channel to permit passage of a cannula for chorionic villi sampling.

ADVANTAGES AND DISADVANTAGES

The desire for earlier diagnosis of fetal genetic disorders and inherited metabolic derangements in pregnancy, as well as the accuracy of the procedure were the impetus for widespread use of CVS.[31] The earlier diagnosis and the shorter waiting period for results (24 to 48 hours rather than the 7 to 10 days for amniocentesis) are especially appealing to patients. A diagnosis can therefore be forthcoming before macroscopic changes associated with pregnancy are apparent and deeper psychological attachment of the patient to the growing fetus is established. The earlier timing of CVS testing, between the 9th and 12th weeks after the last menstrual period, is a benefit over the later timing of the amniocentesis procedure. Preliminary laboratory results are obtainable within 48 hours by the short-term culture method.[32] Confirmation of the results occurs through the long-term culture method, which become available 4 to 7 days later.

LIMB DEFECTS

The possibility of a diagnosis of a severely affected fetus before the 40th day of pregnancy would have made termination, if desired, a more acceptable option to some orthodox Jewish religious groups.[33] However, many reports from 1991 onward[34-38] have discouraged this practice by raising the issue of the association of CVS, both transcervical and transabdominal, with transverse limb deficiencies. CVS was found to carry an increased risk for transverse limb deformities at 10 weeks' gestation (70 to 76 days), either solely or as part of the oromandibular-limb hypogenesis syndrome, which is about three times the background population rate of 0.3 per 1,000 for similar defects.[39] The limb defect was found to decrease in frequency and severity as gestational age increases. Although the risk may be higher at later gestational ages than the general population rate in non-CVS patients, it is thought to be very small, not as well defined, and much smaller than the risk of the procedure itself. The recommendation is, therefore, that patients should be counseled regarding the increased risk for transverse limb defects at least up to 76 postmenstrual days (10 weeks).[19,39]

Until recently, the fetal loss rate after CVS was reported to be 4%, compared to the 0.3% to 1.0% loss

rate after amniocentesis.[12] More recent information from the compilation of the CVS registry data[40] indicate a significant reduction in fetal loss in centers with the largest experience, making the risk for this procedure comparable to that of amniocentesis.[31,41]

The problem of discordance in the chromosome results among cells obtained from the chorion, amniotic fluid, and the newborn has yet to be resolved. A recent report by Callen and coworkers[42] noted a discordance in 22 karyotypes of 1,312 diagnostic CVS procedures, an incidence 20-fold higher than that reported for amniocentesis. Chorionic cells may therefore not always be a true representation of the fetus.

ULTRASOUND-GUIDED SAMPLING

In all methods of prenatal fetal evaluation, ultrasound visualization has become a *sine qua non* whether the prenatal procedure is for diagnostic or operative guidance purposes. More important than the equipment used is the training and experience of the sonographer, who must be able to work in coordination with the operator obtaining a tissue sample. For CVS, the type of real-time equipment used is secondary.[43] Ultrasound scanning and sampling can be performed simultaneously by the same person, or one person can scan while the other obtains the tissue. A third alternative is for the obstetrician to scan while manipulating the cannula and then to hand the transducer to the sonographer, leaving both of the obstetrician's hands free to obtain the specimen.

Transcervical Technique

Like amniocentesis, CVS is an outpatient procedure performed in an ultrasound laboratory. The aim is to obtain a small sample of viable chorionic tissue uncontaminated with maternal cells and without injuring the pregnancy. Early identification of at-risk patients allows identification of genetic problems, proper counseling, and procedure scheduling between the 10th and 11th gestational weeks.

Before scheduling a patient for testing, the clinician must obtain a comprehensive obstetric and gynecologic history. Among the contraindications to CVS are active infection of the vagina or any part of the genital tract, the presence of an intrauterine device, and stenosis of the cervical os. The patient's bladder may be full or empty, depending on which allows a better view of the pelvic organs. A distended bladder at times can cause undesirable distortion of the uterine contents. Inform the patient of an abnormal gestational sac or absence of fetal heart tones before proceeding.

Ultrasound examination before CVS is essential, not only to confirm pregnancy and the presence of a viable fetus in the uterus but also to evaluate the gestational age and location of the placenta. Vaginal and cervical smears are usually taken for culture to rule out *Neisseria*

PATHOLOGY BOX 31-2

Advantages and Disadvantages of Chorionic Villus Sampling

Advantages	Disadvantages
• Accurate	• Limb defects
• Early genetic diagnosis	• Fetal loss
	• False-positive result

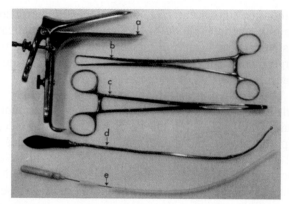

Figure 31-6 Instruments used in endovaginal chorionic villus sampling: **(A)** vaginal speculum, **(B)** tenaculum, **(C)** ring forceps, **(D)** uterine sound, **(E)** plastic catheter enclosed in plastic sleeve with the malleable obturator withdrawn slightly from the catheter.

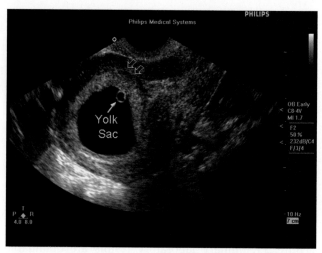

Figure 31-8 Vaginal ultrasound scan of the target area for CVS (open arrows). (Image courtesy of Philips Medical Systems, Bothell, WA.)

gonorrhoeae and other pathogens before preparing the vagina and cervix with povidone iodine solution. A vaginal speculum is inserted; upon visualization, the clinician carefully grasps the cervix with a tenaculum (Fig. 31-6). Ultrasound imaging then confirms the position of the internal cervical os.

Different clinicians use a variety of rigid instruments and flexible catheters or cannulas. Regardless of the tools or procedures, ultrasound visualizes the instrument's course into the uterus and through the cervix. The thickest part of the trophoblast, the chorion frondosum, where the umbilical cord is attached, is the target area for obtaining samples (Figs. 30-7–8). Many clinicians use the yolk sac as a landmark. The crown-rump length is measured, and the shape and direction of the uterine axis determined. A flexible polyethylene catheter with a metal obturator is inserted into the cervix.

When the catheter tip has reached the proper site, the clinician removes the malleable aluminum obturator. A 20-ml syringe, previously prepared and containing 3 to

5 ml of sterile culture medium and a small amount of heparin, attaches to the outer end of the catheter, and the specimen is obtained through aspiration. Negative pressure is generated by sharply withdrawing the barrel of the syringe either once or repeatedly as the catheter is slowly withdrawn. During the procedure, constant ultrasound visualization documents catheter placement and removal.

An average of 20 to 30 mg of tissue transfers to a sterile Petri dish containing a culture medium. After washing the specimen with sterile culture media or saline solution, the pathologist examines the sample under a low-power dissecting microscope to verify the presence of chorionic villi. Maternal cell contamination removal occurs with a dissecting needle under the dissecting microscope. The tissue culture laboratory then processes the washed chorionic tissue specimen.

After collecting the specimen and removing the instruments, reexamine the patient sonographically before release. The examiner observes the sampling site for evidence of hematoma formation or other complications that may have occurred because of the procedure. Any follow-up ultrasound examinations occur at intervals of a few days to a week later.

TRANSABDOMINAL TECHNIQUE

Currently, most of the CVS procedures are performed transabdominally. The transabdominal approach differs from the transcervical only in the anatomic access route and the instrument used to obtain the specimen. The preparation of the patient, the treatment place, and the goals are the same in both approaches. In the transabdominal approach, the patient is in the supine rather than the lithotomy position. Identify the placenta and measure the thickness. A povidone iodine solution cleans the abdomen at the elected site. A 20-gauge, 3.5-inch spinal needle with a stylet, like the one used in amniocentesis, is introduced into the

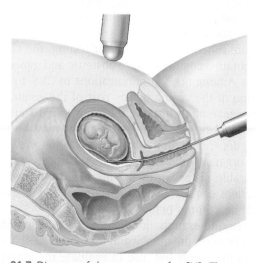

Figure 31-7 Diagram of the target area for CVS. The vaginal approach uses a pliable plastic catheter. The abdominal approach uses a spinal needle introduced transabdominally.

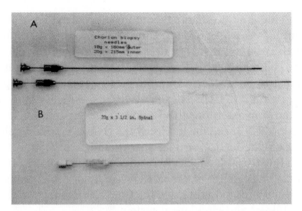

Figure 31-9 A: Double-needle set with stylets for transabdominal CVS. The larger-bore needle is inserted first through the abdominal wall to just proximal to the target site. The stylet is withdrawn and the second, smaller (20-gauge) needle is inserted through the first one to the site of sampling, and the specimen obtained as described in the text. **B:** Spinal needle with stylet partially withdrawn. This needle may be used for both amniocentesis and for transabdominal CVS.

placenta (Fig. 31-9) and held by the sonographer. The physician–operator removes the stylet, holding the needle steadily in place, attaches a 20-ml Luer-lok syringe containing 3 ml of Hanks culture medium mixed with a few drops of heparin, and collects the specimen. Withdrawal of the plunger of the syringe creates a negative pressure. Slow movement of the needle tip obtains a specimen of about 30 mg of tissue. The needle is then withdrawn and the patient is treated as described previously for amniocentesis and transcervical CVS. In both transcervical and transabdominal CVS, the informed patient realizes that amniocentesis may be necessary with the return of equivocal results.

Transcervical versus Transabdominal Technique

Until recently, the more accepted method of CVS was the transcervical technique introduced by Brambati and coworkers.[44] This method uses a flexible plastic catheter with a malleable inner obturator inserted into the cervix *per vaginum*, guided by an abdominally placed transducer (see Fig. 31-7). The transabdominal method first introduced in 1984[45] has gained wide acceptance because of the reported decreased chance of infection and the greater success rate in obtaining specimens. The transabdominal approach is successful in situations in which the transcervical method has failed, as, for example, in the case of the anteriorly implanted placenta or hyperflexion of the uterus.

There have been a few large, prospective, randomized studies comparing transabdominal and transcervical CVS done worldwide. In the United States, a report on a randomized study population in which 1,944 women were in a transcervical group and 1,929 in a transabdominal group found that first-attempt abdominal sampling success was 94% with a 90% success rate using the cervical route.[46] Maternal complications such as fluid leakage and vaginal spotting and bleeding

were statistically significantly higher in the group that underwent transcervical CVS. The rate of spontaneous miscarriage was 2.3% in the transabdominal group and 2.5% in the transcervical group. This confirmed the safety of both methods. Comparing the two approaches in 2,882 women, the sampling success for the first attempt was 98.1% in the transabdominal group and 96% in the transcervical group.[47] They found that the rate of unintentional pregnancy loss was significantly higher in the transcervical group (7.7%) compared to the transabdominal group (3.7%). Contamination with blood and maternal cells was greater with transcervically obtained specimens. These investigators have abandoned transcervical CVS because of the associated high pregnancy loss rate.

The data from these and other randomized trials[44] lead to a conclusion that transabdominal CVS is a better procedure because of the higher sampling success, fewer minor complications, and fewer pregnancy losses.

AMNIOCENTESIS VERSUS CHORIONIC VILLUS SAMPLING

Rhoads and colleagues[41] compared the safety and efficacy of transcervical CVS in 2,278 women to amniocentesis in 671 women. They obtained cytogenetic diagnoses in 97.8% of CVS cases and 99.4% of amniocentesis cases. Due to an inadequate tissue sample obtained by CVS, the procedure was repeated up to four times. The overall pregnancy loss rate was 7.2% in the CVS group and 5.7% in the amniocentesis group. This included spontaneous and missed abortions, termination of abnormal pregnancies, stillbirths, and neonatal deaths. There was a greater number of minor complications in the CVS group, including cramping, spotting, bleeding, and leakage of amniotic fluid. Seventeen patients underwent amniocentesis after CVS because the diagnosis was ambiguous. Comparison of transabdominal and transcervical CVS to amniocentesis exemplified that the transcervical CVS group had the highest postprocedure fetal loss rate (7.63%), followed by the transabdominal CVS group (2.34%), and finally by the amniocentesis group (1.16%).[47]

Studies suggest that amniocentesis is the safest and most accurate of the three procedures. CVS, by whichever route chosen, carries a higher risk of repeated procedures, maternal cell contamination, sampling failures, and multiple insertions because of inadequate amounts of tissue, and a higher incidence of false-positive and false-negative results.

EARLY AMNIOCENTESIS VERSUS TRANSABDOMINAL CHORIONIC VILLUS SAMPLING

There has been an attempt to perform amniocentesis earlier than the traditional 15 weeks. A prospective study of women with pregnancies at 10 to 13 weeks of gestation who requested fetal karyotyping included 731 women undergoing early amniocentesis and 570 undergoing transabdominal CVS.[18] The successful sampling rate was the same for both groups (97.5%). The rate of fetal loss was significantly higher in the early amniocentesis group (5.3%) than in the CVS group (2.3%). In the subgroups of randomized women (238 randomized to amniocentesis group and 250 randomized to transabdominal CVS group), the fetal loss rates were 5.9%, and 1.2% respectively. There were more culture failures after early amniocentesis (2.3%) versus CVS (0.53%). Result confirmation occurred in 120 early amniocenteses, with 8 fetal losses compared to none in 64 women who underwent transabdominal CVS.[48]

The main advantages of early amniocentesis are the decreased rate of mosaicism, decreased need for repeat testing, and the ability to do direct AFP determinations. The principal disadvantages are the increases in the rates of fetal loss and culture failure when performing the procedure before the 13th week. This leads to the recommendation that early amniocentesis should not be attempted before 14 weeks of gestation. Transabdominal CVS appears to be superior to early amniocentesis based on the information obtained from the studies mentioned here.

COELOCENTESIS

During the first 10 weeks of pregnancy, coelomic fluid surrounds the amniotic sac. Coelocentesis is a new technique that involves the ultrasound-guided insertion of a needle into the extra-amniotic cavity through the vagina, from as early as 6 weeks of gestation (Fig. 31-10).[49] This method helps investigation of early fetal physiology and pathophysiology. Moreover, it offers the possibility for very early prenatal diagnosis, from at least 7 weeks of gestation.[49,50] There are three main limitations that have prevented coelocentesis from becoming an alternative to amniocentesis and CVS for fetal karyotyping. First, it is difficult to culture coelomic cells. Analyzing the nuchal translucency thickness and first- or second-trimester biochemistry also helps in screening for chromosomal defects. Finally, there is a concern regarding the safety of the procedure. The most likely mechanisms by which coelocentesis could cause fetal demise or fetal abnormalities are hypovolemia due to hemorrhage, hypoxia due to uterine contractions, and release of vasoactive substances in response to intrauterine trauma, leading to direct damage of the fetal heart and circulatory system.[50]

FETAL BLOOD SAMPLING

By the end of the 20th century, the commonest indications for fetal blood sampling were the diagnosis of hemoglobinopathies and red blood cell disorders; the diagnosis and management of Rh isoimmunization, platelet disorders, and intrauterine congenital infections; and rapid karyotype. The development of new molecular biology techniques, such as polymerase chain reaction (PCR) following CVS and amniocentesis, resulted in the limitation of fetal blood sampling to cases with mosaicism on amniocentesis, Rh isoimmunization, hydrops of unknown origin, alloimmune thrombocytopenia, fetal infections, fetal blood grouping, thyroid disease, and rapid karyotype in delayed diagnosis of congenital anomalies.[51] The anterior placenta requires transplacental cordocentesis, whereas the posterior placenta allows sampling of the cord approximately 1 cm from the placental umbilical cord insertion, always avoiding free cord loops. Before initiating the procedure, perform a preliminary ultrasound examination to determine fetal viability, position, and amniotic fluid volume and localize the placenta and umbilical cord insertion. Color and/or power Doppler may assist in fetal blood sampling because it facilitates visualization of the vein insertion into the placenta. The intrahepatic umbilical vein allows for sampling at this site but is considered a second-choice technique because of the higher rate of fetal losses (6.2%), compared to cordocentesis (1% to 5%).[51,52] The volume of blood during fetal blood sampling procedure varies with the gestational age and number of tests required. Usually up to 4 ml (during the second trimester), and 6 ml (during the third trimester) is considered sufficient. Check the puncture site for bleeding 10 minutes after the procedure completion. Assess and document the fetal heart rate prior to and 30 to 60 minutes after the procedure. The most common complications of fetal blood sampling are failure to obtain fetal blood, fetal loss, bleeding, cord hematoma, and chorioamnionitis.[52] To prevent Rh sensitization in Rh-negative patients with Rh positive or unknown Rh of the fetus, administer 300 mg of anti-D globulin.

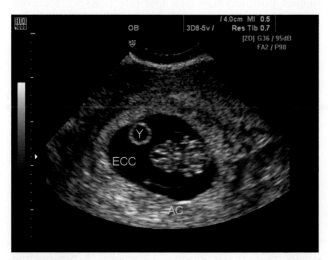

Figure 31-10 The coelocentesis samples fluid from the exocoelomic cavity (ECC). *Y,* yolk sac; *AC,* amniotic cavity.

Fetal Transfusion

The widespread use of Rh immune globulin has significantly reduced the incidence of hemolytic disease in newborns. Efforts in intrauterine treatment of Rh isoimmunization started in the 1960s with intraperitoneal transfusions and were continued with intravascular transfusions via cordocentesis.[53,54] Previous monitoring of pregnancies complicated by isoimmunization included maternal indirect Coombs titers, ultrasound markers, amniocentesis, and fetal blood sampling. Introduction of the peak systolic velocity assessment of the middle cerebral artery (PSV MCA) has significantly reduced the need for invasive diagnostic methods.[55] Fetal blood sampling and intrauterine transfusions now occur only in patients with abnormal PSV MCA.

Fetal Therapy

Access to fetal circulation offers the possibility of infusing pharmacologic agents for therapeutic purposes (for example, digoxin in hydropic fetuses with supraventricular tachycardia, therapy of fetal metabolic disorders, fetal hyperthyroidism and hypothyroidism, acute toxoplasmosis infection in pregnancy, etc.). Another promising future application may be intrauterine genetic therapy.

The most common invasive procedures available for direct fetal therapy are treatment of fetal anemia, alloimmune thrombocytopenia, and nonimmune hydrops by cordocentesis. Cases of fetal urinary tract obstruction, severe fetal ascites, and ovarian cysts usually result in a percutaneous procedure. Shunting procedures may be planned for fetuses with urinary tract obstruction, hydrocephalus, and cystic adenomatoid malformation. Intrauterine laser treatment in feto-fetal transfusion syndrome (also known as twin-to-twin transfusion syndrome) permits the selective coagulation of superficial vascular anastomoses of the placenta. Open and endoscopic fetal surgery has been performed in human fetuses with varying degrees of success and is still of experimental nature.

Fetal Tissue Sampling

The methodology of fetal tissue sampling is similar to blood sampling methods and is restricted to a limited number of tertiary centers.[51] To obtain a diagnosis of a specific enzyme deficit, a fetal liver biopsy under ultrasound guidance helps obtain a tissue sample. Fetal skin biopsy permits the diagnosis of genodermatoses. Prenatal diagnosis of Duchenne muscular dystrophy and other hereditary myopathies is made through a muscle biopsy.

Multifetal Pregnancy Reduction

In the past 25 years, the increased use of ovulation-inducing drugs, as well as the increased number of medically assisted reproduction procedures, has

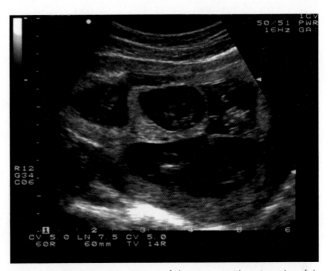

Figure 31-11 Transverse image of the uterus with quintuplets following ovulation induction at 8 to 9 weeks' gestation.

resulted in a large number of multiple gestations (Fig. 31-11). Multiple pregnancies are associated with high mortality and morbidity rates, and the probability of achieving a term pregnancy with healthy neonates is inversely proportional to the number of the fetuses. The aim of multifetal pregnancy reduction is to reduce the number of embryos to improve survival for the remaining ones.[56] Clinicians often offer selective reduction to women with four or more embryos, with the number of embryos usually reduced to two. The procedure is normally delayed until after 8 weeks, when the spontaneous loss is relatively low. Transabdominal approach is preferred for multifetal embryo reduction between 10 and 12 weeks' gestation, whereas the endovaginal approach may be successfully applied between 8 and 10 weeks' gestation.[57,58,59] Advantages of endovaginal ultrasound–guided procedure are the following: shorter puncture route and a more precise needle placement that reduces the risk of inadvertent injury to adjacent gestational sacs or other pelvic structures. Color Doppler may aid in monitoring fetal heart action during and after the sonographically guided procedure (Fig. 31-12).

A brief explanation of techniques for endovaginal multiembryo reduction is as follows:
- a baseline mapping procedure of the chorionic sacs
- detailed evaluation of the heartbeats of the targeted fetus, and placement of the needle with 0.5 to 1 ml of 2 mEq/ml KCl solution.

Observe the heartbeat of each injected fetus for 5–10 minutes to confirm cessation. Rescan the patient at 3 hours and 1 week after the procedure. The disadvantage of endovaginal fetal reduction is that at an early gestational age the final number of fetuses is not yet established. Prospective evaluation of 90 women undergoing early endovaginal selective embryo reduction with KCl injected near the fetal heart at 7.5 weeks' gestation (range 7.0 to 8.0 weeks) reported pregnancy

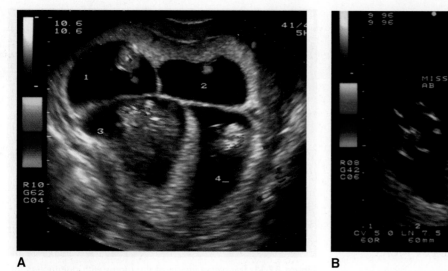

A **B**

Figure 31-12 A: Color Doppler ultrasound of quadruplets at 10 weeks' gestation. Note the color signals indicating regular heart activity of all fetuses. **B:** Image of the 1-week follow-up sonographic exam. At that time, color Doppler detected heart activity of three fetuses and one fetus with absent heart activity.

loss of 11.7%.[60] Similar results occurred in the study evaluating the efficacy of early endovaginal intracardiac embryo puncture.[61] The overall pregnancy loss rate associated with early embryo aspiration is similar to that performed at later gestational age but is significantly lower when the initial number of embryos is four or greater.

In patients undergoing multifetal pregnancy reduction after 11 weeks' gestation, preprocedural noninvasive genetic screening and detailed nuchal translucency measurement help detect fetuses with an increased risk for chromosomal abnormality. Before the procedure, each patient undergoes extensive consultation and assessment of the number and viability of the fetuses, their mutual inter-relationship, and location in relation to the internal cervical os, localization of the placentas, and evaluation of fetal anatomy. Transabdominal procedure is usually performed using a freehand technique.[62] The fetus in the lowest sac is usually not reduced, unless a fetal anomaly was detected. Placement of the needle is into the fetal thorax in the longitudinal plane, with slow injection of 2 to 3 milliequivalents (mEq) of potassium chloride. Carefully observe cardiac activity for at least 2 minutes. Observe the patient an hour after the procedure for evidence of uterine contractions, vaginal bleeding, or leakage of amniotic fluid. Repeat the ultrasound examination to confirm normal cardiac activity in nonreduced fetuses and absence of heart action in reduced fetuses. Current practice recommends termination of no more than three fetuses at each attempt. If all the fetuses are alive and have appropriate size at 12 weeks' gestation, there is no advantage of delaying the procedure because spontaneous losses are not likely to occur. At the same time, the risk of miscarriage and preterm rupture of membranes is increased.[63]

ULTRASOUND-GUIDED ENDOVAGINAL PROCEDURES

With the advances in ultrasonographic equipment settings and technique, guided procedures using endovaginal sonography have replaced abdominally guided puncture in most of the gynecologic interventions. The first who have used ultrasound-guided puncture procedures to achieve both diagnostic and therapeutic goals were Smith and Bartrum, who performed percutaneous aspiration of intra-abdominal abscesses in 1974, and Gerzof et al., who used an abdominal catheter placed sonographically to drain purulent collections.[64,65] The advantages of these procedures over surgery are accurate needle placement, rare injury to adjacent organs, low cost, shorter time of the procedure, portability, and patient comfort. Possible rare complications include bleeding, infection, and unintentional puncture of neighboring organs.

Either a needle guide or freehand technique is used when performing the procedure through the abdominal wall. When puncture procedures are performed endovaginally because of limited mobility of the transducer, the freehand approach is difficult. A fixed needle guide attached to the transducer shaft allows easier visualization of the entire length of the needle within the scanning plane and better control for exact needle placement. An automated puncture device, when mated to the shaft of the endovaginal transducer, provides a high degree of accuracy and precision, and its high-velocity release makes the procedure virtually painless; no anesthesia or analgesia is required. The first use of this technique was for ovum pick-up in assisted reproductive technology programs. The need for reloading with each new follicle aspiration resulted in quick abandonment of this technique. The automated puncture device is crucial in cases where extreme accuracy is required. Manual needle introduction is less accurate and more painful because of the slower forward motion of the needle displacing the mobile targets rather than penetrating them.[66]

The use of a 5.0 to 7.5 MHz endovaginal ultrasound transducer with a needle guide attached to the transducer shaft aids in the performance of the puncture. A software-generated fixed "biopsy guide" line is displayed on the ultrasound monitor screen, which marks the path of the entering needle. The selection of needle gauges ranging from 14 to 21 depends on the nature of the procedure itself; use the narrowest possible needle able to perform the desired task. For better imaging, use the "zoom" feature of the equipment as frequently as possible. After the initial withdrawal, the needle, pelvic structures, and cul-de-sac must be examined sonographically approximately 10 minutes after and rescanned after 2 to 3 hours of observation to check for internal bleeding or previously undetected complications. The most common ultrasound-directed endovaginal puncturing procedures are the following:

1. Endovaginal oocyte retrieval
2. Ovarian cyst aspiration
3. Biopsy of pelvic masses
4. Drainage of pelvic abscesses
5. Culdocentesis
6. Local treatment of ectopic pregnancy

Ultrasound-guided endovaginal nonpuncturing procedures are the following:

1. Embryo transfer and tubal catheterization
2. Hysterosonography and hysterosonosalpingography
3. Evaluation of the position and displacement of an intrauterine contraceptive device
4. Radiotherapy planning and monitoring

ENDOVAGINAL OOCYTE RETRIEVAL

Experience has proven that the endovaginal technique using a needle-guided endovaginal transducer is superior to all other ultrasound-guided techniques.[67] The proximity of the transducer to the pelvic organs allows the use of high-frequency transducers, thereby enhancing the resolution and clinical efficiency. By increasing the pressure of the tip of the transducer to the elastic vault of the vagina, the sonographer can approximate the ovaries. Since there is no need for a full urinary bladder, pelvic anatomy is undistorted and ovaries are beyond the focal zone of the transducer. Obesity or adhesions do not significantly inhibit the visualization of the follicles. Controlled ovarian hyperstimulation is monitored by endovaginal sonography.[68] Additional information may be obtained by hormonal estimation, color Doppler studies of the ovarian and uterine circulation,[69-71] and more recently three-dimensional (3D) ultrasound (Fig. 31-13).

The entire treatment occurs in an outpatient setting. Position the patient on a gynecologic table in lithotomy position. Although anesthesia or any sedative analgesia has been abandoned in about 50% of in vitro fertilization (IVF) programs, sedative medication may be used.[72] Since the mean duration of the oocyte retrieval is 10 minutes, most patients easily tolerate the procedure. However, the operator should be aware of possible drops in blood pressure and discomfort experienced by some patients. Before inserting the transducer into the cover, the operator should apply the ultrasonic coupling gel, then stretch the cover (sterile condom, surgical rubber glove, or specially produced rubber cover) to expel the air from the end of the transducer. This can prevent any artifacts during the procedure. Do not use gel or lubricant while inserting the transducer because of spermicidal action and reported embryotoxicity.[73] Instead, one can use a physiologic saline or culture medium. Use sterile needle guides for endovaginal puncture of the follicles. A sterile keyboard cover of the ultrasound machine enables the operator to make any readjustment under sterile conditions. Sterile drapes then cover the patient's legs and perigenital area. After cleaning the vagina with isotonic saline or cultured medium, the endovaginal transducers is inserted into the vagina. The use of an automatic puncturing device helps to prevent potential risks of the puncture procedures. This device contains a mobile metal tube, the needle carrier into which the aspiration needle is inserted and locked by a twisting movement.[67] Before inserting the transducer with a puncture device into the vagina, the device should be loaded and secured. After insertion, a detailed ultrasound examination is performed to locate the uterus and the ovaries. The biopsy vector indicates the direction of the needle, which is placed into the central part of the nearest follicle. The operator counts the distance on the biopsy vector on the screen and "shoots" the follicle either automatically or manually. After the needle is rapidly advanced into the follicle, the operator begins the suction through the tubing connected to the suction pump. The follicular fluid is pulled into the collecting chamber and the follicle collapses.[67] A flushing procedure may be used to improve the satisfactory rate of the aspirated oocytes. Flushing medium that contains heparin is injected through the tubing or using an automated flushing system. All the follicles along the same line are aspirated without withdrawing the needle. Endovaginal technique for oocyte recovery is a standard technique with low complication rates reported by many authors.[74] Iliac veins may sometimes be confused for a follicle and mistakenly punctured, which may lead to bleeding into the pouch of Douglas. It was observed that filling the bladder might exert pressure on the site and, therefore, stop the bleeding. Color Doppler can easily prevent such a complication, since iliac vessels are easily visualized using this technique.

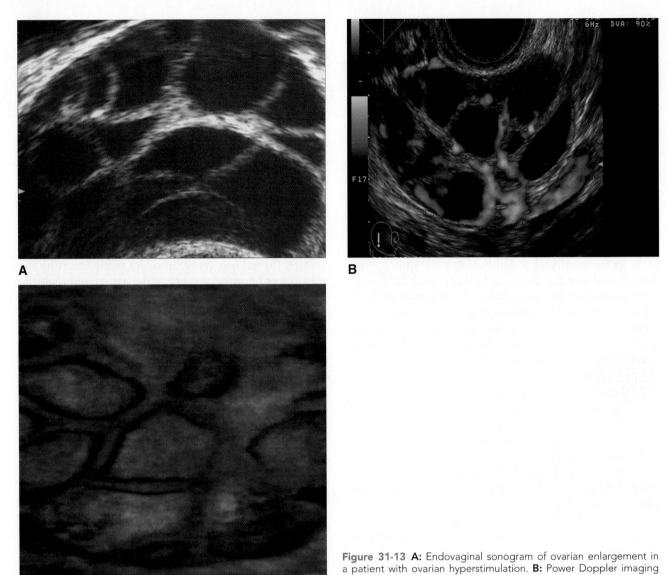

A

B

C

Figure 31-13 A: Endovaginal sonogram of ovarian enlargement in a patient with ovarian hyperstimulation. **B:** Power Doppler imaging of ovarian hyperstimulation. The visualization rate of the perifollicular areas correlates with the number and quality of aspirated oocytes. **C:** 3D ultrasound of ovarian hyperstimulation.

The bleeding from the vaginal vault is easily detectable and can be stopped by compression. Pelvic inflammatory disease (PID) is a rare complication of endovaginal follicle aspiration reported in 0.14% of the patients.[72] The infections were mostly caused by infected semen and occurred in patients with positive history of PID.

Recent technology enables the performance of 3D and four-dimensional (4D) puncture procedures in real time,[73] enabling better anatomic orientation, especially in patients with severe adhesions.

OVARIAN CYST ASPIRATION

Endovaginal guidance permits direct visualization and aspiration of persistent follicular cysts.[74] Such cysts may impair follicular development because of the release of hormones or because of decreased perfusion by compression of the ovarian parenchyma. In the puncture of an ovarian or para-ovarian cyst, the center of the cyst is targeted and the needle is inserted. Such a procedure is highly debated in the literature. The concern of cell spillage from potentially malignant ovarian cysts into the abdominal cavity prevents many from using it more frequently. Although the aspirated fluid is necessarily submitted for cytologic evaluation, a negative cytologic examination may sometimes give a false-negative result. High sensitivity and specificity of endovaginal color Doppler in differentiation between benign and malignant adnexal lesions seems to increase the reliability in determining which cysts should be aspirated (Fig. 31-14).

Another reason that ovarian cyst aspiration is highly debated in the literature is a high recurrence rate (48% in premenopausal patients, and 80% in postmenopausal women).[76,77] An attempt to prevent cyst recurrence by

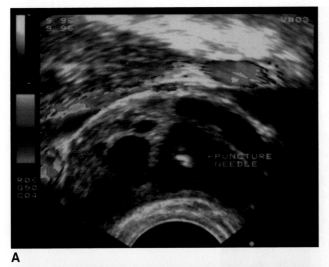

A

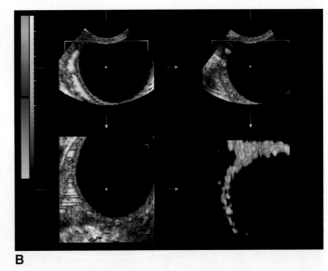

B

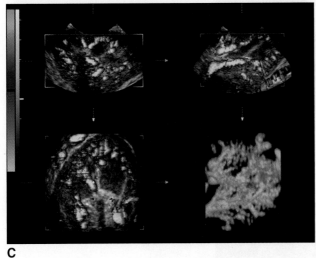

C

Figure 31-14 A: Endovaginal color Doppler scan of the ovary during aspiration procedure. The tip of the needle is advanced into the proximal follicle. Iliac vessels are clearly displayed on color Doppler. **B:** 3D power Doppler ultrasound of a simple ovarian cyst. Note the regularly separated vessel encircling the cyst. **C:** 3D power Doppler scan of a recurrent ovarian carcinoma. Numerous randomly dispersed vessels with irregular branching assists indicate recurrent ovarian malignancy.

injecting alcohol immediately after cyst aspiration was successful in only about 57% of patients.[78]

To diminish the cancellation rate, it may be beneficial to perform ovarian cyst puncture during the early follicular phase in patients with ovarian cysts undergoing IVF. The aspiration of endometriotic cysts is technically simple, however, its overall benefit and safety are still inconclusive.

BIOPSY OF PELVIC MASSES

Ultrasound-guided biopsy of pelvic masses is safe, accurate, and effective. The advantage of ultrasound-guided procedures over CT-guided biopsy is real-time imaging, lack of ionizing radiation, and lower cost (Fig. 31-15).[79] In cases presenting with intra-abdominal masses, both ultrasound-guided needle aspiration and needle core biopsy may be efficiently used for early confirmation and/or exclusion of malignancy. During needle aspiration biopsy, tissue is obtained by suction through a needle attached to a syringe. Needle core biopsy is performed using a large hollow needle that extracts a

core of tissue. In a recent study of 129 abdominal lesions, fine needle aspiration cytology identified 86%, and needle core biopsy detected 80.6%, of malignant lesions.[80]

The combination of these sampling techniques increases diagnostic sensitivity and provides more accurate preoperative classification of intra-abdominal and pelvic tumors.

In patients with a history of multiple abdominal surgeries, transabdominal aspiration of ascites and/or biopsy of pelvic masses have a high complication rate, resulting mainly in bowel injury. In these patients, endovaginal aspiration using ultrasound guidance is particularly suitable.

DRAINAGE OF PELVIC ABSCESS

It has been reported that in patients with a tubo-ovarian abscess, abscess drainage with sonographic guidance can hasten recovery and improve the efficacy of antibiotic therapy. Once the needle is placed into the abscess cavity, the contents can be aspirated as completely as possible

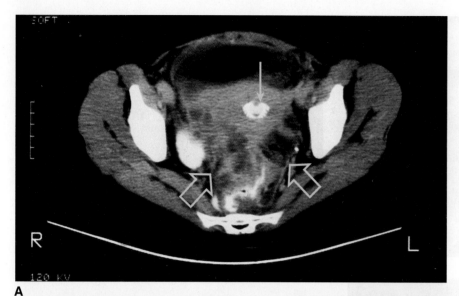

A

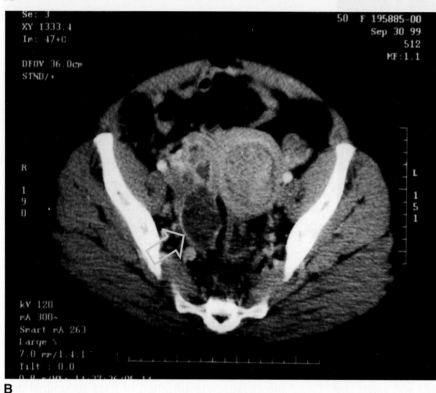

B

Figure 31-15 A: CT scan of tubo-ovarian abscess *(open arrows)* with Dalkon Shield *(arrow)*. **B:** MRI of tubo-ovarian abscess *(open arrow)*.

or a drainage catheter can be placed.[81] Figure 31-16 illustrates ultrasound-guided drainage of pelvic abscess. This technique is accepted as an alternative to open laparoscopy for treating the tubo-ovarian abscess.

DIAGNOSTIC CULDOCENTESIS

The introduction of endovaginal sonography has limited the need for diagnostic culdocentesis. The presence of fluid in the posterior cul-de-sac is easily established by endovaginal ultrasound, but it remains difficult to differentiate different types of effusions (clear fluid,

blood, or pus). The wide availability of endovaginal color Doppler sonography to distinguish the dominant pelvic pathology in the presence of pelvic fluid based on different vascularity patterns is helpful in routine diagnostic procedures. Inserting a needle in the cul-de-sac is a simple technique that can be performed safely and accurately with endovaginal ultrasound guidance (Fig. 31-17). High-quality 2D B-mode endovaginal sonography with superimposed color Doppler flow allows accurate simultaneous identification of the main pelvic vessels and physiologic angiogenesis of the corpus luteum and ectopic peritrophoblastic blood flow.[82] Color

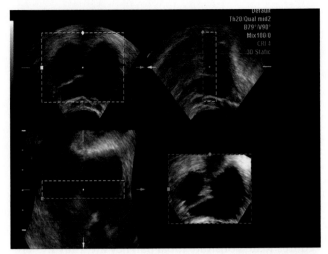

Figure 31-16 3D ultrasound scan of aspiration of the tubo-ovarian abscess. Tip of the needle introduced into the abscess cavity is clearly demonstrated in three orthogonal planes.

helps in accurate needle placement and in diminishing the risk of injury to adjacent vessels, especially in women who have had previous inflammatory disease of the pelvis with an obliterated cul-de-sac.

LOCAL TREATMENT OF ECTOPIC PREGNANCY

In the past, the diagnosis of ectopic pregnancy was usually made at the time of laparotomy, very often in a hemodynamically unstable patient. Little choice was left but to perform a salpingectomy, adnexectomy, or segmental resection of the fallopian tube. At that time, the physician's concern was to save the patient's life and usually not to preserve the function of the affected fallopian tube. Early-stage ectopic pregnancy diagnosis results in simpler surgery and the use of medical therapies. This is due to the use of sensitive pregnancy tests and endovaginal ultrasonography. Systemic use of methotrexate has been documented to be safe, effective, and well tolerated. Data is suggestive that fertility potential after such treatment is comparable to that of conservative surgery.[83–85]

Local treatment of ectopic pregnancy using methotrexate under endovaginal ultrasound guidance may also be used. It was first reported in 1987,[86] and since then was used in many centers in patients with ectopic pregnancy.[87–89] The most common complication reported is concurrent or delayed hemorrhage, occurring in less than 15% of patients.[90] Another reported complication is the persistence of trophoblastic tissue within the fallopian tube, and persistent elevation of the beta human chorionic gonadotropin (beta hCG) levels following the procedure. These cases may successfully be treated nonsurgically using systemic administration of methotrexate.[88]

Since the introduction of endovaginal sonography with color flow imaging within a high-frequency transducer, a more accurate and more rapid diagnosis of

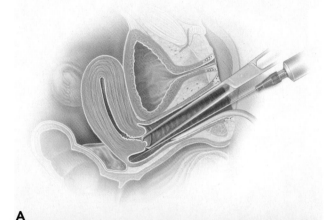

A

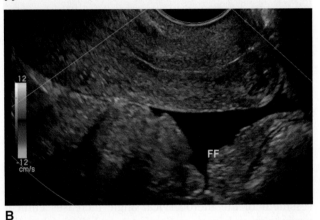

B

Figure 31-17 A: Culdocentesis is easily done if the needle is inserted at the correct level and the vaginal mucosa over the posterior fornix is taut. **B:** Transvaginal scan of free fluid in the posterior cul-de-sac.

ectopic pregnancy is feasible. Color Doppler appears to be useful in diagnosis of ectopic pregnancy with ultrasonography when no adnexal gestational sac is observed.[91] Peritrophoblastic flow is prominent, randomly dispersed inside the solid part of an adnexal mass and clearly separated from ovarian tissue (Fig. 31-18). Low-impedance blood flow signals and a resistance index less than 0.45 extracted from the color-coded area indicate invasive trophoblast. A clinical impression of tubal abortion is probable with lack of color flow, or increased vascular resistance of the peritrophoblastic flow and a beta hCG level less than 1,000 IU/ml. Doppler can identify the vitality and invasiveness of the trophoblast, the most important feature in planning the management of ectopic pregnancy.

Using a similar technique, an injection of potassium chloride guided by endovaginal sonography can be used in patients with cervical and cornual ectopic pregnancy with positive heart action (Fig. 31-19).[92,93]

EMBRYO TRANSFER AND TUBAL CATHETERIZATION

Although intrauterine embryo transfer is not considered a sonographically guided procedure, many centers report that ultrasound-guided embryo transfer

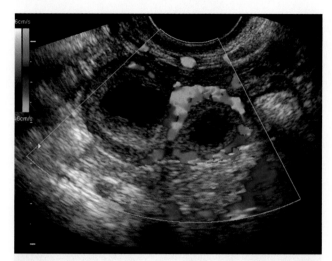

Figure 31-18 Endovaginal color Doppler image of an ectopic pregnancy. Color Doppler facilitates visualization of randomly dispersed tubal arteries encircling the ectopic gestational sac, suggestive of prominent trophoblastic vitality guides the clinician to the location of the ectopic pregnancy. The ipilateral corpus luteum is lateral from the gestational sac.

significantly increases clinical pregnancy and live birth rates compared with the clinical-touch method.[94–97]

It has also been reported that shaping the catheter for embryo transfer according to the ultrasound assessment of the uterocervical angle increases clinical pregnancy and implantation rates and diminishes the incidence of difficult and bloody transfers.[98,99] In patients with cervical abnormalities ultrasound-guided transmyometrial puncture may be performed under the ultrasound guidance.[100]

Tubal catheterization is a diagnostic and therapeutic technique in diagnosing tubal patency via injecting and observing fluid passage into the pelvis. The course

of the procedure can be monitored using the abdominal ultrasound, which enables better positioning of an endovaginally guided catheter. Using ultrasound guidance, fertilized ova may be carried into the ampullary portion of the tube.

HYSTEROSONOGRAPHY AND HYSTEROSONOSALPINGOGRAPHY

The number of cases of tubal sterility is increasing and tubal factors, such as tubal dysfunction or obstruction, account for approximately 35% of the causes of infertility. Imaging plays a key role in diagnostic evaluation of women for infertility.[101] The most frequently used procedures to demonstrate tubal patency are x-ray hysterosalpingography (HSG) and chromopertubation during laparoscopy. Hysteroscopy is a technique that complements hysterosalpingography and accurately differentiates between endometrial polyps and submucous leiomyomas; this technique can be used for minimally invasive treatment of congenital anomalies and intrauterine synechiae. Laparoscopy is the gold standard for establishing the tubal status but requires general anesthesia and carries the risk of anesthesiologic and surgical complications such as bowel or vascular injury, hemorrhage, and infection.

Significant improvement in resolution of ultrasound equipment and use of endovaginal transducers have made sonographic evaluation of the uterine cavity and tubes a feasible option for investigation of uterine and tubal causes of infertility. The benefits of hysterosonography, saline intrauterine infusion for evaluation of the uterine cavity, and hysterosonosalpingography (saline intrauterine infusion to evaluate the uterine cavity and tubal patency) are low cost and avoiding ionization

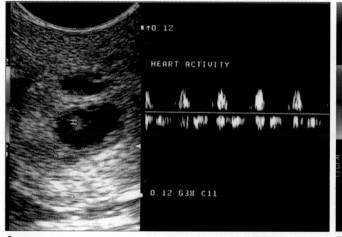

A

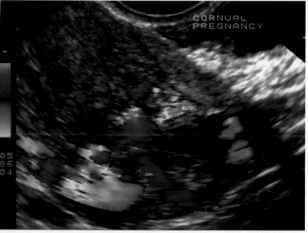

B

Figure 31-19 A: Endovaginal color Doppler image of the cervix in a patient with an ectopic cervical pregnancy. Note the Nabothian cyst superior to the gestational sac. Blood flow signals are derived from the fetal heart and demonstrate regular heart activity. **B:** Endovaginal color Doppler image of a cornual pregnancy. Color Doppler assists in diagnosis of the ectopic pregnancy by exposing peritrophoblastic vessels at the periphery of the gestational sac.

and allergic reactions to contrast media. This method is easily reproducible and enables evaluation of tubal motility. The course of the procedure may be recorded, reviewed, and analyzed in the presence of an infertile couple, which increases their knowledge and understanding of infertility problems. More recently, color/ power and pulsed Doppler and 3D ultrasound have been used to evaluate the uterine cavity and tubal patency. The accuracy of hysterosonosalpingography compared with x-ray HSG varies from 70.37% to 92.20%.[102,103] Depending on the method used (B-mode vs. color Doppler vs. 3D ultrasound), the accuracy of hysterosonosalpingography compared to chromopertubation varies from 81.82% to 100.00%.[104-107]

Accuracy of the method also depends on the contrast medium. Contrast media with different echogenicity from the human body may be used as contrast. Contrast media are divided into two major groups: hypoechogenic and hyperechogenic media. Isotonic saline and Ringer and dextran solutions belong to the first group. Instillation of these media facilitates the detection of echogenic border surfaces, such as endometrium. The use of hyperechogenic contrast media enhances echo signals, allowing detection of the flow by both B-mode and Doppler ultrasound. Commercial echo contrast media contain microbubbles and usually contain special galactose microparticles suspended in either a galactose solution or sterile water.[108] Absolute contraindication for instillation of these fluids is galactosemia, an autosomal recessive disease in which, due to deficiency of galactose-1-phosphate uridyltransferase, galactose cannot be metabolized into glucose.

When ultrasound contrast is administered via the vascular system or into body cavities, it changes the acoustic properties of the body region under investigation. Contrast agents are acoustically heterogeneous, resulting in scattering and rendering the structures visible.[109] These effects are facilitated if analyzed by color, power, or B flow.

A gynecologic and ultrasound examination prior to the procedure is necessary to define the uterine position and anomalies, if present, as well as both adnexal regions. Before any intervention, a pregnancy test should be performed. Local or systemic infections should be excluded by clinical examination and inspection of the genital tract and cervical smears. The procedure should never be performed in women with active pelvic infections, and antibiotic prophylaxis is recommended in patients with a positive history of PID. Hysterosonosalpingography should always be performed during the early follicular phase of the menstrual cycle, after complete cessation of menstrual bleeding. This avoids dispersion of menstrual debris into the peritoneal cavity. Procedures done in this period allow absorption of the media prior to ovulation, thus avoiding the presence of a foreign substance around the time of a forming corpus luteum. This decreases any potential effect the media may have on tubal transport.

The technique for performing hysterosonosalpingography is similar to x-ray HSG. After voiding, the patient is positioned supine on the gynecologic table. With the patient's legs flexed, a speculum is inserted into the vagina and positioned such that the entire cervix is visualized and the os is easily accessible. After washing the cervix and the vagina, a tenaculum is placed on the anterior lip of the cervix, and the cannula is gently guided into the endocervical canal. Application of the contrast medium is performed via a thin uterine catheter fitted with a balloon for stabilization and occlusion of the internal cervical os. The first observation to be made is of the uterine cavity, with verification of the catheter placement. After removal of the tenaculum, the endovaginal transducer is introduced into the posterior fornix of the vagina. The hypoechogenic contrast (i.e., sterile saline) is slowly injected under control of ultrasound. At this stage one can observe the morphology of the uterus and endometrial lining and detect duplication anomalies of the uterus or existence of endometrial polyps or submucous fibroids that are protruding into the uterine cavity, which is marked with anechoic contrast (Fig. 31-20).

Following visualization of the uterine cavity, lateral sweeps of the ultrasound transducer may allow visualization of intratubal flow on each side. Intermittent injections of contrast medium during at least three observation phases for each tube are needed to verify the tubal status. To exclude the formation of iatrogenic hydrosalpinx, both adnexal regions and the retrouterine space are carefully examined. Progressive accumulation of retrouterine fluid on both sides suggests bilateral tubal patency. If present, adhesions are visualized as bright bands in the adnexal region and/ or cul-de-sac.

The addition of pulsed Doppler waveform analysis is recommended as a supplement to gray-scale imaging in cases of suspected tubal occlusion and in cases when intratubal flow is demonstrated only over a short distance. When 152 fallopian tubes were analyzed using hysterosonosalpingography with pulsed Doppler, conventional hysterosalpingography and dye laparoscopy, sonographic evaluation showed 87.5% concordance with other techniques, predicted 100% of tubal occlusions, and detected 86% of patent tubes.[108]

Color Doppler may also aid to the precision of grayscale HSG. Visualization of color and/or power Doppler signals passing through the fallopian tube indicates patency, whereas the absence signifies tubal occlusion.[110] Spillage of the fluid through the fimbrial end, followed by accumulation of the fluid in the cul-de-sac controlled by endovaginal color and pulsed Doppler, is an accurate indicator of tubal patency.

More recently, 3D ultrasound has been introduced in evaluation of tubal patency.[107,111,112] The reduction of

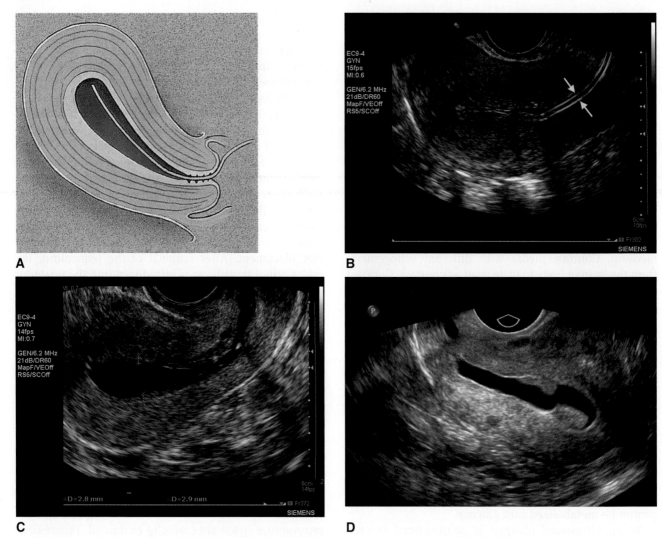

A

B

C

D

Figure 31-20 A: Diagram showing an intrauterine catheter used for distention of lumen with saline for detailed internal evaluation of the endometrium. **B:** Hyperechoic catheter within the cervix and lower uterine segment (LUS). **C:** The anechoic saline outlines the uterine cavity allowing for a single layer measurement of the normal endometrium. **D:** Two focal areas of increased echogenicity within the uterine cavity are two polyps clearly outlined after instillation of anechoic contrast medium. (Images B and C courtesy of Derry Imaging Center, Derry NH, Robin Davies, Ann Smith, and Denise Raney.)

the procedural time is major advantage in addition to multiplanar view, 3D reconstruction, surface rendering, power Doppler facilities, accurate assessment of the volume, and coronal plane assessment of the uterine anatomy, which leads to decreased discomfort of the patients. Figure 31-21 illustrates HSG performed by 3D power Doppler ultrasound.

POSITION AND DISPLACEMENT OF INTRAUTERINE CONTRACEPTIVE DEVICE

Endovaginal, and in particular 3D ultrasound, enables precise evaluation of the uterine anatomy and detection of submucosal fibroids and congenital anomalies before insertion of an intrauterine contraceptive device (IUCD).[113] The same technique may be efficiently used to follow up the IUCD position, orientation of its shaft and branches, and detection of the misplaced IUCD.[114] Figure 31-22 demonstrates 3D ultrasound of T-type of IUCD.

PATHOLOGY BOX 31-3

Advantages and Disadvantages of Hysterosonosalpingography

Advantages	Disadvantages
• Avoids	• Requires technical competence
• Radiation exposure	• Technique mastery requires 10–20 examinations
• Allergic reactions to iodinated contrast media	• Steep learning curve
• General anesthesia	• Tubal spasm may lead to misdiagnosis of tubal occlusion
• May be performed as outpatient procedure	• Tubal flow may give a false impression of tubal patency in the presence of hydrosalpinx
• Short duration	
• Well tolerated with little discomfort and few adverse events	• Lack of visualization of intrapelvic and bowel pathology
• Real-time demonstration of tubal patency	

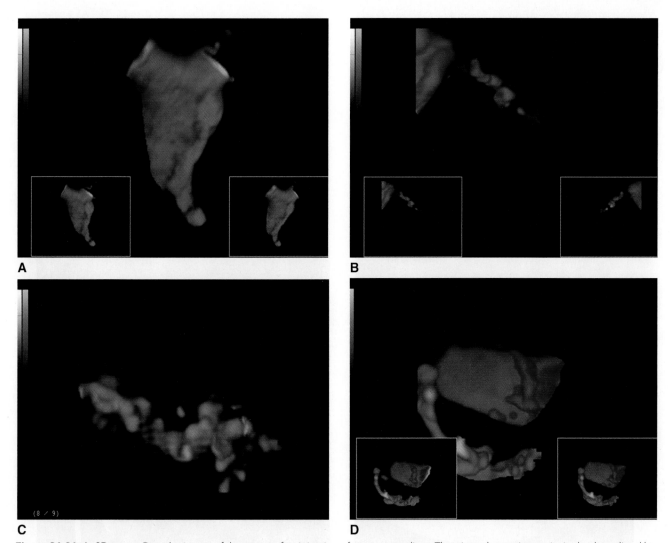

Figure 31-21 **A:** 3D power Doppler image of the uterus after injection of contrast medium. The triangular uterine cavity is clearly outlined by power Doppler imaging. **B:** Simultaneous assessment of the triangular uterine cavity and proximal part of the tube using 3D power Doppler HSG. **C:** 3D power Doppler image of a patent fallopian tube. **D:** Simultaneous assessment of the uterine cavity and entire tubal length. Note free spillage of the contrast medium from the fimbrial end of the tube.

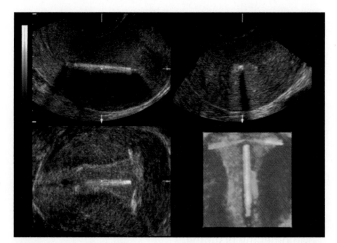

Figure 31-22 3D ultrasound of a T-shaped IUCD. Extension of its branches is best demonstrated in coronal plane.

RADIOTHERAPY PLANNING AND MONITORING

The goal of radiotherapy is to deliver the highest possible radiation dose to the malignant tissue and minimize the damage to the adjacent normal tissue. Noninvasive endovaginal measurements may precisely determine the uterine and cervical size, for example length and width of the uterine cavity, anteroposterior dimensions of the uterus and cervix, and myometrial thickness, which may assist in radiotherapy planning. Prior to radiotherapy, the urinary bladder should be carefully explored for tumor invasion. In patients with cervical cancer, the response to radiotherapy may be sonographically monitored. Following radiotherapy, reduction in size and echogenicity of the cervical and/or endometrial cancer has been reported.[115] Endovaginal ultrasound can also detect sequelae of radiotherapy, such as mucometra or hematometra due to cervical stenosis (Fig. 31-23).

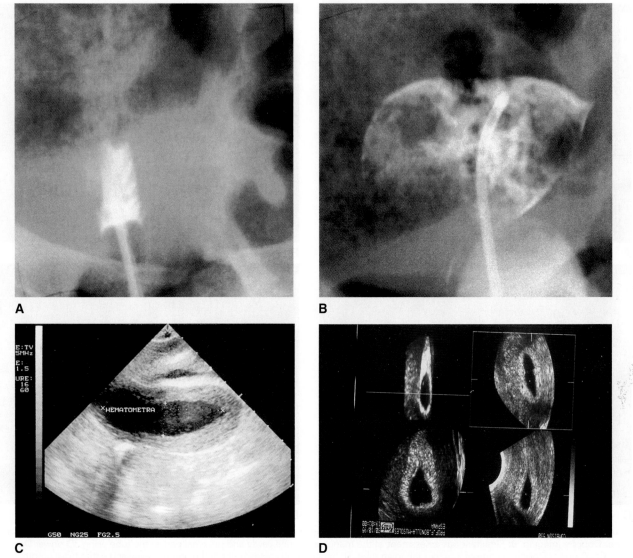

Figure 31-23 A: Attempted HSG in a patient with scarring of the internal os and hematometera. **B:** HSG in the same patient after uterine sound had disrupted adhesions. Dye outlined multiple blood clots. Initial diagnosis was uterine cancer. **C:** Ultrasound demonstrating hematometra in a patient with postcurettage amenorrhea and scarring of the lower uterine segment. **D:** 3D ultrasound image of patient with hematometra.

SUMMARY

- A gestationally adjusted MSAFP value greater than 2.5 times the normal limit raises suspicion for birth defects or multiple fetuses.
- The optimal timing for an amniocentesis is between 14 and 20 gestational weeks.
- To ensure sampling of different amniotic fluid in multiples, an indigo carmine dye injection turns the sampled sac a blue color.
- The optimal timing for a CVS is between the 9th and 12th day after the last menstrual period.
- Coelocentesis removes fluid from the embryonic coelomic fluid surrounding the amniotic sac.

- Coelocentesis, performed vaginally, can provide a sample as early as 6 weeks.
- Fetal blood sampling occurs at the venous cord insertion site.
- Fetal transfusion decrease is due to Rh treatment and development of PSV MCA guidelines.
- An increase in the need for multifetal pregnancy reduction is due to ovulation-inducing drug use.
- Endovaginally directed procedures include oocyte retrieval, ovarian cyst aspiration, pelvis mass biopsy, abscess drainage, culdocentesis, local treatment of ectopic pregnancy, embryo transfer, tubal catheterization, tubal patency studies, IUCD position, and radiotherapy planning.

Critical Thinking Questions

1. A 38-year-old primigravida patient of African descent has the following history:

   1. Sister, cousin, and sister-in-law with sickle cell disease.
   2. Last menstrual period 12 weeks ago.
   3. MSAFP correlating with gestational age.

   What prenatal invasive test could be offered to this patient? Explain your answer.

   ANSWER: Amniocentesis would be best for her gestational age and the blood disorder history in her family. The normal MSAFP correlation helps rule out any congenital defects.

2. An in vitro procedure resulted in a patient with five embryos. Three had diamniotic/dichorionic membrane configurations; the fourth and fifth were a set of twins with monoamniotic/monochorionic membranes. During a selective reduction, which embryos would be selected for reduction?

   ANSWER: In all cases of reduction, the embryo with the best access is used in the procedure. Any malformed embryo or one at high risk of problems, such as the monoamniotic/monochorionic pregnancy, are reduced first.

REFERENCES

1. Daffos F, Capella-Pavlosky M, Forestier F. A new procedure for fetal blood sampling in utero: preliminary results of 53 cases. *Am J Obstet Gynecol.* 1983;146(8):985–987.
2. Shaw MW. Genetic counseling. *Science.* 1974;184(138):751.
3. Shaw MW. Review of published studies of genetic counseling: A critique. In: Lubs HA, de la Cruz F, eds. *Genetic Counseling. A Monograph of the National Institute of Child Health and Human Development.* New York: Raven Press; 1977:252–259.
4. Lambl D. Ein seltener Fall von Hydramnios. *Zentralbl Gynakol.* 1881;5:329–334.
5. Schatz F. Eine besondere Art von ein seitiger Poly bei Zwillingen. *Arch Gynaekol.* 1882;19:329–369.
6. Parvey B. Report of a case of acute hydramnion treated by abdominal puncture. *N Engl J Med.* 1933;208:683–685.
7. Bumm E. Cited by Wormser E. Uber Punktion des Uterus bei Hydramnion. *Zentralbl Gynakol.* 1920;44:137–140.
8. Bevis DCA. Composition of liquor amnii in haemolytic disease of newborn. *Lancet.* 1950;2(6631):443.
9. Walker AHC. Liquor amnii studies in the prediction of haemolytic disease of the newborn. *Br Med J.* 1957;2(5041):376–378.
10. Liley AW. Liquor amnii analysis in the management of the pregnancy complicated by rhesus sensitization. *Am J Obstet Gynecol.* 1961;82:1359–1370.
11. President's Commission for the Study of Ethical Problems in Medicine and Biomedical and Behavioral Science. Screening and Counseling for Genetic Conditions. Washington, DC: U.S. Government Printing Office; 1983.
12. Elias S, Simpson JL. Amniocentesis. In: Milunsky A, ed. *Genetic Disorders and the Fetus: Diagnosis, Prevention and Treatment.* 3rd ed. Baltimore, MD: The Johns Hopkins University Press; 1992:33–57.
13. Dacus JV, Wilroy RS, Summitt RL, et al. Genetic amniocentesis: a twelve years' experience. *Am J Med Genet.* 1985;20(3):443–452.
14. Golbus MS, Loughman WD, Epstein CJ, et al. Prenatal diagnosis in 3000 amniocenteses. *N Engl J Med.* 1979;300:157–163.
15. Merkatz IR, Nitowsky HM, Macri JN, et al. An association between maternal serum alphafetoprotein and fetal chromosome abnormalities. *Am J Obstet Gynecol.* 1984;148:1331–1334.
16. Leek AF. Raised alpha-fetoprotein maternal serum with anencephalic pregnancy. *Lancet.* 1972;2(7825):385.
17. Milunsky A. Maternal serum screening for neural tube and other defects. In: Milunsky A, ed. *Genetic Disorders and the Fetus: Diagnosis, Prevention and Treatment.* 3rd ed. Baltimore MD: The Johns Hopkins University Press; 1992:507–563.
18. Nicolaides K, Brizot ML, Patel F, et al. Comparison of chorionic villus sampling and amniocentesis for fetal karyotyping at 10–13 weeks' gestation. *Lancet.* 1994;344:435–439.
19. Chervenak FA, Farley MA, Walter L, et al When is termination of pregnancy during third trimester morally justifiable? *N Engl J Med.* 1984;310(8):501–504.
20. American Institute of Ultrasound. *Guidelines for Second and Third-Trimester Sonography.* Laurel MD: American Institute of Ultrasound; 1994:1–8.
21. Duff P, Brady WK, Robertson AW. An important medical use for the baggie. *N Engl J Med.* 1986; 315(26):1681.
22. Simpson JL, Elias E. Genetic amniocentesis. In: Sabbagha RE, ed. *Diagnostic Ultrasound Applied to Obstetrics and Gynecology.* 2nd ed. Philadelphia: JB Lippincott; 1987:64–82.
23. Benn PA, Hsu LY. Maternal cell contamination of amniotic fluid cell cultures: results of a U.S. nationwide survey. *Am J Med Genet.* 1983;15(2):297–305.
24. Benn PA, Schonhaut AG, Hsu LY. A high incidence of maternal cell contamination of amniotic fluid cell cultures. *Am J Med Genet.* 1983;14(2):361–365.
25. Hahnemann N. Early prenatal diagnosis: a study of biopsy techniques and cell culturing from extraembryonic membranes. *Clin Genet.* 1974;6(4):294–306.
26. Kullander S, Sandahl B. Fetal chromosome analysis after transcervical placental biopsies during pregnancy. *Acta Obstet Gynecol Scand.* 1973;52(4):355–359.
27. Han A, Zhou B, Wang H. Long-term follow-up results after aspiration of chorionic villi during early pregnancy. In: Fraccaro M, Simoni G, Brambati B, eds. *First-Trimester Fetal Diagnosis.* Berlin: Springer-Verlag; 1985:1–6.
28. Kazy Z, Rozovsky IS, Bakharev VA. Chorion biopsy in early pregnancy: a method of early prenatal diagnosis for inherited disorders. *Prenat Diagn.* 1982;2:39–45.

29. Brambati B, Simoni G. Fetal diagnosis of trisomy 21 in the first trimester of pregnancy. *Lancet.* 1983;1:586.

30. Simoni G, Brambati B, Danesino C, et al. Diagnostic application of first-trimester trophoblast sampling in 100 pregnancies. *Hum Genet.* 1984;66(2–3):252–259.

31. Pergament E, Verlinsky Y, Ginsberg NA, et al. Assessment of the safety and accuracy of chorionic villus sampling in first trimester fetal diagnosis. In: Fraccaro M, Simoni G, Brambati B, eds. *First Trimester Fetal Diagnosis.* Berlin: Springer-Verlag, 1985:314–320.

32. Heaton DE, Czepulkowski BH. Chorionic villi and direct chromosome preparation. In: Liu DTY, Symonds EM, Golbus MS, eds. *Chorionic Villus Sampling.* Chicago: Year Book Medical Publishers, 1987:273–286.

33. Edelman C, Heimler A, Stamberg J. *Acceptability of chorionic villus sampling in view of the Orthodox Jewish views on abortion.* L. I. Jewish Hospital, New York, NY; unpublished manuscript, 1988.

34. Firth HV, Boyd PA, Chamberlain P, et al. Severe limb abnormalities after chorion villus sampling at 56–66 days' gestation. *Lancet.* 1991;337(8744):762–763.

35. Burton BK, Schulz CJ, Burd LI. Limb anomalies associated with chorionic villus sampling. *Obstet Gynecol.* 1992;79(5 (Pt 1)):726–730.

36. Firth HV, Boyd PA, Chamberlain PF, et al. Analysis of limb reduction defects in babies exposed to chorionic villus sampling. *Lancet.* 1994;343(8905):1069–1071.

37. Hsieh F, Shyo M, Sheu B, et al. Limb defects after chorionic villus sampling. *Obstet Gynecol.* 1995;85(1):84–88.

38. Olney RS, Khoury MJ, Botto LD. Limb defects and gestational age at chorionic villus sampling. *Lancet.* 1994;344(8920):476.

39. Chorionic villus sampling and amniocentesis: recommendations for prenatal counseling. Centers for Disease Control and Prevention. MMWR Recomm Rep. 1995;44 (No. RR-9):1–12.

40. Jackson LG. *CVS Newsletter No. 26.* Philadelphia: Jefferson Medical College; 1988.

41. Rhoads GG, Jackson LG, Schlesseiman SE, et al. The safety and efficacy of chorionic villus sampling for early diagnostic abnormalities. *N Engl J Med.* 1989;320(10):609–617.

42. Callen DF, Korban G, Dawson G, et al. Extra embryonic/fetal karyotypic discordance during chorionic villus sampling. *Prenat Diagn.* 1988;8(6):453–460.

43. Richardson RE, Liu DTY. Ultrasound for transcervical chorionic villus sampling. In: Liu DTY, Symonds EM, Golbus MS, eds. *Chorionic Villus Sampling.* Chicago: Year Book Medical Publishers; 1987:107–125.

44. Brambati B, Terzian E, Tognoni G. Randomized trials of transabdominal vs. endovaginal chorionic villus sampling methods. *Prenat Diagn.* 1991;11:285–292.

45. Smidt-Jensen S, Hahnemann N. Transabdominal fine-needle biopsy from chorionic villi in the first trimester. *Prenat Diagn.* 1984;4:163–169.

46. Jackson LG, Zachary JM, Fowler SE, et al. A randomized comparison of transcervical and transabdominal chorionic villus sampling. *N Engl J Med.* 1992;327(9):594–598.

47. Smidt-Jensen S, Permin M, Philip J, et al. Randomized comparison of amniocentesis and transabdominal and transcervical chorionic villus sampling. *Lancet.* 1992;340:1237–1244.

48. Vandenbussche FPHA, Kanbai HHH, Keirse MJNC. Safety of early amniocentesis. *Lancet.* 1994;344:1032.

49. Jurkovic D, Jauniaux E, Campbell S, et al. Coelocetesis: a new technique for early prenatal diagnosis. *Lancet.* 1993;341(8861):1623–1624.

50. Makrydimas G, Georgiu I, Bouba I, et al. Early prenatal diagnosis by coelocentesis. *Ultrasound Obstet Gynecol.* 2004;23(5):482–585.

51. Antsaklis A. Amniocentesis and fetal blood sampling for prenatal diagnosis. In: Kurjak A, Chervenak FA, eds. *Donald School Textbook of Ultrasound in Obstetrics and Gynecology.* New Delhi: Jaypee Brothers; 2008:755–764.

52. Antsaklis AI, Daskalakis G, Papantoniou NE, et al. Fetal blood sampling—indication-related losses. *Prenat Diagn.* 1998;18(9):934–940.

53. Liley AW. Intrauterine transfusion of the fetus in hemolytic disease. *Br. Med. J.* 1963;2:1107–1109.

54. Daffos F, Capella Parlovsky M, Forestier F. A new procedure for fetal blood sampling in utero: preliminary results of fifty-three cases. *Am J Obstet Gynecol.* 1983;146(8):985.

55. Mari G, Deter RL, Carpenter RL, et al. Noninvasive diagnosis by Doppler ultrasonography of fetal anemia due to maternal red-cell alloimmunization. Collaborative Group for Doppler Assessment of the Blood Velocity in Anemic Fetuses. *N Engl J Med.* 2000;342(1):9–14.

56. Berkowitz RI, Lynch L. Selective reduction: an unfortunate misnomer. *Obstet Gynecol.* 1990;75(5):873–874.

57. Dumez Y, Oury JF. Method for first trimester selective abortion in multiple pregnancy. *Contrib Gynecol Obstet.* 1986;15:50–53.

58. Birnholz JC, Dmowski WP, Binor Z, et al. Selective continuation in gonadotropin-induced multiple pregnancy. *Fertil Steril.* 1987;48(5):873.

59. Brandes JM, Itskovitz J, Timor-Tritsch IE. Reduction of the number of embryos in multiple pregnancy. *Fertil Steril.* 1987;48(2):326–327.

60. Coffler MS, Kol S, Drugan A, et al. Early endovaginal embryo aspiration: a safe method for selective reduction in high order multiple gestations. *Hum Reprod.* 1999;14:1875–1878.

61. Iberico G, Navarro J, Blasco L, et al. Embryo reduction of multifetal pregnancies following assisted reproduction treatment: a modification of the endovaginal ultrasound-guided technique. *Hum Reprod.* 2000;15(10):2228–2233.

62. Berkowitz RL, Lynch L, Lapiski R, et al. First trimester transabdominal multifetal pregnancy reduction: a report of two hundred completed cases. *Am J Obstet Gynecol.* 1993;169(1):17–21.

63. Evans J, Krivchenie EL, Gelber SE, et al. Selective reduction. *Am J Obstet Gynecol.* 2003;30:103–111.

64. Smith EH, Bartrum RJ Jr. Ultrasonically guided percutaneous aspiration of abscesses. *Am J Roentgenol Radium Ther Nucl Med.* 1974;122:308–312.

65. Gerzof SG, Johnson WC. Radiologic aspects of diagnosis and treatment of abdominal abscesses. *Surg Clin North Am.* 1984;64(1):53–65.

66. Kupesic S, Ahmed B. Guided procedures using endovaginal sonography. *Ultrasound Review Ob Gyn.* 2005;5:201–209.

67. Feichtinger W. Endovaginal oocyte retrieval. In: Chervenak FA, Isaacson GC, Campbell S, eds. *Ultrasound in obstetrics and gynecology.* London: Little, Brown and Company; 1993:1397–1406.

68. Kupesic S. Sonographic imaging of infertility. In: Kurjak A, Chervenak F, eds. *Donald School Textbook of Ultrasound in Obstetrics and Gynecology*. New Delhi: Jaypee; 2008:865–887.

69. Kurjak A, Kupesic S, Schulman H, et al. Endovaginal color Doppler in the assessment of ovarian and uterine blood flow in infertile women. *Fertil Steril*. 1991;56(5):870–873.

70. Kupesic S, Kurjak A. Uterine and ovarian perfusion during the periovulatory phase assessed by endovaginal color Doppler. *Fertil Steril*. 1993:60(3):439–443.

71. Kurjak A, Kupesic S. Ovarian senescence and its significance on uterine and ovarian perfusion. *Fertil Steril*. 1995;64(3):532–537.

72. Feichtinger W, Putz M, Kemeter P. New aspects of vaginal ultrasound in an in vitro fertilization program. *Ann NY Acad Sci*. 1988;541:125–130.

73. Schwimer SR, Rothman CM, Lebovic J, et al. The effect of ultrasound coupling gels on sperm motility in vitro. *Fertil Steril*. 1984;42:946–950.

74. Hill ML, Nyberg DA. Endovaginal sonography guided procedures. In: Nyberg DA, Hill LM, Bohm-Velez M, Mendelson EB, eds. *Endovaginal ultrasound*. St. Louis: Mosby Year Book; 1992:319–329.

75. Feichtinger W. Follicle aspiration with interactive three-dimensional digital imaging (Voluson): a step toward real-time puncturing under three-dimensional ultrasound control. *Fertil Steril*. 1998;70(2):374–377.

76. Kato O, Takatsuka R, Asch RH. Transvaginal-transmyometrial embryo transfer: the Towako method; experiences of 104 cases. *Fertil Steril*. 1993;59(1):51–53.

77. Bret PM, Guibaud L, Atri M, et al. Endovaginal US-guided aspiration of ovarian cysts and solid pelvic masses. *Radiology*. 1992;185(2):377.

78. Bret P M, Atri M, Guibaud L, et al. Ovarian cysts in postmenopausal women: preliminary results with endovaginal alcohol sclerosis. *Radiology*. 1992;184(4):661.

79. Yarram SG, Nghiem HN, Higgins E, et al. Evaluation of imaging-guided core biopsy of pelvic masses. *Am J Roentgenol*. 2007;188(5):1208–1211.

80. Stewart CJR, Coldewey J, Stewart IS. Comparison of fine needle aspiration cytology and needle core biopsy in the diagnosis of radiologically detected abdominal lesions. *J Clin Pathol*. 2002;55(2):93–97.

81. Teisala K, Heinonen PK, Punnonen R. Endovaginal ultrasound in the diagnosis and treatment of tuboovarian abscess. *Br J Obstet Gynaecol*. 1999;97:178–180.

82. Kupesic S, Kurjak A. Guided procedures using endovaginal sonography. In: Kurjak A, Chervenak F, eds. *Donald School Textbook of Ultrasound in Obstetrics and Gynecology*. New Delhi: Jaypee; 2008:913–922.

83. Stowall TG, Ling FW, Gray LA. Single dose methotrexate for treatment of ectopic pregnancy. *Obstet Gynecol*. 1991;77(5):754–757.

84. Fernandez H, Baton C, Lelaidier C, et al. Conservative management of ectopic pregnancy: prospective randomized clinical trial of methotrexate versus prostaglandin sulphostrone by combined endovaginal and systemic administration. *Fertil Steril*. 1991;55(4):746.

85. Ory SL. Chemotherapy for ectopic pregnancy. *Obstet Gynecol Clin N Am*. 1991;18:123–124.

86. Feichtinger W, Kemeter P. Conservative treatment of ectopic pregnancy by endovaginal aspiration under sonographic control and methotrexate injection. *Lancet*. 1987;1(8529):381–382.

87. Egarter C. Methotrexate treatment of ectopic gestation and reproductive outcome. *Am J Obstet Gynecol*. 1990;62:406–409.

88. Brown DL, Felker RE, Stowall TG, et al. Serial endovaginal sonography of ectopic pregnancies treated by methotrexate. *Obstet Gynecol*. 1991;77(3):406–408.

89. Mottla GL, Rulin MC, Guzick DS. Lack of resolution of ectopic pregnancy by intratubal injection of methotrexate. *Fertil Steril*. 1992;57(3):685.

90. Timor-Tritsch IE, Peisner DB, Monteagudo A. Vaginal sonographic puncture procedures. In: Timor-Tritsch IE, Rottem S, eds. *Endovaginal Sonography*. New York: Elsevier; 1991:427.

91. Kupesic S, Kurjak A. Color Doppler assessment of ectopic pregnancy. In: Kurjak A, Kupesic S, eds. *An Atlas of Endovaginal Color Doppler*. New York: The Parthenon Publishing Group; 2000:137–149.

92. Monteagudo A, Tarricone NJ, Timor-Tritsch IE, et al. Successful endovaginal ultrasound-guided puncture and injection of a cervical pregnancy in a patient with simultaneous intrauterine pregnancy and a history of a previous cervical pregnancy. *Ultrasound Obstet Gynecol*. 1996;8:381–386.

93. Timor-Tritsch IE, Monteagudo A, Lerner JP. A 'potentially safer' route for puncture and injection of cornual ectopic pregnancies. *Ultrasound Obstet Gynecol*. 1996;7(5):353–355.

94. Eskandar M, Abou Setta AM, Almushait MA, et al. Ultrasound guidance during embryo transfer: a prospective, single operator, randomized, controlled trial. *Fertil Steril*. 2008;90:1187–1190.

95. Anderson RE, Nugent NL, Gregg AT, et al. Endovaginal ultrasound guided embryo transfer improves outcome in patients with previous failed in vitro fertilization cycles. *Fertil Steril*. 2002;77(4):769–775.

96. Sallam HN, Sadek SS. Ultrasound-guided embryo transfer: a meta analysis of randomized controlled trials. *Fertil Steril*. 2003;80(4):1942–1946.

97. Buckett WM. A meta-analysis of ultrasound-guided versus clinical touch embryo transfer. *Fertil Steril*. 2003;80(4):1037–1047.

98. Sallam HN, Agameya AF, Rahman AF, et al. Ultrasound measurement of the uterocervical angle before embryo transfer: a prospective controlled study. *Hum Reprod*. 2002;17(7):1767–1772.

99. Li R, Lu L, Hao G, et al. Abdominal ultrasound-guided embryo transfer improves clinical pregnancy rates after in vitro fertilization: experiences from 330 clinical investigations. *J Assist Reprod Genet*. 2005;22(1):3–8.

100. Kato O, Takatsuka R, Asch RH. Endovaginal-transmyometrial embryo transfer: the Towako method; experiences of 104 cases. *Fertil Steril*. 1993;59(1):51–53.

101. Steinkeler JA, Woodfield CA, Lazarus E, et al. Female infertility: a systematic approach to radiologic imaging and diagnosis. *Radiographics*. 2009;29(5):1353–1370.

102. Peters JA, Coulam CB. Hysterosalpingography with color Doppler ultrasonography. *Am J Obstet Gynecol*. 1991; 164(6 Pt 1):1530–1532.

103. Volpi E, Zuccaro A, Patriarca S, et al. Endovaginal sonographic tubal patency testing air and saline solution

as contrast media in a routine infertility clinic setting. *Ultrasound Obstet Gynecol.* 1996;7(1):43–48.

104. Stern J, Peters AJ, Coulam CB. Color Doppler ultrasonography assessment of tubal patency: a comparison study with traditional technique. *Fertil Steril.* 1992;58(5):897–900.

105. Kupesic S, Kurjak A. Gynecological vaginal sonographic interventional procedures–what does color add? *Gynecol Perinatol.* 1994;3:57–60.

106. Deichert U, Schlief R, van de Sandt M, et al. Endovaginal hysterosalpingo-contrast sonography for the assessment of tubal patency with gray scale imaging and the additional use of pulsed wave Doppler. *Fertil Steril.* 1992;57:62–67.

107. Kupesic S, Plavsic MB. 2D and 3D hysterosalpingo-contrast-sonography in the assessment of uterine cavity and tubal patency. *Eur J Obstet Gynecol Reprod Biol.* 2007;133(1):64–69.

108. Deichert U, van de Sandt M. Endovaginal hysterosalpingo-contrast sonography (Hy-Co-Sy). The assessment of tubal patency and uterine abnormalities by contrast enhanced sonography: advances in echo-contrast. *Fertil Steril.* 1993;2:55–58.

109. Kupesic S, Kurjak A. Contrast enhanced three-dimensional power Doppler sonography for differentiation of adnexal lesions. *Obstet Gynecol.* 2000;96(3):452–458.

110. Kurjak A, Kupesic S. The use of echo enhancing contrasts in gynecology. *Ultrasound Rev Obstet Gynecol.* 2001; 1:85–95.

111. Sladkevicius P, Ojha K, Campbell S, et al. Three-dimensional power Doppler imaging in the assessment of Fallopian tube patency. *Ultrasound Obstet Gynecol.* 2000;16(7):644–647.

112. Kiyokawa K, Masuda H, Fuyuki T, et al. Three-dimensional hysterosalpingo-contrast sonography (3D-HyCoSy) as an outpatient procedure to assess infertile women: a pilot study. *Ultrasound Obstet Gynecol.* 2000;16(7):648–654.

113. Kupesic S, Kurjak A. Septate uterus: detection and prediction of obstetrical complications by different forms of ultrasonography. *J Ultrasound Med.* 1998;17(10): 631–636.

114. Kalmantis K, Daskalakis G, Lymberopoulos E, et al. The role of three-dimensional imaging in the investigation of IUD malposition. *Brat Lek Listy.* 2009;110(3): 174–177.

115. Weitman HD, Knocke TH, Waldhausl C, et al. Ultrasound guided interstitial brachytherapy in the treatment of advanced vaginal recurrences from cervical and endometrial carcinoma. *Strahlenter Onkol.* 2006;182(2):86–95.

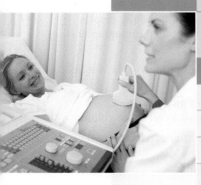

32 | 3-D and 4-D Imaging in Obstetrics and Gynecology

Bridgette Lunsford

OBJECTIVES

Define common terms related to three-dimensional (3D)/four-dimensional (4D) imaging

Describe the differences between two-dimensional (2D), 3D, and 4D imaging

Identify the advantages of 3D/4D imaging

List the benefits and drawbacks of the three data set acquisition techniques

Summarize the basic steps and system settings used to obtain a 3D volume

Recall 3D volume data set manipulation through use of the multiplanar reconstruction (MPR) format

List the advantages of using the MPR format

Describe tomographic or multislice ultrasound imaging and list the benefits of this viewing format

Explain common rendering modes and the clinical application of each

Define virtual organ computer-aided analysis (VOCAL) listing potential clinical applications in both OB and GYN imaging

Describe common clinical applications for 3D ultrasound in obstetric and gynecologic imaging

Identify the concerns surrounding keepsake imaging and describe the current position of the ultrasound community

KEY TERMS

3D | 4D | 3D volume | pixel | voxel | orthogonal planes | region of interest (ROI) | multiplanar reconstruction (MPR) | tomography | rendering mode | virtual organ computer aided analysis (VOCAL) | spatio-temporal image correlation (STIC)

GLOSSARY

3D ultrasound Imaging technology involving the automatic or manual acquisition and display of a series of 2D images

3D volume or volume data set Collection of acquired 2D images

4D imaging Continuously updated display of volume information; also known as real-time 3D ultrasound and live 3D ultrasound

C-plane Coronal plane, also called the Z-plane; often, 2D imaging does not allow imaging on this reconstructed plane

Digital imaging and communication in medicine (DICOM) Standard file format for handling, storing,

printing, and transmitting information in any form of medical imaging (i.e., radiology, pathology, laboratory, etc.)

Multiplanar reconstruction (MPR) Display algorithm for viewing more than one plane simultaneously; frequently sagittal, transverse, and coronal planes that are 90 degrees to each other. Also known as sectional planes or orthogonal planes

Orthogonal planes Planes that are always at right angles (90 degrees) to each other; typically sagittal, transverse, and coronal

Picture archiving and communication system (PACS) Computer or server used to store, retrieve, and display digital images and patient information from a variety of imaging resources

Pixel Smallest unit of a 2D image; has a length and a height

Reference dot Point where all three orthogonal planes intersect within the volume; depicts the same anatomic point in three orthogonal planes; also called the marker dot

Region of interest (ROI) Area of data acquisition for the 3D/4D volume

Spatio-temporal image correlation (STIC) Technique used to acquire and display a volume data set of the fetal heart; the volume displays as a 4D cine sequence of the beating heart

Surface rendering 3D rendering mode that displays the surface or skin of the body without displaying the underlying anatomy

Threshold Filter used to eliminate low-level echoes

Tomographic ultrasound imaging (aka multislice) Display format in which the data is viewed as a series of parallel tomographic images similar to the display methods traditionally used in computed tomography and magnetic resonance imaging

Transparency Determines whether the voxels will be more or less see-through

Virtual organ computer-aided analysis (VOCAL) Software program used to measure volume

Volume ultrasound Term used to describe both 3D and 4D imaging

Voxel Smallest unit of a 3D volume, consisting of a length, width, and depth

---

Ultrasound has changed dramatically over the last 30 years and continues to experience exciting break-throughs. Three-dimensional (3D) ultrasound represents one of the latest innovations in the field. As 3D technology has rapidly evolved over the last decade, it has gained increasing acceptance, especially in the fields of obstetrics and gynecology. A review of the medical literature reveals hundreds of research articles describing clinical applications for 3D and four-dimensional (4D) ultrasound. 3D ultrasound has the potential to overcome some of the limitations inherent in two-dimensional (2D) imaging, and these enhanced diagnostic capabilities are the focus of current research.[1]

As with many emerging technologies, excitement and some skepticism surround the use and application of 3D/4D imaging. Although many practitioners believe "volume" imaging, a term used to describe both 3D and 4D technologies, will change the performance of the sonographic examination, there are also those who believe entertainment is the main purpose of these technologies. As 3D/4D technologies have become widely available on commercial ultrasound machines, a growing number of ultrasound centers have these technologies available. Despite this accessibility, many users are unfamiliar with the techniques and are therefore uncomfortable with their use. In many offices, 3D/4D imaging is only used to demonstrate the fetal face to the parents. This application has popularized 4D imaging with the medical community and the public alike; however, this application is only one small piece of what the technology has to offer.

3D ultrasound represents a major advancement in the field. As with any breakthrough, this advance in technology requires clinicians and sonographers to learn a new set of skills and even a new language.[2] Sonographers have always reconstructed 3D images in their minds from the serially obtained 2D images. This reconstruction has occurred for as long as ultrasound has been performed. 3D ultrasound gives a visual display to these mentally created images. Although the new format for reviewing and manipulating the volumes may seem complicated, the concept should be familiar, as clinicians have been practicing this since the beginning.

Numerous research studies have documented the benefits of volume imaging. 3D ultrasound provides anatomic views that are difficult or even impossible to obtain with 2D ultrasound. Regardless of volume acquisition methods, data manipulation allows viewing of data on any plane or orientation. The volume of data obtained from one 3D acquisition can increase diagnostic confidence by providing an infinite number of images to the clinician rather than the multiple still images included in a traditional examination. The ability to review and reconstruct these volumes offline after the patient has left the exam room opens up the possibility to receive remote consultation from experts in the field. Another advantage is the ability to reconstruct images rapidly in a manner similar to CT or MRI, providing the potential to standardize examinations and increase productivity and efficiency while maintaining diagnostic quality.[5]

This chapter reviews the many applications of this exciting and still evolving technology. This chapter contains information on the volume acquisition process, available data display options, rendering techniques, and the clinical applications in both obstetrics and gynecology. Learning the terminology and techniques involved in 3D/4D imaging helps eliminate some of the apprehension those new to the technology might experience. Developing a familiarity with the available technologies encourages ultrasound practitioners to include 3D/4D imaging in their diagnostic process.

HISTORY OF 3D/4D IMAGING

3D ultrasound has been one of the most rapidly evolving techniques in ultrasound. Engineers and clinicians have been working to make 3D ultrasound a reality since the early 1970s, but the greatest advances have occurred in the last decade.[2] In early 3D technology, large computers separate from the ultrasound scanner processed the data. Additional equipment attached to the ultrasound transducer made it bulky and difficult to use (Fig. 32-1). In the 1980s, the process was still time consuming because of the massive computer processing required to reconstruct a 3D image. This process could take hours, and the resulting image was without the diagnostic information of the original 2D image.[2]

Breakthroughs in 3D technology have paralleled the rapid advancements in computer speed, size, and memory volume.[1,6,7] As computers became faster and smaller, the processing speed needed to make the necessary computations in a timely manner became possible. The ultrasound scanner is essentially a computer; therefore, as faster data manipulation became a reality, image reconstruction moved from separate computers to the scanner itself.[1,2,6,7] This change occurred in the 1990s and made the use of 3D ultrasound possible in clinical practice.[2]

Commercially available ultrasound equipment became available in the mid to late 1990s and has evolved rapidly since its introduction (Fig. 32-2).[7] The most clinically relevant advances have been faster acquisition speeds, higher volume rates, and an ever-increasing number of display options.[13] These improvements made 3D faster, more sensitive, and easier to use and have helped move 3D/4D technologies from experimental techniques to an accepted part of clinical practice.

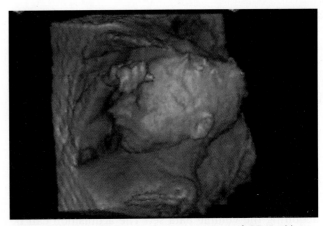

Figure 32-2 Early 3D image. (Images courtesy of GE Healthcare, Wauwatosa, WI.)

WHAT IS VOLUME ULTRASOUND?

2D ultrasound examination consists of acquiring and storing a series of single images. These images of representative anatomy make up the examination. Although some postprocessing of the images is available, what you see is what you get. Resolution of questions regarding the imaged anatomy requires additional imaging of the patient. Sometimes, this involves bringing the patient back to the office. Volume ultrasound has the potential to change the way we evaluate patients.

Volume ultrasound is a term used to describe both 3D and 4D imaging. These technologies are termed "volume ultrasound" because, instead of acquiring and storing single images, they are capable of acquiring entire volumes of data. This leads us to the question of what makes up a volume of data or a volume data set. When discussing a 2D image, the smallest unit that makes up the image is the pixel or picture element (Fig. 32-3).[6] A pixel has an X and Y dimension and is essentially flat. The smallest unit of a 3D data set, or a volume, is the

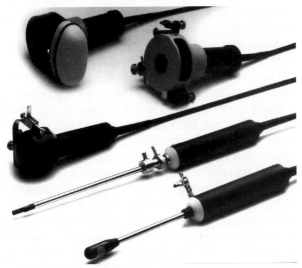

Figure 32-1 Early 3D transducers. (Photograph courtesy of GE Healthcare, Wauwatosa, WI.)

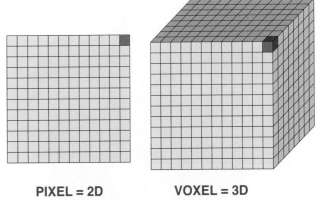

PIXEL = 2D   VOXEL = 3D

Figure 32-3 Pixels are the smallest unit of a 2D image and are made up of an X- and Y-axis. Voxels are the smallest unit of a 3D volume data set and are made up of an X-, Y-, and Z-axis. A voxel has depth. (Diagram courtesy of GE Healthcare, Wauwatosa, WI.)

voxel or volume element.[6] A voxel is a 3D cube composed of X, Y, and Z dimensions, giving the voxel depth. One analogy is to think of a 2D image as a single page in a book, whereas the volume data set is the entire book made up of hundreds of individual pages. Viewing the information found on each page in the book is as easy as flipping through the pages. The same is true of a volume data set; scrolling through the volume allows evaluation of any image or plane within the data set.

ACQUISITION TECHNIQUES

The first step in performing a 3D ultrasound involves acquiring the volume data set. The acquisition can be done in a number of ways. Current methods for acquiring the volume include freehand, sensor-based, and automated acquisition.

Freehand volume acquisition techniques allow the use of conventional 2D transducers. The benefit to this method is that no additional equipment is required. In this method, examiners manually sweep the transducer through the area of interest, as they routinely do with real-time scanning (Fig. 32-4).[2] This method does require some practice, as a slow, steady sweep is required and a fast frame rate must be maintained. When using the 2D

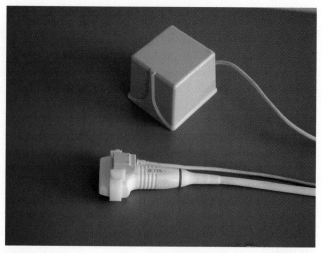

Figure 32-5 Sensor-based 3D requires the use of a separate transmitter to create an electromagnetic field. Sensors placed on the transducer relay the position and orientation of the transducer to the ultrasound scanner. (Photograph courtesy of GE Healthcare, Wauwatosa, WI.)

transducer, the equipment has no knowledge of the transducer's position or orientation; therefore, no measurements can be performed when using this method.[2,4,6,8]

In sensor-based techniques, a separate transmitter creates an electromagnetic field (Fig. 32-5). Sensors placed on the outside of a conventional 2D transducer allow recording of the motion, position, and orientation of the transducer throughout the volume acquisition. This method requires additional equipment and can be bulky; however, the knowledge of position and orientation allows measurements in any plane.[2,8] The volume acquisition process is identical to the technique used in freehand acquisition and requires the user to manually sweep the area of interest with a slow steady sweep.

The third and most common method of obtaining a volume data set involves using a mechanical 3D/4D transducer. These transducers are capable of conventional 2D scanning and can also obtain 3D/4D volumes (Fig. 32-6). A motor contained within the transducer housing provides an automated sweep. The transducer is steered electronically without external moving parts[8] and remains stationary over the area of interest while transducer elements sweep in a fanlike motion.[2] The motor either performs a single static sweep for a 3D volume or continuously sweeps back and forth to acquire a 4D volume. Instead of the external sensors used in the sensor-based transducers, mechanical transducers incorporate the sensor into the transducer housing.[2] The sensors provide spatial information, allowing for precise volume reconstruction and quantitative measurements in all planes.[8] Mechanical transducers provide smooth, consistent data acquisition and have become the industry standard.[2] Mechanical 3D/4D transducers are commercially available for many applications and include abdominal, endovaginal, and high-frequency linear transducers. Transducers for pediatric and cardiac examinations are also available.

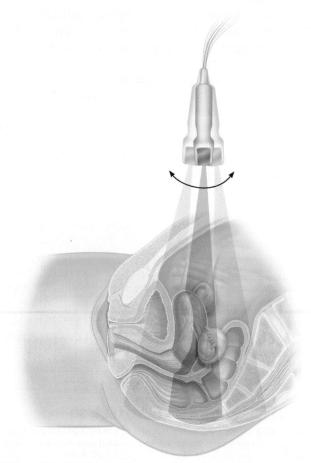

Figure 32-4 This diagram illustrates the freehand method of acquiring a data set.

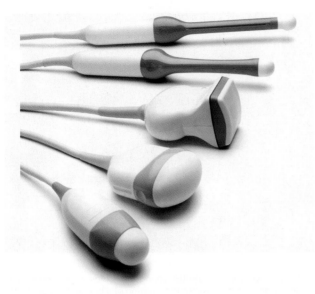

Figure 32-6 Mechanical 3D/4D transducers contain a motor within the transducer housing that provides a consistent automated sweep. Endocavitary, high-frequency linear, abdominal, and pediatric 3D/4D transducers are available. (Photograph courtesy of GE Healthcare, Wauwatosa, WI.)

As transducer technology improves, a new class of 3D/4D transducers called matrix transducers is available for research purposes in obstetric imaging. The primary use for this transducer is with cardiac applications (Fig. 32-7). Matrix technology offers many advantages over the current mechanical transducers.

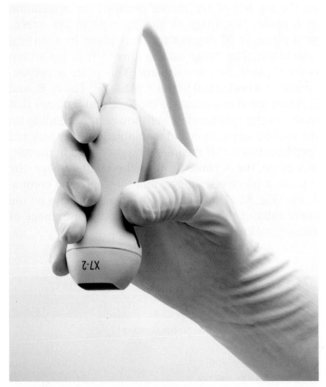

Figure 32-7 The x7-2 transducer has a smaller, square footprint due to the matrix crystal contained within the housing. (Photograph courtesy of Philips Medical Systems, Bothell, WA.)

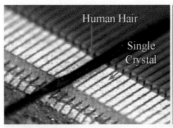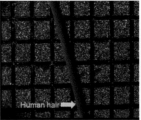

Figure 32-8 The left photograph illustrates the crystal configuration in a conventional transducer. The right image demonstrates the size and positioning of the matrix transducer crystal. (Photograph courtesy of Philips Medical Systems, Bothell, WA.)

Matrix transducers use more transducer crystals to provide greater out-of-plane focus and spatial resolution (Fig. 32-8).[4,8,9] Developments in matrix technology will eventually allow volume rates closer to real-time imaging and may prove especially useful in evaluating the fetal heart (Fig. 32-9).[4,8]

OBTAINING A 3D VOLUME

The following steps describe the method used to store a 3D volume with a mechanical 3D transducer. Although the terminology differs with each ultrasound manufacturer, the basic steps remain the same. When acquiring a 3D volume, the first step is to determine the region of interest (ROI) or the area to include in the volume. Place the ROI box over the structure and include the data acquired on the X and Y-axis (Fig. 32-10). The ROI determines the width and height of the volume data set, but unlike a 2D image, a volume also contains a Z-axis or depth. Adjusting the volume angle controls the amount of information acquired in the Z-axis. The volume angle is equal to the distance the transducer covers during the sweep.[10] When evaluating a smaller organ such as the fetal heart, use a small volume angle; for evaluating a larger organ, such as the uterus, use a larger volume angle.

One user-controlled parameter, the acquisition speed, changes the quality of the resulting data set.[6] Slower acquisition speeds result in more slices, and therefore the acquisition of a larger volume of data.[6] The images will be closer together and less data will need to be filled in or interpolated. This results in a higher-quality volume and higher resolution in the reconstructed planes.[11] Slower acquisitions can be used in gynecologic imaging and in cases where the fetus is not moving.[7,11] Faster acquisition speeds are needed with an active fetus to eliminate motion artifacts.[7,11]

2D image quality is extremely important when acquiring a volume. Poor 2D image quality results in a poor quality volume data set. Optimize the 2D image parameters before beginning the volume acquisition. Optimization of the 3D parameters occurs upon activation of the system 3D option. The ROI box appears on the screen, allowing sizing to include the desired

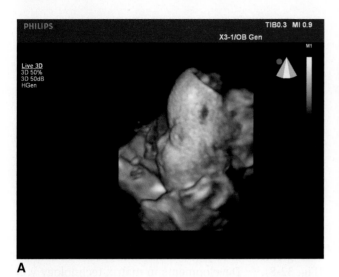

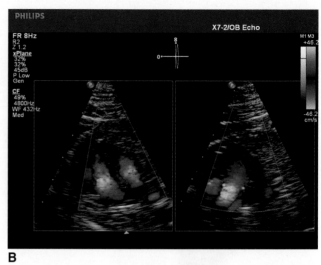

A   **B**

Figure 32-9 A: An image obtained with a matrix transducer of a fetus with Apert syndrome. Note the changes in color to help determine which structures are closer to the viewer. **B:** The crystal configuration of the matrix transducer allows for the creation of a bi-plane image. In this case, two color images of the fetal heart at 90 degrees to each other. (Images courtesy of Philips Medical Systems, Bothell, WA.)

anatomy. The sonographer chooses the correct volume angle and quality setting. With the patient still and respiration suspended, activate the 3D. The transducer is held still, and the array inside the transducer housing performs a slow, single sweep of the ROI (Table 32-1). The orthogonal planes appear on the screen at the conclusion of the acquisition. The volume can be stored to the ultrasound scanner's hard drive. Frequently, several volumes are taken to ensure that the anatomy of interest is included in the data set. Acquiring a 3D volume takes less than a minute and can add crucial information to the ultrasound examination.

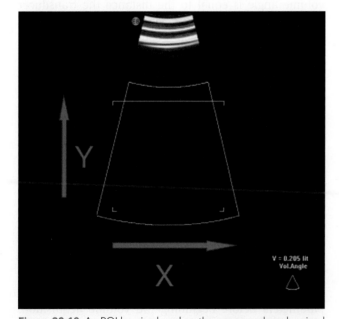

Figure 32-10 An ROI box is placed on the screen and can be sized to include the area of interest. The size of the ROI box determines what data are acquired in the X and Y planes. The icon located in the lower right of the image indicates the angle of data acquisition.

3D MULTIPLANAR RECONSTRUCTION

Once the volume is acquired and stored, a display format is chosen. Many formats exist for viewing the data set; however, the MPR display takes the volume information and displays it in a usable format. With this format, the three orthogonal planes and the rendered image are displayed on the same screen.

The three orthogonal planes are always at right angles (90 degrees) to each other.[2,7] The image displayed on the top left of the screen is called the acquisition or A plane. The image on the top right of the screen, or B plane, is 90 degrees to the A plane in a vertical orientation. The image on the lower left of the screen is the C plane, or coronal plane. This plane is perpendicular and horizontal to the A plane.[10,12] The A, B, and C planes are synonymous to the X, Y, and Z planes that make up the volume data set; however, depending on the volume acquisition and manipulation, they may not correlate directly.[2] If the image was acquired in the sagittal plane, the A plane displays the sagittal image, the B plane a transverse image, and the C plane a coronal image (Fig. 32-11).[6] The rendered image displays on the lower right of the screen and is a composite image of slices contained within the volume.

TABLE 32-1
Basic Steps for a 3D Acquisition

- Optimize your 2D image parameters
- Select ROI
- Adjust volume angle
- Select quality setting
- Have patient hold his or her breath
- Activate 3D mode

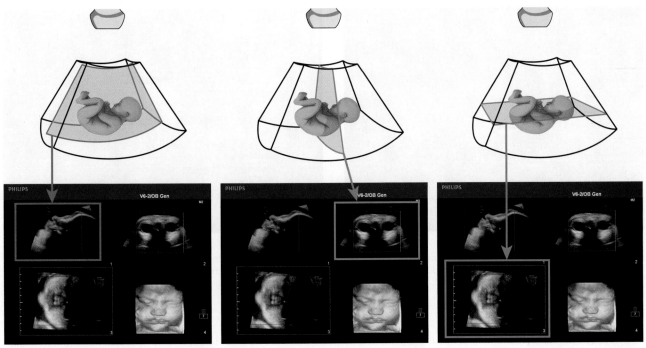

Figure 32-11 The A plane is the acquired plane and in this case is a sagittal image of the fetal face. The B plane is 90 degrees to the A plane and is a transverse image of the fetal orbits. The C plane demonstrates the coronal plane of the face, and the lower right image is a surface rendered view of the face. (Images courtesy of Philips Medical Systems, Bothell, WA.)

The ROI box determines the amount of information displayed in the A and B planes, whereas determination of the amount of information in the C plane is through the size of the volume angle. The A plane, or the acquired plane, has the highest resolution. The B and C planes are reconstructed from the volume data set and have a lower resolution than the A plane. The C plane has the lowest resolution.[2,10]

The point where the three orthogonal planes intersect is marked by a dot, sometimes called the marker dot or reference dot (Fig. 32-12).[4,6,7] This dot represents the same point, or voxel, in all three planes.[6,7] When evaluating pathology, the dot can be placed in the area of interest in one of the planes and the exact same area simultaneously displays in the other planes.[4,6] The marker dot is useful when evaluating the spatial relationships between anatomy and maintaining orientation when reconstructing the volume.

When viewing the MPR display, the user is not limited to the three images that are initially displayed. Manipulation of the data set produces an infinite number of images. Remember, the data is stored as a volume, not as a single slice. This format allows the user to rotate the images along any axis. Each image can be rotated using the X, Y, and Z rotations. Linked planes maintain the orthogonal planes at right angles to each other, and the reference dot marks the same point in all three planes. The translation control, also referred to as parallel shift, sweeps through each plane front to back or side to side. With these controls, the orthogonal planes can be manipulated into virtually

any orientation and give clinicians the benefit of what is often called a "virtual rescan." Manipulating the volume is similar to moving the transducer to obtain a better view. Now this can be done without the patient even in the room. Orientation markers placed on the screen allow the user to maintain orientation, limiting confusion during data set manipulation.

The MPR display provides the option of viewing the anatomy of interest from three different planes simultaneously, giving the clinician the possibility of

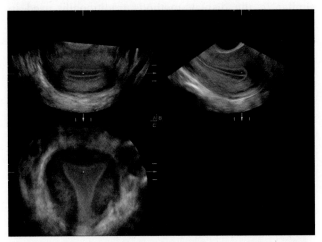

Figure 32-12 The colored marker or reference dot represents the same point in all three planes and can be moved within the volume to identify an area of interest in the three orthogonal planes simultaneously. In this volume, the marker dot is placed within the endometrium. (Image courtesy of GE Healthcare, Wauwatosa, WI.)

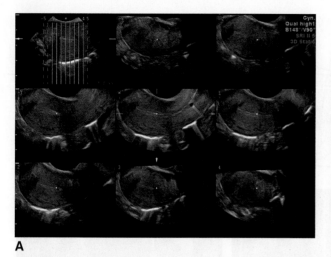
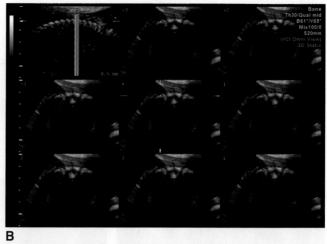

A **B**

Figure 32-13 A,B: Tomographic ultrasound imaging is a quick way to evaluate an organ of interest. The parallel lines in the top left reference image represent the spatial relationship and distance between the slices displayed on the screen. In Figure A, the slices are spaced further apart to evaluate the entire uterus. In Figure B, the slices are tightly spaced to closely interrogate one level on the fetal spine in more detail. (Image courtesy of GE Healthcare, Wauwatosa, WI.)

evaluating anatomic structures from multiple perspectives.[2,4,6] This format displays the traditional planes as well as those that have been unavailable with conventional ultrasound. The C plane, or Z plane as it is sometimes called, is the plane that we are unable to acquire with 2D scanning and can be critical for making certain diagnoses. Understanding this data display enables the clinician to produce diagnostic images quickly from the volume data set.[2] With a little practice, manipulating the volume data set can become as intuitive as manually scanning the patient in real time, and it provides even more possibilities.

TOMOGRAPHIC ULTRASOUND IMAGING

On many ultrasound scanners, the data can also be displayed as a series of parallel tomographic images similar to the display methods traditionally used in computed tomography (CT) and magnetic resonance imaging (MRI).[4,7,13,14] This display format is often called multislice or tomographic ultrasound. A reference or overview image is shown in the upper left hand corner and provides an anatomic reference for the slices displayed (Fig. 32-13).[4] The reference slice shows the position of each individual parallel slice within the volume data set.[4] The user can select the number of slices and the distance between the slices displayed. The X, Y, and Z rotational controls that are available in the MPR display are also available in the tomographic display. The volume can also be acquired using color or power Doppler, and this information can be displayed in the multislice format.[7] Tomographic imaging allows the user to rapidly and efficiently reconstruct images in a format similar to CT or MRI.[5,15] This format could allow ultrasound to implement more uniform protocols similar to other imaging modalities.[5] The tomographic ultrasound

format displays the volume information quickly and thoroughly and can lead to improved comprehension of the anatomic structures.[16]

RENDER MODES

Once the volume is stored, different rendering modes can be applied to the same volume, yielding different information from the same data source. Rendering modes are different algorithms that are used to display the 3D data set on the screen.[2] The wide array of available rendering modes has given sonographers images they never thought possible, and the options continue to expand. The variety of rendering techniques allows the examiner

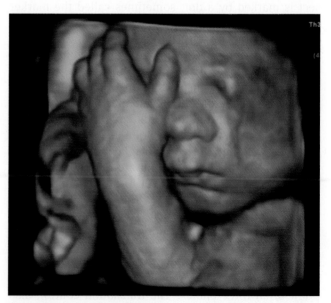

Figure 32-14 In this surface rendering of the fetal face and arm, the skin—or surface—of the fetus is displayed without displaying the underlying anatomy. (Image courtesy of GE Healthcare, Wauwatosa, WI.)

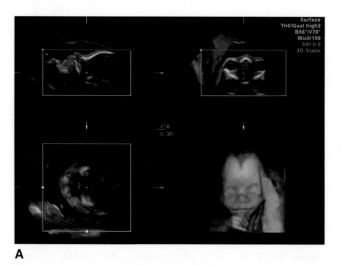
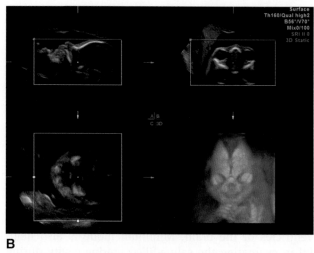

A   **B**

Figure 32-15 A: Applying a low threshold to the surface-rendered image of the fetal face eliminates few echoes, allowing for visualization of the skin of the face. The underlying bony structure is not seen. **B:** Raising the threshold on the same volume eliminates the lower intensity echoes of the skin and highlights the bony structure of the face. (Image courtesy of GE Healthcare, Wauwatosa, WI.)

to highlight different characteristics of the same anatomy, such as the bony structures of the palate or the soft tissue of the lips.[4,16] This section discusses some of the most commonly used render modes and their clinical utility.

Surface rendering techniques are without a doubt the most recognizable of the rendering modes.[6,7] Surface renderings of the fetal face are what have given 3D/4D technologies their popularity with both patients and the medical community (Fig. 32-14). The surface rendering mode displays the surface of the face or body without displaying the underlying anatomy.[13] This allows for better visualization of the soft tissues.

Various controls are available within the surface render mode, such as surface smooth, surface texture, or gradient light. As the names suggest, surface smooth controls how smooth the surface appears. Surface texture adds texture to enhance the details of the surface. The gradient light setting displays the structure as if it were illuminated by a light source.[6] This technique provides an impression of depth that gives the images a more lifelike appearance.[2] The threshold can also be manually adjusted. A low threshold setting rejects fewer low-level echoes. Be careful, as a high threshold could eliminate more echoes but remove valuable information. (Fig. 32-15).[2] The transparency control determines the degree to which we see through the voxel.[2] An electronic eraser or scalpel is available to remove unwanted structures in the image. This technique is similar to editing a digital photo (Fig. 32-16). The restore or initialize button undoes any changes

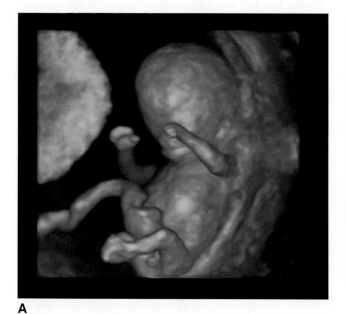
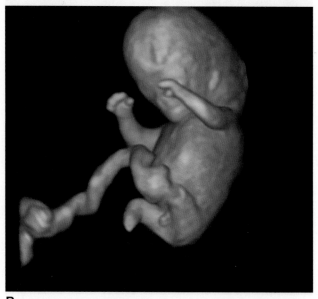

A   **B**

Figure 32-16 An electronic scalpel can be used to remove the placenta, umbilical cord, uterine wall, and other structures surrounding the fetus. (Image courtesy of GE Healthcare, Wauwatosa, WI.)

that have been made and returns the volume to the original saved version.

Maximum, skeletal, or x-ray mode reduces or eliminates the weaker echoes of the soft tissue structures and prominently displays the strong echoes of the bony skeleton (Fig. 32-17).[6,7,13] This rendering mode is useful for evaluating the spine, extremities, cranial sutures, and bones of the face.

Two techniques are used for evaluating hypoechoic structures: minimum mode and inversion mode. Minimum mode is used to evaluate hypoechoic or fluid-filled structures.[13] This mode can be used to evaluate fluid-filled structures in the fetus such as the fetal circulatory system, stomach, urinary tract, and ventricles of the brain. Minimum mode is also helpful in evaluating the saline-filled uterine cavity during sonohysterography. Inversion mode takes the hypoechoic structures and displays them as a solid structure or creates a digital cast of the object.[13] The gray-scale portions of the anatomy are removed and all cystic areas within the entire volume are imaged together as echogenic areas.[17] This improves visualization of complex cystic structures that cannot be imaged in their entirety with a single slice.[7,17] Inversion mode is especially useful in evaluating a dilated fetal urinary tract or hydrocephalus (Fig. 32-18). Pelvic imaging inversion mode is used to investigate complicated hydrosalpinx and polycystic ovaries, and it can be used to count follicles quickly during follicular stimulation.[17] When using both minimum mode and inversion mode, the threshold must be set correctly. If the threshold is set too high, only purely cystic areas are displayed; if the setting is too low, solid areas may be included in the display.[17]

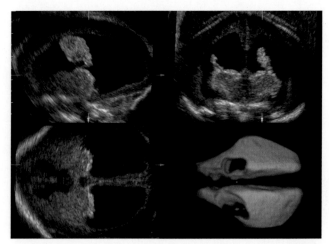

Figure 32-18 Inversion mode is used in this volume to better demonstrate the size and shape of the dilated fetal ventricles. Inversion mode displays fluid-filled structures as solid volumes. (Image courtesy of GE Healthcare, Wauwatosa, WI.)

Glass-body or transparency mode is a rendering mode that is used in conjunction with power or color Doppler (Fig. 32-19).[7] This technique is useful for highlighting the vascular anatomy while still displaying the surrounding tissues.[13] In this mode the tissue is more transparent, allowing the vessels throughout the volume to show through, making the relationship of the blood vessels to the surrounding anatomy more apparent. All gray-scale data can be removed to display only the vascular anatomy to display a color Doppler image similar to an angiography (Fig. 32-20).[7]

Once the volume data set is stored, multiple rendering methods can be applied to the same volume to interrogate different structures. One volume can provide almost limitless diagnostic possibilities. The potential to evaluate the anatomy in a variety of ways after the patient has left the exam room is one of the greatest advantages of 3D technology.

Virtual organ computer-aided analysis or VOCAL is a 3D measurement tool that is used to calculate the volume of an object such as the endometrial cavity, an ovarian cyst, or fetal organs such as the lateral ventricles, lungs, and bladder.[4,13,18,19] VOCAL allows contour mapping of a region of interest, creating a 3D model of the object of interest. The complicated volume calculation supersedes the spheroid formula often used ($L \times W \times H/1.57$). The data set is rotated 180 degrees around a fixed central axis through a preset number of rotation steps. At each step, tracing of the object contours occurs either manually or automatically. After the contours are outlined, the system then reconstructs a contour model and provides a volume measurement.[14]

3D VERSUS 4D

3D and 4D imaging modes are two distinct types of volume imaging. 3D is sometimes referred to as "static 3D." In 3D imaging, the ultrasound transducer makes

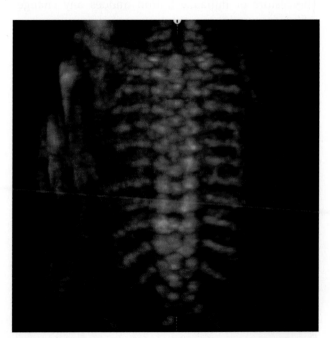

Figure 32-17 Maximum rendering or x-ray mode highlights the maximum intensity echoes in a volume such as the fetal skeleton in this image. (Image courtesy of GE Healthcare, Wauwatosa, WI.)

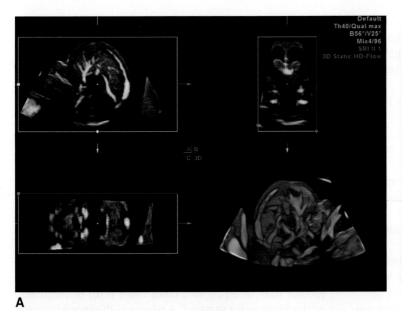

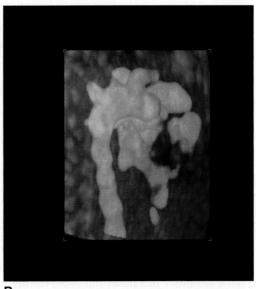

Figure 32-19 Glass-body or transparency mode uses color or power Doppler to provide a 3D visualization of the vasculature of a structure. The surrounding tissue is more transparent so that the anatomic relationships can be better evaluated. **A:** Vasculature of the fetal brain. **B:** Fetal aortic arch. (Image courtesy of GE Healthcare, Wauwatosa, WI.)

a single sweep through the area of interest and the obtained volume is stored and viewed in one of the many available formats. 4D imaging is often called "live or real-time 3D." When obtaining a 4D image, the transducer elements sweep back and forth, continuously acquiring volume data to obtain an image close to real time. The volume rate in 4D imaging is the number of volumes acquired per second, similar to the frame rate in 2D imaging.[2] The higher the volume rate, the closer to real time the images appear.

4D imaging is useful in many aspects of fetal imaging. The volume acquisition process is similar to that of 3D imaging. The ROI box is placed over the region of interest and the 4D mode is activated with the appropriate

control. The transducer is held still while the transducer elements continuously sweep back and forth over the area. Fetal position, amniotic fluid volume, and maternal body habitus affect the image in 3D/4D imaging just as they do in 2D imaging. To acquire a good 4D image of the fetal face, the fetus must be in a good position with amniotic fluid surrounding the face. The face should not be in contact with the uterine wall or placental surface. At least a small amount of fluid must be present between the fetal face and the uterine wall or placenta to obtain a surface rendering. With 4D sonography, fetal movement and facial expressions can be observed. Scanning in 4D allows the user to make changes to the image dynamically. The user can reposition the transducer to obtain a better angle, reposition the ROI, or change gain and other 2D parameters.

USE OF 3D/4D IN GYNECOLOGY

3D ultrasound has proven to be a complementary tool for a number of clinical applications in gynecology (Table 32-2). In particular, visualization of the coronal

Figure 32-20 When using glass-body or transparency mode the surrounding tissue can be completely removed to display only the vasculature, as in this volume of the umbilical cord. (Image courtesy of GE Healthcare, Wauwatosa, WI.)

TABLE 32-2
Clinical Applications of 3D/4D in Gynecology

- Congenital uterine anomalies
- IUD location
- Endometrial lesions
- Determining fibroid number and location
- Origin of adnexal masses
- Saline-infused sonohysterography
- Infertility evaluation

plane of the uterus is one of the greatest advantages of 3D ultrasound in pelvic imaging. The coronal plane cannot be obtained with conventional 2D imaging, and visualizing this plane is crucial to certain diagnoses. Applications include:

- Evaluating the uterine shape and contour for congenital anomalies
- Ovary evaluation
- Identifying the exact location of fibroids or intrauterine contraceptive devices
- Evaluating the endometrium for polyps or other lesions
- Determining the origin of adnexal masses
- Guidance for procedures such as sonohysterography
- Evaluation of the pelvic floor[5,20]

3D pelvic ultrasound is noninvasive and less costly than MRI and should be used whenever possible to make a more definitive diagnosis and avoid further testing.

One of the most useful applications of 3D ultrasound in gynecology is in the evaluation of congenital uterine anomalies. Mullerian duct anomalies occur in 3% to 4% of the general population and are associated with an increased risk of infertility and poor pregnancy outcome.[21,22] 2D ultrasound does not always accurately distinguish between a bicornuate and a septate uterus. Either hysteroscopic and laparoscopic evaluation of uterine morphology and contour or MRI has traditionally been the most reliable way to distinguish between the two conditions.[21,22] Visualizing the coronal plane of the uterus with 3D endovaginal ultrasound is a more efficient and economical way to make this diagnosis and has been shown to be extremely accurate.[7] The coronal plane is beneficial for examining the fundal contour of the uterus as well as the endometrial canal, enabling a more accurate diagnosis of uterine anomalies (Fig. 32-21).[21,22]

Diagnosis of a bicornuate uterus is made through the visualization of two separated uterine cornua on a coronal imaging plane. An external fundal indentation of greater than or equal to 1 centimeter (cm) is diagnostic of the bicornuate uterus.[21] A uterus is diagnosed as septate when a septum dividing the cavity is demonstrated in the presence of a less-than-1-cm notch in the fundal

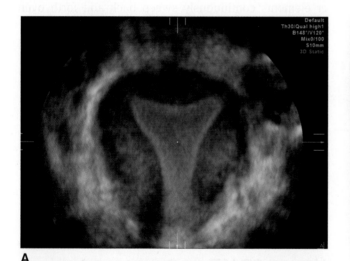

A

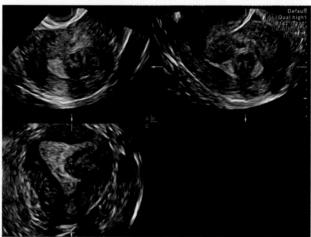

B

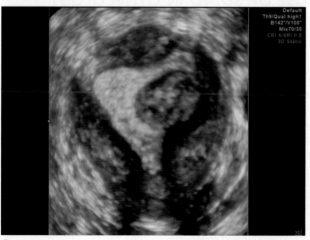

C

Figure 32-21 The coronal plane of the uterus can be used to evaluate fundal and endometrial contour. **A:** Coronal view of the uterus showing normal endometrial contour. **B:** Multiplanar view of the uterus demonstrating a submucosal fibroid distorting the endometrial cavity. **C:** Coronal view of same patient highlighting the fibroid location. (Image courtesy of GE Healthcare, Wauwatosa, WI.)

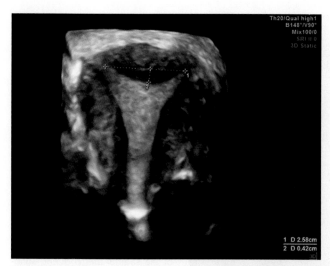

Figure 32-22 Coronal view of the endometrial cavity in an arcuate uterus. The endometrial notch measures less than 1 cm. (Image courtesy of GE Healthcare, Wauwatosa, WI.)

contour.[21] An arcuate uterus has a normal external uterine contour and concave fundal indention of the endometrial cavity of less than 1 cm (Fig. 32-22).[21] Surgical techniques for repairing Mullerian duct anomalies have become more advanced and require a detailed evaluation of the uterus and the endometrium.[23] Making the distinction between a septate uterus and a bicornuate uterus is an important diagnosis and can be helpful for surgical planning.[22] 3D endovaginal ultrasound can provide a more complete evaluation and make additional imaging, such as MRI, unnecessary (Fig. 32-23).[23]

3D ultrasound can also provide additional information during saline-infused sonohysterography. After saline injection, a volume of the uterus can be quickly stored to the hard drive. 3D reconstruction has been shown to offer improved visualization of polyps, fibroids, and adhesions, especially in complex cases.[23] The coronal view offers a better view of any cavity distortion and can provide a better global perspective (Fig. 32-23).[23] One of the greatest benefits, though, is patient comfort. Because the volumes can be stored

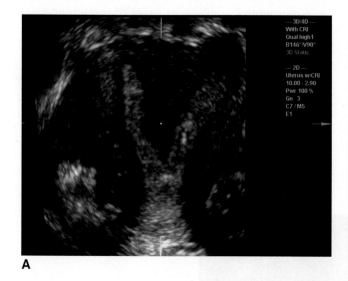

A

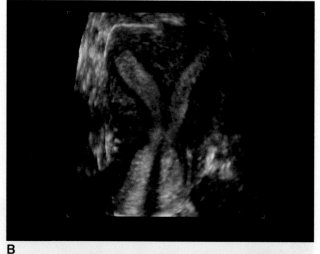

B

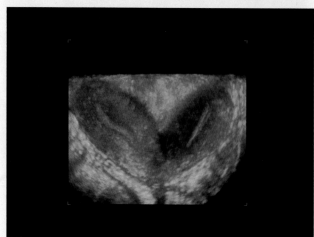

C

Figure 32-23 Congenital uterine anomalies. **A:** Coronal view of a septate uterus. **B:** Septate uterus. **C:** Coronal view of a bicornuate uterus. (Image courtesy of GE Healthcare, Wauwatosa, WI.)

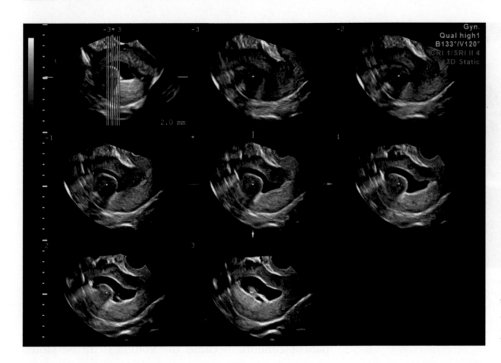

Figure 32-24 Tomographic display of the sagittal uterus during sonohysterography. A polyp is seen projecting into the endometrial cavity. The parallel slices are set close together to evaluate the polyp. (Image courtesy of GE Healthcare, Wauwatosa, WI.)

quickly, the examination can be completed in a shorter amount of time and frequently with less saline, without compromising the results.[7] The volume can be reconstructed once the examination is complete, allowing for a more thorough evaluation of the anatomy. The clinician can scroll through the volume in all three planes and can also magnify or measure any areas of concern. Inversion mode can be used during saline infused sonohysterography to essentially create a cast of the cavity.[7] 3D ultrasound during sonohysterography offers many benefits over conventional 2D ultrasound, from patient comfort to improved diagnostic confidence (Fig. 32-24).

3D imaging of the coronal plane of the uterus can be a meaningful addition in cases of intrauterine device (IUD) location.[24] Frequently, an ultrasound examination is requested to confirm the location of an IUD when the string cannot be located on physical examination. 3D ultrasound has improved the precision of locating IUDs. The coronal view provides a precise view of the location of the IUD, confirming the location of all device parts within the endometrial canal and can many times visualize the string, as well (Fig. 32-25).[24,25] Cases of malposition or perforation can be more easily diagnosed and, because correct positioning has an

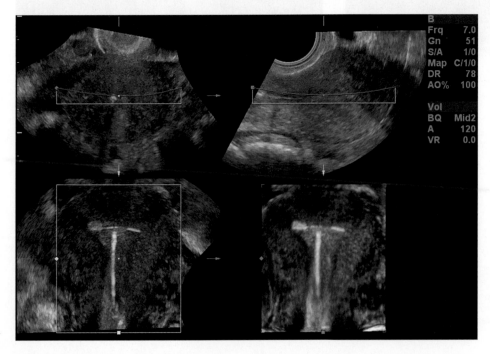

Figure 32-25 Multiplanar display of the uterus showing normal placement of an IUD within the endometrial cavity. (Image courtesy of GE Healthcare, Wauwatosa, WI.)

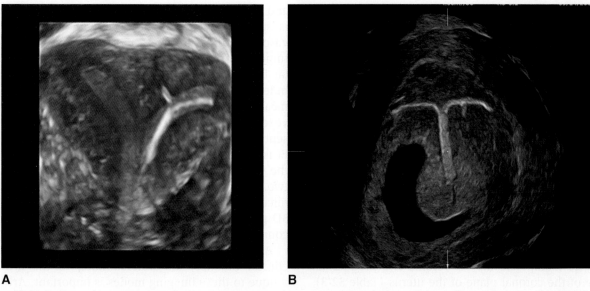

Figure 32-26 A: Coronal reconstruction of a bicornuate uterus containing an IUD within one of the endometrial cavities. **B:** Coronal reconstruction of a septate uterus with an IUP in one endometrial cavity and an IUD in the second cavity. (Image courtesy of GE Healthcare, Wauwatosa, WI.)

impact on the effectiveness of the device, the diagnosis is an important one.[24,25] 3D imaging can diagnose the existence of an intrauterine pregnancy (IUP) in a bicornuate uterus or the coexistence of an IUP and an IUD in a bicornuate uterus (Fig. 32-26).[24,25] Imaging the coronal plane of the uterus for IUD placement and uterine anomalies gives a more definitive diagnosis, instead of the presumptive diagnosis 2D imaging supplies.[24]

A new method of permanent birth control called Essure was approved by the Food and Drug Administration (FDA) in 2002 and is performed by a growing number of gynecologists in the United States.[26] Essure is an attractive alternative to traditional tubal ligation because it is performed without an incision.[26] Using hysteroscopic

guidance, microinsert coils are placed into each fallopian tube. Within 3 to 6 months, the coils stimulate tissue growth that occludes the fallopian tubes.[26] Current protocol calls for a hysterosalpingogram (HSG) to be done at 3 months to confirm successful occlusion of the fallopian tubes.[26] 3D ultrasound could provide a less invasive alternative to HSG to confirm correct placement of the coils in the cornua without exposing the patient to ionizing radiation (Fig. 32-27).[26]

Although it is valuable in many clinical situations, 3D reconstruction does not provide additional information in all examinations. Studies have shown that the coronal view was not helpful in evaluating patients with normal 2D ultrasounds.[22,27] The measurement of

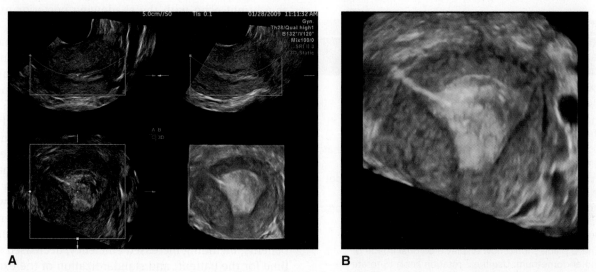

Figure 32-27 A: Mulitplanar reconstruction of a uterus following Essure placement. The echogenic Essure device can be seen in the right cornua on both the coronal and rendered images. **B:** Rendered image of the same patient confirming correct placement of the coils. (Image courtesy of GE Healthcare, Wauwatosa, WI.)

the endometrial lining has been shown to be an important indicator of the usefulness of the coronal view.[27] Reconstructing the coronal view of the endometrium is technically difficult in patients with an endometrial lining measuring less than 5 millimeters (mm).[22,27] When the endometrial lining measures more than 5 mm, the reconstructed view is likely to offer greater clinical benefit. Acquiring the 3D volume, however, is not time consuming and can be added to the 2D scan quickly when clinically indicated.

When implementing a new technology such as 3D, any technique that reduces the learning curve and simplifies the process is appreciated. The Z-technique, introduced by Abuhamad et al., is a step-by-step process used to reconstruct the coronal plane of the uterus from a 3D volume.[28] The Z-technique outlines the steps necessary to manipulate the 3D volume and produce an image of the coronal plane of the uterus (Table 32-3). According to Abuhamad et al., the Z-technique "adds simplification and consistency to the manipulation of 3D volumes of the uterus and thus is a first step along the path of standardization."[28] Physicians and sonographers alike express concern over the lack of standardization in both the acquisition and manipulation of 3D volumes.[5,28] Protocols such as the Z-technique that make using 3D easier increase acceptance and use of the technology in the clinical setting (Fig. 32-28).[5,28]

Acquiring a 3D volume with power Doppler could potentially help distinguish benign adnexal tumors from those that are malignant.[29,30] Power Doppler angiography allows for a 3D reconstruction of a tumor's vascular network and could help reduce the false-positive rate that is associated with tumor diagnosis by 2D ultrasound.[29,30] The vessel patterns between the two types of tumors appear to be different. Malignant tumors tend to have a vascular distribution that is more chaotic with more vessel narrowing, microaneurysms,

and abnormal branching patterns.[29] Once the volume is stored, VOCAL can be used with power Doppler vascular indices to give a more objective view of the tumor's vascularity.[29,30] Three power Doppler vascular indices are used: vascularization index (VI), flow index (FI), and vascularization flow index (VFI). VI measures the percentage of color voxels to grey-scale voxels in the acquired volume, and therefore represents the vessel density in the area of interest.[22,29,30] The FI is a measure of the intensity of the color voxels in the volume, and the VFI is a relationship between the two.[30] Malignant tumors typically demonstrate a higher microvessel density and therefore should have higher 3D power Doppler vascular indices than their benign counterparts (Fig. 32-29).[30]

As 3D/4D imaging becomes more widely used in clinical practice, an understanding of the artifacts unique to these imaging modes is important. Artifacts common to 2D imaging such as shadowing and enhancement are displayed in all three dimensions and can cause confusion.[31] Depending on the orientation and manipulation of the volume, the shadowing and enhancement can appear to reflect upward rather than downward.[31] One such artifact is the echo enhancement artifact from the endometrium.[31] This artifact is more pronounced during the luteal phase of the menstrual cycle and is thought to be the result of increased water content of the endometrium.[31] As the uterus is imaged in the coronal plane, the enhancement artifact can mimic the normal endometrium. In situations such as this, the reference dot enables the user to ensure that the endometrium, not the enhancement artifact, is correctly displayed in the coronal plane.[31] Shadowing from an IUD can also lead to misdiagnosis if the artifact is not fully understood. The strong shadow from the IUD persists through the coronal plane and should not be confused for the actual position of the IUD. As in 2D imaging, the IUD displays as a bright echo with the shadowing posterior to the device (Fig. 32-30).

Volume ultrasound has the potential to change the performance of the pelvic sonographic examination. Currently a pelvic sonogram involves taking 12–30 images of the uterus, ovaries, and adnexa one by one.[20] What if, instead of those individual images, you could simply acquire four 3D volumes?[20] One study by Benacerraf et al. suggested that instead of acquiring the standard protocol of 2D images, four volumes of the pelvis could be acquired and all requisite images could be obtained from those four volumes.[20] In this study, the exam time was reduced by at least half without decreasing the accuracy of the scans or adversely affecting patient care.[9,20] Volume ultrasound has many benefits, including increased efficiency, decreased scan time for the patient, and standardization of the examination.[9,20] Acquiring volumes also reduces some of the operator dependency inherent in ultrasound.[20]

TABLE 32-3

Steps for Obtaining a Coronal Plane of the Uterus Using the Z-Technique[28]

- Obtain a 3D volume of the uterus in the sagittal plane
- Use the MPR display to view the volume
- In the A plane (sagittal image) place the reference dot in the center of the endometrium
- Using the Z rotation knob, align the endometrium so that it is parallel to the horizontal plane
- In the B plane (transverse image) place the reference dot in the center of the endometrium
- Again use the Z rotation knob to straighten the transverse image so that the endometrium is parallel to the horizontal plane
- The C plane should now display a coronal image of the endometrium. Use the Z rotation knob to rotate the C image so that the coronal plane is visualized in the traditional orientation

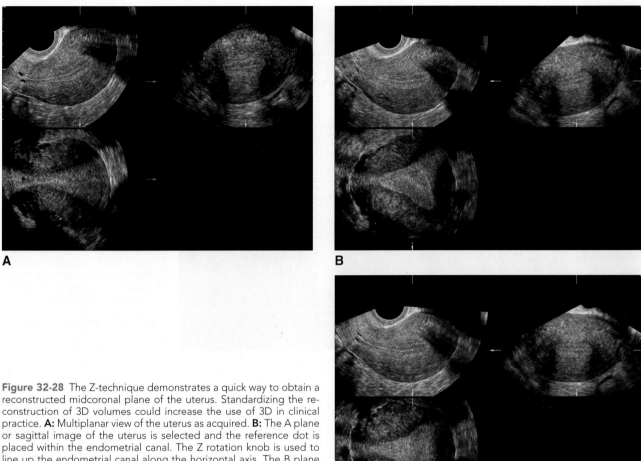

Figure 32-28 The Z-technique demonstrates a quick way to obtain a reconstructed midcoronal plane of the uterus. Standardizing the reconstruction of 3D volumes could increase the use of 3D in clinical practice. **A:** Multiplanar view of the uterus as acquired. **B:** The A plane or sagittal image of the uterus is selected and the reference dot is placed within the endometrial canal. The Z rotation knob is used to line up the endometrial canal along the horizontal axis. The B plane or transverse image of the uterus is selected and again using the Z rotation knob, the image is turned to line up the endometrial canal along the horizontal axis. **C:** The C plane or coronal image of the uterus is chosen and using the Z rotation knob the image is turned to display the coronal view of the uterus in the conventional orientation. (Images courtesy of GE Healthcare.)

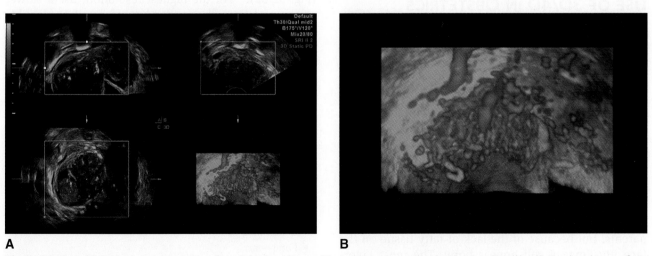

Figure 32-29 A: Multiplanar reconstruction of a solid adnexal mass. The volume was acquired with power Doppler. **B:** Rendered image from the same patient using the glass-body rendering mode to display the vasculature throughout the entire mass. (Images courtesy of GE Healthcare.)

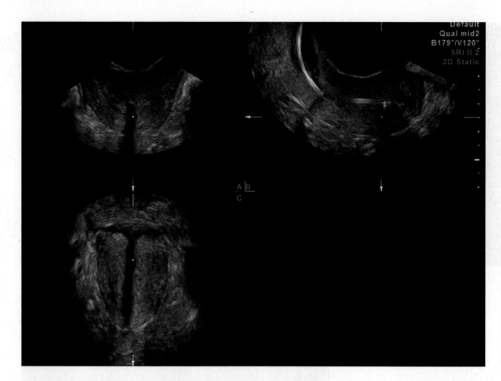

Figure 32-30 Artifacts seen in 3D can be confusing. The marker dot can be used for clarification. A multi-planar view of the uterus. The image in the C plane could be mistakenly called the endometrial canal. Notice in the A and B planes the marker dot is placed outside of the endometrial canal. The image in the C plane demonstrates the endometrial echo enhancement artifact. (Images courtesy of GE Healthcare.)

Although 3D ultrasound has been integrated into practice more slowly in pelvic imaging than in obstetrical ultrasound, 3D ultrasound has proven to be a meaningful addition to 2D ultrasound in gynecologic applications.[7] The 2005 American Institute of Ultrasound in Medicine (AIUM) Consensus Conference on 3D/4D listed numerous applications where 3D was found to provide additional value to the pelvic examination.[5] Obtaining a volume of the uterus at the end of the pelvic ultrasound gives the clinician additional information while adding very little time to the examination. Continuing research will determine what role 3D ultrasound will play in pelvic imaging.

USE OF 3D/4D IN OBSTETRICS

Volume ultrasound is most widely used in the field of obstetrics and has proven to add value to the diagnostic examination. The majority of articles written relating to 3D/4D involve applications in the field of obstetrics. Currently 3D ultrasound has been shown to offer advantages in many different applications throughout the pregnancy (Table 32-4).

One of the earliest applications of 3D ultrasound, imaging of the fetal face, is still the most used today. Anatomic detail of the facial structures can be evaluated with surface rendering techniques as early as 13 to 14 weeks' gestation.[1,32] By 18 to 20 weeks, the facial structures become more recognizable to the parents, but because of the lack of fatty tissue on the face, the images still appear bony. The most favorable time for obtaining a surface rendering of the face is between 23 and 30 weeks; however, just as in 2D

imaging, fetal positioning and fluid volume play a big role, and obtaining images all the way to term is possible if the conditions allow (Fig. 32-31).[1,32] With surface rendering techniques, small details such as the eyebrows, eyelids, mouth, and ears can be seen like never before.[32]

3D ultrasound is especially beneficial in evaluating for cleft lip and palate as well as imaging the fetal ears and other facial abnormalities.[1,4,5,7,13,16,32] Orofacial clefting is the fourth most common birth defect, affecting 1 in 700 infants.[33] Isolated cleft palate is more difficult to diagnose on 2D ultrasound than cleft lip because of shadowing from the anterior palate.[33] To evaluate for cleft lip and palate, a 3D volume is stored in the sagittal plane (Fig. 32-32).[33] For the highest resolution, use a slower sweep and keep the render box as small as possible in the anteroposterior (AP) dimension.[33] A technique called the 3D reverse face view can be used to more

TABLE 32-4
Clinical Applications of 3D/4D in Obstetrics

- Facial anomalies and ears
- Nasal bone
- CNS anomalies
- Cranial sutures
- Spine
- Extremities
- Fetal heart
- Chromosomal abnormalities and syndromes
- Fetal movement and behavior

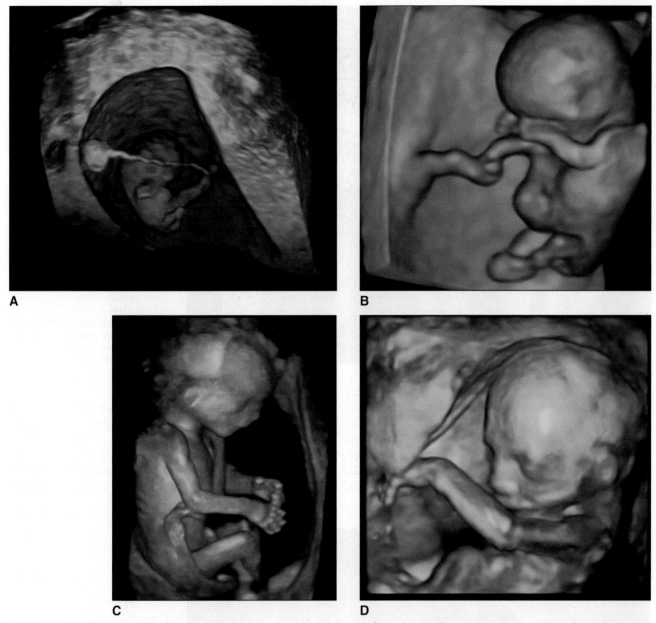

Figure 32-31 Surface rendering of the fetus can be done at any age. **A:** 8-week fetus showing the gestational sac and the yolk sac. **B:** 10-week fetus and umbilical cord. Note the physiologic hernia at the base of the cord. **C:** 13-week fetus. **D:** 20-week fetus. (Image courtesy of GE Healthcare, Wauwatosa, WI.)

accurately diagnose clefts of the posterior palate.[1,32–34] In the MPR format, the surface-rendered face is rotated 180 degrees so that the anatomy is approached from the posterior palate to the anterior palate.[1,32–34] This approach helps overcome shadowing by approaching the palate, nasal cavity, and orbits from the reverse side.[1] Adjusting the threshold levels determines whether the skin or bony structures are highlighted.[32]

A single-volume data set of the fetal face can provide all necessary images for a comprehensive evaluation of the fetal face.[32] Surface-rendering techniques can be applied to evaluate the lips and ears, and maximum mode can be used to evaluate the bony structures of the face. Using the translation or parallel shift control through the transverse plane of the face, one can evaluate the mandible, maxilla, palate, tooth buds, and orbits.[32] The sagittal plane is useful for evaluating the forehead, nasal bone, and the mandible; the coronal view demonstrates facial symmetry, soft tissue, and bony features of the face.[32] This demonstrates how much information can be obtained from a single 3D volume.

An absent nasal bone can indicate the possibility of a chromosomal abnormality, so imaging this structure has become part of many routine examinations. Obtaining a true midline sagittal view is vital to the diagnosis.[1,5,8,32] An off-axis image can lead to either false-positive or -negative results.[1,5,8,32] The 3D

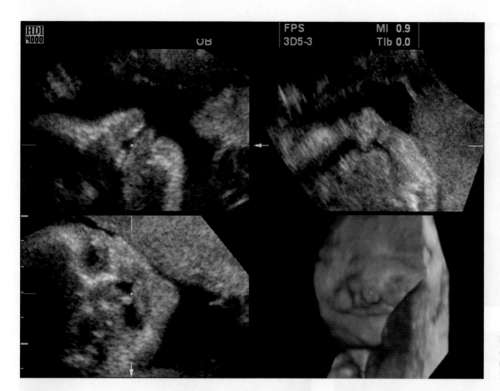

Figure 32-32 This MPR image demonstrates a cleft lip and palate. (Image courtesy of Philips Medical Systems, Bothell, WA.)

multiplanar view can assist the sonographer in ensuring that the correct plane is chosen. A true midline sagittal view confirms the nasal bone in all three planes. Use of the reference dot ensures imaging of the same structure in all three planes (Fig. 32-33). Ear anomalies are also associated with complex congenital syndromes. 3D surface rendering mode can better show the morphological detail, location, and orientation of the ears (Fig. 32-34).[32]

The multiplanar view can also be used to evaluate the fetal chin for micrognathia and retrognathia.[32] Both anomalies carry an increased risk of abnormal

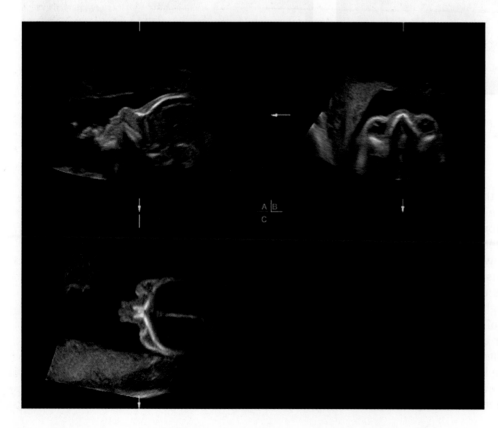

Figure 32-33 Multiplanar view of the fetal face. A true midline sagittal view is obtained by rotating the volume along the X-, Y-, and Z-axis. Place the marker dot on the nasal bone to display the nasal bone in all three planes. (Image courtesy of GE Healthcare, Wauwatosa, WI.)

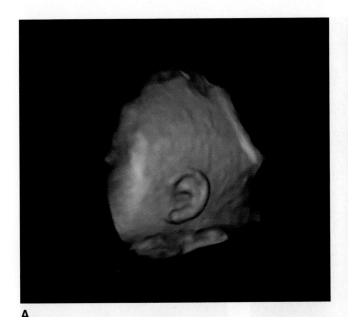

A

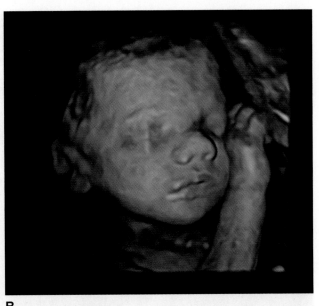

B

Figure 32-34 A,B: The surface-rendering mode can be used to evaluate the structure of the fetal ears in detail. (Image courtesy of GE Healthcare, Wauwatosa, WI.)

karyotype, making the diagnosis an important one. Again, the benefit of the multiplanar view lies in the ability to ensure that a true midsagittal plane of the facial profile is being evaluated.[5,8] A more complete evaluation of the sutures and fontanelles in the fetal skull is also possible with the MPR format.[1,3–7,13,32,34] The cranial bones can be viewed in their entirety in the three orthogonal planes, offering the potential to identify cranial lesions difficult to detect by 2D ultrasound (Fig. 32-35).[4]

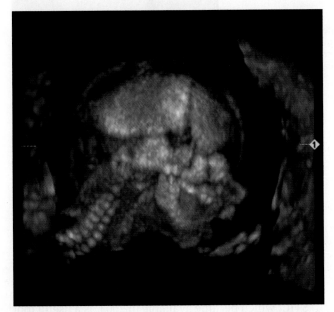

Figure 32-35 Fetal skull displayed using maximum mode to highlight the cranial bones and sutures. (Image courtesy of GE Healthcare, Wauwatosa, WI.)

3D ultrasound can also be valuable in evaluating the fetal central nervous system.[6,8] Using the MPR view allows the clinician to visualize the spine from multiple perspectives, making the evaluation of the spinal column quicker and more comprehensive (Fig. 32-36). In cases of spina bifida, the level of the lesion and the severity is easier to evaluate. Studies have shown that 3D ultrasound offers a more realistic view of the location and severity of the lesion.[8] Once a volume of the spine is stored, the translation or parallel shift can be used to evaluate each level of the spine in all three planes. Maximum intensity mode is useful for evaluating the bony structures, whereas surface rendering mode brings out the skin line.[1,4,5,7,8,13,34] Scoliosis of the spine and hemivertebrae can also be evaluated.[4,34] When evaluating the fetal brain, agenesis of the corpus callosum is a difficult diagnosis to make with conventional 2D ultrasound.[6] Using 3D, a true midsagittal view of the entire corpus callosum is possible, allowing for a more definitive diagnosis (Fig. 32-37).[3–7]

3D ultrasound also provides benefits in the first-trimester scan. The nuchal translucency scan can be very time consuming if the fetus is not in the optimal position. In cases where the fetus is not in the ideal position, 3D multiplanar imaging can be used to obtain an accurate nuchal translucency measurement in less time.[3,4,6,7,13,19]

One area where 3D and 4D have been shown to consistently add clinical value is in the examination of the fetal extremities. 4D imaging demonstrates both the size and shape of the extremities and documents their movement.[1,5,6,13,34] The foot and leg can be evaluated to rule out anomalies such as clubfeet or rocker bottom feet.[1] Hyperdactyly, overlapping fingers, and club

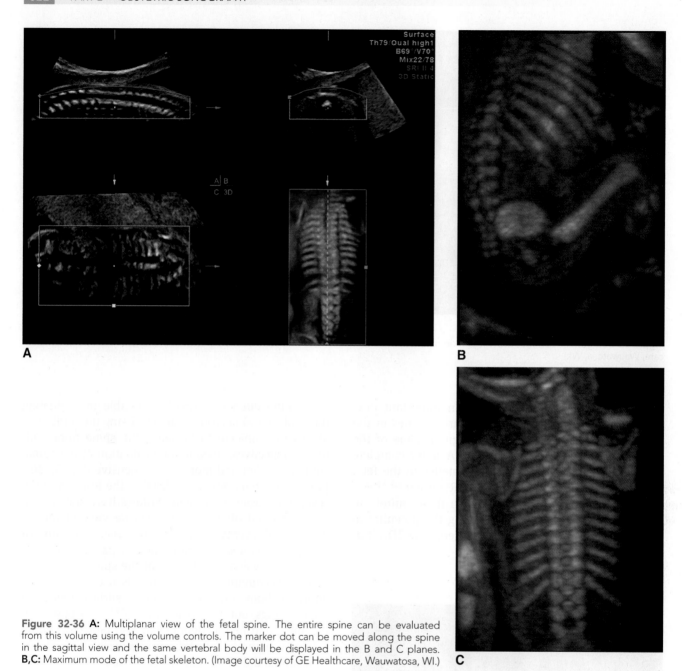

Figure 32-36 A: Multiplanar view of the fetal spine. The entire spine can be evaluated from this volume using the volume controls. The marker dot can be moved along the spine in the sagittal view and the same vertebral body will be displayed in the B and C planes. **B,C:** Maximum mode of the fetal skeleton. (Image courtesy of GE Healthcare, Wauwatosa, WI.)

hands can be better visualized with 3D/4D imaging.[16] 4D can be used to visualize the opening and closing of the hands to rule out the clenched fists frequently seen with trisomy 18 (Fig. 32-38).[16]

Cardiac defects are the most frequently overlooked lesions on prenatal ultrasound scans. Congenital heart disease occurs in 8 of 1,000 live births and is the most common type of congenital malformation.[12] Prenatal diagnosis of cardiac defects increases the chance of survival but only 5% to 22% of cases are detected antenatally.[11,12] The AIUM and American College of Radiology (ACR) guidelines recommend that a basic fetal cardiac examination include a four-chamber view of the heart and, if possible, evaluation of both outflow tracts.[15,35] The outflow tracts become critical in cases of

transposition, aortic coarctation, and other defects that have a normal four-chamber appearance.[12,35] Less than 10% of anomalies requiring the outflow tract and great artery views are detected with ultrasound.[12] The skill and experience of the sonographer plays a big role in the detection of congenital heart disease. Volume imaging offers two tools for evaluating the fetal heart that can reduce operator dependence: spatio-temporal image correlation, more commonly known as STIC, and imaging automation. The use of these techniques could improve the detection rates of congenital heart disease and reduce neonatal morbidity and mortality.[11,36]

STIC, which became available in 2003, is a useful tool for evaluating the fetal heart in an efficient, standardized format. This technique results in better image resolution

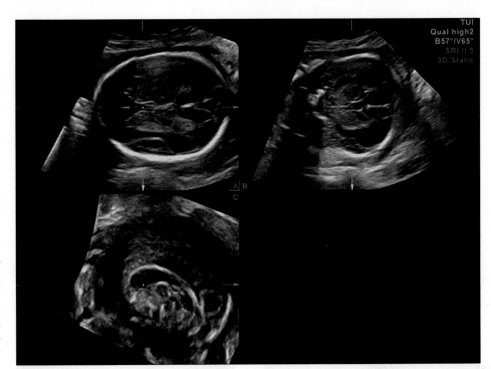

Figure 32-37 Multiplanar view of the fetal head. The marker dot is placed on the corpus callosum and can be visualized in all three planes. The coronal plane can provide a more definitive diagnosis of agenesis of the corpus callosum. (Image courtesy of GE Healthcare, Wauwatosa, WI.)

in all three planes.[10] As with any volume technology, the first step is volume acquisition. Once the STIC mode is activated, a single real-time volume acquisition of the fetal heart begins. According to Falkensammer and Helmut, "the system analyzes the data according to their spatial and temporal domain and processes a 4D cine sequence. This sequence presents the heart beating in real time in a multiplanar display. The examiner can navigate within the heart, reslice, and produce all of the standard planes necessary for comprehensive diagnosis."[37] STIC is a motion-gated scanning mode. During a 10-second volume acquisition, around 1,500 frames of the fetal heart are stored.[1,5,10,12,14] If the fetal heart beats at 150 beats per minute, the heart will beat approximately 20 to 25 times during this acquisition; therefore, there will be 20 to 25 frames demonstrating a systolic peak in the volume. The system performs a spatial and temporal correlation of the data to detect these systolic peaks and calculates the fetal heart rate from the number of peaks present in the volume.[1,5,10,14,38] The images in the volume are rearranged and placed in order according to their spatial and temporal domain. The volume is then displayed as a cine loop containing the functional and anatomic information from one full cardiac cycle (Fig. 32-39).[1,5,10–12,14,38]

The STIC volume can be viewed as a cine loop in the multiplanar view or the image can be frozen and manipulated using the volume controls. The data set contains all planes imaged in a basic and extended fetal echocardiogram, plus additional planes that are not possible with 2D imaging. The only view the operator needs to obtain is the four-chamber view, thus reducing operator variability. The standard heart views such as

outflow tracts, venous connections, and arches as well as the five chamber, three vessel, and three vessel trachea views are achieved by reconstructing the volume data set.[11,12,38–40] STIC provides consistent visualization of the outflow tracts (Fig. 32-40).[12]

Obtaining a good volume, however, is still operator dependent.[39] The same challenges that exist in 2D are present when using STIC. Early gestational age, maternal body habitus, fetal lie, and fetal movement still present challenges.[12,39,40] As with 2D imaging, the outcome is best when the fetal spine is down, but as long as the spine is not between 11:00 and 1:00, good volumes can usually be obtained.[11] Table 32-5 offers more tips for obtaining high-quality STIC volumes (Table 32-5). STIC technology provides many clinical benefits and is especially helpful when evaluating complex anatomy. Scan time is decreased because the entire volume of data and all available views are present in a good STIC volume.[12] The volume can be navigated without the patient present, allowing for more time to review complex cases. Spatial relationships that need to be determined in cases of complex CHD can be easier to see, as the cardiac anatomy can be viewed in transverse and longitudinal planes simultaneously.[10,38,40] The clinician can quickly scroll through the volume to evaluate situs, heart position, four- and five-chamber views, and the three-vessel view.[11,38] The volume can also be viewed frame by frame or placed in motion at any point. One of the greatest benefits of any 3D technology is the ability to review the case offline. Difficult cases can be sent to a specialist across the country for review without having to transport the patient. This could increase access to specialized care, especially in remote areas.

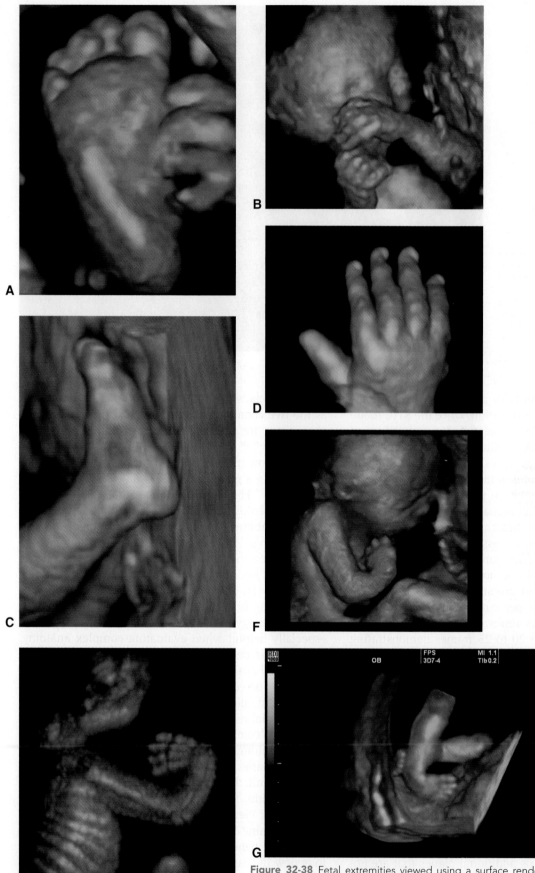

Figure 32-38 Fetal extremities viewed using a surface rendering mode. **A:** Fetal foot. **B:** Fetal hands. **C:** Fetal foot and ankle. **D:** Fetal hand. **E:** Surface rendering of a club hand. **F:** Maximum mode rendering of club hand. (Image courtesy of GE Healthcare, Wauwatosa, WI.) **G:** Surface rendering of a clubfoot. (Image courtesy of Philips Medical Systems, Bothell, WA.)

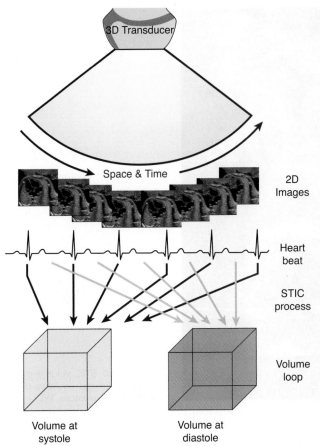

Figure 32-39 This diagram illustrates the acquisition of a STIC data set. The transducer makes a slow automated sweep through the volume. The resolution of the individual 2D images taken during this sweep is much higher than the resolution of images in a conventional 3D or 4D sweep. Because of the length of the sweep there will be many fetal heart cycles contributing to the volume of data. The system analyzes the content of the individual 2D images upon completion of the sweep searching for periodic changes in the data set. The length and frequency of the periodic changes determine the average fetal heart rate. Using the accepted fetal heart rate, the system divides the length (time) of the acquisition by the fetal heart rate.

Individual images are assigned to new groups based on their time in a cardiac cycle. Within the new groups there are many images. The system uses the spatial coordinates of each image to determine the location of that image in the volume of tissue. The spatial and temporal correlation occurs simultaneously. The system knows how to arrange them spatially because they have all occurred at different positions in space with known positional coordinates.

In the example above two volumes are shown: volume at systole and volume at diastole. In reality, there are many volumes between these two locations. (Image courtesy of Philips Medical Systems.)

STIC volumes can also be acquired with color or power Doppler to evaluate hemodynamic information. Using color flow and STIC together is especially helpful in documenting the crossing of the great vessels.[13] Tomographic ultrasound imaging can be applied to the data set to evaluate the vessels in a more efficient manner (Fig. 32-41).[15]

Dr. Greg DeVore and his colleagues introduced the Spin technique to simplify the process of manipulating the STIC volume. The Spin technique uses a combination of STIC and the MPR to evaluate the vessels of the heart.[10,11,35,38] The Spin technique is performed by placing the marker dot in the anatomic structure of interest and then spinning the volume using the X or Y rotation until the image displays the relevant heart anatomy.[7,11,35] To evaluate the outflow tracts and venous connections, identify the vessel of interest in a transverse plane, place the reference dot over the area of interest, and rotate along the X or Y axis until the image displays the full length of the vessel.[10,35,38]

Automated programs for evaluating the fetal heart are also available. The goal of the automated programs is to standardize the fetal cardiac examination, much like CT or MRI.[36] This standardization could improve detection of congenital heart disease by decreasing operator dependence, reducing technologist error, and increasing efficiency.[5,11,14,36,39] As with STIC, the technologist must acquire a volume of the heart in the four-chamber view. The system uses the constant spatial relationships in the heart to automatically manipulate the volume and display the standard views using the tomographic ultrasound imaging display.[36] The system displays the left and right outflow tracts, aortic and ductal arches, venous connections, and the stomach.[15,36] The software program can be used between 18 and 23 weeks' gestation.[36] 3D adds a steeper learning curve and can seem more operator-dependent unless protocols are standardized or automated imaging is used. If 3D applications become easier to use, then the clinical use and applicability of the technology should increase.[36]

The accuracy of fetal weight estimation, especially in macrosomic and IUGR fetuses, has always been low using traditional ultrasound parameters of fetal growth.[4,8] Measurements such as head and abdominal circumference, biparietal diameter, and femur length do not reflect the soft tissue mass that accounts for much of the variation in newborn body composition and weight.[14] Incorporating soft tissue mass into the equation for calculating fetal weight may lead to more accurate predictions of birth weight.[4,8] One study by Lee et al. concluded that fractional thigh volume was the strongest predictor of body fat in the fetus.[41] In newborns, the thigh volume accounted for 46% of the variation in body composition, whereas traditional biometric parameters for fetal weight estimation accounted for only 4% to 14%.[41] Fractional limb volumes may provide the answer.[4,8,14] A 3D volume of the thigh or upper arm can be acquired and the volume of the limb can be calculated using VOCAL software. This technique speeds up the process by measuring the limb in five equidistant segments (Fig. 32-42).[14] Fractional limb volumes could improve fetal weight estimation and evaluation of fetal nutritional status.[14]

VOCAL can be used in a number of situations in the obstetric patient. One instance is in evaluating for pulmonary hyperplasia. Pulmonary hyperplasia is associated with a high mortality rate, especially when coexisting conditions such as premature rupture of membranes or a diaphragmatic hernia exist.[4,14] VOCAL can be used to more accurately measure the volume of the fetal lungs. Volume data sets make the measurements of this irregular organ faster, and the 3D volume

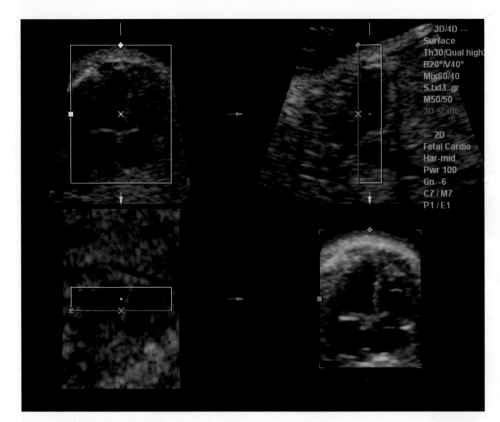

Figure 32-40 STIC volume of the fetal heart. (Image courtesy of GE Healthcare, Wauwatosa, WI.)

measurements were found to be comparable to those calculated using MRI.[1,4,14] Volume measurements have also been reported for the placenta, amniotic cavity, fetal brain, and liver.[1,13,19] VOCAL is useful for quickly measuring the volume of any irregular object.[19]

4D imaging allows the observer to study fetal behavior in more detail than ever before. For the first time, facial expressions such as mouth opening, tongue protrusion, yawning, smiling, scowling, eye opening, and blinking can be studied (Fig. 32-43).[1,4,32] Fetal movement, not only facial movement but also limb and body movement, can be studied in detail. Studying facial and other fetal movement patterns could lead to diagnostic criteria for prenatal brain development, because fetal movement correlates with central nervous system development and maturation.[1,32] Now that visualization of these behaviors is possible, measurable parameters could be used to assess normal central nervous system development.[32]

4D imaging can provide real-time needle guidance in three planes and potentially provide increased accuracy of needle positioning through elimination of the lateralization phenomenon.[1,42] Lateralization occurs when the needle position seen on ultrasound does not depict the exact location of the needle in the body.[42] This occurs because the width of the ultrasound beam is wider than the needle.[1,42] Chorionic villus sampling (CVS) and cordocentesis targets are extremely small and needle placement is critical.[1,42] With current technology, image degradation in the orthogonal planes is an issue, especially in the coronal or C plane.[1] As resolution improves, volume ultrasound will be used for more interventional procedures.

Another benefit to 3D and 4D imaging is increased clinical understanding. Obstetricians and radiologists work closely with neonatologists, surgeons, pediatricians, and other consultants when evaluating complicated cases.[3,13] 2D ultrasound can be difficult for those unfamiliar with the modality to understand. Volume ultrasound techniques can help consulting physicians view complex anatomy in a more complete manner and gain a better understanding of the conditions. By providing a more realistic view, 3D ultrasound can also

---

TABLE 32-5

Tips for Acquiring a STIC Volume[35,36,38]

- Start with an apical four-chamber view of the fetal heart
- Select an ROI as narrow as possible to maximize frame rate and temporal resolution
- Choose a volume angle 5 degrees above the gestational age; for example: in a 25-week fetus choose a volume angle of 30 degrees
- Slower acquisition times will result in volumes with better spatial resolution
- For active fetuses, a faster acquisition time may be needed
- After acquisition, orient volume so that spine is at 6 o'clock with the four-chamber heart in an apical position with the left side of the heart on the left side of the screen

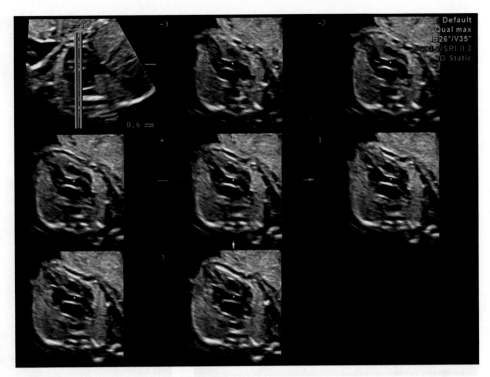

Figure 32-41 Tomographic view of the fetal heart demonstrating the left outflow tract. (Image courtesy of GE Healthcare, Wauwatosa, WI.)

help the family understand the extent of the anomalies and in some cases can lead to better acceptance of the condition.[1,3,32,34,43] A 3D volume helps the consultant make a more thorough diagnosis by providing the entire volume of data rather than still images or cine clips.[3,13] The consultant can manipulate the data and perform a virtual rescan of the patient even when the patient is not physically present.[44]

As with gynecologic imaging, 3D is a useful addition to 2D ultrasound, not a replacement. Although most anomalies can be visualized with 2D imaging, 3D ultrasound has been shown in many instances to aid in diagnosis or help make a more complete diagnosis. 3D ultrasound is not a screening tool, but it is used for more targeted evaluations when indicated. 3D ultrasound has been shown to be consistently advantageous

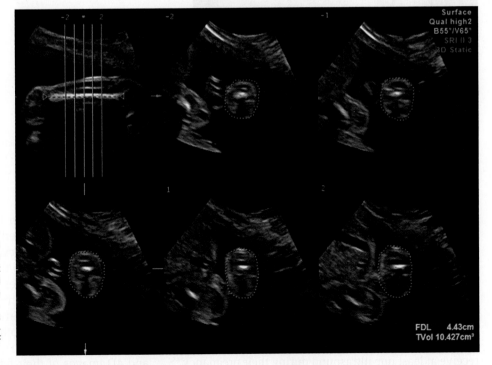

Figure 32-42 Fractional limb volume. A volume of the fetal thigh is stored. VOCAL is used to calculate the limb volume. Five equidistant sections of the thigh are displayed and the contour of the thigh on each image is manually traced. Once all five sections are traced, a fractional limb volume is automatically calculated. (Image courtesy of GE Healthcare, Wauwatosa, WI.)

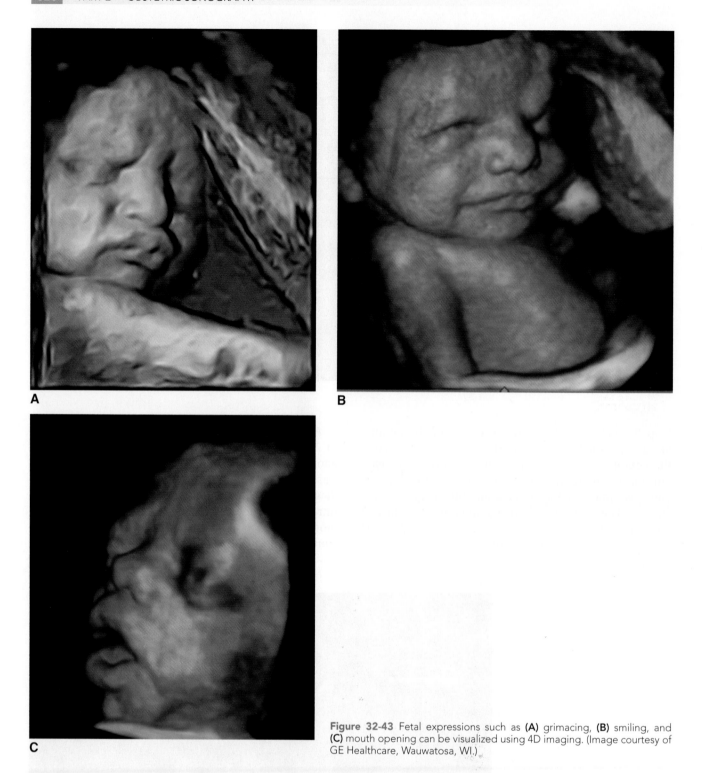

Figure 32-43 Fetal expressions such as **(A)** grimacing, **(B)** smiling, and **(C)** mouth opening can be visualized using 4D imaging. (Image courtesy of GE Healthcare, Wauwatosa, WI.)

in evaluating anomalies of the fetal face, extremities, heart, and central nervous system.[4,34]

ETHICAL CONSIDERATIONS/ PARENTAL BONDING

In today's society, separating the emotional aspect of the ultrasound experience from the medical aspect can be difficult. Patients are better informed and expect to receive at least one ultrasound during their pregnancy.[45]

Parents look forward to having a visual confirmation of the pregnancy, "meeting the baby," and receiving reassurance of normalcy.[45,46] Parents and even their families look forward to the bonding experience the sonographic exam provides.[1,43,45,47] Studies have reported that 2D sonography decreases patient anxiety and can even contribute to positive maternal health behaviors such as encouraging mothers to give up smoking.[1,4,6,43]

There is no question that parents enjoy seeing 3D and 4D images of their fetus, but whether or not these technologies provide an enhanced bonding experience has yet to be determined. Study results seem to be mixed. A few studies have suggested that 4D images of the fetus do provide the parents with more positive feelings about the experience because the images are more realistic and recognizable.[1] Some believe that because the images appear more "lifelike," the parents could form a tighter bond and create stronger positive emotions.[43,45] One study found that when parents received 3D images, they showed the images to significantly more people.[43]

Since 2000, private fetal photo businesses have been expanding as a result of the rise in popularity of 3D imaging.[27] Some argue that the psychosocial indications justify imaging without a diagnostic medical examination; however, most members of the ultrasound community do not condone this use of ultrasound.[3] The AIUM states, "the AIUM advocates the responsible use of diagnostic ultrasound for all fetal imaging."[48] The AIUM and the FDA both discourage the use of ultrasound for reasons not medically indicated.[46] One of the major concerns of the sonographic community is follow-up care. Who takes responsibility for the patient if an anomaly is discovered on a nondiagnostic sonogram? Should the patient be responsible?[46] Another problem lies in who is performing the examination. Untrained users could create a false sense of security or could find false-positive results that could cause unnecessary anxiety.[3]

The medical community agrees that allowing the parents to view images of the fetus in either 2D or 3D and providing keepsake images for the patient during the course of their diagnostic ultrasound is appropriate. Although most sonographers give images to the parents at the end of the exam, an examination for the sole purpose of obtaining keepsake images is not condoned by the medical community.[3]

USE OF THE DATA SET AFTER ACQUISITION

Acquiring the volume data set is only the beginning. As we have discussed, the volume can be manipulated on the scanner itself at any time after the acquisition. As long as the volume is saved on the system, manipulation can occur days or even weeks after the initial examination. Software programs are available that bring the manipulations available on the ultrasound machine to a computer.[7] Currently, most equipment manufacturers that offer 3D/4D technology on their equipment also have offline computer software that accepts volume data sets from their machines.[7] This allows the manipulations and reconstructions to occur off the machine and even in remote locations. The one drawback is that the software is proprietary, meaning that the programs do not accept volumes from other manufacturers' equipment,[7] limiting the exchange of volumes between systems.

2D ultrasound images are stored in the DICOM format. DICOM stands for digital imaging and communications in medicine.[5] According to the AIUM, "the DICOM standard and its supplements are the result of engineers, manufacturers, scientists, and other imaging professionals collaborating to create universal file format definitions and computer communication codes that can be adopted by all vendors for scanners, servers, workstations, printers, and network hardware."[49] The DICOM standard is what allows images from ultrasound scanners of different manufacturers to be viewed and stored on a PACS system from a different vendor. Unfortunately, at this time, a DICOM standard for 3D ultrasound data sets is not available; therefore, most PACS workstations do not accept 3D ultrasound volumes. The DICOM Standards Committee is working toward developing a DICOM standard for 3D ultrasound. This is called the DICOM Supplement 43: Storage of 3D Ultrasound Images.[49] Once all ultrasound equipment and PACS manufacturers adopt the 3D DICOM standard, PACS workstations will accept 3D volumes from the ultrasound scanner. Having the ability to reconstruct the volume data set at the PACS workstation will make incorporating 3D into clinical practice much easier.[5]

The role volume imaging will play in the field of obstetric and gynecologic ultrasound is still evolving. The use of 3D and 4D imaging in daily practice has increased over the last 10 years and interest continues to grow. The 2005 AIUM Consensus Conference on 3D/4D reported that, "when used in conjunction with 2D ultrasound, 3D ultrasound has added diagnostic and clinical value for select indications and circumstances in obstetric and gynecological ultrasound."[5] At least in the near future, 3D imaging will not replace traditional 2D imaging, but will instead serve as a complementary technology.[4,5,34] The ability to display an infinite number of images in both the acquired plane and planes in which direct image acquisition was not possible, such as the coronal plane, adds diagnostic value to conventional 2D imaging.[5,13] 3D ultrasound has been called a problem-solving tool, as the utility of the technology becomes apparent when dealing with complex cases (Table 32-6).[1,5,32]

For 3D to be incorporated into practice, more needs to be done by the ultrasound community to educate sonographers and physicians not only on the clinical applications of 3D ultrasound but also on the techniques.[5,13] The lack of standardization between different manufacturers, however, is a limiting factor in training.[2,5,13,28] For 3D ultrasound to be integrated into daily practice, the techniques must be faster, easier to use, and more intuitive (Table 32-7).[5,13] Protocols need to be developed for the acquisition, display, and manipulation of volumes.[5,13,28] Tools such as the Z-technique for evaluating the coronal plane of the uterus and the Spin technique for evaluating the fetal heart simplify the process. As more techniques such as these become available, 3D will gain more widespread acceptance. As with any

TABLE 32-6
Benefits of 3D/4D Imaging

- A volume of data is obtained instead of single images
- Ability to view any plane in the volume
- Ability to image planes that are not possible with 2D imaging
- Rendering mode options
- Surface rendering
- Accurate volume measurements
- Volumes can be stored electronically for review
- Remote consultation
- Virtual rescan
- Clinical understanding
- Increased diagnostic confidence
- Better visualization of spatial relationships
- Standardization
- Improved productivity
- Teaching normal and abnormal anatomy and standardized views

TABLE 32-7
Limitations of 3D/4D Imaging

- Learning curve
- Protocols and manipulation techniques are not standardized
- 3D cannot overcome poor 2D image
- Image resolution is lower in the reconstructed planes
- Artifacts and orientation can be confusing
- Patient conditions such as low fluid volume, patient body habitus, fetal movement

new technology, learning to acquire and manipulate the volumes takes time, but once this is overcome, the benefits are worth the time spent. As technology continues to advance, so will 3D/4D imaging. There is much to learn, but the research is exciting and encouraging. 3D ultrasound clearly provides distinct advantages and its use will continue to expand.

SUMMARY

- Computer evolution in size, processing speed, and memory capabilities have paralleled 3D imaging development.
- Volume ultrasound (3D and 4D) is the acquisition and storage of a series of 2D images.
- Pixels are part of the flat 2D image; the addition of the voxel creates the volume portion of the image or data set.
- Obtaining the volume data occurs via a freehand, sensor-based, or automated acquisition.
- The ROI determines the amount of data acquired in the X- and Y-axes (2D) and the Z-axis (3D).
- Image quality of the 3D or 4D data depends on the 2D image, requiring optimization *before* beginning volume imaging.
- The most common view for the 3D image is the MPR format.
- The A, B, and C planes display in an orthogonal manner with a dot indicating the intersection of the three images.
- The C plane is a coronal image of anatomy that we have not been able to acquire with conventional 2D imaging.

- Manipulation of the three orthogonal planes allows for the creation of an infinite number of images.
- Multislice or tomographic ultrasound is the serial display of all the acquired 2D images within the data set.
- Rendering the 3D data set allows for specific anatomy of interest such as bony structures or facial features.
- Surface rendering displays the surface of a structure such as in the case of the fetal face or limbs.
- Transparency changes how well we can see through the voxel while the scalpel removes surrounding structures, allowing for increased visualization of desired anatomy.
- Maximum, skeletal, or x-ray mode allows for imaging of the bony skeleton of the fetus.
- Minimum and inversion modes help in the evaluation of hypoechoic structures.
- Glass body, used in conjunction with color Doppler modes, highlights vascular anatomy by decreasing the transparency of the overlying tissue.
- Manipulation of the 3D data set can occur during the exam or after saving of the data set.
- VOCAL aids in measurement of irregular anatomy or cavities such as the internal volume of the uterine cavity or fetal limbs.
- 4D imaging is the addition of time to the data acquisition, resulting in a real-time display.
- The Z-technique is a systematic process to aid in the reconstruction of the coronal plane of the uterus.
- Artifacts occurring in 2D imaging carry over to the 3D data.
- Volume imaging has the potential to change how sonographers perform the examination.
- 3D data set manipulation of fetal exams has the potential to reveal birth defects, as in the case of STIC used in cardiac imaging.
- Volume imaging during pregnancy has shown to increase parental bonding, decrease patient anxiety, and foster positive health behaviors.

Critical Thinking Questions

1. A patient presents for a 3D exam of her 30-week fetus. There is a known cleft palate from a routine size and dates done at the clinician's office. What would be the best method to image this facial malformation? Explain your answer.

   ANSWER: Because of the ability to manipulate the 3D data set, an acquisition with the mechanical transducer would be the best method to obtain images. MPR displays allow for the display of the face on multiple planes as well as the surface rendering.

2. This image is an example of one manner we can display the images from a 3D data set (Fig. 32-44). Philips has called it iSlice, whereas GE calls this feature Tomographic Ultrasound Imaging, and the comparable Siemens feature is called *four*Sight™. What are the benefits and disadvantages to displaying the normal anatomy in this manner? (Fig. 32-44)

   ANSWER: The sequential display of the slices at known intervals allows for a similar display format to CT, MRI, and positron emission tomography (PET) images. This allows the clinician to localize pathology within known slice thicknesses. Sonographers do this routinely during the exam; however, the clinician does not know exactly where within the organ the image acquisition occurred. With a saved 3D data set, this display becomes possible either in real time or at a later date.

   The biggest disadvantage to this format is the compatibility with current PACS systems. The data may be sent either as one single image or each image sent individually. There is also the problem of the large size of the data.

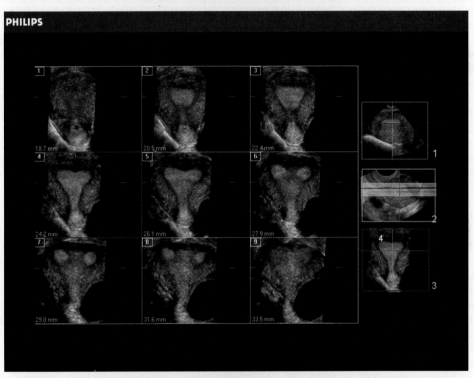

Figure 32-44

REFERENCES

1. Kurjak A, Miskovic B, Andonotopo W, et al. How useful is 3D and 4D ultrasound in perinatal medicine? *J Perinat Med*. 2007;35(1):10–27.
2. Stephenson SR. 3D and 4D sonography: history and theory. *JDMS*. 2005;21:392–399.
3. Benacerraf BR. Three-dimensional fetal sonography: use and misuse. *J Ultrasound Med*. 2002;21(10):1063–1067.
4. Goncalves LF, Lee W, Espinoza J, et al. Three- and 4-dimensional ultrasound in obstetric practice: does it help? *J Ultrasound Med*. 2005;24(12):1599–1624.
5. Benacerraf BR, Benson CB, Abuhamad AZ, et al. Three and 4-dimensional ultrasound in obstetrics and gynecology: proceedings of the American Institute of Ultrasound in Medicine consensus conference. *J Ultrasound Med*. 2005;24(12):1587–1597.

6. Timor-Tritsch IE, Platt LD. Three-dimensional ultrasound experience in obstetrics. *Curr Opin Obstet Gynecol.* 2002;14(6):569–575.

7. Timor-Tritsch IE, Monteagudo A. Three and four-dimensional ultrasound in obstetrics and gynecology. *Curr Opin Obstet Gynecol.* 2007;19(2):157–175.

8. Lee W. 3D fetal ultrasonography. *Clin Obst and Gynecol.* 2003;46(4):850–867.

9. Hagle J, Bicknell SG. Impact of 3D sonography on workroom time efficiency. *AJR Am J Roentgenol.* 2007;188(4):966–969.

10. DeVore GR. Three-dimensional and four-dimensional fetal echocardiography: a new frontier. *Curr Opin Pediatr.* 2005;17(5):592–604.

11. Goncalves LF, Lee W, Espinoza J, et al. Examination of the fetal heart by four-dimensional (4D) ultrasound with spatio-temporal image correlation (STIC). *Ultrasound Obstet Gynecol.* 2006;27(3):336–348.

12. Tuning N. Does spatiotemporal image correlation enhance the diagnostic usefulness of 3D and 4D fetal cardiac imaging? A literature review. *JDMS.* 2007;23:75–84.

13. Chaoui R. Heling KS. Three-dimensional ultrasound in prenatal diagnosis. *Curr Opin Obstet Gynecol.* 2006;18:192–202.

14. Yagel S, Cohen SM, Messing B, et al. Three-dimensional and four dimensional ultrasound applications in fetal medicine. *Curr Opin Obstet Gynecol.* 2009;21(2):167–174.

15. DeVore GR, Polanko B. Tomographic ultrasound imaging of the fetal heart: a new technique for identifying normal and abnormal cardiac anatomy. *J Ultrasound Med.* 2005;24(12):1685–1696.

16. Zheng Y, Zhou XD, Zhu YL, et al. Three- and 4-dimensional ultrasonography in the prenatal evaluation of fetal anomalies associated with trisomy 18. *J Ultrasound Med.* 2008;27(7):1041–1051.

17. Benacerraf BR. Inversion mode display of 3D sonography: applications in obstetric and gynecologic imaging. *AJR Am J Roentgenol.* 2006;187(4):965–971.

18. Kalache KD, Espinoza J, Chaiworapongsa T, et al. Three-dimensional ultrasound fetal lung volume measurement: a systematic study comparing the multiplanar method with the rotational (VOCAL) technique. *Ultrasound Obstet Gynecol.* 2003;21(2):111–118.

19. Shaw SW, Hsieh TT, Hsu JJ, et al. Measurement of nuchal volume in the first trimester down screening using three-dimensional ultrasound. *Prenat Diagn.* 2009;29:69–73.

20. Benacerraf BR, Shipp TD, Bromley B. Improving the efficiency of gynecologic sonography with 3-dimensional volumes: a pilot study. *J Ultrasound Med.* 2005;25(2):165–171.

21. Ghi T, Casadio P, Kuleva M, et al. Accuracy of three-dimensional ultrasound in diagnosis and classification of congenital uterine anomalies. *Fertil Steril.* 2009;92(2):808–813.

22. Wu MH, Pan HA, Chang FM. Three dimensional and power Doppler ultrasonography in infertility and reproductive endocrinology. *Taiwan J Obstet Gynecol.* 2007;46:209–214.

23. Lev-Toaff AS, Pinheiro LW, Bega G, et al. Three-dimensional multiplanar sonohysterography: comparison with conventional two-dimensional sonohysterography and x-ray hysterosalpingography. *J Ultrasound Med.* 2001;20(4):295–306.

24. Wilson M, Whyte-Evans J. The use of volume imaging in the evaluation of intrauterine contraceptive devices. *JDMS.* 2009;25:38–43.

25. Zohav E. Use of three-dimensional ultrasound in evaluating the intrauterine position of a levonorgestrel-releasing intrauterine system. *Reprod BioMed Online.* 2007;14:495–497.

26. Oliveira M, Johnson D, Switalski P, et al. Optimal use of 3D and 4D transvaginal sonography in localizing the essure contraceptive device. *JDMS.* 2009;25:163–167.

27. Benacerraf BR, Shipp TD, Bromley B. Which patients benefit from a 3D reconstructed coronal view of the uterus added to standard routine 2D pelvic sonography? *AJR.* 2008;190:626–629.

28. Abuhamad AZ, Singleton S, Zhao Y, et al. The Z technique: an easy approach to the display of the midcoronal plane of the uterus in volume sonography. *J Ultrasound Med.* 2006;25(5):607–612.

29. Alcazar JL, Cabrera C, Galvan R, et al. Three-dimensional power Doppler vascular network assessment of adnexal masses: intraobserver and interobserver agreement analysis. *J Ultrasound Med.* 2008;27(7):997–1001.

30. Alcazar JL, Rodriguez D. Three dimensional power Doppler vascular sonographic sampling for predicting ovarian cancer in cystic-solid and solid vascularized masses. *J Ultrasound Med.* 2009;21:1105–1111.

31. Abuhamad AZ. Clinical implications of the echo enhancement artifact in volume sonography of the uterus. *J Ultrasound Med.* 2006;25:1431–1435.

32. Kurjak A, Azumendi G, Andonotopo W, et al. Three- and four-dimensional ultrasonography for the structural and functional evaluation of the fetal face. *Am J Obstet Gynecol.* 2007;196:16–28.

33. Platt LD, DeVore GR, Pretorius DH. Improving cleft palate/cleft lip antenatal diagnosis by 3-dimensional sonography: the "flipped face" view. *J Ultrasound Med.* 2006;25(11):1423–1430.

34. Avni FE, Cos T, Cassart M, et al. Evolution of fetal ultrasonography. *Eur Radiol.* 2007;17(2):419–431.

35. DeVore GR, Polanco B, Sklansky MS, et al. The 'spin' technique: a new method for examination of the fetal outflow tracts using three-dimensional ultrasound. *Ultrasound Obstet Gynecol.* 2004;24:72–82.

36. Abuhamad A, Falkensammer P, Reichartseder F, et al. Automated retrieval of standard diagnostic fetal cardiac ultrasound planes in the second trimester of pregnancy: a prospective evaluation of software. *Ultrasound Obstet Gynecol.* 2008;31:30–36.

37. Falkensammer P, Helmut B. 4D fetal echocardiography: spatio-temporal image correlation for fetal heart acquisition. *Ultrasound Technology Update.* http://www.gehealthcare.com/euen/ultrasound/docs/education/whitepapers/UltrasoundTechnologyUpdate-STIC.pdf. Accessed September 25, 2009.

38. Yagel S, Cohen SM, Shapiro I, et al. 3D and 4D ultrasound in fetal cardiac scanning: a new look at the fetal heart. *Ultrasound Obstet Gynecol.* 2007;29:81–95.

39. Zhivora SM. Improving detection of transposition of the great arteries in routine obstetric sonographic screening. *JDMS.* 2008;24:279–283.

40. Gindes L, Hegesh J, Weisz B, et al. Three and four dimensional ultrasound: a novel method for evaluating fetal cardiac anomalies. *Prenat Diagn.* 2009;29(7):645–653.

41. Lee W, Balasubramaniam M, Determ RL, et al. Fetal growth parameters and birth weight: their relationship to newborn infant body composition. *Ultrasound Obstet Gynecol.* 2009;33(4):441–446.

42. Dolkart L, Harter M, Snyder M. Four-dimensional ultrasonographic guidance for invasive obstetric procedures. *J Ultrasound Med.* 2005;24(9):1261–1266.

43. Pretorius DH, Hearon HA, Hollenbach KA, et al. Parental artistic drawings of the fetus before and after 3-/4-dimensional ultrasonography. *J Ultrasound Med.* 2007; 26:301–308.

44. Benacerraf BR, Shipp TD, Bromley B. Three-dimensional US of the fetus: volume imaging. *Radiology.* 2006;238: 988–996.

45. Lee S, Pretorius DH, Asfoor S, et al. Prenatal three-dimensional ultrasound: perception of sonographers, sonologists, and undergraduate students. *Ultrasound Obstet Gynecol.* 2007;30:77–80.

46. Wiseman CS, Kiehl EM. Picture perfect: benefits and risk of fetal 3D ultrasound. *MCN Am J Matern Child Nurs.* 2007;32:102–109.

47. Burlbaw J. Obstetric sonography – that's entertainment? *JDMS.* 2004;20:444–448.

48. AIUM. AIUM official statement on keepsake imaging. http://www.aium.org/publications/viewStatement .aspx?id = 31. Accessed September 25, 2009.

49. AIUM. DICOM–explained. http://www.aium.org/misc/ dicom.aspx. Accessed September 25, 2009.

Index